AF583882

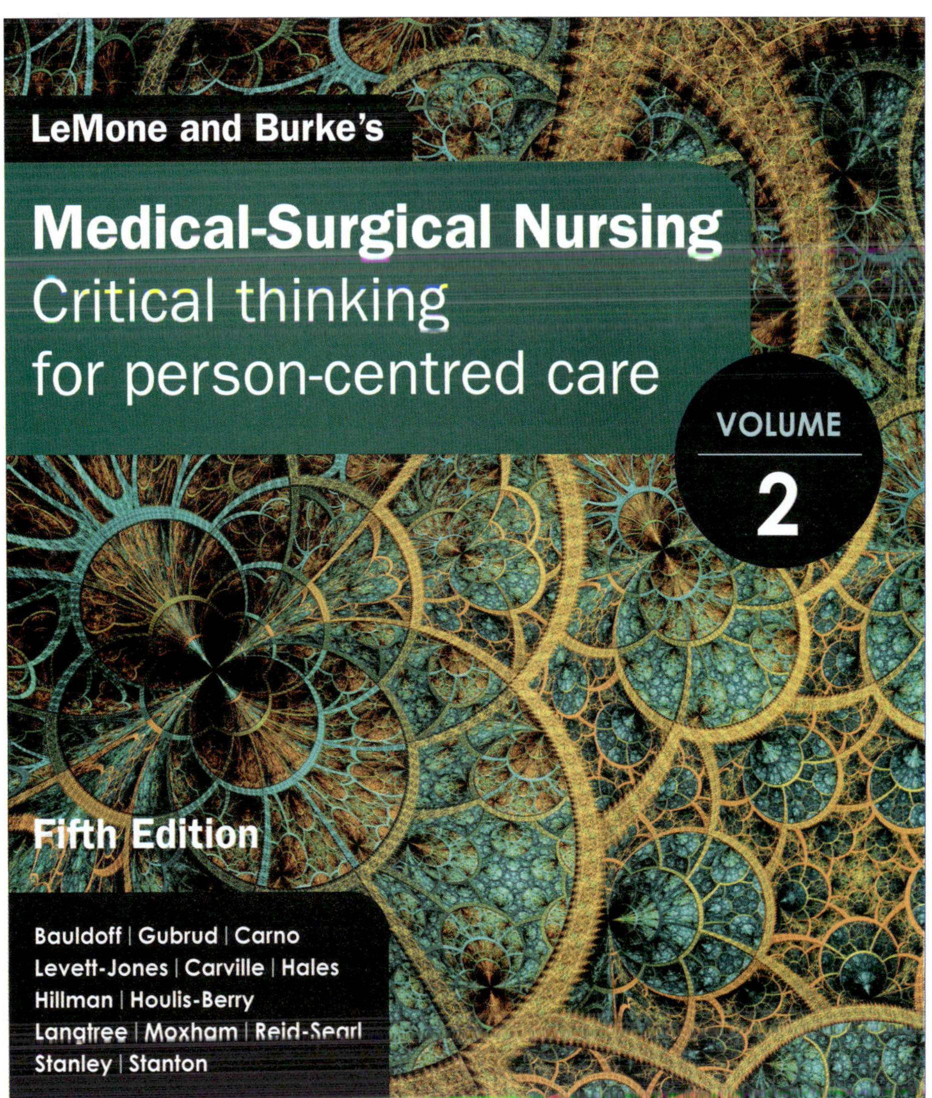
LeMone and Burke's
Medical-Surgical Nursing
Critical thinking
for person-centred care
VOLUME
2
Fifth Edition
Bauldoff | Gubrud | Carno
Levett-Jones | Carville | Hales
Hillman | Houlis-Berry
Langtree | Moxham | Reid-Searl
Stanley | Stanton

Pearson Australia
Building B, Level 1
459–471 Church Street
Richmond Victoria 3121

www.pearson.com.au

Authorised adaptation from the United States edition entitled *LeMone's Medical–Surgical Nursing: Clinical Reasoning in Patient Care*, 7th edition, by LeMone, Priscilla; Burke, Karen; Bauldoff, Gerene, Gubrud, Paula, published by Pearson Education, Inc., Copyright © 2020.

Fifth adaptation edition published by Pearson Australia Group Pty Ltd, Copyright © 2024

Pearson respects and honours Aboriginal and Torres Strait Islander Elders past, present and future. We acknowledge the stories, traditions and living cultures of the Traditional Custodians of the lands on which our company is located and where we conduct our business. Pearson is committed to honouring Australian Aboriginal and Torres Strait Islander peoples' unique cultural and spiritual relationships to the land, waters and seas and their rich contribution to society.

Aboriginal and Torres Strait Islander peoples are advised that this text may contain images, voices and names of deceased persons.

Links to National Patient Safety Standards reproduced with permission from *National Safety and Quality Health Service Standards* (second edition), developed by the Australian Commission on Safety and Quality in Health Care (ACSQHC). ACSQHC: Sydney 2021.

Senior Commercial Product Manager: Mandy Sheppard
Development Editor: Anna Carter
Senior Project Manager: Bernadette Chang
Content Producer: Linda Chryssavgis
Digital Media Production Manager: Paul Ryan
Assistant Manager Rights and Permissions: Samantha Russell-Tulip
Lead Editor/Copy Editor: Katie Millar
Indexer: Integra Software Services
Cover and internal design by Natalie Bowra
Cover image by Sabena Jane Blackbird/Alamy Stock Photo
Typeset by Integra Software Services

Printed in Malaysia (CTP-VVP)

Etext ISBN: 9780655709152
Print ISBNs: 9780655709145 (Vol 1), 9780655709275 (Vol 2), 9780655709282 (Vol 3)
ePUB ISBN: 9780655709169

1 2 3 4 5 28 27 26 25 24

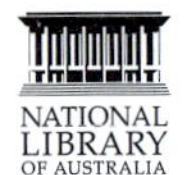

A catalogue record for this work is available from the National Library of Australia

Pearson Australia Group Pty Ltd ABN 40 004 245 943

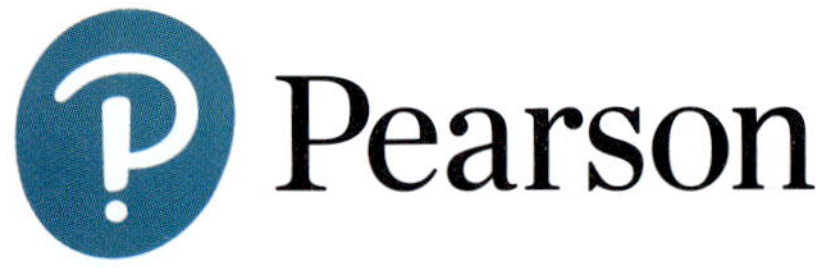

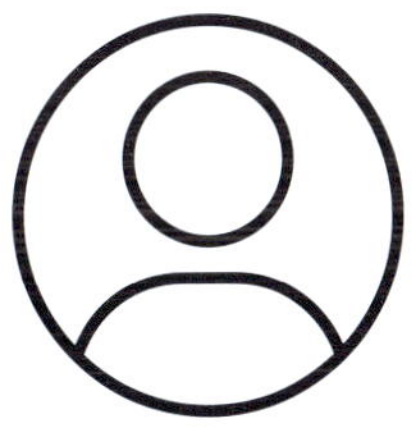

Pearson's Commitment to Diversity, Equity, and Inclusion

Pearson is dedicated to creating bias-free content that reflects the diversity, depth, and breadth of all learners' lived experiences.

We embrace the many dimensions of diversity, including but not limited to race, ethnicity, gender, sex, sexual orientation, socioeconomic status, ability, age, and religious or political beliefs.

Education is a powerful force for equity and change in our world. It has the potential to deliver opportunities that improve lives and enable economic mobility. As we work with authors to create content for every product and service, we acknowledge our responsibility to demonstrate inclusivity and incorporate diverse scholarship so that everyone can achieve their potential through learning. As the world's leading learning company, we have a duty to help drive change and live up to our purpose to help more people create a better life for themselves and to create a better world.

Our ambition is to purposefully contribute to a world where:

- Everyone has an equitable and lifelong opportunity to succeed through learning.
- Our educational content accurately reflects the histories and lived experiences of the learners we serve.
- Our educational products and services are inclusive and represent the rich diversity of learners.
- Our educational content prompts deeper discussions with students and motivates them to expand their own learning (and worldview).

Accessibility

We are also committed to providing products that are fully accessible to all learners. As per Pearson's guidelines for accessible educational Web media, we test and retest the capabilities of our products against the highest standards for every release, following the WCAG guidelines in developing new products for copyright year 2022 and beyond.

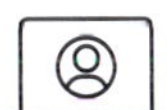

You can learn more about Pearson's commitment to accessibility at **https://www.pearson.com/us/accessibility.html**

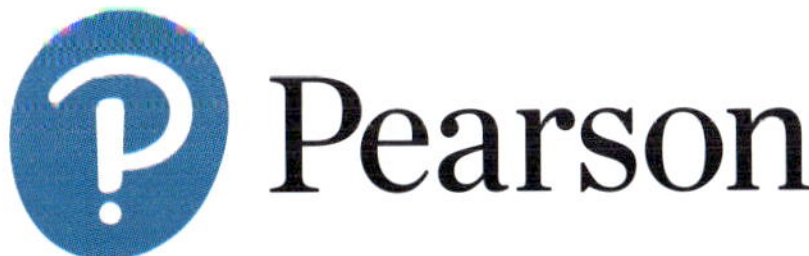

Contact Us

While we work hard to present unbiased, fully accessible content, we want to hear from you about any concerns or needs with this Pearson product so that we can investigate and address them.

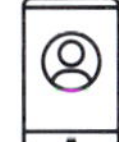

Please contact us with concerns about any potential bias at **https://www.pearson.com/report-bias.html**

For accessibility-related issues, such as using assistive technology with Pearson products, alternative text requests, or accessibility documentation, email the Pearson Disability Support team at **disability.support@pearson.com**

Brief contents

VOLUME 3

Detailed contents

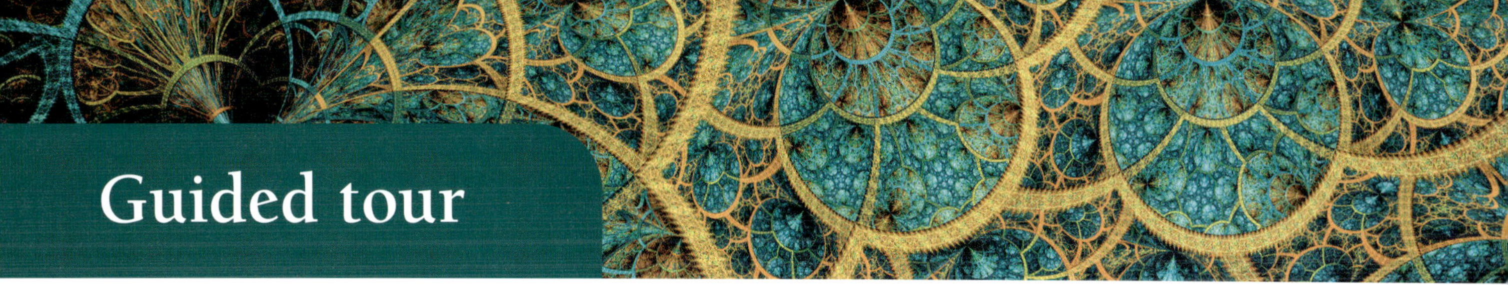

Guided tour

Key features of the Australian edition include:

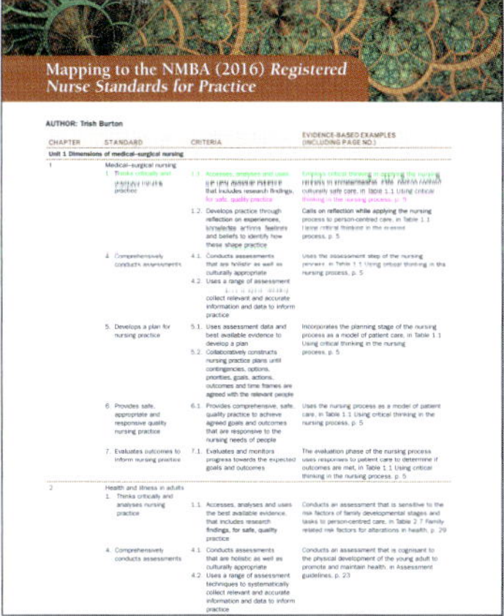

Mapping to the NMBA (2016) *Registered Nurse Standards for Practice* *maps examples from the text to relevant* Registered Nurse Standards for Practice, *thereby aligning the content to contemporary professional practice in Australia.*

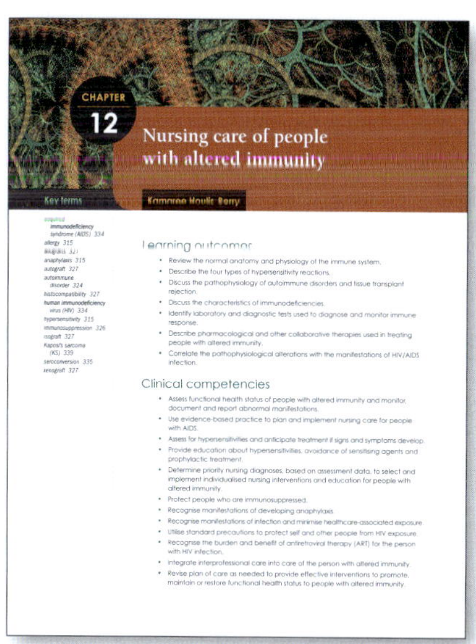

Learning Outcomes *show you the knowledge you'll gain, while*

Clinical Competencies *demonstrate how you will apply that knowledge.*

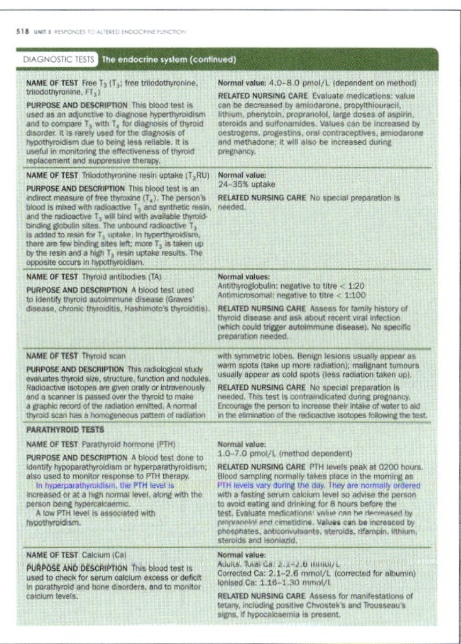

518 UNIT 5 RESPONSES TO ALTERED ENDOCRINE FUNCTION

DIAGNOSTIC TESTS The endocrine system (continued)

NAME OF TEST Free T_3 (T_3; free triiodothyronine, triiodothyronine, FT_3) **PURPOSE AND DESCRIPTION** This blood test is used as an adjunctive to diagnose hyperthyroidism and to compare T_3 with T_4 for diagnosis of thyroid disorder. It is rarely used for the diagnosis of hypothyroidism due to being less reliable. It is useful in monitoring the effectiveness of thyroid replacement and suppressive therapy.	**Normal value:** 4.0–8.0 pmol/L (dependent on method) **RELATED NURSING CARE** Evaluate medications: value can be decreased by amiodarone, propylthiouracil, lithium, phenytoin, propranolol, large doses of aspirin, steroids and sulfonamides. Values can be increased by oestrogens, progestins, oral contraceptives, amiodarone and methadone; it will also be increased during pregnancy.
NAME OF TEST Triiodothyronine resin uptake (T_3RU) **PURPOSE AND DESCRIPTION** This blood test is an indirect measure of free thyroxine (T_4). The person's blood is mixed with radioactive T_3 and synthetic resin, and the radioactive T_3 will bind with available thyroid-binding globulin sites. The unbound radioactive T_3 is added to resin for T_3 uptake. In hyperthyroidism, there are few binding sites left; more T_3 is taken up by the resin and a high T_3 resin uptake results. The opposite occurs in hypothyroidism.	**Normal value:** 24–35% uptake **RELATED NURSING CARE** No special preparation is needed.
NAME OF TEST Thyroid antibodies (TA) **PURPOSE AND DESCRIPTION** A blood test used to identify thyroid autoimmune disease (Graves' disease, chronic thyroiditis, Hashimoto's thyroiditis).	**Normal values:** Antithyroglobulin: negative to titre < 1:20 Antimicrosomal: negative to titre < 1:100 **RELATED NURSING CARE** Assess for family history of thyroid disease and ask about recent viral infection (which could trigger autoimmune disease). No specific preparation needed.
NAME OF TEST Thyroid scan **PURPOSE AND DESCRIPTION** This radiological study evaluates thyroid size, structure, function and nodules. Radioactive isotopes are given orally or intravenously and a scanner is passed over the thyroid to make a graphic record of the radiation emitted. A normal thyroid scan has a homogeneous pattern of radiation	with symmetric lobes. Benign lesions usually appear as warm spots (take up more radiation); malignant tumours usually appear as cold spots (less radiation taken up). **RELATED NURSING CARE** No special preparation is needed. This test is contraindicated during pregnancy. Encourage the person to increase their intake of water to aid in the elimination of the radioactive isotopes following the test.
PARATHYROID TESTS	
NAME OF TEST Parathyroid hormone (PTH) **PURPOSE AND DESCRIPTION** A blood test done to identify hypoparathyroidism or hyperparathyroidism; also used to monitor response to PTH therapy. In hyperparathyroidism, the PTH level is increased or at a high normal level, along with the person being hypercalcaemic. A low PTH level is associated with hypothyroidism.	**Normal value:** 1.0–7.0 pmol/L (method dependent) **RELATED NURSING CARE** PTH levels peak at 0200 hours. Blood sampling normally takes place in the morning as PTH levels vary during the day. They are normally ordered with a fasting serum calcium level so advise the person to avoid eating and drinking for 8 hours before the test. Evaluate medications: value can be decreased by propranolol and cimetidine. Values can be increased by phosphates, anticonvulsants, steroids, rifampin, lithium, steroids and isoniazid.
NAME OF TEST Calcium (Ca) **PURPOSE AND DESCRIPTION** This blood test is used to check for serum calcium excess or deficit in parathyroid and bone disorders, and to monitor calcium levels.	**Normal value:** Adults: Total Ca: 2.1–2.6 mmol/L Corrected Ca: 2.1–2.6 mmol/L (corrected for albumin) Ionised Ca: 1.16–1.30 mmol/L **RELATED NURSING CARE** Assess for manifestations of tetany, including positive Chvostek's and Trousseau's signs, if hypocalcaemia is present.

Diagnostic Tests *include diagnostic test tables and a narrative summary. The tables include the name of the test, the purpose and description of the test, and related nursing care.*

Pathophysiology Illustrated *art brings physiological processes to life.*

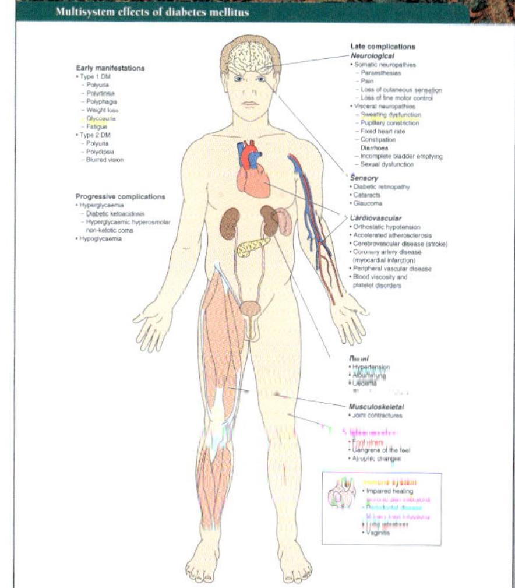

FOCUS ON CULTURAL DIVERSITY **Diabetes in Aboriginal and Torres Strait Islander communities**

Type 2 DM represents a serious public health problem for Aboriginal and Torres Strait Islander communities, occurring at a much higher rate than in the non-Indigenous population, and with a much earlier age of onset of the disease and its micro- and macrovascular complications. It is likely that type 2 DM is an important contributor to the considerably higher circulatory disease mortality rate among Aboriginal and Torres Strait Islander communities at younger ages. Thus type 2 DM imposes significant financial and human costs on Australian society, which are disproportionately borne by Aboriginal and Torres Strait Islander communities.

The National Aboriginal and Torres Strait Islander [illegible] and Torres Strait Islander people reported they had DM (ABS, 2019), the most common being type 2 DM. The prevalence of DM is almost three higher in Aboriginal and Torres Strait Islander communities than in the rest of the population across all age groups. In 2021, diabetes was the second leading cause of death for Aboriginal and Torres Strait Islander people (ABS, 2022). The incidence of GDM in pregnancy is also two to three times higher among Aboriginal and Torres Strait Islander women than in the general Australian population. Living in remote areas also increases the prevalence rates for Aboriginal and Torres Strait Islander groups to six times higher than non-remote areas.

Focus on Cultural Diversity boxes *demonstrate how culture, age and gender produce differences in incidence, prevalence and mortality.*

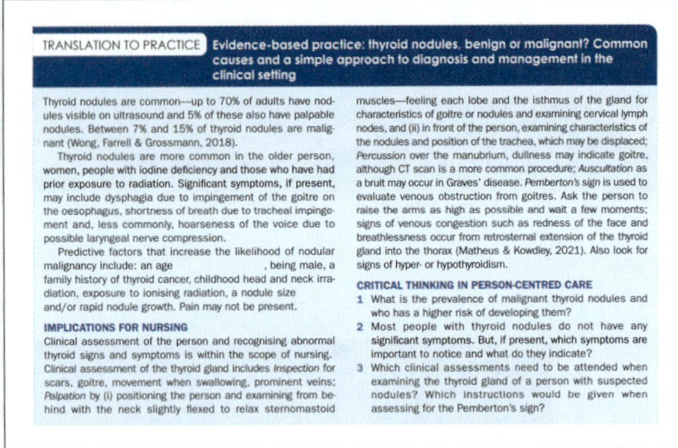

TRANSLATION TO PRACTICE **Evidence-based practice: thyroid nodules, benign or malignant? Common causes and a simple approach to diagnosis and management in the clinical setting**

Thyroid nodules are common—up to 70% of adults have nodules visible on ultrasound and 5% of these also have palpable nodules. Between 7% and 15% of thyroid nodules are malignant (Wong, Farrell & Grossmann, 2018).

Thyroid nodules are more common in the older person, women, people with iodine deficiency and those who have had prior exposure to radiation. Significant symptoms, if present, may include dysphagia due to impingement of the goitre on the oesophagus, shortness of breath due to tracheal impingement and, less commonly, hoarseness of the voice due to possible laryngeal nerve compression.

Predictive factors that increase the likelihood of nodular malignancy include: an age , being male, a family history of thyroid cancer, childhood head and neck irradiation, exposure to ionising radiation, a nodule size and/or rapid nodule growth. Pain may not be present.

IMPLICATIONS FOR NURSING

Clinical assessment of the person and recognising abnormal thyroid signs and symptoms is within the scope of nursing. Clinical assessment of the thyroid gland includes *Inspection* for scars, goitre, movement when swallowing, prominent veins; *Palpation* by (i) positioning the person and examining from behind with the neck slightly flexed to relax sternomastoid muscles—feeling each lobe and the isthmus of the gland for characteristics of goitre or nodules and examining cervical lymph nodes, and (ii) in front of the person, examining characteristics of the nodules and position of the trachea, which may be displaced; *Percussion* over the manubrium, dullness may indicate goitre, although CT scan is a more common procedure; *Auscultation* as a bruit may occur in Graves' disease. *Pemberton's sign* is used to evaluate venous obstruction from goitres. Ask the person to raise the arms as high as possible and wait a few moments; signs of venous congestion such as redness of the face and breathlessness occur from retrosternal extension of the thyroid gland into the thorax (Matheus & Kowdley, 2021). Also look for signs of hyper- or hypothyroidism.

CRITICAL THINKING IN PERSON-CENTRED CARE

1 What is the prevalence of malignant thyroid nodules and who has a higher risk of developing them?
2 Most people with thyroid nodules do not have any significant symptoms. But, if present, which symptoms are important to notice and what do they indicate?
3 Which clinical assessments need to be attended when examining the thyroid gland of a person with suspected nodules? Which instructions would be given when assessing for the Pemberton's sign?

Translation to Practice boxes *focus on how research relates to current nursing care and application of evidence in clinical settings.*

Nursing care

Health promotion

Because of the large stores of calcium in bones, most healthy adults have a very low risk of developing hypocalcaemia. However, a deficit of total body calcium is often associated with ageing, increasing the risk of osteoporosis, fractures and disability. Women have a higher risk of developing osteoporosis than men, due to lower bone density and hormonal influences. Educate women of all ages about the importance of maintaining adequate calcium intake through diet and, as needed, calcium supplements. Stress the relationship between weight-bearing exercise and bone density and encourage women to engage in a regular aerobic and weight-training exercise regimen. Discuss hormone replacement therapy and its potential benefits during and after menopause. See the chapter 'Nursing care of people with musculoskeletal disorders' for more information about osteoporosis.

inspiratory sound indicative of upper airway obstruction), or increased respiratory rate or effort, to the doctor. *These changes may indicate laryngeal spasm due to tetany.*

- Monitor cardiovascular status, including heart rate and rhythm, blood pressure and peripheral pulses. *Hypocalcaemia decreases myocardial contractility, causing reduced cardiac output and hypotension. It also can cause bradycardia or ventricular arrhythmias. Cardiac arrest may occur in severe hypocalcaemia.*
- Continuously monitor ECG in the person receiving intravenous calcium preparations, especially if the person also is taking digitalis. *Rapid administration of calcium salts can lead to hypercalcaemia and cardiac arrhythmias. Calcium administration increases the risk of digitalis toxicity and resultant arrhythmias.*
- Provide a quiet environment. Institute seizure precautions such as raising the side rails and keeping an airway at the bedside. *A quiet environment reduces central nervous system stimuli and the risk of convulsions in the person with tetany.*

Community-based care

In preparing the person with hypocalcaemia for discharge and home care, consider the circumstances leading to low serum

Nursing Care *sections detail the assessment and planning aspects relating to specific conditions and outline potential pain and risks.*

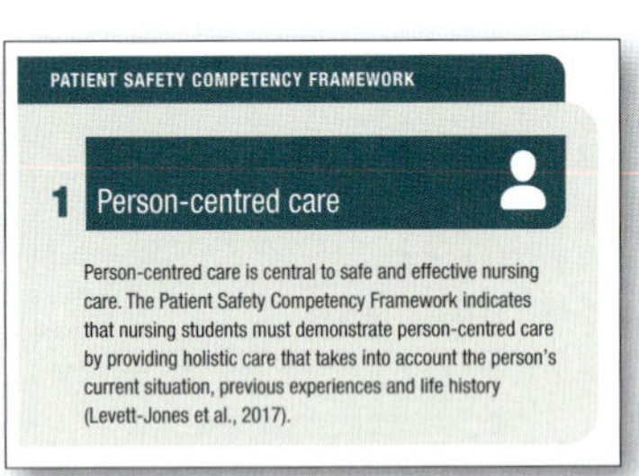

PATIENT SAFETY COMPETENCY FRAMEWORK

1 Person-centred care

Person-centred care is central to safe and effective nursing care. The Patient Safety Competency Framework indicates that nursing students must demonstrate person-centred care by providing holistic care that takes into account the person's current situation, previous experiences and life history (Levett-Jones et al., 2017).

Patient Safety Competency Framework *boxes appear in the chapters where applicable to demonstrate how concepts relate back to the skills and knowledge that underpin patient safety.*

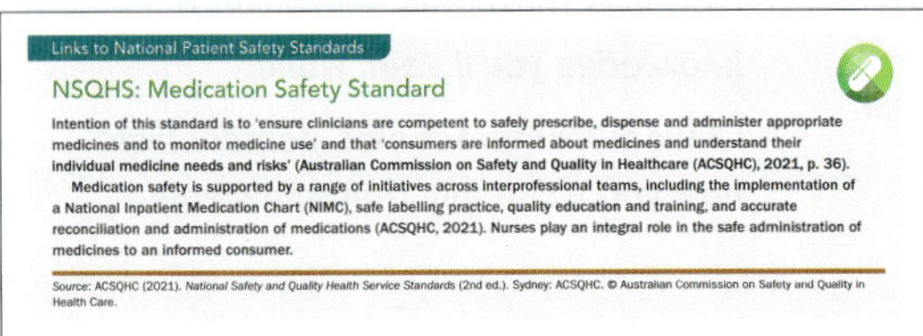

Links to National Patient Safety Standards

NSQHS: Medication Safety Standard

Intention of this standard is to 'ensure clinicians are competent to safely prescribe, dispense and administer appropriate medicines and to monitor medicine use' and that 'consumers are informed about medicines and understand their individual medicine needs and risks' (Australian Commission on Safety and Quality in Healthcare (ACSQHC), 2021, p. 36).

Medication safety is supported by a range of initiatives across interprofessional teams, including the implementation of a National Inpatient Medication Chart (NIMC), safe labelling practice, quality education and training, and accurate reconciliation and administration of medications (ACSQHC, 2021). Nurses play an integral role in the safe administration of medicines to an informed consumer.

Source: ACSQHC (2021). *National Safety and Quality Health Service Standards* (2nd ed.). Sydney: ACSQHC. © Australian Commission on Safety and Quality in Health Care.

Links to National Patient Safety Standards *boxes appear in the chapters where applicable to demonstrate how concepts relate back to patient safety standards.*

FAST FACTS

- Older people have the highest rate of illness and surgical procedures associated with pain; they also have the highest rate of complications associated with surgical interventions.
- Persistent pain is common in older adults. For those over 70 years of age, 50% of those living in the community and 80% of those in residential care suffer persistent pain.
- Musculoskeletal pain affecting major joints and back, or neuropathic pain from diabetic neuropathy and post-herpetic neuralgia have an increased prevalence in the ageing population.
- Concurrent illnesses are common in the elderly, making clinical presentation complex and sometimes difficult.
- Cognitive impairment enhances the risk of poor pain control, negatively influencing the individual's quality of life.

Sources: ANZCA (2020). *Acute pain management: Scientific evidence* (5th ed.). Melbourne: Australian and New Zealand College of Anaesthetists; Youngcharoen (2022). A cross-sectional study of factors associated with nurses' postoperative pain management practices for older patients. *Nursing Open*. https://doi.org/10.1002/nop2.1281

Fast Facts boxes *highlight and summarise important data about the prevalence and incidence of selected disorders in Australia, and of other featured content.*

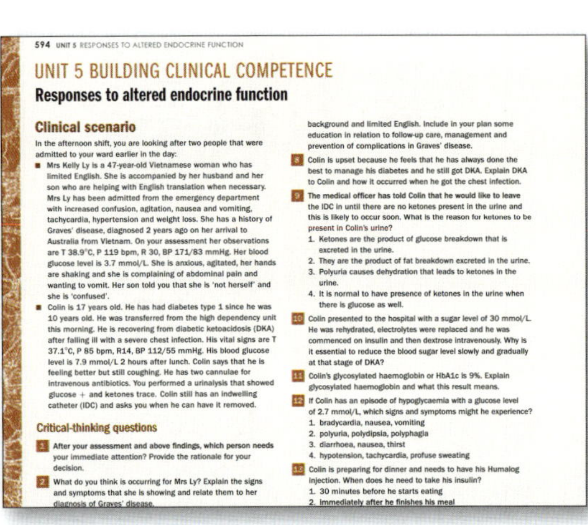

594 UNIT 5 RESPONSES TO ALTERED ENDOCRINE FUNCTION

UNIT 5 BUILDING CLINICAL COMPETENCE

Responses to altered endocrine function

Clinical scenario

In the afternoon shift, you are looking after two people that were admitted to your ward earlier in the day:

- Mrs Kelly Ly is a 47-year-old Vietnamese woman who has limited English. She is accompanied by her husband and her son who are helping with English translation when necessary. Mrs Ly has been admitted from the emergency department with increased confusion, agitation, nausea and vomiting, tachycardia, hypertension and weight loss. She has a history of Graves' disease, diagnosed 2 years ago on her arrival to Australia from Vietnam. On your assessment her observations are T 38.9°C, P 119 bpm, R 30, BP 171/83 mmHg. Her blood glucose level is 3.7 mmol/L. She is anxious, agitated, her hands are shaking and she is complaining of abdominal pain and wanting to vomit. Her son told you that she is 'not herself' and she is 'confused'.
- Colin is 17 years old. He has had diabetes type 1 since he was 10 years old. He was transferred from the high dependency unit this morning. He is recovering from diabetic ketoacidosis (DKA) after falling ill with a severe chest infection. His vital signs are T 37.1°C, P 85 bpm, R14, BP 112/55 mmHg. His blood glucose level is 7.9 mmol/L 2 hours after lunch. Colin says that he is feeling better but still coughing. He has two cannulae for intravenous antibiotics. You performed a urinalysis that showed glucose + and ketones trace. Colin still has an indwelling catheter (IDC) and asks you when he can have it removed.

Critical-thinking questions

1 After your assessment and above findings, which person needs your immediate attention? Provide the rationale for your decision.

2 What do you think is occurring for Mrs Ly? Explain the signs and symptoms that she is showing and relate them to her diagnosis of Graves' disease.

background and limited English. Include in your plan some education in relation to follow-up care, management and prevention of complications in Graves' disease.

8 Colin is upset because he feels that he has always done the best to manage his diabetes and he still got DKA. Explain DKA to Colin and how it occurred when he got the chest infection.

9 The medical officer has told Colin that he would like to leave the IDC in until there are no ketones present in the urine and this is likely to occur soon. What is the reason for ketones to be present in Colin's urine?
1. Ketones are the product of glucose breakdown that is excreted in the urine.
2. They are the product of fat breakdown excreted in the urine.
3. Polyuria causes dehydration that leads to ketones in the urine.
4. It is normal to have presence of ketones in the urine when there is glucose as well.

10 Colin presented to the hospital with a sugar level of 30 mmol/L. He was rehydrated, electrolytes were replaced and he was commenced on insulin and then dextrose intravenously. Why is it essential to reduce the blood sugar level slowly and gradually at that stage of DKA?

11 Colin's glycosylated haemoglobin or HbA1c is 9%. Explain glycosylated haemoglobin and what this result means.

12 If Colin has an episode of hypoglycaemia with a glucose level of 2.7 mmol/L, which signs and symptoms might he experience?
1. bradycardia, nausea, vomiting
2. polyuria, polydipsia, polyphagia
3. diarrhoea, nausea, thirst
4. hypotension, tachycardia, profuse sweating

13 Colin is preparing for dinner and needs to have his Humalog injection. When does he need to take his insulin?
1. 30 minutes before he starts eating
2. Immediately after he finishes his meal

An end-of-unit review for each of the units, called **Building Clinical Competence**, *synthesises what you have learned in the unit and applies the knowledge to specific cases. The feature includes:*

- *A* **clinical scenario** *involving a priority issue reflection piece that synthesises the underlying concepts and includes a variety of questions that allow students to apply different skills.*
- *A* **case study** *with concept map that further synthesises material using the nursing process.*

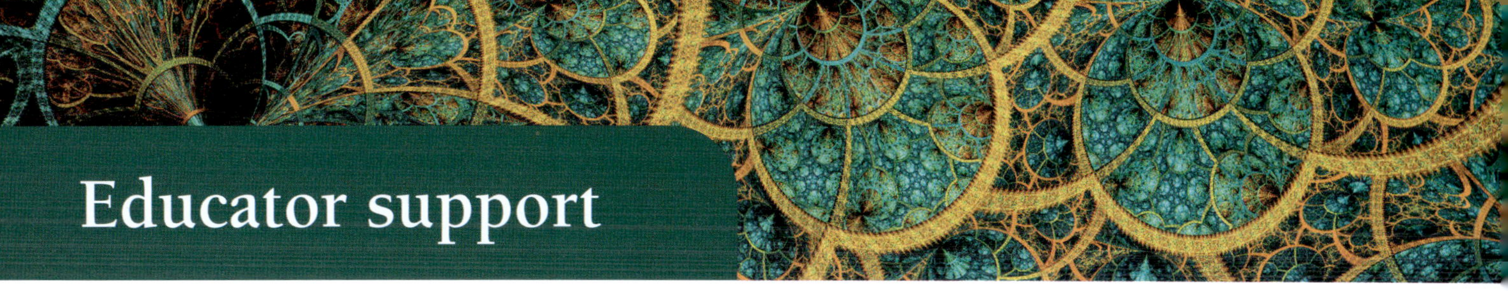

Educator support

A suite of resources is provided to assist with delivery of the text, as well as to support teaching and learning.

Solutions Manual

The Solutions Manual provides educators with detailed, accuracy-verified solutions to in-chapter and end-of-chapter problems in the text.

Test Bank

The Test Bank provides a wealth of accuracy-verified testing material. Updated for the new edition, each chapter offers a wide variety of question types, arranged by learning objective and tagged by NMBA Standards.

Questions can be integrated into Blackboard, Canvas and Moodle Learning Management Systems.

Digital Image Powerpoint slides

All the diagrams and tables from the text are available for lecturer use.

Mapping to the NMBA (2016) *Registered Nurse Standards for Practice*

AUTHOR: Trish Burton

CHAPTER	STANDARD	CRITERIA	EVIDENCE-BASED EXAMPLES (INCLUDING PAGE NO.)
Unit 6 Responses to altered gastrointestinal function			
20 A person-centred approach to assessing the gastrointestinal system	1. Thinks critically and analyses nursing practice	1.6. Maintains accurate, comprehensive and timely documentation of assessments, planning, decision making, actions and evaluations	Provides comprehensive nursing notes in relation to nutritional status assessment, in Sample documentation, p. 608
	4. Comprehensively conducts assessments	4.1. Conducts assessments that are holistic as well as culturally appropriate	Conducts a health history for a person with an alteration or at risk of alterations in nutrition and gastrointestinal function, in Functional health pattern interview, pp. 610–611
		4.2. Uses a range of assessment techniques to systematically collect relevant and accurate information and data to inform practice	Conducts and/or assists in the collection of gastric secretions, blood and tissue samples and radiographical studies, in Diagnostic tests, pp. 612–616 Conducts a physical assessment of nutritional status and the gastrointestinal system, in Nutritional and gastrointestinal assessments, pp. 617–626
	6. Provides safe, appropriate and responsive quality nursing practice	6.1. Provides comprehensive, safe, quality practice to achieve agreed goals and outcomes that are responsive to the nursing needs of people	Provides related nursing care and monitors the results of diagnostic tests, in Diagnostic tests, pp. 612–616
21 Nursing care of people with nutritional disorders	1. Thinks critically and analyses nursing practice	1.3. Respects all cultures and experiences, which includes responding to the role of family and community that underpin the health of Aboriginal and Torres Strait Islander peoples and people of other cultures	Considers the person's cultural background when providing care, in Nursing care plan, p. 646
	2. Engages in therapeutic and professional relationships	2.3. Recognises that people are the experts in the experience of their life	Conducts education that is sensitive to the older adult's age group and experiences, in Meeting individualised needs, p. 639
		2.6. Uses delegation, supervision, coordination, consultation and referrals in professional relationships to achieve improved outcomes	Notifies the doctor in relation to hypersensitivity to iodine or seafood, in Medication administration, p. 642 Includes dietitian in the evaluation of nutritional needs, in Nursing care plan, p. 646
	4. Comprehensively conducts assessments	4.1. Conducts assessments that are holistic as well as culturally appropriate	When caring for a person with obesity, carries out the processes involved in the assessment phase that specifically address the person's needs, in Nursing care plan, p. 637 Provides comprehensive assessment, including cultural practices in relation to nutritional assessment, for the person with malnutrition, in Nursing care plan, p. 646

CHAPTER	STANDARD	CRITERIA	EVIDENCE-BASED EXAMPLES (INCLUDING PAGE NO.)
		4.2. Uses a range of assessment techniques to systematically collect relevant and accurate information and data to inform practice	Monitors vitamin and mineral manifestations, in Medication administration, p. 642
	5. Develops a plan for nursing practice	5.1. Uses assessment data and best available evidence to develop a plan	Plans for safe nursing management of medication to treat obesity, in Medication administration, p. 632
			Uses assessment data to determine priority nursing diagnoses and to select and implement nursing interventions for a person with obesity, in Nursing care plan, p. 637
			Plans and provides family teaching to restore, promote and maintain nutritional status in the older person, in Meeting individualised needs, p. 639
			Adapts cultural values and variations into the plan of care for a person with a nutritional disorder, in Nursing care plan, p. 646
		5.2. Collaboratively constructs nursing practice plans until contingencies, options, priorities, goals, actions, outcomes and time frames are agreed with the relevant people	Integrates interprofessional care into the plan of care for a person with malnutrition, in Nursing care plan, p. 646
	6. Provides safe, appropriate and responsive quality nursing practice	6.1. Provides comprehensive, safe, quality practice to achieve agreed goals and outcomes that are responsive to the nursing needs of people	Implements medication management of the person with obesity, in Medication administration, p. 632
			Conducts education for maintaining nutritional status following bariatric surgery, in Meeting individualised needs, p. 635
			When caring for a person with obesity, carries out the processes involved in the intervention phase that specifically address the person's needs, in Nursing care plan, p. 637
			Administers vitamin and mineral supplements and enteral and parenteral nutrition knowledgeably and safely, in Medication administration, p. 642
			Conducts education for maintaining nutritional status for the older adult, in Meeting individualised needs, p. 639
			Provides comprehensive nursing care for a person with malnutrition, in Nursing care plan, p. 646
	7. Evaluates outcomes to inform nursing practice	7.1. Evaluates and monitors progress towards expected goals and outcomes	Evaluates responses to comprehensive nursing care for a person with obesity, in Nursing care plan, p. 637
			Evaluates medication management of vitamin and mineral supplements, in Medication administration, p. 642
			Provides comprehensive nursing care for a person with malnutrition, in Nursing care plan, p. 646
22 Nursing care of people with upper gastrointestinal disorders	2. Engages in therapeutic and professional relationships	2.6. Uses delegation, supervision, coordination, consultation and referrals in professional relationships to achieve improved outcomes	Includes dietitian in the assessment of nutritional needs for a person with oral cancer, in Nursing care plan, p. 659
			Includes pharmacist in the assessment and delivery of education for pharmacotherapy for peptic ulcer disease, in Nursing care plan, p. 683

CHAPTER	STANDARD	CRITERIA	EVIDENCE-BASED EXAMPLES (INCLUDING PAGE NO.)
	4. Comprehensively conducts assessments	4.1. Conducts assessments that are holistic as well as culturally appropriate	Demonstrates assessment in nursing care for a person with oral cancer, in Nursing care plan, p. 659
			Includes evidence-based practice in relation to the assessment of the person with peptic ulcer disease, in Nursing care plan, p. 683
			When caring for a person with gastric cancer, carries out the processes involved in the assessment that specifically address the person's needs, in Nursing care plan, p. 689
	5. Develops a plan for nursing practice	5.1. Uses assessment data and best available evidence to develop a plan	Plans for safe nursing management of medication for mucositis, in Medication administration, p. 656
			When caring for a person with oral cancer, determines priority nursing diagnoses and interventions based on assessed data, in Nursing care plan, p. 659
			Plans for safe nursing management of medication for GORD, gastritis and peptic ulcer disease, in Medication administration, pp. 663–664
			Plans for safe nursing management of medication for nausea and vomiting, including contraindications, interactions, adverse effects, oral and intravenous routes and monitoring test results, in Medication administration, p. 670
			Plans nursing care using evidence-based research for the person with peptic ulcer disease, in Nursing care plan, p. 683
			Devises a teaching plan for the person with peptic ulcer disease, in Community-based care, p. 684
			When caring for a person with gastric cancer, determines priority nursing diagnoses and interventions based on assessed data, in Nursing care plan, p. 689
		5.2. Collaboratively constructs nursing practice plans until contingencies, options, priorities, goals, actions, outcomes and time frames are agreed with the relevant people	When caring for a person with oral cancer, coordinates and integrates interprofessional care into the plan of care that specifically address the person's energy needs and enteral feeding, in Nursing care plan, p. 659
			When caring for a person with peptic ulcer disease, coordinates and integrates interprofessional care of the pharmacist, which specifically addresses pharmacotherapy, in Nursing care plan, p. 683
			Plans and provides the person with gastric cancer and their family with education to promote, maintain and restore functional health in relation to diet, pain management and diagnosis, in Nursing care plan, p. 689

CHAPTER	STANDARD	CRITERIA	EVIDENCE-BASED EXAMPLES (INCLUDING PAGE NO.)
	6. Provides safe, appropriate and responsive quality nursing practice	6.1. Provides comprehensive, safe, quality practice to achieve agreed goals and outcomes that are responsive to the nursing needs of people	Administers medications knowledgeably and safely for mucositis, in Medication administration, p. 656
			Demonstrates comprehensive nursing care for a person with oral cancer, in Nursing care plan, p. 659
			Administers medications, including oral and intravenous routes, and monitors drug interactions and adverse reactions, in Medication administration, pp. 663–664
			Focuses on education of a person with peptic ulcer disease and their family in relation to medication and stress management, in Nursing care plan, p. 683
			When caring for a person with gastric cancer, carries out the processes involved in the intervention phase that specifically address the person's needs, in Nursing care plan, p. 689
	7. Evaluates outcomes to inform nursing practice	7.1. Evaluates and monitors progress towards expected goals and outcomes	Evaluates responses to comprehensive nursing care for a person with oral cancer, in Nursing care plan, p. 659
			Evaluates responses to comprehensive nursing care for a person with peptic ulcer disease, in Nursing care plan, p. 683
			Evaluates responses to comprehensive nursing care for a person with gastric cancer, in Nursing care plan, p. 689
23 Nursing care of people with bowel disorders	1. Thinks critically and analyses nursing practice	1.2. Practises within a professional and ethical nursing framework	Considers the person's cultural background when providing care for ulcerative colitis, in Nursing care plan, p. 741
	2. Engages in therapeutic and professional relationships	2.2. Communicates effectively and is respectful of a person's dignity, culture, values, beliefs and rights	Communicates effectively to ensure religious and cultural beliefs are incorporated when caring for the person with ulcerative colitis, in Nursing care plan, p. 741
	4. Comprehensively conducts assessments	4.1. Conducts assessments that are holistic as well as culturally appropriate	When caring for a person with appendicitis, carries out the processes involved in the assessment phase that specifically address the person's needs, in Nursing care plan, p. 711
			Provides an assessment for a person having an ileostomy, in Nursing care of the person, pp. 737–738
			Provides an assessment for a person with ulcerative colitis, in Nursing care plan, p. 741
			When caring for a person with colorectal cancer, carries out the processes involved in the assessment phase that specifically address the person's needs, in Nursing care plan, p. 757
		4.2. Uses a range of assessment techniques to systematically collect relevant and accurate information and data to inform practice	During the postoperative phase, fluid status, nasogastric drainage, wound assessment and gastrointestinal assessment are ongoing so the plan of care can be revised to ensure optimal care for a person having bowel surgery, in Nursing care of the person, p. 753

CHAPTER	STANDARD	CRITERIA	EVIDENCE-BASED EXAMPLES (INCLUDING PAGE NO.)
	5. Develops a plan for nursing practice	5.1. Uses assessment data and best available evidence to develop a plan	Plans for safe nursing management of antidiarrhoeal preparations, including contraindications, interactions, adverse effects, response to medication and monitoring test results, in Medication administration, p. 695
			Devises a teaching plan for the person with diarrhoea, in Community-based care, p. 697
			Plans for safe nursing management of laxative medication, including medication preparation, contraindications, monitoring blood profile and adverse reactions, in Medication administration, pp. 699–700
			Devises a teaching plan for the person with an appendectomy, in Community-based care, pp. 710–711
			Plans nursing care using evidence-based research for the person with appendicitis, in Nursing care plan, p. 711
			Revises plan of care when necessary to provide effective interventions restoring functional health status to a person with a bacterial infection of the bowel, in Table 23.3 Selected bacterial infections of the bowel, p. 717
			Plans for effective medication management of protozoal infections of the bowel, in Table 23.5 Common protozoal infections of the bowel, p. 723
			Plans for safe nursing management of antiprotozoal agents, including contraindications, adverse effects, response to medication and monitoring blood test results, in Medication administration, p. 725
			Plans for safe nursing management of inflammatory bowel disease medications, including vital signs, blood tests, contraindications, adverse effects and response to medication, in Medication administration, pp. 734–735
			Plans for comprehensive nursing care for a person having an ileostomy, in Nursing care of the person, pp. 737–738
			Devises a teaching plan for the person with polyps, in Community-based care, p. 750
			Plans for comprehensive nursing care for a person requiring bowel surgery, in Nursing care of the person, p. 753
			Plans for comprehensive nursing care for a person with a colostomy, in Nursing care of the person, p. 755
			Determines priority nursing diagnoses, based on assessed data, to select and implement individualised nursing interventions for a person with colorectal cancer, in Nursing care plan, p. 757
			Devises a teaching plan for the person with a hernia, in Community-based care, p. 760

CHAPTER	STANDARD	CRITERIA	EVIDENCE-BASED EXAMPLES (INCLUDING PAGE NO.)
		5.2. Collaboratively constructs nursing practice plans until contingencies, options, priorities, goals, actions, outcomes and time frames are agreed with the relevant people	Integrates interprofessional care into care of a person with ulcerative colitis, in Nursing care plan, p. 741
	6. Provides safe, appropriate and responsive quality nursing practice	6.1. Provides comprehensive, safe, quality practice to achieve agreed goals and outcomes that are responsive to the nursing needs of people	Administers antidiarrhoeal medications and monitors response, drug interactions and adverse reactions, in Medication administration, p. 695
			Administers laxatives and monitors response and blood profile, in Medication administration, pp. 699–700
			Provides targeted nursing care for a person with appendicitis, in Nursing care plan, p. 711
			Administers antiprotozoal agents and monitors response, adverse reactions and blood test results, in Medication administration, p. 725
			Administers medications used in the management of inflammatory bowel disease knowledgeably and safely, including monitoring vital signs, blood tests, adverse effects and response to medication, in Medication administration, pp. 734–735
			Provides skilled care to a person following the formation of an ileostomy, in Nursing care of the person, pp. 737–738
			Provides comprehensive nursing care for a person with ulcerative colitis, in Nursing care plan, p. 741
			Provides skilled care to a person following bowel surgery, in Nursing care of the person, p. 753
			Provides skilled care to a person following the formation of a colostomy, in Nursing care of the person, p. 755
			When caring for a person with colorectal cancer, carries out the processes involved in the intervention phase that specifically address the person's needs, in Nursing care plan, p. 757
	7. Evaluates outcomes to inform nursing practice	7.1. Evaluates and monitors progress towards expected goals and outcomes	Evaluates responses to nursing care for a person with appendicitis, in Nursing care plan, p. 711
			Evaluates responses to comprehensive nursing care for a person with ulcerative colitis, in Nursing care plan, p. 741
			Evaluates responses to comprehensive nursing care for a person with colorectal cancer, in Nursing care plan, p. 757
		7.3. Determines, documents and communicates further priorities, goals and outcomes with the relevant persons	Communicates to the surgeon abnormal findings for a person having an ileostomy, in Nursing care of the person, p. 737
			Communicates decreased urine output, in Consideration for practice, p. 764
24 Nursing care of people with gallbladder, liver and pancreatic disorders	2. Engages in therapeutic and professional relationships	2.3. Recognises that people are the experts in the experience of their life	Provides verbal and written information about medication and complications of cirrhosis, in Nursing care plan, p. 800

CHAPTER	STANDARD	CRITERIA	EVIDENCE-BASED EXAMPLES (INCLUDING PAGE NO.)
		2.6. Uses delegation, supervision, coordination, consultation and referrals in professional relationships to achieve improved outcomes	Involves the social worker for referral to community services for the person with alcoholic cirrhosis, in Nursing care plan, p. 800
	4. Comprehensively conducts assessments	4.1. Conducts assessments that are holistic as well as culturally appropriate	Assesses the person with pancreatitis, in Nursing care plan, p. 809
		4.2. Uses a range of assessment techniques to systematically collect relevant and accurate information and data to inform practice	Assesses the person with alcoholic cirrhosis, in Nursing care plan, p. 800
	5. Develops a plan for nursing practice	5.1. Uses assessment data and best available evidence to develop a plan	Develops a plan of care for the person for the management of post-laparoscopic cholecystectomy, in Nursing care of the person, p. 780 Integrates psychosocial considerations into the plan of care for a person with cholelithiasis, in Nursing care plan, p. 781 Plans for safe nursing management of medications for cirrhosis, including vital signs, weight, fluid balance, blood tests, electrocardiogram, bowel function, hearing function and other responses to the medication, in Medication administration, p. 796 Plans comprehensive nursing care for a person with a liver transplantation, in Nursing care of the person, p. 799 Plans comprehensive nursing care for a person with a resection of the pancreas, in Nursing care of the person, p. 809
		5.2. Collaboratively constructs nursing practice plans until contingencies, options, priorities, goals, actions, outcomes and time frames are agreed with the relevant people	Integrates a plan for social work support into nursing care of the person with alcoholic cirrhosis, in Nursing care plan, p. 800 Plans for appropriate person and family education to promote, maintain and restore functional health status for the person with post acute pancreatitis, in Nursing care plan, p. 809
	6. Provides safe, appropriate and responsive quality nursing practice	6.1. Provides comprehensive, safe, quality practice to achieve agreed goals and outcomes that are responsive to the nursing needs of people	Educates the person for home care of a laparoscopic cholecystectomy, in Nursing care of the person, p. 780 Monitors for postoperative bleeding with a T-tube, in Nursing care of the person, p. 779 Provides comprehensive nursing care for a person with cholelithiasis, in Nursing care plan, p. 781 Administers medications used in the management of the liver knowledgeably and safely, including monitoring vital signs, weight, fluid balance, blood tests, electrocardiogram, bowel function, hearing function and other responses to the medication, in Medication administration, p. 796 Provides comprehensive nursing care for a person with a liver transplant, in Nursing care of the person, p. 799

CHAPTER	STANDARD	CRITERIA	EVIDENCE-BASED EXAMPLES (INCLUDING PAGE NO.)
			Provides comprehensive nursing care for a person with alcoholic cirrhosis, in Nursing care plan, p. 800
			Conducts education for home-based care post acute pancreatitis, in Nursing care plan, p. 809
			Provides comprehensive nursing care for a person with a resection of the pancreas, in Nursing care of the person, p. 811
	7. Evaluates outcomes to inform nursing practice	7.1. Evaluates and monitors progress towards expected goals and outcomes	Monitors for and documents manifestations of postoperative bleeding, in Nursing care of the person, p. 779
			Evaluates nursing care for a person with cholelithiasis, in Nursing care plan, p. 781
			Evaluates nursing care for a person with alcoholic cirrhosis, in Nursing care plan, p. 800
			Evaluates nursing care for a person with pancreatitis, in Nursing care plan, p. 809
		7.3. Determines, documents and communicates further priorities, goals and outcomes with the relevant persons	Reports manifestations of postoperative bleeding, in Nursing care of the person, p. 779
Unit 7 Responses to altered urinary elimination			
25 A person-centred approach to assessing the renal system	4. Comprehensively conducts assessments	4.1. Conducts assessments that are holistic as well as culturally appropriate	Conducts a health history for a person with an alteration or at risk of alterations in urinary elimination, in Functional health pattern interview, pp. 825–826
		4.2. Uses a range of assessment techniques to systematically collect relevant and accurate information and data to inform practice	Conducts and/or assists in the collection of urine and blood samples and radiographical studies, in Diagnostic tests, pp. 828–833
			Conducts a physical assessment of the renal system, in Renal/Kidney assessments, pp. 833–834
	6. Provides safe, appropriate and responsive quality nursing practice	6.1. Provides comprehensive, safe, quality practice to achieve agreed goals and outcomes that are responsive to the nursing needs of people	Provides related nursing care and monitors the results of diagnostic tests, in Diagnostic tests, pp. 828–833
26 Nursing care of people with urinary tract disorders	2. Engages in therapeutic and professional relationships	2.2. Communicates effectively and is respectful of a person's dignity, culture, values, beliefs and rights	Communicates therapeutically with patient and family member, in Nursing care plan, pp. 871–872
		2.6. Uses delegation, supervision, coordination, consultation and referrals in professional relationships to achieve improved outcomes	Includes the Continence Nurse Advisor in the provision of care that specifically addresses the person's urinary elimination via stoma, in Nursing care plan, p. 860
	4. Comprehensively conducts assessments	4.1. Conducts assessments that are holistic as well as culturally appropriate	Assesses the person with a bladder tumour, in Nursing care plan, p. 860
			Assesses the functional health status of a person at risk of UTI and UI, in Nursing care of the older adult, p. 866
			Assesses the person with urinary incontinence, in Nursing care plan, pp. 871–872

CHAPTER	STANDARD	CRITERIA	EVIDENCE-BASED EXAMPLES (INCLUDING PAGE NO.)
		4.2. Uses a range of assessment techniques to systematically collect relevant and accurate information and data to inform practice	Assesses the person with urinary calculi, in Nursing care plan, p. 853
			During the postoperative phase, provides ongoing assessment for urine output, catheter drainage and wound to ensure optimal care for a person with a bladder neck suspension, in Nursing care of the person, p. 869
	5. Develops a plan for nursing practice	5.1. Uses assessment data and best available evidence to develop a plan	Plans for safe nursing management of urinary anti-infective medication, in Medication administration, p. 841
			Plans for the postoperative phase for a person with a ureteral stent, in Nursing care of the person, p. 842
			When caring for a person with urinary calculi, carries out the processes involved in the planning phase that specifically address the person's needs, in Nursing care of the person, p. 851
			Based on assessment data, determines priority nursing diagnoses and interventions for a person with urinary calculi, in Nursing care plan, pp. 853–854
			In the preoperative phase, provides education, stoma preparation and bowel care, and during the postoperative phase, monitors urine output, catheter drainage, stoma assessment and electrolytes to ensure optimal care for a person with a cystectomy and urinary diversion, in Nursing care of the person, p. 859
			Plans for safe nursing management of medication for the person with a neurogenic bladder, including contraindications, desired effect, drug interactions, vital signs and adverse reactions, in Medication administration, p. 864
			Plans individualised education for the person at risk of UTI and UI, in Nursing care of the older adult, pp. 866–867
			Recognises that the preoperative phase involves education and that, during the postoperative phase, urine output, catheter drainage and wound assessment are ongoing to ensure optimal care for a person with a bladder neck suspension, in Nursing care of the person, p. 869
		5.2. Collaboratively constructs nursing practice plans until contingencies, options, priorities, goals, actions, outcomes and time frames are agreed with the relevant people	Plans education for prevention and self-care of cystitis, in Nursing care plan, p. 844
			Integrates the interprofessional plan of care into care for a person with a bladder tumour, in Nursing care plan, p. 860
			Plans education for prevention and self-care of urinary incontinence, in Nursing care plan, p. 872
	6. Provides safe, appropriate and responsive quality nursing practice	6.1. Provides comprehensive, safe, quality practice to achieve agreed goals and outcomes that are responsive to the nursing needs of people	Knowledgeably and safely administers prescribed medications, including monitoring adverse reactions, for people with urinary tract disorders, in Medication administration, p. 841
			Conducts education for home-based cystitis, in Nursing care plan, p. 844

CHAPTER	STANDARD	CRITERIA	EVIDENCE-BASED EXAMPLES (INCLUDING PAGE NO.)
			When caring for a person with urinary calculi, carries out the processes involved in the intervention phase that specifically address the person's needs, in Nursing care of the person, p. 851
			Provides comprehensive nursing care for a person with urinary calculi, in Nursing care plan, p. 853
			In the preoperative phase, provides education, stoma preparation and bowel care, and during the postoperative phase, monitors urine output, catheter drainage, stoma assessment and electrolytes to ensure optimal care for a person with a cystectomy and urinary diversion, in Nursing care of the person, p. 859
			Provides comprehensive nursing care for a person with a bladder tumour, in Nursing care plan, p. 860
			Knowledgeably and safely administers oral and subcutaneous prescribed medications and monitors vital signs and adverse reactions for people with urinary tract disorders, in Medication administration, p. 864
			Conducts education for home-based urinary incontinence, in Nursing care plan, p. 872
	7. Evaluates outcomes to inform nursing practice	7.1. Evaluates and monitors progress towards expected goals and outcomes	Evaluates responses to home care for a person with cystitis, in Nursing care plan, p. 844
			Evaluates responses to nursing care for a person with urinary calculi, in Nursing care plan, pp. 853–854
			Evaluates responses to nursing care for a person with a bladder tumour, in Nursing care plan, p. 860
			Evaluates responses to home care for a person with urinary incontinence, in Nursing care plan, p. 872
27 Nursing care of people with kidney disorders	2. Engages in therapeutic and professional relationships	2.2. Communicates effectively and is respectful of a person's dignity, culture, values, beliefs and rights	Involves the person with end-stage kidney disease in the decision making for health management, in Nursing care plan, p. 919
		2.6. Uses delegation, supervision, coordination, consultation and referrals in professional relationships to achieve improved outcomes	Consults the dietitian for menu planning that specifically addresses the nutritional needs of a person with end-stage kidney disease, in Nursing care plan, p. 919
	4. Comprehensively conducts assessments	4.1. Conducts assessments that are holistic as well as culturally appropriate	When caring for a person with end-stage kidney disease, carries out the processes involved in the assessment phase that specifically address the person's needs, in Nursing care plan, pp. 887–888
		4.2. Uses a range of assessment techniques to systematically collect relevant and accurate information and data to inform practice	Collects assessment data related to traumatic injuries and complications for a person with acute kidney injury, in Nursing care plan, pp. 887–888

CHAPTER	STANDARD	CRITERIA	EVIDENCE-BASED EXAMPLES (INCLUDING PAGE NO.)
		4.3. Works in partnership to determine factors that affect, or potentially affect, the health and wellbeing of people and populations to determine priorities for action and/or referral	When caring for a person with end-stage kidney disease, involves the person and the interprofessional team when addressing the person's needs, in Nursing care plan, p. 919
	5. Develops a plan for nursing practice	5.1. Uses assessment data and best available evidence to develop a plan	Plans appropriate care for a person with acute kidney injury, including weight, vital signs, laboratory results, oral and intravenous administration, hearing assessment, drug interactions and adverse reactions, in Medication administration, p. 885
			Based on assessment data, determines priority nursing diagnoses and interventions for a person with acute kidney injury, in Nursing care plan, p. 888
			In the preoperative phase, monitors blood results and provides person-focused teaching, and in the postoperative phase, monitors urine output and drainage tubes, addressing loss of kidney for a person having a nephrectomy, in Nursing care of the person, p. 891
			Plans that pre-, intra- and post-dialysis care ensures optimal management for a person requiring intermittent haemodialysis, in Nursing care of the person, p. 910
			Plans evidence-based practice care for a person undergoing peritoneal dialysis, in Nursing care of the person, p. 913
			In the preoperative phase, plans for education, dialysis and immunosuppressive medication, and in the postoperative phase, monitors urine output, catheter drainage, fluid and electrolyte balance, vital signs and wound assessment to ensure optimal care for a person receiving a kidney transplant, in Nursing care of the person, p. 916
			Devises a teaching plan for the person with chronic kidney and end-stage kidney disease, in Community-based care, pp. 920–921
		5.2. Collaboratively constructs nursing practice plans until contingencies, options, priorities, goals, actions, outcomes and time frames are agreed with the relevant people	Collaborates with the person and other members of the interprofessional team to prioritise and implement care, in Nursing care plan, p. 919
	6. Provides safe, appropriate and responsive quality nursing practice	6.1. Provides comprehensive, safe, quality practice to achieve agreed goals and outcomes that are responsive to the nursing needs of people	When caring for a person with trauma and acute kidney injury, carries out the processes involved in the care of the trauma victim, in Nursing care plan, p. 888
			Monitors blood results and provides person-focused teaching, and in the postoperative phase, monitors urine output and drainage tubes and addresses loss of kidney for a person having a nephrectomy, in Nursing care of the person, p. 891

CHAPTER	STANDARD	CRITERIA	EVIDENCE-BASED EXAMPLES (INCLUDING PAGE NO.)
			Ensures optimal management for a person requiring intermittent haemodialysis, in Nursing care of the person, p. 910
			Provides evidence-based care for a person undergoing peritoneal dialysis, in Nursing care of the person, p. 913
			Provides education, dialysis and immunosuppressive medication, and during the postoperative phase, monitors urine output, catheter drainage, fluid and electrolyte balance, vital signs and wound assessment for the optimal care of a person receiving a kidney transplant, in Nursing care of the person, p. 916
			When caring for a person with end-stage kidney disease, carries out the processes involved in the intervention phase that specifically address the person's needs, in Nursing care plan, p. 919
	7. Evaluates outcomes to inform nursing practice	7.1. Evaluates and monitors progress towards expected goals and outcomes	When caring for a person with acute kidney injury, carries out the processes involved in the evaluation phase that specifically address the person's needs, in Nursing care plan, p. 888
			Evaluates all responses to care for a person with end-stage kidney disease, in Nursing care plan, p. 919
Unit 8 Responses to altered cardiovascular function			
28 Responses to altered cardiovascular function	4. Comprehensively conducts assessments	4.1. Conducts assessments that are holistic as well as culturally appropriate	Conducts a health history for a person with an alteration or at risk of alterations in cardiac, haematological or lymphatic function, in Functional health pattern interview, pp. 946–947
		4.2. Uses a range of assessment techniques to systematically collect relevant and accurate information and data to inform practice	Conducts and/or assists in the collection of blood and fluid samples and electrocardiograph and radiographical studies for cardiac disorders, in Diagnostic tests, pp. 948–952
			Conducts an electrocardiograph and interprets tracing, in Box 28.2 Electrocardiogram, pp. 952–954
			Conducts and/or assists in the collection of blood, fluid and tissue samples for haematological, peripheral vascular and lymphatic disorders, in Diagnostic tests, pp. 957–958
			Conducts a physical assessment of the cardiac, haematological, peripheral vascular and lymphatic systems, in Cardiac assessments, pp. 961–971
	5. Develops a plan for nursing practice	5.1. Uses assessment data and best available evidence to develop a plan	Plans the nursing management of the processes involved before, during and after the procedure of cardiac catheterisation, in Nursing care of the person, p. 956
			Plans the nursing management of the processes involved before, during and after the procedure of pericardiocentesis, in Nursing care of the person, p. 956
			Plans the nursing management of the processes involved before, during and after the procedure of bone marrow studies, in Nursing care of the person, p. 958

CHAPTER	STANDARD	CRITERIA	EVIDENCE-BASED EXAMPLES (INCLUDING PAGE NO.)
	6. Provides safe, appropriate and responsive quality nursing practice	6.1. Provides comprehensive, safe, quality practice to achieve agreed goals and outcomes that are responsive to the nursing needs of people	When caring for a person having cardiac catheterisation, carries out the processes involved before, during and after the procedure, in Nursing care of the person, p. 956 When caring for a person having pericardiocentesis, carries out the processes involved before, during and after the procedure, in Nursing care of the person, p. 956 Provides related nursing care and monitors the results of diagnostic tests for cardiac disorders, in Diagnostic tests, pp. 948–952 Provides related nursing care and monitors the results of diagnostic tests for haematological, peripheral vascular and lymphatic disorders, in Diagnostic tests, pp. 957–958 When caring for a person having bone marrow studies, carries out the processes involved before, during and after the procedure, in Nursing care of the person, p. 958
29 Nursing care of people with coronary heart disease	2. Engages in therapeutic and professional relationships	2.6. Uses delegation, supervision, coordination, consultation and referrals in professional relationships to achieve improved health outcomes	Advises consultation with the doctor if adverse reaction occurs for a cholesterol-lowering drug, in Medication administration, p. 984 When caring for a person with acute myocardial infarction, notifies medical team of abnormal bleeding and dangerous arrhythmias, in Nursing care plan, p. 1007 When caring for a person with supraventricular tachycardia, notifies doctor of changes in vital signs and ECG, in Nursing care plan, p. 1029
	4. Comprehensively conducts assessments	4.1. Conducts assessments that are holistic as well as culturally appropriate	When caring for a person with coronary heart disease, carries out the processes involved in the assessment phase that specifically address the person's needs for undergoing PTCA, in Nursing care of the person, p. 993 When caring for a person with acute myocardial infarction having a coronary artery bypass surgery, carries out the processes involved in the assessment phase that specifically address the person's needs, in Nursing care plan, p. 998 When caring for a person with acute myocardial infarction, carries out the processes involved in the assessment phase that specifically address the person's needs, in Nursing care plan, p. 1007 When caring for a person with cardiac arrhythmias, carries out the processes involved in the assessment phase that specifically address the person's age-related needs, in Nursing care of the older adult, p. 1011 When caring for a person with supraventricular tachycardia, carries out the processes involved in the assessment phase that specifically address the person's needs, in Nursing care plan, p. 1029

CHAPTER	STANDARD	CRITERIA	EVIDENCE-BASED EXAMPLES (INCLUDING PAGE NO.)
		4.2. Uses a range of assessment techniques to systematically collect relevant and accurate information and data to inform practice	Recognises that the preoperative phase involves education and laboratory and diagnostic tests, and during the postoperative phase, monitoring vital signs, haemodynamic monitoring, heart sounds, urine output, chest drainage and fluid and electrolyte balance, and administration of drugs are ongoing to ensure optimal care for a person with a coronary artery bypass graft, in Nursing care of the person, pp. 995–997
	5. Develops a plan for nursing practice	5.1. Uses assessment data and best available evidence to develop a plan	In the preoperative phase, plans for education and laboratory and diagnostic tests, and during the postoperative phase, monitors vital signs, haemodynamic monitoring, heart sounds, urine output, chest drainage and fluid and electrolyte balance and administration of drugs to ensure optimal care for a person with a coronary artery bypass graft, in Nursing care of the person, pp. 995–997
			Plans appropriate nursing interventions for a person having coronary artery bypass surgery, in Nursing care plan, p. 998
			Plans the pre-infusion, during infusion and post-infusion care for the person receiving thrombolytic therapy, in Nursing care of the person, p. 1004
			Plans appropriate nursing interventions for a person with acute myocardial infarction, in Nursing care plan, p. 1007
			Plans the health education that addresses the older person's needs in relation to cardiac arrhythmias, in Nursing care of the older adult, p. 1011
			Plans for safe nursing management of anti-arrhythmic drugs, in Medication administration, pp. 1021–1022
			In the preoperative phase, plans for education and cardiac monitoring, and during the postoperative phase, undertakes a chest x-ray, positioning, range of movement exercises, cardiac monitoring, identification of potential complications and appropriate health education for a person requiring a permanent pacemaker implant, in Nursing care of the person, pp. 1027–1028
			Devises a teaching plan for the person with arrhythmias, in Community-based care, p. 1030
		5.2. Collaboratively constructs nursing practice plans until contingencies, options, priorities, goals, actions, outcomes and time frames are agreed with the relevant people	Integrates multidisciplinary care into nursing care planning and implementation for a person with supraventricular tachycardia, in Nursing care plan, p. 1029

CHAPTER	STANDARD	CRITERIA	EVIDENCE-BASED EXAMPLES (INCLUDING PAGE NO.)
	6. Provides safe, appropriate and responsive quality nursing practice	6.1. Provides comprehensive, safe, quality practice to achieve agreed goals and outcomes that are responsive to the nursing needs of people	Delivers safe nursing management and health education of anti-anginal medications, in Medication administration, pp. 987–988
			Delivers safe nursing management and health education of antiplatelet drugs, in Medication administration, pp. 991–992
			When caring for a person who has had coronary artery bypass surgery, carries out the processes involved in the implementation phase that specifically address the person's needs, in Nursing care plan, p. 998
			Undertakes pre-infusion care assessment and diagnostic tests, during the infusion monitors vital signs, body position and haemodynamic monitoring, and post infusion monitors vital signs, blood tests, body position, puncture sites, bleeding, platelet drugs and cardiac monitoring for the optimal care of a person receiving thrombolytic therapy, in Nursing care of the person, p. 1004
			When caring for a person with acute myocardial infarction, carries out the processes involved in the implementation phase that specifically address the person's needs, in Nursing care plan, p. 1007
			Conducts education for cardiac arrhythmias, in Nursing care of the older adult, p. 1011
			Delivers safe nursing management and health education of anti-arrhythmic drugs, in Medication administration, pp. 1021–1022
			In the preoperative phase, conducts person-centred education and cardiac monitoring, and during the postoperative phase, undertakes a chest x-ray, positioning of the body, range of movement exercises, cardiac monitoring, the identification of potential complications and appropriate health education for a person requiring a permanent pacemaker implant, in Nursing care of the person, pp. 1027–1028
			When caring for a person with supraventricular tachycardia, carries out the processes involved in the implementation phase that specifically address the person's needs, in Nursing care plan, p. 1029
	7. Evaluates outcomes to inform nursing practice	7.1. Evaluates and monitors progress towards expected goals and outcomes	Evaluates the effectiveness of nursing interventions for coronary artery bypass surgery, Nursing care plan, p. 998
			Evaluates the ongoing nursing interventions for a person with acute myocardial infarction, in Nursing care plan, p. 1007
		7.3. Determines, documents and communicates further priorities, goals and outcomes with the relevant persons	Reports manifestations of bleeding and arrhythmias, in Nursing care plan, p. 1007
			Evaluates the effectiveness of nursing interventions and reports vital signs and cardiac monitoring assessment for the person with supraventricular tachycardia, in Nursing care plan, p. 1029
30 Nursing care of people with cardiac disorders	2. Engages in therapeutic and professional relationships	2.6. Uses delegation, supervision, coordination, consultation and referrals in professional relationships to achieve improved outcomes	Collaborates with the medical staff, dietitian and physiotherapist in the care of a person with heart failure, in Nursing care plan, p. 1048

CHAPTER	STANDARD	CRITERIA	EVIDENCE-BASED EXAMPLES (INCLUDING PAGE NO.)
	4. Comprehensively conducts assessments	4.1. Conducts assessments that are holistic as well as culturally appropriate	Makes appropriate assessments for home care for the older adult with heart failure, in Nursing care of the older adult, p. 1038
			When caring for a person with heart failure, carries out the processes involved in the assessment phase, in Nursing care plan, p. 1048
		4.2. Uses a range of assessment techniques to systematically collect relevant and accurate information and data to inform practice	Includes evidence-based assessment in relation to providing nursing care for mitral valve prolapse, in Nursing care plan, p. 1074
	5. Develops a plan for nursing practice	5.1. Uses assessment data and best available evidence to develop a plan	Plans appropriate education and community-based care for the person with heart failure, in Nursing care of the older adult, p. 1038
			Plans appropriate and safe nursing management of medication for the person with heart failure, in Medication administration, pp. 1045–1046
			Devises a teaching plan for the person with infective endocarditis, in Community-based care, p. 1059
			Devises a teaching plan for the person with myocarditis, in Community-based care, p. 1060
			Devises a teaching plan for the person with pericarditis, in Community-based Care, p. 1064
			Devises a teaching plan for the person with valvular disease, in Community-based care, p. 1074
		5.2. Collaboratively constructs nursing practice plans until contingencies, options, priorities, goals, actions, outcomes and time frames are agreed with the relevant people	Actively participates in planning and coordinating interprofessional care for the person with heart failure, in Nursing care plan, p. 1048
			Plans evidence-based care with the cardiologist for the person with mitral valve prolapse, in Nursing care plan, pp. 1074–1075
	6. Provides safe, appropriate and responsive quality nursing practice	6.1. Provides comprehensive, safe, quality practice to achieve agreed goals and outcomes that are responsive to the nursing needs of people	Conducts education for heart failure, in Nursing care of the older adult, p. 1038
			Administers prescribed medications to individuals with heart failure, including monitoring fluid volume status, blood pressure, electrolyte levels, blood cell count, weight, abnormal bleeding, persistent cough, vital signs, renal function, pulse, cardiac monitoring, toxicity and renal function, and conducts health education, in Medication administration, pp. 1045–1046
			When caring for a person with heart failure, carries out the processes involved in the intervention phase that specifically address the person's medication, dietary and physiotherapy requirements, in Nursing care plan, p. 1048
			Includes evidence-based practice in relation to providing nursing care for mitral valve prolapse, in Nursing care plan, pp. 1074–1075
	7. Evaluates outcomes to inform nursing practice	7.1. Evaluates and monitors progress towards expected goals and outcomes	Evaluates evidence-based nursing care for mitral valve prolapse, in Nursing care plan, p. 1075

CHAPTER	STANDARD	CRITERIA	EVIDENCE-BASED EXAMPLES (INCLUDING PAGE NO.)
		7.3. Determines, documents and communicates further priorities, goals and outcomes with the relevant persons	Evaluates the effectiveness of nursing interventions and reports laboratory results for the person with heart failure, in Nursing care plan, p. 1048
31 Nursing care of people with vascular and lymphatic disorders	2. Engages in therapeutic and professional relationships	2.6. Uses delegation, supervision, coordination, consultation and referrals in professional relationships to achieve improved outcomes	Consults the dietitian for the person with hypertension dietary requirements, in Nursing care plan, p. 1098
			Consults the dietitian for the person with peripheral vascular disease dietary requirements, in Nursing care plan, p. 1111
			Consults the interprofessional team for assessments and interventions for the person with deep venous thrombosis, in Nursing care plan, p. 1123
	4. Comprehensively conducts assessments	4.1. Conducts assessments that are holistic as well as culturally appropriate	When caring for a person with hypertension, carries out the processes involved in the assessment phase that specifically address the person's requirements, in Nursing care plan, pp. 1097–1098
			Undertakes a holistic assessment of the person with peripheral vascular disease, in Nursing care plan, p. 1111
			Assesses evidence-based practice in relation to providing nursing care for deep venous thrombosis, in Nursing care plan, p. 1123
	5. Develops a plan for nursing practice	5.1. Uses assessment data and best available evidence to develop a plan	Plans person-centred teaching for antihypertensive therapy, in Medication administration, pp. 1091–1092
			Devises a teaching plan for the person with hypertension, in Community-based care, p. 1097
			In the preoperative phase, plans for education and reducing risk of rupture, and during the postoperative phase, monitors vital signs, fluid balance and adverse changes, and provides appropriate health education for a person requiring surgery to the aorta, in Nursing care of the person, p. 1105
			Devises a teaching plan for the person with an aneurysm, in Community-based care, pp. 1106–1107
			Devises a teaching plan for the person with peripheral vascular disease, in Community-based care, p. 1112
			Devises a teaching plan for the person with arterial occlusion, in Community-based care, p. 1114
			Plans person-centred teaching for anticoagulant therapy, in Medication administration, pp. 1120–1121
			Uses research and evidence-based plans to provide individualised care for the person with deep venous thrombosis, in Nursing care plan, p. 1123
			Devises a teaching plan for the person with venous thrombosis, in Community-based care, p. 1125

CHAPTER	STANDARD	CRITERIA	EVIDENCE-BASED EXAMPLES (INCLUDING PAGE NO.)
		5.2. Collaboratively constructs nursing practice plans until contingencies, options, priorities, goals, actions, outcomes and time frames are agreed with the relevant persons	Collaborates with the dietitian in planning care for a person with hypertension, in Nursing care plan, p. 1098 Collaborates with the dietitian to establish a healthy diet for the person with peripheral vascular disease, in Nursing care plan, p. 1111
	6. Provides safe, appropriate and responsive quality nursing practice	6.1. Provides comprehensive, safe, quality practice to achieve agreed goals and outcomes that are responsive to the nursing needs of people	Administers prescribed medications to individuals with hypertension, including monitoring blood pressure, pulse, blood count, electrolytes, renal function, adverse reactions, contraindications, adverse effects and fluid volume, and conducts health education, in Medication administration, pp. 1091 1092 When caring for a person with hypertension, carries out the processes involved in the intervention phase that specifically address the person's medication and exercise requirements, in Nursing care plan, p. 1098 In the preoperative phase, conducts person-centred education about reducing risk of rupture, and during the postoperative phase, monitors vital signs, fluid balance and adverse changes, and conducts appropriate health education for a person requiring surgery to the aorta, in Nursing care of the person, p. 1105 For the person with peripheral vascular disease, addresses diet, exercise, cessation of smoking and leg and foot care, in Nursing care plan, p. 1111 Administers prescribed anticoagulant medications orally, subcutaneously or intravenously, including monitoring blood results, test dose, adverse reactions and contraindications, in Medication administration, pp. 1120–1121 Includes evidence-based practice in relation to providing nursing care for deep venous thrombosis, in Nursing care plan, p. 1123
	7. Evaluates outcomes to inform nursing practice	7.1. Evaluates and monitors progress towards expected goals and outcomes	Evaluates the medication and exercise outcomes for a person with hypertension, in Nursing care plan, p. 1098 When caring for a person with peripheral vascular disease, evaluates diet, exercise, cessation of smoking and leg and foot care outcomes, in Nursing care plan, p. 1111 Evaluates evidence-based nursing care for deep venous thrombosis, in Nursing care plan, p. 1123
32 Nursing care of people with haematological disorders	2. Engages in therapeutic and professional relationships	2.6. Uses delegation, supervision, coordination, consultation and referrals in professional relationships to achieve improved outcomes	Notifies the performance of handwashing as per protocol, in Nursing care plan, p. 1164

CHAPTER	STANDARD	CRITERIA	EVIDENCE-BASED EXAMPLES (INCLUDING PAGE NO.)
	4. Comprehensively conducts assessments	4.1. Conducts assessments that are holistic as well as culturally appropriate	Assesses for education for folic acid deficiency anaemia, in Nursing care plan, p. 1150
			When a person has a definitive diagnosis of acute myelocytic leukaemia, ensures further assessment is conducted, in Nursing care plan, p. 1164
			When caring for a person with haemophilia, carries out ongoing assessment, in Nursing care plan, p. 1182
	5. Develops a plan for nursing practice	5.1. Uses assessment data and best available evidence to develop a plan	Plans for safe nursing management of medication that treats anaemia, in Medication administration, p. 1148
			Plans for appropriate education for the person with folic acid deficiency anaemia, in Nursing care plan, p. 1150
			Devises a teaching plan for the person with anaemia, in Community-based care, p. 1151
			Uses continuing assessment data to revise the plan of care as needed to restore, maintain or promote functional health in the person with acute myelocytic leukaemia, in Nursing care plan, p. 1164
			Devises a teaching plan for the person with leukaemia, in Community-based care, p. 1166
			Based on knowledge of pathophysiology, prescribed treatment and assessed data, identifies and prioritises nursing diagnoses for a person with Hodgkin's disease, in Nursing care plan, p. 1172
			Devises a teaching plan for the person with a malignant lymphoma, in Community-based care, p. 1173
			Devises a teaching plan for the person with multiple myeloma, in Community-based care, pp. 1175–1176
			Includes evidence-based practice in plan for providing nursing care for a person with haemophilia, in Nursing care plan, p. 1182
			Devises a teaching plan for the person with a bleeding disorder, in Community-based care, p. 1183
	6. Provides safe, appropriate and responsive quality nursing practice	6.1. Provides comprehensive, safe, quality practice to achieve agreed goals and outcomes that are responsive to the nursing needs of people	Safely and knowledgeably administers prescribed medications orally, intramuscularly and intravenously for anaemia, including monitoring drug interactions, adverse reactions, blood counts and electrolyte levels, in Medication administration, p. 1148
			Conducts education for folic acid deficiency anaemia, in Nursing care plan, p. 1150
			When a person has a definitive diagnosis of acute myelocytic leukaemia, ensures further intervention is conducted, in Nursing care plan, p. 1164
			Uses nursing research and evidence-based practice to implement individualised nursing interventions for a person with Hodgkin's disease, in Nursing care plan, p. 1172

CHAPTER	STANDARD	CRITERIA	EVIDENCE-BASED EXAMPLES (INCLUDING PAGE NO.)
			Implements nursing care that focuses on providing haematasis for a person with haemophilia, in Nursing care plan, p. 1182
	7. Evaluates outcomes to inform nursing practice	7.1. Evaluates and monitors progress towards expected goals and outcomes	Evaluates outcomes for reduction in folic acid deficiency anaemia and weight increase, in Nursing care plan, p. 1150
			When a person has a definitive diagnosis of Hodgkin's disease, ensures further evaluation is conducted, in Nursing care plan, p. 1172
			Evaluates the progression of haematasis for a person with haemophilia, in Nursing care plan, p. 1182

Source: Nursing and Midwifery Board of Australia (NMBA) (2016). *Registered Nurse Standards for Practice*. © Nursing and Midwifery Board of Australia, www.nursingmidwiferyboard.gov.au/.

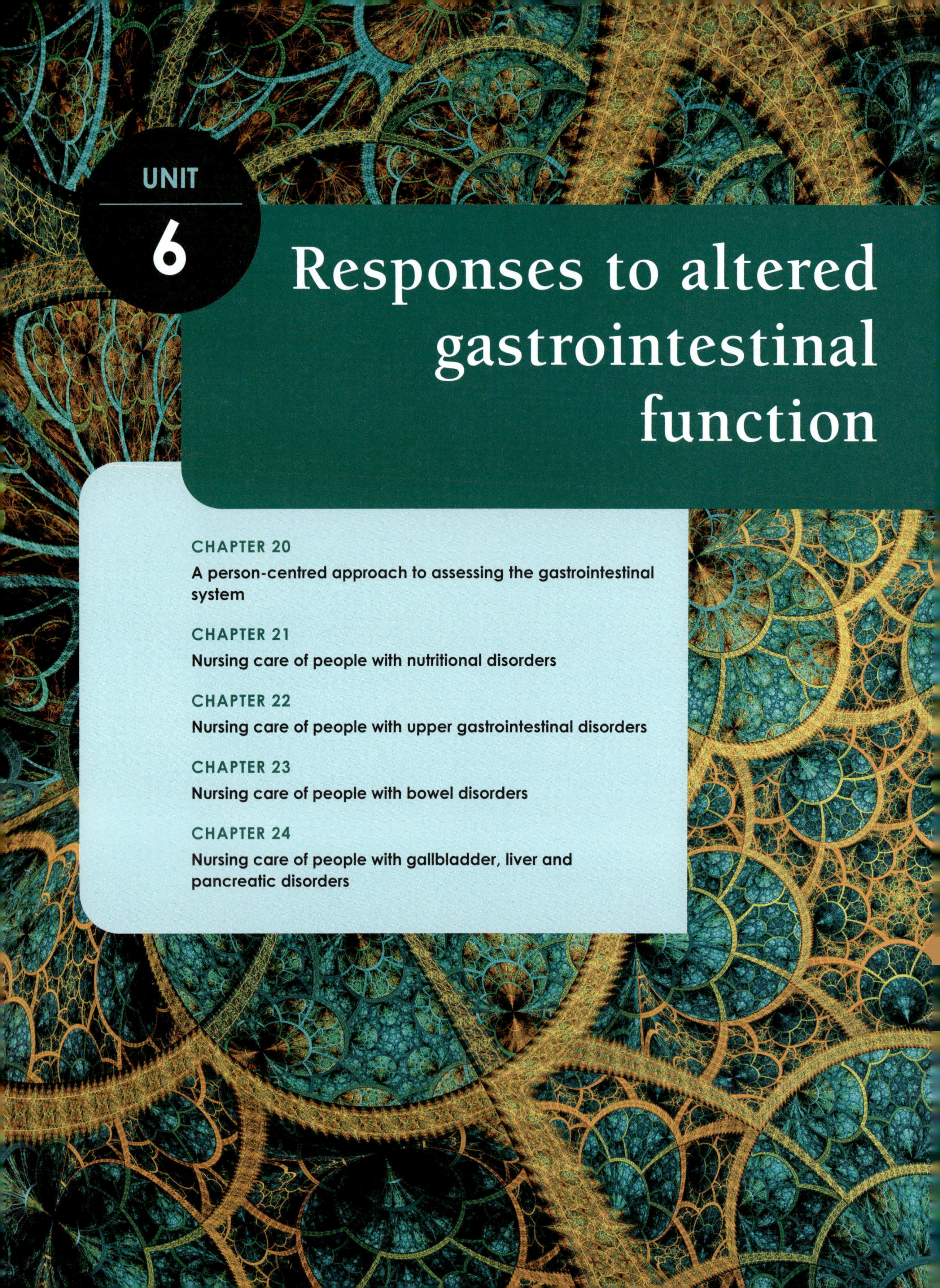

UNIT 6

Responses to altered gastrointestinal function

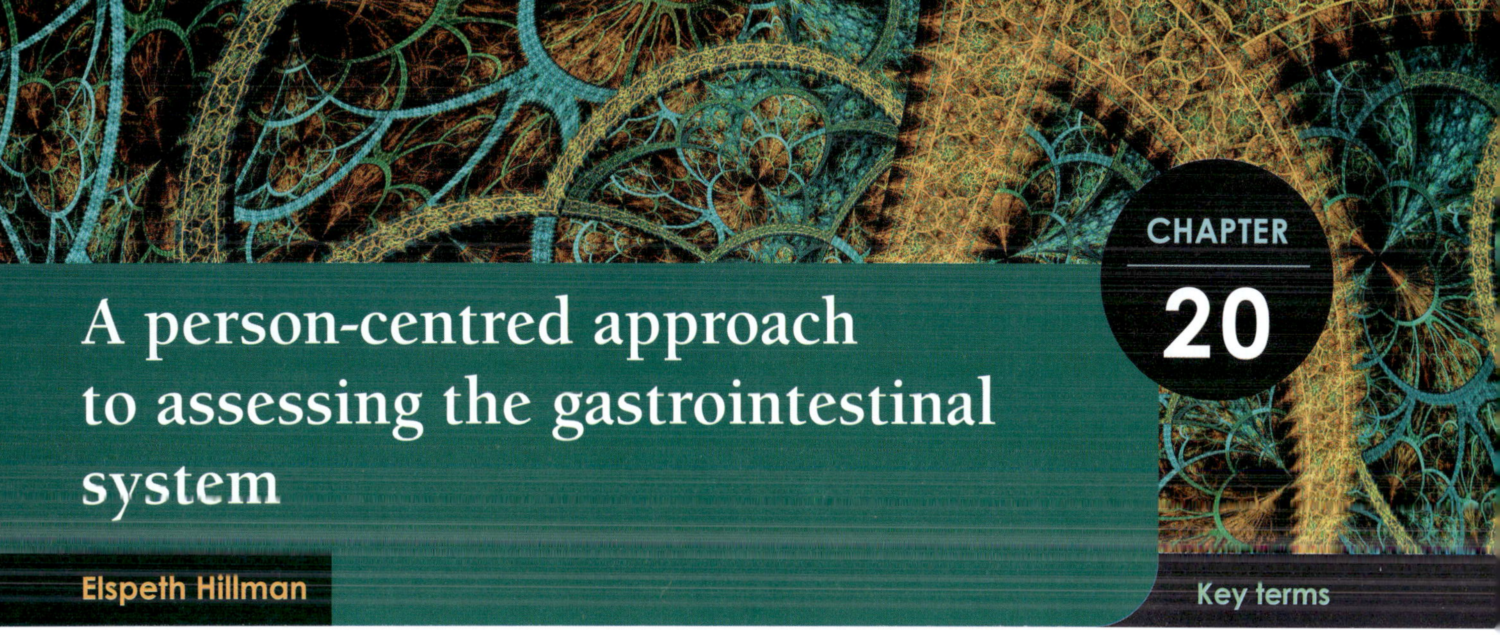

CHAPTER 20

A person-centred approach to assessing the gastrointestinal system

Elspeth Hillman

Key terms

bariatric care 607
bile 606
borborygmus 621
bruit 622
cheilosis 619
constipation 606
diarrhoea 608
flatus 609
gingivitis 620
glossitis 619
halitosis 620
hernia 625
leucoplakia 620
melaena 626
metabolism 607
nutrition 598
ostomy 609
peristalsis 603
steatorrhoea 626
striae 621
Valsalva manoeuvre 606

Learning outcomes

- Describe sources of nutrients and their functions in the human body.
- Describe the anatomy, physiology and functions of the gastrointestinal system and accessory digestive organs.
- Discuss rationales for questions included in a health assessment interview of a person with nutritional and gastrointestinal disorders.
- Explain techniques used for assessing nutritional status and gastrointestinal function.

Clinical competencies

- Conduct and document a health history for people who have or are at risk of alterations in nutrition and gastrointestinal function.
- Conduct and document a physical assessment of nutritional status and the gastrointestinal system.
- Monitor the results of diagnostic tests and report abnormal findings.

Equipment needed

- Stethoscope
- Weight scale with height measuring attachment
- Tape measure
- Skinfold callipers
- Water soluble lubricant
- Faecal occult blood test kit (FOBT)
- Disposable gloves

Nutrition is the sum total of the processes involved in the taking in and the utilisation of food substances by which growth, repair and maintenance of the body are accomplished. It involves ingestion, digestion, absorption/assimilation and elimination. Nutrients are stored by the body in various forms and drawn upon when the food intake is not sufficient.

The digestive organs responsible for these processes are the gastrointestinal tract (also called the alimentary canal) and the accessory digestive organs. The gastrointestinal tract consists of the mouth, pharynx, oesophagus, stomach, small intestine and large intestine. The accessory digestive organs include the liver, gallbladder and pancreas (see Figure 20.1). This chapter discusses the assessment of these organs.

NUTRIENTS

Nutrients are substances found in food and are used by the body to promote growth, maintenance and repair. The categories of nutrients are carbohydrates, proteins, fats, vitamins, minerals and water. Dietary guidelines for nutrients specific to Australians are summarised in Table 20.1.

Nutritional deficits are common in people who are obese. All treatments, including bariatric surgery (see the chapter 'Nursing care of people with nutritional disorders'), consist of lifelong dietary control, exercise and behaviour change. These procedures contribute to nutritional deficiencies by restricting food intake and/or limiting intestinal absorption. The most commonly described nutritional deficiencies include thiamine (B_1), B_{12}, folate (B_9), vitamin D, vitamin E and copper deficiencies (Tardy et al., 2020). The incidence of neurological complications in this group of people is estimated at around 16% and includes encephalopathy, optic neuropathy, myelopathy and polyneuropathy. Risk factors for nutritional complications include vitamin non-adherence, protracted vomiting and excessive alcohol consumption.

Carbohydrates

The primary sources of carbohydrates (which include sugars and starches) are plant foods. Monosaccharides and disaccharides come from milk, sugar cane, sugar beets, honey and fruits. Polysaccharide starch is found in grains, legumes and root

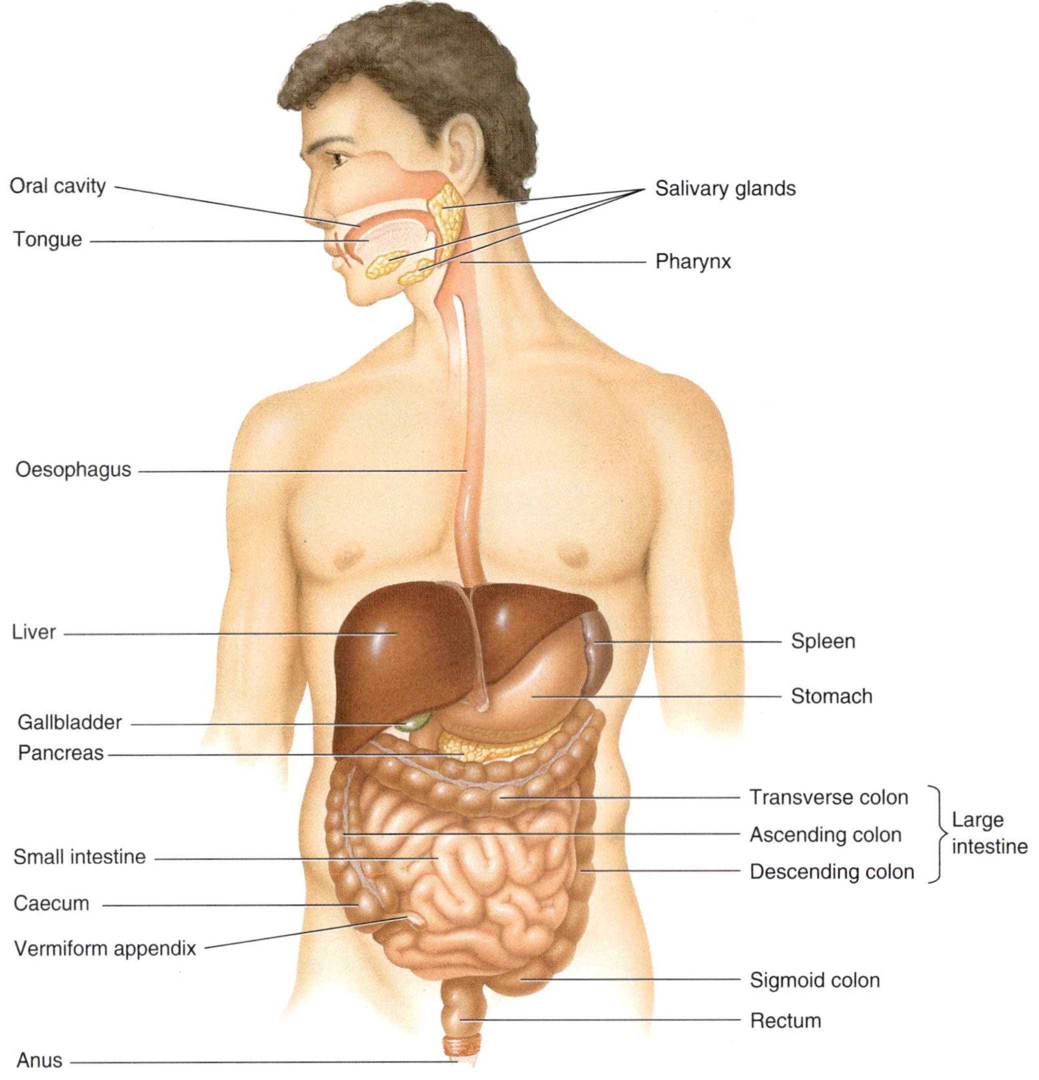

FIGURE 20.1 *Organs of the gastrointestinal tract and accessory digestive organs*

TABLE 20.1 Dietary guidelines for Australians

<table>
<tr><th>FOR ADULTS</th><th>FOR CHILDREN AND ADOLESCENTS</th></tr>
<tr><td>

Enjoy a wide variety of nutritious foods

Adults should be encouraged to:

- Eat mostly vegetables and legumes/beans
- Include grain (cereal) foods, mostly wholegrain and/or high cereal fibre varieties (including breads, rice, pasta and noodles)
- Include lean meat and poultry, fish, eggs, tofu, nuts and seeds, and legumes/beans
- Include milks, yoghurts, cheeses and/or alternatives, mostly reduced fat
- Include 2 servings of fruit per day
- Drink plenty of water

and take care to:

- Limit foods with saturated fat and moderate total fat intake
- Limit foods with added salt
- Limit your alcohol intake if you choose to drink
- Limit foods and drinks containing added sugars

Prevent weight gain: be physically active and eat according to your energy needs

Care for your food: prepare and store it safely

Encourage and support breastfeeding

</td><td>

Encourage and support breastfeeding

Children and adolescents need sufficient nutritious foods to grow and develop normally

- Growth should be checked regularly for young children
- Physical activity is important for all children and adolescents

Enjoy a wide variety of nutritious foods

Children and adolescents should be encouraged to:

- Eat plenty of vegetables and legumes/beans
- Eat moderate amounts of fruit (whole fruit is preferred to fruit juice)
- Eat plenty of cereal foods, mostly wholegrain and/or high cereal fibre varieties (including breads, rice, pasta and noodles)
- Include lean meats and poultry, fish, eggs, tofu, nuts and seeds, and legumes/beans
- Include milks, yoghurts, cheese and/or alternatives. Reduced-fat milks are not suitable for young children under 2 years, because of their high energy needs, but reduced-fat varieties should be encouraged for older children and adolescents
- Choose water as a drink. Alcohol is not recommended for children

and care should be taken to:

- Limit foods with saturated fat and moderate total fat intake. Low-fat diets are not suitable for infants
- Limit foods high in salt
- Limit foods and drinks containing added sugars

Care for your child's food: prepare and store it safely

</td></tr>
</table>

Source: Based on material provided by the National Health and Medical Research Council (NHMRC) (2013). *Eat for health educator guide: Information for nutrition educators*, https://www.eatforhealth.gov.au/sites/default/files/2022-09/n55b_educator_guide_140321_1.pdf. Licensed under a Creative Commons Attribution 4.0 International Licence, https://creativecommons.org/licenses/by/4.0/.

vegetables. Following ingestion, digestion and metabolism, carbohydrates are converted primarily to glucose, the molecule body cells use to make adenosine triphosphate (ATP). Excess glucose in the healthy person is converted to glycogen or fat. Glycogen is stored in the liver and muscles; fat is stored as adipose tissue. Carbohydrate use by the body is shown in Figure 20.2A.

Regardless of the source, all carbohydrates supply 16.7 kilojoules (kJ) per gram. The recommended dietary intake is 125 to 175 g, most of which should be complex carbohydrates (such as fruits, starchy vegetables and whole grains). Excessive intake of carbohydrates over time can result in obesity, tooth decay and elevated plasma triglycerides. Over extended periods of time, carbohydrate deficiencies lead to tissue wasting from protein breakdown and metabolic acidosis from an excess of ketones as a by-product of fat breakdown.

Proteins

Proteins are classified as either complete or incomplete. Complete proteins are found in animal products such as eggs, milk, milk products and meat. They contain the greatest amount of amino acids and meet the body's amino acid requirements for tissue growth and maintenance. Incomplete proteins are found in legumes, nuts, grains, cereals and vegetables. These sources are low in or lack one or more of the amino acids essential for building complete proteins.

The body uses proteins to build many different structures, including skin keratin and the collagen and elastin in connective tissues and muscles. They also are used to make enzymes, haemoglobin, plasma proteins and some hormones. Protein use by the body is shown in Figure 20.2B.

Proteins provide 16.7 kJ per gram. The recommended dietary intake of protein is 64 g for men and 46 g for women. (This is higher for adults over 70 years of age.) Healthy people with adequate energy intake have an equal rate of protein synthesis and protein breakdown and loss, reflected as nitrogen balance. If the breakdown and loss of proteins exceed intake, a negative nitrogen balance results. This may be due to starvation, altered physical states (e.g. from injury or illness) and altered emotional states (such as depression or anxiety). A positive nitrogen balance, which results when protein intake exceeds breakdown, is normal during growth, tissue repair and pregnancy. Anabolic steroids affect the rate of protein use; for example, the adrenal corticosteroids are released in times of stress to increase protein breakdown and conversion of amino acids to glucose. Excessive intake of proteins may lead to obesity, whereas deficits cause weight loss and tissue wasting, oedema and anaemia.

Fats (lipids)

Fats, or lipids, include phospholipids; steroids, such as cholesterol; and neutral fats, more commonly known as triglycerides. Neutral fats are the most abundant fats in the diet. They may be either saturated or unsaturated. Saturated fats are found in animal products (milk and meats) and in some plant products (such as coconut). Unsaturated fats are found in seeds, nuts and most vegetable oils. Sources of cholesterol include meats, milk products and egg yolks. Fat use by the body is shown in Figure 20.2C.

Fats supply 37.7 kJ per gram. When a person consumes more than the body requires, the excess is stored as adipose tissue, increasing the risk of obesity and heart disease. A deficit of fats may cause excessive weight loss and skin lesions.

Fats are a necessary part of the structure and function of the body. For example:

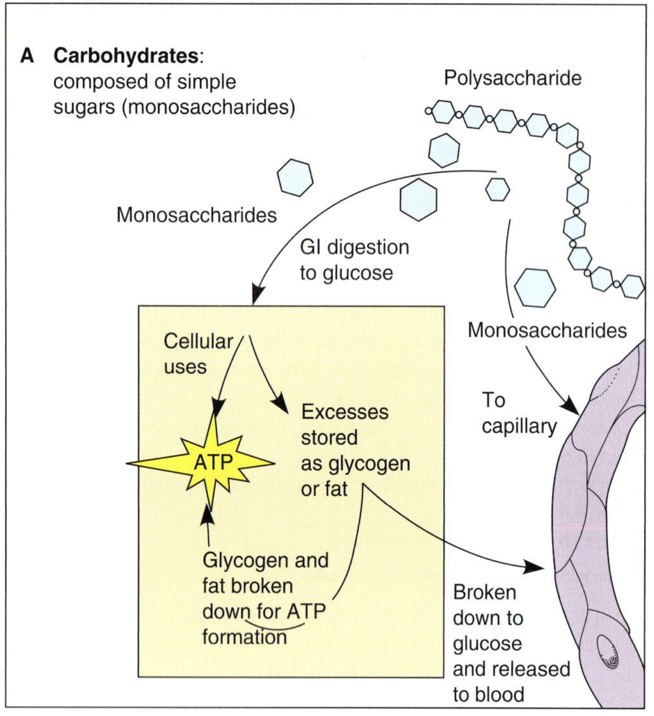

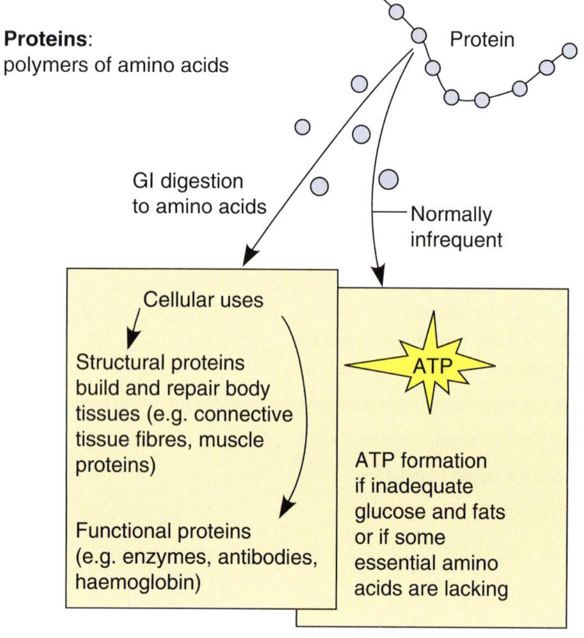

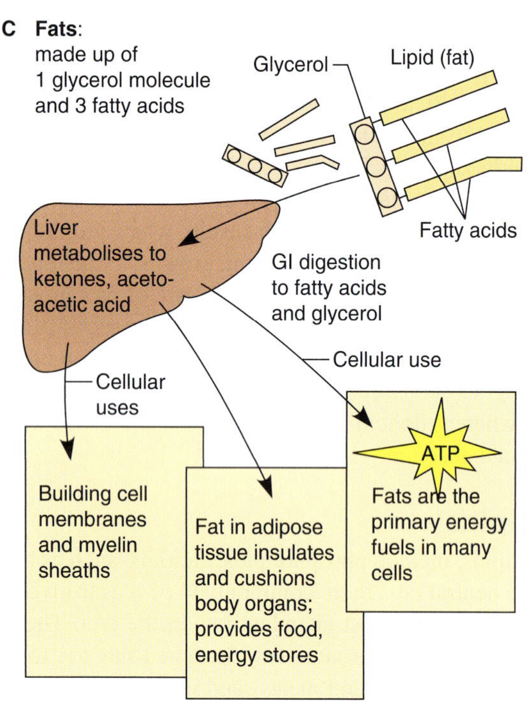

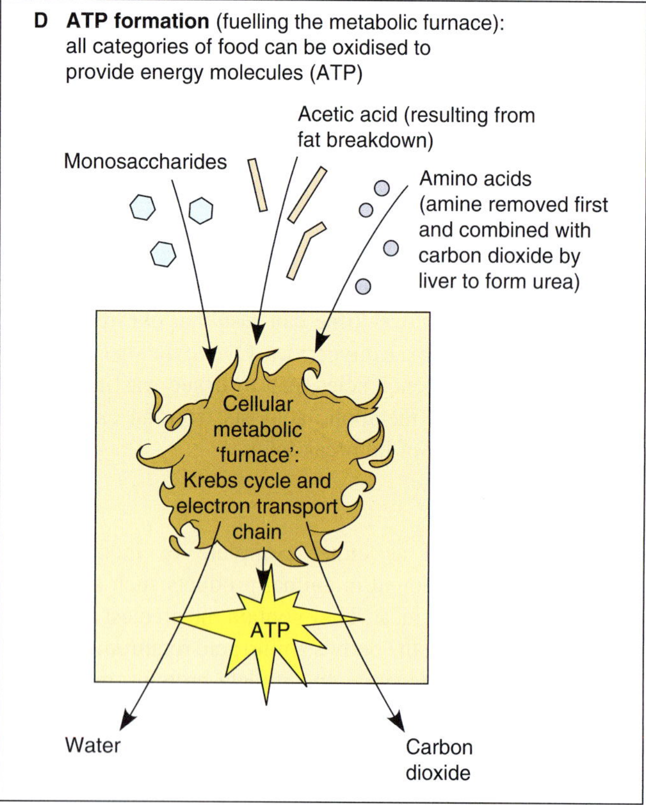

FIGURE 20.2 *A schematic overview of nutrient use by body cells, including A, carbohydrates; B, proteins; C, fats; and D, ATP formation*

- Phospholipids are a part of all cell membranes.
- Triglycerides are the major energy source for hepatocytes and skeletal muscle cells.
- Dietary fats facilitate absorption of fat-soluble vitamins.
- Linoleic acid, an essential fatty acid, helps form prostaglandins, regulatory molecules that assist in smooth muscle contraction, maintenance of blood pressure and control of inflammatory responses.
- Cholesterol is the essential component of bile salts, steroid hormones and vitamin D.
- Adipose tissue serves as a protection around body organs, as a layer of insulation under the skin and as a concentrated source of fuel for cellular energy.

Vitamins

Vitamins are organic compounds that facilitate the body's use of carbohydrates, proteins and fats. All the vitamins except vitamins D and K must be ingested in foods or taken as supplements. Vitamin D is made by ultraviolet irradiation of cholesterol molecules in the skin and vitamin K is synthesised by bacteria in the intestine.

Vitamins are categorised as either fat soluble or water soluble. The fat-soluble vitamins (A, D, E and K) bind to ingested fats and are absorbed as the fats are absorbed. Water-soluble vitamins (the B complex and C) are absorbed with water in the gastrointestinal (GI) tract. (However, vitamin B_{12} must become attached to the intrinsic factor (a protein) to be absorbed.) Fat-soluble vitamins are stored in the body and excesses may cause toxicity; water-soluble vitamins in excess of body requirements are excreted in the urine.

The recommended daily dietary intake (RDI) or adequate intake (AI) and the source and function of vitamins, as stated by the National Health and Medical Research Council (NHMRC), are listed in Tables 20.2 and 20.3.

Minerals

Minerals work with other nutrients to maintain the structure and function of the body. An adequate supply of calcium, phosphorus, potassium, sulfur, sodium, chloride and magnesium—as well as other trace elements such as iron, iodine, copper and zinc—is necessary to health. Most minerals in the body are found in body fluids or are bound to organic compounds. The best sources of minerals are vegetables, legumes, milk and some meats. Dietary sources for the major minerals are discussed in the chapter 'Nursing care of people with altered fluid, electrolyte and acid–base balance'. The recommended dietary intake for minerals is outlined in Table 20.4.

Dietary fibre

Food Standards Australia New Zealand (FSANZ) defines dietary fibre as:

> *that fraction of the edible parts of plants or their extracts, or synthetic analogues, that are resistant to the digestion and absorption in the small intestine, usually with complete or partial fermentation in the large intestine and promote one or more of the following beneficial physiological effects—(i) laxation; (ii) reduction in blood cholesterol; (iii) modulation of blood glucose.* (FSANZ, 2021, p. 6)

Adequate intake of dietary fibre has been linked to a reduction in the occurrence of several chronic diseases and is essential to maintain functioning of the GI tract. An adequate intake for women is 25 g/day and for men is 30 g/day.

TABLE 20.2 Recommended dietary intake/adequate intake of fat-soluble vitamins

NAME	SOURCE	FUNCTION	MINIMUM RECOMMENDED DIETARY INTAKE/ADEQUATE INTAKE (AI) (M = MEN, W = WOMEN)
Vitamin A (retinol)	• Fish liver oils • Egg yolk • Liver • Fortified milk • Margarine	Necessary for vision, integrity of skin and mucous membranes, cell membrane function and reproductive function	M = 900 micrograms W = 700 micrograms
Vitamin D	• The action of sunshine on cholesterol in the skin	Necessary for blood calcium homeostasis (in turn, necessary for blood clotting), bone formation and neuromuscular function	M and W = 5 micrograms M and W 51–70 = 10 micrograms M and W > 70 = 15 micrograms
Vitamin E (as a tocopherol)	• Vegetable oils • Margarine • Whole grains • Dark green leafy vegetables	As an antioxidant, helps prevent the oxidation of vitamins A and C in the intestines and decreases the oxidation of unsaturated fatty acids to facilitate cell membrane integrity	M = 10 mg W = 7 mg
Vitamin K	• Synthesised by coliform bacteria in the large intestine • Green leafy vegetables • Cabbage • Cauliflower • Pork	Essential for the formation of clotting proteins in the liver	M = 70 micrograms W = 60 micrograms

TABLE 20.3 Recommended dietary intake of water-soluble vitamins

NAME	SOURCE	FUNCTION	MINIMUM RECOMMENDED DIETARY INTAKE/ ADEQUATE INTAKE (A1) (M = MEN, W = WOMEN)
Vitamin B_1 (thiamine)	• Lean meats • Liver • Eggs • Green leafy vegetables • Legumes • Whole grains	An essential coenzyme for carbohydrate metabolism and use; also for healthy function of nerves, muscles and the heart	M = 1.2 mg W = 1.1 mg
Vitamin B_2 (riboflavin)	• Liver • Egg white • Whole grains • Meat • Poultry • Fish • Milk	Involved in the catabolism and use of carbohydrates, fats and proteins; the use of other B vitamins; and is important for the production of adrenal hormones	M = 1.3 mg M > 70 years = 1.6 mg W = 1.1 mg W > 70 years = 1.3 mg
Vitamin B_6 (pyridoxine)	• Meat • Poultry • Fish • Potatoes • Tomatoes • Sweet potatoes • Spinach	Necessary for amino acid metabolism, and formation of antibodies and haemoglobin	M and W < age 51 = 1.3 M > age 51 = 1.7 mg W > age 51 = 1.5 mg
Vitamin B_{12} (cyano-cobalamin)	• Liver • Meat • Poultry • Dairy foods (except butter) • Eggs	Essential for the production of nucleic acids and red blood cells in the bone marrow; also plays an important role in the use of folic acid and carbohydrates and in healthy function of the nervous system	M and W = 2.4 micrograms
Vitamin C (ascorbic acid)	• Citrus fruits • Potatoes • Tomatoes • Green leafy vegetables	Acts as an antioxidant and vasoconstrictor; also serves in the formation of connective tissue, conversion of cholesterol to bile salts, iron absorption and use and conversion of folic acid to an active form	M and W = 45 mg
Vitamin B_3 (niacin; nicotinamide)	• Meat • Poultry • Fish • Liver • Peanuts • Green leafy vegetables	Plays an important role in the metabolism of carbohydrates and fats; inhibits cholesterol synthesis; important for integumentary, nervous and digestive system health; assists in the manufacture of reproductive hormones	M and W = 35 mg (as nicotinic acid)
Biotin (B_7)	• Liver • Eggs • Nuts • Legumes	Essential for the catabolism of fatty acids and carbohydrates and helps dispose of the waste products of protein catabolism	M = 30 micrograms W = 25 micrograms
Pantothenic acid (B_5)	• Meats • Whole grains • Egg yolk • Liver • Yeast • Legumes	Assists in the synthesis of steroids and of the haem in haemoglobin; is essential for the metabolism of carbohydrates and fats, and for the manufacture of reproductive hormones	M = 6 mg W = 4 mg
Folic acid (folate; B_9)	• Liver • Dark green vegetables • Lean beef • Eggs • Veal • Whole grains • Synthesised by bacteria in the intestine	The basis of a coenzyme necessary to the manufacture of nucleic acids and so is essential for the formation of red blood cells, growth and development, and nervous system health	M and W = 400 micrograms

TABLE 20.4 Recommended dietary intake of minerals

NAME	MINIMUM RECOMMENDED DIETARY INTAKE/ADEQUATE INTAKE (A1) (M = MEN, W = WOMEN)	NAME	MINIMUM RECOMMENDED DIETARY INTAKE/ADEQUATE INTAKE (A1) (M = MEN, W = WOMEN)
Calcium	M and W = 1,000 mg M > 70 and W > 51 = 1,300 mg	Chromium	M = 35 micrograms W = 25 micrograms
Phosphorus	M and W = 1,000 mg	Iodine	M and W = 150 micrograms
Iron	M = 8 mg W = 18 mg W > 51 = 8 mg	Selenium	M = 70 micrograms W = 60 micrograms
Zinc	M = 14 mg W = 8 mg	Magnesium	M = 400–420 mg W = 310–320 mg
Manganese	M = 5.5 mg W = 5 mg	Copper	M = 1.7 mg W = 1.2 mg
Molybdenum	M and W = 45 mg	Sodium	M and W = 460–920 mg

Anatomy, physiology and functions of the gastrointestinal system

The gastrointestinal tract is a continuous hollow tube, extending from the mouth to the anus. Foods are placed in the mouth, then they are subjected to a variety of processes that move them and break them down into usable elements, and nutrients are absorbed from the lumen of the small intestine into the blood or lymph, while indigestible materials are eliminated. Bowel elimination is the end process in digestion. The digestive processes are as follows:

- ingestion of food
- movement of food and wastes
- secretion of mucus, water and enzymes
- mechanical digestion of food
- chemical digestion of food
- absorption of nutrients from digested food
- elimination of wastes.

The mouth

The mouth, also called the oral or buccal cavity, is lined with mucous membranes and is enclosed by the lips, cheeks, palate and tongue (see Figure 20.3).

The lips and cheeks are skeletal muscle covered externally by skin. Their function is to keep food in the mouth during chewing. The palate consists of two regions: the hard palate and the soft palate. The hard palate covers bone in the roof of the mouth and provides a hard surface against which the tongue forces food. The soft palate, extending from the hard palate and ending at the back of the mouth as a fold called the uvula, is primarily muscle. When food is swallowed, the soft palate rises as a reflex to close off the oropharynx.

The tongue, composed of skeletal muscle and connective tissue, is located in the floor of the mouth. It contains mucous and serous glands, taste buds and papillae. The tongue mixes food with saliva during chewing, forms the food into a mass (called a *bolus*) and initiates swallowing. Some papillae provide surface roughness to facilitate licking and moving food; other papillae house the taste buds.

Saliva moistens food so it can be made into a bolus, dissolves food chemicals so they can be tasted and provides enzymes (such as amylase) that begin the chemical breakdown of starches. Saliva is produced by salivary glands, most of which lie superior or inferior to the mouth and drain into it. The salivary glands include the parotid, the submaxillary and the sublingual glands.

The teeth chew (masticate) and grind food to break it down into smaller parts. As the food is masticated, it is mixed with saliva. Adults have 32 permanent teeth. The teeth are embedded in the gingiva (gums), with the crown of each tooth visible above the gingiva.

The pharynx

The pharynx consists of the oropharynx and the laryngopharynx (see Figure 20.3). Both structures provide passageways for food, fluids and air. The pharynx is made of skeletal muscles and is lined with mucous membranes. The skeletal muscles move food to the oesophagus via the pharynx through **peristalsis** (alternating waves of contraction and relaxation of involuntary muscle). The mucosa of the pharynx contains mucus-producing glands that provide fluid to facilitate the passage of the bolus of food as it is swallowed.

The oesophagus

The oesophagus, a muscular tube about 25 cm long, serves as a passageway for food from the pharynx to the stomach (see Figures 20.1 and 20.3). The epiglottis, a flap of cartilage over the top of the larynx, keeps food out of the larynx during swallowing. The oesophagus descends through the thorax and

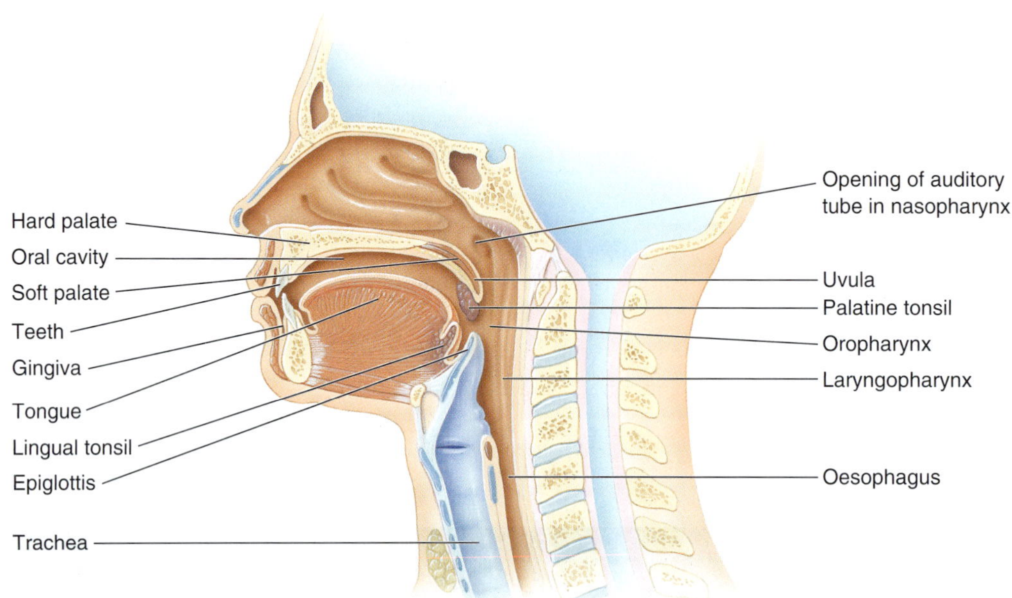

FIGURE 20.3 ***Structures of the mouth, the pharynx and the oesophagus***

diaphragm, entering the stomach at the cardiac orifice. The gastro-oesophageal sphincter surrounds this opening. This sphincter, along with the diaphragm, keeps the orifice closed when food is not being swallowed.

For most of its length, the oesophagus is lined with stratified squamous epithelium; simple columnar epithelium lines the oesophagus where it joins the stomach. The mucosa and submucosa of the oesophagus lie in longitudinal folds when the oesophagus is empty.

The stomach

The stomach, located high on the left side of the abdominal cavity, is connected to the oesophagus at the upper end and to the small intestine at the lower end (see Figure 20.4). Normally about 25 cm long, the stomach is a distensible organ that can expand to hold up to 4 L of food and fluid. The concave surface of the stomach is called the lesser curvature; the convex surface is called the greater curvature. The stomach may be divided into regions extending from the distal end of the oesophagus to the opening into the small intestine. These regions are the cardiac region, fundus, body and pylorus (see Figure 20.4). The pyloric sphincter controls emptying of the stomach into the duodenal portion of the small intestine. The stomach is a storage reservoir for food, continues the mechanical breakdown of food, begins the process of protein digestion and mixes the food with gastric juices into a thick fluid called chyme.

The stomach is lined with columnar epithelial, mucus-producing cells. Millions of openings in the lining lead to gastric glands that can produce 4 to 5 L of gastric juice each day. The gastric glands contain a variety of secretory cells, including the following:

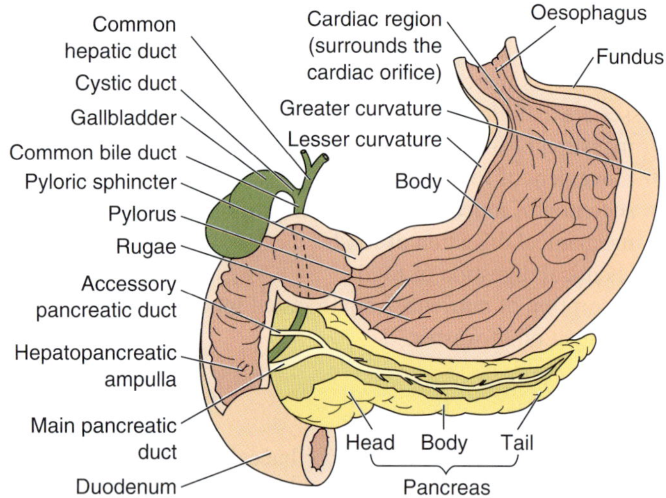

FIGURE 20.4 ***The internal anatomical structures of the stomach, including the pancreatic, cystic and hepatic ducts, the pancreas and the gallbladder***

- Mucous cells produce alkaline mucus that clings to the lining of the stomach and protects it from being digested by gastric juice.
- Zymogenic cells produce pepsinogen (an inactive form of pepsin, a protein-digesting enzyme).

- Parietal cells secrete hydrochloric acid and intrinsic factor. Hydrochloric acid activates and increases the activity of protein-digesting cells and also is bactericidal. Intrinsic factor is necessary for the absorption of vitamin B_{12} in the small intestine.
- Enteroendocrine cells secrete gastrin, histamine, endorphins, serotonin and somatostatin. These hormones or hormone-like substances diffuse into the blood. Gastrin is important in regulating secretion and motility of the stomach.

The secretion of gastric juice is under both neural and endocrine control. Stimulation of the parasympathetic vagus nerve increases secretory activity; in contrast, stimulation of sympathetic nerves decreases secretions. The three phases of secretory activity are the cephalic phase, the gastric phase and the intestinal phase.

- The cephalic phase prepares for digestion and is triggered by the sight, odour, taste or thought of food. During this initial phase, motor impulses are transmitted via the vagus nerve to the stomach.
- The gastric phase begins when food enters the stomach. Stomach distension (stimulating stretch receptors) and chemical stimuli from partially digested proteins initiate this phase. Gastrin-secreting cells produce gastrin, which in turn stimulates the gastric glands (especially the parietal cells) to produce more gastric juice. Histamine also stimulates hydrochloric acid secretion.
- The intestinal phase is initiated when partially digested food begins to enter the small intestine, stimulating mucous cells of the intestine to release a hormone that promotes continued gastric secretion.

Mechanical digestion in the stomach is accomplished by peristaltic movements that churn and mix the food with the gastric juices to form chyme. Gastric motility is either enhanced or retarded by the same factors that affect secretion—namely, distension and the effect of gastrin. After a person eats a well-balanced meal, the stomach empties completely in approximately 4 to 6 hours. Gastric emptying depends on the volume, chemical composition and osmotic pressure of the gastric contents. The stomach empties large volumes of liquid content more rapidly, while solids and fats slow gastric emptying.

The small intestine

The small intestine begins at the pyloric sphincter and ends at the ileocaecal junction at the entrance of the large intestine (see Figure 20.1). The small intestine is about 6 m long but only about 2.5 cm in diameter. This long tube hangs in coils in the abdominal cavity, suspended by the mesentery and surrounded by the large intestine. The small intestine has three regions: the duodenum, the jejunum and the ileum. The duodenum begins at the pyloric sphincter and [illegible] around the head of the pancreas for about 25 cm. Both pancreatic enzymes and bile from the liver enter the small intestine at the duodenum. The jejunum, the middle region of the small intestine, extends for about 2.4 m. The ileum, the terminal end of the small intestine, is approximately 3.6 m long and meets the large intestine at the ileocaecal valve.

Food is chemically digested, and most of it is absorbed, as it moves through the small intestine. Circular folds (deep folds of the mucosa and submucosa layers), villi (finger-like projections of the mucosa cells) and microvilli (tiny projections of the mucosa cells) increase the surface area of the small intestine to enhance absorption of food. Although up to 10 L of food, liquids and secretions enter the GI tract each day, less than 1 L reaches the large intestine.

Enzymes in the small intestine break down carbohydrates, proteins, lipids and nucleic acids. Pancreatic amylase acts on starches, converting them to maltose, dextrins and oligosaccharides; the intestinal enzymes dextrinase, glucoamylase, maltase, sucrase and lactase further break down these products into monosaccharides. Pancreatic enzymes (trypsin and chymotrypsin) and intestinal enzymes continue to break down proteins into peptides. Pancreatic lipases digest lipids in the small intestine. Triglycerides enter as fat globules and are coated by bile salts and emulsified. Nucleic acids are hydrolysed by pancreatic enzymes and then broken apart by intestinal enzymes. Both pancreatic enzymes and bile are excreted into the duodenum in response to the secretion of secretin and cholecystokinin, hormones produced by the intestinal mucosa cells when chyme enters the small intestine.

Nutrients are absorbed through the mucosa of the intestinal villi into the blood or lymph by active transport, facilitated transport and passive diffusion. Almost all food products and water, as well as vitamins and most electrolytes, are absorbed in the small intestine, leaving only indigestible fibres, some water and bacteria to enter the large intestine.

The large intestine

The large intestine, or colon, begins at the ileocaecal valve and terminates at the anus (see Figure 20.5). It is about 1.5 m long. The large intestine frames the small intestine on three sides and includes the caecum, the appendix, the colon, the rectum and the anal canal.

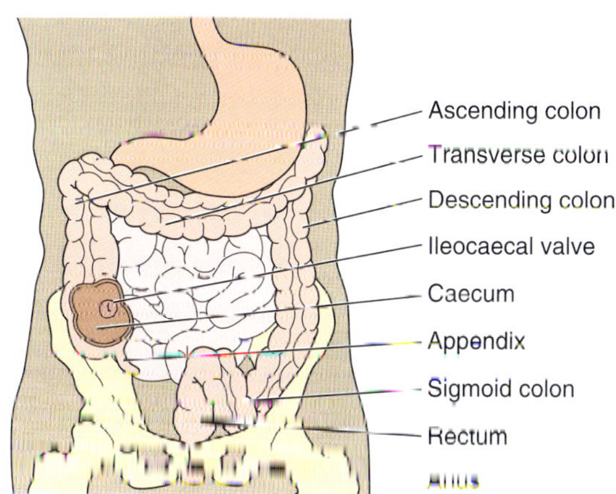

FIGURE 20.5 *Anatomy of the large intestine*

The first section of the large intestine is the caecum. The appendix is attached to its surface as an extension. The appendix, a twisted structure in which bacteria can accumulate, may become inflamed.

The colon is divided into ascending, transverse and descending segments. The ascending colon extends along the right side of the abdomen to the hepatic flexure, where it makes a right-angled turn. The next segment, called the transverse colon, crosses the abdomen to the splenic flexure. At this juncture, the descending colon descends down the left side of the abdomen and ends at the S-shaped sigmoid colon. The sigmoid colon terminates at the rectum.

The rectum is a mucosa-lined tube approximately 12 cm in length (see Figure 20.6). The rectum has three transverse folds (valves of Houston) that retain faeces yet allow flatus to be passed through the anus. The rectum ends at the anal canal, which terminates at the anus.

The anus is a hairless opening at the end of the digestive system, from which bowel motions (stools) are passed. It has both an internal involuntary sphincter and an external voluntary sphincter. The sphincters are usually open only during defecation. The anorectal junction separates the rectum from the anal canal and may be the site of internal haemorrhoids (clusters of dilated veins in swollen anal tissue).

The major function of the large intestine is to eliminate indigestible food residue from the body. The large intestine absorbs water, salts and vitamins formed by the food residue and bacteria. The semiliquid chyme that passes through the ileocaecal valve is formed into faeces as it moves through the large intestine. Faeces are moved along the intestine by peristalsis, waves of alternating contraction and relaxation. Goblet cells lining the large intestine secrete mucus that facilitates the lubrication and passage of faeces.

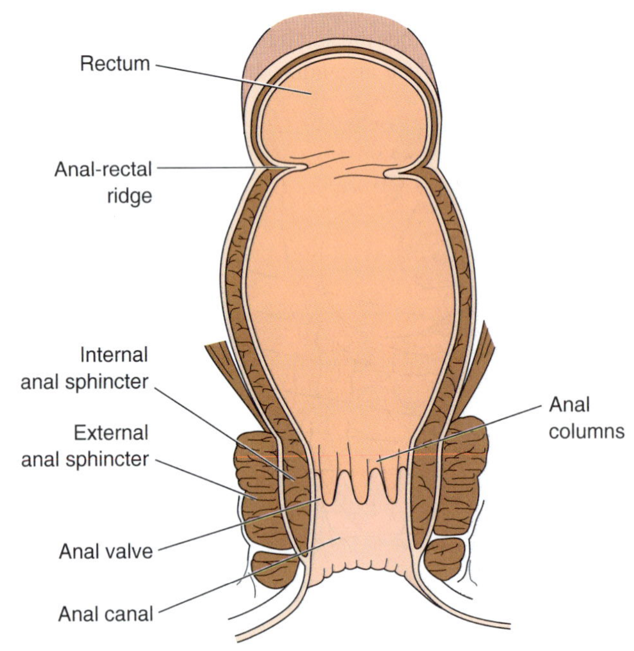

FIGURE 20.6 ***Structure of the rectum and anus***

The defecation reflex is initiated when faeces enter the rectum and stretch the rectal wall. This spinal cord reflex causes the walls of the sigmoid colon to contract and the anal sphincters to relax. This reflex can be suppressed by voluntary control of the external sphincter. Closing the glottis and contracting the diaphragm and abdominal muscles to increase intra-abdominal pressure (**Valsalva manoeuvre**) facilitate expulsion of faeces. Prolonged suppression of defecation can result in a weakened reflex that may in turn lead to **constipation** (infrequent and often uncomfortable passage of hard, dry stool). Frequent bouts of constipation may lead to external haemorrhoids at the area of the external haemorrhoidal plexus.

The accessory digestive organs

The liver, gallbladder and exocrine pancreas secrete substances necessary for the digestion of chyme. The liver produces bile, necessary for fat digestion and absorption, and stores it in the gallbladder. The liver also receives nutrients absorbed by the small intestine and metabolises or synthesises these nutrients so they are in a form that can be used by the cells of the body. The exocrine pancreas produces enzymes necessary for digestion of fats, proteins and carbohydrates.

The liver and gallbladder

The liver weighs about 1.4 kg in the average-size adult. It is located in the right side of the abdomen, inferior to the diaphragm and anterior to the stomach (see Figure 20.1). The liver has four lobes: right, left, caudate and quadrate. A mesenteric ligament separates the right and left lobes and suspends the liver from the diaphragm and anterior abdominal wall. The liver is encased in a fibroelastic capsule, called the Glisson capsule. This capsule contains blood vessels, lymphatics and nerves. When the liver is diseased or swollen, distension causes pain and the lymphatics may ooze fluid into the peritoneal cavity.

Liver tissue consists of units called lobules, which are composed of plates of hepatocytes (liver cells). A branch of the hepatic artery, a branch of the hepatic portal vein and a bile duct communicate with each lobule. Sinusoids, blood-filled spaces within the lobules, are lined with Kupffer cells. These phagocytic cells remove debris from the blood.

Bile production is the liver's primary digestive function. **Bile** is a greenish, watery solution containing bile salts, cholesterol, bilirubin, electrolytes, water and phospholipids. These substances are necessary to emulsify and promote the absorption of fats. Liver cells make from 700 to 1,200 mL of bile daily. When bile is not needed for digestion, the sphincter of Oddi (located at the point at which bile enters the duodenum) is closed and the bile backs up the cystic duct into the gallbladder for storage.

Bile is concentrated and stored in the gallbladder, a small sac cupped in the inferior surface of the liver. When food containing fats enters the duodenum, hormones stimulate the gallbladder to secrete bile into the cystic duct. The cystic duct joins the hepatic duct to form the common bile duct, from which bile enters into the duodenum (see Figure 20.4).

The major digestive and metabolic functions of the liver are outlined in Box 20.1. These functions require a large amount of blood, with the liver receiving blood from both venous and arterial blood vessels. The hepatic artery, branching from the

BOX 20.1 Major digestive and metabolic functions of the liver

- Secretes bile.
- Stores fat-soluble vitamins (A, D, E and K).
- Metabolises bilirubin.
- Stores blood and releases blood into the general circulation during haemorrhage.
- Synthesises plasma proteins to maintain plasma oncotic pressure.
- Synthesises prothrombin, fibrinogen and factors I, II, VII, IX and X, which are necessary for blood clotting.
- Synthesises fats from carbohydrates and proteins to be either used for energy or stored as adipose tissue.
- Synthesises phospholipids and cholesterol necessary for the production of bile salts, steroid hormones and plasma membranes.
- Converts amino acids to carbohydrates through deamination.
- Releases glucose during times of hypoglycaemia.
- Takes up glucose during times of hyperglycaemia and stores it as glycogen or converts it to fat.
- Alters chemicals, foreign molecules and hormones to make them less toxic.
- Stores iron as ferritin, which is released as needed for the production of red blood cells.

abdominal aorta, provides oxygenated blood at the rate of 400 to 500 mL/min. The hepatic portal vein delivers about 1,000 to 1,200 mL/min of deoxygenated blood to the liver from the inferior and superior mesenteric veins and the splenic vein.

The exocrine pancreas

The pancreas, a gland located between the stomach and small intestine, is the primary enzyme-producing organ of the digestive system. It is a triangular gland extending across the abdomen, with its tail next to the spleen and its head next to the duodenum (see Figure 20.4). The body and tail of the pancreas are retro-peritoneal, lying behind the greater curvature of the stomach. The pancreas is actually two organs in one, having both exocrine and endocrine structures and functions. The exocrine portion of the pancreas, through secretory units called acini, secretes alkaline pancreatic juice containing many different enzymes. The acini, clusters of secretory cells surrounding ducts, drain into the pancreatic duct. The pancreatic duct joins with the common bile duct just before it enters the duodenum (so that pancreatic juice and bile from the liver enter the small intestine together). The pancreas also has endocrine functions, discussed in the chapter 'A person-centred approach to assessing the endocrine system'.

The pancreas produces from 1 to 1.5 L of pancreatic juice daily. Pancreatic juice is clear and has a high bicarbonate content. This alkaline fluid neutralises the acidic chyme as it enters the duodenum, optimising the pH for intestinal and pancreatic enzyme activity. The secretion of pancreatic juice is controlled by the vagus nerve and the intestinal hormones secretin and cholecystokinin. Pancreatic juice contains enzymes that aid in the digestion of all categories of foods: lipase promotes fat breakdown and absorption; amylase completes starch digestion; and trypsin, chymotrypsin and carboxypeptidase are responsible for half of all protein digestion. Nucleases break down nucleic acids.

METABOLISM

After nutrients (carbohydrates, fats and proteins) are ingested, digested, absorbed and transported across cell membranes, they must be metabolised to produce and provide energy to maintain life. **Metabolism** is the process of biochemical reactions occurring in the body's cells. Metabolic processes are either catabolic or anabolic. Catabolism involves the breakdown of complex structures into simpler forms—for example, the breakdown of carbohydrates to produce ATP, an energy molecule that fuels cellular activity. In the process of anabolism, simpler molecules combine to build more complex structures—for example, amino acids bond to form proteins.

The biochemical reactions of metabolism produce water, carbon dioxide and ATP (see Figure 20.2D). The energy value of foods is measured in calories or joules; in Australia, the preferred unit of measure is kilojoules (kJ). One kilojoule is equivalent to 0.24 kilocalorie. A kilocalorie is defined as the amount of heat energy needed to raise the temperature of 1 kilogram (kg) of water 1°C.

ASSESSING NUTRITIONAL STATUS AND GASTROINTESTINAL FUNCTION

Nutritional status and the function of the gastrointestinal system are assessed by findings from a health assessment interview to collect subjective data, a physical assessment to collect objective data and diagnostic tests. The obesity epidemic has put **bariatric care** in the forefront for all healthcare providers. Bariatric nurse specialists reveal that obese individuals are often the target of prejudice, bullying and ridicule, and that misunderstanding by the community, media and health professionals is common. People affected in this way are often reluctant to seek care or to follow medical advice. Person-centred care and collaboration with the affected person and their family is essential to positive long-term outcomes. Sensitive attention to health assessment interviews and physical assessment of overweight and obese people is required to identify those at risk of nutritional and neurological deficits and in need of specialist support.

Health assessment interview

A health assessment interview to determine problems with nutrition and GI function may be conducted during a health screening, may focus on a chief complaint (such as nausea or unexplained weight loss) or may be part of a total health assessment. People may feel embarrassed to talk about weight, digestion and bowel elimination patterns. Remember to request permission to conduct the interview. Due to the sensitive nature of many of the questions, ask about the presence of others during the assessment. To promote effective rapport, ask about less personal information first. It is important to identify whether the problem is acute (less than 3 months) or chronic (more than 3 months). If there has been a change in the person's normal

SAMPLE DOCUMENTATION

Assessment of nutritional status

28/02/2023 NURS 1100 hrs A 22-year-old female visiting her GP for a regular check-up. Height 165 cm; weight 58 kg. BMI: 24. MAC: 28 cm. Waist-to-hip ratio: 0.6. Skin is warm, moist and smooth without lesions other than well-healed scar on RLQ of abdomen from appendectomy, age 15. Oral mucosa and tongue pink and moist. No breath odour. All teeth present with evidence of dental care. Abdomen slightly concave when lying on back, bowel sounds present in all four quadrants, liver non-palpable, tympany over lower abdomen on percussion. ________ S Brown

(SHANE BROWN, RN)

GI function lasting for 4 weeks or longer, ask if this is related to any change in their lifestyle. Questions could cover diet, fluids, medication (prescribed, complementary and over-the-counter medicines), personal stresses such as a change in job, recent foreign travel (especially if a person has diarrhoea) and surgery.

If the person has a health problem involving nutrition and GI function, analyse its onset, characteristics and course, severity, precipitating and relieving factors, and any associated symptoms, noting the timing and circumstances. For example, the nurse may ask the person:

- Have you had any episodes of indigestion, nausea, vomiting, diarrhoea or constipation? If so, describe the appearance of what was vomited or the stools and anything that makes these problems better or worse. How long have you had these problems?
- What do you usually eat and drink (include alcohol) during a 24-hour period? Has your dietary pattern changed recently? If so, please describe.
- Are you generally happy with your diet? If necessary, ask person to describe what they believe to be a 'healthy' diet.

Also consider red-flag symptoms for bowel cancer, such as blood mixed in with stools, an increase in mucus and wind, weight loss without dieting, feeling tired and a family history. For example, ask the person:

- Do you have cramping or abdominal pain? If so, please ask for a description of type, frequency and quality.
- Have you ever had any bleeding from your rectum? If so, please describe the amount and colour of the blood (for example, was it bright red or dark?).

When collecting information about the person's current health status, ask about any changes in weight, appetite and the ability to taste, chew or swallow. What is the person's perception of the role of nutrition in maintaining health? Who buys and prepares the food? What medications (prescribed, over-the-counter or complementary) is the person currently taking? Does the person take any vitamins, herbal supplements or other 'health food' items? Does the person consume alcohol or recreational drugs (how much, what type, how often)?

If the person has experienced nausea or vomiting, ask whether the vomitus contains bright red blood, dark (old) blood, bile or faecal material. If the person is very thin or expresses concerns about body size incongruent with the ratio of height to weight, ask whether the person induces vomiting or uses laxatives to control weight. Ask whether the person has dental appliances, such as braces, bridges or dentures, and what self-care measures are used for them, as well as oral hygiene practices and frequency of dental visits.

CONSIDERATION FOR PRACTICE

Culture influences all aspects of one's life. It is a learned system of beliefs, values and rules that people use to guide their activities. Culture shapes behaviours, attitudes and beliefs about being overweight, being thin, eating, food nutrition, activity and exercise. Culture provides the foundation for how you view your own body as well as someone else's body. The term 'fat' is influenced by culture. Body weight is looked at differently from one culture to another.

Ask the person to describe any heartburn, indigestion, abdominal discomfort or pain. Explore the location of the pain, the type of pain, the time it occurs, foods that aggravate or relieve it, and how it is relieved. Abdominal pain is often referred to other sites (see the chapter 'Nursing care of people in pain' for further information on pain assessment). For example, a person with a liver disorder may experience pain over the right shoulder (Kehr's sign). Epigastric (middle upper abdominal) pain is experienced in cases of acute gastritis, obstruction of the small intestine and acute pancreatitis. Pain in the right upper quadrant is associated with cholecystitis.

Pain in the left upper quadrant may be related to a gastric ulcer. Sudden onset of lower abdominal cramping often occurs in obstruction of the colon. Left lower abdominal pain may be associated with diverticulitis. Rectal pain may occur with stool retention and/or haemorrhoids. Determine whether the person has had any lower abdominal pain or rectal pain, which may be associated with a distended colon filled with gas or fluid. Crampy, colicky pains occur with diarrhoea and/or constipation. Ask about any medical conditions that may influence the person's bowel elimination pattern, such as stroke or spinal cord impairment, inflammatory gastrointestinal diseases, endocrine disorders, cancer, allergies and reactions to allergen.

Note any recent travel to other countries or to remote areas in northern Australia. Information about the person's psychosocial history and cultural background is also important. Assess the person's lifestyle for any patterns of psychological stress and/or depression, which may alter bowel elimination. Depression may be associated with constipation, whereas **diarrhoea** (frequent passage of loose, watery stools) may occur in situations of high stress and anxiety. Explore the person's activities of daily living (ADLs), including exercise, sleep–rest patterns and dietary and fluid intake. Changes in ADLs can influence bowel elimination patterns.

More women than men seek help for constipation, suggesting that hormonal changes may play a role. Ask about history of diarrhoea, constipation or bleeding from the rectum, and collect information about the use of medications, laxatives, suppositories or enemas. For example, anticholinergic drugs, antihistamines, tranquillisers or narcotics may cause constipation.

The health history should include questions about any prior surgeries or GI tract trauma. Explore with the person their personal and family history of any medical condition that may affect the person's ingestion, digestion and/or metabolism (e.g. Crohn's disease, diabetes mellitus, irritable bowel syndrome, peptic ulcers or pancreatitis). Other areas significant to the assessment of nutritional status and the gastrointestinal system are food allergies (especially to milk, which is evidenced as lactose intolerance with abdominal cramping, excessive flatus and loose stools), and a family history that may provide clues to increased risk of health problems.

If the person has an **ostomy** (surgical opening into the bowel), ask about skin care management, skin integrity, consistency of stool, foods causing diarrhoea or **flatus** (intestinal gas), the number of times that the person empties the appliance bag daily and irrigation habits. It is also important to explore the person's feelings about the appliance.

To obtain information about the person's nutritional status, ask about changes in weight, appetite, food preferences, fibre content, food intolerances (wheat or dairy products—possible intolerance), special or supplementary diets (may cause diarrhoea), spicy foods (often increase gut motility) and any cultural or ethnic influences on dietary intake. The person could complete a food diary before attending a clinic or outpatient visit. Ask about regular fluid intake—for example, amount of coffee, diet drinks, sports drinks, excess alcohol; these may increase gut motility, giving a loose stool. Ask whether the person experiences nausea and vomiting; if so, determine any relation to food intake and ask the person to describe the character of the emesis.

In addition, ask about indigestion, the use of antacids or other over-the-counter medications, herbal preparations and episodes of diarrhoea and its character. Also ask about the use of analgesic medications or other medications prescribed; for example, opioid analgesia decreases bowel motility and can lead to chronic constipation, and anti-inflammatory drugs can irritate the gut and bowel.

Explore any family history of colon cancer, colitis, gallbladder disease or malabsorption syndromes, such as lactose intolerance and coeliac disease. Assess the person's risk factors for cancer, including age greater than 50; family member with colon cancer; history of endometrial, ovarian or breast cancer; and previous diagnoses of inflammatory bowel disease, polyps or cancer.

People with cognitive problems require careful assessment. For example, if a person is unable to retain information or change behaviour, there is little point in teaching anal exercises to improve the strength of the pelvic floor muscles as these are unlikely to be carried out. An assessment of cognitive function should include the person's ability to understand what is being explained, retain information and learn, change behaviour and carry out instructions at home.

In addition to other factors assessed in the health history, culture and ethnicity are important components of nutritional status and gastrointestinal health. Australia is culturally and ethnically diverse and, as such, numerous cultural food customs can be seen throughout the country. Nutritional diversity is common among cultural and ethnic groups, and questions should be included to identify specific customs, food likes and dislikes, and how foods are prepared and served. In some ethnic groups, for example, dietary substances are used to protect health, such as eating raw garlic or onions (Spector, 2016). In Aboriginal and Torres Strait Islander peoples' culture, food is often depicted in art and stories, highlighting how important food and the collecting and sharing of it are in this culture. In other cultures, dietary balance is believed to be necessary to keep the body in balance or harmony. It is therefore necessary for nurses to be mindful of specific culturally related nutritional values and practices and to ask questions to identify health-related concerns specific to individualised dietary intake.

If English is not the person's first language, it is important to assess oral and written language fluency, ask in which language they prefer to receive their health information and use interpreters where necessary.

Interview questions categorised by functional health patterns are listed in the accompanying box.

Physical assessment

Begin by explaining what will happen during the physical examination, and encourage the person to take deep, regular breaths to increase relaxation. If a rectal examination is included, explain that it may be uncomfortable, they may feel as though they might be about to have a bowel movement, and sometimes flatus (gas) is passed. Assure the person that this is normal. Ensure that the examination area is private and the person is draped properly to prevent unnecessary exposure. Remember to ask the person's permission to proceed with a physical examination.

Physical assessment of gastrointestinal and nutritional status may be performed as part of a total health assessment, as a focused assessment of people with known or suspected health problems, in combination with assessment of the urinary and reproductive systems (problems that may cause manifestations similar to those of the gastrointestinal system), or alone for people with known or suspected health problems. The techniques of inspection, auscultation, percussion and palpation are used. Palpation is the last method used in assessing the abdomen.

> **CONSIDERATION FOR PRACTICE**
>
> **When assessing the abdomen, use palpation last, because pressure on the abdominal wall and contents may interfere with bowel sounds and cause pain, ending the examination.**

Collect objective data by obtaining anthropometric measurements (height, weight, triceps skin folds and midarm circumference) and by examining the mouth and abdomen. Prior to the examination, collect all necessary equipment and explain techniques to the person to decrease anxiety. The person may

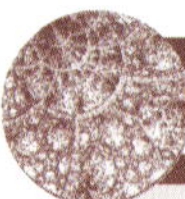

FUNCTIONAL HEALTH PATTERN INTERVIEW Nutritional status and gastrointestinal system

FUNCTIONAL HEALTH PATTERN	INTERVIEW QUESTIONS AND LEADING STATEMENTS
Health perception–Health management	■ Have you had any illness or surgery affecting your nutrition and gastrointestinal (GI) function? If so, how were these treated?
	■ Describe your current problem; how long has it lasted; what have you done to treat it?
	■ What medications do you take? Do you take antacids? If so, what do you use them for and how often do you take them?
	■ Are you currently taking alternative or complementary medicines, such as herbs, homeopathics, traditional medicines? If so, what do you use them for and how often do you take them?
	■ Do you have allergies to foods? What are they and how do you react? How do you manage these?
	■ Do you have your own teeth? If not, please describe any gaps, replacement teeth/dentures.
	■ Do you have tooth or gum problems or pain that interferes with your ability to eat?
	■ When was your last dental examination?
	■ Describe what you do each day to take care of your teeth.
Nutritional–Metabolic	■ Describe what you eat and how much (and type) of fluids you drink in a 24-hour period.
	■ Describe dietary supplements, such as vitamins, minerals, tonics, herbs, that you currently are taking.
	■ Have you noticed any change in your appetite recently? Explain.
	■ What is your current weight? What do you feel your ideal weight would be? Have you had a recent gain or loss? Explain.
	■ Describe your food likes and dislikes.
	■ Do you have any of the following: indigestion, belching, nausea, vomiting, difficulty swallowing? If so, what causes this and how do you manage it?
	■ Do you drink alcohol? If so, what type? Describe your average daily number of alocholic drinks.
	■ Questions specific to the person's culture and ethnic group is included in this functional health pattern area, such as what types of food are preferred or not eaten, what types of foods are never eaten together and what types of foods are eaten to remain healthy.
Elimination	■ What is the pattern of your bowel movements? Has it been affected by your condition/illness?
	■ Ask women of reproductive age if their menstrual cycle affects their bowel movements. If so, how?
	■ Do you use laxatives, suppositories, enemas or other substances to help the regularity of your bowel movements? Please describe.
	■ Are your bowel movements affected by what you eat? Explain.
	■ Have you noticed any change in the colour of your urine or bowel movements? Explain.
	■ Have you ever used laxatives or made yourself vomit to control your weight? Explain.
Activity–Exercise	■ Describe your activities on a typical day.
	■ What type of exercise do you get, and how often?
	■ Do you smoke? If so, what and how many cigarettes per day?
	■ Do you use recreational drugs? If so, what type, amount and how often?
Sleep–Rest	■ Do you wake up hungry during the night?
	■ Does abdominal pain, cramping, nausea or diarrhoea ever interfere with your sleep? Explain.
Cognitive–Perceptual	■ Describe the amount and type of foods you should eat each day.
	■ Rate your ability to taste and smell foods on a scale of 1 to 10 (with 10 being excellent).
	■ Describe any pain you have had in your mouth, stomach or abdomen. What type of pain was it (dull, crampy, achy, burning)? What seems to cause it? What do you do to relieve it?

FUNCTIONAL HEALTH PATTERN INTERVIEW **Nutritional status and gastrointestinal system (continued)**

FUNCTIONAL HEALTH PATTERN	INTERVIEW QUESTIONS AND LEADING STATEMENTS
	■ How do you prefer to receive your health information? Written, verbal, internet, mixture? Please explain.
	■ Do you have any difficulties reading and understanding health information? If so, what or who helps you to understand and feel well informed?
Self-perception–Self-concept	■ How does this problem/condition make you feel about yourself?
	■ Are you satisfied with your appearance in terms of weight? If not, why?
	■ Have you tried gaining or losing weight? If so, what worked or didn't work for you?
Role–Relationships	■ How does this condition affect your relationships with others?
	■ Who normally buys food and prepares your meals?
	■ Do you eat with others regularly? If so, who? Where do you normally eat your meals?
Sexuality–Reproductive	■ Has this condition affected your usual sexual activities? Can you describe your concerns and what you do to manage?
	■ Ask women of reproductive age if their menstrual cycle is affected by this condition. If so, please describe what happens, and how you manage it.
Coping–Stress tolerance	■ Have you experienced any type of stress that may have worsened this condition?
	■ Has having this condition created stress for you?
	■ Describe what you do when you feel stressed.
Value–Belief	■ Tell me how specific relationships or activities help you cope with this problem.
	■ Do you have specific cultural beliefs or practices that affect how you care for and feel about this condition? Please describe.
	■ Are there any specific treatments that you would not use to treat this condition?
	■ Are your spiritual beliefs, needs or practices affected by this condition/illness? Please describe.

be seated during assessment of the mouth but is supine during the abdominal assessment. Older adults or those with limited mobility may need assistance with positioning.

Physical assessment of the integumentary system, nervous system, musculoskeletal system, cardiovascular system and respiratory system may also reflect the person's nutritional status. Table 20.5 summarises abnormal nutritional assessment findings related to these body systems. Normal age-related findings for the older adult are summarised in Table 20.6.

Diagnostic tests

The results of diagnostic tests of nutritional status and gastrointestinal function are used to support the diagnosis of a specific disease, to provide information to identify or modify the

TABLE 20.5 Assessment findings due to malnutrition

BODY SYSTEM	ASSESSMENT FINDINGS
Nails	Soft and spoon shaped in iron deficiency. Splinter haemorrhages in vitamin C deficiency.
Hair	Dry, dull and scarce in zinc, protein and linoleic acid deficiencies.
Skin	Flaky and dry in vitamin A, vitamin D and/or linoleic acid deficiency. Cracks and/or hyperpigmentation in niacin deficiency. Bruising in vitamin C or vitamin K deficiency.
Eyes	Eyes become dry and soft with decrease in vitamin A. Conjunctiva is pale with a decrease in iron and red with a decrease in riboflavin.
Nervous system	Reflexes are decreased and person may have peripheral neuropathies with thiamine deficiency. Person may be irritable and/or disoriented with thiamine deficiency.
Musculoskeletal system	Muscle wasting is seen with deficits in protein, carbohydrate and fat metabolism. Calf pain occurs with thiamine deficiency; joint pain may occur with vitamin C deficiency.
Cardiovascular system	Heart size and rate may increase with thiamine deficiency. Blood pressure may be increased with a high intake of fat. Lowered cardiac output and decreased blood pressure may occur with kilojoule deficiencies over a long time period.
Gastrointestinal system	Cheilosis (sores at corner of mouth) seen in vitamin-B-complex deficiencies, especially riboflavin. Stomatitis and spongy, bleeding gums may also be seen in malnutrition.

TABLE 20.6 Age-related gastrointestinal changes

AGE-RELATED CHANGE	SIGNIFICANCE
Teeth: ↑ number of root cavities and cavities around existing dental work; tooth enamel harder and more brittle; dentin is more fibrous; tooth cusps flatten; root pulp shrinks; ↑ loss of bone supporting teeth	Increase in periodontal disease and tooth loss Increase in fractures of teeth Increased incidence of dentures, caps, tooth implants
Gums: gingiva retracts	Increase in periodontal disease
Taste: less acute as tongue atrophies, especially for sweet sensations	Excessive seasoning of foods
Saliva: ↓ amount is produced (one-third of that produced in younger years)	Decreased ability to break down starches Swallowing may take longer
Oesophageal motility: ↓ intensity of propulsive waves and slower emptying time, weaker gag reflex	Discomfort when swallowing food Increased risk of aspiration
Stomach: mucosa atrophies, ↓ production of hydrochloric acid and pepsin leading to higher pH in stomach	Increase in incidence of gastric irritation
Liver: less efficient handling of cholesterol	Increased incidence of gallstones

appropriate medication or therapy used to treat the disease and to help nurses monitor the person's responses to treatment and nursing care interventions. More information, including specific laboratory tests, is included in the discussion of disorders in the chapters 'Nursing care of people with nutritional disorders', 'Nursing care of people with upper goastorintestinal disorders', 'Nursing care of people with bowel disorders' and 'Nursing care of people with gallbladder, liver and pancreatic disorders'.

Regardless of the type of diagnostic test, the nurse is responsible for explaining the procedure and any special preparation needed, for supporting the person during the examination as necessary, for documenting the procedure as appropriate and for monitoring the results of the test.

Genetic considerations

When conducting a health assessment interview and physical assessment, it is important for the nurse to consider genetic influences on the health of the adult. During the health assessment interview, ask about family members with known abnormalities of copper accumulation in the body, hypercholesteraemia, abnormal cholesterol or fat metabolism, obesity or cancer of the pancreas. During the physical assessment, assess for any manifestations that might indicate a genetic disorder (see the 'Genetic considerations' box). If data are found to indicate genetic risk factors or alterations, ask about genetic testing and refer for appropriate genetic counselling and evaluation. The chapter 'Genetic implications of adult health nursing' provides further information about genetics in medical–surgical nursing.

DIAGNOSTIC TESTS Gastrointestinal disorders

OESOPHAGEAL AND STOMACH TESTS

NAME OF TEST Oesophageal acidity, Oesophageal manometry, Acid perfusion (Bernstein test)

PURPOSE AND DESCRIPTION Oesophageal acidity is measured to diagnose problems of the lower oesophageal sphincter and chronic reflux oesophagitis. A catheter with a pH electrode is inserted into the oesophagus through the mouth. The measurement may be one time or over a 24-hour period.

Oesophageal manometry is done to measure oesophageal sphincter pressure and peristaltic contractions for diagnosis of oesophageal motility problems, such as achalasia. A manometric catheter with a pressure transducer is inserted into the oesophagus through the mouth and oesophageal pressure is measured before and after swallowing.

Acid perfusion (Bernstein test) tests are performed to distinguish between gastric acid reflux and cardiac involvement. A nasogastric tube is inserted through the nose into the oesophagus. A saline solution, followed by a mild hydrochloric acid (HCl) solution, is dripped into the catheter and the person is asked to indicate when pain occurs. Normal oesophageal pH is 5 to 6.

RELATED NURSING CARE Advise the person to be nil by mouth (NBM) and to avoid alcohol intake for 8–12 hours prior to the exam. Assess medications: results of the tests may be affected by antacids, anticholinergics and H2-receptor antagonist medications, which increase the pH, reducing acidity and causing false test results.

DIAGNOSTIC TESTS Gastrointestinal disorders (continued)

NAME OF TEST Barium swallow or Upper GI series (see Figure 20.7)

PURPOSE AND DESCRIPTION To diagnose oesophageal varices, inflammation, ulcerations, hiatal hernia, foreign bodies, polyps, diverticula and tumours of the oesophagus, stomach and duodenal bulb. These radiological studies are done by observing the movement of a contrast medium with a fluoroscope.

RELATED NURSING CARE Advise the person to be NBM and avoid smoking for 8–12 hours before the exam; person will drink 450–550 g of barium sulfate (a non-water-soluble chalky liquid) or meglumine diatrizoate (Gastrografin, a water-soluble liquid) before the exam. Withhold medications for 8 hours before the exam, according to the medical officer's directions. Following the exam, ensure the person eliminates the barium by giving laxatives and encouraging increased fluids as appropriate.

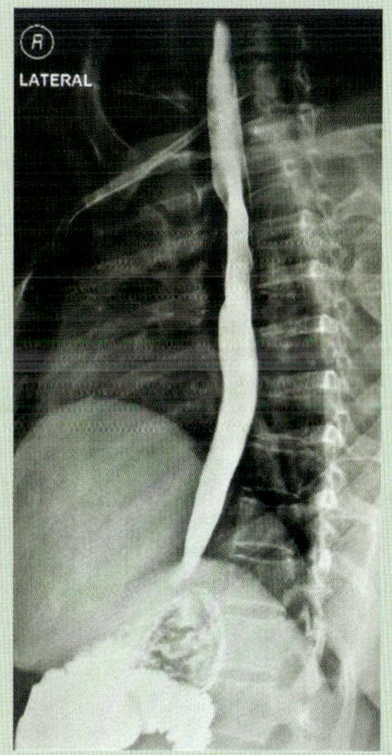

FIGURE 20.7 ***A barium x-ray of a healthy stomach***

Source: Karan Bunjean/Shutterstock.

NAME OF TEST Barium enema

PURPOSE AND DESCRIPTION A lower gastrointestinal (GI) tract x-ray is used to diagnose inflammation, ulcerations, structural changes, diverticula and lower GI tumours and for investigations of pain and anaemia. These radiological studies are done by observing the movement of a contrast medium, which is inserted through a tube in the rectum into the colon.

RELATED NURSING CARE Preparation for the test requires emptying of the large intestine. The nurse will advise the person to follow a clear fluid diet for 1–3 days prior to the examination. The day prior to the test the person will be required to take a combination of oral laxatives and an enema (an additional enema may be required on the day). Following the exam, the person will resume a normal diet. If the person has not eliminated the barium, a laxative may be required.

NAME OF TEST Faecal occult blood test (FOBT)

PURPOSE AND DESCRIPTION A bowel cancer screening test that can be performed every 2 years from the age of 40. It can detect a miniscule amount of blood in stool that is not visible to the eye. It is an early screening tool that may lead to further investigation for bowel cancer or polyps.

RELATED NURSING CARE Advise people over the age of 50 without a family history or symptoms to perform a home FOBT every 2 years.

NAME OF TEST Colonoscopy

PURPOSE AND DESCRIPTION An examination of the lower GI tract, used to diagnose cancer, inflammation, ulcerations, structural changes and investigations of pain, bowel changes and anaemia. The colonoscope is used to directly visualise the colon and rectum; a biopsy can be taken during the examination if an abnormal growth is visualised.

RELATED NURSING CARE Preparation for the test requires emptying of the large intestine. The nurse will advise the person to follow a clear fluid diet for 1–3 days prior to the examination. The day prior to the test the person will be required to take a combination of oral laxatives and an enema (an additional enema may be required on the day). Inform the person a light sedative is given during the exam. Following the exam, the person will resume a normal diet; inform the person flatus is quite common post procedure. The person will require someone to drive them home following the [illegible] during the examination.

(continued)

DIAGNOSTIC TESTS Gastrointestinal disorders (continued)

NAME OF TEST Upper GI endoscopy (Oesophagogastroduodenoscopy (OGD))

PURPOSE AND DESCRIPTION To directly visualise mucous membrane lining of the oesophagus, stomach and duodenum. A flexible fibre-optic endoscope is used to visualise inflammations, ulcerations, tumours or varices; and video imaging may illustrate gastric motility. May also be combined with an ultrasound examination by attaching an ultrasound transducer to the endoscope.

RELATED NURSING CARE Schedule at least 2 days after barium swallow or upper gastrointestinal series. Ensure the informed consent is signed prior to premedication. Encourage questions and provide answers and support.

Keep the person NBM for 6–8 hours before the procedure. Remove dentures and eyewear. Follow routine preoperative checklist.

HEALTH EDUCATION FOR THE PERSON AND FAMILY

- Do not eat or drink anything for 6–8 hours before the procedure.
- The procedure is somewhat uncomfortable and requires 20–30 minutes to complete.
- A local anaesthetic will be used in your throat and you will be given a sedative during the procedure.
- After the procedure, you will be allowed to eat and drink as soon as your gag reflex returns and you are able to swallow.
- You may experience mild bloating, belching or flatulence following the procedure.
- Contact your doctor immediately if you develop any of the following: difficulty swallowing; epigastric, substernal or shoulder pain; vomiting blood; black tarry stools; or fever.

NAME OF TEST Magnetic resonance imaging (MRI)

PURPOSE AND DESCRIPTION A scan that uses magnetic and radio waves to identify a source of gastric bleeding, tumours or cysts.

RELATED NURSING CARE Inform the person of need to lie still during the examination. Remove any metallic objects (such as hair clips, jewellery) and assess for any metallic implants (such as pacemakers, body piercings, shrapnel). If present, test is not performed due to the danger caused by the magnetic field from the machine. Explain the need to be NBM for at least 6 hours prior to the exam.

NAME OF TEST Gastroscopy

PURPOSE AND DESCRIPTION See Upper GI endoscopy.

RELATED NURSING CARE See Upper GI endoscopy.

NAME OF TEST Gastric analysis

Normal values:

Fasting: 1.0–5.0 mEq/L/per hour

Stimulation: 10–25 mEq/L/per hour

PURPOSE AND DESCRIPTION To evaluate gastric secretions and detect an increase or decrease of free hydrochloric acid. To conduct the gastric analysis, a nasogastric tube is inserted into the stomach and specimens are aspirated to evaluate gastric acidity. A stimulation gastric analysis may follow, with a gastric stimulant (such as Histalog or pentagastrin) administered and several gastric samples aspirated.

RELATED NURSING CARE Advise person to remain NBM with no smoking for 8–12 hours prior to the exam. Assess medications and fluid intake: anticholinergics, cholinergics, adrenergic blockers, antacids, steroids, alcohol and coffee can alter results. Remove loose dentures. Insert nasogastric tube. Aspirate gastric contents at 15- to 20-minute intervals as ordered.

NAME OF TEST Gastric emptying studies

PURPOSE AND DESCRIPTION To evaluate the ability of the stomach to empty liquids or solids. In this nuclear imaging study, the person is asked to eat a cooked egg containing ^{99m}Tc (solids) or to drink orange juice with ^{99m}Tc (liquids). Sequential images are recorded with a gamma camera every 2 minutes for up to an hour. Emptying should occur within 70–125 minutes.

RELATED NURSING CARE Explain to the person that the substances contain only very small amounts of radioactivity and are not hazardous.

DIAGNOSTIC TESTS Gastrointestinal disorders (continued)

GALLBLADDER AND PANCREAS TESTS

NAME OF TEST Abdominal ultrasound, Hepatobiliary ultrasound, Gallbladder ultrasound

PURPOSE AND DESCRIPTION Abdominal ultrasound is used to detect abdominal tumours, cysts and ascites.

Hepatobiliary ultrasound is used to visualise the biliary ducts and to detect subphrenic abscesses, cysts, tumours and cirrhosis of the liver. Gallbladder ultrasound is used to detect gallstones.

These non-invasive procedures record ultrasound waves as they are reflected off body structures. A conductive gel is applied to the skin and a transducer placed on the area.

RELATED NURSING CARE Advise the person to remain NBM for 8–12 hours prior to the test.

NAME OF TEST Cholecystography (oral) (GB series) If the gallbladder cannot be visualised with an oral contrast substance, an IV cholangiography may be ordered. *If the person is also having GI x-rays with barium, the GB tests should be done first, because barium would interfere with the test.*

PURPOSE AND DESCRIPTION To detect gallbladder stones, inflammation or tumours and obstruction of the cystic duct. The evening before the test, radiopaque tablets (e.g. iopanoic acid (Telepaque), sodium ipodate (Oragrafin), iodoalphionic acid (Priodax) or iodipamide meglumine (Cholografin)) are given; the following morning x-rays are taken. A high-fat meal may be given after the fasting x-rays are completed and further x-rays taken to determine how fast the GB expels the dye.

RELATED NURSING CARE Advise person to eat a fat-free diet 24 hours prior to the test. Other than sips of water, no food or fluids should be taken 12 hours before the test. Assess person for allergy to iodine, seafood or x-ray dye (many contain iodine).

NAME OF TEST Cholangiography

- Percutaneous transhepatic cholangiogram (PTC)
- Surgical cholangiogram

PURPOSE AND DESCRIPTION A PTC is done to evaluate filling of the hepatic and biliary ducts. Using local anaesthesia, the liver and bile duct is entered with a long needle (using fluoroscopy), bile is withdrawn and a contrast medium is injected into the bile duct.

During a surgical cholangiogram with general anaesthesia, contrast medium is injected into the common bile duct to evaluate filling of the common bile duct.

RELATED NURSING CARE Assess person for allergy to iodine, seafood or x-ray dye (many contain iodine). Monitor for bile leakage or haemorrhage following the tests. Normal preoperative routine is required for the surgical procedure.

NAME OF TEST Magnetic resonance cholangiopancreatography (MRCP)

PURPOSE AND DESCRIPTION This non-invasive MRI study is done to evaluate the biliary and pancreatic ducts.

RELATED NURSING CARE Assess for metal implants or pregnancy. (Test will not be done if present.)

NAME OF TEST Computed tomography (CT)

PURPOSE AND DESCRIPTION A non-invasive procedure, using radiofrequency waves and a magnetic field; used to evaluate disorders of the gallbladder, pancreas, biliary tract and liver.

RELATED NURSING CARE No special preparation is needed.

NAME OF TEST Endoscopic retrograde cholangiopancreatography (ERCP)

PURPOSE AND DESCRIPTION To directly visualise gastrointestinal structures and retrieve gallstones from the distal common bile duct, dilate structures and biopsy tumours. A fibre-optic endoscope is inserted (under fluoroscopy) through the mouth down the oesophagus, stomach and descending duodenum, and the common bile ducts and pancreatic ducts are cannulated. Contrast medium is injected into the ducts and structures are visualised.

RELATED NURSING CARE Advise the person to be NBM for 8 hours before the test. Following the test, assess vital signs and gag reflex and monitor for complications (such as pancreatitis).

NAME OF TEST Serum lipase

PURPOSE AND DESCRIPTION This blood test is used to measure the secretion of lipase by the pancreas.

Normal value:
0–160 Unit/L

RELATED NURSING CARE No special preparation is needed.

(continued)

DIAGNOSTIC TESTS Gastrointestinal disorders (continued)

NAME OF TEST Serum amylase

PURPOSE AND DESCRIPTION This blood test is used to measure the secretion of amylase by the pancreas. It is used to diagnose acute pancreatitis, when amylase level peaks in 24 h and then returns to normal in 48 to 72 h.

Normal value:
0–130 Unit/L

RELATED NURSING CARE No special preparation is needed.

LIVER TESTS

NAME OF TEST Liver biopsy

PURPOSE AND DESCRIPTION To rule out metastatic cancer or to detect a cyst or cirrhosis of the liver. Using ultrasound, a biopsy needle is inserted into the liver and guided to the pathological site. See Figure 20.8.

RELATED NURSING CARE Related nursing care of the person having a liver biopsy is described below.

PREPARATION OF THE PERSON

- Review chart for signed consent form.
- Keep the person NBM as per policy, usually 4–6 hours pre-procedure.
- Assess and record baseline vital signs.
- Review prothrombin time (PT) and platelet count; administer vitamin K as ordered.
- Instruct to empty bladder immediately before the biopsy.
- Place in supine position on far right side of bed; turn head to left and extend right arm above head to improve access to the biopsy site.

HEALTH EDUCATION FOR THE PERSON AND FAMILY

- Discuss preparation for the biopsy and expected sensations during the procedure.
- Hold your breath following expiration during needle insertion to keep diaphragm and liver high and stabilised in the abdominal cavity.
- Obtaining the tissue sample usually requires only 10–15 seconds; there may be some pain or discomfort during this time.
- Direct pressure is applied to the site immediately after the needle is removed; you will be placed on your right side to maintain site pressure.
- You may develop pain in the right shoulder as the anaesthetic loses effect.
- You will be monitored for bleeding after the procedure.
- Food and fluids are withheld for 2 hours after the biopsy; you then can resume your usual diet.
- Avoid coughing, lifting or straining for 1–2 weeks.

Note: A wide variety of blood tests are used to diagnose and monitor liver disease. These are discussed in appropriate interprofessional care sections in the chapter 'Nursing care of people with gallbladder, liver and pancreatic disorders'.

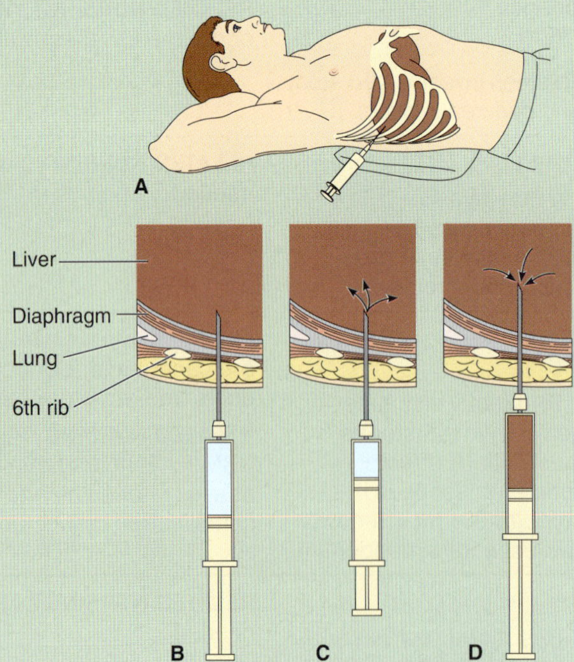

FIGURE 20.8 *Liver biopsy. A, The person exhales completely, and then holds their breath. This brings the liver and diaphragm to their highest position. B, The biopsy needle is inserted into the liver. C, Approximately 1 mL of saline is injected to clear the needle of blood and tissue. D, The needle is advanced and a tissue sample is aspirated. Pressure is applied to the site immediately after the needle is withdrawn. The specimen is sent to the laboratory for analysis*

GENETIC CONSIDERATIONS

Nutritional and gastrointestinal system

- Cleft lip and/or palate are influenced by genetic factors.
- An autosomal recessive disorder, Wilson's disease is an abnormality of copper transport, resulting in copper accumulation and toxicity to the liver and brain, resulting in neurological disease in adults.
- Colon cancer is one of the most common inherited cancer syndromes.
- Tangier disease is a disease of cholesterol transport, leading to characteristic orange tonsils, very low levels of high-density lipoprotein and an enlarged liver and spleen.
- Hypercholesterolaemia has a familial tendency.
- About 90% of human pancreatic cancers show a chromosome defect.
- Obesity is believed to result from a variety of factors, including genetics.
- Gaucher disease, more common in descendants of Jewish people from Eastern Europe, results in the lack of an enzyme to break down fats. Fats accumulate in the liver, spleen and bone marrow, causing pain, fatigue, jaundice, bone damage, anaemia and even death.
- Coeliac disease is a genetic, inherited disease responsible for the malabsorption of nutrients resulting in malnutrition. If people with coeliac disease eat certain types of proteins (glutens, found in wheat, barley, rye and oats) an autoimmune response causes damage to the small intestine, so that nutrients are not absorbed.
- Due to a rapid change in diet, Aboriginal and Torres Strait Islander peoples are prone to a group of conditions identified as 'insulin-resistant syndrome' (also known as syndrome X). It includes renal disease, heart disease, obesity and type 2 diabetes (Australian Institute of Health and Welfare, n.d.).

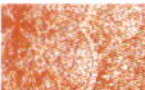

NUTRITIONAL AND GASTROINTESTINAL ASSESSMENTS

Technique/normal findings	Abnormal findings
Anthropometric assessment	
Weigh the person and measure the person's height. Compare the person's actual weight to ideal body weight (IBW) (see Table 20.7). *Weight should be appropriate to height as indicated on a standardised table.*	■ A weight 10–20% less than ideal body weight indicates malnutrition. ■ A weight 10% above ideal body weight is considered overweight. ■ A weight 20% above ideal body weight is considered obese.

TABLE 20.7 Example of a height and weight table (IBW)

HEIGHT (CM)	WEIGHT (KG)	HEIGHT (CM)	WEIGHT (KG)
148	44-55	173	59-74
150	45-56	175	61-76
152	46-58	178	63-79
155	48-60	180	65-81
158	50-62	183	66-83
160	51-64	185	68-85
162	52-66	188	71-88
165	54-68	190	72-90
168	56-71	193	74-92
170	58-72	196	77-96

(continued)

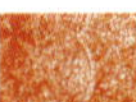

NUTRITIONAL AND GASTROINTESTINAL ASSESSMENTS (continued)

Technique/normal findings	Abnormal findings

Calculate the person's percentage of ideal body weight (%IBW). Use the formula in Table 20.8 to determine the presence of obesity and/or malnutrition based on %IBW. *Ideal body weight should be within normal range.*

TABLE 20.8 Indications of nutritional status by body weight

%IBW	%UBW	NUTRITIONAL STATUS
> 120	–	Obese
110–120	–	Overweight
80–90	85–95	Mildly undernourished
70–79	75–84	Moderately undernourished
< 70	< 75	Severely undernourished

UBW = usual body weight

Calculate the person's percentage of usual body weight (%UBW) to determine weight change, using this formula:

$$\frac{\text{Current weight}}{\text{Usual weight}} \times 100$$

Refer to Table 20.8 to determine nutritional status based on %UBW.

- Using %IBW may result in overlooking malnutrition in a very obese person.

Measure body mass index (BMI). Determine BMI by using one of the following formulas. *BMI should be between 20 and 25.*

$$\frac{\text{Weight in kilograms}}{\text{Height in metres}^2} = \text{BMI}$$

$$\frac{\text{Weight in pounds} \times 705}{\text{Height in inches}^2} = \text{BMI}$$

- A BMI of 25–29.9 kg/m^2 indicates overweight.
- A BMI of 30 kg/m^2 and above indicates obesity.

Measure triceps skinfold thickness (TSF). Find the midpoint between the person's olecranon and acromion processes. Grasp the skin and fat and pull it away from the muscle. Apply skinfold calipers for 3 seconds and record reading (see Figure 20.9). Repeat three times and average the three readings. Compare the person's reading with the standard values shown in Table 20.9. *TSF should be within normal range as compared to standard values.*

- Triceps readings are 10% or more below standards in malnutrition and 10% or more above standards in obesity or overnutrition.

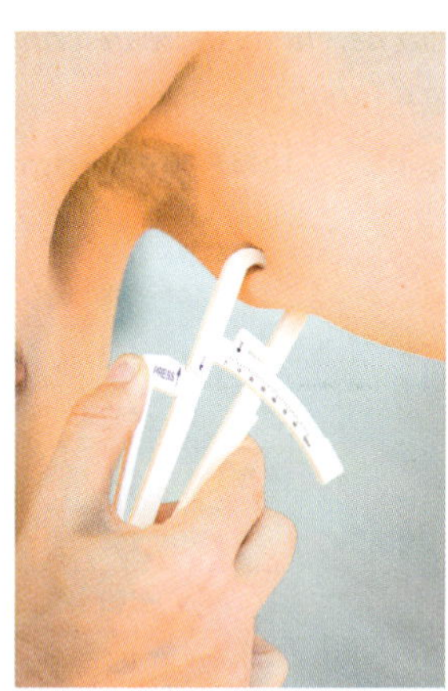

FIGURE 20.9 ***Measuring TSF with calipers***

Source: Edward Olive/Alamy Stock Photo.

TABLE 20.9 Values for anthropometric measurements

	STANDARD VALUE	
MEASUREMENT	MALE	FEMALE
Triceps skinfold thickness	12.5 mm	16.5 mm
Midarm circumference	29.3 cm	28.5 cm
Midarm muscle circumference	25.3 cm	23.2 cm

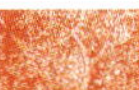

NUTRITIONAL AND GASTROINTESTINAL ASSESSMENTS (continued)

Technique/normal findings	Abnormal findings
Measure midarm circumference (MAC). Find the midpoint between the person's olecranon and acromion processes. Wind tape measure around arm (see Figure 20.10). Compare the person's reading to the standard values shown in Table 20.9. *MAC should be within normal range as compared with standard values.*	■ MAC decreases with malnutrition and increases with obesity.
Calculate midarm muscle circumference (MAMC). Use the person's triceps skinfold measurement and midarm circumference readings to calculate the person's MAMC: $\text{MAMC} = \text{MAC} - (0.314 \times \text{TSF})$ **Compare the result to the standard values shown in Table 20.9.** *MAMC should be within normal range as compared to standard values.*	■ In mild malnutrition, the MAMC is 90% of the standard; in moderate malnutrition, 60–90%. In severe malnutrition (muscle wasting), the MAMC is less than 60% of the standard.
Determine waist-to-hip ratio. With the person standing, measure the waist and then measure the hips midway between the iliac crest and the greater trochanter. Use the formula below to calculate the waist-to-hip ratio. *Normal findings: females, waist ratio less than or equal to 0.80; males, waist ratio less than or equal to 1.0.* $\frac{\text{Waist circumference}}{\text{Hip circumference}} = \text{waist-to-hip ratio}$	■ Females with a ratio greater than 0.80 and males with a ratio greater than 1.0 have a greater risk of mortality from a cardiac-related death.
Oral assessment	
Inspect and palpate the lips. *Lips should be of normal colour for race without lesions.*	■ **Cheilosis** (painful lesions at corners of mouth) is seen with riboflavin and/or niacin deficiency. ■ Cold sores or clear vesicles with a red base are seen in herpes simplex 1.
Inspect and palpate the tongue. *Tongue should be pink, smooth and have good turgor.*	■ Atrophic smooth glossitis is characterised by a bright red tongue. It is seen in B_{12}, folic acid and iron deficiencies. ■ Vertical fissures are seen in dehydration.

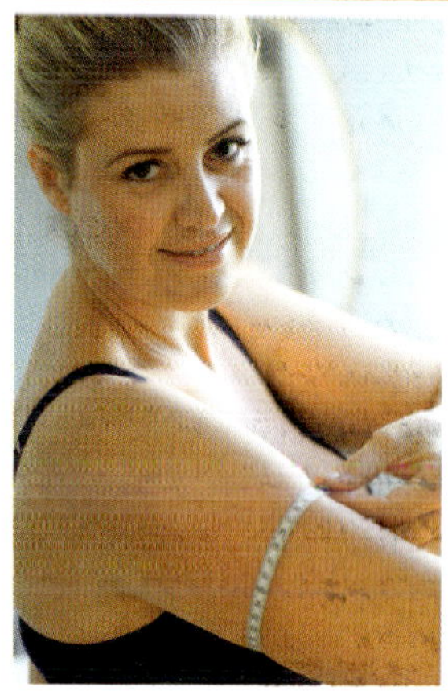

FIGURE 20.10 ***Measuring MAC with a tape measure***

Source: Cultura Creative (RF)/Alamy Stock Photo.

CONSIDERATION FOR PRACTICE

Always wear gloves when assessing the oral cavity.

(continued)

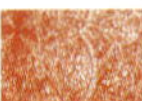

NUTRITIONAL AND GASTROINTESTINAL ASSESSMENTS (continued)

Technique/normal findings	Abnormal findings
	■ A white or pale coated tongue during or after treatment with oral antibiotics can be caused by *Candida albicans* (the same pale fungus responsible for most vaginal yeast infections). ■ Black hairy tongue, also known as lingua villosa nigra, results from hyperkeratosis of the tongue. It may have different colours varying from white, yellow or brown to black depending upon the involved extrinsic factors (i.e. tobacco, coffee, tea, food or drugs) and intrinsic factors (i.e. chromogenic organisms in the normal flora).
Inspect and palpate the buccal mucosa. *Mucosa should be moist, without lesions and of appropriate colour.*	■ **Leucoplakia** (small white patches) may be a sign of a premalignant condition. ■ A reddened, dry, swollen mucosa may be seen in stomatitis. ■ Candidiases (white cheesy patches that bleed when scraped) may be seen in immunosuppressed people receiving antibiotics or chemotherapy, and in terminally ill people.
Inspect and palpate the teeth. *Teeth should be in a state of good hygiene without caries.*	■ Cavities and excessive plaque are seen with poor nutrition and/or poor oral hygiene.
Inspect and palpate the gums. *Gums should be of even colour without swelling.*	■ Swollen, red gums that bleed easily (**gingivitis**) are seen in periodontal disease, vitamin C deficiencies or with hormonal changes.
Inspect the throat and tonsils. *Tonsils (if present) should be of appropriate colour and size.*	■ In acute infections, tonsils are red and swollen and may have white spots.
Note the person's breath. *Breath should not have unusual or foul odours* **(halitosis).**	■ Sweet, fruity breath (like the smell of apples which are 'past their prime' or even downright rotten) is noted in diabetic ketoacidosis. A person on a high-protein diet can suffer from halitosis. ■ Acetone breath (smells like nail polish remover) may be a sign of uraemia or diabetes. ■ Foul breath may result from respiratory infections, postnasal drip, liver disease and anorexia. ■ Poor dental/oral health (e.g. untreated cavities, oral candidiasis and poor oral hygiene—inadequate brushing and flossing) may result in bad breath.

Abdominal assessment

The quadrants of the abdomen, with related internal structures, are illustrated in Figure 20.11. Box 20.2 provides guidelines for abdominal assessment.

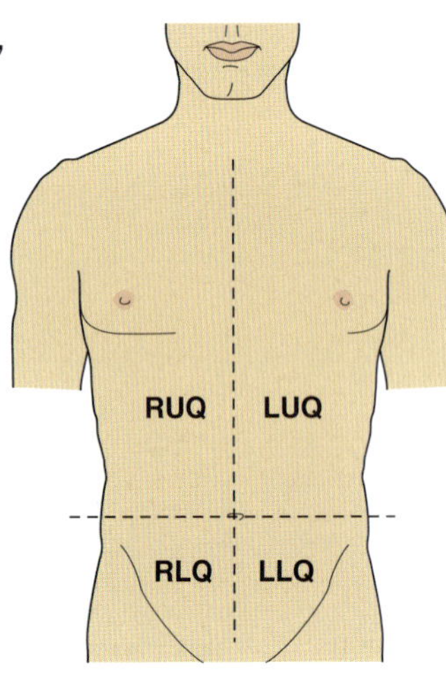

FIGURE 20.11 *The four quadrants of the abdomen, with anatomical location of organs within each quadrant*

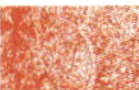

NUTRITIONAL AND GASTROINTESTINAL ASSESSMENTS (continued)

Technique/normal findings | **Abnormal findings**

BOX 20.2 Guidelines for assessing the abdomen

Ask the person to empty their bladder before beginning the examination. Assist the person to the dorsal recumbent (supine) position, with a small pillow under the head, a pillow under the knees (if desired) and the arms at the sides of the body. Warm the stethoscope before applying it to the person's skin. Ask the person to point to areas that are painful and explain that those areas will be examined last. Expose the abdomen from below the breasts to the pubic symphysis and drape the person's thoracic and genital areas. When you document your findings, specify the location by abdominal quadrant.

General guidelines for abdominal assessment are as follows:

1. Inspect the abdomen under a good light source that is shining across the abdomen. Sit at the right side of the person and note symmetry, distension, masses, visible peristalsis and respiratory movements. If masses are detected, ask the person to take a deep breath, which decreases the size of the abdominal cavity and makes any abnormality more visible.
2. Auscultate each quadrant of the abdomen, using the diaphragm of the stethoscope. Listen for bowel sounds, arterial bruits, venous hums and friction rubs.
3. Percuss several areas within each quadrant of the abdomen, using a systematic path (e.g. always begin in the lower left quadrant, then proceed to the lower right quadrant, upper right quadrant and upper left quadrant, respectively). The predominant percussion tones for the entire abdomen are tympany and dullness. Tympany is present over gas-filled intestines. Dullness is present over the liver, the spleen, an enlarged kidney or a full stomach. Percuss for fluid, gaseous distension and masses.
4. Palpate each quadrant of the abdomen for shape, position, mobility, size, consistency and tenderness of the major abdominal organs. Begin this part of the assessment with light palpation and increase the depth of palpation to elicit tenderness or better identify organ size and shape. Deep palpation should be conducted only by nurses with considerable experience. Remember to palpate areas of indicated tenderness last and to use gentle pressure. Palpation may be difficult or impossible if the person exhibits muscle guarding from pain or is ticklish. The gallbladder and the spleen are normally not palpable.

Inspect abdominal contour, skin integrity, venous pattern and aortic pulsation. *Abdomen should be slightly concave or rounded with intact skin. There should not be distended veins or obvious aortic pulsations.*

- Generalised abdominal distension may be seen in gas retention or obesity.
- Lower abdominal distension is seen in bladder distension, pregnancy or ovarian mass.
- General distension and an everted umbilicus are seen with ascites and/or tumours.
- A scaphoid (sunken) abdomen is seen in malnutrition or when fat is replaced with muscle.
- **Striae** (whitish silver), commonly called stretch marks, may result from rapid growth at puberty, during or after pregnancy, or significant weight gain. Striae may also occur as a result of abnormal collagen formation or a result of medications or chemicals that interfere with collagen formation.
- Spider angiomas may be seen in liver disease.
- Dilated veins are prominent in cirrhosis of the liver, ascites, portal hypertension or venocaval obstruction.
- Pulsation is increased in aortic aneurysm.

Auscultate all four quadrants of the abdomen with the diaphragm of the stethoscope (see Figure 20.12). Begin in the lower right quadrant, where bowel sounds are almost always present. Normal bowel sounds (gurgling or clicking) occur every 5 to 15 seconds. *Listen for at least 5 minutes in each of the four quadrants to confirm the absence of bowel sounds.*

- **Borborygmus** (hyperactive high-pitched, tinkling, rushing or growling bowel sounds) is heard in diarrhoea or at the onset of bowel obstruction.
- Bowel sounds may be absent later in bowel obstruction, with an inflamed peritoneum and/or following surgery of the abdomen.

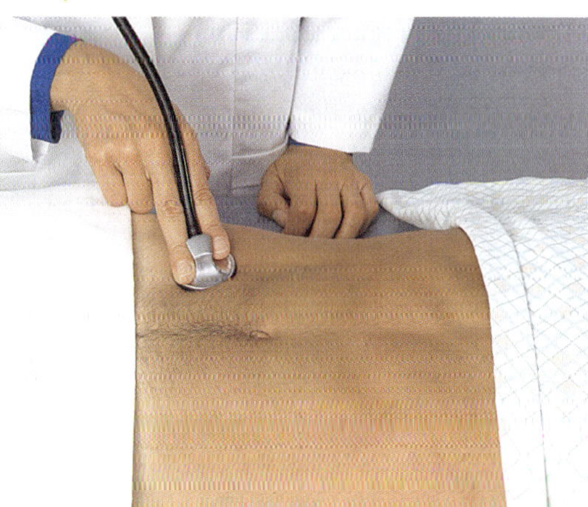

FIGURE 20.12 *Auscultating the abdomen with the diaphragm of the stethoscope*

(continued)

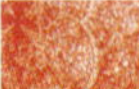

NUTRITIONAL AND GASTROINTESTINAL ASSESSMENTS (continued)

Technique/normal findings	Abnormal findings
Auscultate the abdomen for vascular sounds with the bell of the stethoscope (see Figure 20.13). *No sounds (bruits, venous hum or friction rub) other than bowel sounds should be auscultated.*	■ **Bruits** (blowing sound due to restriction of blood flow through vessels) may be heard over constricted arteries. A bruit over the liver may be heard in hepatic carcinoma. ■ A venous hum (continuous medium-pitched sound) may be heard over a cirrhotic liver. ■ Friction rubs (rough grating sounds) may be heard over an inflamed liver or spleen.

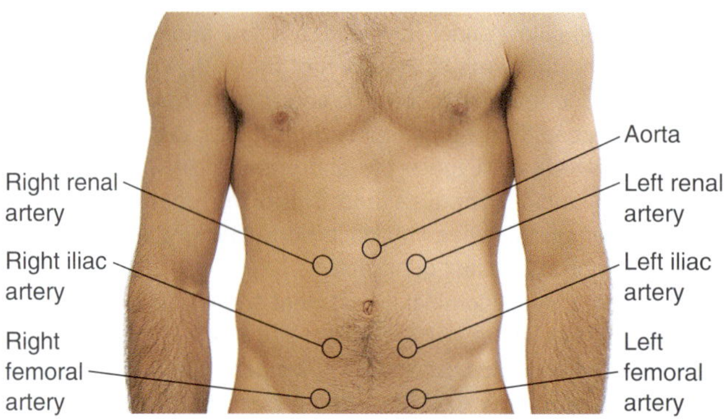

FIGURE 20.13 *Location of placement of the stethoscope for auscultation of arteries of the abdomen*

Technique/normal findings	Abnormal findings
Percuss the abdomen in all four quadrants (see Figure 20.14). *Normally, tympany is heard over the stomach and gas-filled bowels.*	■ Dullness is heard when the bowel is displaced with fluid or tumours, or filled with a faecal mass.

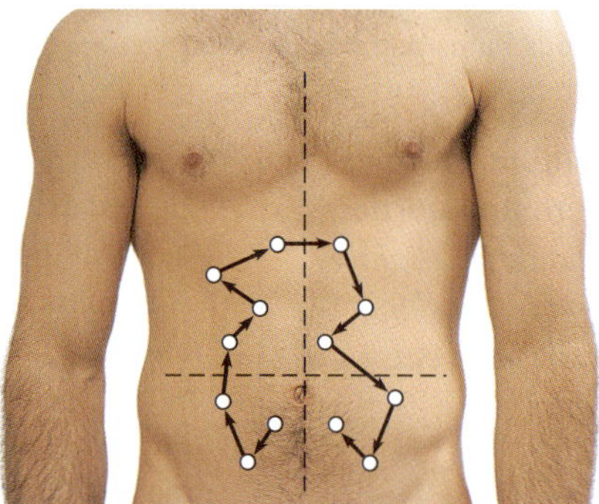

FIGURE 20.14 *Location of sites for systematic percussion of all four quadrants*

Technique/normal findings	Abnormal findings
Percuss the liver (see Box 20.3 for guidelines for liver percussion and palpation; see Figure 20.15 for landmarks). *The lower border of liver dullness is located at the costal margin to 1–2 cm below.*	■ In cirrhosis and/or hepatitis, the liver span is greater than 6–10 cm in the MCL and greater than 4–8 cm in the MSL.

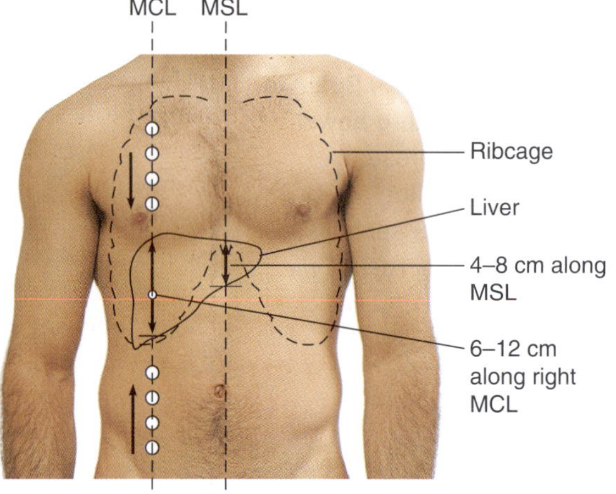

FIGURE 20.15 *Anatomical location of the liver, with the midclavicular line (MCL) and midsternal line (MSL) superimposed. The normal liver span is 6–12 cm at the MCL*

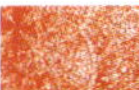

NUTRITIONAL AND GASTROINTESTINAL ASSESSMENTS (continued)

Technique/normal findings | **Abnormal findings**

BOX 20.3 Guidelines for percussing and palpating the liver

The size of the liver may be determined by percussion and palpation, as follows:

1. Percuss in the midclavicular line (MCL), beginning below the umbilicus (see Figure 20.15). Begin to percuss over a region of tympany and move upwards. The first dull percussion tone occurs at the lower border of the liver. Determine the upper liver border by beginning percussion over an area of lung resonance (in the MCL) and percussing downwards to the first dull tone, usually at the 5th to 7th interspace. Mark each of these locations and measure the distance from one mark to the other to determine liver size. The normal liver size is 6–12 cm at the MCL; however, men have larger livers than women.
2. Conduct bimanual palpation of the liver (see Figure 20.19) by placing your left hand under the person at the level of the 11th to 12th ribs and applying upward pressure. Place your right hand below the costal margin, ask the person to take a deep breath and palpate for the liver border. The liver is not normally palpable in a healthy adult, although it may be in very thin people.

Percuss the spleen for dullness posterior to the midaxillary line at the level of the 6th to 11th rib (see Figure 20.16). *The spleen is percussed as an oval area of dullness approximately 7 cm wide near the left 10th rib and slightly posterior to the midaxillary line.*

- A large area of dullness that extends to the left anterior axillary line on inspiration is associated with an enlarged spleen and may be related to trauma, infection or mononucleosis.

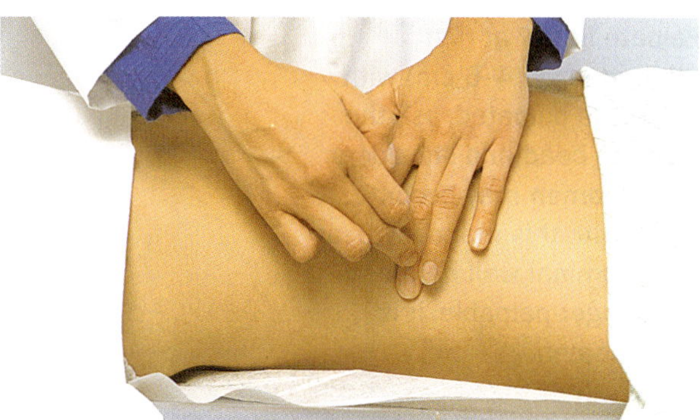

FIGURE 20.16 *Percussing the spleen*

Percuss for shifting dullness (see Figure 20.17). *If ascites is not present, the borders between tympany and dullness remain relatively constant despite position changes.*

- In a person with ascites, the level of dullness increases when the person turns to the side.

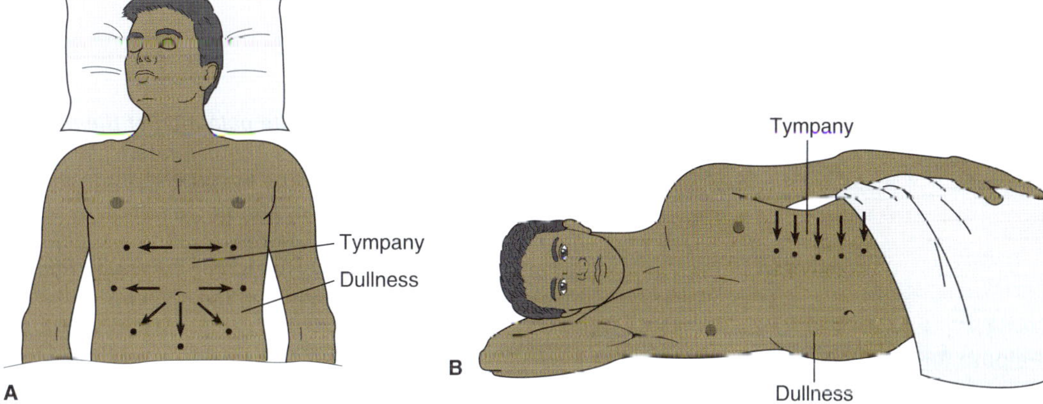

FIGURE 20.17 *Percussing for shifting dullness in ascites. A, Common percussion tones when the person is lying supine. B, Changes in percussion tones (shifting dullness) when the person turns to the side*

(continued)

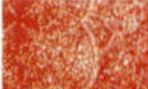

NUTRITIONAL AND GASTROINTESTINAL ASSESSMENTS (continued)

Technique/normal findings	Abnormal findings
Palpate the abdomen in all four quadrants. *There should be no abdominal masses or pain on palpation.*	■ In cases of peritoneal inflammation, palpation causes abdominal pain and involuntary muscle spasms. ■ Abnormal masses include aortic aneurysms, neoplastic tumours of the colon or uterus, and a distended bladder or distended bowel due to obstruction. ■ A rigid, board-like abdomen may be palpated when the person has a perforated duodenal ulcer.

CONSIDERATION FOR PRACTICE

Never use deep palpation in a person who has had a pulsatile abdominal mass, renal transplant or polycystic kidneys, or is at risk of haemorrhage.

Use a circular motion to move the abdominal wall over underlying structures (see Figure 20.18). Feel for masses and note any tenderness or pain the person may have during this part of the exam. Palpate lightly at first (1.3–2 cm), then deeply (4–5 cm) with caution. If a mass is palpated, ask the person to raise the head and shoulders. A mass in the abdomen may become more prominent with this manoeuvre, as will a ventral abdominal wall hernia. If the mass is no longer palpable, it is deeper in the abdomen.

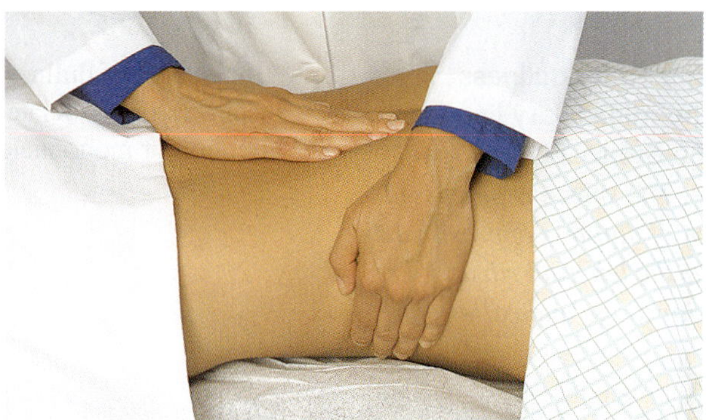

A

B

FIGURE 20.18 *Light to moderate palpation of the abdomen. A, In light palpation, the examiner, keeping the fingers approximated, gently depresses the abdominal wall about 1 cm to assess for large masses, slight tenderness and muscle guarding. B, The examiner performs moderate palpation by using the palm or the side of the hand to depress the abdominal wall to a slightly greater depth than in light palpation. This technique is useful for assessing abdominal organs that move with respiration (such as the liver and the spleen)*

Technique/normal findings	Abnormal findings
Palpate for rebound tenderness. Press the fingers into the abdomen slowly and release the pressure quickly. *Releasing pressure should not cause or increase pain.*	■ In peritoneal inflammation, pain occurs when the fingers are withdrawn. ■ Right upper quadrant pain occurs with acute cholecystitis. ■ Upper middle abdominal pain occurs with acute pancreatitis. ■ Right lower quadrant pain occurs with acute appendicitis. ■ Left lower quadrant pain is seen in acute diverticulitis.

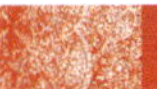

NUTRITIONAL AND GASTROINTESTINAL ASSESSMENTS (continued)

Technique/normal findings	Abnormal findings
Palpate the liver (see Figure 20.19). Note whether the person guards the abdomen or reports any sharp pain, especially on inspiration. *The abdomen should be non-tender and the liver is usually non-palpable.*	■ An enlarged liver with a smooth, tender edge may indicate hepatitis or venous congestion. ■ An enlarged, non-tender liver may be felt in a malignant condition. ■ The person with inflammation of the gallbladder feels sharp pain on inspiration and stops inspiring. This is called Murphy's sign.

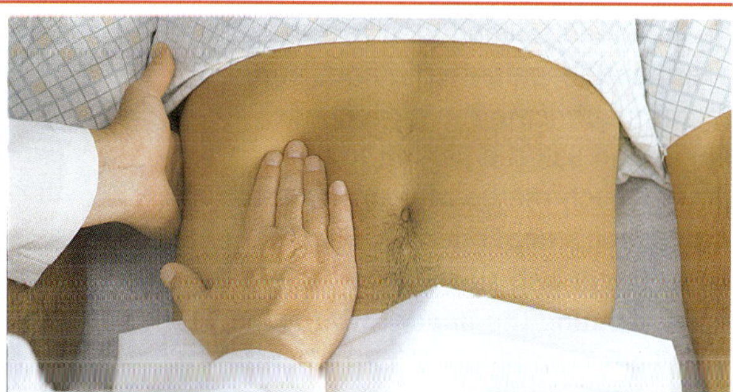

FIGURE 20.19 *Palpating the liver with the bimanual method*

Inguinal area assessment

Technique/normal findings	Abnormal findings
Inspect the inguinal area for bulges after asking the person to bear down. *The inguinal area is normally free of bulges.*	■ Bulges that appear in the inguinal area when the person bears down may indicate a **hernia** (a defect in the abdominal wall that allows abdominal contents to protrude outward).

CONSIDERATION FOR PRACTICE

Nurses need to be culturally alert and competent when working with people with disorders of the bowel, bowel cancer and undergoing faecal testing. Ways of raising issues and talking about them will depend on a person's cultural worldview about health, bodies and elimination practices. Being well informed and engaging in ongoing cultural education, together with close collaboration with Indigenous or migrant health professionals, will assist nurses to provide relevant, timely and culturally safe care.

Technique/normal findings	Abnormal findings
Palpate the inguinal area with a gloved hand. Ask the person to shift weight to the left to palpate the right inguinal area and vice versa. Place your right index finger upward into the inguinal area and ask the person to bear down or cough. *Bulging or masses are normally not palpable.*	■ A bulge or mass may indicate a hernia.

Perianal assessment (performed only by experienced nurses or under supervision)

Technique/normal findings	Abnormal findings
Inspect the perianal area. Wearing gloves, spread the person's buttocks apart. Observe the area and ask the person to bear down as if trying to have a bowel movement. *The perianal area should be intact, without obvious lesions.*	■ Swollen, painful, longitudinal breaks in the anal area may appear in people with anal fissures. (These are caused by the passing of large, hard stools or by diarrhoea.) ■ Dilated anal veins appear with haemorrhoids. ■ A red mass may appear with prolapsed internal haemorrhoids. ■ Doughnut-shaped red tissue at the anal area may appear with a prolapsed rectum. ■ Movable, soft masses may be polyps.

(continued)

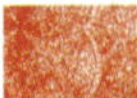

NUTRITIONAL AND GASTROINTESTINAL ASSESSMENTS (continued)

Technique/normal findings	Abnormal findings
If accredited to conduct a rectal examination, palpate the anus and rectum. Lubricate the gloved index finger and ask the person to bear down. Touch the tip of your finger to the person's anal opening. Flex the index finger and slowly insert it into the anus, pointing the finger towards the umbilicus (see Figure 20.20). Rotate the finger in both directions to palpate any lesions or masses. *There should be no masses in the anus or rectum.*	■ Hard, firm, irregular embedded masses may indicate carcinoma.

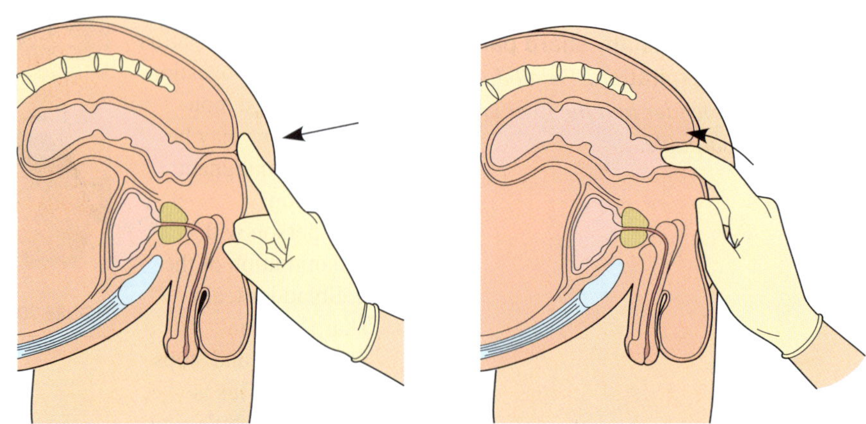

FIGURE 20.20 *Digital examination of A, the anus; and B, the rectum*

Technique/normal findings	Abnormal findings
Faecal assessment	
Inspect the person's faeces. After palpating the rectum, withdraw your finger gently. Inspect any faeces on the glove. Note colour and/or presence of blood. Also use gloved fingers to note consistency. *Stool should be soft with no blood present, either on the stool or as occult blood.*	■ See Box 20.4 for information about stool characteristics.
Test the faeces for occult blood. Use a testing kit such as Occultest or Hemoccult II. *There should be no blood in the faeces.*	■ A positive occult blood test requires further testing for colon cancer or gastrointestinal bleeding due to peptic ulcers, ulcerative colitis or diverticulosis.
Note the odour of the faeces. *No distinctly foul odours should be present.*	■ Distinctly foul odours may be noted with stools containing blood, infections, parasites or extra fat, or in cases of colon cancer.

BOX 20.4 Assessing stool characteristics

Inspect faeces for colour, odour and consistency after the rectal exam or after defecation. Both hands are gloved.

Colour

- Blood *on* the stool results from bleeding from the sigmoid colon, anus or rectum. Blood *within* the stool indicates bleeding from the colon due to ulcerative colitis, diverticulosis or tumours. Black, tarry stools, called **melaena**, occur with upper gastrointestinal bleeding. Oral iron may turn stools black and mask melaena.
- Greyish or whitish stools can result from biliary tract obstruction due to lack of bile in stool.
- Greasy, frothy, yellow stools, called **steatorrhoea**, may appear with fat malabsorption.

Odour

- Distinct, foul odours may be noted with stools containing blood or extra fat, or in cases of colon cancer.
- Consistency:
  - Hard stools or long flat stools may result from a spastic colon or bowel obstruction due to a tumour or haemorrhoids. Hard stools may also result from dehydration or ingestion of oral iron.
  - Mucusy, slimy faeces may indicate inflammation and occur in irritable bowel syndrome.
  - Watery, diarrhoea stools appear with malabsorption problems, irritable bowel syndrome, emotional or psychological stress, ingestion of spoiled foods or lactose intolerance.

CONCEPT CHECK

1 A person you are caring for asks you what type of foods are complete proteins. What would be your best response?
1 none
2 eggs and milk
3 fruits and vegetables
4 butter and oils

2 Following minor surgery, a nurse would assess a person who is deficient in vitamin K for what possible complication?
1 infection
2 blood clotting
3 keloid formation
4 slow peristalsis

3 On monitoring a person's lab results, you notice a greatly elevated serum amylase level. What disease does this indicate?
1 cheilosis
2 gastric reflux
3 gallstones
4 acute pancreatitis

4 While assessing an older adult, you notice her teeth have obvious cavities and she has difficulty swallowing. She says, 'My mouth is so dry.' What health problem might result from these findings?
1 nutritional deficit
2 acute pain
3 altered elimination
4 risk of infection

5 What percussion sound would a nurse expect to hear when assessing the abdomen of a person with ascites?
1 inaudible bowel sounds
2 resonance
3 alternating amplitude
4 shifting dullness

6 A person asks you to tell her what internal haemorrhoids are. What would you say?
1 'They are part of the arteries of the body.'
2 'They are just bits of tissue that occur for no reason.'
3 'They are swollen veins in the anal canal.'
4 'They are part of the lymphatic system.'

7 Which of the following questions or statements would be appropriate for the person with an ostomy?
1 'Have you had any bleeding from your haemorrhoids?'
2 'Has your appetite changed lately?'
3 'Tell me about your family.'
4 'Describe the consistency of your stools.'

8 Why is removal of polyps from the colon during a colonoscopy important?
1 to identify genetic disorders
2 to prevent the development of cancer
3 to facilitate further examination of the bowel
4 to decrease future problems with constipation

9 What term is used to describe black, tarry stools?
1 occult blood
2 haematemesis
3 melaena
4 steatorrhoea

10 You are caring for a person the first day following bowel surgery. You do not hear bowel sounds during your initial assessment. What would you do?
1 Immediately call the doctor and report this abnormal finding.
2 Repeat the assessment in 30 minutes to ensure accuracy of findings.
3 Document the assessment as normal following abdominal surgery.
4 Ask another nurse to check your assessment before reporting it.

BIBLIOGRAPHY

Australian Institute of Health and Welfare (n.d.). *Health risk factors—Indigenous people: Nutrition*. Retrieved from https://www.aihw.gov.au/

Food Standards Australia New Zealand (FSANZ) (2021). *Australia New Zealand Food Standards Code, approval report—Application A1178*. Retrieved from https://www.foodstandards.gov.au

National Health and Medical Research Council (NHMRC) (2013). *Eat for health educator guide: Information for nutrition educators*. Retrieved from https://www.eatforhealth.gov.au/

Spector, R. (2010). *Cultural diversity in health and illness* (9th ed.). Sydney: Pearson Australia.

Tardy, A.-L., Pouteau, E., Marquez, D., Yilmaz, C. & Scholey, A. (2020). Vitamins and minerals for energy, fatigue and cognition: A narrative review of the biochemical and clinical evidence. *Nutrients*, *12*(1), 228–263. doi: 10.3390/nu12010228

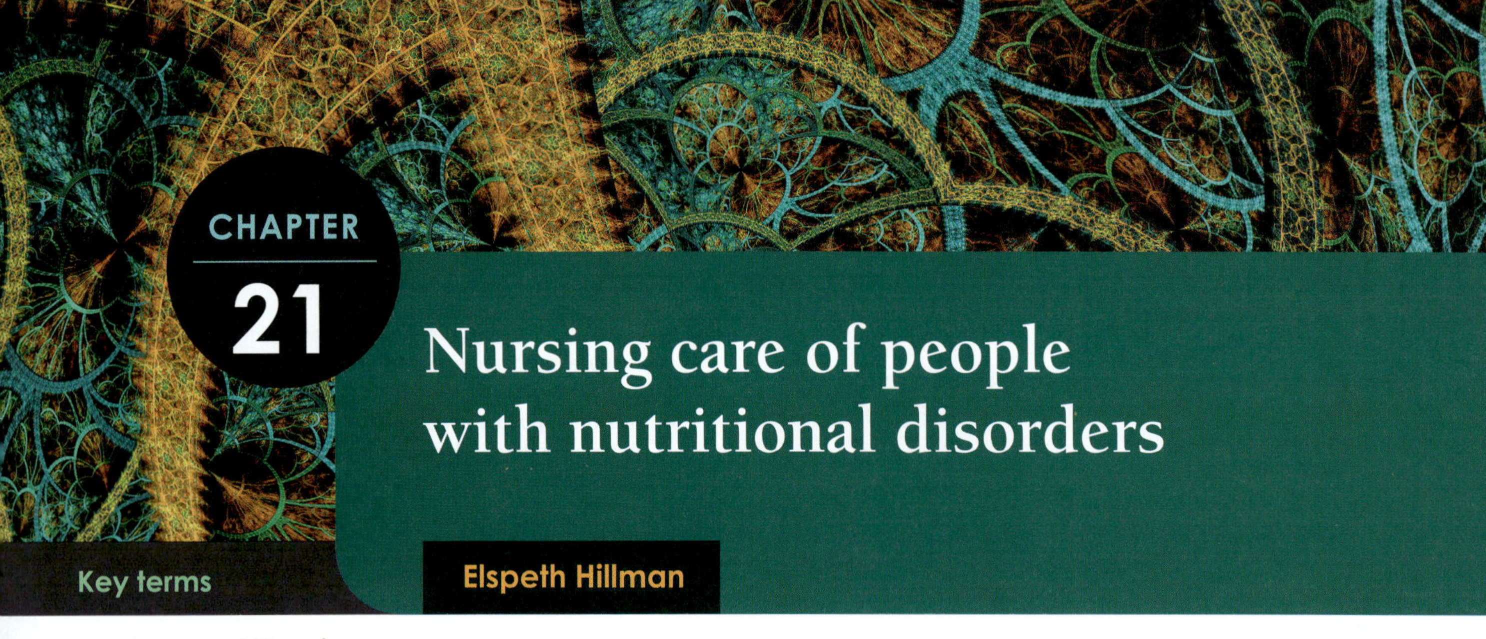

Nursing care of people with nutritional disorders

Elspeth Hillman

Key terms

Learning outcomes

- Describe the pathophysiology, complications and interprofessional care associated with the nutritional disorder of obesity.
- Describe the pathophysiology, complications and interprofessional care associated with the eating disorder malnutrition.
- Compare and contrast the three nutritional eating disorders of anorexia nervosa, bulimia nervosa and binge-eating disorder.

Clinical competencies

- Assess a person's functional health status with nutritional disorders.
- Monitor a person's nutritional status and responses to care; document and report abnormal or unexpected responses.
- Use assessment data to determine priority nursing diagnoses and select and implement nursing interventions.
- Administer medications; enteral and parenteral nutrition knowledgeably and safely.
- Integrate interprofessional care in the plan of care.
- Incorporate a person's cultural values and variations into the plan of care of a person with nutritional disorders.
- Plan and provide family teaching to restore, promote and maintain a person's functional health status.
- Evaluate a person's responses to care and use data to revise a plan of their care as needed.

Obesity and malnutrition are global major nutritional disorders, increasingly affecting different age groups. A person with nutritional disorders requires complex, skilled nursing care. Developmental, socioeconomic, cultural, psychological and physiological factors and living in rural or remote locations may play a role in these disorders: a holistic approach to nursing care is vital. Nursing care focuses on identifying causes, meeting nutritional and physiological needs, providing education and meeting the psychological needs of the person and their family. Before proceeding with the discussion of obesity and malnutrition, review the sections on metabolism and nutrients in the chapter 'A person-centred approach to assessing the gastrointestinal system'.

THE PERSON WITH OBESITY

Obesity, an excess of adipose tissue, is one of the most common, preventable non-communicable health problems worldwide, with more than 1.9 billion adults classified as overweight and over 650 million considered obese (World Health Organization (WHO), 2021). Being overweight or obese increases a person's likelihood of developing many chronic conditions (Australian Institute of Health and Welfare (AIHW), 2022a). Health-related problems associated with obesity are listed in Table 21.1.

In 2018–2019, 381,800, or 71% of, Aboriginal and Torres Strait Islander people aged 15 and over were overweight or obese (AIHW, 2022b). This was higher than in 2012–2013 (66%). The rise was driven by an increase in non-remote areas (AIHW, 2022b).

While obesity is often defined by body weight, it is more accurately measured by the **body mass index (BMI)**, the international standard measurement of the amount of body fat or adipose tissue compared to height, and the waist-to-hip ratio. (See Box 21.1 to calculate BMI.) A BMI of 25 to 29.9 kg/m^2 is classified as *overweight but not obese*; class 1 obese is a BMI between 30 and 34.9 kg/m^2, class 2 obese is a BMI between 35 and 39.9 kg/m^2 and class 3 is a BMI greater than 40 (AIHW, 2020). Class 3 obesity is also known as **morbid obesity**.

Incidence and prevalence

Australia ranks sixth highest among 22 OECD member countries for the proportion of overweight or obese people aged 15+ (AIHW, 2020). In 2017–2018, almost 67% of Australian adults were estimated to be either overweight or obese and, of these, 36% were estimated as being obese (AIHW, 2020). The prevalence of overweight and obese Australian adults aged 18 years and over has continued to rise. More than 1 in 4 children and adolescents aged 2–17 were overweight or obese in 2017–2018. One challenge in obtaining accurate prevalence data is the tendency for people to underestimate their self-reported weight (Robinson et al., 2022).

Table 21.2 shows estimations of overweight and obesity in Australia. It indicates that in 2014–2015, Western Australia had the greatest percentage of Australian adults who were overweight, but Tasmania had the greatest percentage who were obese. The Australian Bureau of Statistics (ABS) (2018a) identified that adults with higher qualifications were less likely to be obese, while those in low-income households were more likely to be obese. Many overweight and obese individuals suffer from sarcopenic malnutrition (high fat mass, low muscle mass) due to the overconsumption of nutrient-poor, high-fat diets.

TABLE 21.1 Health-related problems associated with obesity

BODY SYSTEM	OBESITY-RELATED PROBLEMS
Cardiovascular	Atherosclerosis, hypercholesterolaemia, dyslipidaemia Coronary artery disease Congestive cardiac failure Hypertension Stroke Varicosities Venous thrombosis, hypercoagulopathy, pulmonary embolism
Respiratory	Sleep disorders Asthma Sleep apnoea
Gastrointestinal	Gallbladder disease Diverticular disease Hiatal hernia Non-alcoholic fatty liver (steatohepatitis) Colorectal cancer Oesophageal cancer
Genitourinary	Cancer of the prostate Kidney cancer Obesity-induced glomerulopathy Stress incontinence
Musculoskeletal	Chronic lower back pain Muscle strains and sprains Osteoarthritis of hips and knees
Endocrine and reproductive	Metabolic syndrome Insulin sensitivity and/or resistance Diabetes mellitus, type 2 Pancreatic cancer Postmenopausal breast cancer Ovarian, uterine and endometrial cancers Amenorrhoea and infertility Complications of pregnancy, gestational diabetes mellitus Polycystic ovarian syndrome
Other	Depression Binge-eating disorder Postoperative complications, infection Obesity-related sarcopenia

BOX 21.1 Calculating body mass index (BMI)

BMI = weight (kg)/height^2 (m^2)
Normal = BMI 18.5–24.9 kg/m^2
[illegible]
Class 1 obese = BMI between 30 and 34.9 kg/m^2
Class 2 obese = BMI between 35 and 39.9 kg/m^2
Class 3 morbid obesity = BMI > 40 kg/m^2

TABLE 21.2 Estimations of overweight and obesity by Australian state or territory

STATE/TERRITORY	OVERWEIGHT	OBESE
South Australia	37.6%	32.6%
Western Australia	37.9%	28.7%
Tasmania	36%	34.8%
Australian Capital Territory	37.6%	26.4%
Victoria	36.6%	31.8%
New South Wales	34.9%	30.8%
Northern Territory	35.1%	29.8%
Queensland	33.5%	32.4%

Source: Adapted from ABS (2018b). *Overweight and obesity*. Canberra: ABS.

Risk factors

Adipose tissue is created when energy consumption exceeds energy expenditure. Research has identified that adipose tissue is not a passive store of energy but plays a complex role in endocrine, metabolic and immune regulation, which can contribute to the development of cancer, insulin resistance and type 2 diabetes mellitus (WHO, 2021). Genotype technologies associated with the Human Genome Project have found specific genes related to the development of obesity, which has led to the view that some individuals are genetically predisposed to obesity (Locke et al., 2015).

Physical inactivity is probably the most important factor contributing to obesity. Inactive people may consume fewer kilojoules than active people but continue to gain weight due to a lack of energy expenditure. Contemporary cultural and environmental factors such as increased work and time pressures encourage the use of labour-saving devices and reliance on the car for transportation. Increased sedentary time spent watching television and using the computer also contribute to decreased energy expenditure (Dunstan et al., 2012). Environmental influences, such as an abundant and readily accessible food supply, fast-food restaurants, advertising and inappropriately stocked vending machines contribute to increased food intake. Magnusson (2010) suggested the imperative within the Australian food industry is the maintenance of profits through unhealthy purchasing patterns.

Sociocultural influences contributing to obesity in Australia include the social appetite, which is the social, cultural, political, religious and economic contexts in which food is eaten. Examples are overeating at family meals, rewarding behaviour with food, religious and family gatherings that promote increased food intake, a tendency to eat meals away from home or eat takeaway meals from fast-food restaurants, and sedentary lifestyles (Germov & Williams, 2016). Economic pressures encourage low-income consumers towards higher-calorie, energy-dense food options (AIHW, 2022a).

Low self-esteem may precipitate unhealthy eating behaviours such as seeking comfort foods (e.g. chocolate) and the resulting weight gain in turn may diminish self-image even further. A person may overeat as a result of anxiety, depression, guilt or boredom, or as a means of getting attention. Some experts characterise overeating as a food addiction and as a coping mechanism for stressful life events (Vainik, García-García & Dagher, 2019).

Overview of normal physiology

All body activities require energy, including activities of daily living and those necessary to maintain cell and tissue function. **Nutrients** in food (or enteral or parenteral feedings) provide this energy and are the building blocks for growth and tissue repair. The body stores excess nutrients and energy (measured as kilojoules) to meet its needs when required nutrients are unavailable. More than 70% of the energy expended each day goes to maintaining the **basal metabolic rate (BMR)**, essentially the 'cost' (in kilojoules) of being alive. Physical activity accounts for only 5–10% of the energy spent daily.

Fat cells store excess energy as **triglycerides**, formed from dietary fats and carbohydrates. The body breaks down the triglycerides in fat cells when needed to provide energy (Porth, 2019).

Pathophysiology

Obesity occurs when excess kilojoules are stored as fat. It can result from excess energy intake, decreased energy expenditure or a combination of both.

Appetite, which affects food intake, is regulated by the central nervous system and by emotional factors (Cifuentes & Acosta, 2021). The hunger centre in the hypothalamus stimulates appetite in response to stimuli such as hypoglycaemia. As nutrient levels rise, the satiety centre (also in the hypothalamus) sends the message to stop eating. Gastrointestinal filling and hormonal factors also signal *satiety* (a sensation of fullness). Several hormones are involved in regulating obesity and body fat distribution including thyroid hormone, insulin, leptin (a peptide produced by adipocyte tissue that suppresses appetite and increases energy expenditure) and ghrelin (a peptide that originates within the lining of the stomach to induce hunger) (Cifuentes & Acosta, 2021). The two main types of body fat distribution are central (visceral) obesity and peripheral (subcutaneous) obesity. Each type of body fat distribution is characterised by a different metabolic profile and degree of cardiovascular risk (Porth, 2019).

Central (or visceral) **obesity** (apple shaped) is identified by a waist circumference greater than 80 cm in women and 94 cm in men or, alternatively, a waist-to-hip ratio of greater than 1 in men or 0.8 in women. (See the chapter 'A person-centred approach to assessing the gastrointestinal system' for a method to calculate the waist-to-hip ratio.) People with central body obesity tend to have more intra-abdominal fat within the mesentery and omentum which surrounds the abdominal organs, generate higher levels of circulating free fatty acids and have a greater uptake of glucose due to insulin resistance (Porth, 2019). As a result, central obesity is associated with a greater risk of complications such as hypertension, abnormal blood lipid profile, heart disease, stroke and elevated insulin levels. Men tend to have more intra-abdominal fat than women, although women tend to develop a central fat distribution pattern after menopause due to oestrogen deficiency (Marieb & Hoehn, 2019).

Peripheral (or subcutaneous) **obesity** (pear shaped), in which the waist-to-hip ratio is less than 0.8, is more commonly seen in women. The risk of hyperinsulinaemia, abnormal lipids and heart disease is lower in people with peripheral obesity than in those with central obesity.

Complications of obesity

Obesity is a significant risk factor for cardiovascular disease, including hypertension, coronary heart disease (CHD) and heart failure. The prevalence of hypertension and hypercholestrolaemia in obese men and women is higher than in people with a BMI of less than 25 (Bauset et al., 2022). The increases in blood pressure seen with obesity increase the risk of CHD and stroke. Approximately 60% of obese individuals have **metabolic syndrome**, including insulin resistance, hypertension, low high-density lipoprotein (HDL) cholesterol and an elevated plasma triglyceride level (Bauset et al., 2022). The metabolic syndrome is an identified risk factor for atherosclerosis and CHD. Obesity-associated obstructive sleep apnoea also contributes to the risk of CHD and heart failure.

Obesity increases the risk of insulin resistance and type 2 diabetes mellitus. Both weight gain in adulthood and abdominal (central) obesity are positively correlated with the risk of developing insulin resistance and type 2 diabetes mellitus (AIHW, 2022a). Obesity affects reproductive function in both men and women. Androgen (male sex hormone) levels are reduced in obese men; menstrual irregularities and polycystic ovarian syndrome (PCOS) are more common in obese women. PCOS is an additional risk factor for hyperinsulinaemia and insulin resistance. Increased weight also increases the risk of developing gallstones in both men and women. The risk of developing several types of cancer, including colon, breast and endometrial, increases in obesity (AIHW, 2022a). A link between obesity and chronic kidney disease has been attributed to the increased metabolic demands of the kidney, leading to higher glomerular capillary pressures with resultant glomerular hypertrophy (AIHW, 2022a). Increased weight places abnormal stress on joints, increasing the prevalence of joint pain and osteoarthritis, particularly in the weight-bearing joints of the knees and hips. Other health-related problems associated with obesity are listed in Table 21.1.

INTERPROFESSIONAL CARE

Because obesity has many contributing factors, its treatment is far more complex than just reducing the amount of food consumed. Most experts recommend an individualised program of moderate exercise, diet and behaviour modification designed to meet that person's specific capabilities and needs.

Diagnosis

Although body weight may be used to identify obesity, measures of body fat are more accurate. Males at ideal body weight have 10–20% body fat, whereas females at ideal body weight have 20–30% body fat.

- *Body mass index* is used to identify excess adipose tissue (WHO, 2021). BMI is calculated by dividing the weight (in kilograms) by the height in metres squared (m^2) (see Box 21.1). BMI calculations may not as accurately reflect the extent of adipose tissue in people who are highly muscular (e.g. body builders) or in those who have lost muscle mass (e.g. older adults). Table 21.3 provides a tool for determining adult BMIs.
- *Anthropometry* includes measurements of height, weight, bone size and skinfold to estimate subcutaneous fat. See the

TABLE 21.3 Body mass index table for BMIs

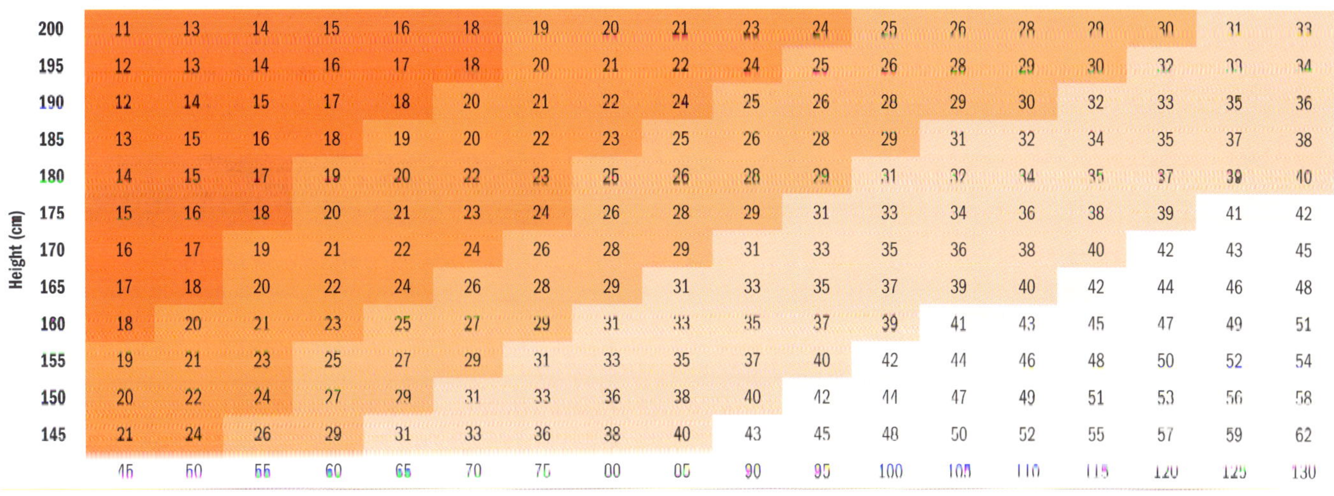

Height (cm)	45	50	55	60	65	70	75	80	85	90	95	100	105	110	115	120	125	130
200	11	13	14	15	16	18	19	20	21	23	24	25	26	28	29	30	31	33
195	12	13	14	16	17	18	20	21	22	24	25	26	28	29	30	32	33	34
190	12	14	15	17	18	20	21	22	24	25	26	28	29	30	32	33	35	36
185	13	15	16	18	19	20	22	23	25	26	28	29	31	32	34	35	37	38
180	14	15	17	19	20	22	23	25	26	28	29	31	32	34	35	37	39	40
175	15	16	18	20	21	23	24	26	28	29	31	33	34	36	38	39	41	42
170	16	17	19	21	22	24	26	28	29	31	33	35	36	38	40	42	43	45
165	17	18	20	22	24	26	28	29	31	33	35	37	39	40	42	44	46	48
160	18	20	21	23	25	27	29	31	33	35	37	39	41	43	45	47	49	51
155	19	21	23	25	27	29	31	33	35	37	40	42	44	46	48	50	52	54
150	20	22	24	27	29	31	33	36	38	40	42	44	47	49	51	53	56	58
145	21	24	26	29	31	33	36	38	40	43	45	48	50	52	55	57	59	62

Weight (kg)

- Underweight
- Healthy
- Overweight
- Obese
- Morbid obesity

chapter 'A person-centred approach to assessing the gastrointestinal system' for more information about anthropometric measurements.

- *Waist circumference* is an additional measurement to determine body fat distribution. The measurement is taken halfway between the last rib and the top of the iliac crest. Men with a waist measurement of 94 cm or greater and women with a waist measurement of 80 cm or greater have a higher risk of complications of obesity.

Other diagnostic tests may be done to help identify a physiological cause of obesity, as well as complications of obesity.

- *A thyroid profile*, including a total T_3 and T_3 uptake, free T_4 (FT_4) and total T_4, free thyroxine index (FTI) and thyroid-stimulating hormone (TSH), rules out thyroid disease (see the chapter 'A person-centred approach to assessing the endocrine system').
- *Serum glucose* is measured to identify coexisting diabetes mellitus.
- A *lipid profile* is ordered; high-density lipoprotein (HDL) ('good cholesterol') levels may be reduced in obese people, whereas low-density lipoprotein (LDL) ('bad cholesterol') levels are elevated.
- An *electrocardiogram* (ECG) is performed to detect effects of obesity on the heart, such as rate or rhythm disruptions, myocardial infarction or ventricular hypertrophy.

Medications

When used in combination with diet and moderate exercise, medications can assist in promoting weight loss. While physical activity and lifestyle modifications have been a cornerstone in controlling obesity and overweight, a range of anti-obesity medications are recommended along with lifestyle modifications. Pharmacotherapy is particularly important for those who are within obese range (BMI $\geq$ 30) or are overweight (BMI $\geq$ 27) and have at least one weight-associated comorbidity (type 2 diabetes mellitus, hypertension, hyperlipidaemia) (Magtoto, 2022). Long-term efficacy is questionable—rebound weight gain following medication cessation is common. Additionally, tolerance, addiction and side effects may occur. Long-term pharmacological weight loss interventions should be provided with behaviour-based interventions (Magtoto, 2022).

Orlistat (Xenical) inhibits GI tract fat absorption, leading to weight loss. It has the added benefit of lowering blood glucose and cholesterol. See the 'Medication administration' box for the nursing implications of this medication.

Methylcellulose and other bulk-forming products may decrease appetite by producing a sensation of fullness. A person taking these products may experience flatulence or diarrhoea and may need to increase fluid intake to prevent constipation.

Treatments

Successful treatment of obesity (sustained achievement of normal body weight without adverse consequences) is rarely achieved. Treatment focuses on reducing the health risks associated with obesity by changing lifestyle in both eating and exercise habits. A combination of treatments including a reduction in sedentary behaviour and an increase in physical activity, dietary therapy, behaviour modification, pharmacology and, in some cases, surgery is required to achieve and maintain the person's weight loss.

EXERCISE Exercise is a critical element in weight loss and maintenance. Physical activity improves physical fitness, decreases appetite, promotes self-esteem and increases the basal metabolic rate. An exercise or activity program should reflect the person's physical condition, interest, lifestyle and abilities (Ortega-Arroyo, 2022). Evaluation by a healthcare practitioner is important before beginning an exercise program. The practitioner instructs the person to progressively increase the duration and intensity of activity but to stop exercising and report symptoms if chest pain or shortness of breath occurs. A moderate aerobic exercise program of 30–40 minutes, 5 or more days a week promotes weight loss while reducing adipose tissue, increasing lean body mass and promoting long-term weight control. Table 21.4 presents examples of kilojoule use per hour for moderate physical activities.

MEDICATION ADMINISTRATION Medications to treat obesity

APPETITE SUPPRESSANTS

LIPASE INHIBITOR (Xenical)

Orlistat inhibits lipases necessary for the breakdown and absorption of fat, thus decreasing the absorption of dietary fat. Its action is primarily local, within the GI tract, with few systemic effects.

Nursing responsibilities

- Administer with meals or up to 1 hour following a meal.
- Provide a fat-soluble vitamin supplement (A, D, E and K) daily.
- Separate administration time from orlistat by at least 2 hours.

Health education for the person and family

- Take as directed; do not increase dose. You may skip a dose if you do not consume a meal containing fat.
- Use in conjunction with a low-kilojoule, low-fat diet.
- Common gastrointestinal side effects include oily or fatty stools, flatulence, oily discharge or frequent stools with difficulty controlling defecation. These side effects may diminish with time or increase if a meal high in fat is consumed.
- Notify your healthcare provider if you become pregnant while taking this medication.

TABLE 21.4 Kilojoule use per hour for moderate physical activities

TYPE OF EXERCISE	KILOJOULES/HOUR	TYPE OF EXERCISE	KILOJOULES/HOUR
Sleeping	230	Walking	1,170
Eating	360	Table tennis	1,210
Sewing	360	Gardening	1,470
Knitting	360	Tennis	1,470+
Sitting	360	Water aerobics	1,670
Standing	420	Skating	1,760+
Driving	460	Dancing, aerobic	1,760+
Office work	590	Aerobics	1,880+
Housework, moderate	670+	Bicycling, moderate	1,880+
Golf, with trolley	750	Jogging	2,090
Golf, without trolley	1,000	Gardening, digging	2,090
Gardening, planting	1,050	Swimming, active	2,090+
Dancing, ballroom	1,090		

NUTRITION The diet is planned to create a daily 2,000 to 4,000 kJ deficit off the recommended 8,700 kJ/day currently recommended in Australia. Ideally, the diet should be low in kilojoules and fat, and contain adequate nutrients, minerals and fibre. The person should eat regular meals with small servings. A gradual, slow weight loss of no more than 0.5 kg per week is recommended. For most people, this means a diet of 4,186 to 5,020 kJ/day for women and 5,020 to 6,700 kJ/day for men. Fewer than 5,020 kJ each day may lead to loss of lean tissue and nutritional deficiencies. 'Yo-yo' dieting (repeated cycles of weight loss and gain) may lead to a metabolic deficiency that makes subsequent weight loss efforts increasingly difficult. Therefore, it is critical that a person take any weight loss effort seriously and include plans for long-term maintenance. The best approach is to modify dietary intake without severe restrictions, eating a well-balanced diet and developing improved eating habits.

Very-low-kilojoule diets (VLKDs), otherwise known as very-low-energy diets (VLEDs), are generally reserved for people who have a BMI greater than 30 (Asher, Burrows & Collins, 2013). Between 1,674 and 3,349 kJ/day is consumed. This type of weight loss regimen must be undertaken for any length of time under close medical supervision. Exercise, nutrition and behaviour modification counselling should accompany the diet (Ortega-Arroyo, 2022). Adverse effects generally are minor, but could include fatigue, constipation, nausea and diarrhoea. Recently, the development of gallstones formation requiring cholecystectomy has been attributed to VLKDs (Gudzune et al., 2015).

BEHAVIOUR MODIFICATION People wishing to lose weight quickly readily accept dangerous regimens to achieve rapid weight loss. Behaviour modification is the critical component of a successful long-term weight loss management program. Strategies such as keeping food records of the type and amount of foods eaten, eliminating cues that precipitate eating such as television advertisements, and changing the type of food eaten and the speed of eating are often helpful.

Researchers have found that most overweight people are stimulated to eat by external and emotional cues, such as the proximity to food and the time of day. In contrast, hunger and satiety are the cues that regulate eating in adults of normal weight. Strategies to control food cues include keeping food out of view, controlling portion size, reducing or eliminating the habit of consuming snack foods, and eating only in designated areas. See Box 21.2 for a list of behavioural modification strategies.

Other behaviour modification approaches focus on helping a person examine factors that affect their eating behaviours (Robinson et al., 2022). The goal is to empower the person who is stimulated to eat to choose non-food-related activities. Weight loss services such as Weight Watchers, SureSlim and Lite n' Easy promote weight loss success through coaching and peer support. Most organised programs require participants to pay a fee, which may improve compliance.

SURGERY Surgical treatment of obesity, otherwise known as *bariatric surgery* or *metabolic surgery*, is limited to morbidly obese people (BMI of over 40 kg/m^2 or 200% ideal body weight) who have a documented failure of non-surgical weight loss or those with a BMI over 35 kg/m^2 who have serious obesity-related health problems such as metabolic syndrome, type 2 diabetes mellitus, hypertension or heart disease (Atieno Odhiambo, 2021). In addition, a person must be able to tolerate surgery and be free of addiction to alcohol or other drugs such as nicotine. The benefits of surgery include major weight loss, improved blood pressure, improved blood lipid profile, a remission of type 2 diabetes mellitus and reduced risk of sleep apnoea, angina and heart failure (Atieno Odhiambo, 2021). However, bariatric surgery is not without risk, and some people regain some of the lost weight over time. Surgical problems, such as a stretched pouch or separated stitches, may also affect

BOX 21.2 Behavioural modification strategies for the obese person

Controlling the environment

- Encourage participation in reading and analysing food labels so as to purchase nutritious low-kilojoule foods.
- Shop from a prepared list and on a full stomach.
- Keep all foods in the kitchen.
- Store all foods in the refrigerator or the cabinets in opaque containers.
- Prepare exact portions of food to eliminate leftovers.
- Limit portion size of foods.
- Ensure two serves of fresh fruit and five serves of vegetables are eaten each day (Department of Health, 2013).
- Eat all foods in the same place; avoid eating in the kitchen or in the car.
- Avoid eating when watching television or reading.
- Reduce frequency of eating out at fast-food restaurants.

Controlling physiological responses to food

- Have set times for meals; avoid grazing behaviour.
- Eat slowly by taking small bites, allowing 20 minutes for a meal.
- Eat a salad or drink a hot beverage before a meal.
- Put eating utensils or food down between bites.
- Concentrate on the eating process; savour the food.
- Stop eating with the first feelings of fullness.

Controlling psychological responses to food

- Appreciate the aesthetic experience of eating.
- Use attractive dinnerware and prepare a formal setting for eating.
- Use small plates and cups to make servings of food look larger.
- Concentrate on conversations and socialisation during the meal.
- Use non-food rewards for meeting a goal.
- Acknowledge small successes and improvements in all behaviour.
- Substitute other activities for eating (e.g. reading, exercise, hobbies).

the amount of weight loss. Although bariatric surgery procedures have been listed on the Australian Medicare Benefits Schedule (MBS) since 1992. Approximately 89% of bariatric surgical procedures are performed in private hospitals with significant out-of-hospital expenses, thereby exacerbating existing Australian health inequalities in obesity due to the socioeconomic gradient (AIHW, 2017).

Bariatric surgery takes two forms: malabsorptive and restrictive. The three most common procedures in Australia are all performed laparoscopically: adjustable gastric banding, sleeve gastrectomy and Roux-en-Y gastric bypass (AIHW, 2017). In restrictive banding procedures such as adjustable gastric banding (AGB) (see Figure 21.1), a hollow band of silicone rubber is placed around the upper (proximal) portion of the stomach. The band is inflated with saline solution to create a small stomach pouch with a narrow passage through to the rest of the stomach, which restricts the amount of food that can be consumed. The amount of band inflation can be adjusted

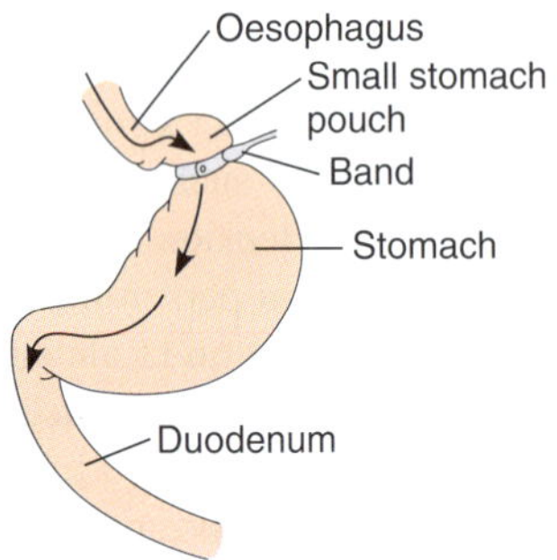

FIGURE 21.1 *Adjustable gastric banding*

using a port implanted under the skin. Sleeve gastrectomy is performed by resecting the stomach to the size of a tubular sleeve in the lesser curvature of the stomach (Rosenthal et al., 2012). The Roux-en-Y gastric bypass involves the stomach being made smaller, with the duodenum being bypassed to reduce absorptive capacity. This procedure was found to achieve a greater total weight loss and for up to 5 years (Thaher et al., 2022).

Few nutritional deficiencies are associated with restrictive bariatric procedures. Postprandial vomiting is a common postoperative complication (Lim et al., 2018). The band may slip or break, necessitating a return to surgery.

Although the risk of postoperative complications is high, the mortality rate for bariatric procedures is low; possible postoperative complications include anastomosis leak with peritonitis, haemorrhage, abdominal wall hernia, gallstones, wound infections, deep venous thrombosis, nutritional deficiencies and gastrointestinal symptoms (Lim et al., 2018). In dumping syndrome, stomach contents move rapidly through the small intestine, drawing fluid into the intestine by osmosis. The person experiences nausea, bloating, abdominal pain, weakness, sweating and possibly syncope. See the chapter 'Nursing care of people with upper gastrointestinal disorders' for more information about dumping syndrome.

Nursing care for the person who has undergone bariatric surgery is substantially the same as for a person who has undergone a gastric resection. See the chapter 'Nursing care of people with upper gastrointestinal disorders' for more information about gastric resection and associated nursing care. People undergoing bariatric surgery have some additional nursing care needs related to the effects of the surgery on gastrointestinal function (see the 'Meeting individualised needs' box).

MEETING INDIVIDUALISED NEEDS **Recommended diet following bariatric surgery**

A person undergoing bariatric surgery to restrict stomach capacity and/or nutrient absorption has unique learning needs to prevent discomfort and nutritional complications after surgery:

- Ensure slow, progressive transitions in food texture from liquids to solid foods over the first 8 postoperative weeks. A restricted liquid diet is prescribed in the first 2 weeks of the postoperative period. Fruit juices and other concentrated sugars are avoided. *The person is at risk of developing dumping syndrome in the early postoperative period; simple carbohydrates increase the risk.*
- When clear liquids are tolerated, non-fat or low-fat milk is added to the diet. *Milk provides a protein source. Lactose-free or soy milk is recommended to reduce the risk of diarrhoea. People with a lactase deficiency may not be able to digest the natural lactose sugar in milk.*
- Pureed foods are introduced into the diet in approximately 1–2 weeks and the diet is advanced to include soft foods within about 2 months after surgery. *Gradual increases in food textures preserve the staple line and allow the restricted stomach to adapt.*
- Increasing fluid intake and maintaining protein intake are priorities during the healing process. *Fluid intake is necessary to maintain fluid balance and protein for nitrogen balance and tissue healing.*
- Instruct the person to eat regularly, consume smaller portions, cut food into small pieces, chew food well and eat slowly. *Failure to thoroughly chew food and eat slowly can lead to regurgitation, vomiting and abdominal discomfort.*
- Advise the person to take an adult multiple vitamin and mineral supplement after restrictive surgery. *Because the overall quantity of food consumed is reduced, the person may develop a micronutrient deficiency.*
- Advise the person to avoid sugar and concentrated sweets (fruit juice, sugar-containing beverages, honey) and to separate consumption of solid foods and liquids by at least 30 minutes. *Concentrated sugars can precipitate dumping syndrome.*

Source: Adapted from Sherf Dagan et al. (2017). Nutritional recommendations for adult bariatric surgery patients: Clinical practice. *Advances in Nutrition*, *8*(2), 382–394.

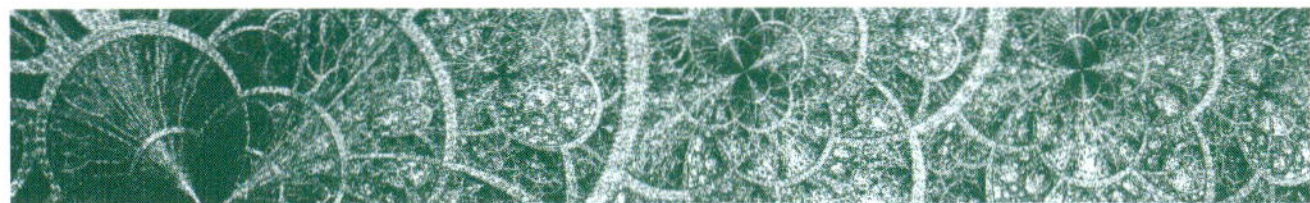

Nursing care

Health promotion

Maintaining a healthy weight throughout the lifespan begins in childhood. Obese children and teenagers become obese adults. Promote healthy eating with education to reduce consumption of highly processed high-sugar, high-fat, high-salt foods and increase the exposure to low-processed nutrient-rich foods such as high-fibre whole grains, lean protein-rich meats, fresh fruits and a variety of vegetables (National Health and Medical Research Council, 2013b). The Health at Every Size (HAES) movement shifts the focus from weight loss to increasing health-promoting behaviours (Bacon & Aphramor, 2011). This healthy eating approach to health and thus weight loss has been supported by the Dietary Approaches to Stop Hypertension (DASH) diet, which has been repeatedly demonstrated to protect against cardiovascular disease, stroke and heart failure (Anginga, 2021). The *Australian Guide to Healthy Eating* provides visual guidance for appropriate food choices to maintain a healthy, well-balanced diet.

Adults commonly gain about 10 kg between early and middle adulthood. Encourage the person to reduce the number of kilojoules consumed as energy needs change.

Assessment

Collect the following data through the health history and physical examination (see the chapter 'A person-centred approach to assessing the gastrointestinal system'):

- *Health history*: risk factors; current and usual weight; recent weight gains or losses; perception of weight and effect on health; usual diet and food intake; exercise/activity patterns; prior weight loss efforts and results; current medications; coexisting disorders such as cardiovascular disease and type 2 diabetes mellitus; tobacco use; family history of overweight and weight-related morbidity.
- *Physical examination*: vital signs; weight and height; anthropometric skinfold measurements; waist circumference; waist-to-hip ratio; BMI; inspect skin under the breasts and abdominal folds.

Nursing diagnoses and interventions

Nursing care for overweight and obese people is community based and holistic, focusing on both physiological and psychological responses to weight and appearance. See the accompanying nursing care plan for the person with obesity.

CONSIDERATION FOR PRACTICE

Use of an inappropriate-sized sphygmomanometer is a common source of error in measuring blood pressure in obese people, resulting in a falsely high blood pressure. Choose a cuff on which the width of the bladder is 40% of the circumference of the arm and the length of the bladder is sufficient to cover at least 65% of the upper arm.

Activity intolerance

People who are obese may experience excess fatigue, tachycardia and shortness of breath with activity due to the physiological effects of excess weight and a sedentary lifestyle. A medical evaluation may be needed before beginning an exercise program.

- Assess current activity level and tolerance to that activity. Assess vital signs. *This provides baseline information to plan an activity program and assess response to that activity.*
- After medical clearance, plan with the person a program of regular, gradually increasing exercise. Consider a consultation with an exercise physiologist. *An individualised exercise program promotes activities within that person's physical capabilities.*

Imbalanced nutrition: more than body requirements

Although many factors contribute to obesity, it always involves an imbalance of kilojoule consumption to energy expenditure.

- Encourage the person to identify the factors that contribute to excess food intake. *Identification of cues to eating helps the person eliminate or reduce these cues.*
- Establish realistic weight loss goals and exercise/activity objectives. *Small, reasonable goals, such as loss of 0.5 kg per week, increase the likelihood of success.*
- Encourage participation in reading and analysing food labels on processed and packaged foods. *Increased decision making encourages healthier food choices.*
- Assess knowledge and discuss well-balanced diet plans. Provide necessary teaching about the recommended inclusion of two fruit and five vegetable serves in the diet. *Knowledge empowers the person to participate and make appropriate food choices.*
- Discuss behaviour modification strategies, such as self-monitoring and environmental management. *Behaviour modification, diet and exercise are critical to promoting successful, long-term weight loss.*
- Monitor weight loss and blood pressure weekly with annual laboratory data, including blood glucose and lipid levels. *Continuing assessment is important not only to evaluate the safety of weight loss strategies, but also to reinforce positive benefits of weight loss.*

Ineffective therapeutic regimen management

Most people who are overweight or obese experience some difficulty integrating all the components of a weight loss program into their daily routine. For a weight loss and maintenance program to be successful, the person must modify dietary intake in a world of daily temptations. There may be many obstacles to exercise, including a busy schedule, activity intolerance, impaired physical mobility, lack of equipment and the embarrassment of being overweight.

- Discuss ability and willingness to incorporate changes into daily patterns of diet, exercise and lifestyle. *This provides data from which to set realistic goals with the person.*
- Beginning with gentle non-weight-bearing exercise such as swimming may encourage participation. Increase activity levels based on physical ability. *Exercise success increases likelihood of continuation.*
- Establish strategies for dealing with 'stress' eating or interruptions in the therapeutic regimen. *A sense of failure associated with overeating or lack of exercise can lead to further overeating. Identifying positive strategies to deal with these situations promotes self-acceptance and limits self-punishment through overeating.*

Chronic low self-esteem

Although many people who are obese may have accepted their weight and body appearance on some level, most people who are overweight or obese verbalise that they experience 'fat prejudice' or stigma in their family, workplace or community. People who are obese may experience ridicule, prejudice and health problems attributed to being 'fat'. These experiences, coupled with day-to-day problems such as finding attractive clothing or a chair large enough to sit on can affect self-esteem. Many report that 'fat' jokes or comments contribute to a sense of negative self-worth.

- Encourage the person to verbalise the experience of being overweight and validate their experiences. *This provides baseline data to use in developing individualised interventions to address self-esteem issues.*
- Set small goals with the person and offer positive feedback and encouragement. Small goals provide more opportunities for success. *Positive feedback and encouragement provide a comfortable environment in which to develop self-esteem.*
- Refer for counselling as appropriate. *Many people benefit from counselling for issues related to reduced self-esteem.*

Community-based care

Weight reduction usually occurs in community-based settings. Weight loss and maintenance require a long-term commitment by the person, their family and supportive environmental systems that encourage healthy choices and lifestyles. Address the following topics with the person and their family:

- Small, subtle lifestyle modifications are more effective than dramatic diets. Fad diets promote rapid weight loss but often are not nutritionally sound or may be difficult to maintain for a lifetime (Robinson et al., 2022).
- All household members should also consume a diet that is nutritionally sound. Encourage participation in analysing nutrient food labels prior to purchasing processed or packaged foods.
- Set realistic goals to increase levels of incidental exercise.
- Establish realistic weight loss goals and a system of non-food rewards for achieving each goal.
- Identify an 'exercise buddy' or support system to promote continued physical activity.
- Expect occasional failures. Resume prescribed diet and exercise routine as soon as possible; the goal is long-term weight management.
- Community resources such as Weight Watchers or healthcare-based programs provide information, strategies and social support for successful weight management.

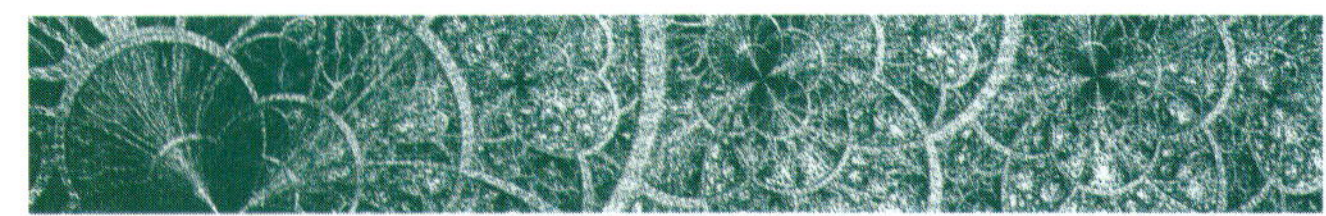

NURSING CARE PLAN A person with obesity

Sam Elliott, aged 57, has gained 20 kg since his retirement 2 years ago. The most active thing he does each day is 'pottering around the garden'. His diet includes apple juice, oatmeal porridge, 2 slices of white toast with strawberry jam and white coffee with 2 sugars for breakfast; 2 donuts or a blueberry muffin and coffee with friends mid-morning; a ham-and-cheese sandwich with a bag of potato chips and a soft drink for lunch; and cheese, biscuits and wine before a dinner of meat, potatoes, vegetables and dessert. He tells the nurse, 'I have never had to diet. I just don't know how to get this weight off.'

ASSESSMENT

Mr Elliott is 173 cm tall and weighs 91.2 kg. His BMI is 30.1 kg/m^2. His cholesterol is 6.14 mmol/L (normal $<$ 5.13 mmol/L) with an HDL of 1.00 mmol/L (normal 1.5 mmol/L) and an LDL of 4.85 mmol/L (normal $<$ 3.31 mmol/L). His BP is 138/90 mmHg. His fasting blood glucose is normal at 5.0 mmol/L. His ECG shows normal sinus rhythm. He reports fatigue and shortness of breath with activity. His healthcare provider has advised a weight loss of 13 kg and a regular exercise program.

DIAGNOSES

- *Imbalanced nutrition* related to food intake in excess of nutritional energy requirements.
- *Risk of ineffective therapeutic regimen* related to knowledge deficit.
- *Activity intolerance* related to sedentary lifestyle evidenced by fatigue when attempting gentle exercise.

PLANNING

- Enter into an agreement with Mr Elliott to meet once each week to assess progress.

Expected outcomes

- Lose 0.5 kg each week.
- Increase levels of moderate exercise up to walking 30 minutes for 5 days each week.
- Verbalise an understanding of the relationship between weight loss, weight control and exercise.
- Identify support systems for behaviour modification.
- Increase knowledge level of healthier food choices.

IMPLEMENTATION

- Assess weight and blood pressure each week.
- Discuss current eating habits and strategies to reduce fat and kilojoule intake.
- Discuss cues such as boredom that promote eating. Identify strategies to eliminate or reduce eating cues.
- Teach to keep a food diary to examine and change eating habits.
- Discuss the role of regular exercise in weight loss and weight control. Instruct to maintain an exercise record to track the intensity and duration of activity.
- Discuss lifestyle and behaviour modification strategies to promote successful weight loss and control.

EVALUATION

Two weeks after changing his diet and beginning to exercise, Mr Elliott has lost 1 kg. He has maintained a food diary. He has identified boredom as a cue to eating. In light of that fact, he has started volunteering at the local hospital. He is walking for 30 minutes, 5 days a week. He plans to increase his activity periods to 45 minutes. He verbalises commitment to a lifelong plan of exercising and eating a high-fibre, low-fat diet. His BP has ranged from 132/76 to 136/84 mmHg. He plans to have the employee health nurse at the hospital check his weight and BP each week and to join Weight Watchers for ongoing support.

CRITICAL THINKING IN THE NURSING PROCESS

1. What are some possible pathophysiological bases for Mr Elliott's abnormal cholesterol, HDL and LDL levels?
2. Develop a teaching plan for a group of overweight men and women.
3. Identify potential barriers to losing weight and strategies to reduce or eliminate these barriers.

REFLECTION ON THE NURSING PROCESS

1. How achievable is a non-surgical weight loss intervention program over the long term?
2. What other nursing interventions would you consider utilising if Mr Elliott's weight loss does not meet the expected outcome?

THE PERSON WITH MALNUTRITION

Malnutrition results from an inadequate intake of nutrients and can be defined as the state of being poorly nourished due to an imbalance in nutrition (Tuso & Beattie, 2015). There may be a lack of macronutrients (kilojoules, carbohydrates, proteins and fats) or micronutrients such as vitamins and/or minerals. Malnutrition is associated with a high burden of illness, depression of the immune system, poor wound healing, bone and muscle weakness, longer lengths of hospital stay with higher treatment costs and increased morbidity and mortality (Scholes & Judd, 2022). Malnutrition may be caused by inadequate nutrient intake; impaired absorption and use of nutrients; or loss of nutrients due to diarrhoea, haemorrhage, renal failure or increased metabolic needs due to an underlying illness (e.g. infection or physiological stressors such as cancer).

Protein energy malnutrition (PEM) is the state of decreased body pools of protein with or without fat depletion or a state of diminished functional capacity, caused at least partly by inadequate nutrient intake relative to nutrient demand, and/or which is improved by nutritional repletion (Scholes & Judd, 2022).

Incidence and prevalence

PEM is a widespread cause of disease and mortality throughout the world. It affects many children and is most common in developing nations (Ashi, 2022). Groups at risk of malnutrition in Australia include children of Aboriginal and Torres Strait Islander heritage, culturally and linguistically diverse people, families with low socioeconomic status, older adults, the homeless and people undergoing complex medical treatments such as chemotherapy or dialysis. Even when food is plentiful, a person may be undernourished due to poor food choices. Food insecurity in Australia is a risk factor for malnutrition due to limited access, either financially or geographically, to healthy nutritious food. Malnutrition is associated with the anorexia of ageing due to decreased appetite or increased food insecurity (Scholes & Judd, 2022). Malnutrition may be present on admission to hospital or may develop as a result of surgery or serious illness. Malnutrition increases both mortality and the incidence of complications in both medical and surgical situations.

See Box 21.3 for conditions commonly associated with malnutrition.

Risk factors

Risk factors for malnutrition include the following:

- age—older adults are at greater risk of malnutrition due to a variety of factors (see the 'Meeting individualised needs' box)
- poverty, homelessness, inadequate food storage and preparation facilities
- functional health problems that limit mobility or vision
- history of rapid weight loss of more than 10% of usual weight over the past 6 months
- oral or gastrointestinal problems that affect food intake, digestion and absorption
- chronic pain or chronic diseases such as pulmonary, cardiovascular, renal and endocrine disorders, or cancer
- dementia, mental health disorders such as depression
- medications or treatments that affect appetite
- alcohol or drug addiction
- acute problems such as infection, surgery or trauma
- dieting behaviours such as anorexia nervosa or bulimia
- inability to obtain food such as would occur in famine or disaster.

BOX 21.3 Conditions associated with malnutrition

- Acute respiratory failure
- Ageing
- AIDS
- Alcoholism
- Burns
- COPD
- Dementia
- Eating disorders
- Ear disease in Aboriginal and Torres Strait Islander children
- Gastrointestinal disorders
- Neurological disorders
- Renal disease
- Short bowel syndrome
- Surgery
- Trauma

Pathophysiology

Carbohydrates and fats in the diet are the body's primary energy sources. Approximately 15–25% of the body is fat, the body's energy reservoir. Fat-free mass includes muscles, bones, skin and organs, which are metabolically active tissues. Proteins in the diet primarily are used to maintain these tissues. Glycogen and proteins in this lean body mass also act as energy stores.

When dietary intake of nutrients does not meet the body's energy needs, the body uses glycogen, body proteins and lipids (fats) to support metabolism. Neurones in the brain depend completely on a constant source of glucose for normal function; importantly, glucose is unable to be stored within the brain and needs to be delivered via the bloodstream.

In **starvation** (inadequate dietary intake), glycogen initially is used to provide energy. After the first 24 hours of starvation, gluconeogenesis (formation of new glucose from proteins) is the major source of energy. As starvation continues, the body breaks down fats into free fatty acids and ketones, which provide glucose for the brain. The size of all body compartments is reduced as body fats and muscle proteins are used to meet this glucose demand. As lean body mass is reduced, metabolically active tissue is lost and energy expenditure decreases.

The stress of acute illness or trauma produces a different response. The acute stress response produces a state of hypermetabolism and **catabolism** (cell and muscle breakdown). This hypermetabolic state increases energy expenditure and nutrient needs. If untreated, up to half of the body's protein stores can be used up within 3 weeks.

Many hospitalised people are malnourished (starved) on admission. Surgery or illness promotes a stress response, resulting in protein energy malnutrition. In PEM, both protein and kilojoules are deficient. The intake of adequate kilojoules but with a chronic reduction in protein intake is called *kwashiorkor*. When both proteins and kilojoules are insufficient to meet the body's needs, PEM is also known as *marasmus*.

Manifestations

Weight loss is the most apparent manifestation of malnutrition. The malnourished person may have a body weight of less than 90% of ideal. Body mass also is reduced (see Box 21.1), as is anthropometric skinfold thickness. Other manifestations include a wasted appearance, dry and brittle hair, and pale mucous membranes. Abdominal or bipedal peripheral oedema may be present. Older adults may present with general symptoms of frailty, falls, weakness, slow walking speed, reduced physical activity capacity, pressure ulcers, unintentional weight loss and exhaustion (Marin & Ndegwa, 2021). Manifestations of specific nutrient deficiencies may be present (see the 'Manifestations' box). See also 'Multisystem effects of malnutrition'.

MEETING INDIVIDUALISED NEEDS Nutrition for the older adult

Older adults are at greater risk of malnutrition. Body fat mass increases up to about 75 years of age, then begins to decrease. Age-related changes that contribute to malnutrition include a loss of appetite due to changes in taste and smell, a higher incidence of gastrointestinal disease such as dysphagia or delayed gastric emptying, poor oral health, loss of teeth or ill-fitting dentures, anorexia caused by medications and functional limitations that contribute to food insecurity by impairing the ability to shop and cook. Psychosocial issues such as depression or dementia also contribute to the problem. Older adults living on fixed incomes may not be able to afford to purchase food. Lifestyle factors such as social isolation and loneliness contribute to the issue (Scholes & Judd, 2022). Eating is a social event and older adults who eat alone may not eat as well as those who share meals with companions.

Conduct a thorough assessment to determine nutritional status. Assess psychological factors that influence eating habits, such as loneliness, isolation and depression. Note the person's general appearance and obtain a diet history, including information about foods and nutrients the person consumes and any recent weight losses or gain. Review laboratory values, including complete blood count, total protein, albumin and prealbumin.

HEALTH EDUCATION FOR THE PERSON AND FAMILY

To maintain nutritional status, the older person should be advised to:

- Eat a well-balanced diet.
- Keep a food diary.
- Eat two serves of fresh fruit and five serves of vegetables each day.
- Consume soft foods if chewing difficulties are present.
- Increase consumption of micronutrient-dense dairy products if tolerated.
- Shop wisely to get the most value for money.
- Avoid high-fat, high-salt processed foods.
- Drink adequate fluids.
- Take regular gentle exercise to maintain muscle tone.
- Take body weight each week and contact local doctor if weight has further decreased.
- Contact local organisations for the availability of congregate meals (e.g. at local senior centres) or home-delivered meals (e.g. Meals on Wheels).

MANIFESTATIONS Specific nutrient deficiencies

DEFICIENCY	ASSESSMENT DATA	DEFICIENCY	ASSESSMENT DATA
Kilojoules	Weight loss	Dry beriberi	Polyneuritis, convulsions, confusion, apathy, muscle weakness, ataxia, nystagmus, sleeplessness, anxiety
Protein (marasmus*)	Weakness, listlessness Loss of subcutaneous fat Muscle wasting	Riboflavin (vitamin B_2)	Cheilosis (crusting and ulceration at the corner of the mouth), stomatitis Neuropathy, glossitis Normocytic anaemia
Protein (kwashiorkor†)	Thin or sparse hair Flaking skin Loss of cardiac muscle Hepatomegaly Peripheral oedema	Vitamin C (scurvy)	Swollen, bleeding gums Delayed wound healing Weakness, depression Easy bruising
Vitamin A	Night blindness Altered taste and smell Dry, scaling, rough skin Impaired immune function	Iron	Smooth tongue Listlessness, fatigue Dyspnoea Anaemia
Thiamine (vitamin B_1‡) Wet beriberi	Confusion, apathy Cardiomegaly, dyspnoea Muscle cramping and wasting Paraesthesias, neuropathy Ataxia		

* Marasmus is a physiological adaptation to severe protein energy malnutrition (PEM) which involves the gradual breakdown of fat and muscle to provide energy and amino acids for protein synthesis, essential for continued homeostasis (Bender, 2014).

† Kwashiorkor is a similar response to severe protein energy malnutrition (PEM) but is associated with more complex and pathological changes due to the inefficient mobilisation and utilisation of adipose tissues together with impaired muscle breakdown processes (Bender, 2014).

‡ Thiamine, vitamin B_1, is a water-soluble vitamin that is absorbed primarily in the jejunum. The thiamine deficiency disease known as beriberi can have neurological or cardiac manifestations. Beriberi may be seen in developed nations where the diet contains excessive carbohydrates as thiamine is a requirement of carbohydrate metabolism. Bariatric beriberi occurs from the rearrangement of the absorptive areas of the intestinal tract resulting in a decreased surface area of the jejunum (Frank, 2011). Diuretics may also contribute to beriberi due to the losses through the urinary system (Misumida, Hisashi Umeda & Iwase, 2014).

Multisystem effects of malnutrition

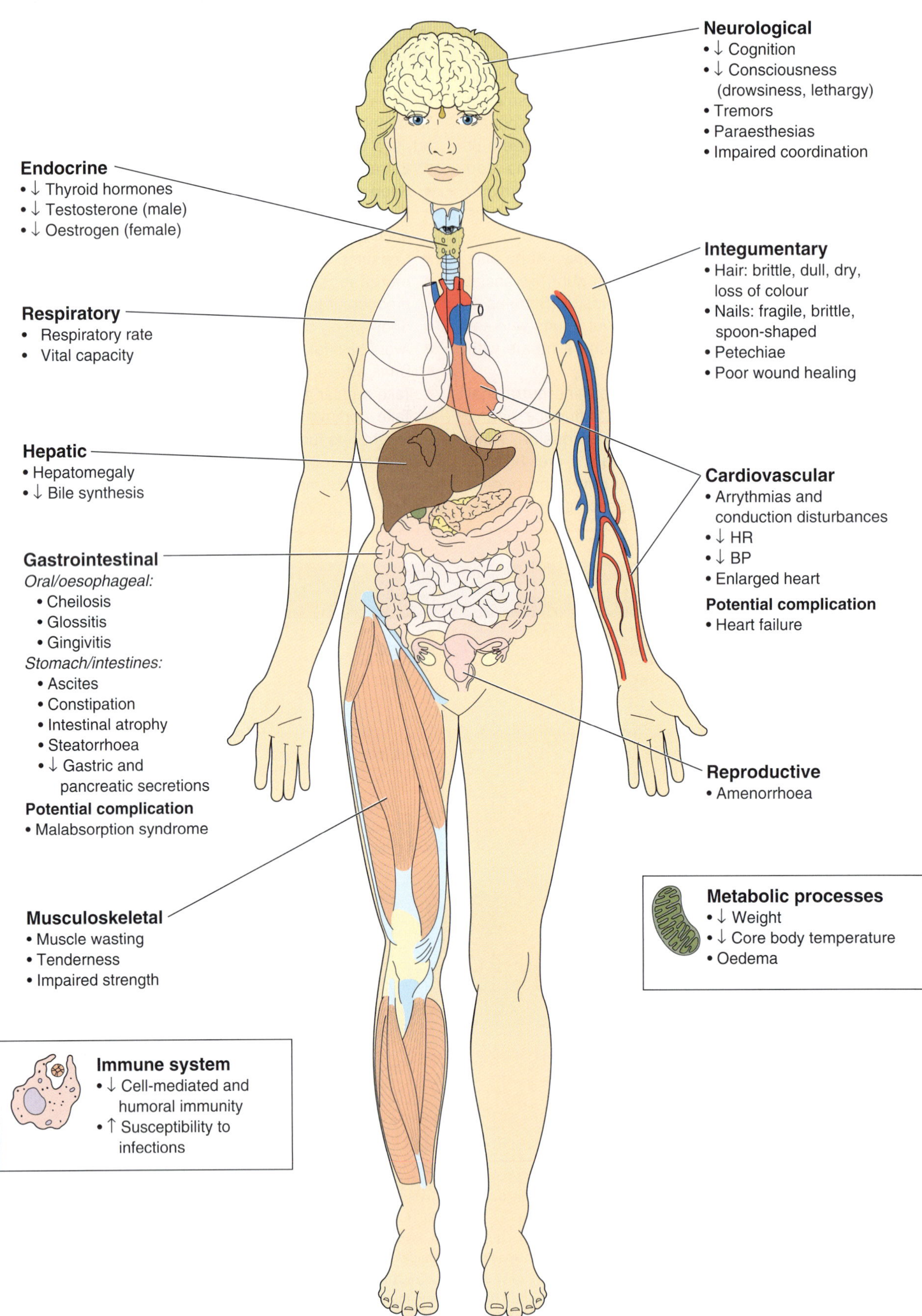

Subcutaneous fat and muscle proteins are broken down in PEM, impairing mobility and increasing the risk of skin and tissue breakdown (pressure ulcers). A lack of physical activity results in further muscle loss known as sarcopenia. Protein synthesis is inhibited in PEM and wound healing is delayed. Serum albumin levels fall, leading to abdominal oedema, diarrhoea and impaired nutrient absorption. Cachexia is characterised by severe muscle loss with increased protein catabolism due to an underlying disease such as chronic kidney disease or cancer (Barker, Gout & Crowe, 2011). Immune function is impaired in cachexia with an increased risk of infection. Cardiac output falls and the risk of postural hypotension increases.

INTERPROFESSIONAL CARE

The goal of treatment for the malnourished person is to restore ideal body weight while replacing and restoring depleted nutrients and minerals. The person's age, severity of malnutrition and coexisting health problems help determine interventions. Treatment may include oral supplementation, tube feedings or parenteral nutrition.

Diagnosis

Nutrition screening tools such as those discussed in Box 21.4 can help identify a person at risk of malnutrition. Their use has been suggested as best practice guidelines for all acute hospital settings by the Dietitians Association of Australia. Marin and Ndegwa (2021) identified a number of validated screening and assessment tools for malnutrition. These include the Malnutrition Screening Tool (MST), the Malnutrition Universal Screening Tool (MUST), the Mini Nutrition Assessment (MNA), the Nutritional Risk Screening (NRS-2002), the four-item Short Nutrition Assessment Questionnaire (SNAQ) and the Subjective Global Assessment (SGA). As with obesity, the standard measurements to assess for malnutrition include diet history, height, weight, calculation of BMI and anthropometric skinfold measurements. A BMI of less than 18–20 kg/m^2 may indicate malnutrition. Other assessments include questioning on any history of unintentional weight loss and the severity of any illnesses that have impacted on oral food intake. The following laboratory studies also may be ordered:

- *Serum albumin* is reduced in PEM and may be below 32 g/L.
- *Prealbumin* (also known as transthyretin) should be measured for any person at risk of malnutrition and anyone with a serum albumin of less than 30 g/L. Prealbumin, which has a short (2-day) half-life, is a better measure of nutritional status than albumin because it is sensitive to acute changes in nutritional status despite the presence of multiple-organ disease (Smith, 2017). See Table 21.5 for normal prealbumin levels and the implications of reduced prealbumin levels.
- *Transferrin* is a protein that transports iron. It decreases in the presence of protein energy malnutrition.

TABLE 21.5 Normal and high-risk prealbumin levels

PREALBUMIN LEVEL	IMPLICATIONS	SUGGESTED INTERVENTIONS
150–360 mg/L	Within normal limits	None
100–150 mg/L	High risk of nutritional deficit	Monitor level biweekly
100–50 mg/L ≤ 50 mg/L	Significant risk of malnutrition Malnourished	Aggressive nutritional support (e.g. enteral feedings or parenteral nutrition)

BOX 21.4 Nutrition screening tools

NUTRITION SCREENING TOOL	SUMMARY/USES	LIMITATIONS
Malnutrition Screening Tool (MST)	• Easy three-question tool which can be used by non-trained staff • Assesses recent weight and appetite losses • Useful in medical, surgical and oncology environments	• Further nutritional assessment is needed for those identified at severe risk of malnutrition
Mini Nutrition Assessment (MNA)	• Used in aged care environments • Has an abbreviated two-step questionnaire which identifies those at risk of malnutrition who then can be referred to the complete 18-step MNA	• Limited scope – developed for use in aged care
Nutritional Risk Screening (NRS-2002)	• Uses BMI, recent weight and appetite losses together with a subjective analysis of disease • Recommended by the European Society for Clinical Nutrition and Metabolism (ESPEN) for hospital use • Is useful in prompting the initiation of nutritional support	• Subjectivity of the tool • Does not allow for definitive diagnosis
The four-item Short Nutrition Assessment Questionnaire (SNAQ)	• Quick and easy screening tool • Developed to diagnose malnutrition in hospitalised people • Does not require calculation of BMI	• Further nutritional assessment is needed for those identified at severe risk of malnutrition

Source: Based on Barker et al. (2011). Hospital malnutrition: Prevalence, identification and impact on patients and the healthcare system. *International Journal of Environmental Research and Public Health*, 8, 514–527.

- The *total lymphocyte count* is evaluated by multiplying the WBC by the percentage of lymphocytes. The total lymphocyte count is reduced in PEM.
- *Serum electrolytes* are measured. Potassium levels are low in severe malnutrition.

Medications

Malafarina et al. (2012) found vitamin D demonstrated increased strength and was associated with fewer falls. Malnourished people generally require supplemental vitamins and minerals to restore essential micronutrients (Travers, 2021). A multivitamin and mineral supplement may be given or therapy may be tailored to correct specific deficiencies. See the 'Medication administration' box for nursing implications of vitamin and mineral supplements.

Nutrition

Fluids and nutrients should be carefully reintroduced in severely malnourished people to prevent life-threatening refeeding syndrome (Redgrave et al., 2015). First, fluid and electrolyte imbalances are corrected, with particular attention paid to restoring normal potassium, phosphate, magnesium and calcium levels, as well as acid–base balance. Once fluid and electrolyte imbalances are corrected, oral protein and kilojoules are gradually reintroduced. Initial feedings are in limited amounts (100 mL) of liquid formula to prevent diarrhoea. Vitamin and mineral supplements at about twice the Nutrient Reference Values (NRVs) are provided along with refeeding. Lactose intolerance may develop in severely malnourished people; lactose-free dairy products or yoghurt may be tolerated better.

MEDICATION ADMINISTRATION Vitamin and mineral supplements

FAT-SOLUBLE VITAMINS

Vitamin A
Vitamin D
Vitamin E
Vitamin K

The fat-soluble vitamins are absorbed in the gastrointestinal tract. Vitamins A and D are stored in the liver. Fat-soluble vitamins A, D, E and K should be taken with food.

All fat-soluble vitamins may become toxic if taken in excess amounts.

Nursing responsibilities

- Monitor for manifestations of vitamin excess as well as for adverse effects from vitamin administration.
- Monitor carefully for hypersensitivity reactions during parenteral administration. Have emergency equipment available.

Health education for the person and family

- Teach the importance of eating a well-balanced diet. If indicated, provide lists of foods high in specific vitamins.
- Caution that excessive intake of these vitamins may lead to vitamin toxicity.

WATER-SOLUBLE VITAMINS

Vitamin C (ascorbic acid)
Vitamin B complex:
Thiamine (B_1)
Riboflavin (B_2)
Niacin (nicotinic acid)
Pyridoxine hydrochloride (B_6)
Pantothenic acid
Biotin

If the diet is deficient in one vitamin, it is usually deficient in other vitamins as well; therefore, multivitamin preparations are often administered. Most of these water-soluble vitamins are well absorbed from the gastrointestinal tract.

Nursing responsibilities

- Monitor for responses to replacement therapy.
- Monitor for hypersensitivity reactions from parenteral administration. Have emergency equipment available.

Health education for the person and family

- Do not exceed the recommended daily allowances for the specific vitamin.

MINERALS

Copper
Manganese
Phosphorus
Chromium
Iodine
Iron
Selenium
Calcium
Zinc

Minerals are inorganic chemicals that are vital to a variety of physiological functions. Also called trace elements, these minerals are part of a balanced diet. Recommended daily intakes have not been established for all mineral substances. The dosage of prescribed minerals depends on the specific deficiency, route of administration and the person's general health.

Nursing responsibilities

- Monitor for manifestations of mineral imbalance.
- Prior to administration, dilute oral mineral preparations. Administer minerals with fruit juice to increase absorption.
- Prior to the administration of iodine, assess for history of hypersensitivity to iodine or seafood; if hypersensitive, notify the doctor.

Health education for the person and family

- Encourage the person to avoid exceeding the known recommended daily intake of the mineral.
- Instruct the person to take minerals on an empty stomach, which will increase their ability to be fully absorbed. Zinc can be taken with or after meals.

Gradual refeeding is necessary to prevent electrolyte imbalances from developing as potassium, magnesium, phosphorus and glucose move into the cells. Heart failure may occur due to depressed cardiac function (Abed et al., 2014). Abnormalities in gastrointestinal function can lead to malabsorption and diarrhoea with refeeding. Food intake is gradually increased in increments of 1,000 kJ twice a week until the person is able to consume about 10,000 kJ per day and is gaining 1.5–2.0 kg weekly. Commercially available nutritional supplements (such as Carnation Instant Breakfast, Ensure and Sustacal) may supplement protein and kilojoule intake.

ENTERAL NUTRITION **Enteral nutrition**, or tube feeding, may be used to meet kilojoule and protein requirements in those unable to consume adequate food. The indication for tube feedings is when the lower gastrointestinal tract is still able to absorb nutrients, such as where there is difficulty swallowing, loss of gag reflex in victims of cerebrovascular accident, unresponsiveness, and oral or neck surgery (Lockwood & Queiroz, 2022). Enteral nutrition is also indicated in the presence of severe trauma where the lower gastrointestinal tract is unaffected, anorexia or serious illness such as Crohn's disease, or malignancy. Tube feedings may provide part or all of the person's nutritional needs. Enteral nutrition is the preferable method of feeding when oral intake is not possible, as this method provides nutrients directly to the stomach and other digestive organs, reduces the incidence of enteric pathogens, promotes blood flow to the gastrointestinal tract and supports other functions of the GI tract such as the release of hormones and epidermal growth factors (Preiser et al., 2015). There is a growing trend in Australia to offer enteral nutrition in the home for long-term serious illnesses (Ishaque, 2022).

Enteral tube feeding is the delivery of a liquid, nutritionally complete formula through a soft, small-calibre tube such as a nasogastric tube into the stomach, or a nasoduodenal or nasojejunal tube into the small intestine (see Figure 21.2). Large-bore gastric (Salem sump) tubes can be used for the dual purposes of gastric decompression and feeding. Fine-bore gastric tubes are more comfortable for the person and cause less trauma and tissue irritation. Jejunal tubes are associated with much better absorption of feeds and a lower risk of regurgitation and subsequent aspiration compared to gastric tubes. A transgastric–jejunal feeding tube allows for simultaneous jejunal feeding and gastric decompression. Feeds can also be administered through a gastrostomy or jejunostomy tube. Percutaneous endoscopic gastrostomy (PEG) tubes are becoming the method of choice for long-term enteral feeding regimens, palliative enteral nutrition for terminal malignancies of the upper gastrointestinal tract or for decompression of malignant obstructions (Lockwood & Queiroz, 2022).

Tube placement must be checked by x-ray prior to initiating any fluids or feeds to confirm that the end of the tube is correctly placed within the stomach and not in the lungs (Singh, 2021). Singh (2021) highlighted that there is insufficient evidence to support ultrasonography as a low-radiation alternative for determining correct placement. Periodical aspiration of the tube and checking the pH of aspirated contents is necessary to verify continued correct placement. A pH of < 4 indicates the presence of gastric acid and confirms placement in the stomach; pH > 6 indicates the tube is in the jejunum. See Box 21.5.

Most tube feeding formulas provide 4 kJ/mL with approximately 14% of the kilojoules from protein, 60% from carbohydrates and 25–30% from fat. Administering 1,500 mL per day provides the recommended daily intake of all vitamins and minerals. Formulas that provide more kilojoules per millilitre, more grams of protein, added fibre or lower fat are also available (see Table 21.6). Commercial products provide instructions

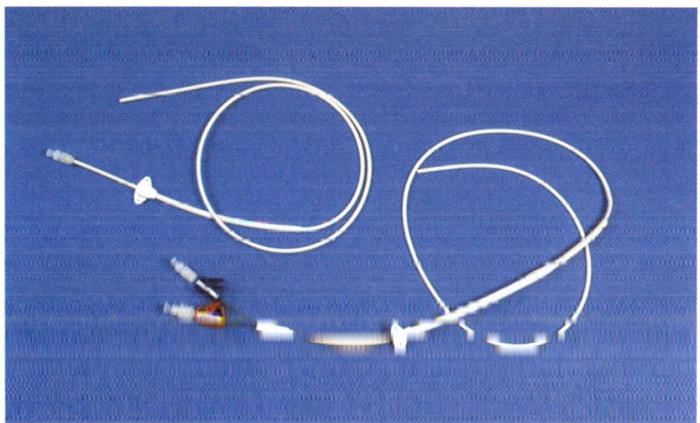

FIGURE 21.2 ***A nasoduodenal tube and a jejunostomy tube***

Source: Courtesy of Michal Heron.

BOX 21.5 Measures to verify feeding tube placement

After inserting the feeding tube and verifying appropriate placement through pH of the aspirate and an x-ray, mark the feeding tube position near the nose with an indelible marker. Prior to each feeding (or every 8 to 12 hours if continuous feedings are being administered), assess the person's abdomen and tube placement. Use the following steps to assess tube placement:

- Assess the abdomen for distension, bowel sounds and tenderness using the sequence of inspection, auscultation, percussion and palpation.
- Assess tube condition and placement by verifying that the indelible mark remains at the same position and that the feeding tube is securely fastened to the nose. Ask the person to open their mouth and inspect the position of the tube in the oropharynx. Do not administer a feeding if the person is having difficulty speaking or is coughing.
- Using a 60 mL syringe, inject 30 mL of air into the feeding tube, then aspirate a small amount of stomach contents and check the pH of the aspirate.

Reassess tube placement if the person vomits or retches, requires oropharyngeal suctioning, complains of discomfort or reflux into the mouth, or develops signs of respiratory distress (Lockwood & Queiroz, 2022).

TABLE 21.6 Selected enteral feeding formulas

FORMULA TYPE	CONTAINS	EXAMPLES
Complete–suitable for most people requiring enteral feedings	• 4 kJ/mL • Protein: ~ 14% total kJ • Fat: ~ 30% total kJ • Carbohydrate: ~ 60% total kJ • Recommended daily intake of all minerals and vitamins is 1,500 mL/day	Compleat, Ensure, Isocal, Nutren, Isolan Sustacal, Resource
High-kilojoule complete–appropriate for those on a fluid restriction	As above; provides 6-8 kJ/mL	Ensure Plus, Sustacal HC, Comply, Nutren 1.5, Resource Plus, Isocal HCN, Magnacal, TwoCal HN
Complete lactose-free, high-residue–used to prevent/treat diarrhoea, constipation	As above; provides fibre	Jevity, Profibre, Nutren 1.0 with fibre, Fibrelan, Sustacal with fibre, Ultracal, Ensure with fibre, Fibresource, Accupep HPF, Reabfin, others
Disease-specific formulas: Renal failure Respiratory failure Liver failure with hepatic encephalopathy	 Essential amino acids Fat: > 50% total kJ High amounts of branched-chain amino acids	 Amin-Aid, Travasorb Renal, Aminess Pulmocare, NutriVent Hepatic-Acid II, Travasorb Hepatic

for initiating therapy. Enteral feedings should be started with small volumes of water then small volumes of feed to prevent diarrhoea, with the volume gradually increased to provide the required kilojoules for maintenance and healing. Formulas may be administered as a bolus feeding or as a continuous drip feeding regulated by a kangaroo feeding pump (see Figure 21.3).

Aspiration pneumonia and diarrhoea are the most common complications of enteral feedings. Continuous infusion of the formula reduces the risk of aspiration. The risk also is reduced by placing the feeding tube in the jejunum rather than the stomach. Unless contraindicated (e.g. spinal injury), position the person at least 30 degrees during feeding and for at least 1 hour after feeding. Formulas containing fibre can reduce the incidence of diarrhoea. The person's fluid and electrolyte status is monitored carefully and additional water is regularly administered as needed to provide fluid replacement.

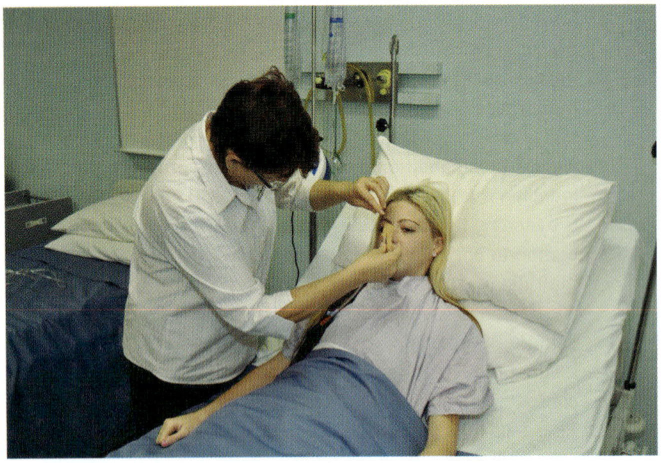

FIGURE 21.3 ***The nurse secures the feeding tube of a person receiving a continuous enteral feeding***

Source: Courtesy of Trudy Dwyer.

A 30 mL water flush administered 4-hourly will ensure tube patency.

PARENTERAL NUTRITION **Parenteral nutrition (PN)** is the intravenous administration of carbohydrates (high concentrations of dextrose), protein (amino acids), electrolytes, vitamins, minerals and fat emulsions. These hypertonic solutions usually are administered through a central vein, such as the subclavian or external jugular vein (see Figure 21.4). A peripherally inserted central catheter (PICC) line may be used for short-term total parenteral nutrition (TPN).

Parenteral nutrition is initiated when a person's nutritional requirements cannot be met through diet, enteral feedings or peripheral vein infusions. A person who has undergone major surgery or trauma where the lower intestinal tract is non-functioning or who is seriously undernourished is often a candidate for PN. PN is used for both short- and long-term management of nutritional deficiencies. Many people are discharged to home with PN and monitored by home health nurses.

To begin therapy, a medical officer inserts the central venous catheter under aseptic conditions. The location of the catheter tip is confirmed by x-ray. A triple-lumen catheter is most commonly used. This type of catheter permits concomitant administration of medications, intralipids or blood through other lumens. Parenteral nutrition solutions are either purchased commercially or mixed in the pharmacy using sterile technique under a laminar-flow airhood. A commonly used solution includes 500 mL of 50% dextrose, 500 mL of an 8.5% amino acid solution, electrolytes, minerals and vitamins. The sterility of the solution is maintained and no medication, other than intralipids, is added to the solution after it is mixed or to the lumen through which the PN is administered. Most hospitals have specific policies and procedures for hanging new containers and changing the tubing. Parenteral nutrition solutions are always administered with an infusion pump to ensure the correct rate of infusion.

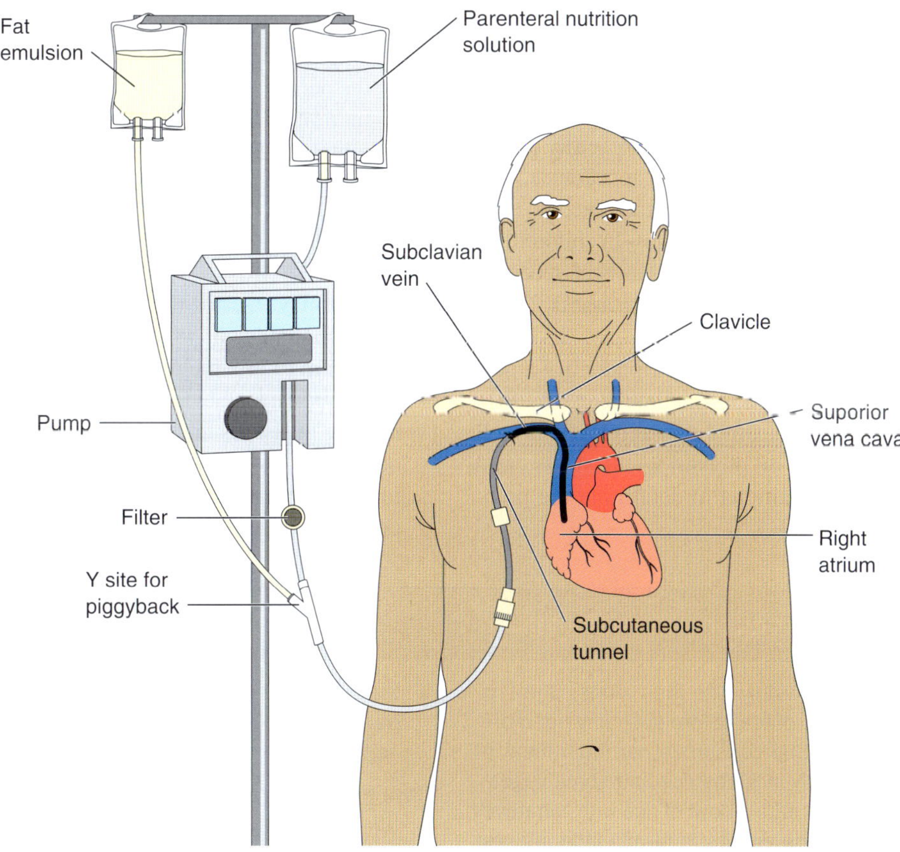

FIGURE 21.4 *Parenteral nutrition through a catheter in the right subclavian vein*

The person receiving parenteral nutrition is at risk of mechanical, metabolic and infectious complications. Pneumothorax, haemothorax, brachial plexus injury and incorrect position are possible complications of central venous catheter insertion. Once in place, the catheter may dislodge, leak or break and become an embolus. Clots also may form within or around the catheter.

Fluid overload is a risk with parenteral nutrition, particularly in older adults. The high-glucose formulas can lead to osmotic diuresis or shifts of electrolytes—potassium and phosphorus in particular—into the cells, leading to hyperglycaemia, hypokalaemia or hypophosphataemia. Blood glucose and serum electrolyte levels are carefully monitored during treatment. In addition to electrolyte imbalances, acid–base disturbances may develop, as well as refeeding oedema or heart failure (Johal, 2022). Long-term use of parenteral nutrition can lead to gallstone formation and liver disease. Nutrient deficiencies may develop, including deficiencies of vitamins, iron and other minerals when parenteral nutrition is continued for three or more months (Johal, 2022).

Disruption of the skin barrier and administration of a solution high in glucose presents a risk of infection in a person receiving PN. Infection may be local, limited to the exit site or surrounding a tunnelled catheter, or may lead to sepsis. The person's temperature and other manifestations of infection must be carefully monitored. Meticulous surgical ANTT is used for catheter exit site care and container and tubing changes (Johal, 2022).

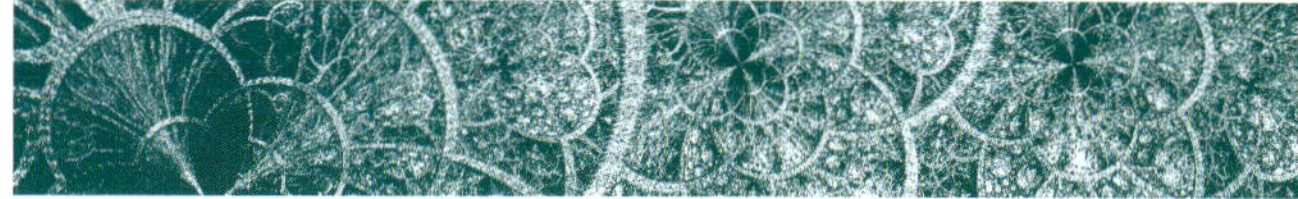

Nursing care

Health promotion

Aggressive nursing assessment and interventions can help prevent malnutrition associated with hospitalisation or long-term care. In hospitalised people, carefully monitor any food intake (Johal, 2022). Document the nutrition plan and report if nutrition intake does not meet with that plan. When the person is placed on nil by mouth (NBM) status for surgery or tests, ask the doctor to restore diet orders as soon as possible. If allowed, encourage family members to provide favourite or culturally appropriate foods to promote intake. In long-term care settings, promote socialisation during meals. Assess food likes and dislikes and provide foods the person is more likely to eat.

Assessment

Collect nutritional assessment data on admission and periodically (once or twice a week) during long-term institutionalisation.

- *Health history*: usual daily dietary pattern (type and amount of foods consumed); usual weight and recent changes; appetite and food tolerance; specific food likes and dislikes;

specific cultural foods; difficulty swallowing; problems such as anorexia, nausea, diarrhoea or constipation; history of surgery and/or chronic diseases (e.g. chronic lung disease) and medications.
- *Physical examination*: height, weight, anthropometric skinfold thickness, BMI; vital signs; general appearance, evidence of muscle wasting, mobility; skin and mucous membranes; bowel sounds; laboratory studies. In children, the mid upper arm circumference (MUAC) has been recently endorsed by the WHO as a validated method to assess malnutrition (Blackwell et al., 2015).

Use of a nutritional assessment tool can help identify a person (older adults in particular) at risk of malnutrition (see Box 21.4). Such tools assess food intake, mobility and BMI, as well as weight loss, psychological or physiological stress, and dementia or psychological conditions to determine the presence or risk of malnutrition.

Nursing diagnoses and interventions

The complex effects of malnutrition on multiple body systems place the person at high risk of a number of other health issues. This section addresses problems with nutrition, infections, fluid volume and skin integrity. See the accompanying nursing care plan for the person with malnutrition.

Imbalanced nutrition: less than body requirements

The nurse plays a critical role in the ongoing assessment of the malnourished person, while collaborating with the multidisciplinary team to provide nutritional therapies.

- If the person is able to eat, provide an environment and nursing measures that encourage eating. Eliminate foul odours, provide oral hygiene before and after meals, make meals appetising and offer frequent, small meals including preferred cultural foods. Consult with the nutrition support

NURSING CARE PLAN A person with malnutrition

Rose Chow is an 88-year-old widow who lives alone. She typically rises early and has a cup of tea before spending her morning pottering in her garden. She consumes her main meal of the day at lunch, which usually includes rice and some vegetables. For dinner, she generally eats a bowl of rice with 'whatever seems to be in the fridge'. She admits to having little interest in cooking or eating since her husband died 10 years ago, and her group of friends has been 'dying off too'.

ASSESSMENT

Mrs Chow weighs 43.1 kg and is 160 cm tall, with a BMI of 16.8.kg/m^2. She reports weighing 53.5 kg 5 years ago. Her triceps anthropometric skinfold thickness measurement is 11 mm. (Normal values for a female: 713 mm.) Her skin is pale and she appears thin and wasted. Her temperature is 36.1°C. Diagnostic test results include serum albumin 30 g/L (normal 38–50 g/L) and serum cholesterol 3.0 mmol/L (normal 3.5–5.4 mmol/L). A diagnosis of protein energy malnutrition is made and a 6,280 kJ per day diet is recommended.

DIAGNOSES

- *Imbalanced nutrition* related to food intake less than nutritional energy requirements.
- *Risk of ineffective therapeutic regimen* related to knowledge deficit.
- *Risk of infection* related to protein energy malnutrition.
- *Impaired social interaction* related to widowhood and reduced social support group.

PLANNING

Plan to meet with Mrs Chow once each week to assess progress.

Expected outcomes

- Gain at least 0.5 kg per week.
- Verbalise understanding of nutritional requirements and identify strategies to incorporate requirements into daily diet after discharge.
- Remain infection-free, evidenced by normal vital signs.
- Identify strategies to increase social interaction, such as participating in senior citizens' lunches at local senior centre.

IMPLEMENTATION

- Weigh weekly at a consistent time of day.
- Refer to dietitian for evaluation of nutritional needs.
- Teach about nutritional requirements and plan an eating program that includes high-kilojoule, high-protein foods and supplements and reflects her food preferences.
- Encourage small, frequent meals.
- Encourage keeping a food intake diary.
- Teach strategies to reduce risks for infection.
- Provide information about communal meals available to seniors in the community and help Mrs Chow develop a plan to participate.

EVALUATION

One month later, Mrs Chow has gained 1.5 kg and reports feeling 'more energetic'. A friend is helping her shop to ensure that she purchases foods to maintain her protein, kilojoule and nutrient intake. She has begun attending senior lunches twice a week and is enjoying 'being around people again'. Although she still doesn't enjoy cooking like she used to, she is using prepared foods and supplements to maintain her nutrient intake.

CRITICAL THINKING IN THE NURSING PROCESS

1. What is the physiological basis for Mrs Chow's low albumin and cholesterol levels?
2. Mrs Chow asks, 'Can I get better by just taking more vitamins?' How will you respond?
3. Design a teaching plan for a person with protein energy malnutrition.

REFLECTION ON THE NURSING PROCESS

1. What role did culture have on Mrs Chow's risk of protein malnutrition?
2. What role did being an older person have on Mrs Chow's nutritional intake?

team to provide adequate protein, kilojoules, minerals and vitamins. *Oral hygiene and a pleasant environment make food more appetising. Small, frequent meals are generally more appealing and less overwhelming to a person with anorexia. Many require complicated nutritional therapy, such as enteral or parenteral therapy, to meet nutritional needs.*

- Provide a rest period before and after meals. *Eating requires energy and the malnourished person may have decreased physical strength and energy.*
- Assess knowledge and provide appropriate teaching. *Lack of knowledge often contributes to undernutrition. Education empowers the person to make healthy choices.*

Risk of infection

Malnourished people have a much higher risk of infection than well-nourished people. Malnutrition affects many components of the immune system, including the skin, mucous membranes, and lymph tissue and cells.

- Monitor temperature and assess for manifestations of infection every 4 hours. *Although the baseline temperature may be subnormal in malnourished people, any elevation from baseline may indicate infection. Manifestations of infection may include chills, malaise, erythema and leukocytosis. Early detection of infection may prevent complications.*
- Maintain medical asepsis when providing care and surgical asepsis when carrying out procedures. *Handwashing is the best strategy to prevent the spread of pathogens. Sterile technique is required for procedures such as inserting central lines and changing dressings.*
- Teach the signs and symptoms of infection, good handwashing technique and factors that increase the risk of infection. *Knowledge empowers the person to participate in self-care, thus reducing exposure to infectious pathogens.*

Risk of fluid volume deficit

The person with malnutrition may also have a fluid volume deficit due to difficulty swallowing fluids. Administration of hyperosmolar nutritional solutions may lead to dehydration or electrolyte disturbances.

- Monitor oral mucous membranes, urine specific gravity, level of consciousness and laboratory findings every 4 to 8 hours. *Dry mucous membranes, increased urine specific gravity, decreased level of consciousness and electrolyte imbalances may indicate dehydration.*
- Weigh daily and monitor intake and output on fluid balance chart. *Daily weights and intake and output measurements help monitor fluid balance.*
- If allowed, offer fluids frequently in small amounts, considering the person's preferences. *Frequent, small amounts of fluids are better tolerated and promote adequate intake.*

Risk of impaired skin integrity

Skin integrity depends on adequate nutrition. Loss of subcutaneous tissue and muscle increase the risk of pressure ulcers. In addition, healing is impaired in malnourished people.

- Assess skin every 4 hours. *Baseline and ongoing assessments allow prompt identification of early skin breakdown.*
- Turn and position at least every 2 hours. Encourage passive and active range-of-motion exercises. *These measures reduce pressure and promote oxygenation of cells.*
- Keep skin dry and clean and minimise shearing forces. Keep linen smooth, clean and dry. Provide therapeutic beds, air mattresses or pads. *These nursing measures promote comfort and reduce the risk of skin breakdown.*

Community-based care

A person with malnutrition may be cared for at home or in the hospital with oral diet, enteral or parenteral therapy. Each year, it is more common to see people managing tube feeding or TPN at home. Health education for the person and their family includes the following topics:

- Diet recommendations and use of nutritional supplements.
- Where to obtain recommended foods and nutritional supplements.
- If continuing enteral or parenteral nutrition, how to: (1) prepare and/or handle solutions, (2) add them to either the feeding tube or central line, (3) manage infusion pumps, (4) care for the feeding tube or central catheter, (5) recognise and manage problems and complications, and (6) how and when to notify the healthcare provider of problems.

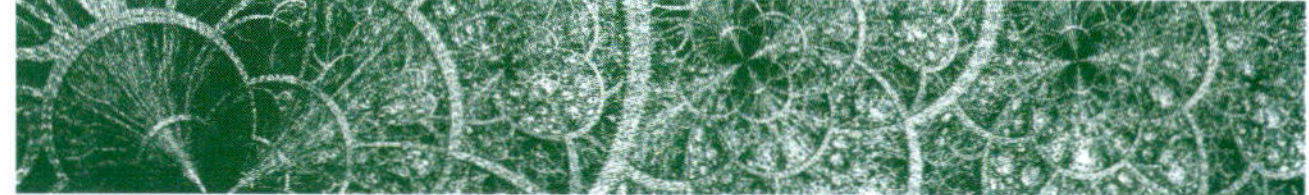

THE PERSON WITH AN EATING DISORDER

Eating disorders are characterised by severely disturbed eating behaviour and weight management. The three most common eating disorders in Australia are anorexia nervosa, bulimia nervosa and binge-eating disorder (BED). Eating disorders are increasing in Australia and are more common in affluent societies that are exposed to mass media advertising and plentiful food. Eating disorders are the third most common chronic illness in adolescents in Australia after obesity and asthma. It is estimated that eating disorders affect nearly 1 million Australians. Premature death from physical causes and by suicide in young adults who suffer from an eating disorder is higher than in the general population (Eating Disorders Victoria, 2022).

The *Diagnostic and Statistical Manual of Mental Disorders* (DSM-5) advises that the diagnosis of **anorexia nervosa** is characterised by: (1) the persistent restriction of oral energy intake leading to a significantly low BMI or BMI-for-age, (2) an intense fear of gaining weight or of becoming fat, or persistent ritualistic behaviour that interferes with weight gain despite having a lower than normal BMI, and (3) a disturbance in the way one's body weight or shape is experienced, undue influence of body shape and weight on self-evaluation or a persistent lack of recognition of the seriousness of the low BMI

(Eating Disorders Victoria, 2022). **Bulimia nervosa** is characterised by recurring episodes of binge eating followed by purge behaviours such as self-induced vomiting, use of laxatives or diuretics, fasting or excessive exercise at least twice a week for a period of greater than 3 months. A third eating disorder, **binge-eating disorder**, is believed to affect many more people than either anorexia or bulimia. Binge-eating disorder is characterised by recurrent episodes of binge eating—eating an excessive amount of food during a defined period of time and a sense of lack of control overeating during binge episodes (Lizarondo, 2022).

Anorexia nervosa

Anorexia nervosa typically begins during puberty in an attempt to cope with a perceived stress (Lock, Le Grange & Russell, 2016). People with anorexia nervosa are usually high achievers who have a distorted body image and an irrational fear of gaining weight. Refusal to maintain body weight at or above a minimally normal level for height and body type is a common manifestation of anorexia nervosa. The person will maintain weight loss by restricted kilojoule intake, often accompanied by excessive exercise. Some may exhibit binge–purge behaviour. Although its cause is unknown, a number of risk factors, both biological and psychosocial, have been identified for anorexia nervosa. Abnormal levels of neurotransmitters and other hormones may play a role. Current research suggests genetic factors linked with environmental factors may influence the development of eating disorders (Eating Disorders Victoria, 2022). Women who develop anorexia nervosa tend to be obsessive and perfectionist and often feel inadequate or unable to maintain control in their lives. Family, social or occupational (e.g. a career in modelling, television or ballet) pressures contribute to maintain low body weight. People with anorexia often experience depression or anxiety.

Bulimia nervosa

Bulimia nervosa is an eating disorder in which people binge on food and then, in an attempt to counteract this behaviour, take extreme measures such as making themselves vomit, taking laxatives or starving themselves (Lizarondo, 2022). Bulimia nervosa develops in late adolescence or early adulthood, often following failed attempts to lose weight through dieting. Foods consumed during a binge often are high in kilojoules and fat. After binge eating, the person induces vomiting (usually by stimulating the gag reflex) or may take excessive quantities of laxatives or diuretics. In contrast to anorexia, the person's weight is often normal. Fluid and electrolyte balance, in contrast, may be severely disrupted by loss of fluid and gastrointestinal secretions. The complications of bulimia nervosa primarily result from the purging behaviour.

Binge-eating disorder

Binge-eating disorder (BED) was identified as a condition distinct from overeating in 1992 (Eating Disorders Victoria, 2022). While many of the characteristics of bulimia and binge-eating disorder are similar with feelings of guilt, disgust and depression, a person with BED usually binges in private and does not purge. The disorder commonly affects middle-aged adults and is slightly more common in women than in men. People with BED usually eat when not hungry and are overweight or obese, often morbidly obese. Psychosocial factors contribute: up to half of people with BED either are depressed or have experienced depression in the past. Alcohol abuse and impulsivity are common behavioural traits in a person with BED.

Links to National Patient Safety Standards

NSQHS: Comprehensive Care Standard

The intention of this standard is 'to ensure that patients receive comprehensive care—that is, coordinated delivery of the total health care required or requested by a patient. This care is aligned with the patient's expressed goals of care and healthcare needs, considers the effect of the patient's health issues on their life and wellbeing, and is clinically appropriate. To ensure that risks of harm for patients during health care are prevented and managed. Clinicians identify patients at risk of specific harm during health care by applying the screening and assessment processes required in this standard' (Australian Commission on Safety and Quality in Health Care (ACSQHC), 2021, p. 44).

Patients with poor nutrition are at an increased risk of pressure injuries and these are usually more severe. They have an increased risk of healthcare-associated infections, with increased mortality during and after hospital admission. Length of stay is increased for patients with malnutrition and they often require readmission.

Nurses should identify patients at risk of poor nutrition and put in place strategies to reduce these risks. Health services need evidence-based food preparation and distribution practices, and nutrition care plans to ensure patients' nutritional needs are met. Patients at risk of malnutrition need their nutritional needs monitored and nutritional support must be supplied to those who cannot meet their nutritional requirements with food alone. Patients should be assisted with their eating and drinking.

Source: ACSQHC (2021). *National Safety and Quality Health Service Standards* (2nd ed.). Sydney: ACSQHC. © Australian Commission on Safety and Quality in Health Care.

MANIFESTATIONS AND COMPLICATIONS **Eating disorders**

DISORDER	MANIFESTATIONS	COMPLICATIONS
Anorexia nervosa	■ Weight < 85% of normal; muscle wasting ■ Fear of weight gain, refusal to eat ■ Disturbed body image, excessive exercise ■ Amenorrhoea (loss of menses) ■ Skin and hair changes (fine hair–lanugo–over body) ■ Hypotension, bradycardia ■ Hypothermia ■ Constipation ■ Insomnia	■ Electrolyte and acid-base disturbances ■ Reduced cardiac muscle mass, low cardiac output, arrhythmias ■ Anaemia ■ Hypoglycaemia, elevated serum uric acid levels ■ Osteoporosis ■ Enlarged salivary glands ■ Delayed gastric emptying ■ Abnormal liver function
Bulimia nervosa	■ Weight often normal; may be slightly overweight ■ Binge-purge behaviour ■ Oligomenorrhoea or amenorrhoea ■ Lacerations of palate; callus on fingers or dorsum of hand	■ Enlarged salivary glands ■ Stomatitis, loss of dental enamel ■ Fluid, electrolyte and acid-base imbalances ■ Arrhythmias ■ Oesophageal tears, stomach rupture

Binge-eating disorder	■ Usually overweight or obese
	■ Recurrent episodes of binge eating (2 or more days a week for 6 months)
	■ Episodes characterised by:
	  ■ Eating more rapidly than usual
	  ■ Eating until uncomfortably full
	  ■ Eating large amounts of food when not physically hungry
	  ■ Eating alone due to embarrassment over quantity
	  ■ Disgust, depression or guilt following a binge episode
	  ■ Marked distress about binging behaviour
		■ Type 2 diabetes mellitus
		■ Hypertension, hyperlipidaemia
		■ Coronary heart disease, heart failure
		■ Gallbladder disease
		■ Depression, social isolation

INTERPROFESSIONAL CARE

Eating disorders, anorexia nervosa in particular, are difficult to treat effectively. Because of the intense fear of weight gain and distorted body image, these people strongly resist increasing food intake. In all cases, a comprehensive treatment plan for eating disorders includes medical care and monitoring, psychosocial interventions and nutrition counselling (Lizarondo, 2022).

Diagnosis

There is no specific diagnostic test for anorexia, bulimia or binge-eating disorder. Laboratory studies of a person with anorexia or bulimia may show anaemia and leucopenia, abnormal serum electrolyte levels and elevated blood urea nitrogen (BUN) and serum creatinine. In people with BED, the blood glucose and lipid levels may be elevated. The BMI is usually above the normal range and may identify the person as obese or morbidly obese.

A mental health evaluation is indicated for people with eating disorders to identify contributing factors and help direct treatment.

Treatment

A multidisciplinary approach that includes psychology, psychiatry, medicine, dietetics, family therapy and social work is used in Australia (Lizarondo, 2022). The aims of treatment are to restore weight, reverse malnutrition and relieve the mental anguish associated with eating.

Treatment is usually as an outpatient but some may require hospitalisation, particularly if their weight is less than 75% of normal. Refeeding is gradually introduced to avoid complications such as heart failure. Oral intake is the preferred option in refeeding. Meals must be supervised and a firm but empathetic attitude conveyed about the importance of adequate food intake. Enteral or intravenous feeding may be required to supplement oral intake. Psychological treatment, initiated when malnutrition has been corrected and weight gain begun, focuses on providing emotional support and helping the person base their self esteem on factors other than weight (e.g. personal relationships, satisfaction with achieving occupational goals) (Lizarondo, 2022). Cognitive–behavioural therapy or psychotherapy may be used; families may be included in the treatment program. Pharmacotherapy such as low dose antipsychotic medications (e.g. olanzapine) may be helpful in extremely anxious individuals to assist in reducing their anxiety.

The goal of bulimia treatment is to reduce or eliminate binge eating and purging behaviour. A combination of nutritional counselling and therapy, psychosocial interventions and medications may be used. Nutritional counselling is directed at establishing a regular meal pattern and encouraging an appropriate amount of regular exercise. Cognitive–behavioural therapy also is used to treat bulimia, focusing on excessive concerns about weight, persistent dieting and binge–purge behaviours.

Treatment for those with BED focuses on establishing healthy eating patterns, psychosocial therapy (including cognitive–behavioural therapy and group counselling) to address underlying issues and management of obesity and its complications. A person with BED may also benefit from pharmacotherapy.

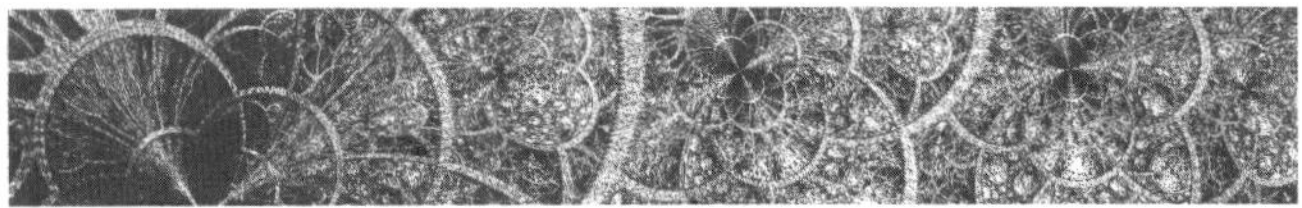

Nursing care

Nurses can be instrumental in identifying a person with an eating disorder and referring for treatment. It is particularly important to identify these disorders early to prevent adverse effects on growth and increase the success of treatment.

The nurse is an integral part of the eating disorders treatment team. *Imbalanced nutrition: less than body requirements* is a primary nursing diagnosis for a person with anorexia or bulimia, and *Imbalanced nutrition: more than body requirements* is a priority nursing diagnosis for people with binge-eating disorder (BED). The following nursing diagnoses also should be considered:

- *Ineffective sexuality patterns* related to body image concerns.
- *Chronic low self-esteem* related to tendency to binge eat.
- *Disturbed body image* related to altered eating pattern.
- *Ineffective therapeutic regimen* related to knowledge deficit.

When planning and implementing care, consider the following nursing activities:

- Ensure a commitment from the person that they wish to alter their eating patterns.
- Regularly monitor weight each week using standard conditions. *Weight gain or loss provides information about the effectiveness of care, as well as the person's risk of complications.*
- Monitor food intake during meals, recording percentage of meal and snacks consumed. Maintain close observation for at least 1 hour following meals; do not allow the person to be alone in the bathroom. *Observing the person during and after meals helps prevent disposal of food and purging behaviour after eating. Recording actual food intake allows accurate calculation of kilojoule intake.*
- Serve balanced meals, including all nutrient groups. Increase serving size gradually. The person may find 'normal' food servings overwhelming, reducing the desire to eat. *Kilojoule intake is initially limited to prevent complications associated with refeeding, then gradually increased.*
- Administer a multivitamin and mineral supplement to replace losses.

Involvement of the family and social support people is vital to success. Encourage family members to participate in teaching and nutritional counselling sessions. Discuss the value of family therapy to address issues that have contributed to the disorder. Emphasise the need to provide consistent messages of support for healthy eating habits. Discuss using rewards for food and kilojoule intake rather than weight gain. Provide referrals to a dietitian, nutritional support team, counselling and support groups for people with eating disorders.

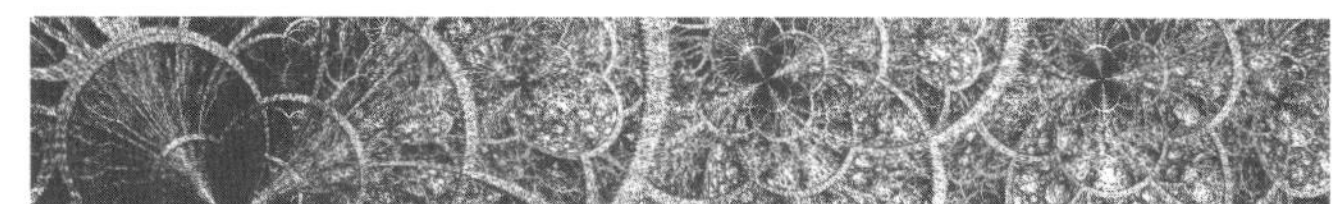

CHAPTER HIGHLIGHTS

- **Nutritional disorders are common, affecting people worldwide and contributing significantly to mortality and morbidity. While malnutrition is a serious problem in underdeveloped nations, obesity and its consequences are more prevalent in Australia and other industrialised societies.**
- **Obesity, defined as excess adipose tissue and a BMI greater than 30 kg/m^2, is linked with many disorders, including type 2 diabetes mellitus, coronary heart disease, gallbladder disease and osteoarthritis.**
- **Exercise and reduced kilojoule intake are the mainstays of obesity treatment. Drugs that suppress the appetite or interfere with fat absorption in the gut may be used to facilitate weight loss in a person with multiple risk factors for obesity complications or people who have had difficulty achieving weight loss through diet and exercise.**
- **Bariatric surgery is a viable treatment option for the morbidly obese. The primary types of bariatric surgery used in Australia are restrictive and malabsorptive procedures that limit stomach capacity and nutrient absorption.**
- **Nursing care for obese people focuses on health promotion, education and support of the prescribed treatment plan.**
- **In Australia, protein energy malnutrition is a common problem among the elderly and hospitalised people. Malnutrition increases the risk of complications and impairs healing. Early identification and prevention are the primary focuses of treatment; nurses can be instrumental in identifying at-risk people (e.g. the elderly, a person living alone, people on extended NBM status).**
- **Refeeding of malnourished people is a gradual process. Enteral feedings (oral or by feeding tube) are preferred whenever possible. Parenteral nutrition may be required when enteral feeding is not possible or not tolerated.**
- **Eating disorders, including anorexia nervosa, bulimia nervosa and binge-eating disorder, can be difficult to effectively treat and maintain in remission. While a person with anorexia typically is underweight and malnourished, resisting efforts to achieve a normal weight, a person with bulimia is more likely to be of normal weight and those with binge-eating disorder tend to be overweight or obese.**
- **Treatment for eating disorders is multifaceted, including physical care to restore electrolyte balance and treat complications, nutritional counselling and therapy, psychosocial therapy, family support and possibly medications.**

CONCEPT CHECK

1 Of the following noted in a person's history, which does the nurse identify as risk factors for obesity?
1 adopted at 2 months of age
2 usual diet includes 'fast-food' meals twice a week
3 does not engage in regular activity
4 allergic to chocolate and strawberries

2 A person on a reduced-kilojoule diet asks the nurse what she can do to lose weight faster because most weeks she loses no more than 0.2 kg. 'At this rate, it will take me years to get to my goal!'
1 'Let's re-evaluate your long-term goal. Perhaps it was set too low for you.'
2 'A kilogram of body fat equals 14,650 kJ. Let's re-evaluate your diet and exercise plan for kilojoule intake and expenditure.'
3 'Perhaps we should look into a diet supplement since you are unable to stick with your prescribed diet plan.'
4 'You sound frustrated. Would you like to take some time off from your diet and exercise plan?'

3 An expected finding in a person admitted with a diagnosis of protein energy malnutrition would be:
1 recent 5 kg weight loss
2 increased anthropometric skinfold thickness measurements
3 hyperactive bowel sounds
4 anxiety and agitation

4 Before administering an intermittent enteral feeding, the nurse confirms placement of the small-bore feeding tube in the stomach by:
1 instilling water and listening for the gastric gurgle
2 withdrawing the tube slightly, then reinserting it
3 aspirating gastric contents and checking for a pH of < 4
4 obtaining an x-ray of the chest and stomach

5 The nurse identifies which of the following as realistic goals for a person with anorexia nervosa?
1 will consume 100% of a 10,465 kJ diet
2 will gain 0.5 kg per week
3 will rest alone in room following meals
4 will participate in family counselling

6 The nurse identifies which nursing diagnosis as high priority for a person with a BMI of 30.4 kg/m^2 and a waist-to-hip ratio of 1.1?
1 *Health-seeking behaviours: weight loss*
2 *Risk of impaired cardiovascular tissue perfusion*
3 *Ineffective coping*
4 *Deficient knowledge regarding diet*

7 The nurse teaching a person about sibutramine (Reductil) includes which of the following instructions?
1 You may skip a dose of the drug if you skip a high-fat meal.
2 Do not consume alcohol while taking this drug.
3 Do not drive while taking this drug because the drug may increase sleepiness.
4 Increase your intake of water and other fluids while taking this drug.
5 Continue to follow your prescribed diet while taking this drug.

8 The nurse caring for a home-bound older adult who is losing 1 to 2 kg monthly plans for which of the following?
1 Meals on Wheels deliveries
2 ensure nutritional supplements
3 placement in a residential care facility
4 transportation to congregate senior meals
5 follow-up by primary care physician
6 referral for diagnostic studies

9 Which of the following is a high-priority nursing intervention to prevent malnutrition in the person undergoing surgery?
1 aggressive pain management
2 daily weighing
3 maintaining intravenous flow
4 requesting early restoration of oral intake

10 Three days after gastric bypass surgery, the person complains of increasing abdominal pain. Bowel sounds are absent; the abdomen is firm and very tender. The nurse should:
1 report findings to the surgeon
2 ambulate the person to promote peristalsis
3 chart assessment data and continue to monitor
4 evaluate the effectiveness of analgesia

BIBLIOGRAPHY

Abed, J., Judeh, H., Abed, E. et al. (2014). 'Fixing a heart': The game of electrolytes in anorexia nervosa. *Nutrition Journal*, *13*, 90.

Aginga, C. (2021). *Evidence summary. Cardiovascular diseases (primary and secondary prevention): Dietary approaches to stop hypertension (DASH) style diet*. The Joanna Briggs Institute EBP Database. JBI-ES-3380-2.

Asher, R. C., Burrows, T. L. & Collins, C. E. (2013). Very low-energy diets for weight loss in adults: A review. *Nutrition & Dietetics*, *70*(2), 101–112.

Ashi, R. S. (2022). Protein energy malnutrition: An overview on first national disorder. *International Journal of Community Health Nursing*, *5*(1), 50–57. https://doi.org/10.37628/ijchn.v5i1.2086

Atieno Odhiambo, M. (2022). *Evidence summary. Type 2 diabetes mellitus (T2DM): Bariatric metabolic surgery*. The Joanna Briggs Institute EBP Database. JBI-ES-2137-1.

Australian Bureau of Statistics (ABS) (2018a). *National health survey: First results methodology 2017–18 financial year*. Canberra: ABS.

Australian Bureau of Statistics (ABS) (2018b). *Overweight and obesity*. Canberra: ABS.

Australian Commission on Safety and Quality in Health Care (ACSQHC) (2021). *National Safety and Quality Health Service Standards* (2nd ed.). Sydney: ACSQHC.

Australian Institute of Health and Welfare (AIHW) (2017). *Weight loss surgery in Australia 2014–15: Australian hospital statistics*. Retrieved from https://www.aihw.gov.au/

Australian Institute of Health and Welfare (AIHW) (2020). *Overweight and obesity: An interactive insight*. Canberra: AIHW.

Australian Institute of Health and Welfare (AIHW) (2022a). *Overweight and obesity*. Canberra: AIHW. Retrieved from https://www.aihw.gov.au/

Australian Institute of Health and Welfare (AIHW) (2022b). *Determinants of health for Indigenous Australians*. Canberra: AIHW. Retrieved from https://www.aihw.gov.au/

Bacon, L. & Aphramor, L. (2011). Weight science: Evaluating the evidence for a paradigm shift. *Nutrition Journal*, *10*(9), 2–13.

Barker, L. A., Gout, B. S. & Crowe, T. C. (2011). Hospital malnutrition: Prevalence, identification and impact on patients and the healthcare system. *International Journal of Environmental Research and Public Health*, *8*, 514–527.

Bauset, C., Martínez-Aspas, A., Smith-Ballester, S., García-Vigara, A., Monllor-Tormos, A., Kadi, F., Nilsson, A. & Cano, A. (2022). Nuts and metabolic syndrome: Reducing the burden of metabolic syndrome in menopause. *Nutrients*, *14*(8), 1677. https://doi.org/10.3390/nu14081677

Bender, A. (2014). *A dictionary of food and nutrition* (4th ed.). Oxford: Oxford University Press.

Blackwell, N., Myatt, M., Allafort-Duverger, T. et al. (2015). Mothers Understand And Can do it (MUAC): A comparison of mothers and community health workers determining mid-upper arm circumference. *Archives of Public Health*, *73*(26), 1–7.

Cifuentes, L. & Acosta, A. (2021). Homeostatic regulation of food intake. *Clinics and Research in Hepatology and Gastroenterology*, *46*(2), 101794. https://doi.org/10.1016/j.clinre.2021.101794

Department of Health (2013). *Australian dietary guidelines*. Canberra: Australian Government.

Dunstan, D. W., Howard, B., Healy, G. N. & Owen, N. (2012). Too much sitting—A health hazard. *Diabetes Research and Clinical Practice*, *97*(3), 368–376.

Eating Disorders Victoria (2022). *Overview of eating disorders today*. Retrieved from https://www.eatingdisorders.org.au

Frank, L. (2011). Bariatric beriberi: Thiamin deficiency in the bariatric patient. *Bariatric Times*, *8*(1), 14.

Germov, J. & Williams, L. (2016). *A sociology of food & nutrition. The social appetite* (4th ed.). Melbourne: Oxford University Press.

Gudzune, K. A., Doshi, R. S., Mehta, A. K. et al. (2015). Efficacy of commercial weight-loss programs: An updated systematic review. *Annals of Internal Medicine*, *162*, 1–14.

Ishaque, S. (2022). *Evidence summary. Enteral tube feeding (nasogastric and gastrostomy): Discharge education*. The Joanna Briggs Institute EBP Database. JBI-ES-445-3.

Johal, J. (2022). *Evidence summary. Total parenteral nutrition: Monitoring*. The Joanna Briggs Institute EBP Database. JBI-ES-5016-1.

Lim, R., Beekley, A., Johnson, D. C. & Davis, K. A. (2018). Early and late complications of bariatric operation. *Trauma Surgery & Acute Care Open*, *3*, e000219. doi: 10.1136/tsaco-2018-000219

Lizarondo, L. (2022). *Evidence summary. Bulimia nervosa or binge eating disorder: Telehealth*. The Joanna Briggs Institute EBP Database. JBI-ES-897-1.

Lock, J., Le Grange, D. & Russell, G. (2016). *Treatment manual for anorexia nervosa: A family-based approach* (2nd ed.). New York: Guildford Publications.

Locke, A. E., Kahali, B., Berndt, S. I. et al. (2015). Genetic studies of body mass index yield new insights for obesity biology. *Nature*, *518*(7538), 197–206.

Lockwood, C. & Queiroz, A. (2022). *Evidence summary. Percutaneous endoscopic gastronomy (PEG) tube: Administration of enteral feed*. The Joanne Briggs Institute EBP Database. JBI-ES-1912-2.

Magnusson, R. S. (2010). Obesity prevention and personal responsibility: The case of front-of-pack food labelling in Australia. *BMC Public Health*, *10*, 662.

Magtoto, L. (2022). *Evidence summary. Obesity and overweight: Long-term pharmacotherapy*. The Joanna Briggs Institute EBP Database. JBI-ES-2028-3.

Malafarina, V., Úriz-Otanoa, F., Iniesta, R. et al. (2012). Sarcopenia in the elderly: Diagnosis, physiopathology and treatment. *Maturitas*, *71*, 109–114.

Marieb, E. N. & Hoehn, K. (2019). *Human anatomy and physiology* (11th ed.). International edition. San Francisco: Pearson.

Marin, T. & Ndegwa, M. (2021). *Evidence summary. Malnutrition risk assessment (older people): Long-term aged care facilities*. The Joanna Briggs Institute EBP Database. JBIES-3182-2.

Misumida, N., Hisashi Umeda, H. & Iwase, M. (2014). Shoshin beriberi induced by long-term administration of diuretics: A case report. *Case Reports in Cardiology*, *2014*. Article ID 878915.

National Health and Medical Research Council (NHMRC) (2013). *Eat for health: Australian dietary guidelines, summary*. Canberra: NHMRC Publications.

Ortega-Arroyo, A. (2022). *Evidence summary. Obesity (older adults): Deliberate weight loss*. The Joanna Briggs Institute EBP Database. JBI-ES-407-2.

Porth, C. M. (2019). *Essentials of pathophysiology: Concepts of altered health states* (5th ed.). Philadelphia: Wolters Kluwer.

Preiser, J.-C., van Zanten, A. R. H., Berger, M. M. et al. (2015). Metabolic and nutritional support of critically ill patients: Consensus and controversies. *Critical Care*, *19*(1), 35.

Redgrave, G. W., Coughlin, J. W., Schreyer, C. C. et al. (2015). Refeeding and weight restoration outcomes in anorexia nervosa: Challenging current guidelines. *The International Journal of Eating Disorders*, *48*(7), 866–873. doi: 10.1002/eat.22390

Robinson, K., Muir, S., Newbury, A., Santos-Merx, L. & Appleton, K. M. (2022). Perceptions of body weight that vary by body mass index: Clear associations with perceptions based on personal control and responsibility. *Journal of Health Psychology*, *27*(1), 147–165. doi: 10.1177/1359105320916540

Rosenthal, R. J. et al. (2012). International Sleeve Gastrectomy Expert Panel consensus statement: Best practice guidelines based on experience of 12,000 cases. *Surgery for Obesity and Related Diseases*, *8*, 8–19.

Scholes, G. & Judd, J. (2022). Protein-energy malnutrition in older Australians: A narrative review of the prevalence, causes and consequences of malnutrition, and strategies for prevention. *Health Promotion Journal of Australia*, *33*(1), 187–193.

Sherf Dagan, S., Goldenshluger, A., Globus, I., Schweiger, C., Kessler, Y., Kowen Sandbank, G., Ben-Porat, T. & Sinai, T. (2017). Nutritional recommendations for adult bariatric surgery patients: Clinical practice. *Advances in Nutrition*, *8*(2), 382–394. doi: 10.3945/an.116.014258

Singh, A. (2021). *Evidence summary. Nasogastric feeding tubes: Methods used to verify tube position*. The Joanna Briggs Institute EBP Database. JBI-ES-1559-1.

Smith, S. H. (2017). Using albumin and prealbumin to assess nutritional status. *Nursing*, *47*(4), 65–66. doi: 10.1097/01.NURSE.0000511805.83334.df

Thaher, O., Tallak, W., Hukauf, M. & Stroh, C. (2022). Outcome of sleeve gastrectomy versus Roux-en-Y gastric bypass for patients with super obesity (body mass index > 50 kg/m^2). *Obesity Surgery*, *32*(5), 1546–1555. https://doi.org/10.1007/s11695-022-05965-6

Travers, C. (2021). *Evidence summary. Vitamin D status: Weight loss*. The Joanna Briggs Institute EBP Database. JBI-ES-3875-2.

Tuso, P. & Beattie, S. (2015). Nutrition reconciliation and nutrition prophylaxis: Toward total health. *The Permanente Journal*, *19*(2), 80–86.

Vainik, U., García-García, I. & Dagher, A. (2019). Uncontrolled eating: A unifying heritable trait linked with obesity, overeating, personality and the brain. *The European Journal of Neuroscience*, *50*(3), 2430–2445. https://doi.org/10.1111/ejn.14352

World Health Organization (WHO) (2021). *Obesity and overweight*. Retrieved from https://www.who.int/

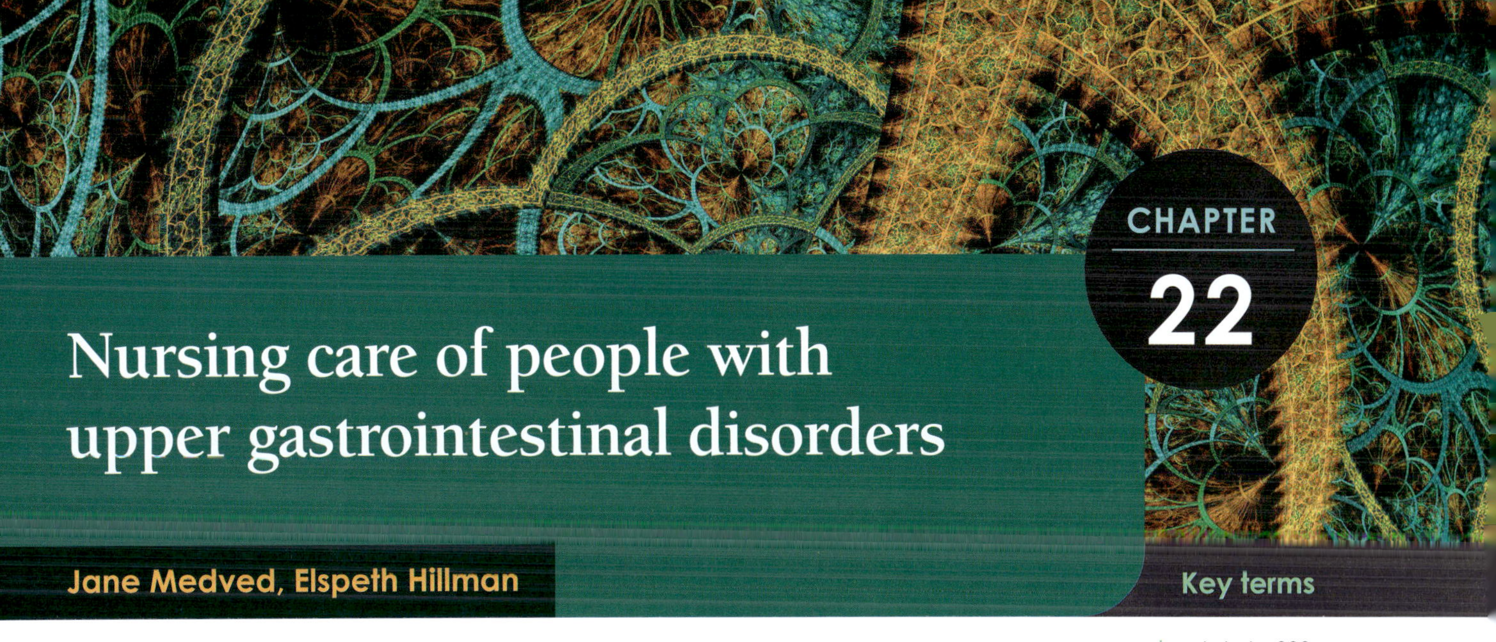

CHAPTER 22

Nursing care of people with upper gastrointestinal disorders

Jane Medved, Elspeth Hillman

Learning outcomes

- Describe the pathophysiology, manifestations and complications associated with common disorders of the mouth.
- Discuss the pathophysiology, manifestations and nursing care of a person with a disorder of the oesophagus.
- Describe the pathophysiology, manifestations and complications associated with common disorders of the stomach and duodenum.

Clinical competencies

- Assess the functional health status of people with upper gastrointestinal disorders.
- Monitor, document and, as needed, report manifestations of upper gastrointestinal disorders and their complications.
- Plan nursing care using evidence-based research.
- Determine priority nursing diagnoses and interventions based on assessed data.
- Administer medications and prescribed care knowledgeably and safely.
- Coordinate and integrate interprofessional care into the plan of care.
- Construct and revise individualised plans of care, considering the culture and values of the person.
- Plan and provide the person and family with teaching to promote, maintain and restore functional health.

Key terms

achalasia 666
acute gastritis 673
anorexia 669
cachectic 685
chronic gastritis 673
Cushing's ulcers 674
diffuse oesophageal spasm 666
dumping syndrome 686
duodenal ulcers 676
dysphagia 665
erosive (stress-induced) gastritis 674
gastric mucosal barrier 668
gastric outlet obstruction 677
gastric ulcers 676
gastritis 673
gastroduodenostomy (Billroth I) 685
gastrojejunostomy (Billroth II) 685
gastro-oesophageal reflux 661
gastro-oesophageal reflux disease (GORD) 661
haematemesis 671
haematochezia 671
haemorrhage 677
hiatal hernia 665
nausea 669
occult bleeding 671
oesophagojejunostomy 686
oral mucositis 654
partial gastrectomy 685
peptic ulcer disease (PUD) 676
peptic ulcers 676
perforation 680
total gastrectomy 686
ulcer 677
vomiting 669
Zollinger–Ellison syndrome 680

The upper gastrointestinal (GI) tract includes the mouth, oesophagus, stomach and proximal small intestine (duodenum and jejunum). Food and fluids, ingested through the mouth, move through the oesophagus to the stomach. The stomach, duodenum and jejunum are responsible for the majority of food digestion. When an acute or chronic disease process interferes with the function of this portion of the GI tract, nutritional status can be affected and the person may experience symptoms that interfere with their lifestyle.

Nurses provide both acute care for the hospitalised person and education about the skills and knowledge needed to manage these conditions at home.

Disorders of the mouth

Inflammations, infections and neoplastic lesions of the mouth affect food ingestion and nutrition. Oral lesions may have a variety of causes, including infection, mechanical trauma, irritants such as alcohol, and hypersensitivity. Appropriate treatment of the disorder, any underlying factors and associated symptoms is essential.

THE PERSON WITH ORAL MUCOSITIS

Oral mucositis refers to inflammation and ulceration of the oral mucosa (Isozaki & Brant, 2022). It may be caused by viral (herpes simplex) or fungal (*Candida albicans*) infections, mechanical trauma (e.g. poorly fitting dentures, cheek biting) or irritants such as tobacco or chemotherapeutic agents. Risk factors for oral mucositis include old age, female gender, increased bodyweight, reduced clearance of drugs and genetic susceptibility (Pulito et al., 2020). Oral mucositis is a very common side effect of cancer treatment, occurring in 40% of people receiving standard dose chemotherapy, 60–85% of patients undergoing hematopoietic stem cell transplantation (HSCT) and almost 90% of head and neck cancer patients receiving combination radiation and chemotherapy (Pulito et al., 2020).

Box 22.1 outlines risk factors for oral mucositis.

BOX 22.1 Risk factors for oral mucositis

- Age > 65 years
- Impaired immune status (HIV disease, cancer, diabetes)
- Chronic renal failure or heart failure
- Chemotherapy, radiation therapy, stem cell transplant
- Oxygen therapy, mouth breathing
- Medications (antibiotics, phenytoin, anticholinergics, corticosteroids)
- Poor oral hygiene, ill-fitting dentures
- Tobacco or alcohol use

Pathophysiology and manifestations

Radiotherapy and chemotherapy damage the DNA of basal epithelial cells, resulting in necrosis and death of some cells. This stimulates the release of inflammatory cytokines such as tumour necrosis factor alpha (TNF-α) and interleukins that further damage tissues, causing additional epithelial cells to die and greater injury to the mucosa (Isozaki & Brant, 2022). The injury to the mucosa is manifested in extremely painful lesions, which are portals for bacteria, viruses and fungi. This may lead to bacteraemia and sepsis; ultimately, however, healing of the mucosa will occur (Isozaki & Brant, 2022).

The clinical manifestations of oral mucositis vary according to its cause; however, the main symptom is pain. Pain may vary from a mild burning through to severe pain and may be associated with nausea, hypersalivation and infection (Isozaki & Brant, 2022). Table 22.1 outlines common causes of oral mucositis with their manifestations and treatment.

Oral mucositis can lead to malnutrition, fluid and electrolyte imbalance, an increased risk of infection (especially for neutropenic patients), a reduction in quality of life and increased hospital stays.

FAST FACTS

- Specific chemotherapy treatments, high-dose and dose-dense chemotherapy protocols increase the risk of oral mucositis.
- Repetitive radiation to the head and neck or radiation directly to the oral mucosa contributes to oral mucositis.
- Adherence to an oral healthcare protocol can reduce the severity and duration of oral mucositis.
- Healing time can take from 2–3 weeks unless there is a complicated infection or repeated doses of chemotherapy or radiation.

INTERPROFESSIONAL CARE

Oral mucositis is diagnosed by direct physical examination and, if indicated, cultures, smears and evaluation for systemic illness. Assessment tools such as the World Health Organization Oral Toxicity Tool are available to assist with diagnosis.

Treatment addresses both the underlying cause and any coexisting illnesses. An undiagnosed oral lesion present for more than 1 week and which does not respond to therapy must be evaluated for malignancy.

Direct smears and cultures of lesions may be obtained to identify causative organisms. If systemic illness is suspected, a variety of diagnostic tests may be ordered to identify the underlying cause.

TABLE 22.1 Manifestations and treatment of common oral mucositis conditions

TYPE	CAUSE	MANIFESTATIONS	TREATMENT
Cold sore, fever blister	Herpes simplex virus	• Initial burning at site • Clustered vesicular lesions on lip or oral mucosa	• Self-limiting • Aciclovir, valaciclovir to shorten course
Aphthous ulcer (canker sore, ulcerative oral mucositis)	Unknown; may be type of herpes virus	• Well-circumscribed, shallow erosions with white or yellow centre encircled by red ring • Less than 1 cm in diameter • Painful	• Topical steroid ointment • Oral prednisone
Candidiasis (thrush)	*Candida albicans*	• Creamy white, curd-like patches • Red, erythematous mucosa	• Fluconazole (Diflucan) • Ketoconazole (Nizoral) • Clotrimazole pessaries • Nystatin mouth rinse
Necrotising ulcerative gingivitis (trench mouth, Vincent's infection)	Infection with spirochetes and bacilli or systemic infection	• Acute gingival inflammation and necrosis • Bleeding, halitosis • Fever • Cervical lymphadenopathy	• Correct any underlying disorders • Oral penicillin
Chemotherapy- or radiation-therapy-induced oral mucositis	Damage to epithelial cells and stem cells in the submucosa caused by chemotherapy or radiation therapy	• Erythema and inflammation of oral mucosa • Painful, irregularly shaped ulcerations, initially superficial, progressing to deep ulcers that may be confluent (overlapping with one another) • Pseudomembranes covering ulcers • Tissue necrosis with spontaneous bleeding, potential sepsis	• Regular oral hygiene with brushing and flossing • Sodium bicarbonate solution or normal saline mouth rinses after and between meals • Lignocaine viscous gel before meals for analgesia • Cryotherapy before, during and after chemotherapy administration

The best management for oral mucositis due to chemotherapy or radiation is prevention through education on oral care and diet. Oral care reduces the amount of microbial flora and reduces pain and bleeding, which assists in preventing infection. General treatment measures include providing meticulous oral hygiene four times a day with a soft toothbrush or sponge swab and flossing. Bland oral mouth rinses such as 0.9% sodium chloride or water and sodium bicarbonate mixed together can be used to loosen debris in the mouth, reduce the acidity of oral fluids, dilute accumulating mucus and discourage yeast colonisation. The person should be instructed to take a tablespoon of the rinse, swish it in their mouth for at least 30 seconds, and then expectorate (Cancer Council, 2020).

Cryotherapy, the use of ice chips or ice-cold water for the prevention of oral mucositis, is recommended for use in chemotherapy agents with a short half-life. Cryotherapy is based on the theory that vasoconstriction decreases exposure of the oral mucous membranes to the chemotherapy agent. The person sucks on ice or holds ice-cold water in their mouth prior to, during and after rapid infusion of the chemotherapy agent. It is not recommended for the person receiving oxaliplatin as a chemotherapy agent (Cancer Council, 2020).

Medications

Topical treatments are applied directly to the mucosa or the ulcer and may help to reduce pain and accelerate healing of oral mucositis. They are available in the form of gel, spray or mouthwash, and aim to reduce symptoms of pain, enabling the person to eat, drink and speak in comfort. Topical treatments include corticosteroids and anaesthetics. Anaesthetics should not be swallowed as they can affect swallowing and cough reflex. It is recommended that if there is no improvement after 7 days of treatment, further medical advice should be sought. See the 'Medication administration' box.

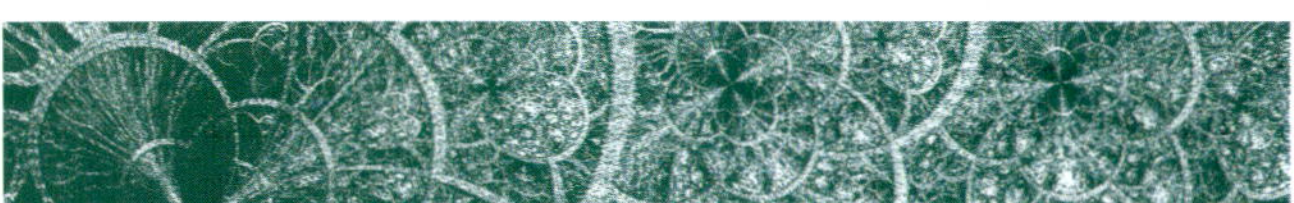

Nursing care

Health promotion

Nurses can help prevent oral mucositis by identifying people at risk and suggesting measures to reduce the likelihood that oral mucositis will develop. Educate and encourage all people to regularly perform mouth care, including teeth brushing and flossing. Written information sheets or posters that can be displayed in the person's bathroom outlining an oral care regimen, with symptoms that should be reported to clinicians, may promote compliance and reduce risk of oral mucositis occurring. Verify the person's understanding with return explanation and demonstration (Cancer Council, 2020).

Encourage people with ill-fitting dentures or other dental prostheses (such as partial plates) to see a qualified dentist or dental prosthetist. Suggest people taking an extended course of antibiotic therapy or who have impaired immune function consume yoghurt containing live bacterial cultures unless contraindicated. Discuss dietary modifications, such as limiting consumption of highly spiced or acidic foods and avoiding very hot beverages. A high-protein diet and increased oral fluids will assist in mucous membrane regeneration. People undergoing chemotherapy or radiation therapy should avoid use of alcohol and tobacco because these substances further damage oral mucosa, increasing the risk of oral mucositis.

Assessment

Oral assessment is important not only for people who have been diagnosed with oral mucositis but also for those with risk factors, manifestations or evidence of possible complications (e.g. recent weight loss).

MEDICATION ADMINISTRATION Medications used to treat oral mucositis based on patient's symptoms

TOPICAL ORAL ANAESTHETICS
Viscous lignocaine
Triamcinolone acetonide (Kenalog in Orabase®)
These drugs reduce the pain associated with mucous membrane lesions or oral mucositis. They provide temporary relief of pain.

Nursing responsibilities
- Instruct the person to seek medical attention for any oral lesion that does not heal within 1 week.
- Monitor for local hypersensitivity reactions and discontinue use if they occur.
- Instruct the person not to swallow the drug as it may impair the swallow reflex.

Health education for the person and family
- Apply every 1 to 2 hours as needed.
- Perform oral hygiene after meals and at bedtime.

TOPICAL ANTIFUNGAL AGENTS
Clotrimazole
Nystatin
These products help in the topical treatment of candidiasis. They are available in oral suspension or as lozenges. Their effects are primarily local rather than systemic.

Nursing responsibilities
- Instruct the person to dissolve lozenges in the mouth.
- Instruct the person to rinse mouth in a 'swishing' motion with oral suspension for at least 2 minutes and expectorate or swallow as directed.
- These medications are contraindicated in pregnancy.

Health education for the person and family
- Take medication as prescribed.
- Do not eat or drink 30 minutes after taking medication.
- Contact doctor if symptoms worsen.
- Perform good oral hygiene after meals and at bedtime; remove dentures at bedtime.

ANTIVIRAL AGENTS
Aciclovir (or acyclovir)
Valaciclovir
Aciclovir and valaciclovir are antiviral agents useful in the treatment of infections caused by the herpes simplex virus, which commonly causes cold sores, and herpes zoster virus, which causes shingles. They help reduce the severity and frequency of infections by interfering with the DNA synthesis of a virus.

Nursing responsibilities
- Start therapy as soon as herpetic lesions are noted.
- Administer with food or on an empty stomach.
- May be taken long term for prevention of further infections.

Health education for the person and family
- The virus remains latent and can recur during stressful events, fever, trauma, sunlight exposure and treatment with immunosuppressive drugs.
- Take the medication as ordered and contact the doctor if symptoms worsen.

- *Health history*: complaints of mouth pain, altered taste, dysphagia, lack of appetite, malaise; presence of dentures, regularity of dental care; current health status including chronic diseases; current medications; use of alcohol or tobacco.
- *Physical examination*: inspect lips, gums, teeth, interior cheeks, tongue and base of tongue, soft and hard palate; tonsils, oral pharynx and the amount of saliva. Observe and assess general health status including temperature and weight.
- *Diagnostic tests*: WBC, erythrocyte sedimentation rate (ESR), serum albumin.

Nursing diagnoses and interventions

Nursing care for the person with oral mucositis or oral mucositis focuses not only on the oral inflammation, but also on any underlying systemic diseases and the effects of the condition on the person's comfort and nutrition.

Impaired oral mucous membrane related to loss of integrity of oral mucous membrane

Regardless of cause, the pain and symptoms must be relieved to promote comfort as well as food and fluid intake.

- Assess and document oral mucous membranes and the character of any lesions every 4 to 8 hours. *Baseline and ongoing assessment data provide the basis for evaluation.* Teach the person or their caregiver to perform daily oral assessments in the outpatient setting and to report findings to clinicians as required.
- Assist with thorough mouth care after meals and at bedtime. Brush all tooth surfaces for at least 90 seconds twice daily with soft toothbrush and floss at least once daily. Allow toothbrush to air dry before storing. If unable to tolerate a toothbrush, offer sponge swabs. Avoid using alcohol-based mouthwashes or lemon-glycerin swabs as these may dry and irritate mucous membranes, causing pain and further tissue damage. *Providing bland rinses such as sodium bicarbonate and 0.9% sodium chloride after meals promotes comfort and reduces risk of infection (Cancer Council, 2020).*
- Assess knowledge and teach about condition, mouth care and treatments. Instruct to avoid alcohol, tobacco and spicy or irritating foods. *Knowledge promotes the person's participation in the plan of care and compliance. Alcohol, tobacco and hot, spicy or rough foods may injure the inflamed mucous membranes.*

Risk of imbalanced nutrition (less than body requirements) related to oral pain

Oral lesions and pain may limit oral intake, which may in turn lead to nutritional deficits. Anorexia and general malaise may also contribute to decreased intake.

- Assess food intake as well as the person's ability to chew and swallow. Weigh daily. Provide appropriate assistive devices such as straws or feeding syringes. *Adequate nutrition is essential for healing. Daily weights allow monitoring of the adequacy of food intake. Assistive devices may allow food intake while avoiding irritation of ulcerations or lesions.*

- Encourage a high-kilojoule, high-protein diet considerate of food preferences. Offer soft, lukewarm or cool foods or liquids, such as milkshakes, nutritional supplements, ice blocks and puddings, frequently in small amounts. Obtain nutritional consultation. *Oral intake may be limited and enriched foods and liquids enhance nutrition. A nutritional consultation can help ensure an adequate diet and assist in meeting nutritional needs.*
- Provide analgesics for pain relief as needed. *Significant pain associated with oral mucositis or oral mucositis can interfere with effective mouth care and food and fluid intake. Pain management is a vital part of nursing care.*

Community-based care

People with mild oral mucositis generally provide self-care. While people with cancer-treatment-related oral mucositis may require more aggressive therapy, the person and caregivers are often able to manage the regimen in home or community-based settings. Include the following topics in teaching for home care:

- management of underlying health conditions and ongoing treatments such as chemotherapy
- the recommended diet and oral hygiene regimen, including foods and substances to avoid (e.g. alcohol, tobacco products)
- nutritional supplements to help meet nutritional requirements
- prescribed medication, its route, side effects, frequency of administration and signs and symptoms to report
- the importance of completing the full course of antibiotic, antiviral or antifungal treatment
- manifestations to report and the importance of follow-up care.

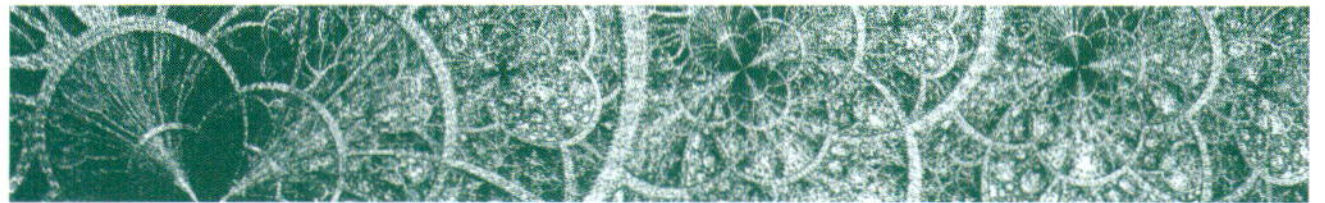

THE PERSON WITH ORAL CANCER

Head and neck cancers usually begin in squamous cells lining the inside of mouth, nose and throat. In Australia, head and neck cancer is one of the 10 most common cancers in both women and men (Cancer Australia, 2022a). Oral cancer, malignancy of the oral mucosa, may develop on the lips, tongue, floor of the mouth or other oral tissues. Oral cancer accounts for approximately 6.5% of all cancers diagnosed in Australia. It has, however, a high rate of morbidity and mortality. The stage of an oral cancer determines the prognosis, treatment and degree of disability. The primary risk factors for oral cancer are smoking, drinking alcohol, chewing tobacco and human papillomavirus (HPV). Marijuana use and occupational exposures to chemicals may also contribute to the risk of oral cancer.

Pathophysiology and manifestations

Oral cancer is usually a squamous cell carcinoma. Although a cancerous lesion can develop in any area of the mouth, the most common sites are the lower lip, tongue and floor of the mouth. Most early cancers present as inflamed areas with irregular, ill-defined borders. These lesions are not typically painful. More advanced cancers appear as deep ulcers that are fixed to deeper tissues. Early lesions involve the mucosa or submucosa, whereas more advanced tumours may invade and destroy underlying tissues, including muscles and bones of the face. Tumours frequently metastasise to regional lymph nodes. Other cancerous lesions, including lymphoma, malignant melanoma and Kaposi's sarcoma, may also develop in the mouth, although less frequently than squamous cell carcinoma.

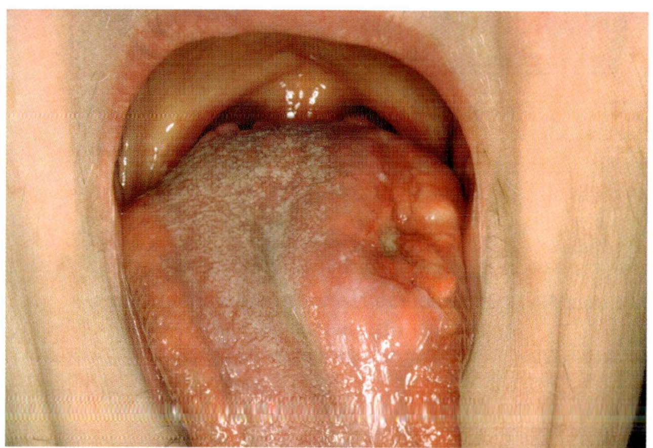

FIGURE 22.1 *Oral cancer*

Source: Mediscan/Alamy Stock Photo.

The person may be asymptomatic with oral cancer in the early stages and detection is through routine screening or referral when symptoms develop. The earliest symptom of oral cancer is a painless oral ulceration or lesion (see Figure 22.1). Later symptoms vary and may include mass lesions, difficulty in speaking, swallowing or chewing; loose teeth, ear ache, bleeding, swollen lymph nodes and sensory or motor nerve compromise. See the 'Manifestations' box for other manifestations of oral cancer. Any oral lesion that does not heal or respond to treatment within 1 to 2 weeks should be evaluated for malignancy.

MANIFESTATIONS Oral cancer

- White patches (leucoplakia)
- Red patches (erythroplakia)
- Ulcers
- Masses
- Pigmented areas (brownish or black)
- Fissures
- Asymmetry of the head, face, jaws or neck

INTERPROFESSIONAL CARE

The first component of treatment is eliminating any causative factors such as smoking, drinking alcohol or chewing tobacco. Tumour staging then determines therapy. The Tumour, Nodes, Metastasis (TNM) classification is used to stage oral cancer (see Box 22.2). A biopsy of the oral lesion allows direct visualisation of cells to determine the presence or absence of cancerous cells. Staging may require additional diagnostic studies such as computed tomography (CT) scans or magnetic resonance imaging (MRI).

BOX 22.2 Oral cancer staging

Stage 0	Carcinoma in situ
Stage I	Tumour ≤2 cm; no regional node involvement
Stage II	Tumour >2 cm to ≤4 cm; no regional node involvement
Stage III	Tumour ≤2 cm to >4 cm; one involved lymph node
Stage IVA & B	Tumour may invade adjacent structures; one or more nodes involved
Stage IVC	Distant metastasis present

Radiation and chemotherapy may be considered based on the person's age, tumour stage, general condition and preferences. Radiation therapy may be used preoperatively to 'shrink' the tumour or postoperatively to limit the risks of metastasis. Chemotherapy may be indicated depending on the stage of the tumour. See the chapter 'Nursing care of people with cancer' for more information about radiation and chemotherapy to treat cancer.

Following the biopsy and staging of the tumour, surgery is generally indicated, although an advanced or extensive tumour may be considered unresectable. If the tumour involves surrounding tissues, the cosmetic effects of surgery are important considerations. The goal of surgery is removal of the lesion and potentially cancerous surrounding tissue or lymph nodes. Advanced carcinomas may require extensive excision or a *radical neck dissection*, a potentially disfiguring procedure in which the lymph nodes and muscles of the neck are removed. A tracheostomy is sometimes performed at the time of surgery to maintain airway patency. The tracheostomy may be temporary but is often permanent. See the chapter 'Nursing care of people with upper respiratory disorders' for more information about caring for a person following radical neck dissection and a tracheostomy.

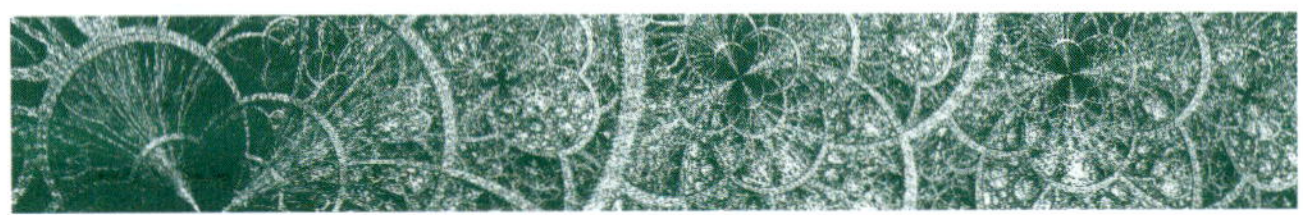

Nursing care

Health promotion

Reducing or eliminating tobacco use (smoking and smokeless tobacco) and excess alcohol consumption can significantly reduce the incidence of oral cancer. Teach children and adolescents about the dangers of using tobacco and alcohol. Emphasise the relationship between smokeless tobacco and oral cancer. Discuss strategies to deal with peer pressure to use tobacco and alcohol.

To promote early identification of and intervention for oral cancer, teach people about the risk factors for and manifestations of the disease. With the link between HPV and oral cancer, promoting vaccination against HPV should also be considered.

Assessment

Early precancerous oral lesions are very treatable. Unfortunately, these lesions usually are painless, so diagnosis and treatment often is delayed. Assess the oral cavity of all people, particularly those with risk factors for oral cancer.

- *Health history*: complaints of oral lesions that fail to heal; use (current or past) of tobacco products or excess alcohol.
- *Physical examination*: inspect and palpate lips and oral mucosa (including tongue and floor of mouth under the tongue) for tumours or lesions. Lesions may appear as velvety red or white patches that do not scrape off or as ulcers or areas of necrosis.

Nursing diagnoses and interventions

The mouth allows food ingestion and the lips are integral to verbal and non-verbal expression. The head, mouth and lips are important to self-perception and body image. Nursing diagnoses discussed in this section consider such problems as airway clearance, nutrition, communication and body image. See the accompanying nursing care plan.

Risk of ineffective airway clearance related to potential oral obstruction by the cancer

The location and the extent of an oral cancer and its excision may compromise the airway. Swelling of adjacent tissues, increased oral secretions or difficulty swallowing may contribute to respiratory distress. If extensive surgery is performed, a tracheostomy is usually performed to maintain airway patency.

CONSIDERATION FOR PRACTICE

In the initial postoperative period, assess airway patency and respiratory status at least hourly. A patent airway is vital to maintain respirations and oxygenation of tissues. Frequent assessment allows early identification of possible airway compromise.

- Unless contraindicated, place in high-Fowler's position, supporting arms. Assist the person to turn, cough and deep breathe at least every 2 to 4 hours. *High-Fowler's position promotes lung expansion. Turning, coughing and deep breathing help maintain a patent airway by preventing pooling of secretions.*
- Maintain adequate hydration (2,000 to 3,000 mL per day unless contraindicated) and humidity of inspired air. *Adequate hydration helps thin and loosen secretions.*

Risk of imbalanced nutrition (less than body requirements) related to inability to tolerate oral intake

Surgery affects oral food and fluid intake. Enteral feedings or total parenteral nutrition may be required. A gastrostomy tube usually is inserted during surgery to maintain nutrition. If an oral diet is permitted, anorexia or pain may affect intake.

- Weigh daily. Assess oral intake for adequacy of protein, kilojoules and nutrients. *Daily weights and nutritional assessments provide information about the adequacy of diet.*
- Offer soft, bland foods with supplements as indicated. Provide small, frequent feedings, making mealtimes pleasant. *Soft, bland foods may be better tolerated following oral surgery. Large meals may be overwhelming; small, frequent meals promote food and nutrient intake.*

NURSING CARE PLAN A person with oral cancer

Gavin Sandford, a married 44-year-old farmer, has two adult children. He and his wife grow and sell fruit and vegetables. Two months ago, Mr Sandford developed a sore on his tongue that would not heal. Mr Sandford tells his admission nurse, Sara Bucklin, 'The doctor says he will have to remove part of my tongue', and anxiously asks, 'Will I look the same? How will I be able to talk?'

ASSESSMENT

Mr Sandford's admission history reveals that he has been healthy but has smoked two packets of cigarettes a day for more than 20 years and usually drinks two to four beers per day. He admits to being anxious and fearful of surgery and its outcomes. He says he quit smoking and drinking 2 weeks ago. The biopsy report is positive for squamous cell carcinoma of the tongue. Mr Sandford has no enlarged cervical nodes and says he has no bloody sputum or saliva, difficulty swallowing, chewing or talking. His weight is in the normal range for his height. A wide excision of the oral lesion is planned.

DIAGNOSES

- *Risk of ineffective airway clearance* related to oral surgery.
- *Risk of imbalanced nutrition (less than body requirements)* related to oral surgery.
- *Impaired verbal communication* related to excision of a portion of the tongue.
- *Disturbed body image* related to surgical excision of the tongue.

PLANNING

- Teach the importance of activity, turning, coughing and deep breathing prior to the surgery.
- Encourage Mrs Sandford to visit at mealtimes to assist with and encourage oral intake.
- Demonstrate and allow practising using magic slate and flash cards prior to surgery.
- Arrange for a dietician review prior to surgery to assess energy needs and plan appropriate enteral feeding.
- Discuss the grief process with Mr Sandford and his family and encourage expression of feelings.

Expected outcomes

- Maintain a patent airway and remain free of respiratory distress.
- Maintain a stable weight and level of hydration.
- Effectively communicate with staff and family using a magic slate and flash cards.
- Communicate an increased ability to accept changes in body image.

IMPLEMENTATION

- Assess airway patency and respiratory status every hour until stable.
- Maintain semi-Fowler's position, supporting arms. Encourage to turn, cough and deep breathe every 2 to 4 hours.
- Monitor daily weights.
- Assess response to enteral feedings.
- Allow adequate time for communication efforts using magic slate and flash cards where necessary.
- Keep nurse call bell in reach at all times and answer promptly. Alert all staff of inability to respond verbally.
- Provide emotional support and encourage self-care and participation in decision making.

EVALUATION

At the time of discharge, Mr Sandford has maintained his weight and has started on oral liquids, including supplements and enriched liquids. His airway has remained clear and he is effectively coughing and deep breathing. He has used the magic slate to communicate throughout his hospital stay. He is regaining use of his tongue and can speak a few words. Although initially distressed, he is communicating an increased ability to cope with loss of part of his tongue. Mr Sandford and his wife say they understand his discharge instructions, including diet, activity, follow-up care and signs and symptoms to report.

CRITICAL THINKING IN THE NURSING PROCESS

1. What measures can you, as a nurse, implement to reduce the incidence of oral cancer?
2. Plan a health education program for young men who smoke.

REFLECTION ON THE NURSING PROCESS

1. Outline what you have learned from this case study that you will apply to your future practice.
2. Mr Sandford's wife calls you 2 weeks after discharge. She tells you that he refuses to try to talk and is relying on his magic slate to communicate. Reflect on how you will respond.

- Provide enteral feedings per gastrostomy tube as ordered. Elevate the head of the bed 30 to 45 degrees. *Enteral feedings maintain nutritional status in the person who is unable to consume foods orally. Elevating the head of the bed reduces the risk of regurgitation and aspiration of gastric contents.*
- Assess for gastric residual volume per facility protocol for the type of feeding (intermittent or continuous). See the 'Translation to practice' box. Notify the doctor of volumes greater than 200 mL or 50% of previous feeding if feeding is intermittent. *Excess residual volume may increase the risk of aspiration.*
- Consider a nutritional consultation to assess diet and plan appropriate supplements. *A registered dietitian can calculate energy requirements and develop an individualised diet plan to meet nutritional requirements.*

Impaired verbal communication

Oral surgery can interfere with communication. Effective communication is vital to postoperative recovery and prevention of complications.

- Before surgery, establish and practise a communication plan such as using a sketch pad or flash cards. *Practising communication techniques reduces fear and anxiety while promoting communication.*

- Provide ample time for communication efforts and do not answer for the person. Be alert for non-verbal communications. Use yes/no questions and simple phrases. *Providing adequate time allows the person opportunity to express ideas and thoughts. Non-verbal communication provides cues regarding comfort or other needs. Simple yes/no questions are easily answered non-verbally.*
- If indicated, refer to or consult with a speech therapist. *A speech therapist can help promote or restore effective communication.*

Disturbed body image

Radical surgery of the head or neck seriously affects body image. An altered speech pattern and any disfigurement affect the person's ability to feel attractive or effective in work or social roles. People may defer lifesaving surgery to postpone disfiguring interventions or therapies.

CONSIDERATION FOR PRACTICE

Provide a nurse call bell by the bedside and respond promptly. Make all staff aware that the person cannot verbally respond. Non-verbal people rely on nurse call bells to summon help. Answering promptly reduces fear and anxiety and maintains safety.

- Assess coping style, self-perception and responses to altered appearance or function. *This information can be used to identify appropriate interventions and care.*
- Encourage verbalisation of feelings regarding perceived and actual changes. *Non-judgmental acceptance of feelings and fears helps establish trust.*
- Provide emotional support, encourage self-care and provide decision-making opportunities. *Self-care promotes self-acceptance and independence. Giving choices empowers the person to participate in care.*

Community-based care

Discharge planning for the person with oral cancer depends on the type of treatment planned and surgery performed. Depending on the person's age, condition and availability of support systems, referral to community healthcare agencies may be an essential component of care. Visits from home health nurses can assist in meeting healthcare needs.

Discuss the following topics with the person and their family members or care providers:

- diagnosis and prescribed care
- monitoring for new lesions or recurrences
- diet, nutrition and activity
- pain management
- airway management, care of incision and signs and symptoms to report.

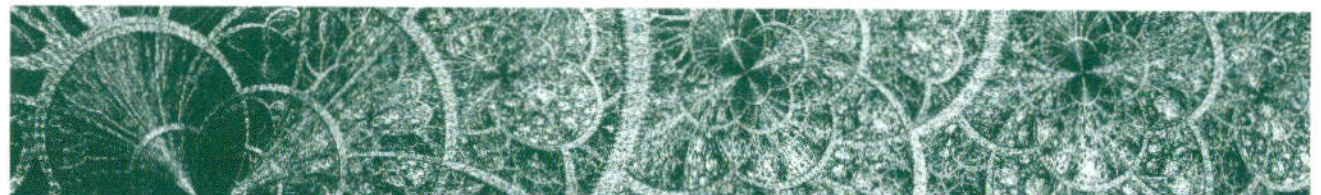

TRANSLATION TO PRACTICE Evidence-based practice for people with enteral feeding tubes

Practices and protocols for caring for enterally fed people and for assessing gastric residual volume have previously been inconsistent. Current recommendations include providing good oral hygiene, elevating the head of the bed 30–45 degrees, administering prokinetic agents such as metoclopramide where indicated, providing continuous feeds, administering the feeds directly to the small bowel via a gastrostomy tube and assessing gastric residual volumes regularly (Joanna Briggs Institute (JBI), 2022).

Gastric residual volumes have been used to determine aspiration risk; when the volume exceeds a predetermined level the tube feed is then withheld. Researchers have come to varying conclusions about the amount of residual volume that is considered safe and does not increase the risk of aspiration. Recent research advocates limits of 200–500 mL as saliva and gastric secretions need to be included in the volume as well as the tube feed (Porritt, 2021). In addition, the withholding of enteral feed should be influenced by assessment of the person. Feelings of fullness, nausea, vomiting, abdominal discomfort or distension indicate when the enteral feed should be withheld (Porritt, 2021).

IMPLICATIONS FOR NURSING

Gastric motility slows following surgery or trauma, in diabetes, sepsis or electrolyte imbalance, and with medications such as narcotic analgesics. Excessive gastric distension may increase the risk of aspiration of gastric contents; however, when enteral feeds are withheld unnecessarily, the nutritional status of the person is at risk. Impaired nutrition affects healing and recovery and may prolong the person's hospital stay. Therefore, it is recommended that a clinical pathway or algorithm is developed which reflects current practice guidelines and is institution-specific to guide nurses with decision making regarding the withholding of feeds (JBI, 2022).

CRITICAL THINKING IN PERSON-CENTRED CARE

1. Which factors might influence the accuracy of residual volume measurements? Which measures can be taken to obtain accurate measurements?
2. What would be the effect of withholding one bolus feeding of 240 mL of a standard enteral formula? If this is repeated daily for a week, what is the cumulative effect?
3. One reason frequently cited for avoiding checking residual volume is the risk of plugging the feeding tube. Identify measures to prevent this potential problem.

Disorders of the oesophagus

The oesophagus plays an essential role in the ingestion of food and liquids. Disorders of the oesophagus can be inflammatory, mechanical or cancerous. Because of its location and neighbouring organs, the symptoms of oesophageal disorders may mimic those of a variety of other illnesses.

THE PERSON WITH GASTRO-OESOPHAGEAL REFLUX DISEASE

Gastro-oesophageal reflux is the backward flowing of gastric contents into the oesophagus. When this occurs, the person experiences heartburn. Many people with gastro-oesophageal reflux have few symptoms, while others develop inflammatory oesophagitis as a result of exposure to gastric juices. **Gastro-oesophageal reflux disease (GORD)** is a common gastrointestinal disorder.

FAST FACTS

- GORD affects up to 10–20% of people in Western countries.
- GORD is increasing in prevalence in Australia (Burton et al., 2020).

Pathophysiology

Normally, the lower oesophageal sphincter (LOS) remains closed except during swallowing. Reflux (backflow) of gastric contents into the oesophagus is prevented by pressure differences between the stomach and the lower oesophagus. The diaphragm, the LOS and the location of the gastro-oesophageal junction below the diaphragm help maintain this pressure difference (see Figure 22.2).

Gastro-oesophageal reflux may result from transient relaxation of the LOS, an incompetent LOS and/or increased pressure within the stomach (see Figure 22.3). Factors contributing to gastro-oesophageal reflux include increased gastric volume (e.g. after meals), positioning that allows gastric contents to remain close to the gastro-oesophageal junction (e.g. bending over, lying down) and increased gastric pressure (e.g. obesity, pregnancy or wearing tight clothing). A hiatal hernia may contribute to GORD.

Gastric juices contain acid, pepsin and bile, which are corrosive substances. Oesophageal peristalsis and bicarbonate in salivary secretions normally clear and neutralise gastric juices in the oesophagus. During sleep, however, and in people with impaired oesophageal peristalsis or salivation, the oesophageal mucosa is damaged by gastric juices, causing an inflammatory response. With prolonged exposure, oesophagitis develops. Superficial ulcers develop and the mucosa becomes red, friable and may bleed. If untreated, scarring and oesophageal stricture may develop.

Manifestations

GORD causes burning, retrosternal pain which may radiate to the jaw or other areas of the chest. These symptoms can be confused with cardiac pain and therefore thorough

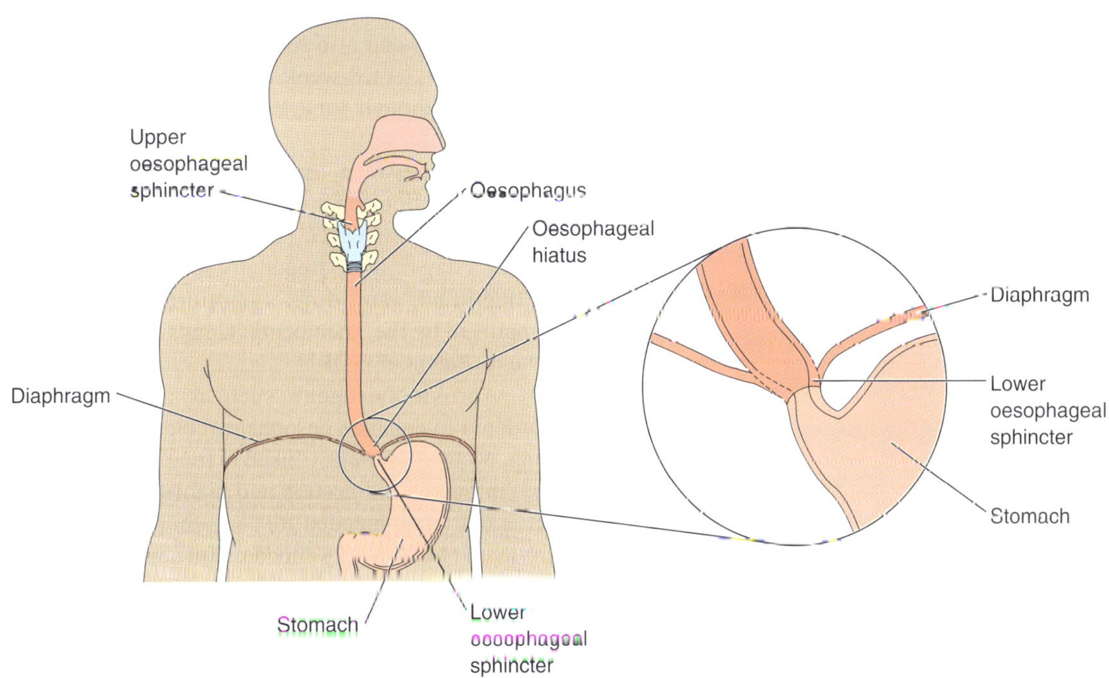

FIGURE 22.2 *The oesophagus. The inset shows a closer view of the lower oesophageal sphincter*

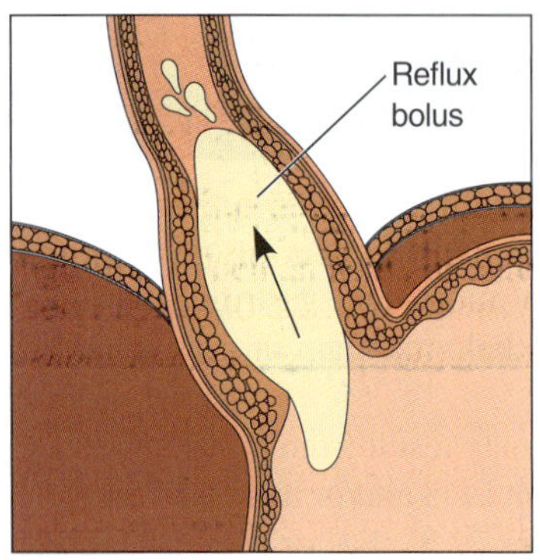

Transient lower oesophageal sphincter relaxation

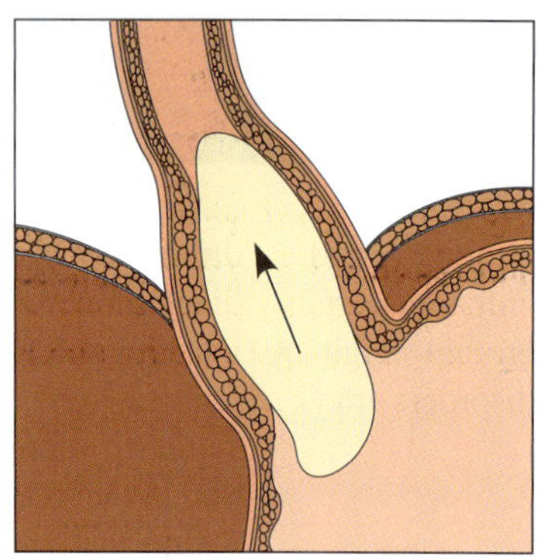
Incompetent lower oesophageal sphincter

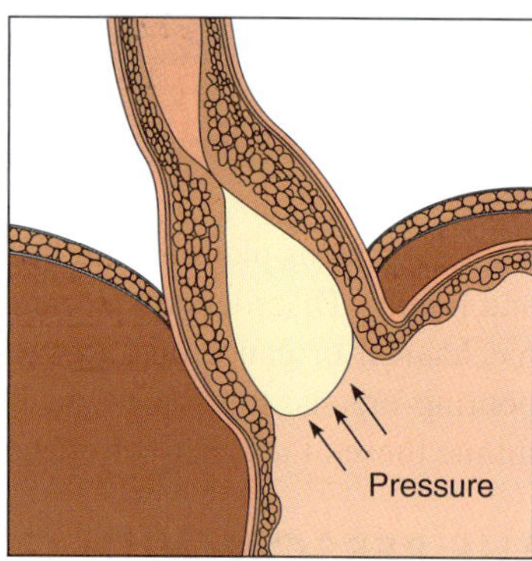

Increased intragastric pressure

FIGURE 22.3 ***Mechanisms of gastro-oesophageal reflux***

assessment, the person's history and investigations are necessary. Regurgitation, or reflux, also occurs in GORD causing gastric acid to enter into the throat leaving a metallic, bitter taste in the mouth. The gastric acid may also irritate the airways, causing the person to develop a chronic cough, or exacerbation of their asthma or chronic obstructive pulmonary disease (Burton et al., 2020).

Complications of GORD include oesophagitis, oesophageal ulcer, peptic stricture, haemorrhage, Barrett's oesophagus and oesophageal cancer. Both symptoms and complications of GORD lead to significant lifestyle disruptions including sleep disturbance, impaired ability to concentrate and inability to undertake physical or social activities (Burton et al., 2020).

INTERPROFESSIONAL CARE

Often the diagnosis of GORD is made by the history of symptoms and predisposing factors. Interprofessional care focuses on lifestyle changes, diet modification and, for more severe cases, drug therapy. Surgery is reserved for people who develop serious complications.

Diagnosis

Diagnostic tests that may be ordered for people with manifestations of GORD include:

- *Barium swallow* to evaluate the oesophagus, stomach and upper small intestine.
- *Upper endoscopy* to permit direct visualisation of the oesophagus. Tissue may be obtained for biopsy to establish the diagnosis and rule out malignancy. See the chapter 'A person-centred approach to assessing the gastrointestinal system' for nursing care of the person undergoing an upper endoscopy.
- *24-hour ambulatory pH monitoring* may be performed to establish the diagnosis of GORD. For this test, a small tube with a pH electrode is inserted through the nose into the oesophagus. The electrode is attached to a small box worn on the belt that records the data. The data are later analysed by computer.
- *Oesophageal manometry* measures pressures of the oesophageal sphincters and oesophageal peristalsis.

Medications

Antacids such as Mylanta® relieve mild or moderate symptoms by neutralising stomach acid. Gaviscon®, which forms a floating barrier between the gastric contents and the oesophageal mucosa when the person is upright, may also be used.

Omeprazole (Losec), lansoprazole (Zoton), pantoprazole (Somac) and esomeprazole (Nexium) are proton-pump inhibitors (PPIs) that reduce gastric secretions. PPIs are the first-line pharmacological treatment as they promote healing of erosive oesophagitis and also relieve symptoms (Miller, Wong & Pollack, 2015). An 8-week course of treatment is initially prescribed, although some people may require 3 to 6 months of therapy.

Histamine$_2$-receptor (H_2-receptor) blockers reduce gastric acid production and are effective in treating GORD symptoms. When treating GORD, H_2-receptor blockers are usually given twice a day or more frequently for a prolonged period of time. Cimetidine, ranitidine, famotidine and nizatidine are all approved by the Therapeutic Goods Administration (TGA) for the treatment of GORD.

A prokinetic agent, such as metoclopramide, may be ordered to enhance oesophageal clearance and gastric emptying. Metoclopramide is used to treat people with regurgitation, symptoms of indigestion and night-time symptoms. However, it is not recommended for long-time use due to unfavourable side effects and only modest efficacy for symptom relief and healing (Miller et al., 2015). See the 'Medication administration' box for the nursing implications of drugs used to treat GORD.

MEDICATION ADMINISTRATION **Medications used to treat GORD, gastritis and peptic ulcer disease**

PROTON-PUMP INHIBITORS
Esomeprazole
Lansoprazole
Omeprazole
Pantoprazole
Rabeprazole
Proton-pump inhibitors are the drugs of choice for GORD. PPIs inhibit the hydrogen–potassium–ATP pump, reducing gastric acid secretion. Initially, the PPI may be given twice a day, with the dose reduced to once daily (at bedtime) after 8 weeks.

Nursing responsibilities
- Administer before breakfast and at bedtime if ordered twice a day; at bedtime if once a day.
- Do not crush tablets.
- Monitor liver function tests for possible abnormal values, including increased AST, ALT, alkaline phosphatase and bilirubin levels.

Health education for the person and family
- Take the medication as ordered for the full course of therapy, even if symptoms are relieved.
- Do not crush, break or chew tablets.
- Avoid cigarette smoking, alcohol, aspirin and NSAIDs while taking this drug because these substances may interfere with healing.
- Report black tarry stools, diarrhoea or abdominal pain to your primary care provider.

H_2-RECEPTOR BLOCKERS
Cimetidine
Ranitidine
Famotidine
Nizatidine
H_2-receptor blockers reduce acidity of gastric juices by blocking the ability of histamine to stimulate acid secretion by the gastric parietal cells. As a result, both the volume and concentration of hydrochloric acid in gastric juice are reduced. H_2-receptor blockers are given orally or intravenously. Both prescription and over-the-counter preparations are available.

Nursing responsibilities
- To ensure absorption, do not give an antacid within 1 hour before or after giving an H_2-receptor blocker.
- When administered intravenously, do not mix with other drugs. Administer in 20 to 100 mL of solution over 15 to 30 minutes. Rapid intravenous injection as a bolus may cause arrhythmias and hypotension.
- Monitor for interaction with such drugs as oral anticoagulants, beta-blockers, benzodiazepines, tricyclic antidepressants and others. H_2-receptor blockers may inhibit the metabolism of other drugs, increasing the risk of toxicity.

Health education for the person and family
- Take the medication as directed, even if pain and gastric discomfort are relieved early in the course of therapy.
- Take at bedtime if once-a-day dosing is ordered. If spaced through the day, take before meals. Avoid taking antacids for 1 hour before and 1 hour after taking this drug.
- To promote healing, avoid cigarette smoking (which increases gastric acid secretion) and gastric mucosal irritants such as alcohol, aspirin and NSAIDs.
- Long-term use of these drugs can lead to gynaecomastia (breast enlargement) and impotence in men, and breast tenderness in women. Discontinuing the drug will reverse these effects.
- Report adverse effects such as diarrhoea, confusion, rash, fatigue, malaise or bruising to your care provider.

ANTI-ULCER AGENT
Sucralfate
Sucralfate reacts with gastric acid to form a thick paste that adheres to damaged gastric mucosal tissue. It protects gastric mucosa and promotes healing through this local action.

Nursing responsibilities
- Administer on an empty stomach, 1 hour before meals and at bedtime.
- Do not crush tablets.
- Separate administration time from antacids by at least 30 minutes.

Health education for the person and family
- Take as directed, even after symptoms have been relieved.
- Do not crush or chew tablets; shake suspension well.
- Increase your intake of fluids and dietary fibre to prevent constipation.

ANTACIDS
Gaviscon®
Gelusil
Gastrogel
Mylanta®
Antacids buffer or neutralise gastric acid, usually acting locally. Antacids are used in GORD, gastritis and peptic ulcer disease to relieve pain and prevent further damage to oesophageal and gastric mucosa.

Nursing responsibilities
- Antacids interfere with the absorption of many drugs given orally; separate administration times by at least 2 hours.
- Monitor for constipation or diarrhoea resulting from antacid therapy. Notify the doctor should either develop; a different antacid may be ordered.
- Although most antacids have little systemic effect, electrolyte imbalances can develop. Monitor serum electrolytes, particularly sodium, calcium and magnesium levels.

Health education for the person and family
- Take your antacid frequently as prescribed, 1 to 3 hours after meals and at bedtime. To be effective, the antacid must be in your stomach.
- Avoid taking an antacid for approximately 2 hours before and 1 hour after taking another medication.
- Shake suspensions well prior to administration.
- Chew tablets thoroughly and follow with a glass of water.
- Report worsening symptoms, diarrhoea or constipation to your primary care provider.
- Continue taking the antacid for the duration prescribed. Although pain and discomfort often are relieved soon after treatment begins, healing takes 6 to 8 weeks.

(continued)

MEDICATION ADMINISTRATION **Medications used to treat GORD, gastritis and peptic ulcer disease (continued)**

PROKINETIC AGENT

Metoclopramide

By acting on the central nervous system, metoclopramide stimulates upper gastrointestinal motility and gastric emptying. As a result, nausea, vomiting and symptoms of GORD are reduced.

Nursing implications

- Do not administer metoclopramide to children or to people with possible gastrointestinal obstruction or bleeding, or a history of seizure disorders, pheochromocytoma or Parkinson's disease.
- Monitor for extrapyramidal side effects (e.g. difficulty speaking or swallowing, loss of balance, gait disruptions, twitching or twisting movements, weakness of arms or legs) or manifestations of tardive dyskinesia (uncontrolled rhythmic facial movement, lip smacking, tongue rolling). Report immediately.
- Give oral doses 30 minutes before meals and at bedtime.
- May be given by direct intravenous push over 1 to 2 minutes.

Health education for the person and family

- Take this drug as directed. If you miss a dose, take as soon as you remember unless it is close to the time for the next dose.
- Do not drive or engage in other activities that require alertness if this drug makes you drowsy.
- Avoid using alcohol or other CNS depressants while you are taking this drug.
- Immediately contact your healthcare provider if you develop involuntary movements of your eyes, face or limbs.

Nutrition and lifestyle management

GORD is a chronic condition. Dietary and lifestyle changes are important to reduce symptoms and long-term effects of the disorder. Contributing factors to GORD include obesity, smoking, alcohol and certain foods, and therefore lifestyle interventions are an essential adjunct to pharmacological therapy for GORD (Whiteman & Kendall, 2016). Dietary modifications such as the avoidance of acidic or fatty foods, avoiding large meals and waiting 2 hours after dinner before going to bed may be beneficial; however, there is limited clinical evidence to support this (Miller et al., 2015). Smoking cessation, alcohol avoidance, stress reduction, weight loss and elevating the head of the bed are recommended for symptom relief (Miller et al., 2015).

Surgery

Surgery may be used for people who do not respond to pharmacological and lifestyle management. Antireflux surgeries increase pressure in the lower oesophagus, inhibiting gastric content reflux. Laparoscopic fundoplication, a procedure in which the gastric fundus is wrapped around the distal oesophagus, is the treatment of choice for GORD. An open surgical procedure known as Nissen fundoplication may also be done (see Figure 22.4). Other laparoscopic procedures to tighten the LOS may include use of an endoscopic suturing system or burning spots on the muscle surrounding the sphincter to create scar tissue. Surgery or ablation therapy also is recommended to reduce the risk of oesophageal cancer in people with persistent cell changes in the distal oesophagus.

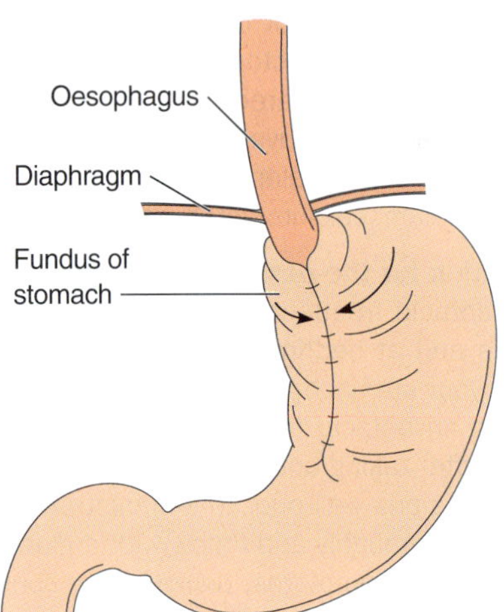

FIGURE 22.4 *Nissen fundoplication. The fundus of the stomach is wrapped around the lower oesophagus and the edges are sutured together*

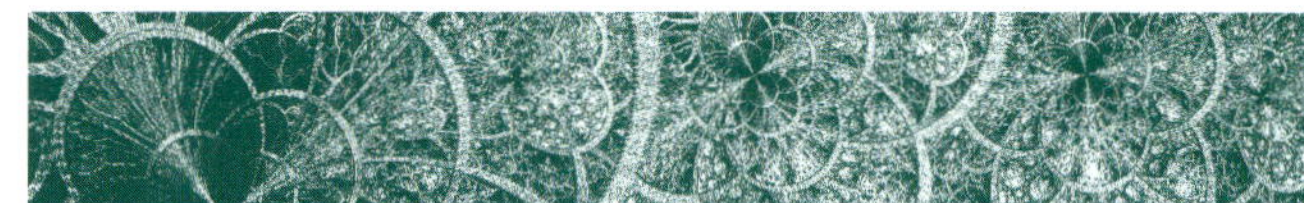

Nursing care

Assessment

Assessment data related to GORD include the following:

- *Health history*: manifestations such as frequent heartburn; intolerance of foods that are acidic, spicy or fatty; regurgitation of acidic gastric juice; increased symptoms when bending over, lying down or wearing tight clothing; difficulty swallowing.
- *Physical assessment*: epigastric tenderness, weight.

Nursing diagnoses and interventions

Relieving the discomfort associated with GORD is the priority of nursing care. Education focuses on preventing symptoms and long-term consequences of the disorder.

Pain related to reflux

The epigastric pain associated with GORD can be severe, interfering with rest and causing anxiety.

- Provide small, frequent meals. Restrict intake of fat, acidic foods, coffee and alcohol. *Limiting the size of meals reduces pressure in the stomach, reducing oesophageal reflux. Fatty, acidic foods, coffee and alcohol increase gastric acidity and interfere with gastric emptying, increasing the incidence of gastro-oesophageal reflux.*

- Encourage the person to consider stopping smoking. Refer to a smoking cessation clinic or program as needed. *Cigarette smoking increases gastric acidity and interferes with healing of damaged mucosa.*
- Administer antacids, H_2-receptor blockers and PPIs as ordered. Instruct the person to continue therapy as prescribed, even after symptoms have been relieved. *These medications neutralise or reduce gastric acid secretion, relieving symptoms and promoting healing.*
- Discuss the long-term nature of GORD and its management. *Lifestyle changes need to be continued after healing and symptom relief to manage the long-term effects of GORD.*

Community-based care

GORD is a lifelong condition best managed by the person. Teach the person and family about continuing management strategies which may be of benefit, including dietary changes, remaining upright after meals and avoiding eating for at least 2 hours before bedtime. Suggest elevating the head of the bed on 15 to 20 cm wooden blocks placed under the legs. Discuss the need for continued gastric acid reduction using antacids, H_2-receptor blockers or PPIs. All are effective to reduce the acidity of gastric juices. Antacids, the most cost-effective measure, require frequent doses to neutralise gastric acid. H_2-receptor blockers, also available over the counter, are a cost-effective management strategy that requires only twice-a-day dosing.

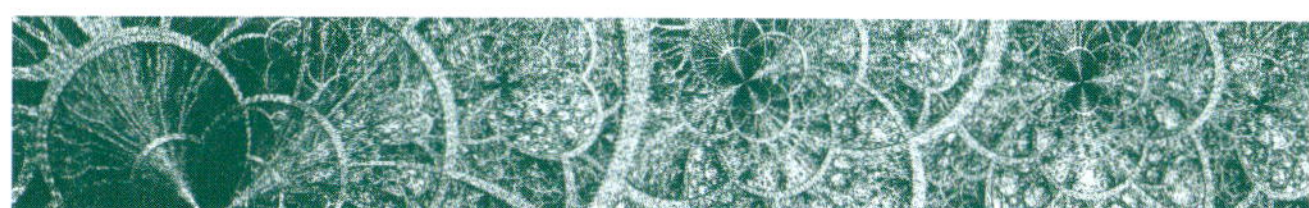

THE PERSON WITH A HIATAL HERNIA

A **hiatal hernia** occurs when part of the stomach protrudes through the oesophageal hiatus of the diaphragm into the thoracic cavity. Although hiatal hernia is thought to be a common problem, most affected individuals are asymptomatic. The incidence of hiatal hernia increases with age.

In a *sliding hiatal hernia*, the gastro-oesophageal junction and the fundus of the stomach slide upward through the oesophageal hiatus (see Figure 22.5A). Several factors may contribute to a sliding hiatal hernia, including weakened gastro-oesophageal diaphragmatic anchors, shortening of the oesophagus or increased intra-abdominal pressure. Small sliding hiatal hernias produce few symptoms.

In a *paraoesophageal hiatal hernia*, the junction between the oesophagus and stomach remains in its normal position below the diaphragm while a part of the stomach herniates through the oesophageal hiatus (see Figure 22.5B). A paraoesophageal hernia can become incarcerated (constricted) and strangulate, impairing blood flow to the herniated tissue. People with paraoesophageal hernia may develop gastritis or chronic or acute gastrointestinal bleeding. See the 'Manifestations' box.

A barium swallow or an upper endoscopy may be done to diagnose hiatal hernia. Many people with hiatal hernia require no treatment. If symptoms are present, treatment

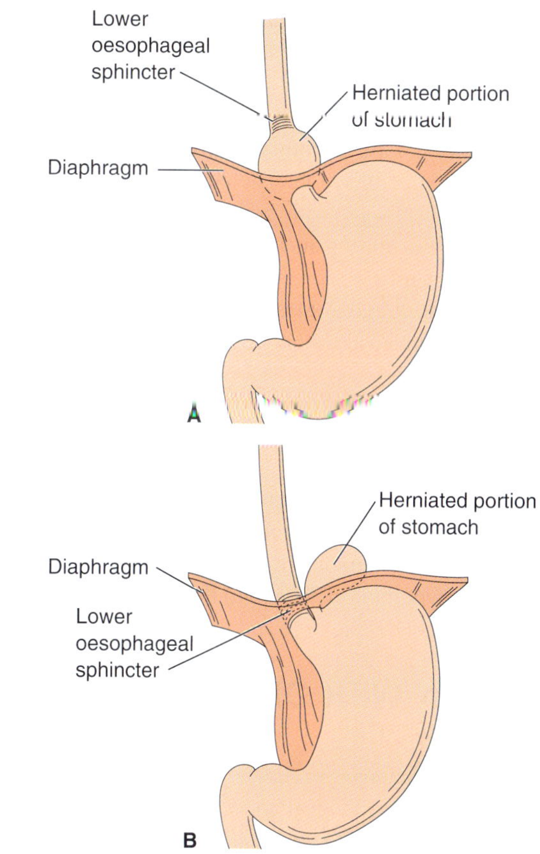

FIGURE 22.5 ***Hiatal hernias. A, Sliding hiatal hernia. B, Paraoesophageal hiatal hernia***

MANIFESTATIONS Hiatal hernia

- Reflux, heartburn
- Feeling of fullness
- Substernal chest pain
- Dysphagia
- Occult bleeding
- Belching, indigestion

measures such as those for people with GORD may be ordered. If medical management is ineffective or the hernia becomes incarcerated, surgery may be required. The most common surgical procedure is the Nissen fundoplication (see Figure 22.4). This surgery, which may be done laparoscopically, prevents the gastro-oesophageal junction from slipping into the thoracic cavity.

Nursing care for the person with a hiatal hernia is similar to that for the person with GORD. If surgery is performed, nursing care is similar to that for people undergoing gastric or thoracic surgery (see the chapter 'Nursing care of people having surgery').

THE PERSON WITH IMPAIRED OESOPHAGEAL MOTILITY

Disorders of oesophageal motility can cause **dysphagia** (difficult or painful swallowing) or chest pain. It is estimated that nearly 75% of people hospitalised with stroke experience dysphagia.

Neurological disorders such as Parkinson's disease, motor neurone disease and Alzheimer's disease also can cause dysphagia.

Primary disorders of swallowing are less common. **Achalasia**, a disorder of unknown aetiology, is characterised by impaired peristalsis of the smooth muscle of the oesophagus and impaired relaxation of the LOS. The person experiences gradually increasing dysphagia with both solid foods and liquids. Fullness in the chest during meals, chest pain and night-time cough are additional manifestations. Other people may experience **diffuse oesophageal spasm** that causes non-peristaltic contraction of oesophageal smooth muscle. This disorder causes chest pain and/or dysphagia. The chest pain can be severe and usually occurs at rest.

Treatment of achalasia may include endoscopically guided injection of botulinum toxin into the LOS or balloon dilation of the LOS. Botulinum toxin injection lowers LOS pressure but may need to be repeated every 6 to 9 months. Balloon dilation tears muscle fibres in the LOS, reducing its pressure (see Figure 22.6). A laparoscopic myotomy (incision into the circular muscle layer of the LOS) also reduces pressure and relieves symptoms.

THE PERSON WITH OESOPHAGEAL CANCER

Cancer of the oesophagus is a relatively uncommon malignancy in Australia. Most oesophageal cancers commence where the lower oesophagus meets the stomach. If oesophageal cancer is not diagnosed and treated early, it invades nearby structures and metastases in other parts of the body, such as the liver (Cancer Australia, 2022b).

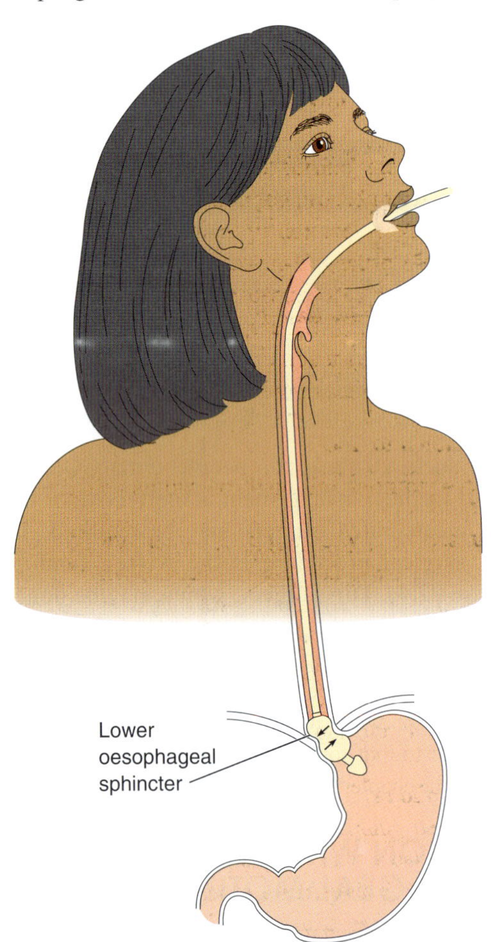

FIGURE 22.6 ***Balloon dilation of the lower oesophageal sphincter***

Pathophysiology

There are two types of oesophageal tumours: adenocarcinoma and squamous cell carcinoma. Cigarette smoking and chronic alcohol use are strong risk factors for squamous cell oesophageal tumours in Western countries. In Asian countries, chewing betel nuts and eating certain pickled vegetables are risk factors.

Adenocarcinoma has been linked to obesity, GORD and Barrett's oesophagus. Combining any of these comorbidities with tobacco use further increases the risk of oesophageal cancer developing (Cancer Australia, 2022b). Box 22.3 lists major identified risk factors for oesophageal cancer.

BOX 22.3 Risk factors for oesophageal cancer

- Excess alcohol consumption
- Cigarette smoking
- Ingested carcinogens such as nitrates and industrial chemicals
- Smoked opiates
- Physical mucosal damage (e.g. lye ingestion, radiation damage, chronic achalasia)
- Congenital disorders
- Chronic gastric reflux
- Obesity

Only about 15% of oesophageal tumours develop in the upper portion of the oesophagus; about 35% develop in the mid portion. The lower third of the oesophagus is the most common site, accounting for about 50% of tumours. Adenocarcinomas tend to develop in dysplastic (abnormal) columnar epithelium in the distal oesophagus. They are commonly associated with Barrett's oesophagus, a possible complication of chronic GORD and achalasia.

The disease usually spreads to adjacent and supraclavicular lymph nodes, the liver, lungs and the pleura.

Manifestations

Dysphagia is the most common symptom of oesophageal carcinoma, typically accompanied by weight loss (Cancer Australia, 2022b). Other manifestations are listed in the 'Manifestations' box.

MANIFESTATIONS Oesophageal cancer

- Dysphagia
- Anaemia
- Unintentional weight loss
- GORD-like symptoms
- Regurgitation
- Anorexia
- Chest pain
- Persistent cough
- Hoarseness
- Vomiting blood
- Black or bloody stools

Tracheoesophageal fistulas may develop as the disease progresses, leading to aspiration, pneumonia and shortness of breath. Paraneoplastic symptoms such as hypercalcaemia also may accompany advanced oesophageal cancer.

INTERPROFESSIONAL CARE

Controlling dysphagia and maintaining nutritional status are essential goals of therapy for people with oesophageal cancer, regardless of the stage of the disease. Treatment may involve surgery, radiation therapy and/or chemotherapy.

Diagnosis

Diagnostic and staging procedures for oesophageal cancer may include endoscopy, bronchoscopy and scans to detect metastasis. The following diagnostic tests may be performed (see the chapter 'A person-centred approach to assessing the gastrointestinal system'):

- *Barium swallow* to identify irregular mucosal patterns or narrowing of the lumen, which suggest oesophageal cancer.
- *Upper endoscopy* to allow direct visualisation of the tumour and obtain tissue for biopsy.
- *Chest x-ray*, *CT scans* or *MRI* to identify possible tumour metastases to other organs or tissues.
- *Full blood count (FBC)* may indicate anaemia due to chronic blood loss. *Serum albumin* levels may be low due to malnutrition and liver function tests (*ALT*, *alkaline phosphatase*, *AST* and *bilirubin*) are elevated if liver metastases are present.

Treatments

The treatment of oesophageal cancer depends on the stage of the disease, as well as factors such as the person's condition and preference.

People with early oesophageal cancer usually are treated with surgery alone. Surgery involves resection of the affected portion of the oesophagus (*oesophagectomy*) and possible anastomosis of the stomach to the remaining oesophagus. Mediastinal lymph nodes may be resected at the time of surgery. Oesophagectomy is not without risk; potential surgical complications include anastomosis leak, respiratory complications such as pneumonia or acute respiratory distress syndrome, gastric necrosis or bleeding, cardiac arrhythmias, and infection and sepsis. Postoperative recovery is usually in the intensive care unit (ICU) for 12 days before transfer to a surgical ward (Low et al., 2019).

Other approaches to early oesophageal cancer include combined radiation and chemotherapy or radiation therapy or chemotherapy alone prior to surgical resection of the tumour. Although the prognosis of oesophageal cancer is poor, current evidence suggests significant benefit from preoperative chemotherapy or chemoradiotherapy prior to resection of local, operable cancer. However, more research in this area is needed.

When the tumour is too advanced or if surgery is considered too risky, palliative measures such as brachytherapy, chemotherapy and oesophageal stenting may be considered (Low et al., 2019). Approximately 50% of people with oesophageal cancer are considered incurable at time of diagnosis; therefore, palliative treatments focus on maintaining good quality of life through relief of dysphagia, providing nutritional support, administering pain relief and offering psychological support (Low et al., 2019).

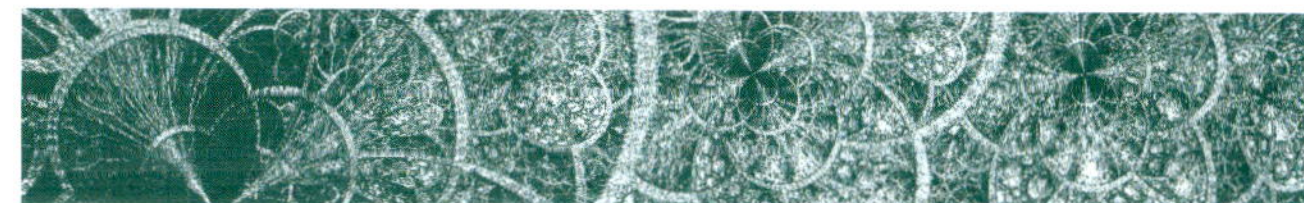

Nursing care

Health promotion

Health promotion measures to reduce the risk and incidence of oesophageal cancer include educating people (especially young people) about the dangers of cigarette smoking and excess alcohol use. Refer to smoking cessation and alcohol treatment programs as indicated. Educate people with GORD about the relationship between chronic damage to the oesophagus due to reflux and oesophageal cancer, and stress the importance of effective disease management.

Assessment

Early diagnosis and treatment of oesophageal cancer can make a difference in the person's prognosis. Collect the following assessment data related to oesophageal cancer:

- *Health history*: current symptoms such as chest pain, dysphagia, odynophagia (pain with swallowing), coughing or hoarseness; duration of symptoms; recent weight loss; smoking history; current and past patterns of alcohol consumption.
- *Physical examination*: weight; general health status; skin colour; supraclavicular and cervical lymph nodes for lymphadenopathy.

Nursing diagnoses and interventions

Disruption of the integrity and function of the oesophagus and the discomfort associated with swallowing in people with oesophageal cancer affect the person's ability to maintain adequate nutritional status and, potentially, a patent airway.

Risk of imbalanced nutrition (less than body requirements) related to dysphagia

The person diagnosed with oesophageal cancer may already suffer from some degree of malnutrition because of difficulty and pain with swallowing. Enteral nutrition via nasogastric feeding tube or gastrostomy tube or parenteral nutrition maintains nutritional status after surgery or if the tumour is inoperable and obstruction occurs. See the chapter 'Nursing care of people with nutritional disorders' for nursing interventions related to enteral and parenteral feedings.

Risk of ineffective airway clearance due to surgery

After surgery for oesophageal cancer, the person is at high risk of aspiration and difficulty maintaining a patent airway due to disruption of the oesophagus and incision into the thoracic cavity.

- Assess mental and respiratory status (including rate, depth, breath sounds and oxygen saturation levels) at least every hour during the initial postoperative period. *Altered mental status increases the risk of aspiration. An increased respiratory rate, dyspnoea, diminished breath sounds or decreased oxygen saturation levels may indicate impaired airway clearance or possible aspiration pneumonia.*
- Provide aggressive pulmonary hygiene measures, including endotracheal suctioning and chest physiotherapy as indicated or ordered. Following extubation, encourage frequent coughing, deep breathing and use of the incentive spirometer. *Respiratory complications are a frequent complication of oesophagectomy. Aggressive nursing care helps mobilise secretions and prevent atelectasis and possible pneumonia.*
- If present, monitor chest tube function and drainage. Promptly report drainage that is bright red and excessive in amount (> 70 mL/hour) or purulent. Maintain patency of chest tubes as per unit protocol or doctor's order. If a thoracic incision has been used, chest tubes are placed to promote lung reinflation. *Proper chest tube function is necessary to prevent pneumothorax and impaired lung inflation.*
- Monitor cardiopulmonary status and haemodynamic pressures. Administer intravenous fluids and fluid boluses as ordered. Fluid volume imbalances that compromise cardiopulmonary status may develop following oesophagectomy. *Maintaining adequate fluid intake and preventing fluid overload are important postoperatively. The person also is at risk of acute respiratory distress syndrome, a critical complication that can further compromise ventilation, gas exchange and circulation.*
- Do not move or manipulate the nasogastric tube. Maintain low gastric suction as ordered. *Manipulating or moving the nasogastric tube may disrupt suture lines, resulting in a leak into the mediastinum.*
- Verify enteral tube feeding placement by x-ray (see the chapter 'Nursing care of people with nutritional disorders'). Stop enteral feedings if feelings of fullness or nausea occur. Suction gastrointestinal contents as needed, positioning the person on the side. *Over-distension of the stomach or delayed gastric emptying may result in regurgitation of stomach contents. Nausea or a feeling of fullness may indicate stomach over-distension. Suctioning and positioning limit the risk of aspiration.*

Anticipatory grieving

Upon a cancer diagnosis, the person and family may experience a grief reaction. The pessimistic prognosis associated with oesophageal cancer and the disruptions in relationships may result in an intense sense of loss. The chapter 'Nursing care of people experiencing loss, grief and death' discusses care of the person experiencing grief and loss.

Community-based care

Most care for people with oesophageal cancer is provided in community-based and home settings. Include the following topics in person and family teaching for home care:

- planned treatment options, including the risks, benefits and potential adverse effects of each
- wound and follow-up care following surgery
- prevention and manifestations of complications such as wound or chest infection, anastomosis leak, deep vein thrombosis
- how to prepare, implement and care for tube feedings or home parenteral nutrition.

Based on the person's needs and prognosis, referral to a home health agency and/or hospice may be appropriate.

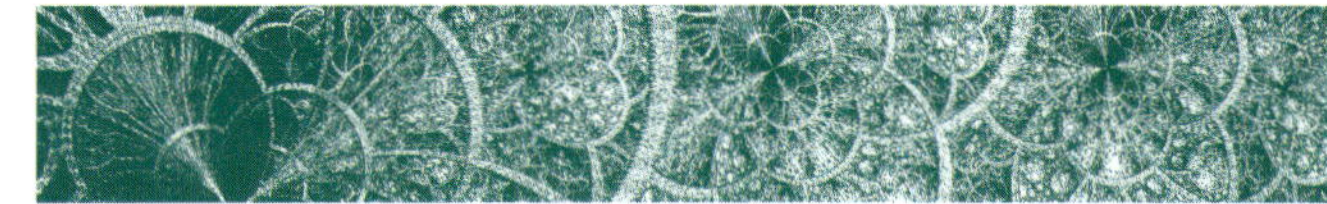

Disorders of the stomach and duodenum

The stomach and upper small intestine (duodenum and jejunum) are responsible for the majority of food digestion. The major disorders that affect digestion are nausea and vomiting, gastritis, peptic ulcer disease and cancer of the stomach. Nursing roles in managing these disorders include both acute care for the hospitalised person and teaching to give the person the skills and knowledge to manage these conditions at home.

OVERVIEW OF NORMAL PHYSIOLOGY

Normally, the stomach is protected from the digestive substances it secretes—namely, hydrochloric acid and pepsin—by the **gastric mucosal barrier**. The gastric mucosal barrier includes:

- An impermeable hydrophobic lipid layer that covers the gastric epithelial cells. This lipid layer prevents diffusion of water-soluble molecules, but substances such as aspirin and alcohol can diffuse through it.
- Bicarbonate ions secreted in response to hydrochloric acid secretion by the parietal cells of the stomach. When bicarbonate (HCO_3^-) secretion is equal to hydrogen ion (H^+) secretion, the gastric mucosa remains intact. Prostaglandins, chemical messengers involved in the inflammatory response, support bicarbonate production and blood flow to the gastric mucosa.
- Mucous gel that protects the surface of the stomach lining from the damaging effects of pepsin and traps bicarbonate to neutralise hydrochloric acid. This gel also acts as a lubricant, preventing mechanical damage to the stomach lining from its contents.

When an acute or chronic irritant disrupts the mucosal barrier, or when disease alters the processes that maintain the barrier, the gastric mucosa becomes irritated and inflamed. Lipid-soluble substances such as aspirin and alcohol penetrate the gastric mucosal barrier, leading to irritation and possible inflammation. Bile acids also break down the lipids in the mucosal barrier, increasing the potential for irritation (Norris, 2018). In addition, aspirin and other non-steroidal anti-inflammatory drugs (NSAIDs) inhibit prostaglandins. Aspirin and NSAIDs also alter the nature of gastric mucus, affecting its protective function.

THE PERSON WITH NAUSEA AND VOMITING

Nausea and vomiting are common gastrointestinal symptoms. **Nausea** is a subjective, unpleasant sensation of sickness or queasiness. It may or may not be accompanied by (and possibly relieved by) vomiting. **Vomiting** is the forceful expulsion of the contents of the upper gastrointestinal tract resulting from contraction of muscles in the gut and abdominal wall. Nausea and vomiting without abdominal pain are commonly associated with food poisoning, infectious gastroenteritis (discussed in the chapter 'Nursing care of people with bowel disorders'), gallbladder disease or ingestion of toxins (such as drugs or alcohol). When associated with severe abdominal pain, they may indicate a serious disorder such as peritonitis, acute gastrointestinal obstruction or pancreatitis.

Pathophysiology

Nausea occurs when the vomiting centre in the medulla of the brain is stimulated. Distension of the duodenum is a common stimulus for nausea. The vomiting centre can be stimulated by input from several different sources:

- the gastrointestinal tract, produced by distension, irritation or infection
- the vestibular system of the ear
- higher central nervous system centres in response to certain sights, smells or emotional experiences
- chemoreceptors outside the blood–brain barrier that are stimulated by drugs, chemotherapeutic agents, toxins, systemic disorders and pregnancy
- disorders such as acute myocardial infarction and heart failure commonly produce nausea and vomiting, possibly due to direct stimulation of the vomiting centre by hypoxia
- increased intracranial pressure (e.g. due to intracranial bleeding or a tumour) produces vomiting that may or may not be accompanied by nausea.

Anorexia—loss of appetite—commonly precedes nausea, just as nausea frequently precedes vomiting. Vomiting, a response that requires coordinated movements of the thorax and abdominal wall, the gut, the pharynx and the muscles of the mouth and face, is coordinated by the brainstem. *Emesis* (or *vomitus*) is produced when inspiratory muscles of the thorax (including the diaphragm) and abdomen contract, increasing intrathoracic and intra-abdominal pressures. The gastro-oesophageal sphincter relaxes and the larynx moves upward to facilitate oral expulsion of gastric contents.

In addition to the subjective sensation of queasiness, nausea frequently is accompanied by autonomic nervous system manifestations such as pallor, sweating, tachycardia and increased salivation. Vomiting, which stimulates the vagus nerve and parasympathetic nervous system, may be accompanied by dizziness, light-headedness, hypotension and bradycardia.

Potential complications of vomiting include dehydration, hypokalaemia, metabolic alkalosis (from loss of hydrochloric acid from the stomach) and aspiration resulting in pneumonia or rupture or tears of the oesophagus (known as a Mallory–Weiss tear).

INTERPROFESSIONAL CARE

In most cases, nausea and vomiting are self-limited and require no treatment. If vomiting is severe or accompanied by other symptoms, acute care may be required to determine the underlying problem and prevent or treat complications such as dehydration.

Diagnostic tests may include serum electrolytes; pregnancy testing if indicated; liver, pancreatic and renal function studies; and imaging studies (x-ray of the abdomen, abdominal CT scan) to detect gastrointestinal obstruction. An upper endoscopy may be performed (see the chapter 'A person-centred approach to assessing the gastrointestinal system'). CT scan or MRI of the head may be ordered if an intracranial problem is suspected as the cause. Specialised testing, such as gastrointestinal motility studies, may be indicated when other diagnostic studies are negative for an anatomical cause of nausea and vomiting.

Food is initially withheld, although clear liquids in small quantities are encouraged to prevent dehydration. Dry foods such as crackers may reduce nausea and promote comfort.

Medications

Unless vomiting is associated with pregnancy, anti-emetic medications may be prescribed to prevent or control nausea and vomiting. These drugs fall into several different classes and often are more effective when given in combination.

- Serotonin receptor antagonists are the most effective medications available for people experiencing nausea and vomiting due to chemotherapy. They are effective when given only once or twice a day, an additional advantage. Medications within this class include ondansetron, granisetron and tropisetron.
- Dopamine antagonists include the phenothiazines (e.g. prochlorperazine (Stemetil) and promethazine (Phenergan)), butyrophenones (haloperidol and droperidol) and other drugs such as metoclopramide. These drugs, while effective, can produce extrapyramidal symptoms, sedation and hypotension.
- Antihistamines such as betahistine (are primarily used to treat nausea and vomiting arising from vestibular centre stimuli (e.g. motion sickness).
- While corticosteroids are not approved as a class for treating nausea and vomiting, two drugs in this class, methylprednisolone and dexamethasone, may be used in combination to treat vomiting associated with cancer treatment.

- Lorazepam (is a benzodiazepine drug approved for use as an anti-emetic. It produces a degree of sedation, but can suppress anticipatory vomiting (e.g. before chemotherapy). It also helps control extrapyramidal symptoms associated with the phenothiazine anti-emetics (dopamine antagonists).

Nursing responsibilities and person education for anti-emetic drugs are outlined in the accompanying 'Medication administration' box.

Complementary and alternative medicine

Mind–body interventions such as biofeedback, guided imagery, music therapy and hypnosis may be effective for some people with nausea. Biofeedback uses machinery to translate physiological processes into audible or visible signals to teach the person to exert conscious control over those processes. In guided imagery, the person uses imagination to invoke specific images to modify physiological responses. Music therapy involves the person in

MEDICATION ADMINISTRATION Medications used to prevent and treat nausea and vomiting

SEROTONIN RECEPTOR ANTAGONISTS

Ondansetron
Granisetron
Tropisetron

The serotonin receptor antagonists suppress nausea and vomiting by blocking the effect of serotonin on vagal afferent nerves that stimulate the vomiting centre. Their primary uses are to prevent vomiting associated with chemotherapy, radiation therapy and surgery.

Nursing responsibilities

- Administer 30 to 60 minutes prior to chemotherapy or surgery as directed.
- May be given orally, sublingually (Ondansetron wafers) or intravenously (push or infusion; follow directions specific to the drug used).
- Monitor liver function and clotting studies; report abnormal levels to the medical officer.

Health education for the person and family

- Take this medication exactly as directed.
- This medication may be taken without regard to food intake.
- Headache is a common side effect of these medications. Use paracetamol or another mild analgesic as directed by your doctor.

DOPAMINE ANTAGONISTS

Prochlorperazine
Promethazine
Haloperidol
Droperidol
Metoclopramide

These medications act by blocking dopamine receptors in the chemoreceptor trigger zone (CTZ). Their primary uses are to suppress nausea and vomiting associated with surgery, cancer chemotherapy and toxins. The major adverse effects associated with these medications are sedation, hypotension and extrapyramidal reactions. Older adults are more sensitive to these effects; a lower dose often is indicated.

Nursing responsibilities

- Administer orally or parenterally as ordered before surgery, or before meals and procedures known to produce nausea and vomiting.
- These medications may interact with a number of other medications, often increasing their sedative and hypotensive effects.
- Administer with caution to older adults, closely monitoring for adverse effects such as confusion, agitation and changes in vital signs.
- Monitor for evidence of extrapyramidal symptoms, including tremor, restlessness, hyperactivity, anxiety and impaired coordination; notify medical officer if these clinical manifestations develop.

Health education for the person and family

- Use the medications as prescribed; do not increase your dose without consulting your primary care provider.
- These medications may cause drowsiness. Avoid using other central nervous system (CNS) depressants such as alcohol while taking these medications.
- Change positions from lying to sitting and sitting to standing slowly because these medications can cause light-headedness or dizziness.
- Promptly report changes in coordination, tremors, difficulty speaking or swallowing, or weakness to your doctor.

ANTIHISTAMINES

Betahistane

Antihistamines are primarily used to treat nausea and vomiting associated with motion sickness. These act by blocking histamine and acetylcholine (muscarinic) receptors in the neural pathway from the inner ear to the vomiting centre in the brainstem.

Nursing responsibilities

- Do not administer these medications to people for whom anticholinergic drugs are contraindicated: people with narrow-angle glaucoma, urinary retention, bowel obstruction.
- May be administered orally, parenterally or rectally, depending on the preparation and the person's ability to tolerate oral preparations.
- Use with caution in people who are taking other CNS depressants or antihistamine preparations, tricyclic antidepressants or monoamine oxidase inhibitors.

Health education for the person and family

- These medications frequently cause drowsiness. Use caution when operating machinery or performing tasks requiring mental alertness.
- Avoid using alcohol or other substances that cause drowsiness or sedation while taking these medications.
- The medication may cause dry mouth. Sips of water, ice chips, boiled lollies or sugarless gum can be used for comfort.
- Use sunscreen and protective clothing to protect from sunburn while using these medications.

creating or listening to music to affect physiological and psychological responses. In hypnosis, an altered mind state is induced to make the person receptive to suggestions.

Ginger, an aromatic root frequently used in cooking and also available in capsule form, may also be helpful in relieving nausea and vomiting, particularly when due to pregnancy and chemotherapy (Edwards, 2021). Ginger can inhibit platelet aggregation and may increase the risk of bleeding in people taking antiplatelet or anticoagulant medications.

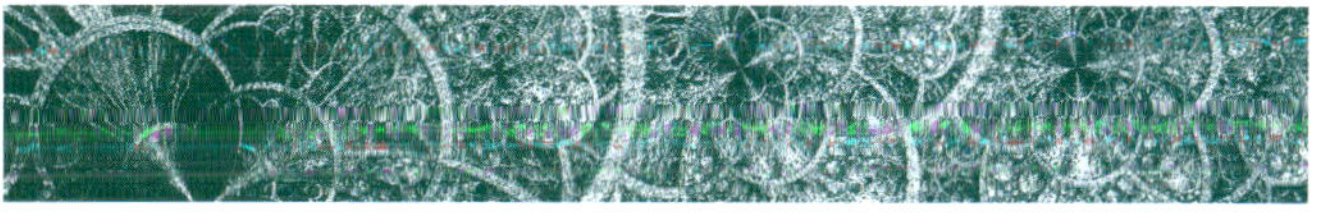

Nursing care

Assessment of the person is vital to help determine the cause of nausea and vomiting and to rule out underlying systemic disease or acute conditions that require immediate care (e.g. bowel obstruction). When the cause is known or no other acute symptoms are present, nursing interventions can promote comfort and prevent complications.

Nausea

An unpleasant sensation in the epigastric or abdominal region, nausea is a subjective sensation best described by the person.

- Monitor subjective complaints of nausea, vital signs, skin turgor and condition, and weight. Maintain accurate intake and output records. Monitor amount, colour and specific gravity of urine. *Nausea can cause aversion to food and fluids, leading to dehydration even when it is not accompanied by vomiting.*
- Administer anti-emetic medication as ordered, prior to meals and before treatments or procedures known to stimulate nausea. *Preventing nausea is particularly important for people receiving chemotherapy, to avoid the association between the treatment and nausea.*
- Instruct to deep breathe to voluntarily suppress the vomiting reflex. *Controlling vomiting helps prevent dehydration and other complications associated with prolonged or severe vomiting.*
- Instruct to consume small quantities of clear fluids and dry foods at separate times. *Separating the intake of dry foods and fluids helps reduce the nausea stimulus.*

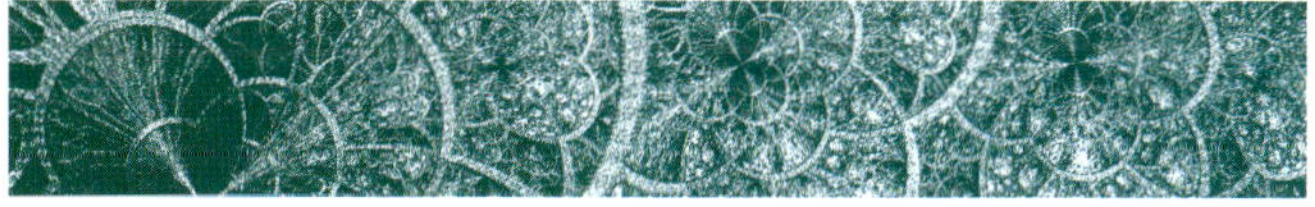

THE PERSON WITH GASTROINTESTINAL BLEEDING

Because of its constant exposure to the environment, the gastrointestinal tract can be subjected to trauma and exposed to toxins, infection with pathogens such as *Helicobacter pylori* (*H. pylori*), inflammatory processes and insults such as ischaemia due to systemic diseases. While the mucosal lining of the GI tract is remarkably able to withstand these insults and heal rapidly, its rich supply of blood can result in significant bleeding when a vessel is eroded or abnormally distended (*varices*). Gastrointestinal haemorrhage is a relatively common cause of admission and complication of critical illnesses. It is a medical emergency requiring aggressive medical and nursing care.

Although bleeding and haemorrhage can occur anywhere in the GI tract, the upper portion of the tract is more commonly affected. The three primary disorders leading to upper gastrointestinal (UGI) haemorrhage are erosive gastritis, peptic ulcer disease and oesophageal varices. Erosive gastritis and peptic ulcer disease are discussed in the following sections of this chapter, oesophageal varices, usually seen as a complication of cirrhosis of the liver, are discussed in the chapter 'Nursing care of people with gallbladder, liver and pancreatic disorders'.

> **FAST FACTS**
> - UGI bleeds are associated with increasing non-steroidal anti-inflammatory drug (NSAID) use.
> - Approximately 64% are associated with *H. pylori* infection in people with peptic ulcer bleeding.
> - UGI bleeding is twice as common in men as in women.
> - Prevalence increases with age (Ryan et al., 2021).

Pathophysiology

Blood in the GI tract has several effects. It is irritating to the stomach and typically leads to nausea and vomiting (**haematemesis**, vomiting blood). If the blood has been present in the stomach for a period of time and is partially digested, it may have a 'coffee-grounds' appearance, rather than presenting as bright red blood. The accumulation of blood in the GI tract stimulates peristalsis, leading to hyperactive bowel sounds and diarrhoea. Stools may be black and tarry (melaena) or frankly bloody (**haematochezia**); stool containing partially digested blood has a characteristic odour. With significant upper GI bleeding, digestion of blood proteins increases blood urea nitrogen (BUN) levels.

Physiological responses to an upper GI bleed depend on the rapidity and magnitude of the blood loss. GI bleeding resulting from erosion of a small vessel typically is slow and may not be identified until the person presents with manifestations of blood loss anaemia due to depletion of iron stores. (See the chapter 'Nursing care of people with haematological disorders' for further discussion of blood loss anaemia.) Although no visible blood may be present in the stool, **occult** (or hidden) **bleeding** may be detected by chemical means.

GI haemorrhage, with loss of a significant amount of blood within a few hours, rapidly depletes blood volume, producing manifestations of decreased cardiac output: tachycardia, hypotension, pallor and decreased urine output. Peripheral blood vessels constrict to maintain perfusion of vital organs. Unless the blood volume is restored, hypovolaemic shock progresses, leading to re-bleeds, renal failure, bowel infarction, acute coronary syndrome, coma and death. See the chapter 'Nursing care of people experiencing trauma and shock' for more information about shock and its management.

INTERPROFESSIONAL CARE

The acuity of the bleed and the person's condition dictate the timing and extent of diagnostic testing and interventions. A person with a massive GI haemorrhage is admitted to the critical care unit and aggressively treated to stem bleeding, restore blood volume and stabilise the cardiovascular system. Identifying the cause of the bleeding is postponed in many cases until the person's condition has been stabilised.

When the bleeding is slow or chronic, diagnostic testing and treatment may be managed in a community-based setting.

Diagnosis

Diagnostic testing focuses on determining the extent and effects of the bleed, as well as its cause.

- A *full blood count (FBC) with haemoglobin and haematocrit* is obtained. In an acute bleed, the FBC, haemoglobin and haematocrit may not initially indicate the extent of blood loss because plasma is lost along with blood cells.
- *Blood type and crossmatch* are performed to prepare for transfusion as necessary.
- *Serum electrolytes*, *osmolality* and *BUN* are obtained to determine the effects of the blood loss and protein digestion on blood chemistries.
- *Liver function tests* and a *coagulation profile* may be obtained to help determine the cause of the bleeding.
- An *upper endoscopy* is performed as soon as possible to identify and, if possible, treat the source of bleeding. See the chapter 'A person-centred approach to assessing the gastrointestinal system' for nursing care of the person undergoing upper endoscopy.

Treatments

In acute GI haemorrhage, initial treatment focuses on stemming the bleeding, restoring cardiovascular stability and maintaining the person's airway. Intravenous fluids such as normal saline are administered through a large-bore intravenous catheter. Fresh whole blood, which contains clotting factors, is administered to restore blood volume and components in an acute haemorrhage. In less acute situations, packed red cells may be administered to restore the oxygen-carrying capacity of the blood. Intubation may be required to protect against aspiration of blood into the airways (Ket et al., 2021).

Haemostasis is achieved using upper endoscopy whenever possible. A sclerosing agent may be injected into the bleeding vessel or the vessel may be sealed using a heated probe, diathermy or laser. Rarely, emergency surgery is required to stop haemorrhage.

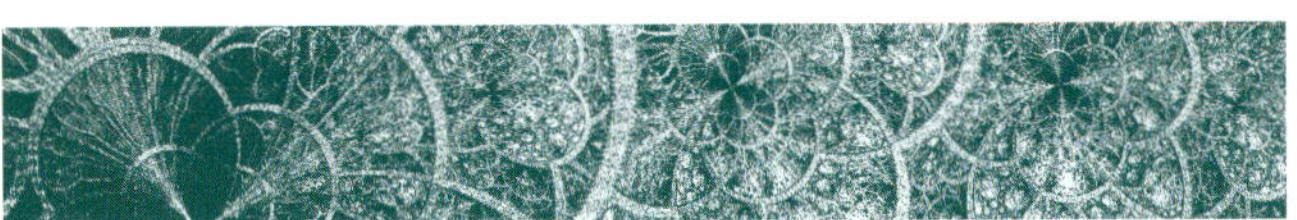

Nursing care

Health promotion

Preventing gastrointestinal bleeding is the most important step in reducing the mortality and morbidity associated with an acute GI haemorrhage. Identifying people at risk and instituting regular gastric pH monitoring and maintenance of drug therapy to reduce gastric acidity are important preventive measures. All critically ill people should be considered to be at risk of stress-related erosive gastritis.

Assessment

Assessment of the person experiencing an acute GI haemorrhage is very focused on the immediate crisis. The ability to obtain subjective information may be limited; however, it is important to identify possible contributing factors such as use of aspirin, NSAIDs, other platelet inhibitors or anticoagulant medications, and the presence of any acute or chronic conditions that may contribute to bleeding (e.g. hypertension, a clotting disorder, peptic ulcer disease, excessive alcohol use, chronic hepatitis or cirrhosis of the liver). If possible, identify all current medications and their purpose, as well as any allergies to medications or other substances. If possible, obtain any history of abdominal pain, black tarry stools, vomiting, dysphagia, rectal bleeding or chest pain (Ket et al., 2021).

Physical examination focuses on the effect of the bleeding on cardiovascular status. Obtain vital signs and orthostatic vital signs (an early sign of hypovolaemia). Place the acutely ill person on a cardiac monitor and obtain a rhythm strip. Obtain oxygen saturation level. Assess peripheral pulse strength, as well as colour, temperature and capillary refill of extremities. Evaluate mental status, including level of consciousness and orientation. An indwelling catheter may be inserted to evaluate urine output.

Nursing diagnoses and interventions

Nursing care priorities for the person with an acute GI bleed focus on restoring and maintaining an effective cardiac output and tissue perfusion, and on stopping the haemorrhage and preventing further bleeding.

Risk of decreased cardiac output related to haemorrhage

Significant amounts of blood may be lost in a very short time with an acute GI haemorrhage. Because some of the blood enters the bowel, it may be difficult to accurately estimate the amount of blood lost by measuring emesis, gastric suction return and blood expelled as faeces. As blood volume drops, venous return decreases. The heart rate increases to maintain the cardiac output, and peripheral blood vessels constrict to improve venous return and cardiac output.

- Frequently assess and document vital signs, including blood pressure, pulse rate and cardiac rhythm, respiratory rate and oxygen saturation levels. Obtain haemodynamic pressure measurements as ordered, reporting trends and changes. *The vital signs, oxygen saturation levels and haemodynamic pressure values provide indicators of the effectiveness of peripheral tissue perfusion, oxygenation and fluid replacement.*
- Monitor for and report changes in skin colour, temperature and moisture, or slow capillary refill. *Peripheral vasoconstriction and activation of the sympathetic nervous system typically cause pale, cool and moist or diaphoretic*

skin. Development of cyanosis or mottling indicates a further decrease in tissue perfusion and oxygenation.

- Insert an indwelling urinary catheter and measure urine output hourly. Report an output of less than 30 mL for two consecutive hours. *A fall in urine output may indicate further reduction in cardiac output. As cardiac output falls, the kidneys become ischaemic and acute renal failure may develop.*
- Unless contraindicated, insert a nasogastric tube to assess for presence of blood or coffee ground material. *Acute blood in the stomach implies UGI bleeding is likely and predicts that the bleeding is caused by a high-risk lesion (Ket et al., 2021).*
- Maintain two peripheral intravenous *lines with large-bore catheters or a central venous catheter for fluid and blood administration as ordered.* Frequently monitor vital signs, respiratory status and haemodynamic pressure measurements, reporting changes in status. *Rapid administration of isotonic intravenous fluids, blood and blood products can lead to fluid overload and potential heart failure.*

Risk of impaired tissue integrity related to nasogastric tube insertion

- Maintain drainage and patency of nasogastric tube. Connect to low suction if ordered. *Blood is irritating to the GI tract, precipitating vomiting and stimulating peristalsis, leading to diarrhoea. In addition, digested blood can increase BUN levels, potentially leading to confusion and altered mental status.*
- Irrigate the nasogastric tube with room-temperature saline or tap water as ordered. Calculate intake and output, subtracting the amount of irrigant from gastric output. *Irrigation of the nasogastric tube helps remove irritating blood from the gut and produces a degree of vasoconstriction in stomach mucosa, slowing bleeding.*
- Prepare for upper endoscopy or surgery as planned. *Endoscopy or emergency surgery may be performed to repair the bleeding site or sclerose bleeding vessels.*
- Following an acute bleed and in people at risk of GI bleeding, monitor gastric pH as ordered and check vomitus and faeces for the presence of occult blood. Maintain infusions of drugs to reduce gastric acidity as ordered. *The person remains at risk of GI bleeding. Monitoring for occult blood helps identify slow bleeding or recurrent haemorrhage. Reducing the acidity of gastric secretions reduces irritation of the gastric mucosa, reducing the risk of bleeding.*

Community-based care

Following an acute GI haemorrhage, continuing care focuses on resolving the underlying disease process if possible and preventing future episodes of GI bleeding. If a bleeding gastric ulcer was identified, testing for *H. pylori* infection will be done and a treatment regimen prescribed to eradicate the infection. (See the section on peptic ulcer disease later in this chapter.) The person who experienced an episode of erosive stress gastritis will often be discharged with instructions to continue taking a gastric-acid-reducing medication and avoid known gastric irritants such as aspirin, NSAIDs and alcohol. The person with oesophageal varices due to cirrhosis or chronic hepatitis needs additional instructions (see the chapter 'Nursing care of people with gallbladder, liver and pancreatic disorders').

People with minor or slow GI bleeding often are managed in the community. Provide teaching about the cause of the bleeding and measures to prevent future episodes. Provide verbal and written instructions for prescribed medications such as acid reducers and oral iron supplements. Discuss appropriate nutrition; while a special diet to 'soothe the stomach' rarely is indicated, foods rich in iron may be recommended to treat the resulting anaemia.

Discuss indicators of GI bleeding to be reported to the doctor. If the source of bleeding has not been identified, provide instructions about prescribed follow-up diagnostic testing.

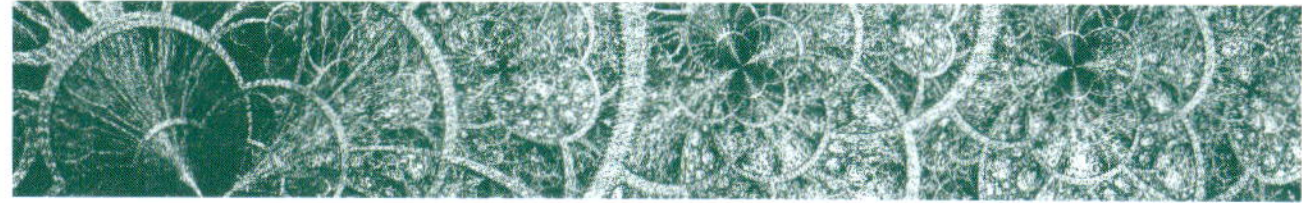

THE PERSON WITH GASTRITIS

Gastritis, inflammation of the stomach lining, results from irritation of the gastric mucosa. Gastritis is common and may be caused by a variety of factors. The most common form of gastritis, **acute gastritis**, is generally a benign, self-limiting disorder associated with the ingestion of gastric irritants such as aspirin, NSAIDs, alcohol, caffeine or foods contaminated with certain bacteria. Manifestations of acute gastritis may range from asymptomatic to mild heartburn to severe gastric distress, vomiting and bleeding with haematemesis (vomiting blood).

Chronic gastritis is a separate group of disorders characterised by progressive and irreversible changes in the gastric mucosa (Norris, 2018). It is more common in older adults, chronic alcoholics and cigarette smokers. When symptoms of chronic gastritis occur, they are often vague, ranging from a feeling of heaviness in the epigastric region after meals to gnawing, burning, ulcer-like epigastric pain unrelieved by antacids.

Pathophysiology

Acute gastritis

Acute gastritis is characterised by disruption of the mucosal barrier by a local irritant. This disruption allows hydrochloric acid and pepsin to come into contact with the gastric tissue, resulting in irritation, inflammation and superficial erosions. The gastric mucosa rapidly regenerates, generally making acute gastritis a self-limiting disorder, with resolution and healing occurring within several days.

The ingestion of aspirin or other NSAIDs, corticosteroids, alcohol and caffeine is commonly associated with the development of acute gastritis. Accidental or purposeful ingestion of a corrosive alkali (such as ammonia, disinfectant and other cleaning agents) or acid leads to severe inflammation and possible necrosis of the stomach. Gastric perforation, haemorrhage and peritonitis are possible results. Iatrogenic causes of acute gastritis include radiation therapy and administration of certain chemotherapeutic agents.

Erosive gastritis

A severe form of acute gastritis, **erosive** or **stress-induced gastritis**, occurs as a complication of other life-threatening conditions such as shock, severe trauma, major surgery, sepsis, burns or head injury. When these erosions follow a major burn, they are called Curling's ulcers, after Thomas Curling, a British physician who first described them in 1842. When stress ulcers occur following head injury or CNS surgery, they are referred to as **Cushing's ulcers**, after Harvey Cushing, a US surgeon.

The primary mechanisms leading to erosive gastritis appear to be ischaemia of the gastric mucosa resulting from sympathetic vasoconstriction and tissue injury due to gastric acid. As a result, multiple superficial erosions of the gastric mucosa develop. Maintaining the gastric pH at greater than 3.5 and inhibiting gastric acid secretion with medications help prevent erosive gastritis.

MANIFESTATIONS The person with acute gastritis may have mild symptoms such as anorexia or mild epigastric discomfort relieved by belching or defecating. More severe manifestations include abdominal pain, nausea and vomiting. Gastric bleeding may occur, with haematemesis or melaena (black, tarry stools that contain blood). Erosive gastritis is not typically associated with pain. The initial symptom often is painless gastric bleeding occurring 2 or more days after the initial stressor. Bleeding typically is minimal but can be massive. Corrosive gastritis can cause severe bleeding, signs of shock and an *acute abdomen* (severely painful, rigid, board-like abdomen) if perforation occurs. See the 'Manifestations' box.

Chronic gastritis

Unrelated to acute gastritis, chronic gastritis is a progressive disorder that begins with superficial inflammation and gradually leads to atrophy of gastric tissues. The initial stage is characterised by superficial changes in the gastric mucosa and a decrease in mucus. As the disease evolves, glands of the gastric mucosa are disrupted and destroyed. The inflammatory process involves deep portions of the mucosa, which thins and atrophies. There appear to be at least two different forms of chronic gastritis, classified as type A and type B.

Type A gastritis, the less common form of chronic gastritis, usually affects people of Northern European heritage. This type of gastritis is thought to have an autoimmune component. In type A or autoimmune gastritis, the body produces antibodies to parietal cells and to intrinsic factor. These antibodies destroy gastric mucosal cells, resulting in tissue atrophy and the loss of hydrochloric acid and pepsin secretion. Because intrinsic factor is required for the absorption of vitamin B_{12}, this immune response also results in pernicious anaemia. For further discussion of pernicious anaemia, see the chapter 'Nursing care of people with haematological disorders'.

Type B gastritis is the more common form of chronic gastritis. Its incidence increases with age, reaching nearly 100% in people over the age of 70. Type B gastritis is caused by chronic infection of the gastric mucosa by *H. pylori*, a Gram-negative spiral bacterium. *H. pylori* infection causes inflammation of the gastric mucosa, with infiltration by neutrophils and lymphocytes. The outermost layer of gastric mucosa thins and atrophies, providing a less effective barrier against the auto-digestive properties of hydrochloric acid and pepsin.

Infection with *H. pylori* also is associated with an increased risk of peptic ulcer disease. *H. pylori* infection significantly increases the risk of developing gastric cancer. See the sections that follow for more information about these disorders.

MANIFESTATIONS Chronic gastritis is often asymptomatic until atrophy is sufficiently advanced to interfere with digestion and gastric emptying. The person may complain of vague gastric distress, epigastric heaviness after meals or ulcer-like symptoms. These symptoms typically are not relieved by antacids. In addition, the person may experience fatigue and other symptoms of anaemia. If intrinsic factor is lacking, paraesthesias and other neurological manifestations of vitamin B_{12} deficiency may be present. See the 'Manifestations' box.

MANIFESTATIONS Acute and chronic gastritis

ACUTE GASTRITIS

Gastrointestinal	*Systemic*
▪ Anorexia ▪ Nausea and vomiting ▪ Haematemesis ▪ Melaena ▪ Abdominal pain	▪ Possible shock

CHRONIC GASTRITIS

Gastrointestinal	*Systemic*
▪ Vague discomfort after eating; may be asymptomatic	▪ Anaemia ▪ Fatigue

INTERPROFESSIONAL CARE

Acute gastritis is usually diagnosed by the history and clinical presentation. In contrast, the vague symptoms of chronic gastritis may require more extensive diagnostic testing.

People with acute and chronic gastritis are generally managed in community settings. The person requires acute care only when nausea and vomiting are severe enough to interfere with their normal fluid and electrolyte balance and nutritional status. If haemorrhage results, surgical intervention may be required.

Diagnosis

Diagnostic tests that may be ordered for the person with gastritis include the following:

- *Haemoglobin, haematocrit* and *red blood cell (RBC) indices* are evaluated for evidence of anaemia. The person with gastritis may develop pernicious anaemia because of parietal cell destruction or iron-deficiency anaemia because of chronic blood loss.

- *Serum vitamin B_{12} levels* are measured to evaluate for possible pernicious anaemia. Normal values for vitamin B_{12} are 200 to 1,000 pictograms per mL, with lower levels seen in older adults.
- *Upper endoscopy* may be done to inspect the gastric mucosa for changes, identify areas of bleeding and obtain tissue for biopsy. Bleeding sites may be treated with electro- or laser coagulation or injected with a sclerosing agent during the procedure. See the 'Diagnostic tests' box in the chapter 'A person-centred approach to assessing the gastrointestinal system' for preparation and teaching related to an upper endoscopy.

Medications

Medications such as a PPI, H_2-receptor blocker or sucralfate may be ordered to prevent or treat acute stress gastritis. PPIs and H_2-receptor blockers reduce the amount or effects of hydrochloric acid on the gastric mucosa. Lansoprazole, esomeprazole and omeprazole are examples of PPIs. H_2-receptor blockers include cimetidine, ranitidine, famotidine and nizatidine). These medications also are available in non-prescription strength. Sucralfate works locally to prevent the damaging effects of acid and pepsin on gastric tissue. It does not neutralise or reduce acid secretion. Nursing implications for drugs commonly used in managing gastritis are included in the 'Medication administration: drugs used to treat GORD, gastritis and peptic ulcer disease' box.

The person with type B chronic gastritis may be treated to eradicate the *H. pylori* infection. This generally involves combination therapy consisting of two antibiotics (such as metronidazole and clarithromycin or a tetracycline) and a PPI. In some cases, eradication of the infection is not warranted and the person is treated symptomatically.

Treatments

In acute gastritis, gastrointestinal tract rest is provided by 6 to 12 hours of NBM status, then slow reintroduction of clear fluids (broth, tea, jelly, carbonated beverages), followed by ingestion of free fluids (creamy soups, puddings, milk) and finally a gradual reintroduction of solid food.

If nausea and vomiting threaten fluid and electrolyte balance, intravenous fluids and electrolytes are ordered.

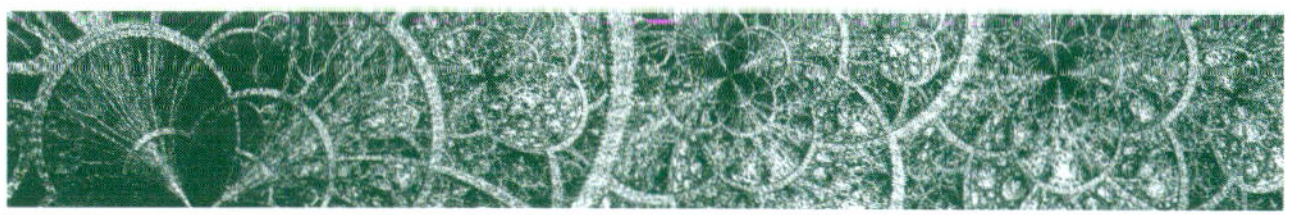

Nursing care

Health promotion

Health promotion aims to educate the person about measures to prevent acute gastritis. Food contaminated with bacteria is a significant cause of acute gastritis. Discuss food safety measures such as fully cooking meats and egg products and promptly refrigerating foods after cooking to avoid bacterial growth. Stress that food contaminated with potential pathogens often looks, smells and tastes good, making it difficult to identify.

Teach people to abstain from eating or drinking anything during an acute episode of vomiting and then to reintroduce clear liquids gradually once vomiting has stopped (2 to 4 hours after the last episode of vomiting). Suggest using a sports drink to replace lost electrolytes and fluid. Instruct people to avoid milk and milk products until they easily tolerate clear liquids and solid foods such as dry toast or crackers.

Assessment

Assessment data to collect for people with acute or chronic gastritis include the following.

- *Health history*: current symptoms and their duration; relieving and aggravating factors; history of ingestion of toxins, contaminated food, alcohol, aspirin or NSAIDs; other medications.
- *Physical examination*: vital signs, including orthostatic vitals if indicated; peripheral pulses; general appearance; abdominal assessment, including appearance, bowel sounds and tenderness.

Nursing diagnoses and interventions

In planning and implementing nursing care for the person with acute or chronic gastritis, consider both the direct effects of the disorder on the gastrointestinal system and nutritional status, as well as its effects on lifestyle and psychosocial integrity. This section focuses on problems of fluid balance and nutrition.

Risk of fluid volume deficit related to gastrointestinal upset

Nausea, vomiting and abdominal distress are the primary manifestations of acute gastritis. The risk of fluid and electrolyte imbalance is high because of inadequate intake of food and fluids and abnormal losses of fluids and electrolytes with vomiting.

> **CONSIDERATION FOR PRACTICE**
>
> **Tachycardia, tachypnoea and hypotension, especially orthostatic hypotension, may indicate fluid volume deficit. Electrolyte or acid–base imbalances resulting from vomiting may cause cardiac arrhythmias or changes in respirations.**

- Monitor and record vital signs at least every 2 hours until stable, then every 4 hours. Check for orthostatic hypotension.
- Weigh daily. Monitor and record intake and output; record urine output every 1 to 4 hours as indicated. *Daily weights are an accurate indicator of fluid volume. Urine output of less than 0.5 mL/kg/hour indicates decreased cardiac output and a need for prompt fluid replacement.*
- Monitor skin turgor, colour and condition and status of oral mucous membranes frequently. Provide skin and mouth care frequently. *Skin turgor and mucous membrane assessments indicate hydration status. Good skin and mouth care are necessary to maintain skin and mucous membrane integrity.*

- Monitor laboratory values for electrolytes and acid–base balance. Report significant changes or deviations from normal. *Electrolytes are lost through vomiting, increasing the risk of electrolyte and acid–base imbalances. These imbalances, in turn, affect multiple body systems.*
- Administer oral or parenteral fluids as ordered. *Oral fluids may be withheld until vomiting has ceased, then gradually reintroduced. Intravenous fluids restore or maintain hydration until adequate oral intake is resumed.*
- Administer anti-emetic and other medications as prescribed to relieve vomiting and facilitate oral feeding. Encourage fluids as soon as feasible. *The oral route is preferred for fluid and nutrient intake; medications may be used to allow earlier resumption of feeding.*

CONSIDERATION FOR PRACTICE

Ensure safety: place nurse call bell within reach, put up the side rails, instruct person to avoid getting up without assistance. Orthostatic hypotension may lead to syncope and to falls if the person attempts to get up without assistance.

Risk of imbalanced nutrition (less than body requirements) related to gastrointestinal upset

Manifestations of chronic gastritis may lead to reduced food intake and malnutrition. The person often associates these unpleasant sensations with eating and may gradually reduce food intake. Associated anorexia also contributes to poor food intake.

- Monitor and record food and fluid intake and any abnormal losses (such as vomiting). *Careful monitoring can help in developing a dietary plan to meet the energy needs of the person. Consultation with a dietitian may prove beneficial.*
- Monitor weight and laboratory studies such as serum albumin, haemoglobin and RBC indices. *Weights and laboratory values provide data regarding nutritional status and the effectiveness of interventions.*
- Arrange for dietary consultation to determine energy and nutrient needs and develop a dietary plan. Consider food preferences and tolerances in menu planning. *A diet high in protein, vitamins and minerals may be prescribed to meet the nutritional needs of the person with chronic gastritis. In addition, specific food intolerances may need to be considered. Planning to include preferred foods in the diet helps ensure consumption of the prescribed diet.*
- Provide nutritional supplements between meals or frequent small feedings as needed. *Many people with chronic gastritis tolerate small, frequent feedings better than three large meals per day.*
- Maintain tube feedings or parenteral nutrition as ordered. Refer to the chapter 'Nursing care of people with nutritional disorders' for further information on enteral and parenteral feedings.

Community-based care

Because acute or chronic gastritis is usually managed in community-based settings, education is vital. For the person with acute gastritis, teaching focuses on managing acute symptoms, reintroducing fluids and solid foods, identifying indicators of possible complications (e.g. continued vomiting, signs of fluid and electrolyte imbalance) and preventing future episodes.

Provide the following information for people with chronic gastritis:

- maintaining optimal nutrition
- helpful dietary modifications
- using prescribed medications
- avoiding known gastric irritants, such as aspirin, NSAIDs, alcohol and cigarette smoking.

Referral to smoking cessation classes or programs to treat alcohol abuse may be necessary.

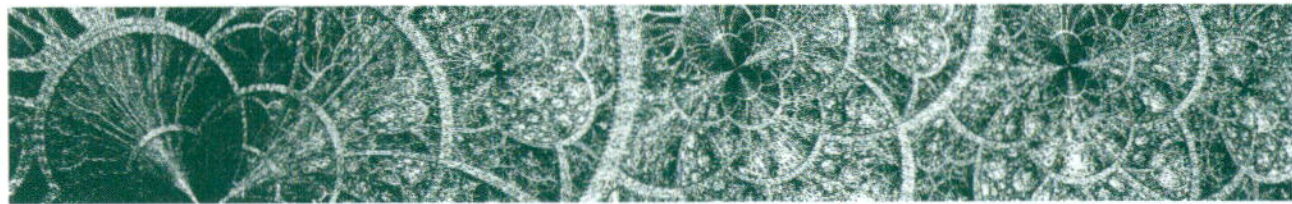

THE PERSON WITH PEPTIC ULCER DISEASE

Peptic ulcer disease (PUD), a break in the mucous lining of the gastrointestinal tract where it comes in contact with gastric juice, is a chronic health problem. In Australia, people presenting to hospital with PUD are likely to be male and aged 60 or above (Eslick et al., 2020). **Peptic ulcers** occur in any area of the gastrointestinal tract exposed to acid–pepsin secretions, including the oesophagus, stomach or duodenum. **Duodenal ulcers** usually develop between the ages of 60 and 69 and are more common in men than women. **Gastric ulcers** usually develop between the ages of 50 and 59 (Eslick et al., 2020).

Risk factors

Chronic *H. pylori* infection and use of aspirin and NSAIDs are the major risk factors for PUD. Contributing risk factors are listed in Box 22.4. Overall, it is estimated that 1 in 6 people infected with *H. pylori* develops PUD. A strong familial pattern suggests a genetic factor in the development of PUD. Cigarette smoking is a significant risk factor, doubling the risk of PUD. Cigarette smoking inhibits the secretion of bicarbonate by the pancreas and possibly causes more rapid transit of gastric acid into the duodenum.

BOX 22.4 Risk factors for peptic ulcer disease

- *H. pylori* infection
- Low socioeconomic status
- Crowded, unsanitary living conditions
- Unclean food or water
- Use of aspirin
- Advanced age
- History of PUD
- Concurrent use of other drugs such as glucocorticoids or NSAIDs
- Cigarette smoking
- Family history of PUD

Pathophysiology

The innermost layer of the stomach wall, the gastric mucosa, consists of columnar epithelial cells supported by a middle layer of blood vessels and glands, and a thin outer layer of smooth muscle. The mucosal barrier of the stomach, a thin coating of mucous gel and bicarbonate, protects the gastric mucosa. The mucosal barrier is maintained by bicarbonate secreted by the epithelial cells, by mucous gel production stimulated by prostaglandins and by an adequate blood supply to the mucosa.

An **ulcer**, or break in the gastrointestinal mucosa, develops when the mucosal barrier is unable to protect the mucosa from damage by hydrochloric acid and pepsin, the gastric digestive juices. See 'Pathophysiology illustrated: peptic ulcer disease'.

H. pylori infection, found in about 70% of people who have PUD, is unique in colonising the stomach. It is spread person to person (oral–oral or faecal–oral) and contributes to ulcer formation in several ways. The bacteria produce enzymes that reduce the efficacy of mucous gel in protecting the gastric mucosa. In addition, the host's inflammatory response to *H. pylori* contributes to gastric epithelial cell damage without producing immunity to the infection. Although the gastric mucosa is the usual site for *H. pylori* infection, this infection also contributes to duodenal ulcers. This is possibly related to increased gastric acid production associated with *H. pylori* infection.

NSAIDs contribute to PUD through both systemic and topical mechanisms. Prostaglandins are necessary for maintaining the gastric mucosal barrier. NSAIDs interrupt prostaglandin synthesis by disrupting the action of the enzyme cyclooxygenase (COX). The two forms of this enzyme are COX-1 and COX-2. The COX-1 enzyme is necessary to maintain the integrity of the gastric mucosa, but the anti-inflammatory effects of NSAIDs are due to their ability to inhibit the COX-2 enzyme. The COX-2-selective NSAIDs may be less damaging to the gastric mucosa because they have less effect on the COX-1 enzyme. In addition to their systemic effect, aspirin and many NSAIDs cross the lipid membranes of gastric epithelial cells, damaging the cells themselves.

The ulcers of PUD may affect the oesophagus, stomach or duodenum. They may be superficial or deep, affecting all layers of the mucosa (see 'Pathophysiology illustrated: peptic ulcer disease'). Duodenal ulcers usually develop in the proximal portion of the duodenum, close to the pylorus (see Figure 22.7). They are sharply demarcated and usually less than 1 cm in diameter (see Figure 22.8). Gastric ulcers often are found on the lesser curvature and the area immediately proximal to the pylorus.

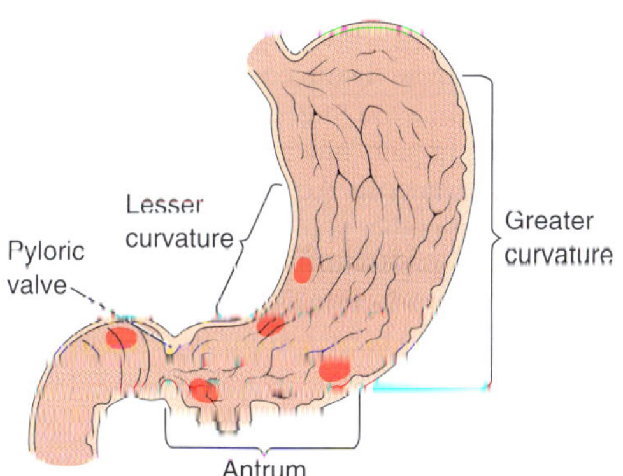

FIGURE 22.7 ***Common sites affected by peptic ulcer disease***

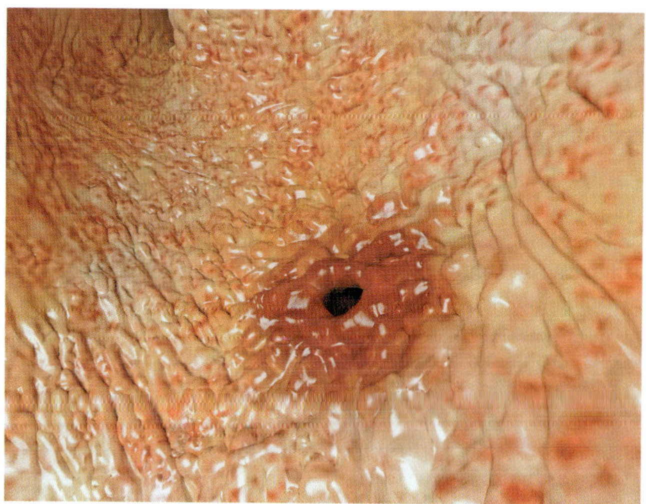

FIGURE 22.8 ***A superficial peptic ulcer***

Source: Juan Gaertner/Shutterstock.

Gastric ulcers are associated with an increased incidence of gastric cancer.

PUD may be chronic, with spontaneous remissions and exacerbations. Exacerbations of the disease may be associated with trauma, infection or other physical or psychological stressors.

Manifestations

Pain is the classic symptom of PUD. The pain is typically described as gnawing, burning, aching or hunger-like and is experienced in the epigastric region, sometimes radiating to the back. The pain occurs when the stomach is empty (2 to 3 hours after meals and in the middle of the night) and is relieved by eating, with a classic 'pain–food–relief' pattern. The person may complain of heartburn or regurgitation and may vomit.

The presentation of PUD in the older adult is often less clear, with vague and poorly localised discomfort, perhaps chest pain or dysphagia, weight loss or anaemia. In the older adult, a complication of PUD, such as upper GI haemorrhage or perforation of the stomach or duodenum, may be the presenting symptom.

Complications

The complications associated with peptic ulcers include haemorrhage, obstruction and perforation. See the 'Manifestations' box for the manifestations of these complications.

Among people with PUD, 10–20% experience **haemorrhage** as a result of ulceration and erosion into the blood vessels of the gastric mucosa. In the older adult, bleeding is the most frequent complication. When small blood vessels erode, blood loss may be slow and insidious, with occult blood in the stool the only initial sign. If bleeding continues, the person becomes anaemic and experiences symptoms of weakness, fatigue, dizziness and orthostatic hypotension. Erosion into a larger vessel can lead to sudden and severe bleeding with haematemesis, melaena or haematochezia (blood in the stool) and signs of hypovolaemic shock.

Gastric outlet obstruction may result from oedema surrounding the ulcer, smooth muscle spasm or scar tissue.

Peptic ulcer disease

Normal gastric mucosa

In the stomach and duodenum, the mucosal barrier protects the gastric mucosa (including the epithelial, vascular and smooth muscle layers) from damage. Specialised mucous cells throughout the gastric mucosa produce a mucus (a mixture of water, lipids and glycoproteins) that serves as a barrier to the diffusion of ions (such as hydrogen ion) and molecules (such as pepsin). A thin layer of bicarbonate, secreted by surface epithelial cells, forms between the mucous and cell membranes. Blood flow to the gastric mucosa is vital to maintain this barrier. Prostaglandins and nitric oxide stimulate mucus and bicarbonate production, helping maintain it as well. The mucosal barrier constantly bathes surfaces of the gastric epithelial lining.

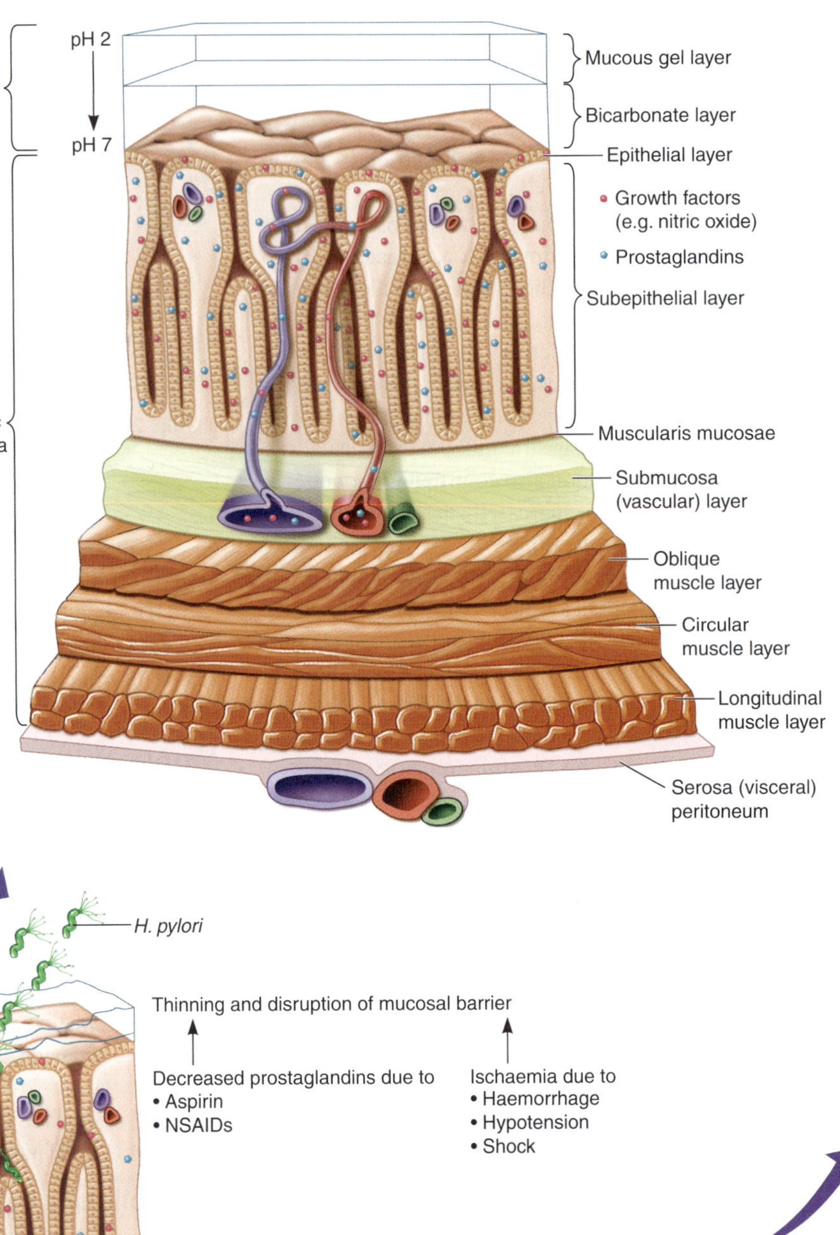

Disruption of mucosal barrier

The mucosal barrier can be disrupted by a number of factors. Ischaemia of the gastric mucosa (e.g. due to haemorrhage, hypotension or shock) impairs mucus production, increasing the risk of damage to the mucosa. Aspirin disrupts the mucosal barrier and, along with other non-steroidal anti-inflammatory drugs, inhibits prostaglandins, which are necessary to maintain mucous production. Alcohol and bile acids also damage the mucous barrier. *H.pylori,* a common pathogen to infect the gastric mucosa, disrupts the mucosal barrier.

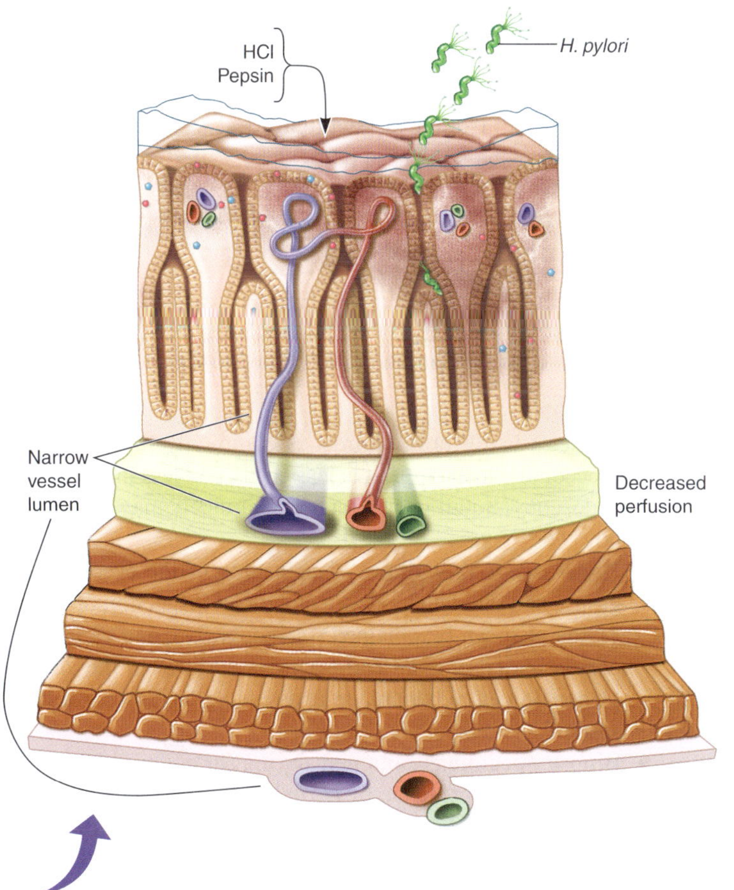

Inflammatory process

When the mucosal barrier is damaged, gastric acid and digestive juices disrupt the epithelial cell membranes, allowing acid to diffuse into cell walls. An acute inflammatory process results. Gastric epithelial cells migrate to the damaged area, a process known as restitution. Adequate blood flow and an alkaline environment are necessary for this repair process. Prostaglandins play an important role in epithelial repair. In the presence of *H. pylori* infection, excess acid production, inadequate blood flow, inhibition of prostaglandins, and other factors that are less clear, the inflammatory process further damages gastric and duodenal epithelial cells, leading to ulceration of the mucosa.

Erosion and ulcer formation

Superficial ulcers (erosions) erode the mucosa, but do not penetrate the muscularis mucosae. True ulcers extend through the muscularis mucosae and into deeper layers of the gastrointestinal wall, damaging blood vessels and potentially penetrating the entire wall. Haemorrhage and peritonitis are potential acute complications of peptic ulcers.

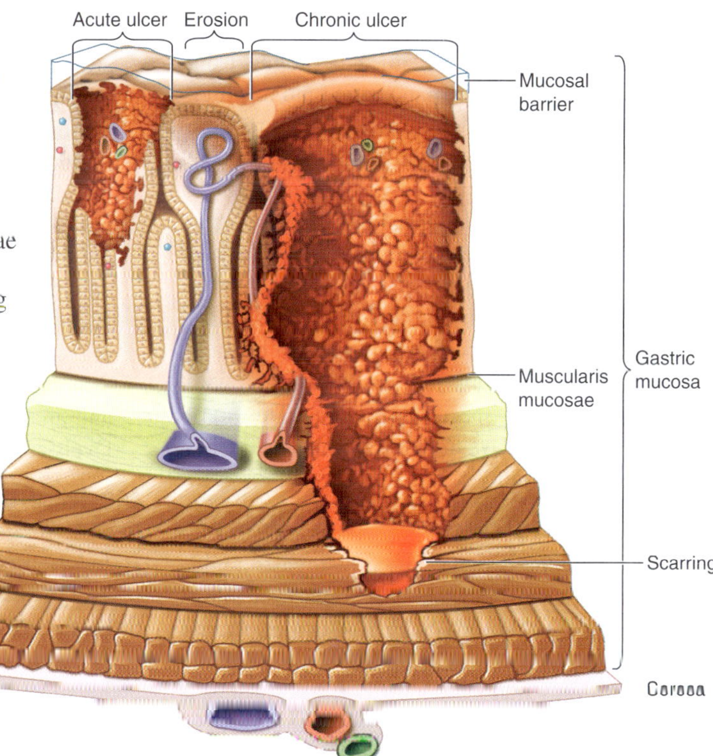

MANIFESTATIONS **PUD complications**

HAEMORRHAGE
- Occult or obvious blood in the stool
- Haematemesis
- Fatigue
- Weakness, dizziness
- Orthostatic hypotension
- Hypovolaemic shock

OBSTRUCTION
- Sensations of epigastric fullness
- Nausea and vomiting
- Electrolyte imbalances
- Metabolic alkalosis

PERFORATION
- Severe upper abdominal pain, radiating to the shoulder
- Rigid, board-like abdomen
- Absence of bowel sounds
- Diaphoresis
- Tachycardia
- Rapid, shallow respirations
- Fever

Generally, obstruction is a gradual rather than an acute process. Symptoms include a feeling of epigastric fullness, accentuated ulcer symptoms and nausea. If the obstruction becomes complete, vomiting occurs. Hydrochloric acid, sodium and potassium are lost in vomitus, potentially leading to fluid and electrolyte imbalance and metabolic alkalosis.

The most lethal complication of PUD is **perforation** of the ulcer through the mucosal wall. When perforation occurs, gastric or duodenal contents enter the peritoneum, causing an inflammatory process and peritonitis. Chemical peritonitis from the hydrochloric acid, pepsin, bile and pancreatic fluid is immediate; bacterial peritonitis follows within 6 to 12 hours from gastric contaminants entering the normally sterile peritoneal cavity. When an ulcer perforates, the person has immediate, severe upper abdominal pain, radiating throughout the abdomen and possibly to the shoulder. The abdomen becomes rigid and board-like, with absent bowel sounds. Signs of shock may be present, including diaphoresis, tachycardia and rapid, shallow respirations. Classic symptoms of perforation may not be present in an older adult. The older adult may instead present with mental confusion and other non-specific symptoms. This atypical presentation can lead to delays in diagnosis and treatment, increasing the associated mortality rate.

Zollinger–Ellison syndrome

Zollinger–Ellison syndrome is PUD caused by a gastrinoma, or gastrin-secreting tumour of the pancreas, stomach or intestines. Gastrinomas may be benign, although 50–70% are malignant tumours. Gastrin is a hormone that stimulates the secretion of pepsin and hydrochloric acid. The increased gastrin levels associated with these tumours result in hypersecretion of gastric acid, which in turn causes mucosal ulceration.

The peptic ulcers of Zollinger–Ellison syndrome may affect any portion of the stomach or duodenum, as well as the oesophagus or jejunum. Characteristic ulcer-like pain is common. The high levels of hydrochloric acid entering the duodenum may also cause diarrhoea and steatorrhoea (excess fat in the faeces) from impaired fat digestion and absorption. Complications of bleeding and perforation are often seen with Zollinger–Ellison syndrome. Fluid and electrolyte imbalances may also result from persistent diarrhoea, with resultant losses of potassium and sodium in particular.

INTERPROFESSIONAL CARE

Treatment for PUD focuses on eradicating *H. pylori* infection and treating or preventing ulcers related to the use of NSAIDs.

Diagnosis

- *CT scan* using oral contrast is commonly the diagnostic procedure chosen first; it is less costly and less invasive than endoscopy. Small or very superficial ulcers may be missed, however.
- *Upper endoscopy* allows visualisation of the oesophageal, gastric and duodenal mucosa and direct inspection of ulcers. Tissue also can be obtained for biopsy. Nursing care of the person undergoing an endoscopy is outlined in the chapter 'A person-centred approach to assessing the gastrointestinal system'.
- Biopsy specimens obtained during an endoscopy can be tested for the presence of *H. pylori* using several different methods. In the *biopsy urease test*, the specimen is put into a gel containing urea. If *H. pylori* is present, the urease that it produces changes the colour of the gel, often within minutes. Biopsy specimen cells also can be microscopically examined or cultured for evidence of *H. pylori*. Although these tests are highly specific for *H. pylori* infection, their invasiveness, cost and lack of availability in some areas limits their usefulness.
- A non-invasive method of detecting *H. pylori* infection is the *urea breath test*. In this test, radio-labelled urea is given orally. The urease produced by *H. pylori* bacteria converts the urea to ammonia and radio-labelled carbon dioxide, which can then be measured as the person exhales.
- If Zollinger–Ellison syndrome is suspected, *gastric analysis* may be performed to evaluate gastric acid secretion. Stomach contents are aspirated through a nasogastric tube and analysed. In Zollinger–Ellison syndrome, gastric acid levels are very high.

Medications

The medications used to treat PUD include agents to eradicate *H. pylori*, drugs to decrease gastric acid content and agents that protect the mucosa. Nursing responsibilities related to selected drugs to treat GORD, gastritis and PUD are found in the 'Medication administration: drugs used to treat GORD, gastritis and peptic ulcer disease' box.

Eradication of *H. pylori* is often difficult. Combination therapies that use two antibiotics with a PPI (e.g. combinations of a PPI, clarithromycin and amoxicillin, or a PPI, a tetracycline and metronidazole) are necessary. With complete eradication of *H. pylori*, reinfection rates are less than 0.5% per year.

In people who have NSAID-induced ulcers, the NSAID in use should be discontinued if at all possible. If this is not possible, twice-daily PPIs enable ulcer healing.

Medications that decrease gastric acid content include PPIs and the H_2-receptor antagonists.

- PPIs bind the acid-secreting enzyme (H^+, K^+ ATPase) that functions as the proton pump, disabling it for up to 24 hours. These medications are very effective, resulting in more than 90% ulcer healing after 4 weeks. Compared with the H_2-receptor blockers, the PPIs provide faster pain relief and more rapid ulcer healing.
- Histamine$_2$-receptor blockers inhibit histamine binding to the receptors on the gastric parietal cells to reduce acid secretion. These medications are very well tolerated and have few serious side effects; however, drug interactions can occur. These medications must be continued for 8 weeks or longer for ulcer healing.

Agents that protect the mucosa include sucralfate, bismuth, antacids and prostaglandin analogues.

- Sucralfate binds to proteins in the ulcer base, forming a protective barrier against acid, bile and pepsin. Sucralfate also stimulates the secretion of mucus, bicarbonate and prostaglandin.
- Antacids stimulate gastric mucosal defences, thereby aiding in ulcer healing. They provide rapid relief of ulcer symptoms and are often used as needed to supplement other anti-ulcer medications. Antacids are inexpensive, but people often have difficulty with a regular regimen because the medications must be taken frequently and may cause either constipation (from the aluminium-type antacids) or diarrhoea (from the magnesium-based antacids). Antacids also interfere with the absorption of iron, digoxin, some antibiotics and other drugs.
- Prostaglandin analogues (misoprostol) promote ulcer healing by stimulating mucus and bicarbonate secretions and by inhibiting acid secretion. Although not as effective as the other medications discussed, misoprostol is used to prevent NSAID-induced ulcers.

Treatments

NUTRITION In addition to pharmacological treatment, people are encouraged to maintain good nutrition, consuming balanced meals at regular intervals. It is important to teach people that bland or restrictive diets are no longer necessary. Mild alcohol intake is not harmful. Smoking should be discouraged because it slows the rate of healing and increases the frequency of relapses.

SURGERY The identification of *H. pylori* as a cause of PUD and the availability of drugs to treat the infection and heal peptic ulcers has all but eliminated surgery as a treatment option for PUD. Older people, however, may have undergone gastric resection surgery for PUD and may have long-term complications related to the surgery. See the section on gastric cancer for more information about gastric surgery and its potential complications.

Treatment of complications

The person hospitalised with a complication of PUD, such as bleeding, gastrointestinal obstruction or perforation, and peritonitis, requires additional interventions to restore homeostasis.

In haemorrhage associated with PUD, initial interventions focus on restoring and maintaining circulation. Crystalloid solutions such as normal saline are administered intravenously to restore intravascular volume if signs of shock (tachycardia, hypotension, pallor, low urine output and anxiety) are present. Whole blood or packed red blood cells may be administered to restore haemoglobin and haematocrit levels. A nasogastric tube is inserted to prevent aspiration of vomited gastric contents.

Endoscopy with direct injection of a clotting or sclerosing agent into the bleeding vessel may be performed. Laser photocoagulation, using light energy, or electrocoagulation, which uses electric current to generate heat, can also be done via endoscopy to seal bleeding vessels.

The person is kept NBM until bleeding is controlled. PPIs are administered intravenously (e.g. 40 mg of esomeprazole per intravenous push or admixture daily) to reduce the risk of rebleeding. Surgery may be necessary if medical measures are ineffective in controlling bleeding. Older adults who experience bleeding as a complication of PUD are more likely to rebleed or require surgery to control the haemorrhage. See 'Nursing care of the person having gastric surgery' later in the chapter.

Repeated inflammation, healing, scarring, oedema and muscle spasm can lead to gastric outlet (pyloric) obstruction. Initial treatment includes gastric decompression with nasogastric suction and administration of intravenous normal saline and potassium chloride to correct fluid and electrolyte imbalance. H_2-receptor blockers are given intravenously as well. Balloon dilation of the gastric outlet may be done via upper endoscopy. If these measures are unsuccessful in relieving obstruction, surgery may be required.

Gastric or duodenal perforation resulting in contamination of the peritoneum with gastrointestinal contents often requires immediate intervention to restore homeostasis and minimise peritonitis. Intravenous fluids maintain fluid and electrolyte balance. Nasogastric suction removes gastric contents and minimises peritoneal contamination. Placing the person in the Fowler's or semi-Fowler's position allows peritoneal contaminants to pool in the pelvis. Intravenous antibiotics aggressively treat bacterial infection from intestinal flora. Laparoscopic surgery or an open laparotomy may close the perforation.

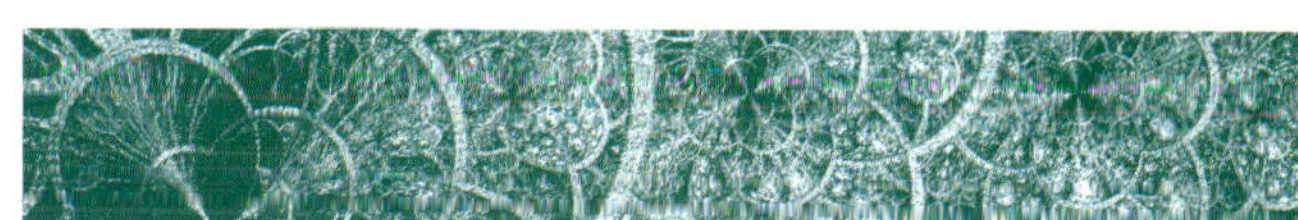

Nursing care

Health promotion

Although it is difficult to predict which people will develop PUD, promote health by advising people to avoid risk factors such as excessive aspirin or NSAID use and cigarette smoking.

In addition, encourage people to seek treatment for manifestations of GORD or chronic gastritis, both of which are also associated with *H. pylori* infection.

Assessment

Collect the following subjective and objective data when assessing the person with PUD:

- *Health history*: complaints of epigastric or left upper quadrant pain, heartburn or discomfort; its character, severity, timing and relationship to eating; measures used for relief; nausea or vomiting, presence of bright blood or 'coffee grounds' appearing material in vomitus; current medications, including use of aspirin or other NSAIDs; cigarette smoking and use of alcohol or other drugs.
- *Physical examination*: general appearance, including height and weight relationship; vital signs, including orthostatic measurements; abdominal examination, including shape and contour, bowel sounds and tenderness to palpation; presence of obvious or occult blood in vomitus and stool.

Nursing diagnoses and interventions

The priorities of nursing care for the person with PUD are reducing discomfort, maintaining nutritional status and preventing or rapidly identifying and intervening for potential complications. See the accompanying nursing care plan.

Pain related to PUD

The pain of PUD is often predictable and preventable. Pain is typically experienced 2 to 4 hours after eating, as high levels of gastric acid and pepsin irritate the exposed mucosa. Measures to neutralise the acid, minimise its production or protect the mucosa often relieve this pain, minimising the need for analgesics.

- Assess pain, including location, type, severity, frequency and duration, and its relationship to food intake or other contributing factors.
- Administer PPIs, H_2-receptor antagonists, antacids or mucosal protective agents as ordered. Monitor for effectiveness and side effects or adverse reactions. *The pain associated with PUD is generally caused by the effect of gastric juices on exposed mucosal tissue. These medications reduce pain and promote healing by reducing acid production, neutralising the acid or providing a barrier for the damaged mucosa.*
- Teach relaxation, stress reduction and lifestyle management techniques. Refer for stress management counselling or classes as indicated. *Although there is no clear relationship between stress and PUD, measures to relieve stress and promote physical and emotional rest help to reduce the perception of pain and may reduce ulcer genesis.*

> **CONSIDERATION FOR PRACTICE**
>
> **Avoid making assumptions about pain. Acute pain may indicate a complication, such as perforation (often heralded by sudden, severe epigastric pain and a rigid, board-like abdomen) or it may be totally unrelated to PUD (e.g. angina, gallbladder disease or pancreatitis).**

Disturbed sleep pattern

Night-time ulcer pain, which typically occurs between 1 and 3 am, may disrupt the sleep cycle and result in inadequate rest. Anticipation of pain may lead to insomnia or other sleep disruptions.

- Stress the importance of taking medications as prescribed. *The bedtime dose of PPI or H_2-receptor blocker minimises hydrochloric acid production during the night, reducing night-time pain.*
- Instruct to limit food intake after the evening meal, eliminating any bedtime snack. *Eating before bed can stimulate the production of gastric acid and pepsin, increasing the likelihood of night-time pain.*
- Encourage the use of relaxation techniques and comfort measures such as soft music as needed to promote sleep. *Once the pain associated with PUD has been controlled, these measures help to reduce anxiety and re-establish a normal sleep pattern.*

Imbalanced nutrition (less than body requirements) related to PUD

In an attempt to avoid discomfort, the person with PUD may gradually reduce food intake, sometimes jeopardising nutritional status. Anorexia and early satiety are additional problems associated with PUD.

- Assess current diet, including pattern of food intake, eating schedule and foods that precipitate pain or are being avoided in anticipation of pain. *The person may not realise the extent of self-imposed dietary limitations, especially if symptoms have persisted for an extended time. Assessment increases awareness and also helps to identify the adequacy of nutrient intake.*
- Refer to a dietitian for meal planning to minimise PUD symptoms and meet nutritional needs. Consider normal eating patterns and preferences in meal planning. *Although no specific diet is recommended for PUD, people should avoid foods that increase pain. Six small meals per day often help increase food tolerance and decrease postprandial discomfort.*
- Monitor for complaints of anorexia, fullness, nausea and vomiting. *Adjust dietary intake or medication schedule as indicated. PUD and resultant scarring can lead to impaired gastric emptying, necessitating a treatment change.*
- Monitor laboratory values for indications of anaemia or other nutritional deficits. Monitor for therapeutic and side effects of treatment measures such as oral iron replacement. Instruct the person taking oral iron replacement to avoid using an antacid within 1 to 2 hours of taking the iron preparation. *Anaemia can result from poor nutrient absorption or chronic blood loss in people with PUD. Oral iron supplements may cause GI distress, nausea and vomiting; if these side effects are intolerable, notify the doctor for a possible change of therapy. Antacids bind with oral iron preparations, blocking absorption.*

NURSING CARE PLAN A person with peptic ulcer disease

Sean O'Donnell is a 47-year-old police officer who lives and works in a metropolitan area. Mr O'Donnell has had 'heartburn' and abdominal discomfort for years, but thought it went along with his job. Last year, after becoming weak, lightheaded and short of breath, he was found to be anaemic and was diagnosed as having a duodenal ulcer. He took omeprazole (Losec) and ferrous sulfate for 3 months before stopping both, saying he had 'never felt better in his life'. Mr O'Donnell has now been admitted to the hospital with active upper GI bleeding.

ASSESSMENT

Rachel Clark is Mr O'Donnell's admitting nurse. On initial assessment, Mr O'Donnell is alert and oriented, though very apprehensive about his condition. Skin pale and cool; BP 136/78, P 98; his abdomen is distended and tender with hyperactive bowel sounds; 200 mL bright red blood is obtained on nasogastric tube insertion. Haemoglobin 82 g/L and haematocrit 23% on admission. Mr O'Donnell is taken to the endoscopy lab where his bleeding is controlled using laser photocoagulation. On his return to the ward, he receives two units of packed RBCs and intravenous fluids to restore blood volume. A 5-day course of high-dose oral omeprazole (40 mg bd) is ordered to prevent rebleeding and Mr O'Donnell is allowed to begin a clear fluid diet 24 hours after his endoscopy. Tissue biopsy obtained during endoscopy confirms the presence of *H. pylori* infection.

DIAGNOSES

- *Deficient fluid volume* related to acutely bleeding duodenal ulcer.
- *Risk of injury* related to acute blood loss.
- *Anxiety* related to threat to wellbeing.
- *Ineffective therapeutic regimen management* related to lack of knowledge regarding PUD and its treatment.

PLANNING

- Ensure nurse call bell is kept by bedside at all times.
- Discuss situation and provide information about all procedures and treatments. Encourage Mr O'Donnell to alert nursing staff immediately if he experiences any signs of blood loss such as dizziness or vomiting.
- Arrange for a pharmacist review to discuss current and planned treatment measures, the importance of completing the prescribed treatment to reduce the risk of further ulcer development and avoiding use of aspirin or NSAIDs in the future.

Expected outcomes

- Maintains normal blood pressure, pulse and urine output (> 0.5 mL/kg/hour).
- Remains injury free.
- Seeks information to reduce anxiety.
- Identifies and uses coping strategies to manage anxiety.
- Describes prescribed therapeutic regimen.
- Verbalises ability to manage prescribed regimen.

IMPLEMENTATION

- Encourage Mr O'Donnell to ask for help when getting up or ambulating. Remind to rise slowly from lying to sitting and sitting to standing.
- Reassure about the effectiveness of treatment in reducing the risk of further bleeding.
- Discuss stress reduction techniques and refer for stress reduction counselling or workshops as indicated.

EVALUATION

Mr O'Donnell is discharged 48 hours after admission. He has had no further evidence of bleeding and has resumed a regular diet. His haemoglobin and haematocrit remain low and he has a prescription for ferrous sulfate. He will complete the prescribed high-dose omeprazole regimen at home and then begin treatment with omeprazole, amoxicillin and clarithromycin to eradicate the *H. pylori* infection detected during endoscopy. After 2 weeks of this regimen, he will continue taking omeprazole at bedtime for 4 to 8 weeks. He verbalises a good understanding of his treatment and of the importance of completing the entire regimen. Mr O'Donnell expresses concern about his ability to 'keep his cool on the inside' when under stress. Registered Nurse Clark provides Mr O'Donnell with several resources to help with stress management in case he wants help.

CRITICAL THINKING IN THE NURSING PROCESS

1. How does *H. pylori* infection contribute to the development of peptic ulcers?
2. Describe the physiological responses to fear and anxiety. Why is it important to alleviate fear and its physical consequences in people with PUD?
3. What suggestions can you make to help Mr O'Donnell manage his complex treatment regimen during the next 3 months?
4. Develop a teaching plan that includes stress reduction techniques Mr O'Donnell can use while carrying out his duties as a police officer.

REFLECTION ON THE NURSING PROCESS

1. Outline what you have learned from this case study that you will apply to your future practice.
2. Reflect on the lifestyle stressors involved in Mr O'Donnell's life. What strategies could he use to reduce stress while carrying out his duties as a police officer?

CONSIDERATION FOR PRACTICE

Advise the person to report increasing or persistent symptoms of anorexia, nausea and vomiting, or fullness to the healthcare provider.

Deficient fluid volume related to haemorrhage

Erosion of a blood vessel with resultant haemorrhage is a significant risk for the person with PUD. Acute bleeding can lead to hypovolaemia and fluid volume deficit, which can lead to a decrease in cardiac output and impaired tissue perfusion.

CONSIDERATION FOR PRACTICE

Monitor and record blood pressure and pulse every 15 to 30 minutes until stable. Monitor central venous pressure or pulmonary artery pressure as indicated. Insert an indwelling catheter and monitor urinary output hourly. Weigh daily. Continuous monitoring of cardiac output parameters is essential in people with an acute haemorrhage to identify possible shock and intervene at an early stage.

- Monitor stools and gastric drainage for overt and occult blood. Assess gastric drainage (vomitus or from a nasogastric tube) to estimate the amount and rapidity of haemorrhage. *Drainage is bright red with possible clots in acute haemorrhage; dark red or the colour of coffee grounds when blood has been in the stomach for a period of time. Haematochezia (stool containing red blood and clots) is present in acute haemorrhage; melaena (black, tarry stool) is an indicator of less acute bleeding. When small vessels are disrupted, bleeding may be slow and not overtly evident. With chronic or slow gastrointestinal bleeding, the risk of a fluid volume deficit is minimal; anaemia and activity intolerance are more likely.*
- Maintain intravenous therapy with fluid volume and electrolyte replacement solutions; administer whole blood or packed cells as ordered. *Both fluids and electrolytes are lost through vomiting, nasogastric drainage and diarrhoea in an episode of acute bleeding. To prevent shock, it is essential to maintain a blood volume and cardiac output sufficient to perfuse body tissues. Whole blood and packed cells replace both blood volume and red blood cells, providing additional oxygen-carrying capacity to meet cell needs.*
- Unless contraindicated, insert a nasogastric tube and maintain its position and patency. Initially, measure and record gastric output every hour, then every 4 to 8 hours. *Nasogastric suction removes blood from the gastrointestinal tract, preventing vomiting and possible aspiration. Gastric output is replaced millilitre for millilitre with a balanced electrolyte solution to maintain homeostasis.*
- Monitor haemoglobin and haematocrit, serum electrolytes, BUN and creatinine values. Report abnormal findings. *Haemoglobin and haematocrit are lower than normal with acute or chronic GI bleeding. In acute haemorrhage, initial results may be within normal range because both cells and plasma are lost. Loss of fluids and electrolytes with gastric drainage and diarrhoea will alter normal levels. Digestion and absorption of blood in the GI tract may result in elevated BUN and creatinine levels.*
- Assess abdomen, including bowel sounds, distension, girth and tenderness, every 4 hours and record findings. *Borborygmi or hyperactive bowel sounds with abdominal tenderness are common with acute GI bleeding. Increased distension, increasing abdominal girth, absent bowel sounds or extreme tenderness with a rigid, board-like abdomen may indicate perforation.*
- Maintain bed rest with the head of the bed elevated. Ensure safety. *Loss of blood volume may cause orthostatic hypotension with resultant syncope or dizziness upon standing.*

Community-based care

PUD is managed in home and community-based settings; only its complications typically require treatment in an acute care setting. Provide the following information when preparing the person for home care:

- prescribed medication regimen, including desired and potential adverse effects
- importance of continuing therapy even when symptoms are relieved
- relationship between peptic ulcers and factors such as NSAID use and smoking. If indicated, refer to a smoking cessation clinic or program
- importance of avoiding aspirin and other NSAIDs; stress the necessity of reading the labels of over-the-counter medications for possible aspirin content
- manifestations of complications that should be reported to the local doctor, including increased abdominal pain or distension, vomiting, black or tarry stools, light-headedness or fainting
- stress and lifestyle management techniques that may help prevent exacerbation. Refer to resources for stress management, such as classes, counselling and formal or informal groups.

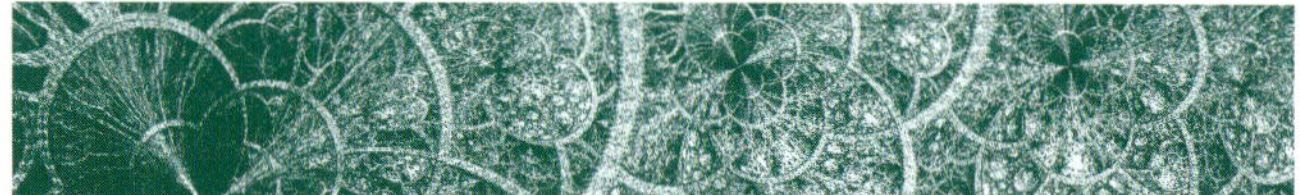

THE PERSON WITH CANCER OF THE STOMACH

Stomach cancer is the third leading cause of cancer deaths worldwide. In Australia, over 2,000 cases are diagnosed every year, with a 28.5% survival rate after 5 years. Stomach cancer affects nearly twice as many men as women and the risk of being diagnosed increases with age (Cancer Australia, 2022c).

Risk factors

H. pylori infection is a major risk factor for cancer of the distal portion of the stomach; from 35% to 89% of cases can be attributed to this infection. Other risk factors are a genetic predisposition, chronic gastritis, pernicious anaemia, gastric polyps and carcinogenic factors in the diet (such as smoked foods and nitrates). Achlorhydria, a lack of hydrochloric acid in the stomach, is a known risk factor. The risk of gastric cancer also is increased in people who have had a partial gastric resection. Socioeconomic factors are also linked with gastric cancer, including occupations that involve exposure to certain chemicals such as dust, asbestos, solvents and pesticides; smoking; and a diet poor in fruit and vegetables and lacking antioxidant mechanisms (Cancer Australia, 2020).

Pathophysiology

Adenocarcinoma, which involves the mucus-producing cells of the stomach, is the most common form of gastric cancer. These carcinomas may arise anywhere on the mucosal surface of the stomach but are most frequently found in the distal portion. Fifty to sixty per cent of gastric cancers occur in the antrum or pyloric region (Norris, 2018). Gastric cancer begins as a

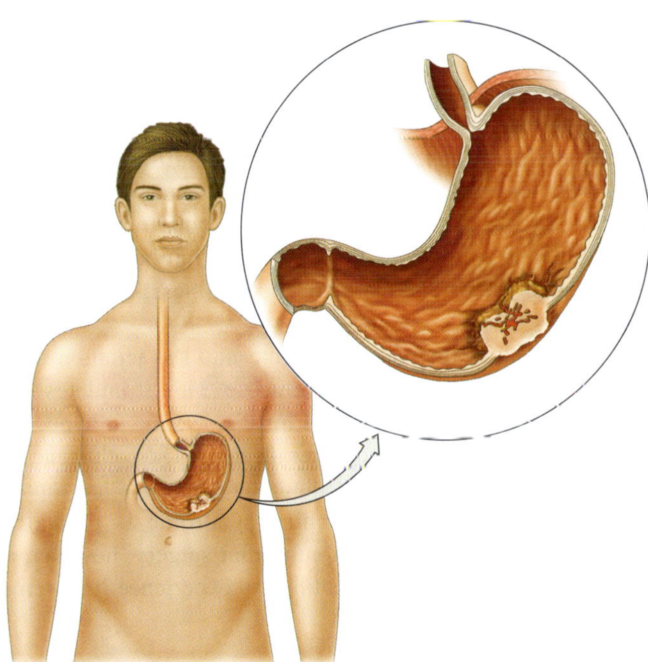

FIGURE 22.9 *Gastric cancer affecting the antrum of the stomach*

localised lesion (in situ), then progresses to involve the mucosa or submucosa (early gastric carcinoma). Lesions may spread by direct extension to tissues surrounding the stomach—the liver, in particular. The lesion may ulcerate or appear as a polypoid (polyp-like) mass (see Figure 22.9). Lymph node involvement and metastasis occur early due to the rich blood and lymphatic supply to the stomach. Metastatic lesions are often found in the liver, lungs, ovaries and peritoneum.

Manifestations

Few symptoms are associated with gastric cancer. Unfortunately, the disease is often quite advanced and metastases are usually present at the time of diagnosis. Early symptoms are vague, including feelings of early satiety, anorexia, indigestion and possibly vomiting. The person may experience ulcer-like pain unrelieved by antacids, typically occurring after meals. As the disease progresses, weight loss occurs and the person may be **cachectic** (in very poor health and malnourished) at the time of diagnosis. An abdominal mass may be palpable and occult blood may be present in the stool, indicating gastrointestinal bleeding.

INTERPROFESSIONAL CARE

Diagnosis

Anaemia detected by a full blood count is often the first indication of gastric cancer. An upper GI x ray with barium swallow is useful to identify lesions and ultrasound or CT scan may identify a mass. Upper endoscopy with visualisation and biopsy of the lesion provides the definitive diagnosis.

Surgery

When gastric cancer is identified prior to the development of metastasis, surgical removal of part or all of the stomach and regional lymph nodes is the treatment of choice. **Partial gastrectomy** involves removal of a portion of the stomach, usually the distal half to two-thirds. In partial gastrectomy, the surgeon constructs an anastomosis from the remainder of the stomach directly to the duodenum or to the proximal jejunum. The **gastroduodenostomy**, or **Billroth I**, and the **gastrojejunostomy**, or **Billroth II**, are commonly used partial gastrectomy procedures (see Figures 22.10A and B).

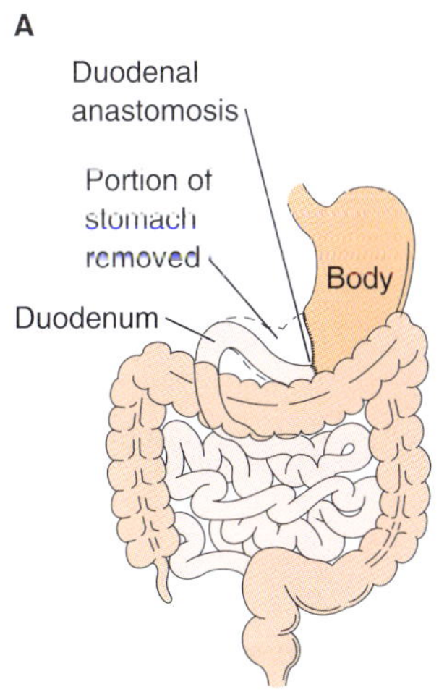

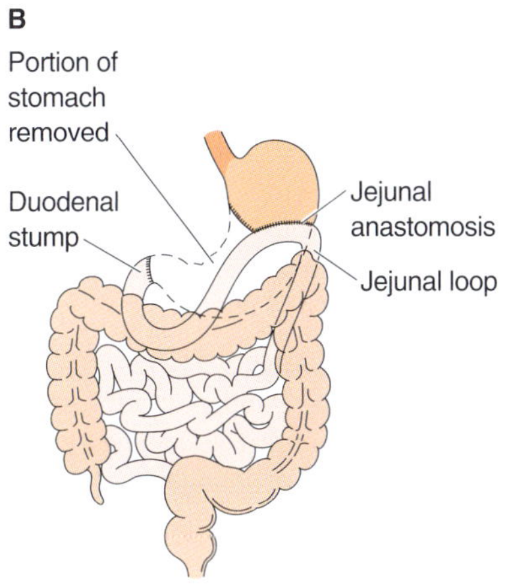

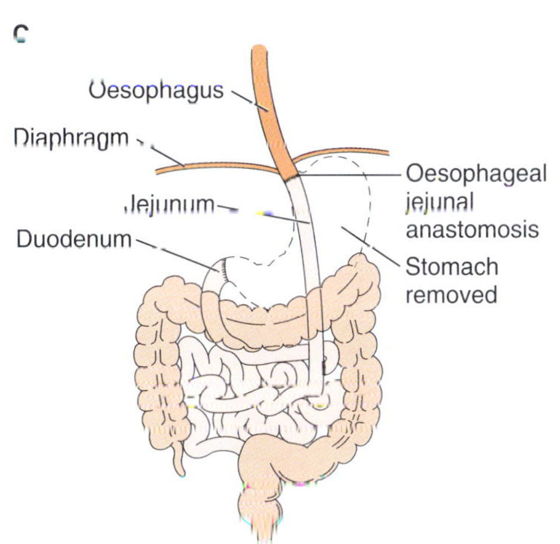

FIGURE 22.10 *Partial and total gastrectomy procedures*
A, Partial gastrectomy with anastomosis to the duodenum.
B, Partial gastrectomy with anastomosis to the jejunum.
C, Total gastrectomy with anastomosis of the oesophagus to the jejunum

A **total gastrectomy**, removal of the entire stomach, may be done for diffuse cancer that is spread throughout the gastric mucosa but limited to the stomach. In a total gastrectomy, the surgeon constructs an anastomosis from the oesophagus to the duodenum or jejunum. Total gastrectomy with **oesophago-jejunostomy** is illustrated in Figure 22.10C.

Nursing care of the person who has undergone gastric surgery is outlined in the accompanying box.

Complications

Several long-term complications may develop following gastrectomy procedures. **Dumping syndrome** is the most common problem. It may follow a partial gastrectomy with duodenal or jejunal anastomosis. When the pylorus has been resected or bypassed, a hypertonic, undigested food bolus may rapidly enter the duodenum or jejunum. Water is pulled into the lumen of the intestine by the hyperosmolar character of the chyme, resulting in decreased blood volume and intestinal dilation. Peristalsis is stimulated and intestinal motility is increased.

Early symptoms of dumping syndrome occur within 5 to 30 minutes after eating. These symptoms result from intestinal dilation, peristaltic stimulation and hypovolaemia caused by undigested food in the proximal small intestine. Manifestations include nausea with possible vomiting, epigastric pain with cramping and borborygmi (loud, hyperactive bowel sounds), and diarrhoea. Systemic symptoms from the hypovolaemia and reflex sympathetic stimulation include tachycardia, orthostatic hypotension, dizziness, flushing and diaphoresis.

The entry of hyperosmolar chyme into the jejunum also causes a rapid rise in the blood glucose. This stimulates the release of an excessive amount of insulin, leading to hypoglycaemic symptoms 2 to 3 hours after the meal. The pathogenesis and clinical manifestations of dumping syndrome are represented in Figure 22.11. Dumping syndrome is typically self-limiting, lasting 6 to 12 months after surgery; however, a small percentage of people continue to experience long-term symptoms.

NURSING CARE OF THE PERSON having gastric surgery

PREOPERATIVE NURSING CARE

- See the chapter 'Nursing care of people having surgery' for routine preoperative care and teaching.
- Insert a nasogastric tube if ordered preoperatively. *Although it is often inserted in the surgical suite just prior to surgery, the nasogastric tube may be placed preoperatively to remove secretions and empty stomach contents.*

POSTOPERATIVE NURSING CARE

- Provide routine care for the surgical person as outlined in the chapter 'Nursing care of people having surgery'.
- Assess position and patency of nasogastric tube, connecting it to low suction. Gently irrigate with sterile normal saline if tube becomes clogged. The nasogastric tube will be placed in surgery to avoid disruption of the gastric suture lines and should be well secured. If repositioning or tube replacement is needed, notify the surgeon. *Patency must be maintained to keep the stomach decompressed, reducing pressure on sutures.*
- Assess colour, amount and odour of gastric drainage, noting any changes in these parameters or the presence of clots or bright bleeding. Initial drainage is bright red. It becomes dark, then clear or greenish-yellow over the first 2 to 3 days. *A change in the colour, amount or odour may indicate a complication such as haemorrhage, intestinal obstruction or infection.*
- Maintain intravenous fluids while nasogastric suction is in place. *The person on nasogastric suction is not only unable to take oral food and fluids but also is losing electrolyte-rich fluid through the nasogastric tube. If replacement fluid and electrolytes are not maintained, the person is at risk of dehydration, imbalances of electrolytes and metabolic alkalosis.*
- Provide anti-ulcer and antibiotic therapy as ordered. *These medications may be ordered for the postoperative person, depending on the procedure performed. Antibiotic therapy is a common preventive measure for infection that may result from contamination of the abdominal cavity with gastric contents.*
- Monitor bowel sounds and abdominal distension. *Bowel sounds indicate resumption of peristalsis. Increasing distension may indicate third spacing, obstruction or infection.*
- Resume oral food and fluids as ordered. Initial feedings are clear fluids, progressing to free fluids and then frequent small feedings of regular foods. Monitor bowel sounds and for abdominal distension frequently during this period. *Oral feedings are reintroduced slowly to minimise trauma to the suture lines by possible gastric distension.*
- Encourage ambulation. *Ambulation stimulates peristalsis.*

HEALTH EDUCATION FOR THE PERSON AND FAMILY

- Begin discharge planning and teaching. Consult with a dietitian for diet instructions and menu planning; reinforce teaching. Teach the person about potential post-operative complications, such as abdominal abscess, dumping syndrome, postprandial hypoglycaemia or pernicious anaemia. Also, teach the person to recognise signs and symptoms and to take preventive measures. *The person's gastric capacity is reduced after partial gastrectomy, necessitating a corresponding reduction in meal size. Changes in gastric emptying and reduction in gastric secretions may change the person's tolerance for many foods, requiring slow reintroduction of these foods. Dumping syndrome, postprandial hypoglycaemia and pernicious anaemia are possible long-term complications of partial gastrectomy. For most people, dietary modifications can control both dumping syndrome and postprandial hypoglycaemia.*

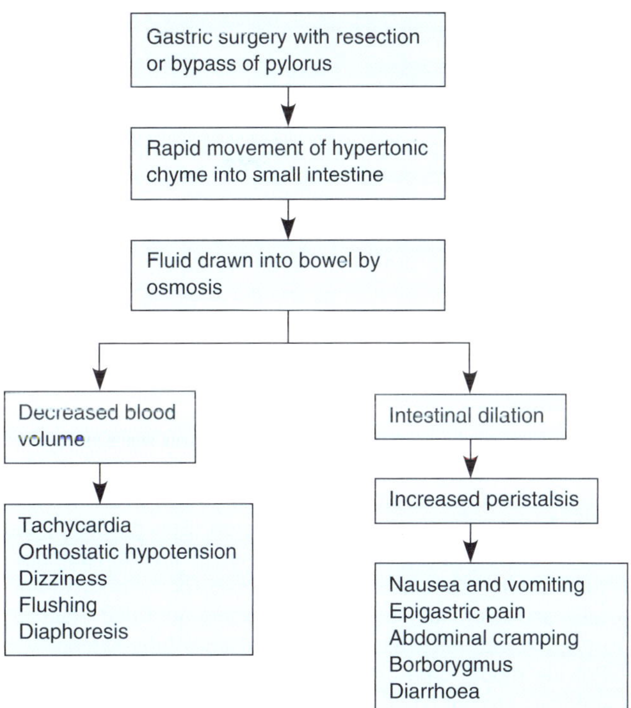

FIGURE 22.11 *The pathogenesis and manifestations of dumping syndrome*

Dumping syndrome is managed primarily by a dietary pattern that delays gastric emptying and allows smaller boluses of undigested food to enter the intestine. Meals should be small and more frequent. Liquids and solids are taken at separate times instead of together during a meal. The amount of proteins and fats in the diet is increased, because they exit the stomach more slowly than carbohydrates. Carbohydrates, especially simple sugars, are reduced. The person is instructed to rest in a recumbent or semi-recumbent position for 30 to 60 minutes after meals. Anticholinergics, sedatives and antispasmodics may be prescribed.

Anaemia may be a chronic problem after a major gastric resection. Iron is absorbed primarily in the duodenum and proximal jejunum; rapid gastric emptying or a gastrojejunostomy may interfere with adequate absorption.

The cells of the stomach produce intrinsic factor, required for the absorption of vitamin B_{12}. Vitamin B_{12} deficiency leads to pernicious anaemia. Because of hepatic stores of vitamin B_{12}, symptoms of anaemia may not be seen for 1 to 2 years after surgery. Vitamin B_{12} levels are routinely monitored following extensive gastric resections.

Other nutritional problems seen following surgery include folic acid deficiency and decreased absorption of calcium and vitamin D. Poor absorption of nutrients, combined with the inability to eat large meals, puts the person at risk of weight loss in addition to the more specific nutrient deficiencies. Nearly 50% of people who have gastric surgery experience significant weight loss, primarily because of insufficient kilojoule intake. Factors contributing to insufficient intake of kilojoules include early satiety (feeling of fullness), decreased stomach size and altered emptying patterns.

Other therapies

Radiation or chemotherapy may be used to eliminate any lymphatic or metastatic spread. For the person with more advanced disease, treatment is palliative and may include surgery and chemotherapy. These people may require a gastrostomy or jejunostomy feeding tube (see Figure 22.12). See the accompanying box for nursing care of the person with a gastrostomy or jejunostomy tube.

Because gastric cancer is generally advanced by the time of diagnosis, the prognosis is poor. The 5-year survival rate of all people treated for gastric carcinoma is 20%.

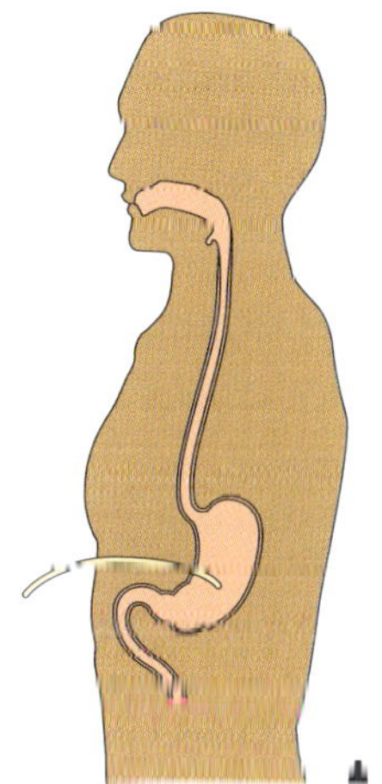

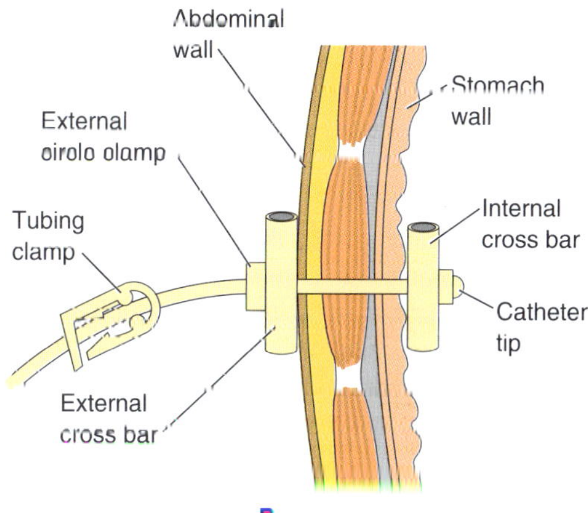

FIGURE 22.12 *Gastrostomy. A, Gastrostomy tube placement. B, The tube is fixed against both the abdominal and the stomach walls by cross bars*

NURSING CARE OF THE PERSON with a gastrostomy or jejunostomy tube

People who have had extensive gastric surgery or who require long-term enteral feedings to maintain nutrition may have a gastrostomy or jejunostomy tube inserted.

PROCEDURE

Gastrostomy tubes are surgically placed in the stomach, with the stoma in the epigastric region of the abdomen (see Figure 22.12). Jejunostomy tubes are placed in the proximal jejunum. Immediately following the procedure, the tube may be connected to low suction or plugged. If the person has been receiving tube feedings, these may be reinitiated shortly after tube placement.

NURSING CARE

- Assess tube placement by aspirating stomach contents and checking pH of aspirate to determine gastric or intestinal placement. A pH of 5 or less indicates gastric placement; the pH is generally 7 or higher with intestinal placement. *Recent studies show auscultation to be ineffective in determining feeding tube placement. Measuring the pH of aspirate from the tube is more reliable as a means of determining tube placement.*
- Inspect the skin surrounding the insertion site for healing, redness, swelling and the presence of any drainage. If drainage is present, note the colour, amount, consistency and odour. *Changes in the insertion site, drainage or lack of healing may indicate an infection.*
- Assess the abdomen for distension, bowel sounds and tenderness *to evaluate functioning of the gastrointestinal tract.*
- Until the stoma is well healed, use sterile technique for dressing changes and site care. Clean technique is appropriate for use once healing is complete. *Sterile technique reduces the risk of wound contamination by pathogens that can lead to infection. Once healing has occurred, clean technique is acceptable because the gastrointestinal tract is not a sterile body cavity.*
- Wearing clean gloves, remove old dressing. Cleanse the site with saline or tap water and rinse as appropriate. A well-healed stoma may be cleansed in the shower with the tube clamped or plugged. Pat dry with 4 × 4 gauze pads and allow to air dry. Apply Stomahesive, karaya or other protective agents around tube as needed to protect the skin. *Gastric acid and other wound drainage is irritating to the skin. Meticulous care is important to maintain the integrity of the skin surrounding the stoma.*
- Re-dress the wound using a stoma dressing or folded 4 × 4 gauze pads. Do not cut gauze pads because threads may enter the wound, causing irritation and increasing the risk of inflammation.
- Irrigate the tube with 30 to 50 mL of water and clean the tube inside and out as indicated or ordered. Soft gastric tubes may require cleaning of the inner lumen to maintain patency. *Tube feeding formulas may coat the inside of the gastrostomy tube and eventually cause it to become occluded. Regular irrigation with water as indicated maintains tube patency.*
- Provide mouth care or remind the person to do so. *When feedings are not being taken orally, the usual stimulus to do mouth care is lost. In addition, salivary fluids may not be as abundant and oral mucous membranes may become dry and cracked.*

HEALTH EDUCATION FOR THE PERSON AND FAMILY

- If indicated, teach the person and family how to care for the tube and feedings. *Refer to a home health agency or community nurse for support and reinforcement of learning. Gastrostomy tubes are often in place long term. When the person and family are able to assume care, independence and self-image are enhanced.*

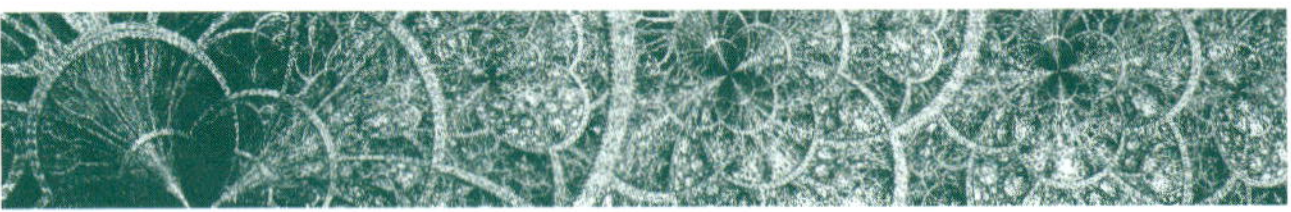

Nursing care

Health promotion

Although the exact causes of gastric cancer are unknown, contributing factors such as *H. pylori* infection and consumption of foods preserved with nitrates have been identified. To reduce their risk of developing gastric cancer, encourage people with known *H. pylori* infection to complete the prescribed course of treatment and verify that it has eradicated the infection. With all people, discuss the relationship between gastric cancer and consumption of foods preserved with nitrates (such as bacon and other processed meats) and encourage limited consumption of these products.

Assessment

Assessment data related to gastric cancer include the following:

- *Health history*: manifestations such as anorexia, early satiety, indigestion or vomiting; epigastric pain after meals; recent unintentional weight loss.
- *Physical assessment*: general appearance, weight for height; abdominal distension or a palpable upper abdominal mass; occult blood in stool or vomitus.

Nursing diagnoses and interventions

Priorities of nursing care for the person with gastric cancer focus on the effects of the disease and its treatment on nutritional status and on the effects of a potentially fatal disease on the person and their family. See the accompanying nursing care plan for a person with gastric cancer.

Risk of imbalanced nutrition (less than body requirements) manifested by unintentional weight loss

The person with gastric cancer may be malnourished because of anorexia, early satiety and increased metabolic needs related to the tumour. Extensive gastric resection also makes it difficult to consume an adequate diet. Malnourishment, in turn, impairs healing and the person's ability to tolerate cancer treatment.

- Consult with dietitian for a complete nutrition assessment and diet planning. *The person is at risk of protein energy malnutrition, which impairs the ability to heal and recover from extensive surgery.*

NURSING CARE PLAN A person with gastric cancer

George Harvey is a 61-year-old lawyer who lives with his wife, Harriet. For the past 3 months, Mr Harvey has had increasing anorexia and difficulty eating. He has lost 4.5 kg. His doctor has diagnosed gastric cancer and Mr Harvey is admitted for a partial gastrectomy and gastrojejunostomy. The oncologist has recommended postoperative chemotherapy and radiation. Mr Harvey reports that the doctor told him, 'That will give me the best chance for a cure.'

ASSESSMENT

On admission before surgery, Mr Harvey tells his nurse, Lauren Walsh, that he has eaten very little in the past few weeks. He asks, 'What will happen to my wife if something happens to me? I'm afraid this cancer will get me.' Mr Harvey weighs 67 kg and is 183 cm tall. He is pale and thin; his vital signs are BP 148/86, P 92, R 18 and T 36.5°C PO. A firm mass is palpable in the left epigastric region. The rest of his physical assessment data are within normal limits. Mr Harvey's haemoglobin is 128 g/L, haematocrit is 39% and serum albumin level is 32g/L, indicating that he is mildly malnourished. All other preoperative laboratory and diagnostic studies are within normal limits.

DIAGNOSES

- *Risk of imbalanced nutrition (less than body requirements)* related to anorexia and difficulty eating.
- *Acute pain* related to surgical incision and manipulation of abdominal organs.
- *Risk of ineffective airway clearance* related to upper abdominal surgery.
- *Anticipatory grieving* related to recent diagnosis of cancer.

PLANNING

- Arrange for dietary education, including strategies to prevent dumping syndrome, prior to surgery.
- Encourage Mrs Harvey to visit at mealtimes to assist with and promote oral intake.
- Discuss the grief process and encourage verbalisation of feelings about diagnosis and perceived losses.
- Establish a schedule to cough, deep breathe and use breathing incentive every 2 to 4 hours and as needed. Demonstrate how to splint abdomen during coughing.
- Ensure the nurse call bell is kept within reach at all times and encourage Mr Harvey to alert nursing staff promptly when he is experiencing pain.

Expected outcomes

- Maintain present weight during hospitalisation.
- Resume a high-kilojoule, high-protein diet by the time of discharge.
- Verbalise effective pain management, maintaining a reported pain level of 3 or less on a scale of 1 to 10.
- Maintain a patent airway and clear breath sounds.
- Verbalise feelings regarding diagnosis and participate in decision making.

IMPLEMENTATION

- Weigh daily.
- Maintain nasogastric tube placement, patency and suction as ordered.
- Maintain intravenous fluids and total parenteral nutrition as ordered until oral food intake is resumed.
- Maintain patient-controlled analgesia until able to take oral analgesics.
- Assess respiratory status, including rate, depth and breath sounds, every hour initially, then every 4 hours.
- Encourage participation in decision making.

EVALUATION

Mr Harvey's weight remained stable through his hospitalisation. On discharge he is taking a high-protein, high-kilojoule diet in six small feedings per day. He and his wife have reviewed his diet with the dietitian and are planning on using some dietary supplements at home to meet protein needs. He verbalises an understanding of measures to prevent dumping syndrome, including separating his intake of solid foods and liquids. Mr Harvey is using oral analgesics in the morning and at bedtime to control his pain. He and his wife have begun to discuss the meaning of his diagnosis. Mrs Harvey tells the discharge nurse, 'We are going to go to a support group called "Coping with cancer" when George is stronger.'

CRITICAL THINKING IN THE NURSING PROCESS

1. What is the rationale for maintaining nasogastric suction after gastrojejunostomy?
2. Develop a preoperative teaching plan for a person undergoing a partial gastrectomy.
3. Design interventions to ensure adequate nutrition for people with advanced gastric cancer.

REFLECTION ON THE NURSING PROCESS

1. Outline what you have learned from this case study that you will apply to your future practice.
2. Mr Harvey calls you just before the initial dose of chemotherapy and says, 'Everyone tells me that chemotherapy will cause vomiting and I don't think I can take being sick again.' Reflect on how you would respond.

- Weigh daily. Monitor laboratory values such as haemoglobin, haematocrit and serum albumin levels. *Daily weights are a valuable measurement of both fluid and nutritional status. Laboratory values provide further evidence of nutritional status.*
- Provide preferred foods; have family prepare meals when possible. Provide supplemental feedings between meals. *Small, frequent feedings and preferred foods encourage intake of nutrients.*
- Arrange for visitors to be present during meals. Eating is a social function as well as a physiological one. *Companionship often improves food intake.*
- Administer pain and anti-emetic medications as needed before meals. *Pain and nausea suppress the appetite; relief promotes food intake.*

CONSIDERATION FOR PRACTICE

Assess ability to consume adequate nutrients. Nausea and feelings of early satiety may impair nutrient consumption, indicating a need to institute enteral or parenteral feedings.

Anticipatory grieving

- Encourage family members to spend as much time as possible with the person. The family may feel helpless and ineffectual. *Supporting family members' presence can encourage this vital interaction.*
- Do not negate denial if present. *Denial is a coping mechanism that protects the person from hopelessness.*
- Allow the person to talk openly if desired about their condition and the prognosis. *Acceptance of the person's fears helps reduce anxiety and promote coping behaviours.*
- Actively listen to the person's and family's expressions of grieving. Avoid interrupting or offering meaningless words of consolation. *Being present and listening actively are often the most effective interventions for the grieving person.*

Community-based care

Although the person with gastric cancer may be hospitalised for surgery, most care is provided in the home and community-based settings such as hospice care. When preparing the person and family for home care, discuss the following topics:

- care of incision and feeding tube (if present) or central venous line
- maintaining nutrition and preventing complications of surgery such as dumping syndrome
- pain management
- provide referrals to home care agencies, hospice and cancer support groups as appropriate
- provide information about services available through the local branch of the Cancer Council.

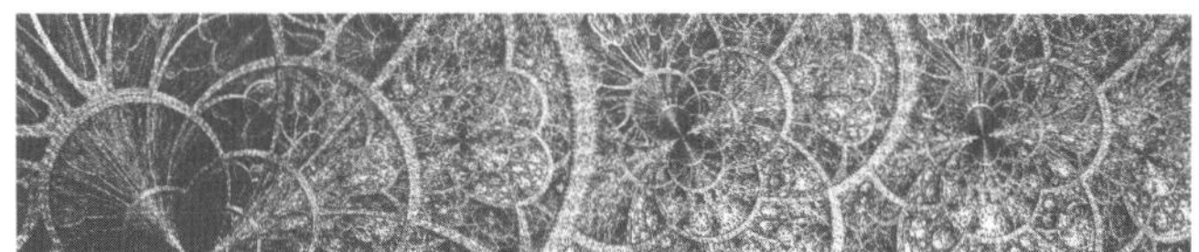

CHAPTER HIGHLIGHTS

- Nausea and vomiting, common GI symptoms, may be indicative of disorders affecting many organ systems, including the GI tract, inner ear, CNS or heart. Complications such as dehydration, electrolyte imbalance and aspiration of gastric contents are primary concerns in treating nausea and vomiting.
- Oral mucositis is a common disorder of the mouth, potentially having a significant effect on comfort and nutrition.
- Tobacco and alcohol use contribute to a number of upper GI disorders, including GORD, oral and oesophageal cancers, and peptic ulcer disease. Encourage all people to stop smoking or use smokeless tobacco and to reduce alcohol to moderate amounts, if at all, to reduce their risk of developing these disorders.
- Gastro-oesophageal reflux disease (GORD) is common. While it often is considered to be a benign condition, prolonged exposure of the lower oesophagus to gastric juices can lead to oesophagitis, haemorrhage and scarring.
- Both oesophageal and gastric cancer are often diagnosed late in the disease because their symptoms may be vague. Encourage people with complaints of dysphagia, a sensation of gastric fullness or heartburn to seek medical evaluation. Surgical resection of the cancerous portion of the oesophagus or stomach is the treatment of choice when the tumour is diagnosed early.
- Upper gastrointestinal bleeding can lead to significant blood loss and shock. Peptic ulcer disease accounts for the majority of UGI haemorrhage, although erosive gastritis and oesophageal varices also are common causes.
- Acute gastritis, often associated with aspirin or NSAID use, is generally benign and self-limited. Erosive gastritis, a complication of critical conditions such as shock, trauma, a major burn or head injury, can lead to unexpected gastric haemorrhage. Chronic gastritis is an unrelated disorder associated with *H. pylori* infection.
- *H. pylori* infection also is a major risk factor for peptic ulcer disease and gastric cancer. Effectively treating the infection can reduce or eliminate the risk of future exacerbations of PUD.
- An acute change in the nature of abdominal pain in a person with PUD, especially when accompanied by vomiting, guarding of the abdomen or a change in bowel sounds, could indicate an obstruction or perforation and release of gastric contents into the peritoneal cavity.

CONCEPT CHECK

1 The nurse assessing for oral cancer risk factors in a person with a persistent sore on his tongue asks about:
1 consumption of highly spiced food
2 thumb sucking or pacifier use as a child
3 regular use of dental floss
4 tobacco use in any form

2 The nurse teaching a person with gastro-oesophageal reflux disease includes which of the following instructions? (Select all that apply.)
1 This is a benign disease requiring no treatment.
2 Elevate the head of the bed.
3 Stop taking the prescribed proton-pump inhibitor once symptoms are relieved.
4 Peppermint and chocolate lollies can help relieve symptoms.
5 Avoid lying down for several hours after eating.

3 The nurse evaluates his teaching of a person with acute stress gastritis as effective when the person states that she will:
1 avoid using aspirin or NSAIDs for routine pain relief
2 consume only bland foods
3 return for yearly upper endoscopy exams
4 fully cook all meat, poultry and egg products

4 The nurse identifies which of the following nursing diagnoses as highest priority for the person admitted with peptic ulcer disease and possible perforation?
1 *Acute pain*
2 *Ineffective health maintenance*
3 *Nausea*
4 *Impaired gastrointestinal tissue integrity*

5 Following a partial gastrectomy for gastric cancer, the person complains of nausea, abdominal pain and cramping, and diarrhoea after eating. Recognising manifestations of dumping syndrome, the nurse recommends:

1 fasting for a period of 6 to 12 hours before meals
2 decreasing the protein content of meals
3 frequent small meals that contain solid foods or liquids, but not both
4 a diet rich in carbohydrates to maintain blood glucose levels

6 The nurse caring for a person with oesophageal cancer affecting the middle portion of the oesophagus would immediately report which of the following?

1 crackles in the base of the right lung
2 bright bleeding from the mouth
3 weight loss
4 difficulty swallowing solid foods

7 The doctor has prescribed omeprazole 20 mg twice daily, clarithromycin 500 mg twice daily and amoxicillin 1 g daily for a person with peptic ulcer disease. It is most important for the nurse to instruct the person to:

1 stop the medications immediately and notify the doctor if a rash, hives or itching develop
2 consume yoghurt daily while taking these drugs
3 take the medications on an empty stomach, 1 hour before breakfast and at least 2 hours after dinner
4 take the medications with a full glass of water

8 When planning care for a person with oral mucositis, the nurse identifies which of the following as a priority intervention?

1 Assist to cleanse mouth with mouthwash following meals.
2 Allow the person to select appealing foods from a menu.
3 Provide viscous lignocaine to relieve mouth pain before meals.
4 Refer the person to a smoking cessation program.

9 The evening following a gastric resection, the nurse notes that there has been no drainage from the nasogastric tube for the past 3 hours. The nurse should:

1 chart the finding
2 reposition the nasogastric tube
3 gently irrigate the tube with normal saline
4 notify the surgeon

10 A person with a history of peptic ulcer disease suddenly reports severe abdominal pain. The nurse should: (Select all that apply.)

1 administer the prescribed proton-pump inhibitor
2 obtain an order for a opioid analgesic
3 withhold oral food and fluids
4 place the person in Fowler's position
5 notify the medical officer

BIBLIOGRAPHY

Burton, L., Beattie, J., Falk, G. L., Van der Wall, H. & Coman, W. (2020.) The burden of gastroesophageal reflux disease on the cost of managing chronic diseases in Australia. The need for a new diagnostic and management paradigm. *Journal of Chronic Disease Management*, 4(1), 1024.

Cancer Australia (2020). *Stomach cancer*. Retrieved from https://www.canceraustralia.gov.au/

Cancer Australia (2022a). *Head and neck cancer*. Retrieved from https://www.canceraustralia.gov.au/

Cancer Australia (2022b). *Oesophageal cancer*. Retrieved from https://www.canceraustralia.gov.au/

Cancer Australia (2022c). *Stomach cancer*. Retrieved from https://www.canceraustralia.gov.au/

Cancer Council (2020). *Mouth health and cancer treatment: Information for people affected by cancer*. Retrieved from https://www.cancercouncil.com.au/

Edwards, D. (2021). *Evidence summary. Chemotherapy-induced nausea and vomiting: Ginger*. The JBI EBP Database. JBI-ES-1129-1.

Eslick, G. D., Tilden, D., Arora, N., Torres, M. & Clancy, R. L. (2020). Clinical and economic impact of 'triple therapy' for *Helicobacter pylori* eradication on peptic ulcer disease in Australia. *Helicobacter (Cambridge, Mass.)*, *25*(6), e12751. https://doi.org/10.1111/hel.12751

Isozaki, A. B. & Brant, J. M. (2022). Clinical updates in mucositis-related symptom management. *Seminars in Oncology Nursing*, *38*(1), 151252.

Joanna Briggs Institute (JBI) (2022). *Recommended practice. Nasoenteric tube: Administration of enteral feed*. The JBI EBP Database. JBI-RP-4814-4.

Ket, S. N., Sparrow, R. L., McQuilten, Z. K., Gibson, P. R., Brown, G. J. & Wood, E. M. (2021). Critical peptic ulcer bleeding requiring massive blood transfusion: Outcomes of 270 cases. *Internal Medicine Journal*, *51*(12), 2042–2050. https://doi.org/10.1111/imj.15009

Low, D. E., Allum, W., De Manzoni, G. et al. (2019). Guidelines for perioperative care in esophagectomy: Enhanced Recovery After Surgery (ERAS®) Society recommendations. *World Journal of Surgery*, *43*, 299–330. https://doi.org/10.1007/s00268-018-4786-4

Millor, G. C., Wong, C. & Pollock, A. J. (2015). Gastro-oesophageal reflux disease (GORD) in Australian general practice patients. *Australian Family Physician*, *44*(10), 701–704.

Norris, T. L. (2018). *Porth's pathophysiology: Concepts of altered health states* (10th ed.). Philadelphia: Lippincott Williams & Wilkins.

Porritt, K. (2021). *Evidence summary. Nasoenteric tube feeding (adults): Monitoring*. The JBI EBP Database. JBI-ES-2153-2.

Pulito, C., Cristaudo, A., Porta, C. L. et al. (2020). Oral mucositis: The hidden side of cancer therapy. *Journal of Experimental & Clinical Cancer Research*, *39*, 210. https://doi.org/10.1186/s13046-020-01715-7

Ryan, K., Malacova, E., Appleyard, M., Brown, A. F. T., Song, L. & Grimpen, F. (2021). Clinical utility of the Glasgow Blatchford Score in patients presenting to the emergency department with upper gastrointestinal bleeding: A retrospective cohort study. *Emergency Medicine Australasia*, *33*(5), 817–825.

Whiteman, D. C. & Kendall, B. J. (2016). Barrett's oesophagus: Epidemiology, diagnosis, and clinical management. *Medical Journal of Australia*, *205*(7), 317–324.

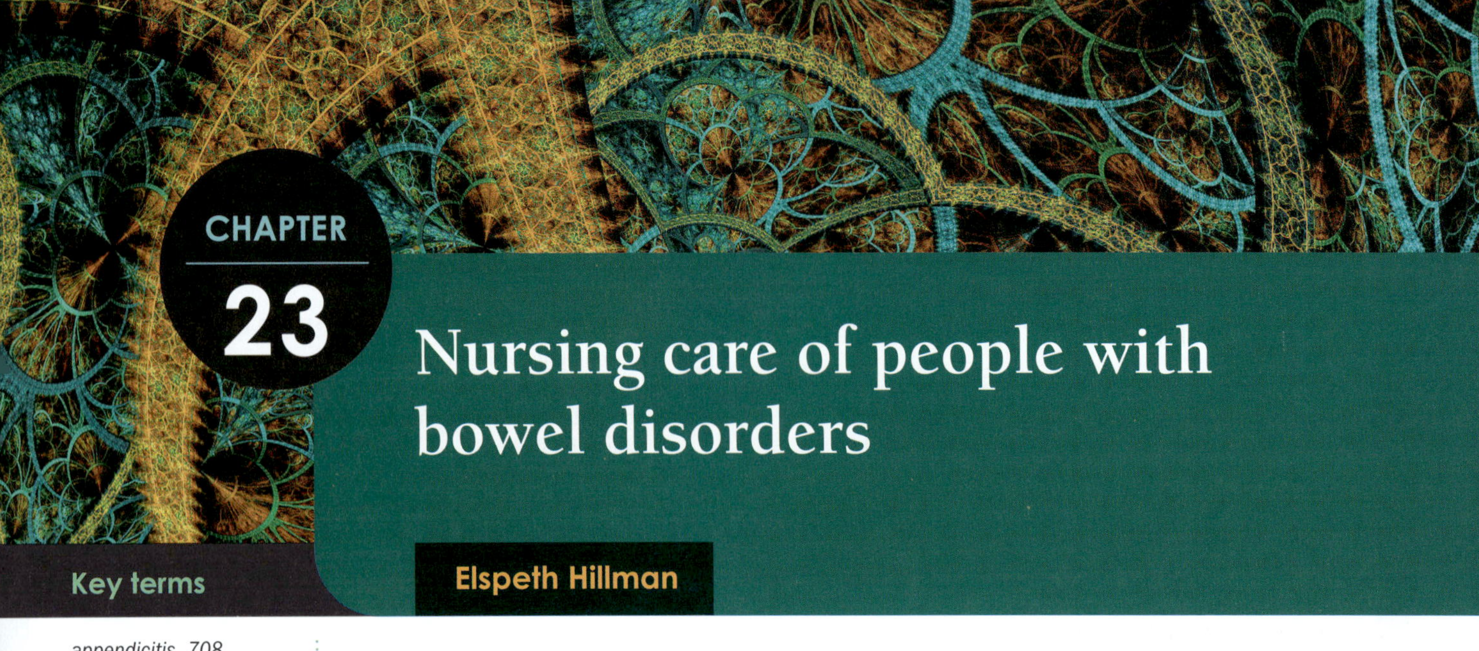

CHAPTER 23

Nursing care of people with bowel disorders

Elspeth Hillman

Key terms

appendicitis 708
colectomy 735
colostomy 753
Crohn's disease 732
diverticulitis 766
diverticulosis 766
faecal impaction 697
gastroenteritis 716
haemorrhoids 768
ileostomy 736
inflammatory bowel disease (IBD) 728
irritable bowel syndrome (IBS) 704
malabsorption 743
paralytic ileus 761
peritonitis 711
sprue 743
stoma 736
ulcerative colitis 729

Learning outcomes

- Explain the pathophysiology, manifestations, interprofessional and nursing care of people with disorders of intestinal motility.
- Explain the pathophysiology, complications and interprofessional care of people with acute inflammatory or infectious bowel disorders.
- Compare and contrast the pathophysiology, manifestations and complications of chronic inflammatory bowel disorders.
- Discuss the risk factors, pathophysiology and interprofessional care associated with neoplastic bowel disorders.
- Discuss the pathophysiology, manifestations and nursing care of people suffering from structural and obstructive bowel disorders.
- Describe the pathophysiology, manifestations and nursing care of a person suffering an anorectal disorder.

Clinical competencies

- Assess the functional status of a person with bowel disorders and monitor, document and report abnormal manifestations.
- Use evidence-based research to prevent aspiration in critically ill individuals with enteral feedings and to make accurate assessments of faecal incontinence in older adults.
- Determine priority nursing diagnoses based on assessed data and select and implement individualised nursing interventions for a person with bowel disorders.
- Administer medications used in the management of bowel disorders knowledgeably and safely.
- Provide skilled care to a person following the formation of an ileostomy or colostomy, or perianal surgery.
- Integrate interprofessional care into care of a person with bowel disorders.
- Provide appropriate teaching to promote nutrition, prevent infectious and helminth infestations, encourage preventive screening for colon cancer and facilitate community-based care for healthcare needs resulting from bowel disorders.
- Revise plan of care when necessary to provide effective interventions promoting, maintaining or restoring functional health status to a person with a bowel disorder.

Disorders of intestinal absorption and bowel elimination do not only affect functional elimination status. Other functional health patterns affected include, but are not limited to, health perception–health management, nutritional–metabolic, activity–exercise, self-perception–self-concept and sexuality–reproductive. Bowel function is affected by inflammations, infections, tumours, obstructions or changes in bowel structure.

A person with an intestinal disorder often faces extensive diagnostic testing, surgery and permanent changes in their physical appearance and lifestyle. Nursing care is directed towards meeting the person's physiological needs, providing emotional support and assisting the person's adaption to lifestyle changes.

Disorders of intestinal motility

Few body functions respond as readily to internal and external influences as defecation. Factors directly affecting the gastrointestinal (GI) tract include food intake and bacterial population, which affect the number and consistency of stools. Indirect factors also affect elimination. Consider the effects psychological stress or voluntary postponement of defecation have on elimination.

'Normal' bowel elimination patterns vary widely. For some people, two to three stools per day is their usual pattern, whereas for other people, their usual pattern is three stools per week. It is important to evaluate each person's bowel elimination against their normal pattern.

THE PERSON WITH DIARRHOEA

Diarrhoea is an increase in the frequency, volume and fluid content of the stool. In diarrhoea, the water content of faeces is increased, usually due to either malabsorption or water secretion in the bowel. It is a clinical manifestation, rather than the primary disorder.

Diarrhoea may be acute or chronic. Acute diarrhoea (lasting less than a week) is usually due to an infectious agent. Chronic diarrhoea (persisting longer than 3 to 4 weeks) may be caused by inflammatory bowel disorders, malabsorption or endocrine disorders.

Pathophysiology

Approximately 1,500 mL of digested material enters the large intestine daily. Normally, most of the water and some solutes are reabsorbed in the bowel, leaving approximately 200 mL of faeces to be eliminated.

Large-volume diarrhoea is characterised by both increased numbers and volume of stools caused by increased water content of the stool. This increased water content results from either osmotic or secretory processes. Water is pulled into the bowel lumen by osmosis when the faeces contain osmotically active molecules. Some stool softeners and laxatives work on this principle. When lactose in milk is not broken down and absorbed, the lactose molecules exert an osmotic pull, causing diarrhoea. The diarrhoea associated with cholera and *Escherichia coli* infection is caused by increased water secretion in the small and large intestines. Unabsorbed dietary fat, some laxatives and drugs cause secretory diarrhoea.

Small-volume diarrhoea, characterised by frequent small stools, is usually caused by inflammation or disease of the colon. Diseases affecting the intestinal mucosa—for example, inflammatory bowel disease—cause exudative diarrhoea. Mucosal inflammation causes plasma, serum proteins, blood and mucus to accumulate in the bowel, increasing faecal bulk and fluidity. An increased propulsion rate within the bowel decreases the amount of water normally absorbed from chyme, leading to diarrhoea. For this reason, laxatives increasing bowel motility and bowel resection or bypass can lead to diarrhoea.

Antibiotic-associated diarrhoea occurs as a result of disruption of normal intestinal flora by antibiotic therapy. Loss of normal flora affects digestion of food leading to diarrhoea, or allows an overgrowth of pathogens (e.g. *Clostridium difficile* (*C. difficile*)). The 'Translation to practice' box provides information about other causes of diarrhoea in hospitalised people.

Manifestations

Clinical manifestations of diarrhoea depend on the cause, duration, severity and area of bowel affected, as well as a person's age and general health. Diarrhoea presents as several large, watery stools daily or very frequent small stools containing blood, mucus or exudates.

Complications

Diarrhoea can have devastating effects. Water and electrolytes are lost in diarrhoeal stools, leading to dehydration, particularly in the very young, older adults or debilitated individuals unable to respond to thirst. With severe diarrhoea, vascular collapse and hypovolaemic shock may occur. Potassium and magnesium are lost, potentially leading to hypokalaemia and hypomagnesaemia. The loss of bicarbonate in the stool can lead to metabolic acidosis. See the chapter 'Nursing care of people with altered fluid, electrolyte and acid–base balance' for further discussion of the effects of fluid and electrolyte imbalances.

INTERPROFESSIONAL CARE

Management of diarrhoea focuses on identifying and treating the underlying cause. Additionally, the diarrhoea itself needs to be treated, [illegible] and complications are prevented. A health history (including the onset and associated circumstances of the diarrhoea) and physical examination often provide enough information to identify its cause. However, precise diagnosis is only achieved with laboratory investigations.

TRANSLATION TO PRACTICE **Evidence-based practice: diarrhoea**

People who have been hospitalised often have a number of risk factors for diarrhoea. *Clostridium difficile* is now recognised as the cause of a significant portion of treatment-related diarrhoea; it does not, however, account for all cases. Previous studies have demonstrated a relationship between diarrhoea and enteral tube feedings, medications containing sorbitol, lactose intolerance and other factors. A review by Odhiambo (2022) looked at the risk of developing diarrhoea during enteral feeding. Findings illustrate the contributory effects of medications, severe illness, infection and enteral tube feeding. Cross-contamination of the enteral nutrition system occurs through poor hand hygiene, inappropriate formulae storage and use, inappropriate cleaning of equipment and ineffective tube maintenance.

IMPLICATIONS FOR NURSING

People who are severely ill often require enteral tube feedings for nutritional support. Healing and immune function require adequate nutrition; other studies point to the beneficial effects of enteral nutrition for the majority of people. Discontinuing enteral feedings due to diarrhoea is not a desirable option. In some cases, changing the enteral feeding formula or adding probiotic (cultures of beneficial yeasts or bacteria) supplements may help normalise bowel function. Other options include antidiarrhoeal medications or soluble fibre supplements.

CRITICAL THINKING IN PERSON-CENTRED CARE

1 Administering medications containing sorbitol, a sugar that is not absorbed by the gut, is associated with an increased risk of developing diarrhoea among people who have been hospitalised. How does sorbitol increase the risk of diarrhoea? What would you do if you realised that a seriously ill person you are caring for was receiving enteral tube feeding and medications containing sorbitol?
2 The position of the feeding tube tip in the gut is also identified as a risk factor for diarrhoea associated with enteral tube feedings. Thinking about the functions of the stomach, pyloric valve, duodenum and jejunum, which type of tube (gastric, duodenal or jejunal) might carry the highest risk of diarrhoea? The lowest? What other enteral tube feeding risk factors are considered in tube placement?
3 A person is being discharged home with a gastrostomy tube and directions for enteral feedings. What teaching will you provide to the person and their family regarding tube care, feeding administration and bowel management?

Diagnosis

Diagnostic tests ordered to help identify the cause of diarrhoea may include a stool specimen analysis, culture and sensitivity. A sigmoidoscopy to visualise the bowel mucosa may be conducted. (See the chapter 'A person-centred approach to assessing the gastrointestinal system' for further information on diagnostic tests.) Tissue biopsy to identify chronic inflammatory processes, infection and other causes of diarrhoea may be obtained. Recently developed and improved diagnostic methods include enzyme immunoassays for faecal antigens and reverse transcriptase-polymerase chain reaction (RT-PCR) to identify some viruses (e.g. norovirus), and ELISA and the fluoresceinlabelled antibody test to detect antigens or oocysts of some protozoa (e.g. *Giardia* and *Cryptosporidium*) (Lee & Bishop, 2016). Additionally, serum electrolytes, serum osmolality and arterial blood gases (ABGs) are collected to assess for adverse effects of diarrhoea. Increased serum osmolality indicates water loss and dehydration.

Medications

Antidiarrhoeal medications are used sparingly or not at all until the cause of diarrhoea is identified. In diarrhoea associated with botulism or bacillary dysentery, giving an antidiarrhoeal agent worsens or prolongs the infection by slowing toxin elimination from the bowel. Once the underlying cause for diarrhoea is established, specific medications, if appropriate, are ordered to treat the underlying cause. Antibiotics are used cautiously as these alter the bowel's normal bacterial population and may actually increase diarrhoea. A balanced electrolyte solution may be required to replace fluid and electrolyte losses. Intravenous or oral potassium preparations may also be prescribed.

Opium and some of its derivatives, anticholinergics, absorbents and demulcents are commonly used as antidiarrhoeal preparations. Specific preparations, their method of action and nursing implications for these medications are outlined in the 'Medication administration' box.

Nutrition

Fluid and electrolyte replacement is of primary importance in managing a person with diarrhoea. If the person is tolerating oral fluids (i.e. the person is not experiencing nausea and vomiting), an oral glucose/balanced electrolyte solution provides the best fluid replacement. Several commercial preparations (e.g. Gastrolyte) are available, as are paediatric solutions, which can be used for adults as well as children.

During acute diarrhoea, the person's diet should be modified to rest the bowel. During the first 24 hours, solid food should be withheld. After this time, frequent, small amounts of starchy foods can be added. Milk and milk products are added last, as these contain lactose, which frequently aggravates the diarrhoea. Raw fruit and vegetables, fried foods, bran, wholegrain cereals, condiments, spices, coffee and alcoholic beverages are avoided during the recovery period as the bowel has difficulty processing these complex materials.

People with chronic diarrhoea may benefit by eliminating specific foods from their diet. Foods and non-food substances aggravating diarrhoea are outlined in Table 23.1. The diet should be high in kilojoules and nutritional value. Vitamin supplements may be necessary, particularly the fat-soluble vitamins (A, D, E, and K). Occasionally, people with severe chronic diarrhoea require parenteral nutrition (see the chapter 'Nursing care of people with nutritional disorders').

MEDICATION ADMINISTRATION Antidiarrhoeal preparations

ABSORBENTS AND PROTECTANTS

Kaolin and pectin (Kaopectate, Donnagel-MB)
Polycarbophil (FigerNorm, Equalactin)

Absorbent preparations act locally in the intestines to bind substances that can cause diarrhoea. Absorbents are safe and are generally available over the counter, although their efficacy has not been proved.

Nursing responsibilities

- Assess for contraindications to antidiarrhoeal therapy, such as some infections or chronic inflammatory bowel disease, including ulcerative colitis.
- If fever is present, check with the doctor before giving the medication.
- Administer these medications at least 1 hour before or 2 hours after other oral medications; these may interfere with the absorption of other medications.
- Observe the person's response to the medication. Constipation is a potential problem.

Health education for the person and family

- Take the recommended dosage at the onset of diarrhoea and after each loose stool.
- Do not take any of these preparations for more than 48 hours. If diarrhoea persists, notify the doctor.
- Do not give antidiarrhoeal medications to debilitated older adults without medical supervision.

ANTISECRETORY

Bismuth subsalicylate (Pepto-Bismol)

Bismuth subsalicylate, available without a prescription, has antisecretory, anti-inflammatory and antibacterial effects. It is widely used to control traveller's diarrhoea. Although it is generally safe at recommended doses, bismuth subsalicylate has potential toxic effects and interacts with medications such as aspirin and oral anticoagulants.

Nursing responsibilities

- Administer as ordered.
- Do not administer within 1 hour of other medications, as it may interfere with their absorption.
- Monitor for increased anticoagulant effect when given with warfarin or aspirin.

Health education for the person and family

- Chew bismuth subsalicylate tablets, rather than swallowing these whole, for maximal effectiveness.
- This medication may cause harmless darkening of your tongue and stools.
- If you are allergic to aspirin, use bismuth subsalicylate with caution. Do not use aspirin while you are taking this medication unless directed to do so by your doctor. Contact your doctor if diarrhoea persists for more than 2 days.

OPIUM AND OPIUM DERIVATIVES

Camphorated tincture of opium (Paregoric)
Tincture of opium (laudanum, opium tincture)
Difenoxin (Motofen)
Diphenoxylate (Lomotil, Lotrol, others)
Loperamide hydrochloride (Imodium)

Opium and its derivatives act on the central nervous system (CNS), decreasing the motility of the ileum and colon, slowing transit time and promoting more water absorption. These medications also decrease the sensation of a full rectum and increase anal sphincter tone.

Difenoxin, diphenoxylate and loperamide hydrochloride are synthetic opioids chemically related to pethidine (Bullock & Manias, 2022). However, they have minimal analgesic, euphoric or abuse-promoting effects and are in more common use today.

Nursing responsibilities

- Assess for contraindications to antidiarrhoeal or narcotic medications prior to giving these drugs.
- Administer paregoric undiluted with water.
- Do not administer difenoxin and diphenoxylate to a person receiving monoamine oxidase inhibitors (MAOIs); hypertensive crises may occur.
- Observe closely for increased effects of other CNS depressants, such as alcohol, narcotic analgesics or barbiturate sedatives.
- Observe for abdominal distension; toxic megacolon may occur if these medications are given to a person with ulcerative colitis.

Health education for the person and family

- Take the medication as recommended at the onset of diarrhoea and after each loose stool.
- These medications may be habit forming; use for no more than 48 hours.
- Avoid using alcohol and over-the-counter cold preparations while taking these medications.
- These preparations may cause drowsiness; avoid driving or operating machinery while taking them.

TABLE 23.1 Foods aggravating chronic diarrhoea

FOODS	REASON
Milk, ice-cream, yoghurt, soft cheeses, cottage cheese	Contain lactose; not tolerated by people with lactase deficiency unable to digest lactose.
Apple juice, pear juice, grapes, honey, dates, nuts, figs, fruit-flavoured soft drinks	Contain fructose; when consumed in large quantities, fructose may not be totally absorbed, causing an osmotic pull of fluid into the bowel.
Table sugar	Contains sucrose; not tolerated by people with sucrase deficiency.
Sugarless gums and mints	May contain sorbitol or mannitol, sugars that are not absorbed, causing an osmotic draw.
Antacids	Magnesium-containing antacids decrease bowel transit time and contain poorly absorbed salts, exerting an osmotic draw.
Coffee, tea, cola drinks, over-the-counter analgesics containing codeine	Contain caffeine, decreasing bowel transit time.

Complementary and alternative therapies

Herbal or homeopathic therapies may be used to help relieve diarrhoea. People with lactose intolerance may use lactase enzymes tablets or drops when consuming milk products. Herbal treatments include a strong tea of black pepper, chamomile, coriander, rosemary, sandalwood or thyme. Ginger tea or capsules are helpful in reducing intestinal inflammation and decreasing the effects of food poisoning.

Probiotics, live microorganisms similar to those normally found in the gut, may be used to prevent or treat antibiotic-associated diarrhoea (Slade, 2021). Probiotics are available as dietary supplements and food (e.g. yoghurt, yoghurt drinks). The person should consult a qualified medical or homeopathic practitioner when choosing to manage their diarrhoea with complementary and alternative therapies.

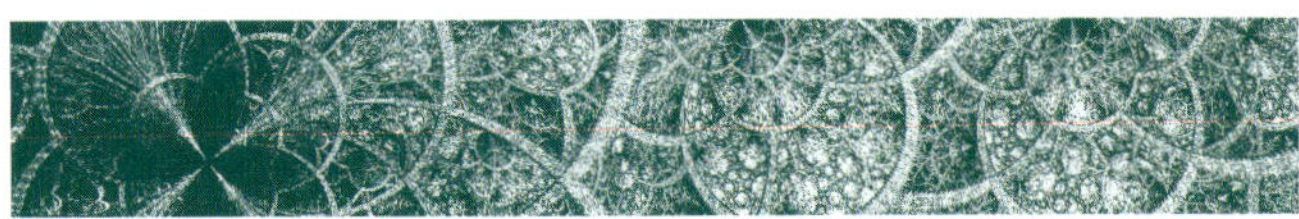

Nursing care

Health promotion

Prevention of diarrhoeal diseases essentially involves avoiding infectious agents (Lee & Bishop, 2016). Educating individuals and their families about the importance of handwashing is a primary measure to prevent and reduce the spread of infectious diseases, including those causing diarrhoea. Educating people about safe food handling techniques prevents bacterial contamination. Discuss measures to ensure safe drinking water. For people planning travel to remote areas or outside Australia, discuss the importance of avoiding the consumption of high-risk foods (especially raw foods) and beverages, and purification methods for drinking and cooking water.

Assessment

The nursing assessment helps identify the cause of the person's diarrhoea, as well as early signs of complications. Collect the following assessment data:

- *Health history*: duration and extent of diarrhoea; associated manifestations; dietary intake; recent visits to remote areas or overseas travel or contact with people recently returned from overseas; previous history of diarrhoea; chronic diseases; prescription and non-prescription medications including complementary supplements.
- *Physical examination*: vital signs (including orthostatic blood pressure); peripheral pulses and capillary refill; skin temperature, moisture and turgor; colour and moisture of mucous membranes; abdominal contour and girth; bowel sounds; stool for obvious or occult blood, pus, mucus or steatorrhoea (bulky, foul-smelling stool).

Nursing diagnoses and interventions

Nursing care of people with diarrhoea focuses on identifying the cause, relieving the clinical manifestations and preventing complications and spread of infection to others.

Diarrhoea

Nursing interventions for diarrhoea are provided to assist a person recover their normal elimination pattern without adverse consequences.

- Use standard precautions, including gloves and handwashing. *Standard precautions help prevent the spread of infection to others.*
- Monitor and record the frequency and characteristics of bowel movements *to provide a measure of the effectiveness of treatment.*
- Measure abdominal girth and auscultate bowel sounds every 8 hours as indicated. *Loud, rushing bowel sounds (borborygmi) indicate increased peristalsis and may be heard in a person with acute diarrhoea. Diminished or absent bowel sounds may indicate a complication of treatment, such as constipation or toxic megacolon.*
- Provide ready access to toilet, commode or bedpan. *The person may have little warning of the need to defecate. Easily accessed toileting facilities reduce the risk of soiling or injury.*
- Administer antimuscarinic medications as prescribed *to promote comfort by reducing colicky pain sometimes associated with diarrhoea.*
- Limit food intake if the diarrhoea is acute, reintroducing solid foods slowly, in small amounts, *allowing the bowel to rest and mucosa to heal in acute diarrhoea states.*

Risk of deficient fluid volume

The increased water content of diarrhoeal stool places the person at risk of fluid deficit.

- Record intake and output; weigh daily; assess skin turgor, mucous membranes and urine specific gravity every 8 hours. *These assessments are used to monitor fluid volume status.*

CONSIDERATION FOR PRACTICE

Assess skin turgor over the sternum of older adults. Loss of subcutaneous fat associated with ageing makes assessment of skin turgor on the arms or hands less reliable.

- Monitor vital signs, including orthostatic blood pressures. *A mild fluid volume deficit results in orthostatic hypotension. This is identified by a 10 mmHg or more drop in BP and increase of 10 beats per minute (bpm) in pulse when changing from a lying to a sitting position or from a sitting to a standing position.*

CONSIDERATION FOR PRACTICE

Remember to institute safety precautions when assisting a person with orthostatic hypotension to ambulate. *The decrease in blood pressure with position changes can cause light-headedness and syncope.*

- Provide fluid and electrolyte replacement solutions as indicated. Ensure ready access to fluids; assist a debilitated person with fluid intake. Notify the doctor if the person is unable to tolerate oral fluids. *Oral fluids are encouraged as tolerated to prevent dehydration. Intravenous fluids are necessary when oral fluids are not tolerated. An intake of 3,000 mL/day or more is often needed to replace fluid losses.*

Risk of impaired skin integrity

Decreased extracellular fluid volume and the irritating effects of diarrhoeal stool increase the risk of skin breakdown.

- Assist with cleaning the perianal area as needed. Use warm water, a gentle cleanser and soft cloths. *Cleansing removes irritating substances in the stool. Gentle cleansing helps maintain integrity of dehydrated skin.*
- Apply protective ointment to the perianal area. *Moisture-barrier ointments or creams protect the skin from excoriation and help prevent tissue breakdown.*

Community-based care

Acute and chronic diarrhoea generally are managed by the person at home. Teach the individual and their family members about the following topics:

- cause of diarrhoea (as directed by the diagnosis)
- importance of handwashing and hygiene measures
- importance of maintaining adequate fluid intake to replace lost water and electrolytes
- use of a balanced electrolyte solution (e.g. Gastrolyte) or a similar product (purchased) for electrolyte replacement
- recommendations to limit food intake during acute diarrhoea and resume food gradually with small meals of foods with a constipating effect: apple sauce, bananas, water crackers, rice and potatoes
- avoiding foods high in fibre, milk products and caffeine
- ways to maintain nutrition if chronic diarrhoea is a problem: frequent small meals, nutritional supplements, vitamin supplements
- precautions and limitations of antidiarrhoeal preparations
- importance of seeking medical intervention if diarrhoea continues or recurs.

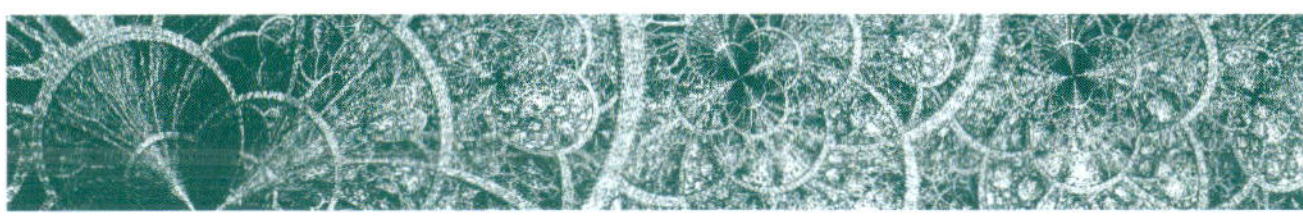

THE PERSON WITH CONSTIPATION

Constipation is defined as the infrequent (less than two bowel movements weekly) or difficult passage of stools. Constipation affects older adults more frequently than younger people. Reports suggest that constipation in older adults ranges between 24% and 30% (Bellman, 2022). Although faecal transit in the large intestine slows with ageing, the increased incidence of constipation is thought to relate more to impaired general health, increased medication use and decreased physical activity in the older adult than to being part of the ageing process.

Pathophysiology

Constipation may be a primary problem or a manifestation of another disease or condition. Acute constipation, a definite change in a person's bowel elimination pattern, is often caused by an organic process. A change in bowel patterns persisting or becoming more frequent or severe may be due to a tumour or other partial bowel obstruction. However, in chronic constipation, functional causes impairing storage, transport and evacuation mechanisms impede the normal passage of stools. Common causes of constipation are listed in Table 23.2.

Psychogenic factors are the most frequent causes of chronic constipation. These factors include postponing defecation when the urge is felt and the perception of satisfaction with defecation. Some people use laxatives and enemas to stimulate a bowel movement when constipation is perceived. Overuse of these leads to intestinal problems, worsening constipation. *Cathartic colon* (impaired colonic motility and changes in bowel structure) mimics ulcerative colitis in that the normal pouch-like or saccular appearance of the colon is lost. *Melanosis coli* is a brownish-black discolouration of the colon mucosa. Both conditions may be caused by long-term laxative use.

Manifestations

Clinical manifestations of constipation include having bowel movements less often than the usual pattern, frequent flatus, abdominal discomfort, anorexia, straining to achieve bowel movement and the passage of hard, dry stools.

Faecal impaction may develop from significant constipation or long-term dependence on laxatives or enemas. Impaction occasionally results after barium administration for radiological exam. The impaction is felt as a rock-hard or putty-like mass of faeces in the rectum. Faecal impaction may result in abdominal cramping and a full sensation in the rectal area. Additionally, watery mucus or foul-smelling liquid stool

TABLE 23.2 Selected causes of constipation

FACTOR	RELATED CAUSE
Activity	Lack of exercise; bed rest
Dietary	Highly refined, low fibre foods; inadequate fluid intake
Medications	Antacids containing aluminium or calcium salts, narcotic analgesics; anticholinergics; many antidepressants, tranquillisers and sedatives; antihypertensives, such as ganglionic blockers, calcium channel blockers, beta-adrenergic blockers, diuretics; iron supplements
Large bowel	Diverticular disease, inflammatory disease, tumour, obstruction, changes in rectal or anal structure or function
Psychogenic	Voluntary suppression of urge; perceived need to defecate on schedule, depression
Systemic	Advanced age; pregnancy; neurological conditions (trauma, multiple sclerosis, tumours, cerebrovascular accident, parkinsonism); endocrine and metabolic disorders (hypothyroidism, hypocalcaemia, uraemia, porphyria)
Other	Chronic laxative or enema use

may be passed around the impaction, causing the person to report diarrhoea.

INTERPROFESSIONAL CARE

Initial evaluation of constipation is based on the health history including diet and medication history, activity level, bowel habits and symptom descriptions (e.g. bloating, straining or pain between passing bowel movements (Bellman, 2022)) and physical examination. The abdomen may appear distended and bowel sounds may be reduced. If faecal impaction is present, digital examination of the rectum reveals a palpable, hard or putty-like faecal mass.

Simple or chronic constipation is treated with education (a daily bowel movement is not necessary for health), modification of diet and increasing fluid intake and exercise routines. If the problem is acute or does not resolve, further diagnostic examination is ordered.

Diagnosis

A barium enema is ordered to identify bowel structure, tumours or diverticula. If the problem is acute, a sigmoidoscopy or colonoscopy may be used for evaluation and biopsy. (See the chapter 'A person-centred approach to assessing the gastrointestinal system' for nursing implications of these tests.)

Medications

Laxatives—occasionally called aperients or purgative preparations—are used to promote stool evacuation. Laxatives are grouped in categories depending on their mechanism of action. These include osmotic laxatives (non-absorbable inorganic salts, polyethylene glycol, sugars and alcohol), stimulant laxatives, faecal softeners, lubricants and bulk-forming laxatives (Bullock & Manias, 2022). Laxatives are indicated for constipation resulting from poor bowel habits, opioid analgesia, medications with anticholinergic side effects and loss of intestinal muscle tone following surgery or bed rest or due to age. Laxatives are often used to reduce straining, reduce pain associated with anorectal disorders and before surgery or diagnostic procedures.

Stimulant laxatives and enemas interfere with normal bowel reflexes and are not recommended for regular use as these may lead to colon dilation and reduced peristalsis, requiring increased amounts. All laxatives are contraindicated if a person has an intestinal obstruction, undiagnosed abdominal pain, nausea or vomiting, paralytic ileus, suspected appendicitis, undiagnosed rectal bleeding, faecal impaction, rectal fissures, ulcerated haemorrhoids, Crohn's disease, ulcerative colitis or chronic inflammatory bowel disease. When the bowel is obstructed, laxatives may cause serious mechanical damage and perforate the bowel.

If a person is unable to consume enough dietary fibre to prevent constipation, the only appropriate laxatives safe for long-term use are bulking agents, such as psyllium seed (e.g. Metamucil), *Plantago ovata* seeds (ispaghula or psyllium husk—e.g. Fybogel) and sterculia and frangula (e.g. Normacol Plus). These agents act by increasing the bulk of the faeces and drawing water into the bowel, softening it. Some bulking agents (e.g. Fybogel and Normafibre) contain aspartame. Therefore, caution is needed if given to a person with phenylketonuria (Tiziani, 2021). Commonly prescribed laxatives are discussed in the 'Medication administration' box.

Nutrition

Foods with high fibre content are recommended. Vegetable fibre is largely indigestible and unabsorbable, so it increases stool bulk. Fibre also helps draw water into the faecal mass, softening the stool and making defecation easier. Raw fruits and vegetables are good sources of dietary fibre, as is cereal bran. Use 2 to 3 teaspoons of unprocessed bran with meals (sprinkled on fruit or cereal) or up to ¼ cup daily to supply adequate fibre.

Fluids are also important to maintain bowel motility and soft stools. If not contraindicated, a person should drink 6 to 8 glasses (i.e. 250 mL each) of fluid per day. It is important to advise the person to increase fluid intake when dietary fibre is initially increased to decrease flatus and help maintain softer stools.

In older adults, constipation may be due to inadequate food and fluid intake. Carefully evaluate the person's diet history and usual daily fluid intake.

Enemas

Significant or chronic constipation or a faecal impaction may require the administration of an enema. As a general rule, enemas should be used only in acute situations and only on a short-term basis. These may also be ordered to prepare the bowel for diagnostic testing or examination. Enema administration is contraindicated in a person with diarrhoea, cardiac dysrhythmias, following recent myocardical infarction, undiagnosed abdominal pains and following recent surgery to the rectum, bowel or prostate gland (Porritt, 2020).

The following types of enemas may be prescribed:

- *Isotonic—saline enemas* using 500 to 1,000 mL of warmed normal saline solution are the least irritating to the bowel. They distend the colon, stimulate peristalsis and soften faeces. The enema solution should be retained for 5 to 10 minutes as tolerated. Evacuation usually occurs within approximately 15 to 20 minutes. Sodium retention is a possible adverse effect of these enemas.
- *Hypotonic—tap-water enemas* use 500 to 1,000 mL of water to soften faeces and irritate the bowel mucosa, stimulating peristalsis. The enema solution should be retained for 5 to 10 minutes as tolerated. Evacuation is within approximately 15 to 20 minutes. Adverse effects include fluid and electrolyte imbalance and water intoxication.
- *Soap-suds enemas*—consist of a tap-water solution (500 to 1,000 mL) to which soap (3 to 5 mL) is added to distend the colon, stimulate peristalsis and soften faeces. The enema solution should be retained for 5 to 10 minutes as tolerated. Evacuation is usually within 10 to 15 minutes. Adverse effects include irritation and damage to mucosa.
- *Hypertonic—phosphate enemas* (e.g. Fleet) use a hypertonic saline (sodium phosphate) solution (90 to 120 mL) to draw fluid into the bowel and irritate the mucosa, leading to evacuation in approximately 5 to 10 minutes. Adverse effect is possible sodium retention.

MEDICATION ADMINISTRATION Laxatives

BULK-FORMING AGENTS

Bran
Psyllium (Metamucil)
Ispaghula (Fybogel)
Sterculia (Normafibe)

Bulk-forming agents are the only safe laxatives for long-term use. These contain vegetable fibre, which is not digested or absorbed in the gut. This natural fibre creates bulk and draws water into the intestine, softening the stool mass, resulting in increased peristalsis (see Figure 23.1).

Nursing responsibilities

- Mix the agent (e.g. one sachet of Fybogel or 1½ to 3 teaspoons of Metamucil one to three times per day) in a 250 mL glass of cool liquid just prior to administering and followed by an additional glass of water. Sterculia (Normafibe) granules (1 to 2 heaped 5 mL teaspoons of granules one or two times per day) can be placed dry on the tongue and swallowed whole with 250 mL of water.
- Do not administer to a person with possible stool impaction or bowel obstruction, or who is dehydrated or on fluid restrictions—for example, a person with chronic kidney disease.

Health education for the person and family

- Drink at least 6 to 8 full glasses (250 mL) of non-alcoholic fluid per day. Adequate hydration is necessary to produce the medication's laxative effect.
- These agents may be mixed with water, milk or fruit juice. Sterculia (Normafibe) granules can be mixed with jam, honey or ice-cream.
- Take the medication in the morning or with meals. To reduce the risk of impaction, do not take at bedtime.
- Because of the increased risk of impaction, check with the doctor before increasing dietary fibre while you are taking these medications.

FAECAL SOFTENERS

Docusate sodium (Coloxyl)
Paraffin liquid (Agarol)

Faecal softeners reduce stool surface tension and form an emulsion of fat and water, softening the stool. These are used primarily to prevent straining and reduce the discomfort of expelling hard stools after rectal and perianal surgery. These medications have limited use in the management of acute or chronic constipation (Bullock & Manias, 2022).

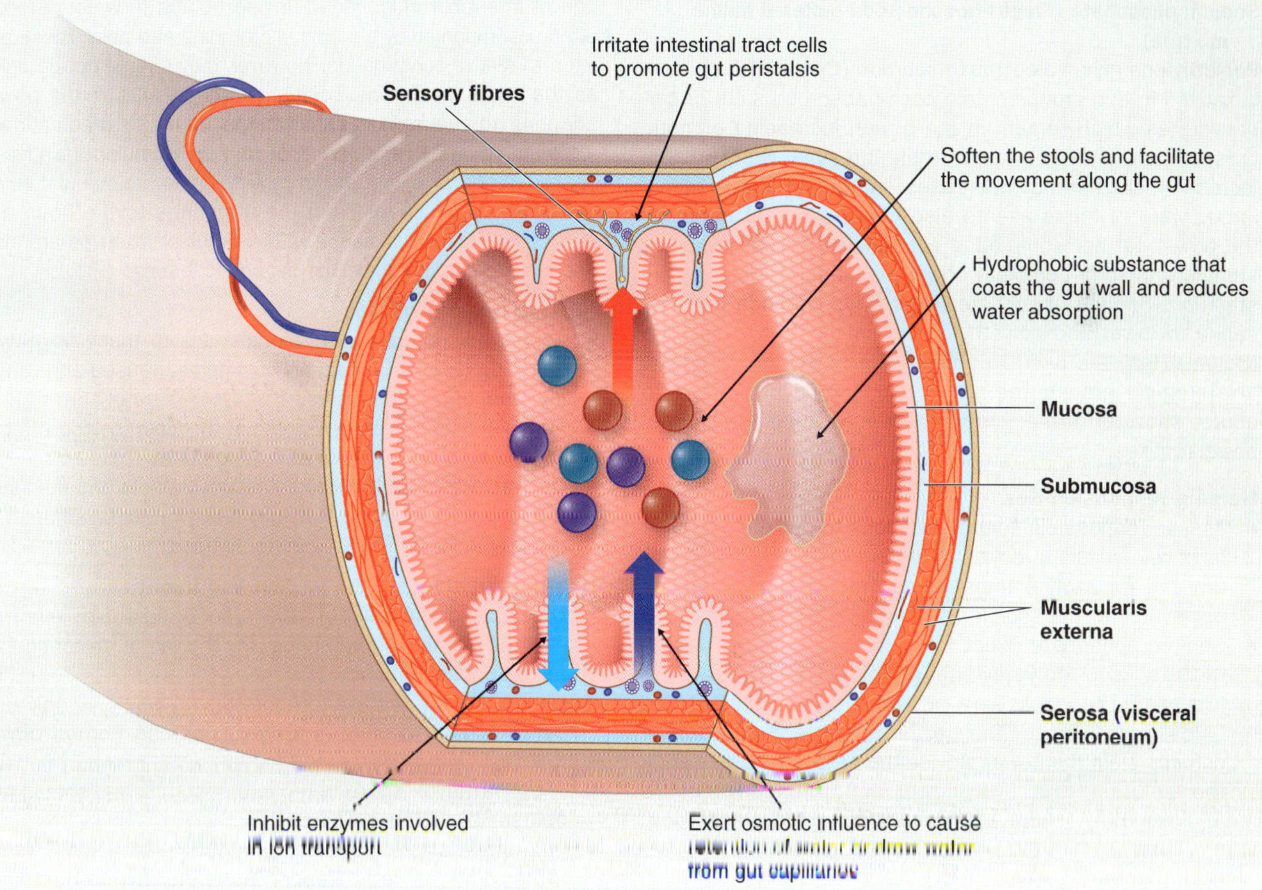

FIGURE 23.1 ***Mechanisms of laxative action***

Source: Bullock & Manias (2014). *Fundamentals of pharmacology* (7th ed.), p. 715, Figure 57.1. Frenchs Forest, NSW: Pearson Australia.

(continued)

MEDICATION ADMINISTRATION Laxatives (continued)

Nursing responsibilities

- Administer with ample fluids to promote softening effect.
- Faecal softening agents may alter the absorption of other drugs. Do not administer within 1 to 2 hours of other oral medications.
- Do not attempt to crush or open capsules; a liquid form is available for a person unable to swallow pills or capsules.
- Caution needs to be taken with the administration of docusate sodium (Coloxyl) tablets in a person with hypertension or congestive cardiac failure, due to the sodium content.

Health education for the person and family

- Do not use for more than 1 week unless specifically recommended by the doctor.
- Take the medication in the morning or evening; remember to avoid taking it with other medications.
- Adequate fluid is necessary to obtain the beneficial effect of the medication. Drink 6 to 8 (250 mL) glasses of non-alcoholic fluid per day.

OSMOTIC AND SALINE LAXATIVES/CATHARTICS

Lactulose (Duphalac)
Sorbitol (Sorbilax)
Magnesium salts (Epsom salts)
Sodium phosphate (Fleet Phospho-Soda buffered saline mixture)
Polyethylene glycol-electrolyte solution (ColonLYTELY)

Laxatives in this group contain poorly absorbed salts or carbohydrates which remain in the bowel, increasing osmotic pressure and drawing water into the intestine. Stool volume increases, consistency decreases and peristalsis is stimulated. Many of these agents also have an irritant effect on the bowel, further stimulating peristalsis. They are used to stimulate rapid or complete bowel evacuation to relieve constipation. Sodium phosphate (Fleet Phospho-Soda buffered saline mixture) and polyethylene glycol-electrolyte solution (ColonLYTELY) are used to prepare the bowel for diagnostic and surgical procedures. Their use should be limited to acute, short-term use; chronic use may suppress normal bowel reflexes.

Nursing responsibilities

- Assess for possible contraindications to osmotic or saline laxatives, including bowel ulceration or obstruction, dehydration, electrolyte imbalances, heart failure (may be aggravated by the sodium content) or kidney injury.
- Sodium phosphate (Fleet Phospho-Soda buffered saline mixture) and polyethylene glycol-electrolyte solution (ColonLYTELY) should have no additional flavouring added unless instructed by the doctor. Red, green and orange cordials stain the bowel. Advise the person to slowly drink the solution: the first bowel action usually occurs approximately 1 hour after commencing the preparation. Preparation is complete when the person is passing clear fluid from the bowels.
- Other osmotic laxatives are administered with a full glass of liquid, preferably in the morning to avoid sleep disturbance.
- Monitor fluid and electrolyte status: skin turgor, mucous membranes, intake and output; daily weight and laboratory studies, such as haemoglobin and haematocrit levels, serum osmolality and electrolytes and urine specific gravity.

Health education for the person and family

- Do not use these agents on a routine basis to treat or prevent constipation. Long-term use can produce electrolyte disturbances.
- Chilling the solution increases its palatability.
- Expect some abdominal cramping.
- Use only as directed. Increase fluid intake to at least 6 to 8 (250 mL) glasses of non-alcoholic fluid.
- Notify the doctor if adverse effects occur, including abdominal pain, bloody stool, excessive skin or mucous membrane dryness, rapid weight loss, dizziness or other unusual symptoms.
- These agents work in 3 to 6 hours; take in the morning or early evening to avoid sleep disturbance.

IRRITANT OR STIMULANT LAXATIVES

Bisacodyl (Durolax, Bisolax)
Sennosides (Sennakot, Laxettes)
Castor oil (no longer in common use)

Stimulant laxatives work by stimulating the motility and secretion of intestinal mucosa. Their use results in watery stools, often accompanied by abdominal cramping and pain. These are used to relieve constipation. However, they should not be used as the initial treatment. Long-term use results in the bowel adapting to the strong stimulations of these medications. Rebound constipation can occur when the stimulant laxative is ceased. A normal diet does not provide adequate stimulation as the afferent messages from the intestines to the brain are ignored (Bullock & Manias, 2022). Stimulant laxatives are also used to prepare the bowel for diagnostic testing.

Nursing responsibilities

- Assess for potential contraindications to these laxatives, including abdominal pain and cramping, nausea and vomiting, anal or rectal fissures.
- Administer on an empty stomach to minimise the effects of food on its dissolution and absorption.
- Do not crush enteric-coated bisacodyl tablets or administer with alkaline products. This may hasten their dissolution in the stomach, leading to gastric distress.

Health education for the person and family

- Discourage the use of this type of laxative, even in over-the-counter preparations, for the initial or continuing relief of constipation.
- Do not use the laxative for more than 1 week; chronic use can be habit forming and may suppress normal bowel reflexes.
- These laxatives are excreted in breast milk and should not be used by lactating women.
- Phenolphthalein-containing products may discolour the urine pink or red. Report possible hypersensitivity manifestations, such as difficulty breathing, dizziness or light-headedness, or skin rashes, to general practitioner and stop taking the medication.

- *Oil retention enemas*—instil 90 to 120 mL mineral or olive or cottonseed oil into the bowel to lubricate the colonic mucosa and the faeces and soften the faecal mass. The instilled oil is retained for as long as possible (30 minutes to 1 hour) before evacuation.

The repeated use of enemas not only leads to impaired bowel function, bowel irritation and loss of muscle tone of the bowel and anal sphincter but also to fluid and electrolyte imbalances (Porritt, 2020). These imbalances are more likely to be caused by tap water and phosphate enemas. In acute conditions with a risk of bowel obstruction, perforation or ulceration, enemas should not be administered until their safe use is established.

Complementary and alternative therapies

Herbal or homeopathic therapies are used to help relieve constipation. Flaxseed oil lubricates the colon for easier passage of stool. Individuals are instructed to take 1 to 2 tablespoons daily. Flaxseed is a highly concentrated source of fibre; 1 to 2 tablespoons of ground flaxseeds can be sprinkled on cereals or salads daily, followed by 300 mL of water.

Biofeedback, sphincter exercises and electrical stimulation can be used to restore normal coordination of the anal sphincter and pelvic floor muscles (Slade, 2021).

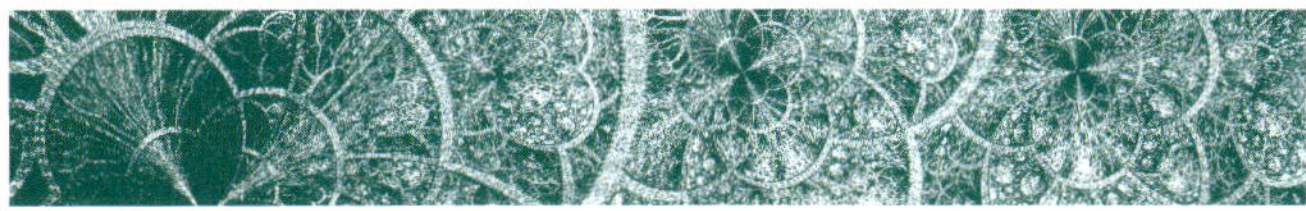

Nursing care

Health promotion

Education can prevent constipation. Highlight to people the importance of maintaining a diet high in natural fibre. Foods such as fresh fruit and vegetables, wholegrain products and bran provide natural fibre. Encourage reducing consumption of meats and refined foods, which are low in fibre and can be constipating. Emphasise the need to maintain a high fluid intake every day, particularly during hot weather and exercise. Discuss the relationship between exercise and bowel regularity. Encourage the person to engage in daily exercise; for example, walking.

Discuss normal bowel habits and explain that a daily bowel movement is not the norm for all people. Highlight that constipation has more to do with ease of a bowel evacuation, rather than the frequency of bowel movements (Bullock & Manias, 2022). Encourage people to respond to the urge to defecate when it occurs. Suggest establishing a routine by setting aside a time, usually following a meal, for elimination.

Assessment

To assess a person with real or perceived constipation, collect the following data:

- *Health history*: usual and current pattern of defecation, including time of day, amount and stool consistency; usual diet, fluid intake and activity pattern. Assess for possible contributing factors such as opioid analgesia, activity limitations, painful haemorrhoids, perianal surgery; chronic diseases such as endocrine or neurological disorders; prescribed and non-prescription medications.
- *Physical examination*: abdominal girth and shape, bowel sounds, tenderness and percussion tone; digital exam of the rectum if impaction is suspected. Maintaining a bowel assessment chart (see Figure 23.2), incorporating, for example, the Bristol Stool Scale, provides a better assessment of potential constipation than the absence of faeces. The Bristol Stool Chart or Bristol Stool Scale developed by Heaton and Lewis at the University of Bristol and first published in the *Scandinavian Journal of Gastroenterology* in 1997 is an aid classifying faeces into seven groups. Types 1 and 2 indicate constipation; 3 and 4 are the 'ideal stools' (especially the latter), as these are the easiest to pass; 5 and 6 are more symptomatic of diarrhoea; and type 7 may be a sign of cholera or food poisoning or urgency (see Figure 23.3). Advising individuals or their carers how to use the Bristol Stool Chart enables appropriate intervention to be implemented, resulting in better management of constipation (Bellman, 2022).

See 'Nursing care of the older adult' for a discussion about constipation in older adults.

Nursing diagnoses and interventions

Nursing interventions for a person with constipation focus chiefly on education.

Constipation

Whether real or perceived, constipation is disruptive to a person's activities of daily living (ADLs) and life satisfaction.

- Monitor pattern of defecation and stool consistency. *This information helps to establish the person's usual pattern of defecation and differentiate between actual and perceived constipation.*
- If not contraindicated, provide additional fluids to maintain an intake of at least 2,500 mL per day. *A generous fluid intake helps to maintain soft stool consistency and promotes intestinal motility.*
- Encourage drinking a glass of warm water before breakfast. Provide time and privacy following breakfast for bowel elimination. *This helps develop a pattern of natural elimination; warm water provides mild stimulation of bowel peristalsis.*
- Consult with the nutritionist to provide a diet high in natural fibre unless contraindicated. Provide foods such as natural bran, prunes or prune juice. *Natural fibre adds bulk to the stool and has a mild stimulant effect.*
- Encourage activities such as ambulation or chair exercises (e.g. range of motion, stretching, wheelchair lifts) as tolerated. *Activity stimulates peristalsis and strengthens abdominal muscles, facilitating elimination.*

Bowel assessment chart

Name *Ian Andrews* Month *Jan* Year *2023*

Date	AM	PM	Nocte	Description of bowel action type: see Bristol stool chart	Continence status C = continent I = incontinent	Comments: use of aperients and results, problems concerning mobility, access to toilet, clothing, mood change etc.
1	$\frac{\cdot}{0}$	$\frac{\cdot}{0}$	$\frac{\cdot}{0}$			*Assessed fluids & diet*
2	$\frac{\cdot}{0}$	$\frac{\cdot}{0}$	$\frac{\cdot}{0}$			*Mobility & toilet access assessed*
3	$\frac{\cdot}{1}$	$\frac{\cdot}{0}$	$\frac{\cdot}{0}$	1^{+}	C	*Aperient as per chart given*
4	$\frac{\cdot}{0}$	$\frac{\cdot}{1}$	$\frac{\cdot}{1}$	1 + 2 2	C	*Encouraged fluid & diet & mob.*
5	$\frac{\cdot}{1}$	$\frac{\cdot}{0}$	$\frac{\cdot}{0}$	3^{+}	C	
6	$\frac{\cdot}{1}$	$\frac{\cdot}{0}$	$\frac{\cdot}{0}$	3^{++}	C	
7	$\frac{\cdot}{0}$	$\frac{\cdot}{0}$	$\frac{\cdot}{0}$			*Drug chart assessed as new Rx*
8	$\frac{\cdot}{1}$	$\frac{\cdot}{0}$	$\frac{\cdot}{0}$	1^{+}	C	*Fluids & dietary fibre encouraged*
9	$\frac{\cdot}{1}$	$\frac{\cdot}{0}$	$\frac{\cdot}{0}$	$1 + 2^{+}$	C	*Fluids, diet & mobility encouraged*
10	$\frac{\cdot}{1}$	$\frac{\cdot}{0}$	$\frac{\cdot}{0}$	2^{++}	C	
11	$\frac{\cdot}{1}$	$\frac{\cdot}{0}$	$\frac{\cdot}{0}$	2^{++}	C	
12	$\frac{\cdot}{0}$	$\frac{\cdot}{0}$	$\frac{\cdot}{0}$			*Away for weekend*
13	$\frac{\cdot}{0}$	$\frac{\cdot}{0}$	$\frac{\cdot}{0}$			*Away for weekend*
14	$\frac{\cdot}{0}$	$\frac{\cdot}{0}$	$\frac{\cdot}{0}$			*Resumed ↑ fluid & ↑ fibre*
15	$\frac{\cdot}{1}$	$\frac{\cdot}{0}$	$\frac{\cdot}{0}$	1^{+}	C	
16	$\frac{\cdot}{1}$	$\frac{\cdot}{0}$	$\frac{\cdot}{0}$	2^{++}	C	
17						
18						
19						
20						
21						
22						
23						
24						
25						
26						
27						
28						
29						
30						
31						

$\frac{\cdot}{0}$ = Bowels not open $\frac{\cdot}{1}$ = the figure below the line indicates the number of times bowels have opened

FIGURE 23.2 ***Bowel assessment chart***

Source: Brown (2007). *Health and illness in older adults*, p. 19. Frenchs Forest, NSW: Pearson Australia.

If indicated, consult with doctor about the use of bulk laxatives, stool softeners or other laxatives as needed. Laxatives may be necessary to relieve acute constipation. *People with long-term activity or nutritional restrictions or impaired abdominal muscle strength may need a bulk-forming laxative to maintain normal elimination patterns and prevent constipation.*

Community-based care

Include the following topics when teaching self-care measures to prevent and manage constipation:

- Increase dietary fibre intake by including fresh fruit and vegetables, whole grains, high-fibre breakfast cereals and unprocessed bran in the diet. (Bran can be sprinkled on cereals, mixed into bread or muffin recipes, or mixed with fruit juice to increase its palatability.)
- Unless contraindicated maintain fluid intake of 6 to 8 (250 mL) glasses of water per day.
- Remain physically active to promote bowel function and maintain muscle tone.
- Respond to the urge to defecate when perceived.

Bristol Stool Scale Form

Type 1	Separate hard lumps, like nuts
Type 2	Sausage-shaped but lumpy
Type 3	Like a sausage but with cracks on the surface
Type 4	Like a sausage or snake, smooth and soft
Type 5	Soft blobs with clear-cut edges
Type 6	Fluffy pieces with ragged edges, a mushy stool
Type 7	Watery, no solid pieces

FIGURE 23.3 *Bristol Stool Chart*

Source: © 2000 Rome Foundation, Inc. All rights reserved.

- Use laxatives appropriately:
  - Do not use laxatives, suppositories or enemas on a regular basis.
  - Bulk-forming agents provide insoluble fibre and are safe for long-term use; it is important to drink at least 6 to 8 (250 mL) glasses of water daily when using these (or any) laxatives.

NURSING CARE OF THE OLDER ADULT

Constipation and older adults

Constipation and perceived constipation are common problems in older adults. Although constipation is not a normal consequence of ageing, factors such as slowed peristalsis, lowered activity levels, reduced food and fluid intake, and decreased sensory perception contribute to the higher incidence of constipation seen in older adults. Chronic diseases such as diabetes mellitus, restricted mobility and medications also increase the risk of constipation in older adults.

Cultural influences and advertising lead many older adults to believe a daily bowel movement is important for health. This belief contributes to an increased incidence of perceived constipation in older adults. Because of this perception, the older adult may come to rely on laxatives, suppositories or enemas to facilitate regular bowel movements. These external aids to defecation further impair the ability to maintain 'normal' bowel habits—a movement of soft stool every 2 to 3 days for older adults. See Box 23.1 for best practice management of constipation in older adults.

BOX 23.1 JBI best practice recommendations for bowel care constipation management

- Prevention is better than cure, so it is recommended that older adults receive advice and education about hydration and a good diet with fibre sources such as cereals, nuts and seeds, wholemeal breads, vegetables and raw vegetables, and fruit. However, careful consideration is required as chewing or swallowing can be difficult for some older people. They may also have a poor tolerance to a high-fibre diet.
- Assessment of the older person should include an initial history of diet, medication, activity level and bowel habits. Also, the person should be asked to describe any symptoms such as bloating or pain when passing movements and associated straining. Screen older adults for the following: history of medication use (especially polypharmacy and taking laxatives) and, where feasible, replacement of constipation-causing medications with alternatives.
- Encourage the person to increase fluids (approximately 2 L per day) and soluble fibre unless contraindicated (e.g. a person with heart or renal failure on fluid restrictions).
- For individuals unable to walk or restricted to bed or otherwise incapacitated, exercises such as low trunk rotation, pelvic tilt and single leg lifts are advised.
- Promote regular bowel activity by assisting the person to the toilet at their preferred time. Encourage the person to use the toilet or commode by sitting upright with their feet resting on a low stool.
- Monitor and record bowel movements for frequency, character and pattern, episodes of constipation/faecal spoiling and use of oral or rectal laxative interventions.
- Set realistic expectations for chronic constipation treatment. Gradually titrate laxative doses (upwards or downwards) to produce one or two soft, formed stools per day.
- Osmotic laxatives such as polyethylene glycol (PEG), lactulose and bulking agents such as psyllium and bran are beneficial in managing constipation in older adults and should be promoted; it is necessary to determine individual requirements.

Sources: Bellman (2022). *Constipation management (older person): Pharmacological interventions*. Adelaide: Joanna Briggs Institute; Fong (2022). *Constipation in hospitalized patients: Management*. Adelaide: Joanna Briggs Institute.

- Other laxatives such as docusate sodium (Coloxyl), bisacodyl (Durolax) and sennosides (Senna) should only be used occasionally to relieve constipation.
- Report any change in bowel habits such as new or persistent constipation or diarrhoea, abdominal pain, black or bloody stools, nausea or anorexia, weakness or unexplained weight loss to your general practitioner.

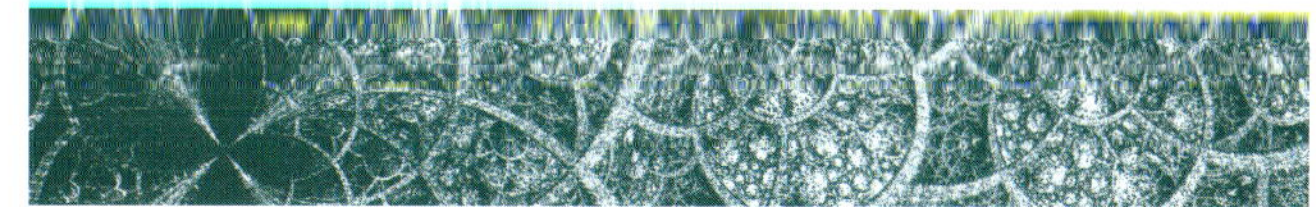

THE PERSON WITH IRRITABLE BOWEL SYNDROME

Irritable bowel syndrome (IBS), also known as *spastic bowel* or *functional colitis*, is a motility disorder of the lower gastrointestinal (GI) tract. It is a functional disorder with no identifiable organic cause. IBS is often characterised by abdominal pain with constipation, diarrhoea or both.

A recent survey estimated that IBS is common, affecting 3.5% of the Australian population and 4.1% globally (Sperber et al., 2021). It usually affects young people, with about 50% of people diagnosed before the age of 35. There is a higher prevalence of IBS in women than in men (Manning, Tuck & Biesiekierski, 2022). IBS can result in reduced quality of life, significant disability and impaired workforce productivity (Lizarondo, 2021).

Pathophysiology

In IBS, it appears the central nervous system regulation of the motor and sensory functions of the bowel is altered. IBS may develop as a sequela of gastroenteritis, particularly when caused by *Camplylobacter*, *Salmonella* or *Shigella.*

People with IBS often experience increased motor reactivity of the small bowel and colon in response to stimuli such as food intake, hormonal influences and physiological or psychological stressors. Manning et al. (2022) suggested IBS is ill defined and includes psychological factors; miscommunication between the gut and central nervous system; altered mucosal, immune and inflammatory function; and genetic susceptibility. IBS is characterised by visceral hypersensitivity and hyperactivity of the GI tract. Hypersecretion of colonic mucus is a common IBS feature.

A lower visceral pain threshold is often found in people with IBS. A person may report pain, bloating and distension even when intestinal gas levels are normal. Serotonin, a neurotransmitter involved in regulating GI motility, and visceral perception may play a role in IBS. Higher than expected postprandial plasma serotonin levels are noted in some individuals with IBS (Chey, Kurlander & Eswaran, 2015). The Rome IV diagnostic criteria divides IBS into three groups: IBS-C (predominant constipation), IBS-D (predominant diarrhoea) and IBS-M (mixed bowel habits) (Marin, 2021).

Manifestations

IBS is characterised by abdominal pain often relieved by defecation and a change in bowel habits (see the 'Manifestations' box). The pain may be colic-like, occurring in spasms, or dull and continuous. Altered patterns of defecation may include:

- a change in frequency
- abnormal stool form (hard or lumpy, loose or watery)
- altered stool passage (straining, urgency or a sensation of incomplete evacuation)
- the passage of mucus.

A person may also describe abdominal bloating and excess gas. Other manifestations include nausea, vomiting and anorexia, fatigue, headache, depression or anxiety. The abdomen is often tender to palpation, particularly over the sigmoid colon.

MANIFESTATIONS Irritable bowel syndrome

ABDOMINAL PAIN
- May be relieved by defecation
- May be intermittent and colicky or dull and continuous

ALTERED BOWEL ELIMINATION
- Constipation
- Diarrhoea
- Mucus stools
- Abdominal bloating and flatulence
- Abdominal tenderness, especially over sigmoid colon
- Possible nausea or vomiting

INTERPROFESSIONAL CARE

Diagnosis of IBS is based on the presence of abdominal pain or discomfort with two of the following three characteristics: (1) relieved by defecation, (2) associated with a change in frequency of elimination, and (3) associated with change in stool frequency or appearance (Lizarondo, 2021). Management is directed towards relieving manifestations and reducing or eliminating precipitating factors. Many people report benefits from psychotherapy and cognitive–behavioural therapy (Lizarondo, 2021).

Diagnosis

The primary purpose of diagnostic testing is to rule out other causes of abdominal pain and altered faecal elimination. The stools may be examined for occult blood, ova, cysts and parasites, and white blood cells. A sigmoidoscopy, colonoscopy and/or a small-bowel series (upper GI series with small-bowel follow-through) and barium enema may be performed to visually examine the bowel mucosa, measure intraluminal pressures and biopsy suspicious lesions. Nursing care for these procedures is outlined in the chapter 'A person-centred approach to assessing the gastrointestinal system'. Laboratory tests include a full blood count (FBC) with differential and erythrocyte sedimentation rate (ESR) to evaluate for anaemia from bleeding or a possible tumour. Increased WBCs indicate a bacterial infection.

Medications

Although not curative, medications are prescribed to manage the manifestations of IBS. Soluble fibres (such as psyllium) may help reduce bowel spasm and normalise the number and form of bowel movements. An anticholinergic medication such as hyoscyamine (Buscopan) may be ordered to inhibit bowel motility by interfering with parasympathetic stimulation of the GI tract (Chey et al., 2015). This relieves postprandial abdominal pain when taken 30 to 60 minutes before meals. Because of side effects, such as dry mouth, blurred vision and urinary hesitancy, these medications are used cautiously in older adults. In a person with diarrhoea, loperamide (Imodium) or diphenoxylate (Lomotil) may be used prophylactically to prevent diarrhoea in selected situations.

Antispasmodic medications are often used to control intestinal muscle spasm associated with IBS. Most antispasmodics are antimuscarinic medications blocking muscarinic receptors on gastrointestinal smooth muscle, inhibiting contractions. One medication used exclusively to manage smooth muscle spasms is mebeverine (Colase). Mebeverine relaxes vascular, cardiac and other smooth muscles. It contains lactose so is contraindicated in a person with lactose intolerance. Additionally, it is used cautiously in a person with cardiac dysrhythmias, angina, ischaemic heart disease and hepatic or renal dysfunction (Tiziani, 2021).

Antidepressant drugs, including tricyclics and selective serotonin reuptake inhibitors (SSRIs), may relieve abdominal pain associated with IBS. Although the anticholinergic side effects of tricyclics (such as amitriptyline (Tryptanol) and imipramine (Tofranil)) may help decrease diarrhoea, these have more adverse effects than SSRIs such as sertraline (Zoloft) and fluoxetine (Prozac). Alosetron (Lotronex) is a serotonin receptor antagonist reducing abdominal pain and diarrhoea in individuals with IBS. Its use is limited, however, by its association with ischaemic colitis.

Nutrition

Diet is an important tool in IBS management. Fermentable oligosaccharide, disaccharide, monosaccharide and polyol (FODMAP) short-chained carbohydrates are poorly absorbed in the small intestine, leading to an osmotic effect in the colon with excessive gas production causing pain and diarrhoea (Manning et al., 2022). When excess gas and flatulence are problems, reduce the intake of gas-forming foods, such as those with fructose (pears and apples), oligosaccharides (wheat and onions), galacto-oligosaccarides (legumes) and sugar polyols (sorbitol and mannitol—stone fruits and artificial sweeteners). A low-FODMAP diet has shown short-term IBS symptom improvement (Marin, 2021). Caffeinated drinks, such as coffee, tea and soft drinks, act as gastrointestinal stimulants; limiting intake of these fluids may also prove beneficial. Some people may benefit from limiting lactose intake (see Table 23.1).

Complementary and alternative therapies

Herbal preparations may provide some benefit for a person with IBS. Herbs with an antispasmodic effect, such as anise, chamomile and sage, may be used to reduce the manifestations of IBS. Peppermint oil targets IBS pathophysiology as it has antimicrobial, anti-inflammatory, antioxidant, immunomodulating and anaesthetic properties. Oral peppermint oil reduces IBS symptoms in adults when taken for more than 3 weeks (Marin, 2022). Dill and aniseed are carminatives included in some commercial preparations to relieve wind or colic in babies (Bullock & Manias, 2022). Ginger root, when consumed as a tea or capsule, assists with reducing gas, bloating and diarrhoea and improves stomach functioning (Braun & Cohen, 2015). According to Manuel (2021), probiotic therapies (such as yoghurt with active bacterial cultures, particularly *Lactobacillus*) improve overall IBS-C symptoms, abdominal pain and flatulence. Urgency and other general symptoms were alleviated by formulations containing *Bifidobacterium lactis*. Manuel (2021) advised informing a person electing to try probiotics to try one preparation at a time for at least 4 weeks and monitor the effects on symptoms of IBS.

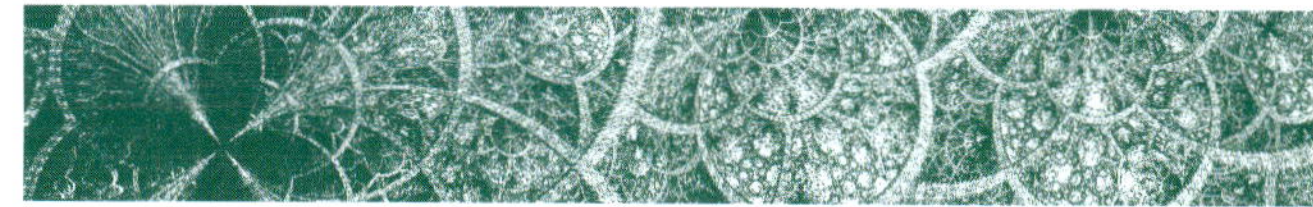

Nursing care

People with IBS rarely require acute care for it as a primary problem. However, nurses frequently interact with individuals with IBS in clinics and other community settings.

Assessment

Careful assessment is important to help identify the effects of IBS on the person. Collect the following assessment data:

- *Health history*: current manifestations, their onset and duration; current treatment measures; effect of manifestations on lifestyle; exploration of mental health status.
- *Physical examination*: apparent general state of health; abdominal shape and contour, bowel sounds, tenderness.

Nursing diagnoses and interventions

The primary nursing responsibility is education; providing referrals and counselling are additional nursing responsibilities to a person with IBS. See the previous sections on diarrhoea and constipation for selected nursing interventions.

Community-based care

Include the following topics in teaching for the person with IBS:

- the nature of the disorder and the reality of the person's manifestations
- the relationship between IBS and stress, anxiety and depression
- stress and anxiety reduction techniques, such as meditation, visualisation, exercise, 'time out' and progressive relaxation
- dietary influences that may contribute to IBS and suggested dietary changes; an increase in intake of insoluble dietary fibre is not recommended
- the use and role of prescribed medications, their adverse effects and when to contact the doctor
- stress the importance of routine follow-up appointments and of notifying the primary care provider if manifestations change (such as blood in the stool, significant constipation or diarrhoea, increasing abdominal pain or weight loss).

If needed, refer the person to a counsellor or other mental health professional for assistance in dealing with psychological factors associated with living with a chronic condition.

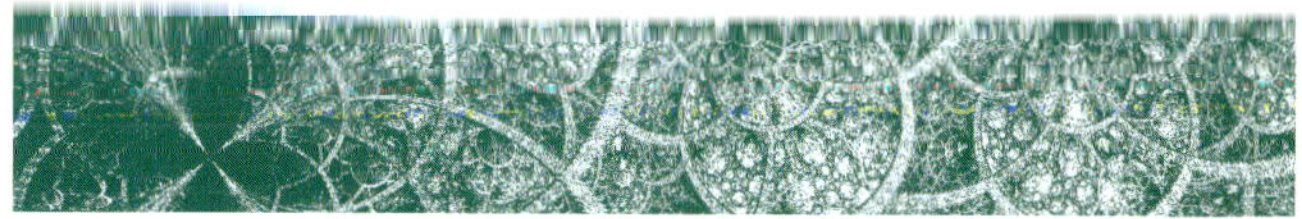

THE PERSON WITH FAECAL INCONTINENCE

Faecal incontinence, the loss of voluntary control of defecation, occurs less frequently than urinary incontinence; however, it is no less distressing to the person. Faecal incontinence has a negative impact on a person's self-esteem and requires an individualised management approach.

Multiple factors contribute to faecal incontinence, including both physiological and psychological conditions (see Box 23.2). Bowel incontinence is usually considered a manifestation of a disorder rather than a disorder in itself. A person often does not reveal faecal incontinence when discussing health concerns. There are approximately 1.3 million Australians (15 years and older) with faecal incontinence (Continence Foundation of Australia (CFA), 2022). The National Continence Management Strategy (NCMS), established in 1998 by the Australian Government Department of Health and Ageing, provides funding to research and service development initiatives aimed at prevention and treatment of this significant problem.

Older adults are more affected by faecal incontinence due to aetiological factors. Le (2018) cited epidemiological data indicating that 1–10% of adults are affected with faecal incontinence and that 0.5–1.0% of adults experience regular faecal incontinence which affects their quality of life.

Pathophysiology

To understand the pathophysiology of faecal incontinence, it is necessary to understand normal defecation mechanisms. The rectum is normally empty. When it is distended by faeces entering from the sigmoid colon, the defecation reflex is stimulated. This reflex causes involuntary relaxation of the internal sphincter and stimulates the urge to defecate. When the external sphincter, which is under both somatic (voluntary) and autonomic (involuntary) control, relaxes, defecation occurs. Adults normally can override the defecation reflex by voluntary contraction of the external sphincter and pelvic floor muscles. The wall of the rectum gradually relaxes and the urge to defecate subsides.

The most common causes of faecal incontinence are those interfering with either sensory or motor control of the rectum and anal sphincters. If the external sphincter is paralysed as a result of spinal cord injury or disease, defecation occurs automatically when the internal sphincter relaxes with the defecation reflex. If sphincter muscles are damaged or excessive pelvic floor relaxation occurs, it may not be possible to override the defecation reflex with voluntary control.

Age-related changes in anal sphincter tone and response to rectal distension increase the risk of faecal incontinence in older adults. Resting and maximal anal sphincter pressures are decreased, particularly in older women. Additionally, older females need less rectal distension to produce sustained relaxation of the anal sphincter.

BOX 23.2 Selected causes of faecal incontinence

Neurological causes
- Spinal cord injury or disease
- Head injury, stroke or brain tumour
- Degenerative neurological disease, such as multiple sclerosis, amyotrophic lateral sclerosis (ALS), dementia
- Diabetic neuropathy

Local trauma
- Obstetric tears
- Anorectal injury
- Anorectal surgery with sphincter damage

Inflammatory processes
- Infection
- Radiation

Other causes
- Diarrhoea
- Stool impaction
- Pelvic floor relaxation or loss of sphincter tone
- Tumours

Psychological causes
- Depression
- Confusion and disorientation

INTERPROFESSIONAL CARE

The diagnosis of faecal incontinence based on the person's history is fraught with difficulty as people are often reluctant to reveal faecal incontinence, or their carer may be unaware of previous continence history (Magtoto, 2022). Physical examination of the pelvic floor and anus evaluates muscle tone and rules out a faecal impaction. Impaired sphincter muscle may be palpable on digital exam. An anorectal manometry or a rectal motility test is used to evaluate the functional ability of the sphincter muscles. In this test, a small, flexible balloon catheter is introduced into the rectum and pressures are measured in the rectum and internal and external sphincters. Normally, rectal dilation causes the internal sphincter to relax and the external sphincter to contract. Sigmoidoscopy may also be used to examine the rectum and anal canal.

Management of faecal incontinence is directed towards the identified cause. Lizarondo (2022) recommended a comprehensive person-centred bowel management program based on formal assessment be developed and then reassessed 6 monthly for a person with faecal incontinence. Medications to relieve diarrhoea or constipation may be prescribed. A high-fibre diet, ample fluids and regular exercise are helpful for many people. Exercises to improve sphincter and pelvic floor muscle tone (Kegel exercises) may be of long-term benefit. See the chapter 'Nursing care of people with urinary tract disorders' for more information about Kegel exercises.

A person may also benefit from using loperamide before meals and prophylactically before leaving home. Lizarondo (2022) suggested antidiarrhoeal medication (e.g. loperamide hydrochloride (Imodium)) can be used long term in doses from 0.5 mg to 16 mg per day, as required. Codeine phosphate may be offered for people who do not tolerate loperamide. Biofeedback therapy is suggested for mentally alert individuals with intact sphincter muscles but low muscle tone. It is thought that, with motivation and reinforcement, the person can achieve improved sphincter control in response to a stimulus. The goal of biofeedback is to improve sensation, coordination and strength of the sphincter muscle (Slade, 2021). Slade (2021) highlighted research findings that support the use of biofeedback and sphincter exercises in the treatment of adults with faecal incontinence.

When damage to the sphincter or rectal prolapse (protrusion of rectal mucous membrane through the anus) is the cause of faecal incontinence, surgical repair is the treatment of choice. Surgery may also be indicated when conservative measures have been ineffective. Permanent colostomy, the creation of an opening from the large bowel on the abdominal wall, is a last-choice option for some people to control faecal output when other measures fail.

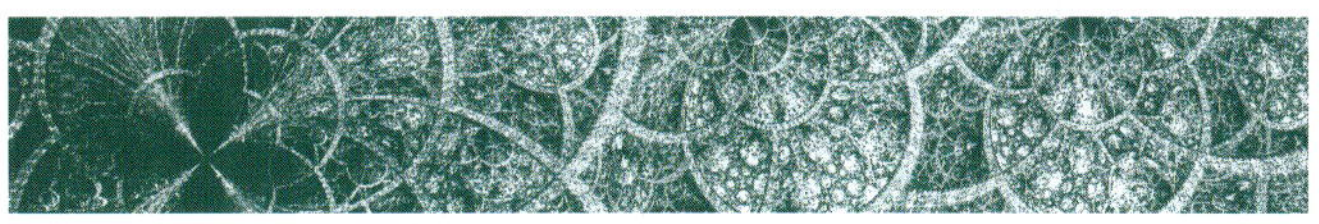

Nursing care

Health promotion

A bowel training program to establish a regular pattern of elimination is often effective in relieving faecal incontinence. Encourage the person to establish a regular time of day for elimination, usually 15 to 30 minutes after breakfast. A stimulant, such as a cup of coffee, a rectal suppository or even a phosphate enema, may be given to prompt defecation. A person with neurological incontinence can learn to stimulate the anal canal digitally to initiate defecation.

Dietary changes may be useful in managing faecal incontinence. If incontinence occurs only with mild loose or liquid stools, increasing dietary fibre or using a bulking agent to increase stool bulk and solidity may be effective. The majority of the fibre should come from a fibre-rich diet because fibre supplements provide only a limited amount of additional fibre (Slade, 2021). When incontinence of solid stool occurs, a low-residue diet of easily digested and absorbed foods may be prescribed to reduce the frequency of defecation.

Assessment

- *Health history*: extent, onset and duration of incontinence; identified contributing factors; history of spinal cord or anorectal injury or surgery; chronic diseases such as diabetes mellitus, multiple sclerosis or other neurological disorders.
- *Physical examination*: mental status; general health; examination of perianal tissues; digital rectal examination.

Nursing diagnoses and interventions

Bowel incontinence

Nurses are often responsible for instituting bowel training programs and other measures to manage faecal incontinence.

- Teach caregivers to place the person on a toilet or commode and provide for privacy at a certain time of day. *Placing the person in the normal position to defecate at a consistent time of day stimulates the defecation reflex and helps re-establish a pattern of stool evacuation.*
- If necessary, insert a glycerin or bisacodyl (Durolax) suppository 15 to 20 minutes before positioning the person on the toilet or commode. This helps to stimulate evacuation. *Once a regular elimination pattern is established, it may be possible to discontinue suppository use.*
- Maintain a caring, non-judgmental manner when providing care. *This promotes a feeling of acceptance when the person may feel unacceptable.*

CONSIDERATION FOR PRACTICE

Provide room odour control with deodoriser tablets, sprays or other devices. Controlling odour is important to preserve the person's self-esteem.

Risk of impaired skin integrity

Good skin care is vital for a person with faecal incontinence. Stools contain enzymes and other irritating substances that promote skin breakdown when not promptly removed. This can lead to pressure ulcers, particularly when a neurological disorder (such as spinal cord injury, dementia or stroke) impairs mobility.

- Clean the skin thoroughly with mild soap and water after each bowel movement. *Toilet paper may be more irritating to the skin and less effective in removing faecal material.*
- Apply a skin barrier cream or ointment after each bowel movement. *These help to protect the skin from irritating substances in the faeces.*
- If disposable pads or briefs are used, check frequently for soiling and change when faeces are noted. *Although these help to protect bedding and clothing from soiling, these contribute to skin breakdown if they are not checked and changed frequently.*

Community-based care

Managing faecal incontinence is a challenging problem for the person and family caregivers. For the person with intact cognition, it can be psychologically devastating. The person may become socially isolated from fear of odour or soiling clothing. Self-esteem may suffer from a sense of lost control over body functions and the inability to provide self-care. It is important to stress that incontinence is never normal (i.e. ageing alone is not a cause of incontinence) and often is treatable. Encourage the person to seek medical evaluation of the problem.

Topics to include in education for the person and their family are:

- Recommended dietary measures — for example, consuming a high-fibre diet and ample fluids to maintain soft, formed stools or a low-residue diet to reduce the number of stools.

- Suggestions for regular exercise stimulating bowel peristalsis and regular evacuation.
- Avoid constipation as straining often to achieve bowel movements stretches and weakens the pelvic floor muscles.
- Use of bulk-forming laxatives, such as psyllium seed (Metamucil), to provide stool bulk and reduce the number of small, liquid stools.
- Bowel training program instructions, including correct sitting position on the toilet or commode; techniques for digital anal stimulation, inserting suppositories or administering enemas as recommended. When sitting on the toilet or commode, advise the person or their carer to position with the feet firmly supported. This helps to fully relax the pelvic floor and sphincter muscles. For digital anal simulation, teach to insert a lubricated gloved finger through the anal sphincter into the rectum 2 to 3 cm while seated on the toilet or commode and then to use a circular side-to-side movement to gently stretch the rectal wall until the internal sphincter relaxes.
- Recommend smoking cessation as chronic coughing associated with smoking weakens the pelvic floor muscles, leading to bowel control problems. Encourage discussion with a doctor or pharmacist for information on quitting smoking and managing chronic coughing.
- Prescribed medications (such as loperamide to reduce the number of stools), their appropriate use and management of adverse effects (such as constipation).
- The importance of good skin care, particularly if the person has a neurological impairment.
- The potential benefits and associated risks of biofeedback and surgical treatment, if recommended.
- Provide referrals to appropriate home care or community health services.

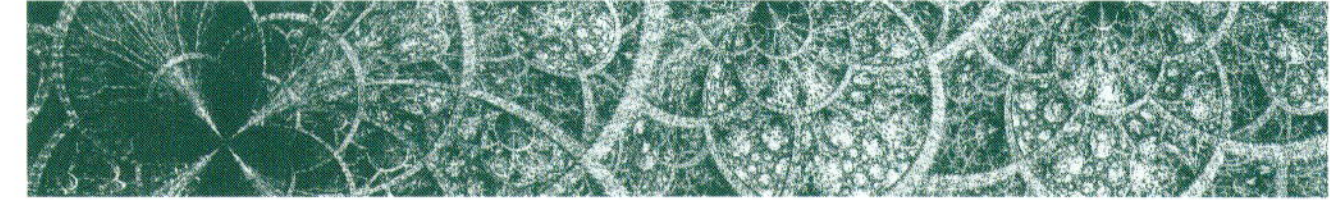

Acute inflammatory and infectious bowel disorders

The GI tract is particularly vulnerable to inflammation and infection because of its continual exposure to the external environment. Although most pathogens affecting the GI tract are ingested in food or water, infection may also be spread by direct contact, possibly by the respiratory route. Pathogens may also be transmitted sexually through anal intercourse.

Acute disease of the GI tract may be caused by the pathogen itself or by a bacterial or other toxin. Acute inflammatory disorders such as appendicitis and peritonitis result from contamination of damaged or normally sterile tissue by the person's own endogenous or resident bacteria.

THE PERSON WITH APPENDICITIS

Appendicitis, inflammation of the vermiform appendix, is a common cause of acute abdominal pain. It is the most common reason for emergency abdominal surgery, affecting 7% to 14% of the population (Nepogodiev et al., 2020). Appendicitis occurs at any age but is more common in adolescents and young adults, and slightly more common in males than females.

Pathophysiology

The appendix is a tube-like pouch attached to the caecum just below the ileocaecal valve. It is usually located in the right iliac region, at an area designated as McBurney's point (see Figure 23.4A). The function of the appendix is not fully understood, although it regularly fills with and empties digested food.

Obstruction of the proximal lumen of the appendix is apparent in most acutely inflamed appendices. The obstruction is often caused by a *faecalith* or hard mass of faeces. Other obstructive causes include a calculus or stone, a foreign body,

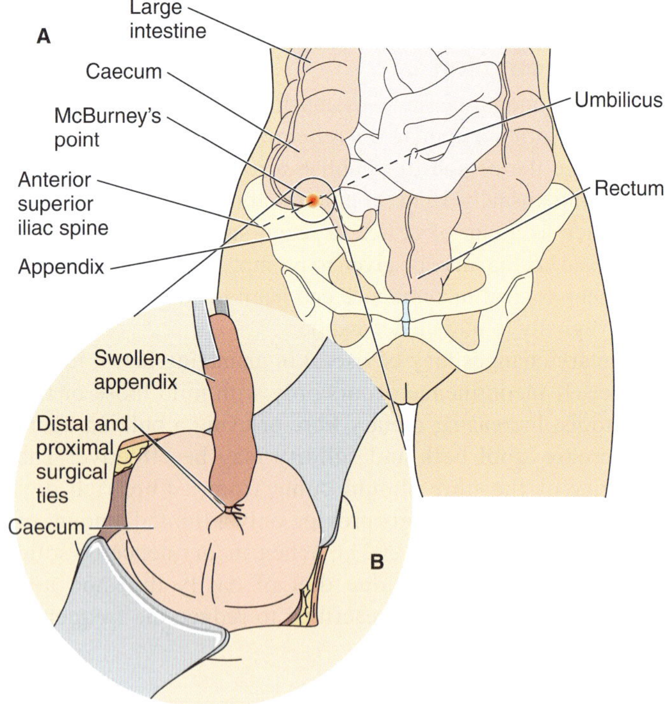

FIGURE 23.4 *A, McBurney's point, located midway between the umbilicus and the anterior iliac crest in the right lower quadrant. It is the usual site for localised pain and rebound tenderness due to appendicitis. B, During an appendectomy, the appendix and caecum are brought through the incision to the surface of the abdomen. The base of the appendix is clamped and ligated; the appendix is then removed*

inflammation, a tumour, parasites (e.g. pinworms) or oedema of lymphoid tissue. Following obstruction, the appendix distends with fluid secreted by its mucosa. As pressure within the lumen of the appendix increases, blood supply is impaired, leading to inflammation, oedema, ulceration and infection. The formation of purulent exudate further distends the appendix. Within 24 to 36 hours, tissue necrosis and gangrene results, leading to perforation if treatment is not initiated. Perforation results in bacterial peritonitis.

Appendicitis is classified as simple, gangrenous or perforated, depending on the stage of the process. In *simple appendicitis*, the appendix is inflamed but intact. When areas of tissue necrosis and microscopic perforations are present in the appendix, it is classified as *gangrenous appendicitis*. A *perforated appendix* shows evidence of gross perforation and contamination of the peritoneal cavity.

Manifestations

Continuous mild generalised or upper abdominal pain is the initial characteristic manifestation of acute appendicitis. Over the next 4 hours, the pain intensifies and localises in the right lower quadrant of the abdomen. It is aggravated by moving, walking or coughing. On palpation, localised and rebound tenderness are noted at McBurney's point. Rebound tenderness is demonstrated by relief of pain with direct palpation of McBurney's point followed by pain on release of pressure. Extension or internal rotation of the right hip increases the pain. Pain and local tenderness in the lower right quadrant as a presenting symptom are absent in approximately 45% of older adults compared with less than 5% of younger adults with appendicitis. This delays diagnosis in older adults, contributing to a 15% mortality of perforated appendicitis in older adults (Papadakis, McPhee & Rabow, 2022). Additionally, acute appendicitis in older adults is more virulent with complications developing sooner.

The classic manifestation of appendicitis is abdominal pain developing over 4 to 48 hours accompanied by nausea, vomiting, anorexia and a low-grade temperature. However, clinical manifestations occur in less than 50% of people developing appendicitis. More commonly, people with appendicitis present with a combination of these symptoms.

Pregnant women may develop right lower quadrant, periumbilical or right subcostal (under the rib cage) pain due to possible displacement of the appendix by the distended uterus. Women in their third trimester are at risk of appendicitis. During pregnancy, abdominal pain, nausea and vomiting are more common and many women developing appendicitis during pregnancy do not experience the classic symptoms, making early identification of appendicitis difficult.

Children, like older adults and pregnant women, often have fewer symptoms, making their diagnosis less obvious and the incidence of complications more frequent.

Complications

Perforation, peritonitis and abscess are possible complications of acute appendicitis. Perforation is manifested by increased pain and a high fever. It can lead to a small, localised abscess, local peritonitis or significant generalised peritonitis. The very young, older adults and those with impaired immune systems—for example, those with diabetes mellitus—generally are at increased risk of complications.

A less common disorder is chronic appendicitis, characterised by chronic abdominal pain and recurrent acute attacks at intervals of several months or more. Other conditions, such as inflammatory bowel disease and renal disorders, cause similar manifestations attributed to chronic appendicitis.

INTERPROFESSIONAL CARE

An acutely inflamed appendix can perforate within 24 hours, so rapid diagnosis and treatment is important. Because of this urgency and the low incidence of surgical complications, diagnostic testing and preoperative treatment are limited. The person is admitted to the hospital and intravenous fluids and antibiotics are initiated. Food and oral fluids are withheld until a diagnosis is confirmed. Once the diagnosis is established, an appendectomy is performed.

Diagnosis

Diagnostic and laboratory tests are used to help confirm the diagnosis and rule out other possible causes for the manifestations. Abdominal ultrasound is the most effective test assisting in diagnosing acute appendicitis, reducing the incidence of exploratory surgery, and is particularly useful in a person with atypical symptoms, such as pregnant women, children and older adults (Nepogodiev et al., 2020). Other diagnostic tests used to accurately diagnose appendicitis include abdominal x-rays, an intravenous pyelogram, a urinalysis and a pelvic examination. Additionally, a WBC count with differential is obtained. With appendicitis, the total white count is elevated (10,000 to 20,000/mm^3), with an increased number of immature WBCs (bands).

Medications

Prior to surgery, intravenous fluids are given to restore or maintain vascular volume and prevent electrolyte imbalance. Antibiotic therapy with a third-generation cephalosporin effective against many Gram-negative bacteria, such as cefotaxime (Cefotaxime Sandoz), ceftazidime (Fortum) or ceftriaxone (Rocephin), is initiated prior to surgery. The antibiotic is repeated during surgery and continued for at least 48 hours postoperatively. (The nursing implications for cephalosporin antibiotics are discussed in the chapter 'Nursing care of people with infections'.) Analgesic medications are administered as prescribed.

Surgery

The treatment of choice for acute appendicitis is an *appendectomy*, surgical removal of the appendix.

Either a laparoscopic approach (insertion of an endoscope to view abdominal contents) or via a laparotomy (surgical opening of the abdomen) are used for appendectomy. Laparoscopic appendectomy requires a very small incision through which the laparoscope is inserted. This procedure has several advantages: (1) direct visualisation of the appendix allows definitive diagnosis without laparotomy, (2) postoperative hospitalisation is short, (3) postoperative complications are infrequent, and (4) recovery and resumption of normal activities is rapid.

An open appendectomy is performed by laparotomy. A small transverse incision is made at McBurney's point (see Figure 23.4A); the appendix is isolated and ligated (tied off) to prevent contamination of the site with bowel contents, and then removed (Figure 23.4B). A laparotomy is generally performed when the appendix has ruptured. It allows removal of contaminants from the peritoneal cavity by irrigation with sterile normal saline. Occasionally the wound may be left unsutured for periodic irrigation. Recovery is generally uneventful. Refer to the chapter 'Nursing care of people having surgery' for specific discussion of preoperative and postoperative nursing care.

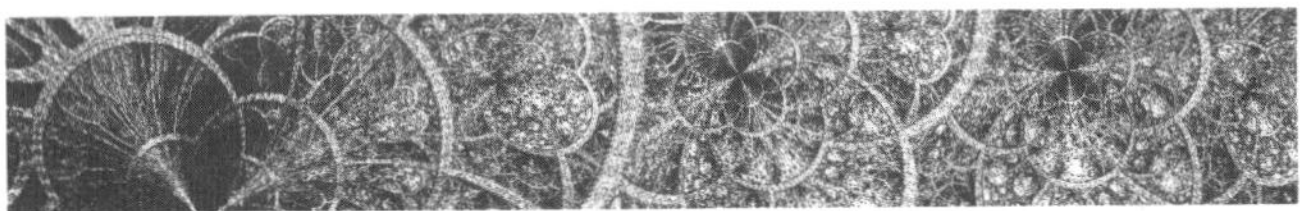

Nursing care

A nursing care plan for a person with acute appendicitis is included below.

Assessment

Because appendicitis rapidly progresses from inflammation to perforation, prompt assessment is vital. Obtain the following assessment data:

- *Health history*: current manifestations, including onset, duration, progression and aggravating or relieving factors; most recent food or fluid intake; known medication or other allergies and reaction to allergen; current medications; history of chronic diseases.
- *Physical examination*: vital signs, including temperature; apparent general health; abdominal shape and contour, bowel sounds, tenderness to light palpation.

Nursing diagnoses and interventions

Preoperative nursing care is directed towards preparing the person physically and psychologically for emergency surgery. Generally, limited time is available for preoperative teaching.

> **CONSIDERATION FOR PRACTICE**
> **Keep the person with suspected appendicitis nil by mouth (NBM). Do not administer laxatives or enemas, which may cause perforation of the appendix. No heat should be applied to the abdomen; this may increase circulation (vasodilation) to the appendix, also causing perforation.**

Risk of infection

Preventing complications during the perioperative period is a primary nursing care goal. Perforation and peritonitis are the most likely preoperative complications; postoperative complications include wound infection, abscess and possible peritonitis.

> **CONSIDERATION FOR PRACTICE**
> **Assess abdominal status frequently, including distension, bowel sounds and tenderness. Increasing generalised pain, a rigid, board-like abdomen and abdominal distension may indicate developing peritonitis.**

- Monitor vital signs, including temperature and pain. Perforation is manifested by increased pain and a high fever. *Tachycardia and rapid shallow respirations may indicate perforation of the appendix with resulting peritonitis. The blood pressure may fall if sepsis is present.*
- Maintain intravenous infusion until oral intake is adequate. *Intravenous fluids are given to maintain vascular volume and to provide a route for antibiotic administration.*
- Assess wound, abdominal girth and postoperative pain. *Swelling of the wound, increased abdominal girth or an increase in pain may indicate infection or peritonitis.*

Acute pain

A person with appendicitis experiences pain before and after surgery. Pain should be controlled preoperatively with anti-inflammatory medications. Postoperative pain is controlled by narcotic or non-narcotic analgesics.

- Assess pain, including its character, location, severity and duration. Report any unexpected changes in the nature of pain. *Both preoperatively and postoperatively, the person's pain provides important clues about the diagnosis and possible complications such as rupture of the appendix or peritonitis.*

> **CONSIDERATION FOR PRACTICE**
> **Sudden relief of preoperative pain may signal rupture of a distended and oedematous appendix.**

- Administer analgesics as ordered. *Preoperatively, pain medication can be given after a diagnosis is established. Postoperatively, provide analgesics to maintain comfort and enhance mobility.*
- Assess effectiveness of medication 30 minutes after administration. Report increasing or unrelieved pain. *Increasing or pain unrelieved by prescribed analgesic may indicate a complication or the need for further assessment. For example, continued abdominal discomfort and distension may indicate excess intestinal gas that may be better relieved by ambulation.*

Community-based care

Often preoperative teaching is limited by pain and the urgent nature of the surgery. Explain why food and fluids are not permitted during this time. If time allows, teach postoperative turning, coughing, deep breathing and pain management.

Following an uncomplicated appendectomy, the person is often discharged either the day of, or the day following, surgery. Postoperative teaching includes:

- wound or incision care, including hand hygiene and dressing change procedures as indicated

NURSING CARE PLAN A person with acute appendicitis

Lynne James is a 19-year-old university student in her first year of a nursing degree. Ms James arrives at the emergency department (ED) at 0100 hrs. She describes a general lower abdominal pain which started the previous evening. By midnight, the pain was more localised over the right lower quadrant. She is also nauseated and reports episodes of vomiting.

ASSESSMENT

Sue Grady, RN, completes the admission assessment in the ED. Ms James reports nausea and abdominal pain, rating it at 9/10 (0 to 10 pain scale) stating, 'Walking makes my stomach hurt worse.' Physical assessment findings include T 37.8°C, P 84, R 16 and BP 110/70; skin warm to touch; abdomen flat and guarded, with marked tenderness in right lower quadrant. Ms James' FBC shows WBC 14,000/mm^3; neutrophils 81.1%; lymphocytes 12.5%. The diagnosis of acute appendicitis is made. Ms James is kept fasting; prepared for theatre, consented and transferred to operating theatre for a laparoscopic appendectomy.

DIAGNOSES

- *Risk of infection* related to impaired skin integrity secondary to surgical incision.
- *Alteration in comfort* related to acute pain secondary to surgical intervention.
- *Anxiety* related to situational crisis.

PLANNING

When planning nursing care with Ms James, it is vital to consider and ensure her religious and cultural beliefs are incorporated into her plan of care.

Expected outcomes

- Ms James' incision will heal without infection or complications.
- Ms James will verbalise adequate pain relief.
- Ms James will verbalise decreased anxiety.
- Ms James will return to preoperative activities.

IMPLEMENTATION

- Assess Ms James' pain using a pain scale; provide analgesics as needed. Monitor Ms James for effectiveness and adverse reactions.
- Teach Ms James pain management following discharge.
- Teach Ms James abdominal splinting during coughing, turning or ambulating as needed.
- Teach Ms James home care of incision.
- Discuss with Ms James activity limitations as ordered.
- Instruct Ms James to report fever or warmth, redness or drainage from the incision, or increasing abdominal pain.

EVALUATION

On discharge the following evening, Ms James was fully mobile. Her appetite had returned and she was tolerating diet and fluids well. Her temperature was 36.3°C. The RN provided Ms James with written and verbal information on postoperative care following an appendectomy.

CRITICAL THINKING IN THE NURSING PROCESS

1. Outline the physiological basis for Ms James' elevated WBC.
2. Describe differences in Ms James' postoperative care and teaching if she had undergone a laparotomy instead of a laparoscopic appendectomy.
3. Outline the teaching plan you would develop with Ms James for home care following a laparoscopic appendectomy.
4. Develop a care plan for Ms James for the nursing diagnosis *Anxiety* related to a situational crisis.

REFLECTION ON THE NURSING PROCESS

1. Reflect on what you learned from completing this section. Outline how you will apply this knowledge to assist you in your clinical reasoning when next on your professional experience placement.
2. Describe nursing interventions you can incorporate into your clinical practice to reduce a person's anxiety levels while they wait for surgery.

- instructions to report fever, increased abdominal pain, swelling, redness, drainage, bleeding or warmth of the operative site to the doctor
- any activity limitations (e.g. lifting, driving)
- when it is appropriate to return to work.

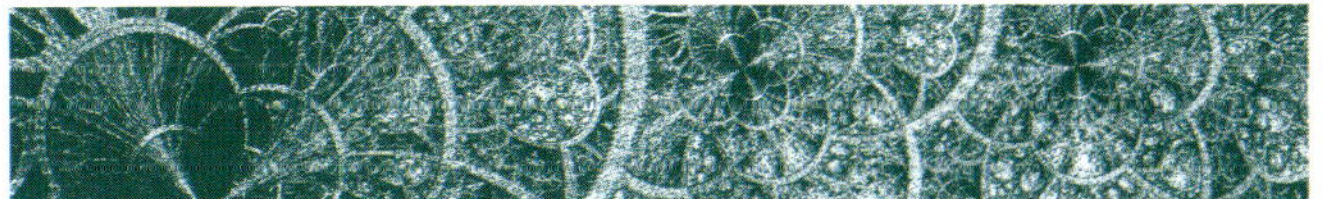

THE PERSON WITH PERITONITIS

Peritonitis, inflammation of the peritoneum, is a serious complication of many acute abdominal disorders. It is usually caused by enteric bacteria entering the peritoneal cavity through a perforated ulcer, ruptured appendix, perforated diverticulum or necrotic bowel, or during abdominal surgery. Pelvic inflammatory disease, gallbladder rupture, abdominal trauma or peritoneal dialysis can also lead to peritonitis.

Pathophysiology

The peritoneum is a double-layered serous membrane lining the walls (parietal peritoneum) and organs (visceral peritoneum) of the abdominal cavity. There is a potential space between the parietal and visceral layers of the peritoneum containing a small amount of serous fluid. This space, the peritoneal cavity, is sterile.

Peritonitis results from contamination of the normally sterile peritoneal cavity by infection or a chemical irritant. Chemical peritonitis often precedes bacterial peritonitis. Perforation of a peptic ulcer or rupture of the gallbladder releases gastric juices (hydrochloric acid and pepsin) or bile into the peritoneal cavity, causing an acute inflammatory response.

Bacterial peritonitis is usually caused by infection by *E. coli*, *Klebsiella*, *Proteus* or *Pseudomonas* bacteria normally inhabiting the bowel. *Neisseria gonorrhoeae* can also cause peritonitis in untreated women with the disease. Inflammatory and immune defence mechanisms are activated when bacteria enter the peritoneal space. These defences can effectively eliminate small numbers of bacteria. However, they are overwhelmed by a massive or continued contamination. When this occurs, mast cells release histamine and other vasoactive substances, causing local vasodilation and increased capillary permeability. Polymorphonuclear leucocytes (a type of WBC) infiltrate the peritoneum to phagocytise bacteria and foreign matter. A fibrinogen-rich plasma exudate, promoting bacterial destruction and forming fibrin clots, seals off and segregates the bacteria. This process helps limit and localise the infection, allowing host defences to eradicate it. Continued contamination, however, leads to generalised inflammation of the peritoneal cavity. The inflammatory process causes fluid to shift into the peritoneal space (third spacing). Circulating blood volume is depleted, leading to hypovolaemia. *Septicaemia*, a systemic disease caused by pathogens or their toxins in the blood, may develop.

Manifestations

Manifestations of peritonitis depend on the severity and extent of the infection, as well as the age and general health of the person. Both local and systemic manifestations are present (see the 'Manifestations' box). A person often presents with evidence of an *acute abdomen*, an abrupt onset of diffuse, severe abdominal pain. The pain may localise and intensify near the area of infection. Movement may intensify the pain. The entire abdomen is tender, with guarding or rigidity of abdominal muscles. The acute abdomen is often described as board-like. Rebound tenderness may be present over the area of inflammation. Peritoneal inflammation inhibits peristalsis, resulting in a paralytic ileus. Bowel sounds are markedly diminished or absent. Progressive abdominal distension is noted. Pooling of GI secretions may cause nausea and vomiting. Systemic manifestations of peritonitis include fever, malaise, tachycardia and tachypnoea, restlessness and possible disorientation. The person may be oliguric (having little urine output) with signs of dehydration and shock.

Older adults or chronically debilitated or immunosuppressed individuals may present with few of the classic manifestations of peritonitis. Increased confusion and restlessness, a decreased urinary output and vague abdominal complaints may be the only clinical manifestations. These individuals are at increased risk of delayed diagnosis, contributing to a higher mortality rate.

Complications

Complications of peritonitis may be life threatening. Abscess formation is common. The very defence mechanisms isolating and localising the infection can protect it from immune responses and systemic antibiotics. Fibrous adhesions in the abdominal cavity are a late complication and may lead to subsequent obstruction.

Without prompt and effective treatment, septicaemia and septic shock develop. Fluid loss into the abdominal cavity leads to hypovolaemic shock. These potentially lethal complications require immediate and aggressive intervention to prevent multiple-organ failure and death. Shock and its management are discussed in the chapter 'Nursing care of people experiencing trauma and shock'.

MANIFESTATIONS Peritonitis

ABDOMINAL/GASTROINTESTINAL MANIFESTATIONS
- Diffuse or localised pain
- Tenderness with rebound
- Board-like rigidity of abdomen
- Diminished or absent bowel sounds
- Distension
- Anorexia, nausea and vomiting

SYSTEMIC MANIFESTATIONS
- Fever
- Malaise
- Tachycardia
- Tachypnoea
- Restlessness
- Confusion or disorientation
- Oliguria

INTERPROFESSIONAL CARE

Care of individuals with peritonitis focuses on establishing the diagnosis and identifying and treating its cause as well as the peritonitis. Preventing complications is a vital aspect of care.

Diagnosis

Diagnostic tests are performed to establish the diagnosis of peritonitis, rule out other disorders and help identify the cause. The tests may include a WBC count (elevated to approximately 20,000/mm^3 in peritonitis), blood cultures, abdominal x-rays, liver and renal function studies, serum electrolytes and an abdominal paracentesis. (In peritonitis, peritoneal fluid contains increased protein and WBCs.) Increased numbers of immature blood cells are present as the bone marrow releases these in response to the infection.

Medications

Until the infecting organism is identified, a broad-spectrum antibiotic effective against organisms commonly implicated in peritonitis is prescribed. Beta-lactum antibiotics such as imipenem (Primaxin) or meropenem (Merrem) are prescribed due

FAST FACTS

Mortality from peritonitis
- The overall mortality rate associated with peritonitis is about 40%.
- People with other medical conditions, older adults and those with greater bacterial contamination have a higher mortality.
- Young people with perforated ulcers or appendicitis, those with less extensive bacterial contamination and those receiving early surgical intervention have mortality rates of less than 10%.

to their broad spectrum of action. Once culture results are obtained, antibiotic therapy is modified to the specific organism(s) responsible.

Other antibiotics ordered may include ampicillin (e.g. Ampicyn), metronidazole (Flagyl), ciprofloxacin (Cipro), clindamycin (Cleocin), a cephalosporin such as ceftriaxone (Rocephin) or an aminoglycoside antibiotic such as gentamicin (Genoptic) or amikacin (Amikin). Nursing implications for antibiotic therapy are discussed in the chapter 'Nursing care of people with infections'. Analgesics are prescribed to promote comfort.

Surgery

If peritonitis is caused by a perforation, gangrenous bowel or inflamed appendix, a laparotomy is done to close the perforation or remove the damaged and inflamed tissue. If an abscess is present, it may be surgically drained or removed.

Peritoneal lavage, washing of the peritoneal cavity with copious amounts of warm isotonic fluid, may be done during surgery. This procedure dilutes residual bacteria and removes gross contaminants, blood and fibrin clots. In rare instances, peritoneal lavage may be continued for several days following surgery. The solution is infused into the upper portion of the peritoneal cavity and removed via drains in the pelvic cul-de-sac. Careful assessment of fluid and electrolyte status and maintaining aseptic techniques are necessary.

Following a laparotomy for peritonitis, the person often returns from surgery with either Penrose or closed drain systems such as a Jackson–Pratt drain. In some cases, the incision is left unsutured. With severe and long-standing peritonitis, the abdomen may be closed temporarily with polypropylene mesh containing a nylon zipper or Velcro, allowing repeated abdominal exploration and drainage of infectious sites.

Nutrition

Intravenous fluids and electrolyte replacements are administered to maintain vascular volume and fluid and electrolyte balance. Parenteral nutrition is given until adequate oral intake resumes.

Other treatments

The person is placed on bed rest in Fowler's position; this helps localise the infection and promotes lung ventilation. Oxygen is often ordered, facilitating cellular metabolism and healing.

INTESTINAL DECOMPRESSION The inflammatory process of peritonitis draws large amounts of fluid into the abdominal cavity and the bowel. Additionally, peristaltic activity of the bowel is slowed or halted by the inflammation, causing *paralytic ileus* (or *ileus*), impaired propulsion or forward movement of bowel contents. Intestinal decompression is used to relieve abdominal distension, facilitate closure and minimise postoperative respiratory complications. A nasogastric or long intestinal tube is inserted and connected to continuous drainage (see Figure 23.5). If prolonged intestinal decompression is anticipated, a jejunostomy may be performed for comfort. Suction is maintained until peristalsis resumes, bowel sounds are present and the person is passing flatus. Food and fluids are withheld until intestinal motility has returned and suction is discontinued.

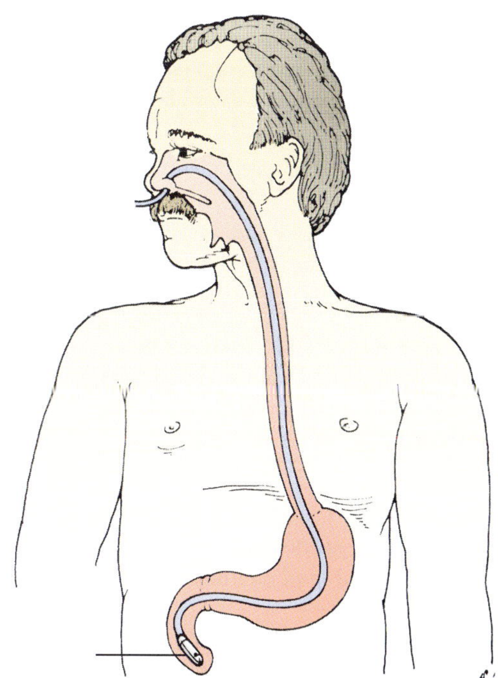

FIGURE 23.5 ***The weighted tip or inflated balloon at the end of an intestinal tube is drawn into the intestine by gravity and peristalsis***

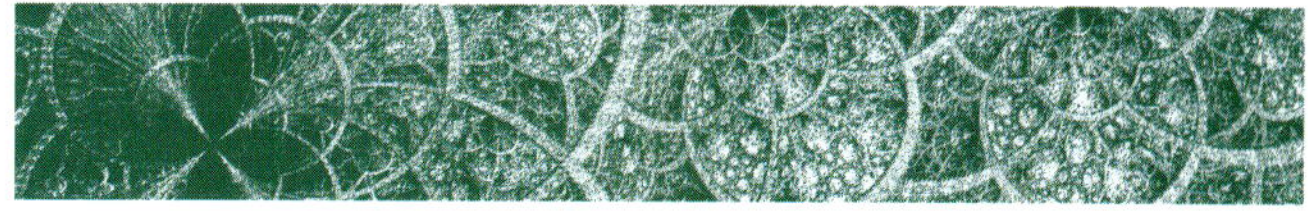

Nursing care

Peritonitis is a serious illness. Early recognition and treatment are important to minimise the risk of complications.

Assessment

- *Health history*: pain, its onset, character, severity, location, aggravating and relieving factors; associated symptoms such as anorexia, nausea, vomiting; current and previous history of peptic ulcer disease, gallbladder disease, chronic diseases; current medications.
- *Physical examination*: vital signs, including temperature; level of consciousness; skin colour, temperature, warmth, capillary refill and turgor; abdominal shape, contour, bowel sounds, tenderness, tympany and guarding.

Nursing diagnoses and interventions

A person with peritonitis requires intensive nursing and medical care to prevent complications and enable a full recovery. Nursing priorities include interventions to relieve pain, restore fluid balance, manage altered protection due to infection and reduce anxiety.

Acute pain

Abdominal distension and acute inflammation contribute to the pain associated with peritonitis. Surgery further disrupts abdominal muscles and other tissues and exacerbates pain. See the chapter 'Nursing care of people in pain' for specific discussion on acute pain and its management. Effective pain management promotes immune function, healing, mobility and recovery.

- Assess pain at rest and on movement, including its location, severity (using a standard pain scale) and type. Monitor analgesic effectiveness. Report adverse changes to the primary care provider.

> **CONSIDERATION FOR PRACTICE**
> **Unrelieved pain or a change in the location, severity or type of pain may indicate spread of infection, abscess formation or other complications of peritonitis.**

- Place in Fowler's or semi-Fowler's position with the knees and feet elevated. *This position reduces stress on abdominal structures and facilitates respirations, promoting comfort.*
- Administer analgesics as ordered on a routine basis or using patient-controlled analgesia (PCA). *Routine analgesic administration maintains a therapeutic blood level and helps maintain comfort, facilitating healing and movement.*
- Teach and assist with adjunctive pain management techniques such as meditation, visualisation, massage and progressive relaxation. *Adjunctive measures augment analgesics and help promote a sense of control over pain.*

Deficient fluid volume

In peritonitis, significant amounts of fluid are drawn into the abdominal cavity and bowel, reducing vascular volume and cardiac output. Fluid is also lost from the body by intestinal suction or through drains placed in the abdomen during surgery. An unsutured incision causes additional significant fluid loss.

- Maintain accurate intake and output records. Measure urine output every 1 to 2 hours; report outputs less than 0.5 mL/kg/hr. *Measure gastrointestinal output at least every 4 hours. Intake and output records provide valuable assessment of fluid volume status.*

> **CONSIDERATION FOR PRACTICE**
> **Urine output of less than 0.5 mL/kg/hr may indicate hypovolaemia, decreased cardiac output and impaired tissue perfusion.**

- Monitor vital signs, peripheral pulses, capillary refill and haemodynamic parameters (such as central venous pressure, cardiac output and pulmonary artery pressures (if Swan–Ganz catheter in situ)) every hour or as indicated. *These measurements provide important information about fluid and vascular volumes and cardiovascular status.*
- Assess skin turgor, colour, temperature and mucous membranes at least every 8 hours. *Warm, dry skin with poor turgor and dry, shiny mucous membranes indicate dehydration.*
- Measure or estimate fluid losses via abdominal drains and on dressings. *Significant amounts of exudative fluid may be lost.*
- Weigh daily. Weight is an accurate indicator of fluid status. *Rapid weight gains or losses reflect changes in fluid volume.*
- Monitor laboratory values, including haemoglobin and haematocrit, urine specific gravity, serum osmolality and electrolytes and ABGs. Report changes to the doctor. *Laboratory results provide information about fluid and electrolyte status and acid–base balance.*
- Administer intravenous fluids and electrolytes as ordered. Gastrointestinal drainage may be replaced millilitre for millilitre with a balanced electrolyte solution. *Intravenous fluids are necessary to meet daily fluid intake needs, as well as to replace continuing losses of water and electrolytes.*
- Provide meticulous skin care and frequent oral hygiene. *Fluid deficit increases the risk of skin breakdown and mucous membrane ulcerations.*

Delayed surgical recovery

Repeated surgeries, an unsutured incision and the presence of drains and intravenous cannula interrupt skin integrity, the body's first line of defence against microorganisms. Additionally, immune defences are stressed by the infection and potential malnutrition. As a result, the risk of impaired healing and further infection is increased.

- Practise meticulous hand hygiene and use standard precautions at all times. *Hand hygiene reduces transient bacteria on the skin. Hand hygiene remains the most important method of controlling infection. Standard precautions reduce the risk of spreading infection to or from the person.*
- Monitor temperature, pulse rate and pain, and for localised signs of infection, such as redness and swelling around incisions and drain sites, increased or purulent drainage, and cloudy or malodorous urine. *Impaired defences increase the risk of extension of the infection or unrelated infections.*
- Use aseptic non-touch technique for dressing changes, wound care and irrigations. *Disruption of the protective barrier of the skin increases the risk of contamination and further infection.*
- Obtain cultures of purulent drainage from any site. *Early identification of any additional infection allows timely intervention.*
- Monitor WBC and differential, serum protein and albumin. *An increased WBC with a higher percentage of immature cells present in the blood is an indicator of infection and normal immune response. Serum albumin and protein levels are indicators of nutritional status as well as immune function.*
- Maintain fluid balance and nutritional status through enteral or parenteral feedings, as indicated. See the 'Translation to practice' box for evidence-based recommendations for care of enterally fed people. *Adequate nutrition and fluid balance are necessary for optimal immune system function.*

TRANSLATION TO PRACTICE Evidence-based practice: malnutrition and the critically ill

A vital component of the treatment and care of critically ill people (such as those with peritonitis) is providing nutritional support, primarily through enteral feedings. Malnutrition is common in critically ill people and is associated with poor clinical outcomes as well as increased healthcare spending. Enteral nutrition (EN) is the method of choice for nutrition delivery for many critically ill people. However, EN delivery practices vary widely, and underfeeding is widespread in critical care. Interruptions in enteral nutrition due to performance of procedures, positioning, technical issues with feeding accesses and gastrointestinal intolerance contribute to underfeeding. Strategies such as head-of-bed positioning, use of prokinetic agents, tolerance of higher gastric residual volumes, consideration of postpyloric feeding access and use of a nutrition support protocol may decrease time spent without nutrition.

Stewart, Biddle and Thomas (2017) highlighted the consequences of malnutrition for critically ill people and current nursing routines contributing to EN interruptions in critically ill people, and described nursing interventions to improve a critically ill person's nutritional support. Despite strong evidence that early enteral feeding is beneficial to critically ill people, only 33% of people had their EN initiated within 48 hours.

Strategies to minimise interruptions include:

- Consider prokinetic agents after two episodes of GRV > 250 mL.
- Consider post-pyloric access when gastric feeding intolerance demonstrated.
- Nutritional support protocols.
- Computerised order sets for EN delivery.

IMPLICATIONS FOR NURSING

Based on Stewart et al.'s (2017) review, further research is warranted into methods to reduce the time a critically ill person spends without EN, such as reduced fasting time before procedures or extubations. Alternative continuous enteral feeding methods, incorporating increased hourly rates to compensate for predicted losses in feeding volumes and compensatory increases in hourly rate to make up for experienced losses in feeding volumes, also requires exploration.

CRITICAL THINKING IN PERSON-CENTRED CARE

1. Malnutrition results when nutritional intake does not meet a person's metabolic demands. Describe the clinical implications when the nutritional intake of a person who is critically ill does not meet their increased metabolic demands.
2. Discuss how routine nursing interventions interrupt administration of enteral nutrition.
3. Outline nursing responses to improve EN to ensure a person's metabolic demands are maintained.

CONSIDERATION FOR PRACTICE

An acute infection such as peritonitis causes a stress response with excess energy expenditure and loss of body proteins and cell mass. Glycogen stores are rapidly depleted and body proteins are used to meet energy needs. Withholding food further complicates this process, leading to rapid development of protein energy malnutrition (PEM). PEM impairs the immune response and delays healing.

Anxiety

The severity and potential threat to life associated with peritonitis present a situational crisis for the individual and their family. Anxiety is a common response.

- Present a calm, reassuring manner. Encourage expression of concerns, listen carefully and acknowledge their validity. *This helps establish trust.*
- Assess the individual and their family's anxiety level and present coping skills. *Interventions need to be tailored to the needs and strengths of the individual and their family.*
- Explain all treatments, procedures, tests and examinations. *An increased understanding of what is being done reduces anxiety.*
- Reinforce and clarify information as needed. *This improves understanding and promotes acceptance.*
- Teach and assist with relaxation techniques such as meditation, visualisation and progressive relaxation. *These measures promote positive coping skills and reduce physical manifestations of anxiety.*
- Maintain consistent caregiver assignments. *Consistency of nursing care and care providers helps reduce anxiety. Complex wound care and irrigation procedures are best performed by people familiar with prescribed techniques.*

Community-based care

Education for home care includes the following topics:

- Wound care procedures, including dressing changes or irrigations. Provide verbal and written instructions on how to change dressings or do irrigations, as well as on where to obtain supplies, and provide opportunities for the person to practise and demonstrate the procedure prior to discharge.
- Prescribed medications, including name and purpose of the drug, dosage, how to take the medication correctly (e.g. not chewing or crushing enteric coated tablets), potential adverse effects and their management.
- Manifestations of further infection (redness, heat, swelling, purulent drainage, chills and fever, and increasing pain) and potential complications to be reported to the care provider.
- Prescribed activity restrictions.
- Instructions for a high-kilojoule, high-protein diet for healing and optimal immune function.

Provide a referral to home health services for assessment, wound care and further assistance, as required.

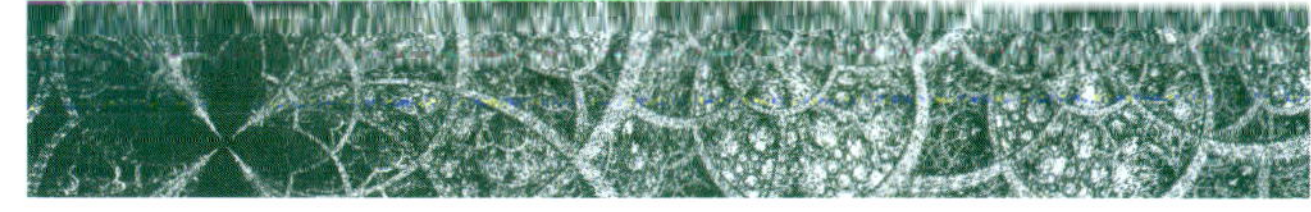

THE PERSON WITH GASTROENTERITIS

Gastroenteritis, or *enteritis*, is an inflammation of the stomach and small intestine. Enteritis may be caused by bacteria, viruses, parasites or toxins. Gastroenteritis is a major health problem throughout the world, particularly in developing countries. Upper GI manifestations such as anorexia, nausea and vomiting are common. Diarrhoea of varying intensity and abdominal discomfort are nearly universal features of gastroenteritis. In Australia, transmission is mainly via contaminated food or water. However, in many remote Indigenous communities, there is a high incidence of gastroenteritis due to poor sanitation facilities and sewage disposal, as is the case in many developing countries, where diarrhoeal diseases are major causes of morbidity and mortality.

Globally there are nearly 1.7 billion cases of diarrhoeal diseases each year (World Health Organization (WHO), 2017a). Diarrhoeal disease is a leading cause of child mortality and morbidity globally, mostly resulting from contaminated food and water sources. The WHO (2017a) statistics highlight that worldwide, 780 million people lack access to improved water and 2.5 billion lack improved sanitation. In low-income countries, children under 3 years experience on average three episodes of diarrhoea every year. Each episode deprives the child of the nutrition necessary for growth. As a result, diarrhoeal diseases are a major cause of malnutrition, and malnourished children are more likely to fall ill from diarrhoea (WHO, 2017b).

The infectious organism is usually acquired by the faecal–oral route, from contaminated water, food or hands. For this reason, gastroenteritis is often called 'food poisoning'. Viruses commonly cause acute diarrhoeal illness. Diarrhoea due to rotaviruses or the noroviruses (formerly known as Norwalk virus) occurs year round (with seasonal peaks in June and December) in both adults and children.

Rotavirus is the most common cause of acute severe gastroenteritis in early childhood and a significant cause of death in young children; more than 500,000 deaths per year (WHO, 2015). Two rotavirus vaccines were added to the Australian National Immunisation Program in July 2007. Immunisation reduces the risk of developing severe rotavirus gastroenteritis by 85–100% and any rotavirus gastroenteritis by around 70% (Queensland Health, 2019). Prior to vaccine introduction, it is estimated the virus was responsible for up to 50% of diarrhoea hospitalisations in childhood, with approximately 10,000 Australian children hospitalised each year. Aboriginal and Torres Strait Islander children have a higher burden of rotavirus illness than non-Indigenous children, more likely to be hospitalised, and for longer periods (Middleton et al., 2020). Most infections occur in children under 2 years of age and are potentially life threatening due to severe dehydration. Older children and adults generally experience a mild self-limiting illness. However, in older adults or those with impaired immune function, as with children less than 2 years of age, rotavirus can also have severe complications.

Pathophysiology

Bacterial or viral infection of the GI tract produces inflammation, tissue damage and manifestations by two primary mechanisms:

1. *The production of exotoxins.* A number of bacteria produce and excrete an exotoxin that enters the surrounding environment (intestinal lumen), causing damage and inflammation. Exotoxins in the GI tract are often referred to as *enterotoxins*. These impair intestinal absorption and can cause secretion of significant amounts of electrolytes and water into the bowel, resulting in diarrhoea and fluid loss. Common bacterial enterotoxins include those produced by *Staphylococcus*, *Clostridium perfringens*, *Clostridium botulinum*, some strains of *E. coli*, *Vibrio cholera* and *C. difficile*.
2. *Invasion and ulceration of the mucosa.* Other bacteria, including some *Shigella*, *Salmonella* and *E. coli* species, damage tissue more directly. These invade the intestinal mucosa of the small bowel or colon, producing microscopic ulceration, bleeding, fluid exudates and water and electrolyte secretion.

In some cases, the mechanism of injury is unclear. It may be a combination of direct and toxic damage. For example, noroviruses damages the mucosa of the jejunum, with fluid and electrolyte secretion.

Manifestations

Although the manifestations of bacterial and viral enteritis vary according to the organism involved, several features are common (see the 'Manifestations' box). Anorexia, nausea and vomiting are caused by distension of the upper GI tract from unabsorbed chyme and excess water. Bowel distension, irritation of the bowel mucosa and gas production from fermentation of undigested food lead to abdominal pain and cramping. *Borborygmi*, excessively loud and hyperactive bowel sounds, are another result. The abdomen is often distended and tender.

Diarrhoea is usually predominant with enteritis. Fluid is secreted into the bowel lumen and the unabsorbed chyme

MANIFESTATIONS Gastroenteritis

GASTROINTESTINAL EFFECTS

- Anorexia, nausea and vomiting
- Abdominal pain and cramping
- Borborygmi
- Diarrhoea

GENERAL EFFECTS

- Malaise, weakness and muscle aches
- Headache
- Dry skin and mucous membranes
- Poor skin turgor
- Orthostatic hypotension, tachycardia
- Fever

and electrolytes create an osmotic pull of fluid into the bowel. Motility is stimulated and stools become watery and frequent. Loss of fluids and electrolytes through diarrhoea can lead to serious manifestations of enteritis. Fluid volume is rapidly depleted, leading to dehydration and hypovolaemia. Initially, orthostatic hypotension and fever may be noted. However, if fluid loss continues, hypovolaemic shock develops.

Complications

Electrolyte and acid–base imbalances may result from gastroenteritis. Extensive vomiting leads to metabolic alkalosis due to the loss of hydrochloric acid from the stomach. When diarrhoea predominates, metabolic acidosis is more likely. Potassium is lost in either case, leading to hypokalaemia. Hyponatraemia may develop if fluids are replaced with pure water. Headache, cardiac irregularities, changes in respiratory rate and pattern, malaise and weakness, muscle aching and signs of neuromuscular irritability are the possible manifestations of disturbances in homeostasis.

Specific types of gastrointestinal infections

Several gastrointestinal infections produce specific effects. These are discussed below and summarised in Table 23.3.

Campylobacter infections

Campylobacter species are a major cause of diarrhoeal illness in humans and are generally regarded as the most common bacterial cause of gastroenteritis worldwide. In Australia, as in other developed and developing countries, they cause more cases of diarrhoea than, for example, food-borne *Salmonella* bacteria. In developing countries, *Campylobacter* infections in children under the age of 2 years are especially frequent, sometimes resulting in death. A fatal outcome is rare and is usually confined to the very young or older adults, or to those already immunosuppressed from another disease (e.g. HIV/AIDS).

The onset of disease symptoms usually occurs 2 to 5 days after infection, but ranges from 1 to 10 days. Usually, *Campylobacter* infections are acquired from eating contaminated and poorly cooked food, especially poultry, red meats and unpasteurised milk. The most common clinical symptoms of *Campylobacter* infections include diarrhoea (frequently with blood in the faeces), abdominal pain, fever, headache, nausea and/or vomiting. The symptoms last typically for 3 to 6 days.

Complications such as bacteraemia, hepatitis, pancreatitis and abortion have been reported with various degrees of frequency. Post-infection complications may include

TABLE 23.3 Selected bacterial infections of the bowel

DISEASE AND ORGANISM	INCUBATION/ DURATION OF ILLNESS	PATHOGENESIS	MANIFESTATIONS	MANAGEMENT
Traveller's diarrhoea: *E. coli*, *Campylobacter*	24–72 hours/5–10 days	Enterotoxin causes hypersecretion of the small intestine.	Abrupt onset of diarrhoea; vomiting rare	Prophylactic bismuth subsalicylate; anti-diarrhoeals such as loperamide or diphenoxylate; 3- to 5-day course of norfloxacin, ciprofloxacin or trimethoprim-sulfamethoxazole
Staphylococcal food poisoning	1–8 hours/12–24 hours	Enterotoxin impairs intestinal absorption and affects vomiting centres in the brain.	Severe nausea and vomiting; abdominal cramping and diarrhoea; headache and fever	Fluid and electrolyte replacement as needed
Cholera: *Vibrio cholerae*	1–3 days/5–7 days	Enterotoxin affects entire small intestine, causing secretion of water and electrolytes into bowel lumen.	Severe diarrhoea with 'rice-water stool', grey, cloudy, odourless, with no blood or pus; vomiting; thirst, oliguria, muscle cramps, weakness; dehydration and vascular collapse	Oral or intravenous rehydration; possible antimicrobial therapy with antimicrobial agents sensitive to specific *V. cholerae* strain
Haemorrhagic colitis (*E. coli*)	1–3 days/5–10 days	Enterotoxin causes direct mucosal damage in large intestine; also toxic to vascular endothelial cells.	Severe abdominal cramping, watery diarrhoea becoming grossly bloody; fever; possible complications: haemolytic uraemic syndrome and thrombotic thrombocytopenic purpura	Supportive care with fluid replacement and bland diet; may require dialysis or plasma-pheresis for complications
Salmonellosis: *Salmonella*	8–48 hours/2–7 days	Superficial infection of the GI tract without invasion or production of toxins.	Diarrhoea with abdominal cramping, nausea and vomiting; low-grade fever, chills, weakness	Treatment of symptoms; trimethoprim sulfamethoxazole, ampicillin or ciprofloxacin for severe illness
Shigellosis (bacillary dysentery): *Shigella*	1–4 days/1–3 days	Local tissue invasion, primarily involving large intestine and distal ileum; endotoxin causes fluid and electrolyte secretion into bowel lumen.	Watery diarrhoea with severe abdominal cramping and tenesmus; lethargy	Fluid and electrolyte replacement; correction of acidosis; antibiotic therapy with trimethoprim sulfamethoxazole, ciprofloxacin or ampicillin
Clostridium difficile colitis (*C. difficile*)	1 day to 8 weeks following antibiotic exposure	Antibiotic therapy interferes with normal protective bacteria in the colon; *C. difficile* colonises and [illegible] toxins causing mucosal inflammation and damage.	Diarrhoea, abdominal cramps, malaise, fever, anorexia	Cessation of the causative antibiotic; antibiotic therapy with vancomycin or metronidazole (specific for *C. difficile*)

reactive arthritis (painful inflammation of the joints lasting for several months) and neurological disorders such as Guillain–Barré syndrome, a polio-like form of paralysis resulting in respiratory and severe neurological dysfunction or death in a small, but significant, number of cases (Lee & Bishop, 2016). In Australia, as in almost all developed countries, the incidence of human *Campylobacter* infections has been steadily increasing for several years. The reasons for this are unknown.

Traveller's diarrhoea

People travelling overseas frequently develop diarrhoea within 2 to 10 days, particularly when there is a significant difference in climate, sanitation standards or food and drink. Strains of enterotoxin-producing *E. coli*, *Shigella* species, *Salmonella* and *Campylobacter* are the most frequent causes of traveller's diarrhoea (Lee & Bishop, 2016). Other bacteria and viruses also cause traveller's diarrhoea.

Up to 10 or more loose stools per day and abdominal cramping are common manifestations. Nausea and vomiting are less frequent; fever is rare. Manifestations usually resolve within 2 to 7 days. Complications are rare.

Staphylococcal food poisoning

Certain foods rich in protein, salt and sugar provide an excellent medium for staphylococcal growth when contaminated and left at room temperature. Examples include ham, fish, salads with mayonnaise and bakery products (e.g. cream-filled cakes). Foods usually become contaminated by resident staphylococci in the nose or on the skin of food handlers (Lee & Bishop, 2016). The organism itself does not affect the bowel. However, the enterotoxin produced impairs intestinal absorption and acts on receptors in the gut, stimulating the medullary centre, inducing vomiting.

The onset of staphylococcal food poisoning is abrupt, occurring within 1 to 6 hours after consuming the contaminated food. Nausea and vomiting are severe. Manifestations typically include abdominal cramping, diarrhoea, headache and fever lasting 12 to 24 hours. Complications such as fluid and electrolyte imbalances are rare; however, they may develop in older adults and people with underlying chronic disease processes.

Cholera

Cholera is an acute diarrhoeal illness caused by strains of *Vibrio cholerae*. It is endemic in South-East Asia, the Middle East, parts of Africa and most of Central and South America. In endemic areas, water is the primary vehicle of cholera transmission, although secondary transmission may occur via food. Transmission of cholera in non-endemic areas is more commonly associated with consumption of foods, such as raw or undercooked seafood, imported from cholera-endemic regions (WHO, 2022). Cholera appears to be increasing worldwide in terms of both the number of cases and their distribution. Epidemics occur periodically, often associated with natural disasters (floods and earthquakes) and situations of social unrest and upheaval.

In Australia, two to six cases (almost all imported from other countries) are reported annually (CDNA–NNDSS, 2018). *V. cholerae* is established in coastal rivers in some parts of Queensland and New South Wales; however, human disease from these sources is rare (Lee & Bishop, 2016). The importance of not eating raw or undercooked seafood from endemic areas was highlighted by Forssman et al. (2007) in their review of the first reported cluster of cholera in Australia for over 30 years, reported in Sydney in November 2006. Three Italian-born women (aged 71, 72 and 84 years) living within a few kilometres of each other but who did not know each other became unwell with severe watery diarrhoea within a 4-day period. It was an unusual outbreak as the women had no history of recent travel or contact with anyone visiting cholera-endemic areas. However, all three women were undergoing long-term therapy with proton-pump inhibitors, which may have contributed to their susceptibility to the disease by reducing their gastric acidity (Forssman et al., 2007). A food trace-back investigation found the only exposure common to all three cases was consumption of raw whitebait imported from Indonesia. All women reported eating cooked seafood before their illness. Forssman et al. (2007) explained that further investigation revealed the women had independently prepared the same dish—whitebait fritters—over the same weekend. During preparation, the women sampled a spoonful of the uncooked fritter mixture of whitebait, eggs, flour and seasoning, for taste and consistency. The mixture was then cooked. As no other food exposures were common to the women, the raw whitebait mixture was considered to be the source of infection.

V. cholerae causes infections only in humans, with symptomatic and asymptomatic carriers being reservoirs of infection (Lee & Bishop, 2016). Cholera is spread by the faecal–oral route through contaminated water or food. The organism produces an enterotoxin, enzymes and other substances affecting the entire small intestine. The cholera toxin increases the levels of cyclic adenosine monophosphate (AMP) in intestinal epithelial cells, resulting in a massive outflow of water and electrolytes into the bowel lumen (Lee & Bishop, 2016). The enzymes and other substances produced by the bacteria may affect mucosal protection of bowel endothelium.

Cholera ranges in severity from very mild, with few or no manifestations, to acute and fulminant. Its onset is typically abrupt, with severe, frequent, watery diarrhoea. Up to 30 L of stool may be passed in a day, rapidly depleting fluid volume. Stool is often described as 'rice-water stool', characteristically grey and cloudy, with no faecal odour, blood or pus. Vomiting may accompany the diarrhoea. Other manifestations related to the loss of fluid and electrolytes include thirst, oliguria, muscle cramps, weakness and significant signs of dehydration. Metabolic acidosis and hypokalaemia develop. Altered fluid, electrolyte and acid–base balance is discussed in the chapter 'Nursing care of people with altered fluid, electrolyte and acid–base balance'.

Among those infected, about 20% develop acute watery diarrhoea, of which 10–20% develop severe watery diarrhoea with vomiting. The mainstay of treatment is rehydration, with up to 80% of cholera cases treated successfully using only oral rehydration salts (WHO, 2022). If untreated, circulatory collapse and acute kidney injury or dysfunction occurs. The WHO (2022) warns that without fluid and electrolyte replacement, mortality can be as high as 30–50%, mostly observed in crisis situations with overcrowding, limited access to healthcare and precarious environmental management. However, with prompt and adequate fluid replacement, mortality is less than 1%. Recovery from cholera usually occurs spontaneously within 3 to 6 days.

The WHO (2022) recommends vaccination when travelling to cholera-endemic areas. It is a live vaccine and therefore is used cautiously in immunocompromised individuals, young children and pregnant women. It contains phenylalanine so caution is needed in those with phenylketonuria. The person should be advised to avoid contact with anyone who is immunosuppressed for at least 8 days after taking the vaccine (Tiziani, 2021). Chloroquine (antimalarial prophylaxis) should not be started within 1 week of taking the vaccine. The vaccine should be separated by at least 8 hours from oral typhoid vaccine (Tiziani, 2021).

Escherichia coli haemorrhagic colitis

Most pathological forms of *E. coli* bacteria cause little more than common traveller's diarrhoea. However, some strains—the most common serotype 0157:H7 and *E. coli* 0111—produce potent enterotoxins in the large intestine after being ingested. These toxins damage bowel mucosa and the endothelial cells of blood vessels in the GI tract. If absorbed, the toxin damages other blood vessels as well, such as those of the kidney.

Cattle provide the reservoir for *E. coli* 0157:H7. It is usually spread through undercooked beef (mince, in particular) and unpasteurised milk or apple juice. It may also be spread by direct contact via the faecal–oral route. The onset of haemorrhagic colitis is abrupt, with severe abdominal cramping and watery diarrhoea that becomes grossly bloody within 24 hours. Fever may be present.

Throughout the world, *E. coli* 0157:H7 is the most common serotype associated with haemolytic uraemic syndrome (HUS) (Lee & Bishop, 2016). HUS is characterised by uraemia, thrombocytopenia and acute kidney injury or dysfunction, occurring within the first few days of the infection. HUS is a severe complication of *E. coli* haemorrhagic colitis, affecting about 5% of people with the disease. HUS can occur in any age group; however, it is most common in children under 4 years. Older adults have the highest risk of developing complications. HUS has been a notifiable disease in Australia since 1999, with approximately 10 to 30 cases notified each year (CDNA–NNDSS, 2018).

Clostridium difficile colitis

Clostridium difficile colitis is associated with antibiotic therapy. While antibiotics are recognised as the main predisposing factor, anything disrupting the intestinal flora of the gut, including another gastrointestinal infection, can lead to *C. difficile* infection. The normal colonic flora of adults and children over the age of 1 year effectively prevent the colonisation by *C. difficile*; however, treatment with antibiotics (especially broad spectrum antibiotics) interferes with the normal protective bacteria of the colon, allowing colonisation of *C. difficile* by the faecal–oral route.

The subsequent release of two exotoxins, A and B, by the bacteria is cytotoxic to a number of cell types, causing mucosal damage and haemorrhage. This induces a local inflammatory response and destruction of the intestinal mucosa, resulting in a pseudomembrane forming consisting of necrotic tissue, mucus, neutrophils and monocytes (Lee & Bishop, 2016) (see Figure 23.6).

C. difficile infection is primarily a problem in hospitalised individuals, in whom infection occurs after ingestion of spores. The spores enable the organism to survive for long periods in the hospital environment. It has been cultured from floors, toilets, bedding, mops and furniture, and also from the hands of healthcare workers (Lee & Bishop, 2016). Transmission of the organism to a susceptible person can readily occur in hospital. It is also being seen in the community in healthy adults.

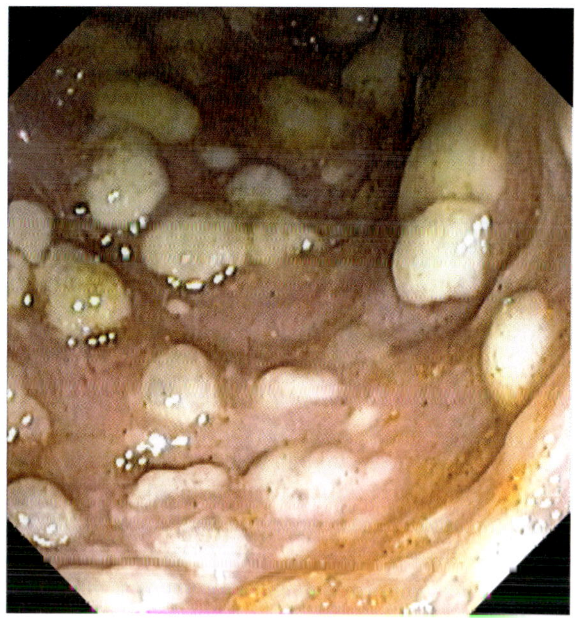

FIGURE 23.6 ***Pseudomembranous colitis***

Source: David M. Martin, MD/Science Photo Library

A hypervirulent strain called ribotype 027, associated with high morbidity and mortality, has emerged and is responsible for hospital outbreaks in North America and Europe.

An infection with *C. difficile* manifests in various ways, from mild diarrhoea and abdominal cramping to the potentially life-threatening pseudomembranous colitis. Perforation of the bowel, abscess formation and vascular thrombi are late complications. Lee and Bishop (2016) advised that *C. difficile* infection should be considered in any person receiving antimicrobial therapy who develops diarrhoea. It commonly begins within 1 to 2 weeks; however, it can commence from 1 day up to 8 weeks after commencing antibiotic treatment (Lee & Bishop, 2016).

The bacteria can be identified in the stool by anaerobic culture and the detection of toxin B in stool filtrate. An enzyme immunoassay method to detect *C. difficile* toxin in the stool sample is also commonly used. It is less sensitive than culture, but a much quicker process (Lee & Bishop, 2016).

Salmonellosis

Salmonellosis is food poisoning caused by ingesting raw or improperly cooked meat, poultry, eggs and dairy products contaminated with *Salmonella* bacteria. In developed countries, salmonellae are the second main cause of diarrhoea; 7,000 to 18,000 cases are reported annually in Australia (CDNA–NNDSS, 2018). These bacteria do not produce a toxin; they cause superficial infection of the GI tract, rarely invading further.

Manifestations develop from 8 to 48 hours after ingesting the bacteria. Diarrhoea may be violent, with abdominal cramping, nausea and vomiting. A low-grade fever, chills and weakness may accompany GI manifestations. The disease is usually self-limiting, resolving within 3 to 5 days. Many people become asymptomatic carriers for weeks to months, continuing to shed organisms in faeces. Bacteraemia, particularly in the very young, older adults or immunosuppressed individuals, may cause arthritis, osteomyelitis, pneumonia or meningitis when the organism invades the mesenteric lymph nodes (Lee & Bishop, 2016).

Shigellosis (bacillary dysentery)

Shigellosis (or bacillary dysentery) occurs worldwide, accounting for 5–10% of diarrhoeal illness in some regions. It may be endemic or it may occur in epidemics. In Australia, shigellosis is more common in disadvantaged communities and more prevalent among Indigenous children than non-Indigenous children. Approximately 500 to 1,700 cases are notified annually, with the highest notifications rates in Aboriginal and Torres Strait Islander children less than 4 years of age (CDNA–NNDSS, 2018). Humans are reservoirs for *Shigella* organisms, which spread directly via the faecal–oral route or indirectly through contaminated food, fomites (inanimate objects) and vectors (such as fleas). The incubation period for shigellosis is 1 to 4 days.

Shigella organisms infect the lower intestine and sometimes the distal ilium. They invade the tissue, causing inflammation and producing an enterotoxin. The result is watery diarrhoea containing blood, mucus and inflammatory exudate. The onset of diarrhoea is abrupt, with severe abdominal cramping and *tenesmus*, a sensation of urgent and continuing need to defecate. Lethargy is common; rarely, neurological manifestations occur.

In adults, shigellosis is usually mild and self-limiting. Older adults and immunosuppressed people are at risk of volume depletion and electrolyte imbalances. Secondary infection is another potential complication, as is acute blood loss from mucosal ulcerations.

INTERPROFESSIONAL CARE

The goals of care for gastroenteritis are to manage the manifestations, prevent complications, identify the cause of the infection and prevent its spread. The history and manifestations provide valuable clues about the cause. Diagnostic testing is used to identify the pathogen and evaluate its effects. In most cases, treatment is supportive, directed towards relieving manifestations, restoring fluid and electrolyte balance, and maintaining function.

Diagnosis

If manifestations are severe or do not resolve within about 48 hours, laboratory testing is used to identify the causative organism and to assess fluid, electrolyte and acid–base balance. A stool specimen for culture, ova, cysts and parasites, and faecal leucocytes usually reveals the infective organism. Some bacteria require up to 6 weeks to be identified. In infections such as botulism, the toxin itself may be isolated in the stool. Contamination of the stool by urine or treatment with antibiotics, bismuth subsalicylate or mineral oil interferes with pathogen growth, altering stool culture results. Use a clean bedpan or collection device to obtain the stool specimen and instruct the person to avoid mixing the stool with urine or toilet paper.

A colonoscopy may be done to differentiate inflammatory bowel disease from infectious processes. It does not replace stool cultures, because the lesions associated with some infectious processes are indistinguishable from those of ulcerative colitis. (Nursing care of a person having a colonoscopy is discussed in the chapter 'A person-centred approach to assessing the gastrointestinal system'.)

Serum osmolality and electrolytes and ABGs are done to assess and monitor fluid, electrolyte and acid–base balance. Common imbalances associated with enteritis and diarrhoea are outlined in Table 23.4.

Medications

Acute enteritis usually resolves spontaneously and no drug treatment is required. If the person is severely ill and manifestations are prolonged, medications may be prescribed.

TABLE 23.4 Laboratory values associated with enteritis and diarrhoea

TEST	NORMAL VALUE	CHANGE WITH SIGNIFICANT DIARRHOEA
Serum osmolality	275–295 mOsm/kg	Increased; levels above 320 mOsm/kg indicate significant dehydration.
Serum potassium	3.5–5.0 mmol/L	Decreased due to loss through stool and vomitus; levels below 2.5 mmol/L are critical.
Serum sodium	136–148 mmol/L	Decreased due to loss through stool and vomitus; may be significant when fluid losses are replaced with pure water; levels below 120 mmol/L are critical.
Serum chloride	96–106 mmol/L	Increased when sodium loss is greater than chloride loss; decreased with severe diarrhoea and with vomiting; possible critical values are below 80 mmol/L or above 115 mmol/L.
Blood gases		
• pH	Arterial: 7.35–7.45	Decreased in metabolic acidosis, a possible result of severe diarrhoea; increased in metabolic alkalosis, a possible result of severe vomiting and chloride loss; values below 7.25 or above 7.55 are critical.
• PCO_2	Arterial: 35–45 mmHg	Typically decreased in metabolic acidosis as the body attempts to eliminate excess acid by 'blowing off' CO_2; increased with metabolic alkalosis as the body retains CO_2 in an attempt to normalise pH.
• Bicarbonate	22–26 mmol/L	Decreased in metabolic acidosis; increased in metabolic alkalosis.
Haematocrit	Male: 40–50% Female: 37–47%	Increased with dehydration and hypovolaemia as a result of concentration of blood cells.
Urine specific gravity	1.010–1.025	Increased with dehydration and hypovolaemia as kidneys attempt to conserve fluid.

Antibiotic therapy specific to the organism is used to treat bacterial colitis, cholera, salmonellosis or shigellosis. Trimethoprim-sulfamethoxazole (Septra, Bactrim), ciprofloxacin (Cipro), ampicillin (Ampicin) or another antibiotic may be prescribed. Stool culture is obtained prior to commencing antibiotics. However, treatment may begin before culture results are available. A presumptive diagnosis based on history and presenting manifestations guides the choice of antibiotic. Multidrug-resistant (MDR) strains of *Salmonella* are now encountered frequently and the rate of multidrug resistance has increased considerably since the 1990s (WHO, 2018). Some variants of *Salmonella* have developed multidrug resistance as an integral part of the genetic material of the organism and are likely to retain their drug-resistant genes even when antimicrobial drugs are no longer used, whereas other resistant strains typically lose their resistance. The emergence of MDR *Salmonella* strains with resistance to fluoroquinolones and third-generation cephalosporins is a serious development, severely limiting possibilities for effective treatment of human infections (WHO, 2018).

An antidiarrhoeal drug may be prescribed to promote comfort and reduce fluid loss. Nursing measures related to antidiarrhoeal medications are outlined in the earlier 'Medication administration' box.

Treatments: nutrition and fluids

Replacing lost fluids and electrolytes is vital when vomiting and/or diarrhoea are severe or prolonged. In many cases of enteritis, fluid and electrolyte replacement are all that is required until the infection resolves.

Oral rehydration is preferred for replacing physiological fluids. An oral glucose–electrolyte solution is often well tolerated in sips, even when vomiting is present. Commercial preparations such as Gastrolyte are available.

Intravenous rehydration may be necessary with severe diarrhoea and fluid loss. In some cases, a combination of oral and intravenous fluids is used to replace lost fluids and maintain vascular volume. Balanced electrolyte solutions, such as dextrose in normal saline and Hartmann's solution, are used. Hartmann's solution or another alkalinising solution may be ordered if metabolic acidosis is present.

GASTRIC LAVAGE Gastric lavage and catharsis—in effect, 'washing out' the stomach and intestines—may be performed to remove unabsorbed toxin from the GI tract if botulism is suspected. A person with botulism is closely observed for clinical manifestations of respiratory distress. Respiratory support with endotracheal intubation or tracheostomy and mechanical ventilation may be required (see the chapter 'Nursing care of people with upper respiratory disorders').

PLASMAPHERESIS Plasmapheresis (plasma exchange therapy) may be performed to remove circulating toxins for haemorrhagic colitis caused by *E. coli*. See the chapter 'Nursing care of people with kidney disorders' for more information on plasmapheresis. Potential complications include those associated with intravenous catheters, shifts in fluid balance and altered blood clotting.

DIALYSIS Acute tubular necrosis and kidney injury associated with haemorrhagic colitis may necessitate dialysis to remove wastes and prevent severe fluid and electrolyte imbalances, and metabolic acidosis. Although acute kidney injury or dysfunction often resolves spontaneously and renal function improves, dialysis can be lifesaving. Either haemodialysis or peritoneal dialysis is used, generally as a temporary measure. Nursing care related to acute kidney injury or dysfunction and dialysis is discussed in the chapter 'Nursing care of people with kidney disorders'.

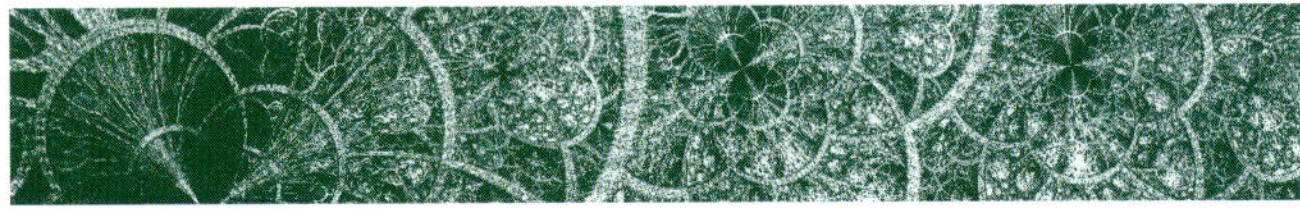

Nursing care

Although *C. difficile* colitis bacterial infections are hospital acquired, few people with acute enteritis require hospitalisation. Most are treated in community settings. Assessment, education and support of self-care measures are the main nursing responsibilities.

Health promotion

Nurses play a significant role in preventing enteritis as educators, community health providers and advocates for environmental safety.

Teach the importance of proper food handling and maintaining appropriate temperatures. Advise those working as food handlers to use disposable paper towels or an air dryer to dry hands rather than cloth towels as cloth towels get dirty quickly and transmit organisms from one person to another.

Adequate cooking of meat products is vital to prevent disorders such as staphylococcal food poisoning, *E. coli* haemorrhagic colitis and salmonellosis. Emphasise the importance of not consuming raw meat products and cooking mince, in particular, to the point where no redness is noted in the meat and the juice from the meat is clear. The highly pathogenic *E. coli* serotype 0157:H7 is present in the gut of infected animals. Meats from the animal may be contaminated with bowel contents. The organism is readily destroyed by heat, so cuts of meat such as steaks or roasts are less likely to cause infection, since the organism is on the outside of the meat. However, the process of mincing meat allows *E. coli* to be mixed throughout the meat. Thorough cooking destroys the organism. This pathogen (and others) may also be spread through unpasteurised milk. Discuss the dangers of consuming unpasteurised milk and encourage people to avoid it. Children should avoid eating unpasteurised and uncooked dairy products, and uncooked meat products such as salami.

Dairy products, eggs and egg products left at room temperature provide a good growth medium for bacteria. Discuss the importance of prompt refrigeration of meats and these products to minimise this risk. Many gastrointestinal infections are spread through contaminated water. Encourage travellers to consume only bottled water and to avoid ice added to drinks unless local water supplies are safe. Water purification tablets are available for bushwalkers and campers and can be used when travelling overseas if local water sources are considered unsafe.

Assessment

- *Health history*: onset, duration and severity of manifestations; recent activities such as attending a picnic or barbecue, camping, international travel or contact with someone recently returned from overseas; other affected members of the household; measures taken to relieve manifestations or replace fluids.
- *Physical examination*: vital signs, including temperature and orthostatic blood pressure; skin colour, temperature, moisture and turgor; peripheral pulses and capillary refill; abdominal shape, contour, bowel sounds, tenderness.

Nursing diagnoses and interventions

Diarrhoea and fluid volume deficit are priority nursing diagnoses. See the earlier section of this chapter on diarrhoea for specific nursing interventions related to these diagnoses. Nausea and vomiting frequently accompany diarrhoea associated with gastroenteritis. Nursing care of a person experiencing nausea and vomiting is discussed in the chapter 'Nursing care of people with upper gastrointestinal disorders'.

Community-based care

Discuss the following topics with the person for self-care:

- the importance of thorough handwashing, with soap and warm running water, for at least 15 seconds, particularly before handling food (preparing food, between handling raw and ready-to-eat foods), before eating, after going to the toilet or changing nappies, and after playing with pets or working in the garden
- the need to wash clothing and linen contaminated with faeces separately in hot water (if available) and detergent
- oral solutions to replace lost fluids and electrolytes
- appropriate use of antidiarrhoeal medications if recommended
- manifestations of complications to report to the healthcare provider.

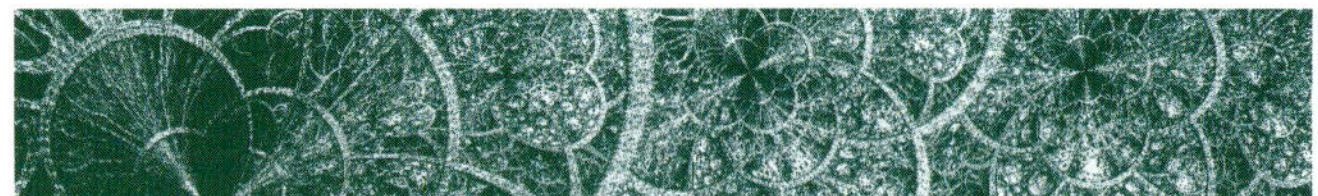

THE PERSON WITH A PROTOZOAL BOWEL INFECTION

Parasites live within, on or at the expense of other organisms. Parasitic intestinal infections are common in developing countries. These include both protozoal and helminthic (parasitic worm) infections. Parasites infecting the bowel usually enter the GI tract through the mouth by the faecal–oral route; some are spread by direct contact or through sexual activity.

Of the protozoal bowel infections, *giardiasis* is the most common in Australia. Cryptosporidiosis, a form of coccidiosis, is an important worldwide cause of sporadic mild diarrhoea, traveller's diarrhoea and severe diarrhoea in immunocompromised people. Amoebiasis (*Entamoeba histolytica*) is found chiefly in the tropics and where sanitation infrastructure is limited.

Pathophysiology and manifestations

The most common protozoal infections of the bowel are discussed below and summarised in Table 23.5.

TABLE 23.5 Common protozoal infections of the bowel

DISEASE AND ORGANISM	INCUBATION	PATHOGENESIS	MANIFESTATIONS	MANAGEMENT
Giardiasis: *Giardia lamblia*	1-3 weeks or more	Trophozoite attaches to mucosa in duodenum and jejunum, causing superficial invasion, inflammation and tissue destruction.	Diarrhoea, mild or severe, daily or intermittent; anorexia, nausea, vomiting; epigastric pain, cramping, distension; flatulence and belching; may be asymptomatic	Metronidazole quinacrine, furazolidone
Amoebiasis: *Entamoeba histolytica*	2-4 weeks	Organisms may reside in large intestine without causing disease or can invade colon wall, causing ulceration; may be carried via blood to liver to produce abscess.	Usually asymptomatic; diarrhoea may be mild with few semi-formed, mucus containing stools per day or severe with 10-20 blood-streaked liquid stools per day; abdominal cramps and flatulence, colic, tenesmus, vomiting, tenderness; fatigue, weight loss; prostration and toxicity	Metronidazole and diloxanide furoate; chloroquine for hepatic abscess
Cryptosporidiosis: *Cryptosporidium*	2-10 days	Organisms attach to epithelial surface of small bowel (jejunum), causing villous atrophy and mild inflammatory changes; may secrete enterotoxin.	In immunocompetent people: asymptomatic to profuse, watery diarrhoea of sudden onset, abdominal cramping; malaise, fever; anorexia, nausea, vomiting. In immunodeficient people: profuse watery diarrhoea with loss of up to 15-20 L/day; severe malabsorption, electrolyte imbalance; weight loss; lymphadenopathy	Self-limiting in immunocompetent people. For immunodeficient people: spiramycin, zidovudine (AZT), paromomycin (Humatin), octreotide, eflornithine; fluid and electrolyte replacement; parenteral nutrition as needed

Giardiasis

Giardiasis is a flagellate protozoal infection of the upper small intestine caused by *Giardia lamblia*, the most common intestinal pathogen worldwide (Bourque et al., 2022). Humans and other mammals are the reservoir for *Giardia*. Giardiasis occurs where there is overcrowding, or inadequate sanitation or treatment of drinking water. In developed countries, the prevalence rates range between 2% and 7%; the faecal–oral route is the most common form of transmission (O'Dempsey & Beeching, 2018). It is also spread by direct contact. *Giardia* is readily transmitted in institutions, such as daycare centres, where there is a higher probability of faecal–oral transmission. Other risk factors for infection include travel to high-risk areas, immunosuppression, unprotected anal sexual intercourse and if a person has achlorhydria. In tropical and temperate countries, children are more frequently infected than adults, particularly those who are malnourished (Bourque et al., 2022).

In Australia, high rates of infection are reported in remote Aboriginal and Torres Strait Islander communities. A high prevalence of the parasite has been found in domestic cats and dogs in Australia. However, it is uncertain if they act as a reservoir for human infection (Lee & Bishop, 2016).

When the cyst form of the organism is ingested, trophozoites emerge in the duodenum and jejunum. These attach to the intestinal mucosa, leading to superficial invasion, inflammation and destruction of the mucosa of the small intestine.

Giardiasis is usually asymptomatic or manifests as acute or chronic diarrhoea associated with abdominal cramps, bloating, nausea, vomiting, fever and fatigue, and weight loss. Other manifestations include weight loss and weakness, anorexia, nausea and vomiting, epigastric pain, abdominal distension and cramping, foul flatulence and belching.

Giardiasis is usually self-limiting with symptoms lasting 1 to 2 weeks; however, it may persist for months. Fat malabsorption leads to steatorrhoea (frequent, copious, frothy, malodorous and greasy stools).

In Australia, Aboriginal and Torres Strait Islander children have high rates of chronic giardiasis (Hanieh et al., 2021). Chronic giardiasis is associated with fat, d-xylose and vitamin A and vitamin B_{12} malabsorption, exacerbating malnutrition which contributes to growth and developmental delays in Aboriginal and Torres Strait Islander children (Hanieh et al., 2021). Those with chronic infections often manifest with symptomatic episodes alternating with periods when asymptomatic.

Amoebiasis

Amoebiasis (amoebic dysentery) is caused by the protozoan *Entamoeba histolytica*, which is thought to infect as much as 10% of the world's population (Kelly, 2014). Several strains of protozoa have been identified. Tropical strains tend to be more virulent and pathogenic than those found in temperate climates. It is endemic in Mexico, India and Africa, where up to 50% of the population may be infected (Kelly, 2014). It is also endemic in northern parts of Australia, with the highest incidence in the Indigenous population (Lee & Bishop, 2016).

Humans are the host for this parasite. It is usually transmitted through food or water contaminated by faeces, and by person-to-person contact. The parasite enters the intestines, where it lives without causing disease, or it invades the intestinal wall, causing ulceration and inflammation. The caecum, appendix, ascending colon, sigmoid colon and rectum are most often affected. Ulcers may deepen to cause haemorrhage, oedema and mucosal sloughing. The trophozoites of some strains may spread via the blood to the liver, lungs or brain.

Amoebiasis is usually asymptomatic. Mild manifestations include abdominal cramps, flatulence and intermittent diarrhoea containing blood and mucus. Severe manifestations of amoebic dysentery include frequent watery stools containing blood, mucus and necrotic tissue; colic, tenesmus and abdominal tenderness; nausea and vomiting; and fever. The liver may be enlarged and tender to palpation.

Complications are rare, and include appendicitis, bowel perforation with peritonitis and fulminating colitis.

Cryptosporidiosis (coccidiosis)

Cryptosporidiosis causes sporadic mild diarrhoea and traveller's diarrhoea in all age groups. In people with impaired immune function, such as those with human immunodeficiency virus (HIV) disease, it causes severe diarrhoea, malabsorption and significant weight loss.

This organism is transmitted by the faecal–oral route. Contaminated water is a frequent source of infection. *Cryptosporidium* is resistant to the usual levels of chlorine in swimming pools, able to survive for days and may be spread through swallowing contaminated swimming pool water (Lee & Bishop, 2016). High doses of chlorine and the cleaning of filters remove *Cryptosporidium* from a contaminated pool.

The organism attaches to bowel epithelium, causing surface damage and inflammation. It does not invade the tissues but secretes an enterotoxin causing characteristic watery diarrhoea. Watery diarrhoea may be accompanied by low-grade fever, nausea, vomiting, abdominal cramps and general malaise.

The disease is self-limiting in people with competent immune systems. In an immunocompromised person, clinical manifestations include profuse watery diarrhoea with significant fluid and electrolyte losses, and severe malabsorption. Lymphadenopathy (enlarged lymph nodes) may also develop.

INTERPROFESSIONAL CARE

Management of protozoal bowel infections includes identifying the causative organism and administering medications.

Diagnosis

Diagnostic testing includes a stool examination for ova, cysts and parasites and possibly for their antigens. Many protozoa are shed intermittently rather than continuously; stools are collected sequentially (e.g. every other day for a total of three specimens). These organisms are often fragile, requiring a fresh stool specimen. Serology testing for an immune response to the suspected parasite may also be performed. A sigmoidoscopy may be performed to examine the bowel mucosa and collect a stool specimen for examination. (In this case, no bowel prep is done prior to the test.) When giardiasis is suspected, duodenal aspirate may be stained and examined microscopically for the protozoa. Small-bowel biopsy can identify giardiasis or *Cryptosporidium* infection.

Medications

Pharmacological treatment includes local and systemic antiparasitic medications—for example, tinidazole (Fasigyn), co-trimoxazole (trimethoprim with sulfamethoxazole (Bactrim)), metronidazole (Flagyl) or albendazole (Eskazole). Treatment is usually provided on an outpatient basis. Severe amoebic dysentery requires hospitalisation for intravenous fluid and electrolyte replacement. Nursing care related to common antiprotozoal drugs is outlined in the 'Medication administration' box.

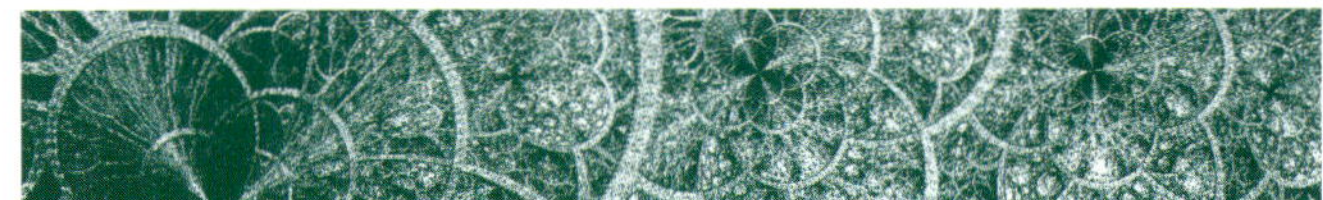

Nursing care

Nursing assessment, diagnoses and interventions for the person with a protozoal GI infection are similar to those indicated for people with bacterial or viral infections. *Diarrhoea* and *Risk of deficient fluid volume* are priority nursing diagnoses. See previous sections of this chapter for specific nursing interventions related to these diagnoses.

Nurses need to teach the public how parasitic diseases are transmitted and how to avoid spreading the infection. Prevention of amoebiasis, cryptosporidiosis and giardiasis infections involves the following:

- Maintain good personal hygiene. Everyone should wash their hands thoroughly with soap and warm running water for at least 15 seconds before preparing food and eating, after going to the toilet or after changing nappies, and after cleaning up when someone has vomited. The towels and face washers of someone diagnosed with protozal GI infections should not be used by others.
- Ensure safe food storage, handling and preparation.
- Instruct people living in high-risk areas (e.g. tropical climates, areas with untreated water supplies) to boil, filter or treat water supplies with iodine to eliminate protozoal contamination, and to avoid foods that cannot be peeled or cooked. Teach the manifestations of protozoal infections and where to obtain treatment.
- Emphasise the importance of keeping toilet areas clean, paying particular attention to cleaning surfaces such as toilet seats and handles, taps and nappy change tables. Ensure all potentially contaminated areas are regularly

MEDICATION ADMINISTRATION Antiprotozoal agents

LOCAL (GASTROINTESTINAL) AGENTS

Tinidazole (Fasigyn)
Co-trimoxazole (trimethoprim with sulfamethoxazole (Bactrim))
Metronidazole (Flagyl)

These medications exert a local amoebicidal effect in the intestines and are poorly absorbed when administered orally. Local agents have the advantage of provoking fewer side effects than systemically active agents.

Nursing responsibilities

- Assess for potential contraindications or hypersensitivity to the drug or drug class.
- Observe for adverse effects: anorexia, nausea, vomiting, abdominal cramping, diarrhoea or constipation, and increased flatulence; report skin rash, visual disturbances, dizziness, somnolence, vertigo, tremor or changes in blood work (leucopenia, neutropenia) to primary care provider.

Health education for the person and family

- Take as prescribed for the full course of therapy.
- Take with food to reduce gastrointestinal effects.
- Advise against driving or operating machinery if drowsy or dizzy.
- Report any of the following adverse effects to doctor:
  a. any change in vision
  b. numbness, tingling or pain in extremities
  c. chills, fever, skin rash or boils
  d. a change in urination or character of urine
  e. diminished hearing or tinnitus
  f. weight loss, diarrhoea, fatty stools
  g. candidiasis of the mouth or vagina.
- Keep follow-up appointments to evaluate the effects of treatment.

SYSTEMIC AGENTS

Metronidazole (Flagyl)
Pentamidine (Pentamidine isethionate for injection)
Albendazole (Eskazole)

A person with symptomatic protozoal infections is generally treated with a systemic antiprotozoal agent. Metronidazole is the most widely used of these antiprotozoal agents and is the medication of choice for treating amoebiasis.

Nursing responsibilities

- Assess for possible contraindications to therapy:
  a. hypersensitivity to the prescribed agent or related medications
  b. liver dysfunction or blood dyscrasias
  c. concurrent use of alcohol or a monoamine oxidase inhibitor (MAOI)
  d. pregnancy.
- Administer as ordered.
  a. Metronidazole may be given orally after meals or as a continuous or intermittent intravenous infusion.
  b. Administer albendazole orally with meals to minimise gastric distress.
- Observe for possible adverse effects; notify the doctor if significant. Gastrointestinal effects are common.
  a. Peripheral neuropathy and CNS effects may occur with metronidazole.
  b. Severe hypotension, syncope, cardiac arrhythmias, including ventricular tachycardia and cardiac arrest, may occur with pentamidine.
  c. Blood dyscrasias may develop with albendazole; monitor FBC and report abnormal results.
  d. Pentamidine can cause severe hypoglycaemia; sometimes followed by hyperglycaemia. Carefully monitor blood glucose levels, particularly in people with diabetes mellitus.
  e. Report abnormal liver function test results and increased serum amylase.
- Monitor the character and number of stools; obtain specimens as ordered to evaluate the effectiveness of therapy.

Health education for the person and family

- Take the drug as prescribed for the full duration of the prescription.
- Taking oral preparations after meals helps minimise gastrointestinal side effects. Notify the doctor if nausea and vomiting continue.
- Report adverse effects to the doctor, including dizziness and other nervous system changes, sore throats, fatigue, bruising or infection.
- Candidiasis of the mouth or vagina may occur with metronidazole therapy. Report symptoms to doctor.
- A harmless change in urine colour to deep yellow, rust or brown (metronidazole or chloroquine) may occur while taking these drugs.
- If you are a diabetic taking pentamidine, carefully monitor blood glucose levels because hypoglycaemia may develop.

ADVICE REGARDING ALCOHOL

Do not use alcohol while taking these drugs and for 72 hours after stopping tinidazole therapy. A disulfiram–alcohol (Antabuse) type response with severe headache, flushing and vomiting, tachycardia, hypertension initially then hypotension, vertigo, blurred vision, chest pain and, in severe cases, cardiopulmonary arrest may occur. Disulfiram reaction is managed by administering 1 g ascorbic acid intravenously, chlorpromazine 5 to 100 mg intramuscularly and resuscitation measures as required (Tiziani, 2021).

cleaned and disinfected using a hypochlorite solution of about 1,000 ppm (250 mL or 1 cup of household bleach diluted in 10 L or one bucket of water) strength.

- Ensure sandpits do not become contaminated with animal faeces and urine: cover the area when not in use, rake the sand frequently and remove any animal faeces.
- Advise the person to avoid rectal contact during sexual activity. Other household members should also have stool specimens examined for parasites. Following a cryptosporidiosis infection, do not use swimming pools for 2 weeks after diarrhoea stops.
- Provide safe water supplies.
- Dispose of human faeces appropriately.

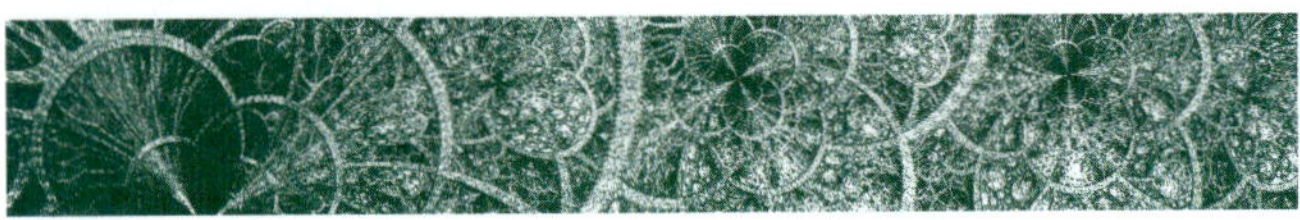

THE PERSON WITH A HELMINTHIC DISORDER

Helminths are parasitic worms capable of causing infectious diseases in humans. Helminths are subclassified as round worms (nematodes), flukes (trematodes) or tapeworms (cestodes). Parasitic helminths are a major cause of morbidity and sometimes death in humans, particularly in the tropics, subtropics and where sanitation is poor. In Australia, helminth infections occur mostly in the northern tropical parts. However, the most common helminth, the pin (or thread) worm (*Enterobius vermicularis*), is found throughout Australia (Lee & Bishop, 2016). Intestinal nematodes are found in northern Indigenous communities with poor sanitation and inadequate health facilities. The WHO (2020) warned that infestations compromise nutritional status, affecting cognitive processes, inducing tissue reactions (e.g. granuloma) and provoking intestinal obstruction or rectal prolapse. Control of helminthiasis is based on drug treatment, improved sanitation and health education.

Pathophysiology

Although all helminths can infect humans, the definitive host and intermediate hosts vary with each organism. In nearly all instances of helminthic disorders, the organism enters the body through the GI tract in contaminated and inadequately cooked foods. Some of these organisms remain in the intestinal tract; others migrate to infect the liver, lungs or other structures. Table 23.6 summarises the most common helminths and their effects.

TABLE 23.6 Selected helminthic diseases

INFECTION	HOST	AREA	PATHOGENESIS	MANIFESTATIONS
Nematode infections				
Ascariasis (roundworm)	Humans	Worldwide, cosmopolitan; warm, moist climates. Common in Australia	Eggs are ingested in faecally contaminated food and drink; motile larvae migrate to lungs and back to small intestine, where they mature to produce more eggs.	Pulmonary: low-grade fever, cough, blood-tinged sputum, wheezing, dyspnoea, substernal chest pain. GI: ulcer-like epigastric pain, vomiting, abdominal distension.
Enterobiasis (pinworm infection)	Humans	Worldwide, cosmopolitan. Common in Australia	Infect caecum; eggs deposit on perianal skin. Organisms may be transmitted to others or reinfect host by oral ingestion.	Nocturnal perianal and perineal pruritus; insomnia, irritability, restlessness.
Hookworm disease	Humans	Tropics and subtropics. Common in remote areas in Australia	Larvae enter through skin or by ingestion and migrate to lungs, up bronchial tree and down oesophagus to mature in upper small bowel, where they attach and suck blood.	Skin: pruritic dermatitis at site of entry. Pulmonary: dry cough, wheezing, blood-tinged sputum. GI: anorexia, diarrhoea, abdominal pain. Systemic: anaemia, pallor, cardiac insufficiency.
Trichinosis	Pigs, dogs, cats, rats, many wild animals	Temperate areas where pork is consumed. Not found in Australian pork	Larvae are ingested in undercooked meat; adult female burrows into mucosa of small intestine to produce larvae that disseminate via blood and lymphatic system to body tissues and become encysted in striated muscle.	GI: diarrhoea, abdominal cramps, malaise. Muscle: fever; muscle pain, tenderness, oedema and spasm. Systemic: periorbital and facial oedema, sweating; photophobia and conjunctivitis; manifestations of inflammation in tissues invaded by larvae.
Cestode infections				
Fasciolopsiasis (intestinal fluke) Tapeworm (beef tapeworm in cattle-raising areas and occasionally dwarf tapeworm found in Northern Australia)	Humans; other mammals and fish Dogs and cats Humans are intermediate host	Worldwide. Sheep-raising areas in mainland Australia	Organism is ingested by eating uncooked fish or meat containing embryo cysts, by faecal contamination or by swallowing infected intermediate hosts, such as arthropods, fleas or lice. Head (scolex) of adult worm attaches in upper small intestine and eggs form in individual segments.	Large tapeworms: often asymptomatic; infection may cause mild nausea, diarrhoea, abdominal pain, anaemia, thrombocytopenia and mild leucopenia. Small tapeworms: may be asymptomatic; diarrhoea, abdominal pain, anorexia, vomiting, weight loss and irritability.
Echinococcus granulosi Hydatid cysts			Eggs of organism transmitted to humans from faeces on fur or tongue of infected animal. Eggs hatch in human intestines, migrating commonly to liver, lungs and brain, forming large fluid-filled sacs–hydatid cysts.	Localised pressure of cyst on the infected organ. Manifestations vary depending on organ involved. Occasional anaphylactic reaction to hydatid antigens when cysts burst.

INTERPROFESSIONAL CARE

The management of helminthic disorders includes diagnostic testing and medications.

Diagnosis

The primary means of diagnosing helminthic disorders is examination of the stool for ova and parasites. Enterobiasis is diagnosed by the presence of the parasite's eggs on the perianal skin or on cellulose tape placed over the anus.

A full blood count may also be ordered. Anaemia may be present, particularly with hookworm disease. *Eosinophilia* (an increased percentage of eosinophils in the blood) is common in helminthic disorders. With trichinosis, serum muscle enzymes such as creatinine kinase (CK) and aspartate aminotransferase (AST) are typically elevated. Serological testing for antibodies to the worm may also be performed. Blood, duodenal washings and cerebrospinal fluid (CSF) may be examined for the presence of the trichinosis larvae. Inflamed muscle may be biopsied.

Medications

Helminthic infections are often treated with a single oral dose or a 3-day course of aldendazole (Eskazole) or mebendazole (Vermox). Doses may need to be repeated every 2 weeks for a person with heavy infections. These medications are generally safe, requiring few precautions. Giving the drug after meals minimises GI side effects. Treatment is followed by a stool culture at 2 weeks to evaluate effectiveness. If necessary, an additional course of the medication is prescribed. Other members of the household are generally also treated.

Trichinosis is a serious infection caused by the roundworm *Trichinella spiralis*, acquired by eating raw or undercooked pork contaminated with cysts of the worm. It is not a problem in Australia as the pork sold is currently free of the parasite, however, it is widespread in North America (Lee & Bishop, 2016). Most people with trichinosis recover spontaneously without long-term effects. Hospitalisation may be required during the muscle invasion phase of the disease if the infection is severe. Corticosteroids may be used to reduce the inflammation and manage the clinical manifestations.

Strongyloides stercoralis is a commonly seen threadworm in tropical and subtropical areas (Lee & Bishop, 2016). It is acquired by larval penetration through the skin (see Figure 23.7). If only a few worms are present, the person may be asymptomatic. Heavy infestations cause abdominal pain; rashes and pruritus also occur (Lee & Bishop, 2016). *Strongyloides* infection is often difficult to diagnose and is done by finding larvae in fresh stools. Serological testing is available; however, this does not identify between a past or current acute infection. It is usually treated with ivermectin or thiabedazole. However, worm eradication is difficult, especially in an immunosuppressed person. Immunocompromised or malnourished individuals often have more severe symptoms and repeated regular treatment is required to eradicate the infection (Lee & Bishop, 2016).

Strongyloides parasites are important causes of morbidity in Aboriginal and Torres Strait Islander communities in northern Australia and their presence is of particular concern in children, contributing to poor weight gain and failure to thrive (Hanieh et al., 2021).

Hookworm infections are caused by *Anclostoma duodenale* and *Nector americanus*. In Australia, hookworms are endemic in some remote areas with poor sanitation (Lee & Bishop, 2016). The Aboriginal and Torres Strait Islander population is particularly susceptible due to chronic malnutrition and the practice of walking barefoot, as the larvae burrow through the skin, enter the blood vessels and are carried to the lungs. The larvae are coughed up in sputum. If swallowed, the larvae finally arrive in the intestine, attaching to mucosal cells and establishing an infection (Lee & Bishop, 2016).

Humans are the intermediate host for *Echinococcus granulosis*, causing a condition known as hydatid cysts. Eggs are shed in the faeces and may be transmitted to humans from faeces on the fur or tongue of animals. Eggs hatch in the

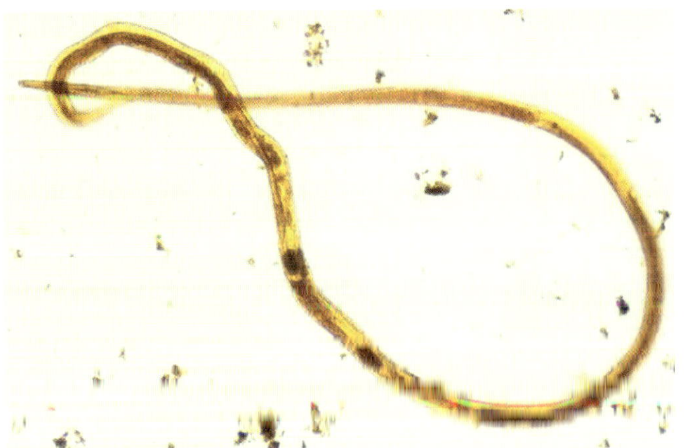

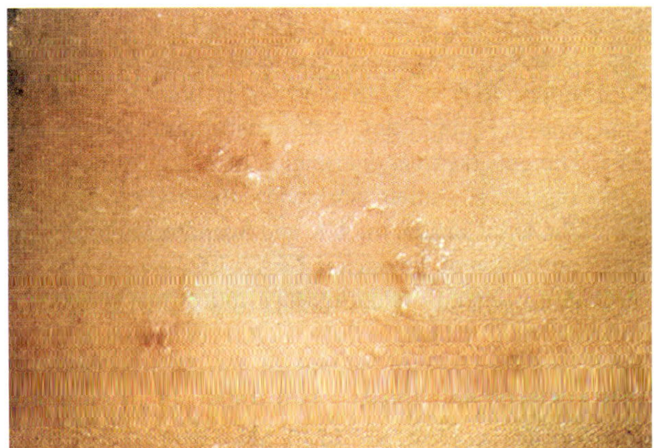

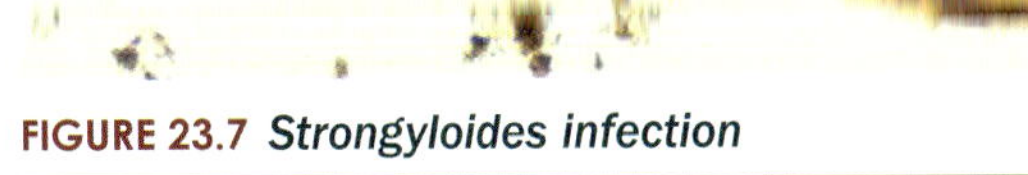

FIGURE 23.7 ***Strongyloides* infection**

Source: © Stephen Neville, Department of Microbiology & Infectious Diseases, Sydney South-West Pathology Service, Liverpool Campus.

intestines and migrate to various parts of the body, forming hydatid cysts—large fluid-filled sacs containing thousands of larvae (O'Dempsey & Beeching, 2018b). These most commonly form in the liver, lungs and brain, with serious consequences. Young children in sheep-farming areas are at greatest risk. In Australia, there are approximately 50 notifications of hydatid infection, with an average of three deaths per year (Lee & Bishop, 2016; Queensland Health, 2017).

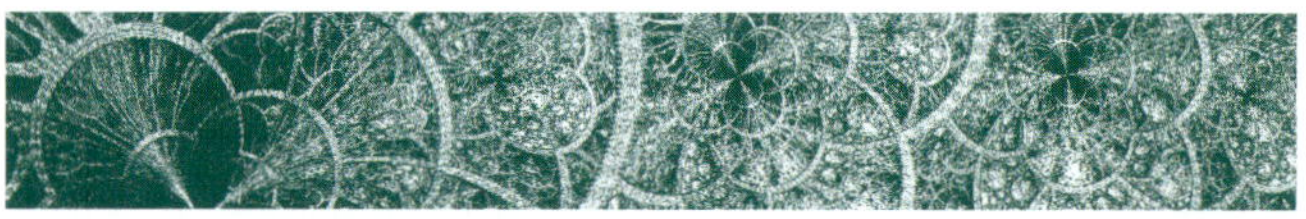

Nursing care

Because many people with these disorders are asymptomatic, nurses need to be alert for histories indicating risk and subtle manifestations of the disorder. Use standard precautions to minimise the risk of spreading these infections to others. Wear gloves and gowns as necessary to prevent faecal contamination of hands and clothing. On rare occasions, parasites may be present in the sputum or vomitus, so handle these secretions with care. Disinfect toilets, toilet seats and commodes after use. Teach the person the importance of washing hands after using the toilet and before handling food to prevent reinfection.

Discuss measures to prevent spread of the disease in the household. Emphasise the importance of hygiene measures, including changing bedding, daily cleaning of toilets with disinfectant and handwashing.

Many helminthic disorders are acquired by consuming faecally contaminated food or food containing larvae of the organism. Explain the importance of not fertilising food or grain crops with faecal material, particularly human faeces. Teach individuals to cook all meats and fish adequately to destroy possible larvae. In general, pickled or salt-preserved meats and fish are no safer than if raw. Smoking, another means of preserving fish and meat, may not achieve temperatures high enough to destroy the organisms. Vegetables grown in soil that may be contaminated with eggs or larvae should be peeled or cooked prior to eating. Hydatids can be avoided by deworming domestic animals regularly and not feeding them uncooked meat.

Emphasise the importance of safe water supplies. Encourage people travelling to areas where water supplies are questionable to drink only bottled water or carry purification tablets. Work with individuals with private water systems to protect water from faecal contamination by either humans or animals.

A person with a helminthic disorder may feel dirty or be ashamed of the disease. Emphasise the prevalence of these disorders, assuring the person that infections can occur despite good health practices when the eggs or larva of the organism are prevalent.

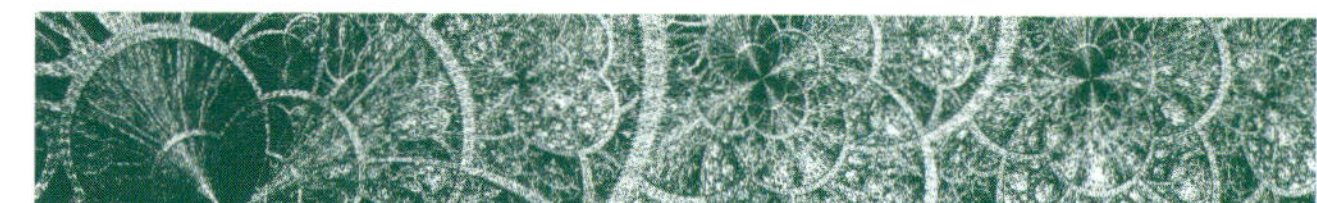

Chronic inflammatory bowel disorders

THE PERSON WITH INFLAMMATORY BOWEL DISEASE

Chronic **inflammatory bowel disease (IBD)** includes two separate but closely related conditions: ulcerative colitis and Crohn's disease. These conditions have a number of similarities. The aetiology of both illnesses is unknown, although current evidence implicates both genetic and environmental factors. The geographical distribution of ulcerative colitis and Crohn's disease is similar worldwide, the highest incidences being in the US, Canada, the UK and Scandinavia (Crohn's & Colitis Foundation of America (CCFA), 2022).

IBD affects certain ethnic groups more than others: it is prevalent among Ashkenazi Jews and decreases progressively in other people of Jewish descent, in non-Jewish Caucasians, Africans, Hispanics and Asians. In Australia, it affects approximately 1 in 250 people aged 5 to 40. More than 100,000 people have Crohn's disease or ulcerative colitis in Australia (Crohn's & Colitis Australia (CCA), 2022).

IBD tends to run in families, with 20–25% of people having a close relative with one of the types of IBD (CCA, 2022). Factors such as an abnormal immune response to microorganisms normally found in the gut are thought to play a role in IBD development. IBD has been linked to the recently discovered TH cell (TH 17), certain cytokines and a deficit of antimicrobial substances (lysoenzyme, defensins and other) secreted by the gut mucosa (Marieb & Hoehn, 2019). Autoimmunity is thought to play a role (see the chapter 'Nursing care of people with altered immunity') and lifestyle factors (such as smoking) may also affect its development. Smoking certainly worsens Crohn's disease. CCA (2022) stressed that those who stop smoking have a 65% lower risk of flare-up (comparable to the benefit conferred by drugs such as Imuran) than continuing smokers. Children developing Crohn's disease are more likely to have been exposed to passive smoking at home (CCA, 2022).

The peak incidence of IBD is in adolescents and young adults between the ages of 15 and 35 years, but it can also affect older adults (CCA, 2022). IBD is a chronic and recurrent disease process. Responses to physiological or psychological stresses do not cause IBD, but often play a role in exacerbations of the disease.

Despite the similarities, ulcerative colitis and Crohn's disease have distinct differences. Ulcerative colitis primarily affects the large bowel in a continuous pattern, progressing distally to proximally. In Crohn's disease, a patchy pattern of involvement is seen, affecting primarily the small intestine. Ulcerative colitis shows mainly mucosal involvement; in Crohn's disease, the submucosal layers of the bowel are affected. A comparison of ulcerative colitis and Crohn's disease is found in Table 23.7. The multisystem effects of IBD are then illustrated.

Ulcerative colitis

Ulcerative colitis is a chronic inflammatory bowel disorder affecting the mucosa and submucosa of the colon and rectum. *Chronic intermittent colitis* (recurrent ulcerative colitis) is the most common form of the disease and affects approximately 40,000 people in Australia each year, resulting in steep hospital and drug costs as well as lost work (CCA, 2022). Most people with ulcerative colitis have mild or moderate disease, with six or fewer stools per day. Its onset is insidious, with attacks lasting 1 to 3 months occurring at intervals of months to years. Typically, only the distal colon is affected, with few systemic manifestations of the disease. Approximately 15% of people with ulcerative colitis develop *fulminant colitis*, with the entire colon involved, severe bloody diarrhoea, acute abdominal pain and fever. Those with fulminant disease are at high risk of complications.

Pathophysiology

The inflammatory process of ulcerative colitis begins at the rectosigmoid area of the anal canal and progresses proximally. In most individuals, it is confined to the rectum and sigmoid colon. It may progress to involve the entire colon, stopping at the ileocaecal junction.

Ulcerative colitis begins with inflammation at the base of the crypts of Lieberkühn in the distal large intestine and rectum. Microscopic, pinpoint mucosal haemorrhages occur and crypt abscesses develop (see Figure 23.8). These abscesses penetrate the superficial submucosa and spread laterally, leading to necrosis and sloughing of bowel mucosa. Further tissue damage is caused by inflammatory exudates and the release of inflammatory mediators, such as prostaglandins and other cytokines (see the chapter 'Nursing care of people with infections' for further discussion of the inflammatory process). The mucosa is red and oedematous due to vascular congestion, friable (easily broken) and ulcerated. It bleeds easily and haemorrhage is common. Oedema creates a granular appearance. Pseudopolyps, tongue-like projections of bowel mucosa into the lumen, may develop as the epithelial lining of the bowel regenerates. Chronic inflammation leads to atrophy, narrowing and shortening of the colon, with loss of its normal haustra.

TABLE 23.7 Characteristics of ulcerative colitis and Crohn's disease

	CHARACTERISTIC	ULCERATIVE COLITIS	CROHN'S DISEASE
Clinical	Gender	Equal	Equal
	Age at onset	15 to 35 years, secondary peak between 60 and 80 years	15 to 30 years; secondary peak between 60 and 80 years
	Course of disease	Typically chronic and intermittent	Slowly progressive, relapsing
	Diarrhoea	5 to 30 stools per day with blood and mucus	Common, usually less severe than colitis, with no obvious blood or mucus in stool
	Abdominal pain	Cramping in left lower quadrant; relieved by defecation	Cramping or steady right lower quadrant or periumbilical pain; tenderness and mass noted in right lower quadrant
	Nutritional deficit	Common; involves anaemia, hypoalbuminaemia and weight loss	Common and significant: involves anaemia, weight loss and multiple vitamin and mineral deficits
	Constitutional manifestations	Fever rare; may have associated arthritic, skin or other organ involvement, such as erythema nodosum or uveitis	Fever, malaise, fatigue; may have some associated conditions plus urinary complications
Pathological	Depth of involvement	Mucosa and submucosa	Transmural (entire bowel wall)
	Portion of bowel involved	Typically rectum and sigmoid colon; may extend to involve entire large bowel	Any portion of GI tract; terminal ileum and ascending colon involvement predominates
	Distribution	Continuous from rectum	Patchy; skip lesions
	Appearance of mucosa	Granular, dull, hyperaemic, friable; disease uniform in affected bowel; pseudopolyps may be seen	Cobblestone appearance, with areas of normal tissue [illegible]
Complications	Acute	Toxic megacolon, perforation, massive haemorrhage	Obstruction, fistulisation, abscess formation, malabsorption
	Long term	Colorectal cancer	Colon cancer

Multisystem effects of inflammatory bowel disease

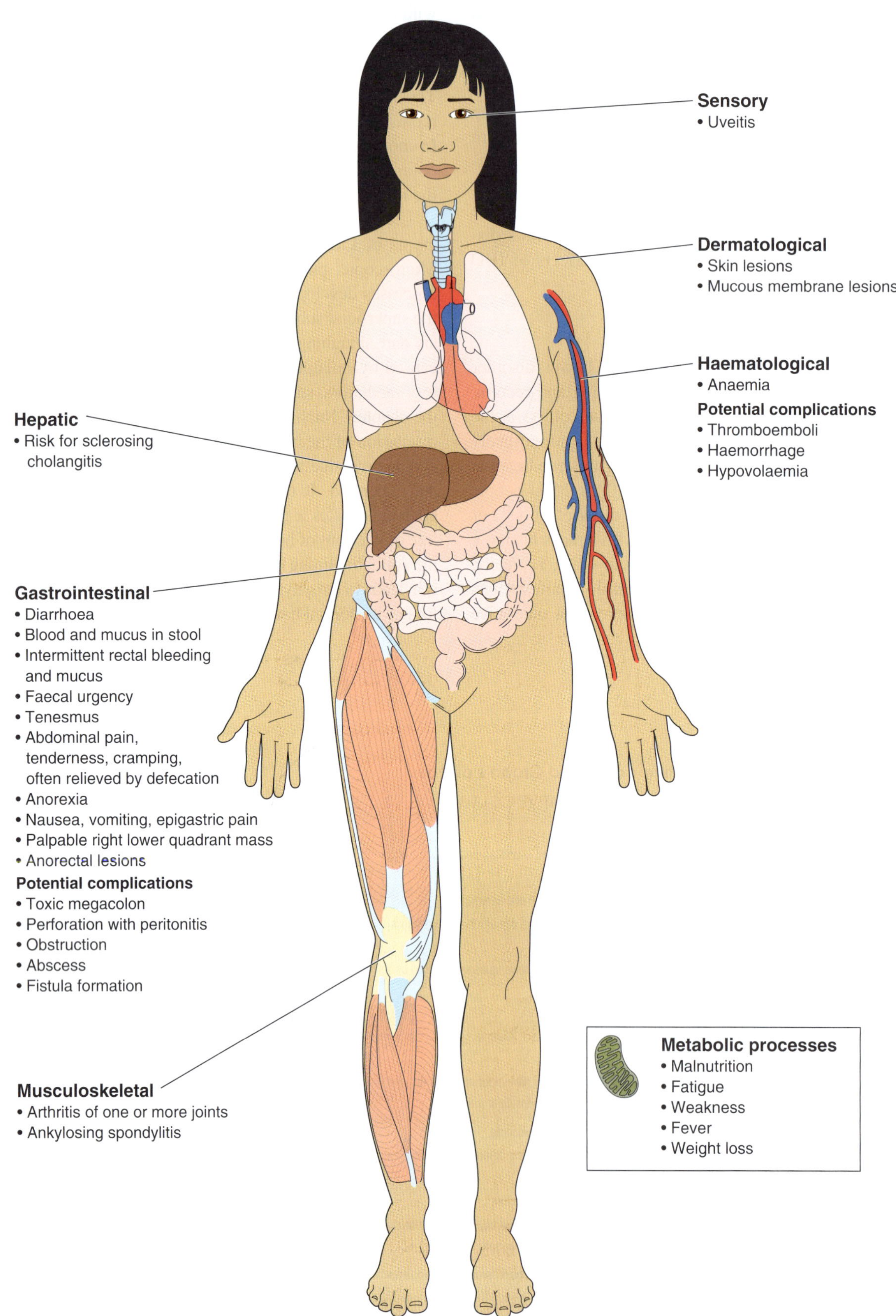

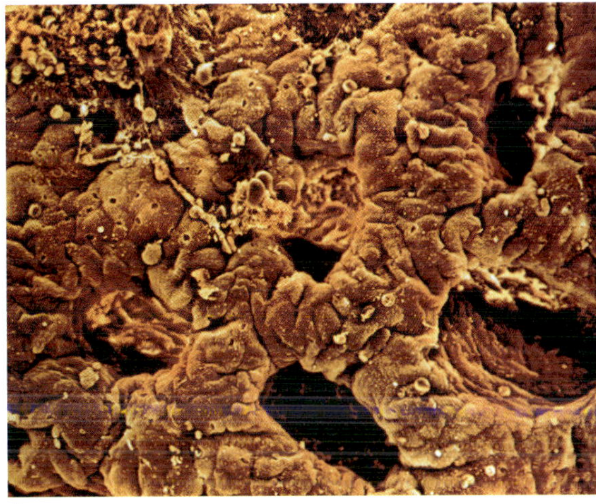
A

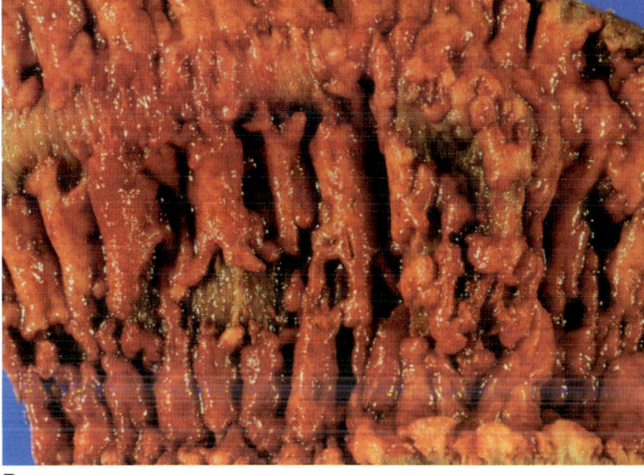
B

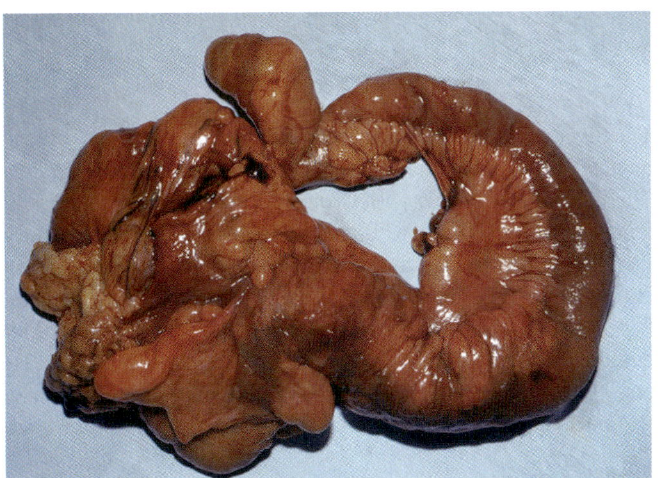
C

FIGURE 23.8 ***A, Photomicrograph of the mucosa of the large intestine showing the entrances to the crypts of Lieberkühn. The crypts are the focal points for B, ulcerative colitis and C, Crohn's disease***

Sources: *A* and *C*, Biophoto Associates/Science Photo Library; *B*, Dr E. Walker/Science Photo Library.

Manifestations

Diarrhoea is the predominant manifestation of ulcerative colitis. Stools contain both blood and mucus. Nocturnal diarrhoea may occur. Mild ulcerative colitis is characterised by fewer than 4 stools per day, intermittent rectal bleeding and mucus, and few systemic manifestations. Severe ulcerative colitis leads to more than 6 to 10 bloody stools per day, extensive colon involvement, anaemia, hypovolaemia and malnutrition. Rectal inflammation causes faecal urgency and tenesmus. Left lower quadrant cramping relieved by defecation is common. Other manifestations include fatigue, anorexia and weakness.

Individuals with severe disease may also have systemic manifestations such as arthritis involving one or several joints, skin and mucous membrane lesions, or *uveitis* (inflammation of the uvea, the vascular layer of the eye, which may also involve the sclera and cornea). Some individuals develop thromboemboli, with blood vessel obstruction due to clots carried from the site of their formation. The liver and biliary system may be affected by the disease as may the kidneys, with an increased risk of gallstones, cirrhosis, renal calculi and ureteral obstruction (Martin, Chan & Hart, 2014).

Complications

Most people with ulcerative colitis (80–90%) respond well to treatment and do not develop complications (CCA, 2022). Acute complications of ulcerative colitis include haemorrhage, toxic megacolon and colon perforation. Massive haemorrhage may occur with severe attacks of the disease. *Toxic megacolon* is a condition characterised by acute motor paralysis and dilation of the colon to greater than 6 cm, affecting part or the entire colon. The transverse segment of the bowel is most commonly affected. Toxic megacolon may be triggered by the use of laxatives, narcotics and anticholinergic drugs, and the presence of hypokalaemia (Devuni, 2014). Manifestations of toxic megacolon include fever, tachycardia, hypotension, dehydration, abdominal tenderness and cramping, and a change in the number of stools per day. Perforation is rare; however, this is a dangerous complication increased with toxic megacolon. Perforation leads to peritonitis.

The risk of colorectal cancer is increased in people with ulcerative colitis. Beginning 8 to 10 years after diagnosis annual or biennial colonoscopies with biopsy to detect masses or cell dysplasia are recommended for individuals with extensive ulcerative colitis (Devuni, 2014).

Crohn's disease

Like ulcerative colitis, **Crohn's disease**, also known as *regional enteritis*, is a chronic, relapsing inflammatory disorder affecting the GI tract. Crohn's disease can affect any portion of the GI tract from the mouth to the anus, but usually affects the terminal ileum and ascending colon. The small bowel only is involved in about 30–40% of people with Crohn's disease. The disease is limited to the colon only in 30% of those affected. Both the small and the large intestine are involved in the remaining 30% of individuals (Marieb & Hoehn, 2019).

Pathophysiology

Crohn's disease typically begins as a small inflammatory *aphthoid lesion* (shallow ulcers with a white base and elevated margin, similar to a canker sore) of the mucosa and submucosa of the bowel. These initial lesions may regress or the inflammatory process can progress to involve all layers of the intestinal wall. Deeper ulcerations, granulomatous lesions and fissures (knife-like clefts extending deeply into the bowel wall) develop. The inflammatory process involves the entire bowel wall (transmural).

The lumen of the affected bowel assumes a 'cobblestone appearance' as fissures and ulcers surround islands of intact mucosa over oedematous submucosa. The inflammatory lesions of Crohn's disease are not continuous; rather, they often occur as 'skip' lesions with intervening areas of normalappearing bowel. Some evidence suggests that, despite its normal appearance, the entire bowel is affected by this disorder.

As the disease progresses, fibrotic changes in the bowel wall cause thickening and decreased flexibility of the bowel (which takes on an appearance likened to a rubber hose). The inflammation, oedema and fibrosis can lead to local obstruction, abscess development and the formation of fistulas between loops of the bowel or the bowel and other organs (see Figure 23.9). Fistulas between loops of the bowel are called enteroenteric fistulas. Enterovesical fistulas occur between the bowel and bladder, and enterocutaneous fistulas occur between the bowel and skin. Perineal fistulas originating in the ileum are relatively common.

Depending on the severity and extent of the disease, malabsorption and malnutrition may develop as the ulcers prevent absorption of nutrients. When the jejunum and ileum are affected, the absorption of multiple nutrients may be impaired, including carbohydrates, proteins, fats, vitamins and folate. Disease in the terminal ileum can lead to vitamin B_{12} malabsorption and bile salt reabsorption. The ulcerations also lead to protein loss and chronic, slow blood loss with consequent anaemia.

Manifestations

The diverse nature of GI system involvement in Crohn's disease means that clinical manifestations vary between individuals. The majority of people with Crohn's disease experience persistent diarrhoea. Stools are liquid or semi-formed and typically do not contain blood, although blood may be passed if the colon is involved. Abdominal pain and tenderness are also common. Pain may be located in the right lower quadrant and relieved by defecation. A palpable right lower quadrant mass is often present. Systemic manifestations such as fever, fatigue, malaise, weight loss and anaemia are common. Anorectal lesions such

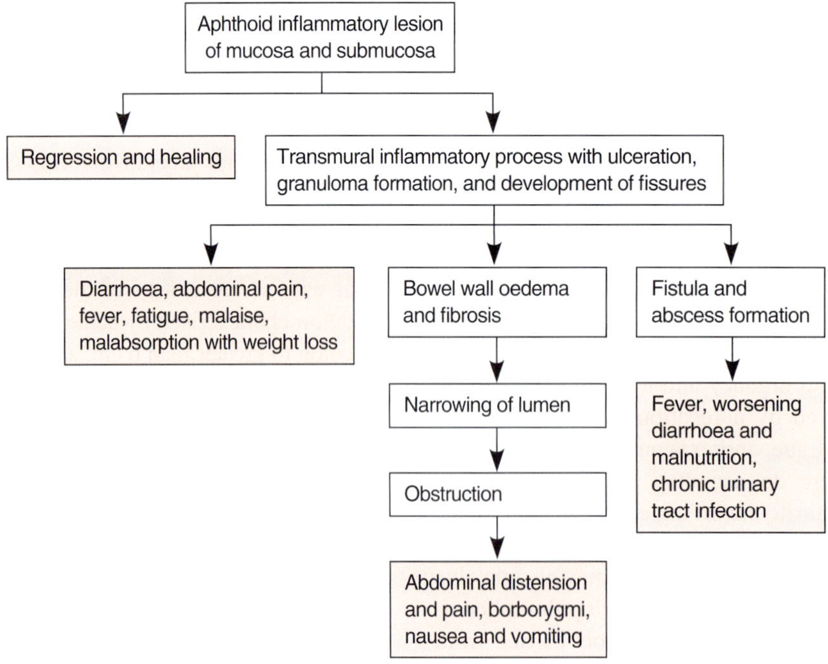

FIGURE 23.9 ***The progression of Crohn's disease***

as fissures, ulcers, fistulas and abscesses are also common and may occur years before intestinal disease is apparent. If the stomach and duodenum are involved, nausea, vomiting and epigastric pain occur.

Complications

Certain complications of Crohn's disease (e.g. intestinal obstruction, abscess and fistula) are so common that they are considered part of the disease process. For many people, the disease initially presents with one of these complications. Intestinal obstruction is a common complication caused by repeated inflammation and scarring of the bowel, leading to fibrosis and stricture. Obstruction of the bowel lumen causes abdominal distension, cramping pain and borborygmi. Nausea and vomiting may occur.

Fistulas may be asymptomatic, particularly those occurring between loops of small bowel. When fistulisation causes an abscess, chills and fever, a tender abdominal mass and leucocytosis develop. A fistula between the small bowel and colon may exacerbate diarrhoea, weight loss and malnutrition. When the bladder is involved, recurrent urinary tract infections occur.

Perforation of the bowel is uncommon. However, it can lead to generalised peritonitis. Massive haemorrhage also is an uncommon complication of Crohn's disease. Long-standing Crohn's disease increases the risk of cancer of the small intestine or colon by five to six times, which is significantly lower than the risk associated with ulcerative colitis.

INTERPROFESSIONAL CARE

Interprofessional care for IBD begins by establishing the diagnosis and the extent and severity of the disease. Treatment is supportive, including medications and dietary measures to decrease inflammation, promote intestinal rest and healing, and reduce intestinal motility. Many people with IBD require surgery at some point to manage the disease or its complications.

Diagnosis

Diagnostic testing is used to establish the diagnosis of IBD, assess the extent of the disease and evaluate the effects of the disorder. A colonoscopy or barium upper and lower x-ray series is performed to inspect the bowel mucosa for characteristic changes of IBD. (Nursing implications for these diagnostic tests are outlined in the chapter 'A person-centred approach to assessing the gastrointestinal system'.)

Laboratory tests to differentiate IBD and identify effects and complications of the disease include a stool examination for blood and mucus, and stool cultures to rule out infectious causes of bowel inflammation and diarrhoea. FBC with haemoglobin and haematocrit shows anaemia from chronic inflammation, blood loss and malnutrition, and leucocytosis due to inflammation and possible abscess formation. ESR and Creactive protein levels are typically elevated during periods of acute inflammation. Serum albumin may be decreased because of malabsorption, malnutrition, protein loss through intestinal lesions and chronic inflammation. Folic acid and serum levels of most vitamins, including A, B complex, C and the fat-soluble vitamins are often decreased due to malabsorption. Liver function tests may show elevated liver enzymes (such as ALT, ALP, AST, GGTP and LDH) and bilirubin levels if sclerosing cholangitis is present.

Medications

The ultimate goal of care is to terminate acute attacks as quickly as possible and reduce the incidence of relapse. Drug therapy plays a key role in achieving this goal. Locally acting and systemic anti-inflammatory drugs are the primary medications used to manage mild to moderate IBD. Medications suppressing the immune response may be used to treat people with severe disease.

Sulfasalazine (Azulfidine) is a sulfonamide antibiotic poorly absorbed from the GI tract and acts topically on the colonic mucosa to inhibit the inflammatory process. The active anti-inflammatory ingredient in sulfasalazine, 5-aminosalicylic acid (5-ASA), is also available in sulfa-free preparations, such as olsalazine and mesalazine. These have the advantage of causing fewer adverse effects than sulfasalazine. Azo compounds, such as balsalazide and olsalazine, are 5-aminosalicylic acid compounds released in the colon and are especially useful to treat ulcerative colitis. Mesalamine is an orally or rectally administered 5-ASA compound providing topical anti-inflammatory action in the colon of individuals with ulcerative colitis. Specific preparations, their method of action and nursing implications for these medications are outlined in the 'Medication administration' box.

For acute exacerbations of IBD, corticosteroids are given to reduce inflammation and induce remission. For ulcerative colitis, the drug may be administered rectally for its local effect and to minimise systemic effects. Hydrocortisone can be administered rectally. Intravenous corticosteroids may be required to treat severe disease; oral preparations are used for less severe manifestations and long-term therapy. Corticosteroids are tapered off once remission is achieved. However, many individuals are unable to withdraw from steroid therapy without experiencing relapse and require long-term, low-dose therapy.

Mercaptopurine (6-MP, Purinethol) and other immunosuppressive agents such as azathioprine (Imuran) and cyclosporin (Sandimmun) are used to treat individuals unresponsive to other treatments or who require long-term steroid therapy. These drugs may allow withdrawal of corticosteroids, maintain remission and facilitate healing. Long-term therapy may be required to produce a beneficial effect. For more information about immunosuppressive medications, see the chapter 'Nursing care of people with altered immunity'.

Newer treatments for IBD employ other immune response modifiers, such as the monoclonal antibody infliximab (Remicade) to suppress tumour necrosis factor (TNF, an inflammatory mediator substance) in those unresponsive to standard

MEDICATION ADMINISTRATION Inflammatory bowel disease

SULFASALAZINE (SALAZOPYRIN)

Sulfasalazine is an anti-inflammatory drug used for its local effect on the intestinal mucosa in IBD. The active part of the drug, 5-aminosalicylic acid, inhibits prostaglandin production in the bowel. Prostaglandin is an important mediator of the inflammatory process; blocking its production reduces inflammation.

Nursing responsibilities

- Assess for contraindications, including pregnancy or a history of hypersensitivity to sulfonamides or salicylates.
- Assess baseline values for renal function tests (serum creatinine, BUN, urinalysis), liver function tests and FBC. Monitor these routinely during therapy.
- Administer as ordered. Suppositories or retention enemas may be administered at bedtime. Administer oral forms with a full glass of water.
- Have resuscitation equipment available, as anaphylactic responses may occur.
- Evaluate for therapeutic response, including reduced number of stools, reduced mucus and blood, and improved stool consistency. Onset of action may take 6 to 12 weeks.
- Monitor for possible adverse responses:
  a. skin rash, dermatitis, urticaria or pruritus
  b. evidence of blood dyscrasias, such as bleeding, easy bruising or fever
  c. leucopenia, thrombocytopenia, haemolytic anaemia or agranulocytosis
  d. changes in urinary output or renal function analysis (including urinalysis)
  e. evidence of hepatitis or myocarditis.

Health education for the person and family

- Take oral preparations after meals to decrease gastric distress.
- Drink at least 2–3 L of fluid per day to reduce the risk of kidney damage.
- Use sunscreen to prevent burns; this drug increases sensitivity to sun.
- Do not take aspirin, vitamin C or any other over-the-counter medications containing aspirin or vitamin C without consulting your doctor.
- This medication may interfere with the effectiveness of oral contraceptives; use alternative methods of contraception.
- Notify your doctor if you develop skin rash or hives, a sore throat or mouth, bleeding gums or joint pain, or bruise easily or develop fever.

MESALAZINE (MESASAL) AND OLSALAZINE (PREDSOL)

Mesalamine and olsalazine contain the same active ingredient, 5-aminosalicylic acid, as sulfasalazine; however, they cause fewer adverse effects. Their mechanism of action is the same as sulfasalazine. These drugs are available as suppositories, suspension for enema or oral tablets.

Nursing responsibilities

- Assess for possible contraindications such as pregnancy, lactation or hypersensitivity to these drugs or aspirin.
- Administer as ordered. If more than one dose per day is ordered, space doses evenly over the 24-hour period.
- Evaluate for desired effects (as for sulfasalazine) and potential adverse effects:
  a. nausea, diarrhoea, abdominal cramps or flatulence
  b. CNS effects, including headache, dizziness, insomnia, weakness or fatigue
  c. rash or itching
  d. flu-like symptoms or general malaise.

Health education for the person and family

- Teach the recommended method of administration, including how to insert rectal suppositories or administer a retention enema.
- Shake suspension forms well prior to using.
- Diarrhoea is the most common side effect of these drugs. Notify your doctor if adverse effects occur.

CORTICOSTEROIDS

Methylprednisolone (Medrol, Solu-Medrol)
Prednisolone (Delta-Cortel)
Prednisone

Glucocorticoids are hormones produced by the adrenal cortex. See the chapter 'Nursing care of people with endocrine disorders' for discussion on hormones and stress response. These hormones are necessary for the stress response. Cortisol, the main glucocorticoid, has potent anti-inflammatory effects. Corticosteroids are used to treat acute episodes of IBD. Because of their multiple and significant side effects, they are not used to maintain remission.

Nursing responsibilities

- Assess for conditions adversely affected by corticosteroid medications: peptic ulcer disease, glaucoma or cataracts, diabetes mellitus or psychiatric disorders.
- Obtain baseline vital signs and weight; monitor both routinely during therapy. Hypertension and weight gain may result from sodium and water retention.
- Monitor for oedema.
- Administer as ordered. For daily or alternate-day dosing, administer in the morning, when physiological glucocorticoid levels are highest, to reduce adrenal cortisone suppression.
- Administering oral preparations with food decreases gastrointestinal side effects. Antacids or histamine H_2-receptor blocking agents may be prescribed during corticosteroid therapy.
- Monitor for desired effects: reduced diarrhoea, less blood and mucus in the stool and less abdominal cramping.
- Monitor for adverse effects:
  a. increased susceptibility to infection and masking of early signs of infection
  b. hyperglycaemia
  c. hypokalaemia, as manifested by muscle weakness, nausea, vomiting and cardiac rhythm disturbances
  d. oedema, hypertension and signs of heart failure
  e. peptic ulcer formation and possible gastrointestinal haemorrhage (abdominal pain, black or tarry stools, and signs of bleeding)

MEDICATION ADMINISTRATION **Inflammatory bowel disease (continued)**

f. changes in mental status, including depression, euphoria, aggression and behavioural changes
g. with long-term use, Cushingoid effects, such as abnormal fat deposits in the face (moon facies) and trunk (buffalo hump), muscle wasting and thin extremities, thinning of the skin and osteoporosis. See the chapter 'Nursing care of people with endocrine disorders' for discussion of nursing care of a person with hypercortisolism (Cushing's syndrome).

Health education for the person and family

- Take as prescribed; do not change the dose or time of day. Do not stop the medication abruptly. The dose will be tapered down gradually when the medication is discontinued.
- Notify the doctor if adverse or Cushingoid effects occur.
- Take with food or at mealtimes to decrease the gastrointestinal effects.
- Monitor weight. If more than 2.5 kg gain is noted, notify the doctor.
- Moderate salt intake and avoid foods and snacks high in sodium, such as processed meats and potato chips. Increase intake of foods high in potassium, such as fruits, vegetables and lean meats.
- Carry a card or wear a MedicAlert® bracelet or tag at all times identifying corticosteroid use.

therapies. Mesalazine (Mesal) is an orally or rectally administered anti-inflammatory medication providing topical anti-inflammatory action in the colon of individuals with ulcerative colitis.

Although antibiotic therapy generally is not indicated in IBD, metronidazole (Flagyl) has active anti-inflammatory effects. It may be prescribed to help prevent remission after ileal resection in Crohn's disease. Ciprofloxacin (Cipro) is an alternative to metronidazole.

Antidiarrhoeal agents, such as loperamide and diphenoxylate, may be given to slow gastrointestinal motility and reduce diarrhoea. These drugs are safe for individuals with mild, chronic manifestations. However, these are not given during acute attacks because they may precipitate toxic dilation of the colon.

Nutrition

Antigens in the diet may stimulate the immune response in the bowel, exacerbating IBD. As a result, dietary management for IBD is individualised. Some people benefit from eliminating all milk and milk products from the diet. Increased dietary fibre may help reduce diarrhoea and relieve rectal manifestations. However, this is contraindicated for individuals with intestinal strictures caused by repeated inflammation and scarring.

All food may be withheld to promote bowel rest during an acute exacerbation of Crohn's disease. Nutritional status is maintained using enteral or total parenteral nutrition (TPN). See the chapter 'Nursing care of people with nutritional disorders' for more information about enteral feedings and TPN. TPN carries a higher risk of complications than does enteral nutrition.

Surgery

Surgical interventions for IBD differ, depending on the primary disease process and the portion of bowel affected. Generally, surgery is performed only when necessitated by complications of the disease or failure of conservative treatment measures.

Bowel obstruction is the leading indication for surgery in Crohn's disease. Other complications requiring surgical intervention include perforation, internal or external fistula, abscess and perianal complications. Resection of the affected portion of bowel with an end-to-end anastomosis to preserve as much bowel as possible is the usual treatment. The disease process tends to recur in other areas following removal of affected bowel segments. There is an increased risk of fistula formation following surgery. Bowel strictures may be treated with a strictureplasty in which longitudinal incisions are made in the narrowed segment, relieving the stricture while preserving bowel.

COLECTOMY Individuals with extensive chronic ulcerative colitis may require a total **colectomy** (surgical resection and removal of the colon) to treat the disease itself; for complications such as toxic megacolon, perforation or haemorrhage; or as a prophylactic measure due to the high colon cancer risk associated with extensive ulcerative colitis.

The surgical procedure of choice for extensive ulcerative colitis is a total colectomy with an *ileal pouch–anal anastomosis (IPAA)*. In this procedure, the entire colon and rectum are removed; a pouch is then formed from the terminal ileum and is brought into the pelvis and anastomosed to the anal canal (see Figure 23.10). A temporary or loop ileostomy (described in the next section) is generally performed at the same time and maintained for 2 to 3 months, allowing the anal anastomosis to heal. When the healing is complete, the ileostomy is closed. The person then has six to eight daily bowel movements through the anus. Advanced age, obesity or other factors may preclude an IPAA. For these individuals, a permanent ileostomy or continent ileostomy may be created.

OSTOMY An intestinal ostomy is a surgically created opening between the intestine and the abdominal wall that

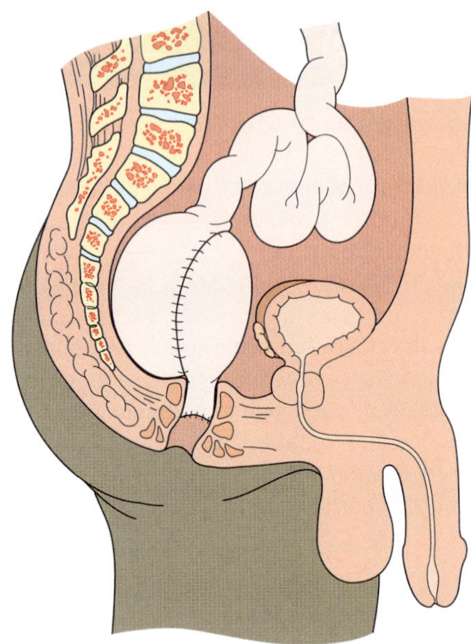

FIGURE 23.10 *Ileal pouch–anal anastomosis (IPAA)*

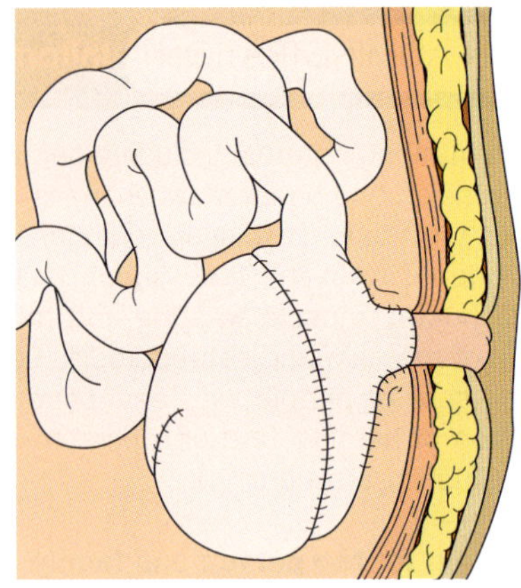

FIGURE 23.12 *Continent (Kock's) ileostomy*

allows the passage of faecal material. The surface opening is called a **stoma** (see Figure 23.11). The precise name of the ostomy depends on the location of the stoma. An **ileostomy** is an ostomy made in the ileum of the small intestine. In an ileostomy, the colon, rectum and anus are usually completely removed (*total proctocolectomy with permanent ileostomy*). The anal canal is closed and the end of the terminal ileum is brought to the body surface through the right abdominal wall to form the stoma. A *temporary* or *loop ileostomy* may be formed to eliminate faeces and allow tissue healing for 2 to 3 months following an IPAA. A loop of ileum is brought to the body surface to form a stoma, allowing stool drainage into an external pouch. When the ileostomy is no longer necessary, surgery is performed to close the stoma and repair the bowel, restoring faecal elimination through the anus.

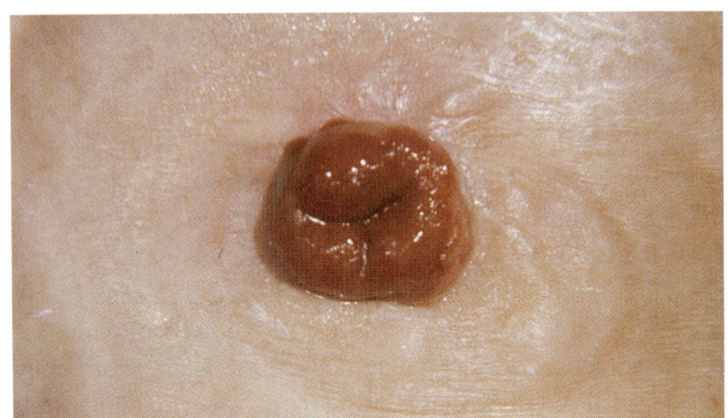

FIGURE 23.11 *A healthy-appearing stoma*

Source: Carol Williams/Pearson Education.

In a *continent ileostomy* (see Figure 23.12), an intra-abdominal reservoir is constructed and a nipple valve formed (the ileum folded back on itself) from the terminal ileum, before it is brought to the surface of the abdominal wall. Stool collects in the internal pouch. The nipple valve prevents leaking through the stoma. A catheter is inserted into the pouch to drain the stool.

Nursing care of a person with an ileostomy is outlined in the accompanying box. When devising nursing care plans for a person requiring stoma care, it is important to incorporate the person's cultural, religious and personal viewpoints into their care plan. Procedure 23.1 describes how to apply one- and two-piece drainable ostomy pouches.

Complementary and alternative therapies

The chronic nature of IBD and the adverse effects of many of the prescribed treatments lead up to 50% of people with IBD to seek or use complementary and alternative therapies. The most common complementary therapies used by people with IBD include herbal therapies, nutritional supplements, probiotics and fish oil (Manuel, 2021). Herbal remedies such as aloe vera gel and curcumin appear to have beneficial effects, as do Chinese traditional medicines including Jian Pi Ling tablets and Yukui tang tablets. Probiotics, bacteria similar to those normally found in the gut, appear to have beneficial antiinflammatory effects in the bowel (Manuel, 2021). Probiotics are available in foods such as yoghurt, miso and soy beverages, as well as in dietary supplements. Results are mixed from studies of the beneficial effects of fish oil or omega-3 fatty acid supplements for IBD. Peppermint tea is an excellent tonic for reducing nausea, relieving abdominal pain and providing a calming effect. Chamomile tea helps to reduce intestinal inflammation (Bullock & Manias, 2022).

NURSING CARE OF THE PERSON having an ileostomy

PREOPERATIVE CARE

- Provide routine pre-operative care and teaching as outlined in the chapter 'Nursing care of people having surgery'.
- Refer to a stomal therapist for marking and teaching about the stoma location, ostomy care and options for ostomy appliances. *It is important to begin teaching prior to surgery to facilitate learning and acceptance of the ostomy postoperatively.*
- Discuss the availability of a local Stoma Association and provide a referral as necessary or desired. *Local branches often have members with ostomies willing to provide both preoperative and postoperative teaching, listening and support.*
- Provide preoperative bowel preparation as ordered. *Laxatives, enemas and preoperative antibiotics are often ordered to reduce the risk of abdominal contamination and infection after surgery.*

POSTOPERATIVE CARE

- Provide routine postoperative care and teaching as outlined in the chapter 'Nursing care of people having surgery'.
- Apply an ostomy pouch over the stoma (see Procedure 23.1). *Stool from an ileostomy is expressed continuously or irregularly and is liquid in nature; continuous use of a pouch to collect the drainage is necessary.*
- Assess frequently for bleeding, stoma viability and function. In the early postoperative period, small amounts of blood in the pouch are expected. *A healthy stoma is pink or red and moist as a result of mucus production (see Figure 23.11) and protrudes approximately 2 cm from the abdominal wall. Frequent assessment is important in the initial postoperative period to ensure stoma health and to monitor for possible complications. A dusky, brown, black or white stoma indicates circulatory compromise. Other possible stoma complications include retraction (indentation or loss of the external portion of the stoma) or prolapse (outward telescoping of the stoma—that is, an abnormally long stoma).*
- As the stoma starts functioning, empty the pouch, explaining the procedure to the person. Initial drainage is dark green, viscid and usually odourless. Drainage gradually thickens and becomes yellow-brown. Empty the pouch when it is one-third full. Measure drainage and include it as output on fluid balance records. Rinse the pouch and reapply the clamp. *Emptying the pouch when it is no more than one-third full helps prevent the skin seal from breaking as a result of the weight of the pouch. Because of the potential for excess fluid loss through ileostomy drainage, it is important to include it as fluid output.*
- Assess the peristomal skin. Skin around the stoma should remain clean and pink and free of irritation, rashes, inflammation or excoriation. *Skin complications may arise from appliance irritation or hypersensitivity, excoriation from a leaking appliance or* Candida albicans *(a yeast infection).*
- Protect peristomal skin from enzymes and bile salts in the ileostomy effluent. Using a skin barrier on the pouch is essential. Change the pouch if leakage occurs or if the person reports burning or itching skin. *Enzymes and bile salts normally reabsorbed in the large intestine are irritating to the skin. Excoriation of skin surrounding the stoma impairs the first line of defence against microorganisms and can interfere with the ability to achieve a tight skin seal and prevent pouch leakage.*
- Report the following abnormal assessment findings to the surgeon:
  a. Allergic or contact dermatitis. *A rash may result from contact with faecal drainage or indicate sensitivity to pouch, paste, tape or sealant.*
  b. Purulent ulcerated areas surrounding the stoma. *Disruption of the protective barrier of the skin allows bacterial entry.*
  c. A red, bumpy, itchy rash or white-coated area. *This is a manifestation of* Candida albicans, *a yeast infection.*
  d. Bulging around the stoma. *This finding may indicate herniation, caused by loops of intestine protruding through the abdominal wall.*
- Apply protective ointments to the perirectal area of people with newly functioning ileoanal reservoirs and anastomoses. This helps protect the skin from the initial stools. *As stools thicken and become fewer per day, the person experiences less perirectal irritation.*

HEALTH EDUCATION FOR THE PERSON AND FAMILY

- While caring for the stoma, explain procedures to the person. *Teaching is immediate and ongoing to assist in acceptance of the stoma and facilitate self-care.*
- Teach to manage the pouch clamp, to empty, rinse and perform pouch changes. *Self-care is vital to independence and self-esteem.*
- Instruct how to use an electric razor to shave the peristomal hair if necessary. *An electric razor prevents accidental cutting of the stoma with a razor blade.*
- Teach to check the stoma and peristomal skin with each pouch change. Ongoing assessment is important for optimal health and function of the stoma and surrounding skin. Stripping of tape or excessively frequent pouch removal may cause mechanical trauma to peristomal skin. *Chronic skin irritation by ileostomy effluent may lead to pseudoverrucous lesions or wartlike nodules.*
- Instruct to report abnormal appearance of the stoma or surrounding skin (as noted previously and below) to the doctor:
  a. Narrowing of the stoma lumen. *This indicates stenosis and may interfere with faecal elimination.*
  b. Lacerations or cuts in the stoma. *The stoma contains no nerves, so trauma may occur without pain.*
  c. Separation of the stoma from the abdominal surface. *This potential complication may require surgical repair.*
- Emphasise the importance of adequate fluid and salt intake; the risk of dehydration and hyponatraemia is increased particularly during hot weather, when fluid is lost through perspiration as well as ileostomy drainage. Water intake should be sufficient to maintain pale urine

(continued)

NURSING CARE OF THE PERSON having an ileostomy (continued)

and an output of at least 2.5 L per day. When exercising in hot weather, the person needs to consume extra water and salt. High-potassium foods, such as bananas and oranges, may also be recommended. *Loss of the reabsorptive surface of the large bowel increases the amount of water and sodium loss in the stool. If the ileostomy is high (more proximal in the ileum), additional potassium losses may also occur.*

- Discuss manifestations of fluid and electrolyte imbalances:
  a. Extreme thirst
  b. Dry skin and oral mucous membrane
  c. Decreased urine output
  d. Weakness, fatigue
  e. Muscle cramps
  f. Abdominal cramps, nausea, vomiting
  g. Shortness of breath
  h. Orthostatic hypotension (feeling faint when suddenly changing positions).
- Discuss dietary concerns. A low-residue diet is recommended initially (see Table 23.8). Foods causing excessive odour or gas are typically avoided as well. Because food blockage is a potential problem, high-fibre foods are limited and foods that may cause blockage, such as popcorn, corn, nuts, cucumbers, celery, fresh tomatoes, figs, strawberries, blackberries and caraway seeds, are avoided. *Symptoms of food blockage include abdominal cramping, swelling of the stoma and absence of ileostomy output for more than 4 to 6 hours.*
- Teach self-care measures to relieve food blockage:
  a. Take a warm shower or bath. *This can help relax the abdominal muscles.*
  b. Assume a knee–chest position. *The knee–chest position reduces intra-abdominal pressure.*
  c. Drink warm fluids or grape juice if not vomiting. *This provides a mild cathartic effect.*
  d. Massage peristomal area. *Massage may stimulate peristalsis and faecal elimination.*
  e. Remove pouch if the stoma is swollen and apply a pouch with a larger opening. *If the stoma swells, the pouch may create a mechanical obstruction to output.*
- Notify the doctor or stomal therapy nurse if:
  a. The above measures fail to relieve the obstruction.
  b. Signs of a partial obstruction persist, including high-volume odorous fluid output, abdominal cramps, nausea and vomiting.
  c. There is no ileostomy output for 4 to 6 hours.
  d. Clinical manifestations of fluid and electrolyte imbalance occur, such as weakness, dizziness, light-headedness or headache.

Should self-care measures not succeed in breaking up a blockage, ileostomy lavage, as described in Procedure 23.2, may be required.

TABLE 23.8 Low-residue diet

FOOD GROUP	ALLOWED	AVOID
Beverages	Coffee, teas, juices, carbonated beverages; milk limited to 300 mL per day	Alcohol, prune juice
Breads and cereals	Products made from refined flours (white bread, water crackers) or finely milled grains (e.g. cornflakes, rice bubbles, puffed wheat)	Wholegrain breads, rolls or cereal; breads or rolls with seeds, nuts or bran
Desserts	Gelatines, tapioca, plain custards or puddings; instant puddings; sponge cake; ice-cream or frozen desserts without fruit or nuts	Any desserts containing dried fruits, nuts, seeds or coconut; rich pastries, pies
Fruits	Fruit juices and strained fruits; cooked or canned apples, apricots, cherries, peaches, pears; bananas	All other raw or cooked fruits
Meats and other protein sources	Roasted, baked or grilled tender or minced beef, veal, pork, lamb, poultry or fish; smooth peanut butter; cottage, creamed cheese or mild cheddar cheeses in small amounts	Tough or spiced meats and those prepared by frying; highly flavoured cheeses; nuts
Potatoes, rice and pasta	Peeled potatoes; white rice; most pasta products	Potato skins, potato chips or fried potatoes; brown rice; wholegrain pasta products
Sweets	Sugar, honey, jelly, hard-boiled lollies and gumdrops, plain chocolates	Jam, marmalade; lollies made with seeds, nuts, coconut
Vegetables	Vegetable juices and strained vegetables; cooked or canned vegetables	Raw or whole cooked vegetables
Other	Salt, ground seasonings; cream sauce and plain gravy	Chilli sauce, horseradish; popcorn, seeds of any kind; whole spices, olives, vinegar

PROCEDURE 23.1 Changing a one- or two-piece drainable ostomy pouch

GATHER SUPPLIES

- Disposable gloves and personal protective equipment (PPE)
- One- or two-piece pouch
- Skin barrier paste
- Skin prep
- Clamp
- Pouch deodorant
- Measuring guide
- Adhesive remover
- Skin cleanser
- Wash cloths
- Plastic bag
- Bed protector
- Air freshener

BEFORE THE PROCEDURE

- Explain the procedure and provide for privacy.
- Position the person (assist as required) in a lying position making removing and applying the pouch easier.
- Use air freshener as required and preferred by the person.
- Follow standard precautions. Don PPE and gloves.

PROCEDURE

1. Remove soiled pouch (and the flange if a two-piece pouch) by gently pulling on the pouch or flange and pushing on skin. Use adhesive remover to remove skin barrier paste.
2. Empty pouch, discarding it and the flange (if applicable) in a plastic bag. Save the tail closure clamp. The pouch from a two-piece system may be cleaned out and reused.
3. Cleanse skin and stoma with warm water and skin cleanser or mild soap. Rinse skin and stoma and pat dry.
4. Note stoma colour and peristomal skin condition.
5. If necessary, clip or shave peristomal hair.
6. Use measuring guide or previous pattern to check size of stoma.
   a. Presized pouch: check to verify size is correct.
   b. Cut-to-fit pouch or flange: trace the correct size of the stoma onto the back of the flange and cut the opening to match the pattern. The opening should be no more than 3 to 4 mm larger than the stoma.
7. Apply skin prep to skin covered by a wafer, pouch or tape. Allow to dry.
8. Remove backings from pouch or flange.
9. Apply a bead of skin barrier paste around the stoma base or around the opening of the pouch or flange. Allow the paste to air dry for 1 to 2 minutes.
10. Centre the pouch or flange over the stoma and press to adhere.
11. For a two-piece pouch, snap the pouch onto the skin barrier flange.
12. Place deodorising powder or a few drops of liquid pouch deodoriser in the pouch. Apply the clamp.
13. 'Picture frame' the pouch with tape to provide extra security.

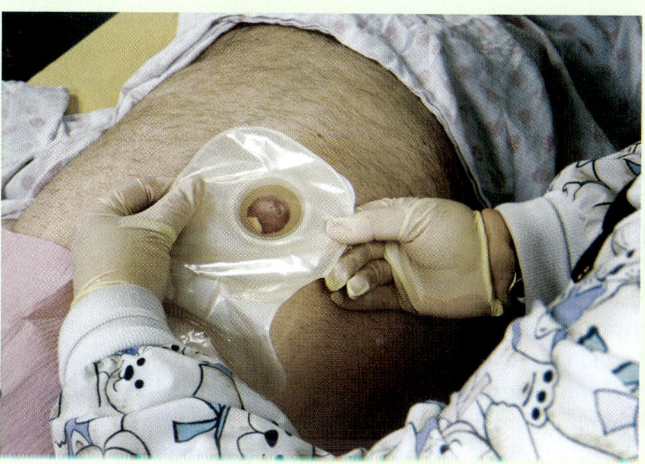

Source: Ron May/Pearson Education.

AFTER THE PROCEDURE

1. Leave the person comfortable.
2. Dispose of equipment correctly.
3. Document assessment of stoma and surrounding skin and the person's response to the procedure.

Anecdotal evidence supports the use of homeopathy to promote comfort in individuals with IBD. Acupuncture improves perceived wellbeing in people with IBD; however it does not appear to effect remission (Aginga, 2021). Many complementary and alternative therapies for IBD may interact with prescribed medications; advise the person to discuss all potential therapies with the primary care provider. Acupressure, body massage, reflexology, aromatherapy and stress reduction therapies can also aid in reducing manifestations of IBD.

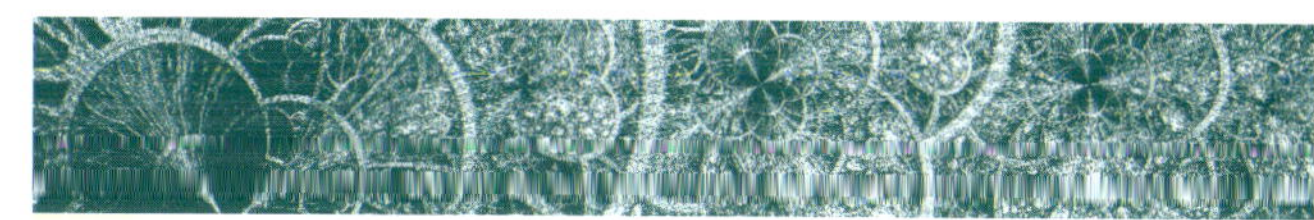

Nursing care

Health promotion

Although IBD cannot, at this time, be predicted or prevented, effective management may help the person avoid complications of the disease. Stress the importance of following the

PROCEDURE 23.2 Ileostomy lavage

GATHER SUPPLIES

- Disposable gloves and PPE
- Disposable irrigation sleeve
- 60 mL catheter-tipped syringe
- #14 Fr. catheter
- Water-soluble lubricant
- Normal saline for irrigation
- Bedpan
- Clean ostomy pouch
- Bed protector
- Air freshener

BEFORE THE PROCEDURE

- Explain the procedure and provide for privacy.
- Follow standard precautions.
- Don PPE and gloves.

PROCEDURE

1. Remove the pouch. Apply disposable irrigation sleeve.
2. Clamp the bottom of the sleeve or place it in the bedpan.
3. Gently examine stoma digitally to break up any faecal mass proximal to stoma and determine direction of the bowel.
4. Lubricate catheter and insert into stoma until blockage is reached. If the catheter does not reach the blockage after 8 to 10 cm, notify the doctor. This may indicate a more proximal obstruction.
5. Instil 30 to 50 mL normal saline.
6. Remove catheter. Allow stoma to drain.
7. Repeat the procedure until the mass is removed.
8. When the blockage is removed, remove the irrigation sleeve.
9. Clean peristomal skin.
10. Apply pouch and clamp.

AFTER THE PROCEDURE

1. Leave the person dry and comfortable.
2. Dispose of equipment correctly.
3. Document the procedure, amount of solution used, consistency of results and the person's response to the procedure.
4. Discuss dietary intake to help determine cause of blockage.

prescribed treatment regimen and promptly reporting manifestations of exacerbations to the doctor.

Assessment

Assessment data related to IBD include the following subjective and objective data:

- *Health history*: current manifestations, including onset, duration, severity (number of stools per day, presence of blood or mucus in stool, abdominal pain or cramping, tenesmus); usual diet, ability to maintain weight and nutrition, smoking habits, food intolerances; associated manifestations such as arthralgias, fatigue, malaise; current medications; previous treatment and diagnostic tests.
- *Physical examination*: general appearance; weight; vital signs, including orthostatic blood pressure, pulse and temperature; abdominal assessment, including shape, contour, bowel sounds, palpation for tenderness and masses, presence of stoma or scars.

Nursing diagnoses and interventions

When planning nursing care for the person with IBD, it is vital to consider the chronic, recurrent nature of the disorder. Religious and cultural beliefs must also be incorporated when planning care for a person with IBD. Teaching is a major aspect of care. Diarrhoea and disturbed body image are significant nursing care problems for a person with IBD. With severe disease, impaired nutrition must also be considered a priority problem. See accompanying nursing care plan for a person with ulcerative colitis.

Diarrhoea

During an acute exacerbation of IBD, diarrhoea can be frequent and painful. The frequency of defecation and associated abdominal pain and cramping may interfere with ADLs and increase the risk of fluid volume deficit and impaired skin integrity.

- Record the frequency, amount and colour of stools using a stool chart. Measure and record liquid stool as output. *The severity of diarrhoea is an indicator of the severity of the disease and helps determine the need for fluid replacement.*
- Monitor vital signs every 4 hours. *Tachycardia, tachypnoea and fever may be indicators of fluid volume deficit.*
- Weigh daily and record. *Rapid weight loss (over days to a week) usually indicates fluid loss, whereas weight loss over weeks to months may indicate malnutrition.*
- Assess for other indications of fluid deficit: warm, dry skin, poor skin turgor, dry shiny mucous membranes, weakness, lethargy, complaints of thirst. *The extent of fluid loss may not be readily evident with diarrhoea, particularly if the person uses the toilet without assistance. Systemic manifestations of fluid volume deficit may be the first indicators of the problem.*
- Maintain bowel rest by keeping NBM or limiting oral intake to elemental feedings as indicated. *Bowel rest during an acute exacerbation of IBD promotes healing and reduces diarrhoea and other manifestations.*

CONSIDERATION FOR PRACTICE

Observe stools for obvious blood and test for occult blood as indicated. Report grossly bloody stools (haematochezia), which may indicate haemorrhage and necessitate emergency surgery.

NURSING CARE PLAN A person with ulcerative colitis

Estelle Lewis is a 42-year-old real estate agent and mother of three school-age children. Mrs Lewis has had ulcerative colitis for 18 years and has been treated with prednisone and sulfasalazine. Over the past 4 months she has been having abdominal pain and cramping and frequent bloody diarrhoeal stools. During the same period, she lost 9 kg and has had difficulty maintaining her career. She recently developed several lesions of the lower leg identified as erythema nodosum. A recent colonoscopy revealed extensive involvement of the entire colon. On admission, Mrs Lewis states, 'I'm tired of fighting this disease. I am a prisoner in my home because of the diarrhoea.' She is admitted for a total proctocolectomy and ileal pouch–anal anastomosis.

ASSESSMENT

Janet Wheeler, RN, completes the admission assessment. Mrs Lewis weighs 52.2 kg. She complains of abdominal cramping, pain and frequent bloody diarrhoeal stools. Several reddened lesions are noted on her lower legs. Physical assessment findings include T 36.6°C, P 72, R 20 and BP 104/72. Skin, peripheries cool and pale. Abnormal laboratory findings include haemoglobin 73 g/L (normal 117 to 157 g/L); haematocrit 23.3% (normal 35–47%); WBC 15,580/mm^3 (normal 3,500 to 11,000/mm^3); platelet count 995,000/mm^3 (normal 150,000 to 450,000/mm^3); serum protein 46 g/L (normal 60 to 80 g/L); serum albumin 24 g/L (normal 35 to 50 g/L). Preparation for surgery is begun.

DIAGNOSES

- *Imbalanced nutrition: less than body requirements* related to impaired absorption.
- *Diarrhoea* related to inflammation of bowel.
- *Risk of deficient fluid volume* related to abnormal fluid loss.
- *Risk of impaired tissue integrity* related to drainage from temporary ileostomy.
- *Alteration in comfort* related to acute pain secondary to surgical intervention.
- *Risk of sexual dysfunction* related to temporary ileostomy.

PLANNING

When planning nursing care with Mrs Lewis, it is vital to consider her preferences. Religious and cultural beliefs are incorporated into her plan of care.

Expected outcomes

- Mrs Lewis will resume prescribed diet within 5 days after surgery.
- Mrs Lewis will demonstrate normal faecal elimination through the temporary ileostomy.
- Mrs Lewis will maintain adequate fluid balance.
- Mrs Lewis will demonstrate appropriate stoma care prior to discharge.
- Mrs Lewis will report a tolerable level of discomfort at rest and during activity.
- Mrs Lewis will verbalise feelings about sexuality and acknowledge importance of discussing sexual issues with partner.

IMPLEMENTATION

- Discuss with Mrs Lewis dietary modifications related to her nutritional status and presence of the ileostomy. Provide Mrs Lewis with a referral to a dietitian for diet planning and teaching.
- Explain to Mrs Lewis the importance of maintaining a high fluid intake and manifestations of dehydration.
- Teach Mrs Lewis to empty and change ileostomy pouch of choice.
- Teach Mrs Lewis stoma and peristomal skin assessment with each pouch change.
- Teach Mrs Lewis food blockage management.
- Provide Mrs Lewis with information about the Australian Stoma Appliance Scheme. It is subsidised by the Australian Government and provides stoma products (medicine and appliances) for people with a permanent or temporary stoma free of charge to members of one of the 22 approved volunteer stoma associations.
- Refer Mrs Lewis to local stoma association.

EVALUATION

On discharge, Mrs Lewis is caring for her ileostomy by demonstrating her ability to empty, rinse and change the pouch. The stomal therapy nurse provided written and verbal instructions on ileostomy care. Mrs Lewis verbalises her understanding of the recommended diet and the need to limit high-fibre food intake and avoid enteric-coated and timed-release medications. The stomal therapy nurse discusses sexual aspects of having an ileostomy and has given Mrs Lewis a booklet, *A Beginning Not an End*, available through the Australian Council of Stoma Associations. Mrs Lewis is looking forward to the planned surgery to close the temporary ileostomy.

CRITICAL THINKING IN THE NURSING PROCESS

1. Why is a person with an ileostomy at risk of dehydration? How can Mrs Lewis monitor her fluid status at home?
2. Why were Mrs Lewis' haemoglobin and haematocrit low on admission? If her haemoglobin had been low but her haematocrit normal on admission, what might be the explanation?
3. Outline a teaching plan Mrs Lewis could be given for home care of her ileostomy.
4. Develop a care plan for Mrs Lewis for the nursing diagnosis *Risk of impaired skin integrity*.

REFLECTION ON THE NURSING PROCESS

1. What are the most important things you feel you have learned from the care planning for Mrs Lewis?
2. If you were caring for a person following the formation of an ileostomy, what additional knowledge and clinical skills do you require to care for a person postoperatively?

- Administer prescribed anti-inflammatory and antidiarrhoeal medications as indicated. *Anti-inflammatory medications reduce the extent of bowel inflammation and diarrhoea. Unless contraindicated, antidiarrhoeal medications help reduce fluid loss and increase comfort.*

CONSIDERATION FOR PRACTICE

When antidiarrhoeal medications are administered to a person with ulcerative colitis, closely observe for manifestations of toxic megacolon: fever, tachycardia, hypotension, dehydration, abdominal pain and cramping, and an abrupt relief of diarrhoea.

- Maintain fluid intake by mouth or intravenously as indicated. *The person with IBD requires fluid to replace ongoing losses, as well as fluid to meet the usual daily needs of the body. If an elemental diet or total parenteral nutrition is prescribed, additional fluids may be required to meet fluid intake needs.*
- Provide good skin care. *Fluid deficit and tissue dehydration increase the risk of skin excoriations or breakdown.*
- Assess perianal area for irritation or denuded skin from the diarrhoea. Use gentle cleansing agents, such as Peri-Wash, nappy wipes or cotton lint-free gauze squares saturated with witch hazel. Apply a protective cream, such as zinc-oxide-based preparations, to protect skin from the irritating effects of diarrhoeal stool. *Digestive enzymes in the stool are very corrosive, increasing the risk of skin breakdown where exposed to diarrhoeal stool.*

Disturbed body image

A person with IBD may experience frustration at not being able to control, or even predict, faecal elimination, particularly when the disease is severe. Diarrhoea interferes with the ability to complete tasks, maintain employment, engage in social activities and even to meet basic needs such as eating, sleeping and sexual activity. Body image can suffer as a result. Treatment of IBD, be it total colectomy with ileal pouch–anal anastomosis, ileostomy or chronic corticosteroid therapy, can affect the view of self.

- Provide care in an accepting, non-judgmental manner. *Acceptance of the person despite potential embarrassment about odours or diarrhoea enhances self-esteem.*
- Accept feelings and perception of self. *Negating or denying the reality of the person's perception impairs trust.*
- Encourage discussion of physical changes and their consequences as they relate to self-concept. *This demonstrates acceptance and provides an opportunity to express the impact of the disease and its treatment on the person's life.*
- Encourage discussion about concerns regarding the effect of the disease or treatment on close personal relationships. *This demonstrates understanding and provides an opportunity for the person to express feelings about the impact of the disease on relationships and significant others.*
- Encourage the person to make choices and decisions regarding care. *This increases the person's sense of control over the disease and their future.*
- Discuss possible treatment options and their effects openly and honestly. *Open discussion allows more informed decisions.*
- Involve the person in their care, teaching and demonstrating as needed. *This encourages and facilitates independence and decision making.*
- Arrange for interaction with other individuals or groups of people with IBD or ostomies. *The person may feel that someone who has not experienced a similar problem cannot understand their feelings.*
- Teach coping strategies (e.g. odour control, dietary modifications) and support their use. *This facilitates healthy adaptation to the disease.*

Imbalanced nutrition: less than body requirements

Crohn's disease can significantly alter the bowel's ability to absorb nutrients. In both forms of IBD, blood and protein-rich fluid may be lost in diarrhoeal stools. With malabsorption and continuing nutrient losses, multiple nutrient deficits can develop, affecting growth and development, healing, muscle mass, bone density and electrolyte balances.

- Monitor laboratory results, including haemoglobin and haematocrit, serum electrolytes, and total serum protein and albumin levels. *These studies provide an indicator of nutritional status.*
- Provide the prescribed diet: high-kilojoule, high-protein, low-fat diet with restricted milk and milk products if lactose intolerance is present. *Kilojoules and protein are important to replace lost nutrients. Fat restriction helps reduce diarrhoea and nutrient loss, particularly when significant portions of the terminal ileum have been resected.*
- Provide parenteral nutrition as necessary if the person is unable to absorb enteral nutrients. *Parenteral nutrition helps reverse nutritional deficits and promotes weight gain and healing in the individual with acute manifestations.*
- Arrange for dietary consultation. Consider food preferences as allowed. *Providing preferred foods in the prescribed diet increases intake and supports nutritional status.*
- Provide or administer elemental enteral nutrition and supplements as ordered. *Elemental enteral nutritional supplements support healing while providing for bowel rest. These replace losses and improve nutritional status more rapidly than diet alone.*
- Include family members—the primary food preparer, especially—in teaching and dietary discussions. *Families can reinforce teaching and help the person maintain required restrictions or kilojoule intake.*

Community-based care

IBD is a chronic condition for which the person provides daily self-management. For this reason, teaching is a vital component of care. Teach the person and their family about:

- the type of IBD affecting the person, including the disease process, short- and long-term effects, the relationship of stress to disease exacerbations and the manifestations of complications
- prescribed medications, including drug names, desired effects, schedules for tapering the doses if ordered (as with corticosteroids), and possible side effects or adverse reactions and their management
- the recommended diet and the rationale for any specific restrictions
- use of nutritional supplements such as Ensure to maintain weight and nutritional status
- indicators of malabsorption and impaired nutrition; recommendations for self-care and when to seek medical intervention

- if discharged with a central venous catheter and home parenteral nutrition, written and verbal instructions on catheter care, troubleshooting and TPN administration (i.e. have the person and a family member demonstrate catheter care and TPN maintenance)
- the importance of maintaining a fluid intake of at least 2 to 3 L per day, and of increasing fluid intake during warm weather, exercise or strenuous work, and when fever is present
- the increased risk of colorectal cancer and the importance of regular bowel exams
- risks and benefits of various treatment options.

If surgery is planned or has been done, include the following topics in home care instructions:

- ileal pouch–anal anastomosis or ileostomy care as indicated
- where to obtain ostomy supplies
- use of non-prescription drugs, such as enteric-coated and timed-release capsules that may not be adequately absorbed before elimination through the ileostomy
- community and national ostomy support groups (see below).

Provide referrals to a nutritionist, a community healthcare agency, home care services and home intravenous care services as indicated. In addition, suggest the following resources:

- Crohn's & Colitis Australia
- Australian Council of Stoma Associations.

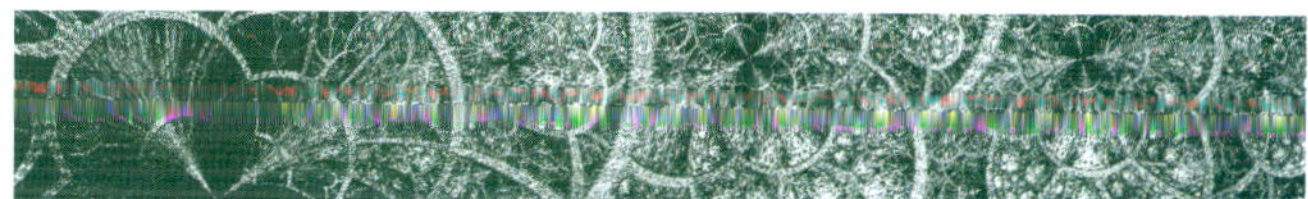

Malabsorption syndromes

Malabsorption is a condition in which the intestinal mucosa ineffectively absorbs nutrients—including carbohydrates, proteins, fats, water, electrolytes, minerals and vitamins—resulting in their excretion in the stool. Multiple bowel disorders can lead to malabsorption.

Diseases of the small intestine often cause malabsorption. Other medical and/or surgical conditions can result in malabsorption if these affect digestion or the intestinal mucosa. Primary diseases of the small-bowel mucosa, such as coeliac disease, Crohn's disease and acute gastrointestional tract infections, can lead to malabsorption. It can also result from maldigestion (inadequate preparation of chyme for absorption). For example, major gastric resections, pancreatic disorders with impaired pancreatic enzyme secretion and biliary disorders affecting bile secretion impair digestion and absorption of chyme. Selected causes of impaired absorption and digestion are listed in Table 23.9.

TABLE 23.9 Selected causes of malabsorption

CAUSE	RELATED FACTORS OR CONDITIONS
Impaired absorption	Tropical sprue
	Short bowel syndrome
	Acute enteritis and other bowel infections or infestations
	AIDS-related opportunistic infections and Kaposi's sarcoma
	Coeliac disease (non-tropical sprue)
	Crohn's disease
	Intestinal ischaemia or infarction
	Scleroderma
Impaired digestion	Lactose intolerance
	Gastrectomy
	Chronic pancreatitis, cancer of the pancreas
	Cystic fibrosis
	Biliary obstruction
	Cirrhosis, hepatitis or liver failure
	Zollinger–Ellison syndrome

Regardless of the cause, malabsorption causes common manifestations resulting from impaired absorption of chyme and the nutrients it contains (see Table 23.10). Predominant GI manifestations include anorexia; abdominal bloating; diarrhoea with loose, bulky, foul-smelling stools; and steatorrhoea (fatty stools). Weight loss, weakness, general malaise, muscle cramps, bone pain, abnormal bleeding and anaemia are common systemic manifestations of malabsorption. These manifestations result from malnutrition and fluid loss due to poor absorption.

Three common malabsorption disorders in adults are coeliac disease (non-tropical sprue), lactose intolerance and short bowel syndrome.

THE PERSON WITH SPRUE

Sprue is a chronic primary disorder of the small intestine in which the absorption of nutrients, particularly fats, is impaired. The severity of the disease depends on the extent of mucosal involvement in the intestine and the duration of the disease. Two major forms of sprue are coeliac disease (coeliac or non-tropical sprue) and tropical sprue.

Pathophysiology

Most absorption of nutrients occurs in the small intestine. The mucosa of the small intestine is arranged in microscopic folds, containing even smaller finger-like projections called *villi*. The cells of the villi are covered with microscopic hairs, *microvilli*, projecting from the cell membrane. The folds, villi and microvilli of the intestinal mucosa provide a huge surface area for nutrient absorption. Cells of the intestines are specialised to absorb different nutrients. Readily digested nutrients are absorbed in the proximal intestine; others are absorbed more distally in the intestines. Nutrients are absorbed by the processes of simple diffusion (water and small lipids), facilitated diffusion (water-soluble vitamins) and active transport

TABLE 23.10 Local and systemic manifestations of malabsorption

CATEGORY	MANIFESTATION	CAUSE
Local (GI)	Diarrhoea	Disruption of bowel mucosa impairing absorption of fluid and electrolytes, leading to excess water in the stool
	Abdominal distension	Gas formation from fermentation of undigested carbohydrates
	Steatorrhoea	Impaired fat absorption, leading to excess fat in faeces
Systemic	Weight loss	Carbohydrate, protein and fat deficit
	Weakness and malaise	Kilojoule deficit, anaemia, fluid and electrolyte losses
	Anaemia	Vitamin B_{12}, folic acid and iron deficits
	Bone pain	Calcium and vitamin D deficits
	Muscle cramps, paraesthesias	Protein wasting, vitamin B_{12} and electrolyte deficits
	Easy bruising and bleeding	Vitamin K deficit
	Glossitis, cheilosis	Iron, folic acid and vitamin B_{12} deficits

(glucose and amino acids). Once absorbed into the cells of the villi, nutrients enter the blood or lymph for systemic distribution.

Sprue is characterised by flattening of the intestinal mucosa with a loss of villi and microvilli. With the loss of villi, intestinal absorptive surface is lost and digestive enzyme production, including disaccharidase and particularly lactase, is reduced.

Coeliac disease

Coeliac disease, also known as *coeliac sprue* or *non-tropical sprue* and *gluten-sensitive enteropathy*, is a chronic immune-mediated malabsorption disorder characterised by sensitivity to the gliadin fraction of gluten, a cereal protein. Gluten is found in wheat, rye, barley and oats. It is also used as filler in many prepared foods and in medications. The cause of coeliac disease is unknown; however, genetic, environmental and immune factors are known to play a role in its development. The development of coeliac disease involves a particular genetic make-up (HLA type), with the genes HLA-DQ2 and HLA-DQ8 being identified as the 'coeliac genes' (Marieb & Hoehn, 2019). Environmental factors also play a role. Coeliac disease was considered a rare malabsorption syndrome manifesting during early childhood; however, it is one of the most common genetic diseases, with a mean prevalence of 1% in susceptible populations (Marieb & Hoehn, 2019).

In coeliac disease, it appears that the intestinal mucosa is damaged by an immunological response. Gliadin acts as an antigen (a substance inducing the formation of antibodies interacting specifically with it), prompting an inappropriate T-cell-mediated immune response. People with coeliac disease have increased antibodies to other antigens as well. The immune response prompts an inflammatory response in the small bowel, resulting in loss of intestinal folds and absorptive surface. Digestive enzyme production, including disaccharidase and particularly lactase, is reduced. The proximal small bowel is affected to the greatest extent, likely due to its greater exposure to dietary gluten.

Manifestations

Manifestations of coeliac sprue may develop at any age. Local manifestations include abdominal bloating and cramps, diarrhoea and steatorrhoea. Systemic manifestations result from the effects of malabsorption and resulting deficiencies. Anaemia is common. People with coeliac disease are often small in stature and may have delayed maturity. Other signs of nutrient deficiencies include tetany, vitamin deficiencies, muscle wasting and osteomalacia (impaired bone development). When gluten is removed from the diet, these manifestations resolve.

Gastrointestinal malignancies and intestinal lymphoma are potential complications of coeliac disease. Other complications include intestinal ulceration and development of refractory sprue or disease no longer responding to a gluten-free diet.

Tropical sprue

Tropical sprue is a chronic disease of unknown cause, although bacterial infection or toxins are thought to contribute. It seems likely that tropical sprue is not a single disease, but rather a pathophysiological process with manifestations resulting from a combination of the initial infection and the person's diet, living standards and genetic predisposition. A milder form of this may lead to asymptomatic abnormalities referred to as tropical enteropathy, while more severe expression leads to debilitating tropical sprue syndrome. The nature and the extent of the nutritional deficiencies are likely to be related to the duration of the disease and the extent of bowel involved (Beeching & Beadsworth, 2018). Tropical sprue occurs chiefly in the Caribbean, south India and South-East Asia. Hanson (2005) described three cases of tropical sprue in Indigenous children living in remote communities in far north Queensland. A number of studies of chronic diarrhoea in Aboriginal and Torres Strait Islander children have documented partial villous atrophy on small bowel biopsy. Additionally, other studies identified higher colony counts and more frequent isolation of Gram-negative organisms in duodenal aspirates from Aboriginal and Torres Strait Islander children with chronic diarrhoea. Some of these studies, Hanson (2005) noted, had similarity with contemporary Indian studies of tropical sprue, suggesting that tropical sprue should be considered in people from remote Aboriginal or Torres Strait Islander communities presenting with weight loss, diarrhoea and nutritional deficiency. The pathophysiological changes in bowel mucosa closely resemble those of coeliac sprue, although gluten intake has no effect on this condition. Its onset may be abrupt or insidious.

Manifestations

Clinical manifestations of tropical sprue include sore tongue, diarrhoea and weight loss. Initially, diarrhoea may be explosive and watery; as the disease progresses, stools become fewer in number and more solid with obvious steatorrhoea. Folic acid deficiency is common. Vitamin B_{12} and iron deficiencies may occur, resulting in glossitis; stomatitis; dry, rough skin; and anaemia.

INTERPROFESSIONAL CARE

With any malabsorptive disorder, the initial focus of management is to identify the cause. Once this has been determined, specific therapy can be prescribed.

Diagnosis

Laboratory and diagnostic testing are used to make the differential diagnosis for various causes of malabsorption syndromes and determine the severity of nutrient deficiencies.

An endoscopy permits direct examination of intestinal mucosa and collection of a tissue specimen for biopsy. Upper GI series with small-bowel follow-through may be done to evaluate the structures of the upper GI tract. With sprue, the typical 'feathery' pattern of barium in the small bowel is lost and the barium may precipitate and clump. Nursing implications of diagnostic tests are included in the chapter 'A person-centred approach to assessing the gastrointestinal system'.

Laboratory tests are used to identify pathophysiological effects and monitor concordance with the prescribed diet. Faecal fat is measured to document the presence of steatorrhoea. The expected result is 2 to 7 g per 24 hours for adults (Kee, 2018). The fat content of stool is increased in many malabsorptive disorders, including coeliac and tropical sprue. Serological testing for IgA endomysial antibodies and IgG and IgA antigliadin antibodies is used to diagnose coeliac disease and evaluate concordance with the prescribed gluten-free diet. Serum levels of protein, albumin, cholesterol, electrolytes and iron may be ordered to evaluate for nutrient deficiencies. The haemoglobin, haematocrit and RBC indices are used to evaluate anaemia. Prothrombin time is increased in vitamin K deficiency.

Medications

Individuals with severe nutritional deficits require vitamin and mineral supplements, as well as iron and folic acid to correct anaemia. Vitamin K may be administered parenterally if the prothrombin time is prolonged. In those whose disease fails to respond to dietary management, corticosteroids may be ordered to suppress the inflammatory response.

Tropical sprue is treated with a combination of folic acid and tetracyclines. This regimen is continued for 3 to 6 months.

Nutrition

An individual with coeliac disease is placed on a gluten-free diet. People with coeliac disease require a strict gluten-free diet irrespective of clinical manifestations of the disease. This treatment is generally successful, as long as the individual avoids gluten totally. However, gluten is so widely used in prepared foods that this is no easy task. In Australia, food labelled gluten-free contains no detectable gluten, oats or malt, and most packaged food containing grain (wheat, rye, oats or barley (Coeliac Australia, n.d.)) must list gluten. Individuals need to be aware of hidden sources of gluten and to analyse dietary labels. Coeliac Australia (n.d.) warns that alcoholic beverage labels are not required to list ingredients derived from gluten-containing grain, and highlights that all regular beers contain gluten. Common sources of gluten and foods to be avoided are indicated in Table 23.11.

Consultation with a nutritionist to obtain detailed dietary instructions is necessary.

TABLE 23.11 Dietary sources of gluten

FOOD GROUP	CONTAINS GLUTEN	MAY CONTAIN GLUTEN
Cereals, grains and grain products	Bread, biscuits, cereal and pasta containing wheat, rye or barley grain or flour	Seasoned rice and potato mixes
Beverages	Malt, Milo, Ovaltine, beers and ales	Commercial chocolate milk, cocoa and other beverage mixes, such as instant tea mix, dietary supplements
Desserts	Cakes, biscuits and pastries made with wheat, rye or barley flour	Commercial ice-cream and gelato
Meats and other protein sources		Meat loaf, manufactured and prepared meats, crumbed meats and fish; cheese products; soy protein meat substitutes; commercial egg products
Fruits and vegetables		Commercial seasoned vegetable mixes or vegetables with sauce, canned baked beans; commercial pie fillings
Miscellaneous		Commercial salad dressings and mayonnaise; tomato sauce and prepared mustard; gravy, white sauce; non-dairy creamer; syrups; commercial pickles

The prescribed diet is high in kilojoules and protein to correct nutrient deficits. Fat content is restricted to minimise steatorrhoea. Initially, the diet is usually restricted in lactose as well to compensate for the loss of lactase-containing microvilli. Foods containing lactose may be reintroduced once remission has occurred (Marieb & Hoehn, 2019).

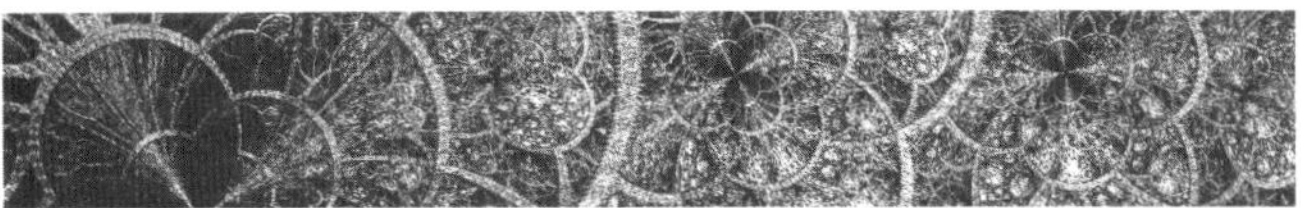

Nursing care

Nursing care of a person with sprue (tropical and non-tropical) focuses on the effects of the disorder on health and nutrition, as well as the person's ability to manage their disease.

Assessment

- *Health history*: onset, duration and severity of manifestations; number and character of stools; history of travel to the Caribbean, southern India or South-East Asia, or living in remote communities in northern Queensland; previous teaching related to the disorder; current treatment and diet.
- *Physical examination*: vital signs; abdominal shape, contour, bowel sounds; manifestations of malnutrition (e.g. anaemia, small stature, muscle wasting, signs of other nutrient deficiencies).

Nursing diagnoses and interventions

Diarrhoea and malnutrition are significant problems for a person with sprue and the priority foci for nursing intervention.

Diarrhoea

Steatorrhoea and diarrhoea typically occur with sprue because fat, water and other nutrients are poorly absorbed, remaining in the bowel to be eliminated in the stool. Diarrhoea interferes with lifestyle, ADLs, skin integrity, and fluid and electrolyte balance.

- Assess and document the frequency and nature of stools. *Bowel elimination reflects the severity of the disease and efficacy of treatment. With effective treatment, stools become less frequent and more normal in colour and appearance.*
- Weigh daily, monitor intake and output, and assess skin turgor and mucous membranes for indications of fluid balance. *Diarrhoea increases the risk of hypovolaemia and dehydration resulting from excess fluid loss in the stool.*
- Assess and document perianal skin condition. *Frequent defecation irritates skin and mucous membranes, increasing the risk of breakdown.*
- Encourage a liberal fluid intake. *Oral fluids help replace fluid lost through diarrhoeal stool.*

Imbalanced nutrition: less than body requirements

Coeliac disease is a chronic condition. With continuing malabsorption, multiple nutrient deficits may occur, resulting in impaired growth and development, impaired healing, muscle wasting, bone disease and electrolyte imbalances.

- Maintain accurate dietary intake records. *Assessment of dietary intake provides information about compliance with the prescribed diet as well as the adequacy of nutrient intake.*
- Monitor laboratory results, including haemoglobin and haematocrit, serum electrolytes, total serum protein and albumin levels. *These studies provide information about nutritional status.*
- Arrange for nutritionist consultation. Provide for food preferences as allowed. *An individualised diet developed to address the person's food preferences as well as nutrient needs will promote appetite and food intake.*
- Provide the prescribed high-kilojoule, high-protein, low-fat, gluten-free diet for the person with coeliac disease. Restrict lactose (dairy product) intake as indicated. *Kilojoules and protein are important to replace lost nutrients. Fat restriction helps reduce diarrhoea and nutrient loss. Lactose may be restricted during initial treatment and then slowly reintroduced into the diet as the gut heals and its normal structure is restored.*
- Provide parenteral nutrition as ordered if the person is unable to absorb enteral nutrients. *Parenteral nutrition can help reverse nutritional deficits and promote weight gain when manifestations are acute.*
- Encourage nutritional supplements. *Nutritional supplements often are necessary to replace losses and restore nutrient levels to normal more rapidly than diet alone can achieve.*
- Include family members—the primary food preparer, in particular—in teaching and dietary discussions. *Families can reinforce teaching and help the person maintain required restrictions or kilojoule intake.*

Community-based care

Although tropical sprue is treated with antibiotic and folic acid therapy, *a person with coeliac sprue has a chronic condition requiring lifelong dietary management.* Encourage the person to join the Coeliac Australia. Coeliac Australia provides information, including the availability of gluten-free foods, recipes and support, for individuals with coeliac disease and their families.

Provide a detailed list of foods containing gluten which need to be eliminated from the person's diet, as well as foods that are allowed. Teach the person and their family how to identify gluten-containing commercial products by reading labels and lists of ingredients. Encourage the purchase and use of a gluten-free cookbook.

If corticosteroids are prescribed, stress the importance of taking the medication as ordered. Emphasise the need to avoid stopping the medication abruptly and to notify all caregivers that a corticosteroid is part of the individual's medication regimen. Instruct to monitor weight frequently. A weight gain of 2.3 kg or more in less than a week usually reflects fluid gain, a possible adverse effect of corticosteroids. Other potential effects include decreased resistance to infection, an impaired inflammatory response and changes in carbohydrates, protein and fat metabolism.

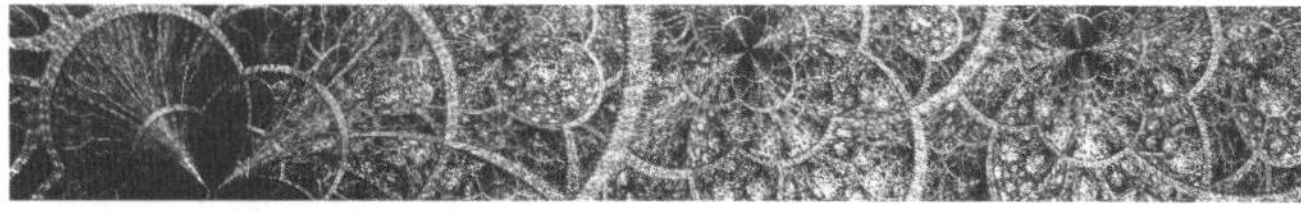

THE PERSON WITH LACTASE DEFICIENCY

For carbohydrates to be absorbed from the small intestine, they first must be broken down into simple sugars (monosaccharides). Lactose is the primary carbohydrate in milk and milk products. It is a disaccharide, requiring the enzyme lactase for digestion and absorption. Lactase deficiency leads to lactose intolerance and manifestations of malabsorption. Lactase deficiency is usually genetic in origin, but also occurs secondarily to coeliac disease, Crohn's disease and other disorders affecting the mucosa of the small intestine. There is a racial/ethnic component to the disorder; it is rare for Caucasians to develop lactose intolerance. However, it is common among people from Asia, Africa, the Middle East and some Mediterranean countries, as well as Aboriginal and Torres Strait Islander people (Alkalay, 2021).

Manifestations

Many people with lactase deficiency are asymptomatic. Small to moderate amounts of milk (250 mL) may be well tolerated. Manifestations of lactose intolerance include lower abdominal cramping, pain and diarrhoea following milk ingestion. Undigested lactose ferments in the intestine, forming gases and contributing to bloating and flatus. Lactic and fatty acids produced by this fermentation irritate the bowel, leading to increased motility and abdominal cramping. The undigested lactose draws water into the intestine, leading to increased motility and diarrhoea. The diarrhoea associated with lactose intolerance may be explosive.

INTERPROFESSIONAL CARE

The diagnosis of lactose intolerance is usually based on a history of intolerance to milk and milk products and a trial of a lactose-free diet. If manifestations resolve when lactose intake is eliminated, the diagnosis of lactose intolerance is confirmed.

Diagnosis

The lactose breath test is a non-invasive test used to diagnose lactose intolerance. Expired hydrogen gas (H_2) is measured following oral administration of 50 g of lactose. If lactose is digested and absorbed normally, then little change occurs in the amount of exhaled H_2 from fasting to post lactose administration. With lactose intolerance, exhaled H_2 increases following lactose administration as the sugar ferments in the bowel.

For the *lactose tolerance test*, 100 g of lactose solution is orally administered, followed by measurement of blood glucose levels at intervals of 30, 60 and 120 minutes. If lactose is digested and absorbed normally, the blood glucose rises more than 20 mg/dL. The expected blood glucose elevation does not occur in lactose intolerance.

Nutrition

A lactose free or reduced lactose diet relieves the manifestations of the disorder. Some people require total elimination of milk and milk products from the diet. Many can tolerate limited amounts of lactose. Avoid low-fat or non-fat milk as they travel quickly through the gut and tend to cause symptoms in those who are lactose intolerant. Also, many low-fat milk products contain skim-milk powder, providing a higher lactose dose. The fat content in full-cream milk slows the absorption of the milk through the intestines, allowing the lactase enzymes more time to break down the sugars. Milk pre-treated with lactase is available. Non-prescription lactase enzyme preparations are available to improve milk tolerance. Yoghurt containing bacterial lactases may be well tolerated. Soy foods are lactose free and provide a good substitute source of calcium. Calcium supplements are often recommended, particularly for women on a reduced-lactose or lactose-free diet.

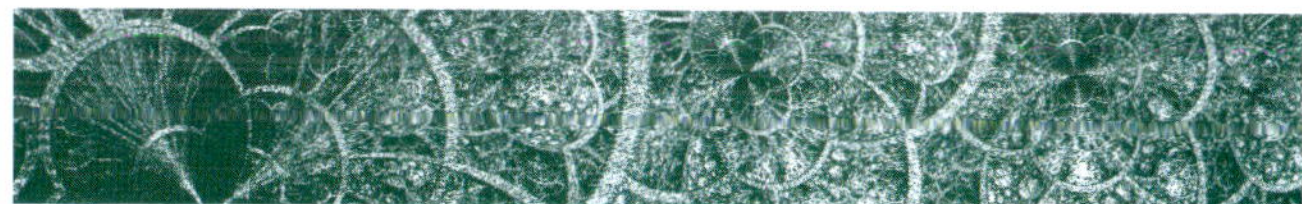

Nursing care

Nursing care for a person with lactose intolerance focuses on providing education and support. Discuss sources of lactose: milk, ice-cream and cottage cheese are high in lactose; aged cheese and yoghurt contain much smaller amounts. Potential hidden sources of lactose include desserts made from milk and milk chocolate, sauces and gravies, and cream soups. Suggest a trial of lactase-treated milk or lactase enzyme supplements. Emphasise the importance of obtaining nutrients contained in dairy products from other sources. Proteins may be obtained from meats, eggs, legumes and grains. Other sources of calcium include soy products, sardines, oysters and salmon, and plant sources such as beans, cauliflower, rhubarb and green leafy vegetables.

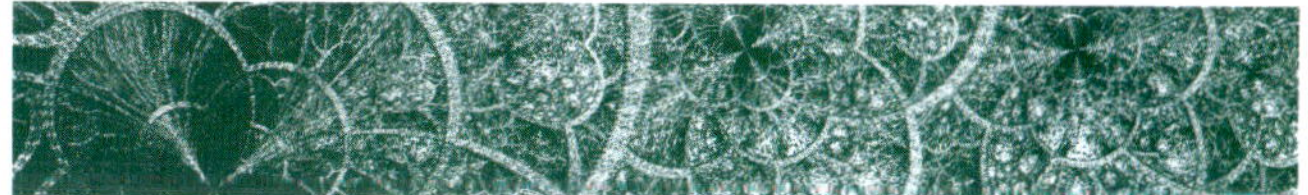

THE PERSON WITH SHORT BOWEL SYNDROME

The small bowel may be resected due to tumours, infarction of bowel mucosa, incarcerated hernias, Crohn's disease, trauma and enteropathy resulting from radiation therapy. Resection of significant portions of the small intestine may result in a condition known as *short bowel syndrome*. The severity of the disorder depends on the total amount of bowel resected, as well as the portions of bowel removed. Removal of the proximal portions, including the duodenum, jejunum and proximal ileum, and of the distal portion of the ileum is associated with more severe malabsorption and manifestations than is resection of mid portions of the ileum.

Resection of the small intestine affects the absorption of water, nutrients, vitamins and minerals. Transit time of ingested foods and fluids is reduced and digestive processes are impaired. The bowel undergoes an adaptive process in which the remaining villi enlarge and lengthen to increase the absorptive surface following resection. For many people, absorption and bowel function return to preoperative or near-normal levels. Others continue to have significant impairment of digestion and absorption, leading to nutrient deficiencies, weight loss and diarrhoea.

INTERPROFESSIONAL CARE

Management of short bowel syndrome focuses on alleviating manifestations. The person often requires frequent, small, high-kilojoule and high-protein meals.

Diagnosis

Laboratory and diagnostic studies are used to evaluate nutrient deficiencies. Total serum proteins and albumin are reduced, as are serum levels of folate, iron, vitamins, minerals and electrolytes. Anaemia and a prolonged prothrombin time (indicative of vitamin K deficiency) may develop.

Medications

Multivitamin and mineral supplementation are also frequently necessary. Antidiarrhoeal medications are used to reduce bowel motility, allowing a greater amount of time for nutrient absorption. Some people are affected by gastric hypersecretion following bowel resection. For these individuals, a proton-pump inhibitor such as omeprazole (Losec) may be ordered. Individuals with severe manifestations of short bowel syndrome may require TPN.

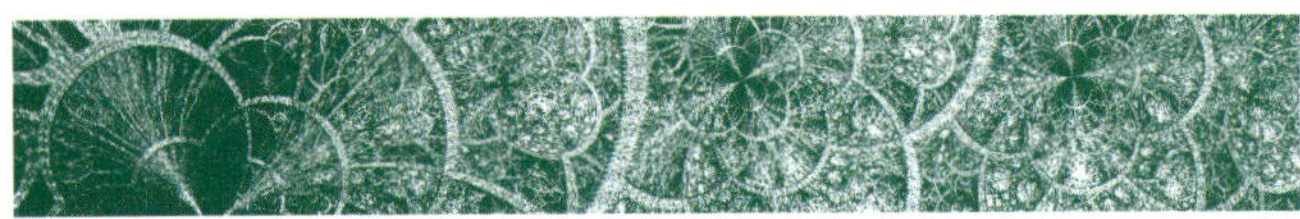

Nursing care

Nursing care for a person with short bowel syndrome focuses on the problems of potential fluid volume deficit, malnutrition and diarrhoea.

Fluid losses are generally greatest in the initial periods following surgery, warranting the closest attention during that time. Close monitoring of vital signs, intake and output, daily weights, skin turgor and condition of mucous membranes is vital. It is important to remember the risk is also high when other abnormal fluid losses occur through, for example, fever, wound drainage or excessive diaphoresis.

Documentation of nutritional status includes weight, anthropometric measurements, laboratory values and kilojoule intake. Provide nutritional supplementation with enteral feedings as needed. Maintain central lines and TPN, using aseptic technique.

For diarrhoea, document the number, volume and character of stools. Administer antidiarrhoeal medications as ordered. If the person is lactose intolerant, limit intake of milk and milk products. Provide good skin care for the perianal region to prevent breakdown from frequent bowel movements. Refer to the discussion of nursing care for a person with coeliac disease for other measures for altered nutrition and diarrhoea.

A person affected by this condition and their family require extensive education. Because there is no way to cure or replace the lost bowel, the individual must manage the disorder on a daily basis. Provide instructions about the recommended diet and medication regimen. Emphasise the importance of maintaining an adequate fluid intake, particularly in hot weather or during strenuous exercise. Teach the person to monitor their weight frequently and report changes. Include teaching about possible manifestations of dehydration and nutrient deficiencies to be reported to the doctor. Referring the person to a nutritionist or counsellor helps the person manage and cope with what will be a lifelong condition.

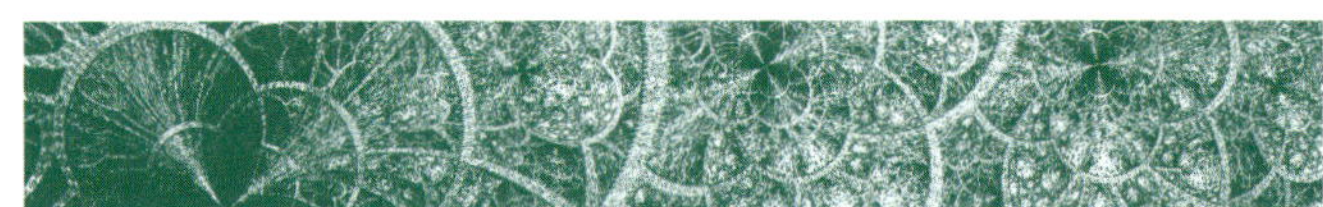

Neoplastic disorders

Cancer is one of the top five causes of death in Australia (Australian Institute of Health and Welfare (AIHW), 2021). Although cancer may affect any portion of the digestive tract, the large intestine and rectum are common sites. Colorectal cancer comprises cancers of the colon and rectum, the two main sections of the large bowel. Colorectal cancer is the third most commonly diagnosed cancer in males and the second most commonly diagnosed cancer in woman, making it a significant healthcare concern (AIHW, 2018).

THE PERSON WITH POLYPS

A *polyp* is a mass of tissue arising from the bowel wall and protruding into the lumen. Polyps may develop in any portion of the bowel, occurring most often in the sigmoid colon and rectum. They vary considerably in size and may be single or multiple. It is estimated that approximately 30% of people over the age of 50 have polyps. Although most polyps are benign, some have the potential to become malignant. Familial adenomatous polyposis (FAP) is a syndrome with a dominant inheritance pattern leading to hundreds to thousands of adenomatous polyps developing. Some of these polyps inevitably become malignant (Loscalzo et al., 2022).

Pathophysiology

Polyps are identified by their structure and tissue type. Most polyps are adenomas, benign epithelial tumours considered premalignant lesions. More than 95% of adenocarcinomas arise from adenomas. However, less than 1% of polyps become malignant (Gastroenterological Society of Australia (GSA), 2022). Of polyps removed during colonoscopy, more than 70% are adenomatous (Shussman & Wexner, 2014).

Adenomatous polyps represent disruption of the normal process of cell proliferation to replace epithelial cells lining the intestine. Cells are constantly being reproduced to replace those shed as faeces move through the colon. Disruption of the normal process of cell division and maturation lead to formation of a polyp composed of tightly packed epithelial cells. The cells may appear grossly normal or show signs of dysplasia. Polyps may develop as tubular, villous or tubulovillous adenomas. Polyps are named by the way they are attached to the bowel wall as either sessile (raised nodules) or pedunculated (attached by a stalk) (see Figure 23.13).

Tubular adenomas (also called pedunculated polyps) are more common than sessile polyps and account for about 65% of benign polyps of the large intestine (Marieb & Hoehn, 2019). A tubular adenoma is a globe-like structure attached to the intestinal wall by a thin, stalk-like stem. The incidence of this type of polyp increases with age, although it occurs in all age groups and in both genders. Most are small, 1 cm or less in diameter, although they may be as large as 4 to 5 cm. The malignant potential of these polyps seems to be related to their size. Adenomas smaller than 1 cm have a low risk of being malignant; adenomas larger than 1 cm have a much higher risk of harbouring malignancy or a high-grade dysplasia. Adenomatous polyps are present in 35% of adults over 50 years of age (Shussman & Wexner, 2014).

Villous adenomas (also called sessile polyps) are broad based with an elevated, cauliflower-like surface (see Figure 23.13B). These typically develop in the rectosigmoid colon. This type of polyp is often larger than tubular adenomas; usually more than 5 cm. Villous adenomas are not common, accounting for about 10% of colon polyps. These have a higher malignant potential than tubular adenomas. Some adenomatous polyps, known as *tubulovillous adenomas*, contain both tubular epithelium and villi.

Manifestations

Most polyps are asymptomatic, found coincidentally during routine examination or diagnostic testing. Intermittent painless bright or dark red rectal bleeding is the most common presenting complaint. A large polyp may cause abdominal cramping, pain or manifestations of obstruction. Diarrhoea and mucus discharge are associated with a large villous adenoma.

INTERPROFESSIONAL CARE

The diagnosis of intestinal polyps is generally based on diagnostic studies such as sigmoidoscopy or colonoscopy. A rectal polyp may be palpable on digital examination. However, further studies are necessary to determine its size and type and the extent of colon involvement and to assess for malignancy.

Once identified, polyps are removed because of the risk of malignancy. Pedunculated polyps and small villous lesions may be removed during colonoscopy using an electrocautery snare or hot biopsy forceps passed through the scope. This relatively safe procedure has less than a 2% risk of complications such as perforation or haemorrhage. Large villous adenomas are completely excised and examined histologically for evidence of malignancy. In some cases, the colon segment containing the polyp is resected. A person with FAP usually undergoes a total colectomy with ileorectal anastomosis before age 20 years to significantly reduce their risk of developing colon cancer.

Treatment following polypectomy depends on histological examination of the excised tissue. Because polyps tend to

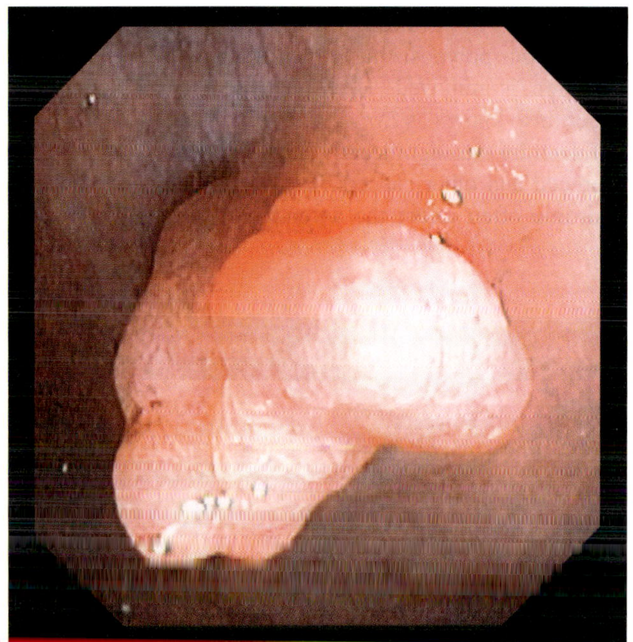

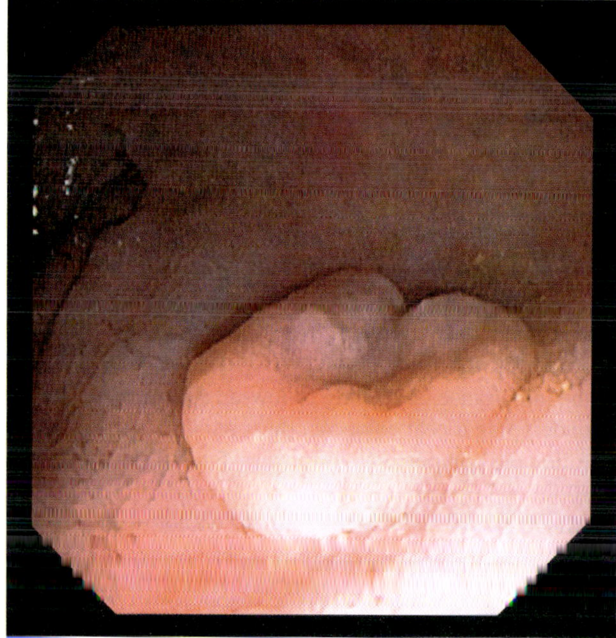

FIGURE 23.13 *A, Tubular (or pedunculated) polyps; B, villous (or sessile) polyps*

Source: © David M. Martin MD/Science Photo Library.

recur, follow-up colonoscopy is recommended in 3 years and then every 5 years if no further polyps are detected. When the polyp is found to be malignant, follow-up care is determined by the tissue type and degree of invasion.

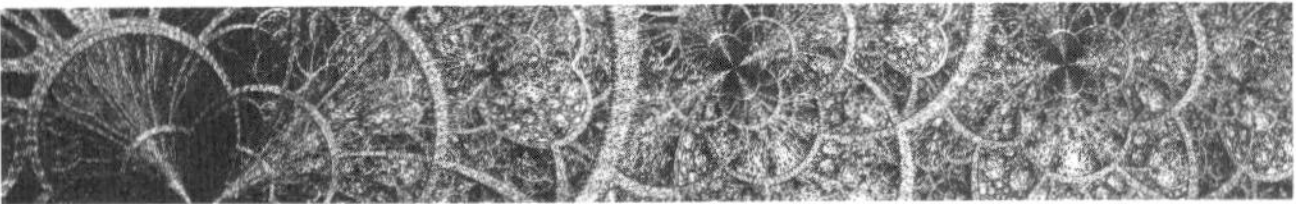

Nursing care

Health promotion

The incidence of intestinal polyps increases with age. They affect men and women equally. It is believed an adenomatous polyp requires more than 5 years of growth to become significant in size and malignant potential. Advise the individual to have a screening for colorectal cancer (with a colonoscopy being the 'gold standard' for diagnosis) at age 50 and as recommended thereafter for early detection of polyps (AIHW, 2021).

Assessment

Polyps are a 'silent' disease, with few or no manifestations.

- *Health history*: rectal bleeding; personal or family history of intestinal polyps or colorectal cancer.

Nursing diagnoses and interventions

Nursing care for a person with polyps focuses on informing and assisting the person through diagnostic testing and polyp removal. Before and after the colonoscopy and polypectomy, provide direct care and teaching about the procedure, expected sensations during the procedure and anticipated postoperative care. Cathartics are prescribed prior to colonoscopy; cleansing enemas may also be ordered. Observe for evidence of fluid and electrolyte imbalance during preoperative preparation. If enemas are ordered, use normal saline (not tap water) to reduce the risk of electrolyte imbalances. Following polypectomy, observe closely for possible complications such as haemorrhage.

Community-based care

Include the following topics when teaching for home care:

- the significance of polyps and their relationship to colorectal cancer
- the importance of keeping follow-up appointments and undergoing repeat colonoscopy as recommended: at 3 years following polypectomy, then every 5 to 10 years unless additional polyps are found
- manifestations to be reported to the doctor, such as diarrhoea, pain, rectal bleeding, light-headedness or other indications of possible blood loss.

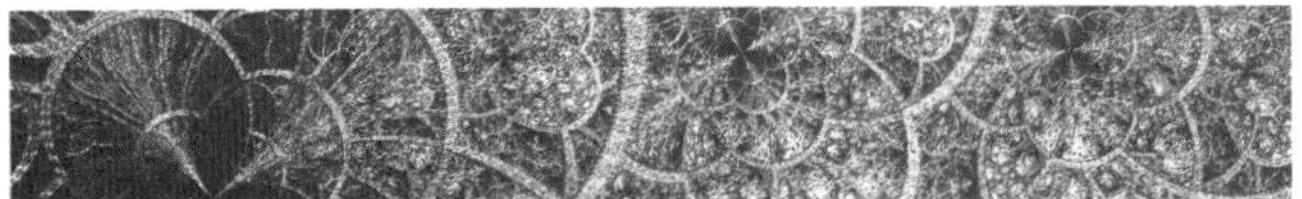

THE PERSON WITH COLORECTAL CANCER

In 2021, it was estimated that almost 16,000 (8,300 males and 7,413 females) were diagnosed with colorectal cancer (AIHW, 2021). Colorectal cancer occurs most frequently after age 50. The incidence continues to rise with increasing age.

Bowel cancer accounts for 8.6% of all deaths from invasive cancers, with 4,114 deaths in 2017, making it the second most common cause of cancer-related death after lung cancer (AIHW, 2018). Unfortunately, there is no national data on the incidence of colorectal cancer in Aboriginal and Torres Strait Islander people as not all states and territories record the incidence of cancer in Indigenous Australians. However, where the incidence of cancer is recorded specifically for Aboriginal and Torres Strait Islander people, colorectal cancer is a commonly occurring cancer in Indigenous men. Cancer has a greater impact on Aboriginal and Torres Strait Islander people, who are less likely to have an early diagnosis and receive adequate treatment such as preventive, curative and palliative services (AIHW, 2021).

Earlier diagnosis and improved treatment have improved the survival rate for colorectal cancer. With early diagnosis and treatment, the 5-year survival rate for colorectal cancer is around 90%; however, only 39% of colorectal cancers are diagnosed at this early stage (AIHW, 2018). Survival varies according to the extent of the cancer development at diagnosis: at stage I colorectal cancer, 90% of individuals are still alive at 5 years; this falls to 87% with stage II, 57% with stage III and 10% for widespread disease (AIHW, 2018).

Although the specific cause of colorectal cancer is unknown, a number of risk factors have been identified (see Box 23.3). Genetic factors are strongly linked to the risk of colorectal cancer. Up to 25% of people developing colorectal cancer have a family history of the disease (GSA, 2022). People with familial adenomatous polyposis inevitably develop colon cancer unless the colon is removed. Hereditary non-polyposis colorectal cancer (also known as *Lynch syndrome*) is an autosomal dominant disorder that significantly increases the risk of developing colorectal and other cancers. Tumours associated with Lynch syndrome often affect the ascending colon and occur at an

BOX 23.3 Risk factors for colorectal cancer

- Age over 50 years
- Polyps of the colon and/or rectum
- Family history and genetic susceptibility for colorectal cancer
- Inflammatory bowel disease
- Exposure to radiation
- Diet: high intake of processed meats and foods high in fat and kilojoules
- Excess body fat and physical inactivity
- Smoking
- Alcohol consumption

earlier age. Inflammatory bowel diseases also increase the risk of colorectal cancer.

Diet plays a role in the development of colorectal cancer. The disease is prevalent in economically prosperous countries where people consume diets high in kilojoules, meat proteins and fats. This dietary pattern, common in Australia, is thought to increase the population of anaerobic bacteria in the gut. These anaerobes convert bile acids into carcinogens. Diets high in fruits and vegetables, folic acid and calcium appear to reduce the risk of colorectal cancer. Cereal fibre, once thought to reduce colorectal cancer risk, does not appear to play a role either way in its development. Other factors that may reduce the risk of colorectal cancer include regular exercise, taking a daily multivitamin and the use of aspirin and other NSAIDs.

Pathophysiology

Nearly all colorectal cancers are adenocarcinomas beginning as adenomatous polyps. Most tumours develop in the rectum and sigmoid colon, although any portion of the colon may be affected (see Figure 23.14). The tumour typically grows undetected, producing few manifestations. By the time manifestations occur, the disease may have spread into deeper layers of the bowel tissue and adjacent organs. Colorectal cancer spreads by direct extension to involve the entire bowel circumference, the submucosa and the outer bowel wall layers.

Neighbouring structures such as the liver, greater curvature of the stomach, duodenum, small intestine, pancreas, spleen, genitourinary tract and abdominal wall may also be involved by direct extension. Metastasis to regional lymph nodes is the most common form of tumour spread. This is not always an orderly process; distal nodes may contain cancer cells while regional nodes remain normal. Cancerous cells from the primary tumour may also spread via the lymphatic system or circulatory system to secondary sites such as the liver, lungs, brain, bones and kidneys. 'Seeding' of the tumour to other areas of the peritoneal cavity can occur when the tumour extends through the serosa or during surgical resection.

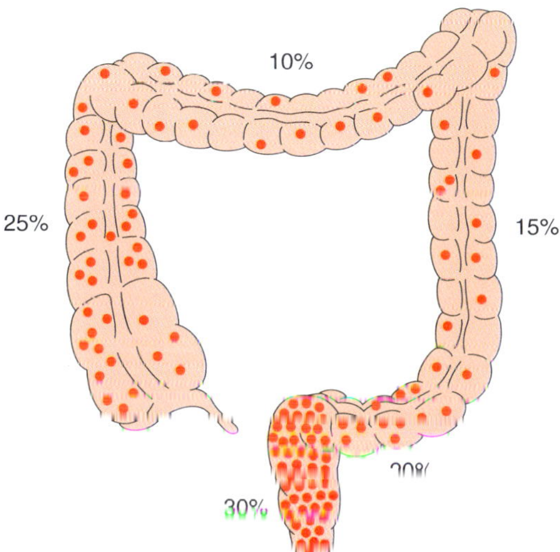

FIGURE 23.14 ***The distribution and frequency of cancer of the colon and rectum***

Manifestations

Bowel cancer often produces no manifestations until it is advanced. Because it grows slowly, 5 to 15 years of growth may occur before manifestations develop. The manifestations depend on its location, type and extent, and complications. Rectal bleeding is often the initial manifestation prompting a person to seek medical care. Other common early manifestations include a change in bowel habits, either diarrhoea or constipation. Pain, anorexia and weight loss are characteristic in advanced disease. A palpable abdominal or rectal mass may be present. Occasionally a person presents with anaemia from occult bleeding.

Complications

The primary complications associated with colorectal cancer are: (1) bowel obstruction due to narrowing of the bowel lumen by the lesion, (2) perforation of the bowel wall by the tumour, allowing contamination of the peritoneal cavity by bowel contents, and (3) direct extension of the tumour to involve adjacent organs.

Most recurrences of colorectal cancer after tumour removal occur within the first 4 years. The size of the primary tumour does not necessarily relate to long-term survival. The numbers of lymph nodes involved, penetration of the tumour through the bowel wall and tumour adherence to adjacent organs are better predictors of the prognosis for the disease.

INTERPROFESSIONAL CARE

The focus of interprofessional care for colorectal cancer is prevention, early detection and intervention. Colorectal cancer is always treated by surgical resection, with chemotherapy and radiation therapy used as adjuncts.

Prevention

Measures to prevent colon cancer considered effective and safe include diets high in fruit and vegetables and low in saturated fat and red meat, regular exercise, avoiding obesity and quitting smoking. Consuming fibre supplements, minerals such as calcium, vitamins and non-steroidal anti-inflammatory medications may help prevent colorectal cancer; however, their effectiveness is not yet proven (Principi & De Censi, 2015). Although considered safe, these measures are the subject of further research to demonstrate conclusive proof of effectiveness (Principi & De Censi, 2015).

Screening

Screening for blood in the faeces (faecal occult blood test (FOBT)) is available through the National Bowel Cancer Screening Program (NBCSP) to Australians turning 50. Since 2020, all Australians aged 50–74 have been offered the test free every 2 years (AIHW, 2018). Abnormal tests are followed up with a colonoscopy. The Cancer Council (2022) recommends one of the following testing schedules for the early detection of colorectal cancer, beginning at age 50. These options are acceptable choices for average-risk adults.

- Yearly FOBT or faecal immunochemical test (FIT). (For FOBT, the take-home multiple sample method should be used.)
- Flexible sigmoidoscopy every 5 years.
- Yearly FOBT or FIT plus flexible sigmoidoscopy every 5 years.
- Double-contrast barium enema every 5 years.
- Colonoscopy every 10 years.

Diagnosis

Diagnostic and laboratory tests are used for screening, diagnosis and monitoring purposes. Diagnostic tests include a sigmoidoscopy or colonoscopy as the primary diagnostic test used to detect and visualise tumours. While flexible sigmoidoscopy detects 50% to 65% of colorectal cancers, many clinicians recommend colonoscopy. Tissue for biopsy is obtained at the time of endoscopy to confirm cancerous tissue and evaluate cell differentiation (see the chapter 'Nursing care of people with cancer').

Laboratory tests used are an FOBT (by guaiac or haemoccult testing) to detect blood in the faeces, an FBC to identify anaemia resulting from chronic blood loss and tumour growth, and a carcinoembryonic antigen (CEA) level, a tumour marker detected in the blood of individuals with colorectal cancer. CEA levels are used to estimate prognosis, monitor treatment and detect cancer recurrence. Newer screening methods for diagnosis of colorectal cancer in the very early stage of development include faecal DNA, immunochemical faecal occult blood tests (iFOBTs) and computed tomographic colonography (CTC) (Leggett & Hewitt, 2015).

Current staging methods primarily use the TNM (tumour, node, metastasis) system, as outlined in Table 23.12. Radiological examinations may include a chest x-ray to detect tumour metastasis to the lung, and computed tomography (CT) scan, magnetic resonance imaging (MRI) or ultrasonic examination may be used to assess tumour depth and involvement of other organs by direct extension or metastasis.

Laser photocoagulation

Laser photocoagulation uses a very small, intense beam of light to generate heat in tissues towards which it is directed. The heat generated by the laser beam can be used to destroy small tumours. It is also used for palliative surgery of advanced tumours to remove obstruction. Laser photocoagulation can be performed endoscopically and is useful for people unable to tolerate major surgery.

Surgery

Stage I and II disease can be treated with surgery to remove the bowel and surrounding lymph nodes. Stage III disease requires surgery and additional chemotherapy to try to prevent recurrence. Widespread disease is treated with chemotherapy. More recently, targeted therapies are being trialled in addition to chemotherapy. Surgical resection of the tumour, adjacent colon and regional lymph nodes is the treatment of choice for colorectal cancer. Options for surgical treatment vary from destruction of the tumour by laser photocoagulation performed during endoscopy to abdominoperineal resection with permanent colostomy. When possible, the anal sphincter is preserved and colostomy avoided.

Other surgical treatment options for small, localised tumours include local excision and fulguration. These procedures may also be performed during endoscopy, eliminating the need for

TABLE 23.12 The TNM classification for colorectal cancer

STAGE	PRIMARY TUMOUR (T)	REGIONAL LYMPH NODES (N)	DISTANT METASTASIS (M)
	TX–Primary tumour cannot be assessed T0–No evidence of primary tumour	NX–Regional lymph node cannot be assessed	MX–Presence of distant metastasis cannot be assessed
		N0–No regional lymph node metastasis	M0–No distant metastasis
Stage 0	Tis–Carcinoma in situ		
Stage I	T1–Tumour invades submucosa T2–Tumour invades muscularis propria		
Stage II	T3–Tumour invades through muscularis propria into subserosa or into non-peritonealised pericolic or perirectal tissues T4–Tumour perforates visceral peritoneum or directly invades other organs or structures		
Stage III	Any T	N1–Metastasis in 1 to 3 pericolic or perirectal lymph nodes N2–Metastasis in 4 or more pericolic or perirectal lymph nodes N3–Metastasis in any lymph node along course of a major named vascular trunk	
Stage IV	Any T	Any N	M1–Distant metastasis

abdominal surgery. Local excision may be used to remove a disk of rectum containing a tumour in a person with a small, well-differentiated, mobile polypoid lesion. *Fulguration* or electrocoagulation is used to reduce the size of some large tumours in a person who is a poor surgical risk. This procedure requires general anaesthesia and may need to be repeated at intervals.

Most people with colorectal cancer undergo surgical resection of the colon with anastomosis of remaining bowel as a curative procedure. The distribution of regional lymph nodes determines the extent of resection because these may contain metastatic lesions. Most tumours of the ascending, transverse, descending and sigmoid colon can be resected.

Tumours of the rectum usually are treated with an abdominoperineal (AP) resection in which the sigmoid colon, rectum and anus are removed through both abdominal and perineal incisions. A permanent sigmoid colostomy is performed to provide for elimination of faeces. Nursing care for a person having bowel surgery is outlined below.

COLOSTOMY Surgical resection of the bowel may be accompanied by a colostomy for diversion of faecal contents. A **colostomy** is an ostomy made in the colon. It may be created if the bowel is obstructed by the tumour, as a temporary measure to promote healing of anastomoses or as a permanent means of faecal evacuation when the distal colon and rectum are removed. Colostomies take the name of the portion of the colon from which they are formed: ascending colostomy, transverse colostomy, descending colostomy and sigmoid colostomy (see Figure 23.15).

A *sigmoid colostomy* is the most common permanent colostomy performed, particularly for cancer of the rectum. It is usually created during an AP resection. This procedure involves the removal of the sigmoid colon, rectum and anus through abdominal and perineal incisions. The anal canal is closed and a stoma formed from the proximal sigmoid colon. The stoma is usually located on the lower left quadrant of the abdomen.

When a *double-barrel colostomy* is performed, two separate stomas are created (see Figure 23.16). The distal colon is not

NURSING CARE OF THE PERSON requiring bowel surgery

PREOPERATIVE NURSING CARE

- Provide routine preoperative care for a person undergoing surgery as outlined in the chapter 'Nursing care of people having surgery'.
- Arrange for consultation with stomal therapy (ST) specialist if appropriate. *The ST nurse is trained to identify and mark an appropriate stoma location, taking into consideration the level of stoma, skinfolds and the person's clothing preferences. Initial stomal care teaching also is provided by the ST nurse during the preoperative visit.*
- Insert a nasogastric tube if ordered. *Although it is often inserted in the operating theatre just prior to surgery, the nasogastric tube may be placed preoperatively to remove secretions and empty stomach contents.*
- Perform bowel preparation procedures as ordered. *Oral and parenteral antibiotics as well as laxatives and enemas may be prescribed preoperatively to clean the bowel and reduce the risk of peritoneal contamination by bowel contents during surgery.*

POSTOPERATIVE NURSING CARE

- Provide routine care for the person postoperatively (see the chapter 'Nursing care of people having surgery').
- Monitor bowel sounds and degree of abdominal distension. *Surgical manipulation of the bowel disrupts peristalsis, resulting in an initial ileus. Bowel sounds and the passage of flatus indicate a return of peristalsis.*
- Assess the position and patency of the nasogastric tube, connecting it to low suction. If the tube becomes clogged, gently irrigate with sterile normal saline. *A nasogastric or gastrostomy tube is used postoperatively to provide gastrointestinal decompression and facilitate healing of the anastomosis. Ensuring its patency is important for comfort and healing.*
- Assess colour amount and odour of drainage from surgical drains and the colostomy (if present), noting any changes or the presence of clots or bright bleeding. Initial drainage may be bright red and then become dark and finally clear or greenish yellow over the first 2 to 3 days. *A change in the colour, amount or odour of the drainage may indicate a complication such as haemorrhage, intestinal obstruction or infection.*
- Alert all personnel caring for the person with an AP resection to avoid rectal temperatures, suppositories or other rectal procedures. *These procedures could disrupt the anal suture line, causing bleeding, infection or impaired healing.*
- Maintain intravenous fluids while nasogastric suction is in place. *A person on nasogastric suction is unable to take oral food and fluids and is losing electrolyte-rich fluid via the nasogastric tube. If replacement fluid and electrolytes are not maintained, the person is at risk of dehydration; sodium, potassium and chloride imbalance; and metabolic alkalosis.*
- Provide antacids, H_2-receptor antagonists and antibiotic therapy as ordered. *The above medications may be ordered for the person postoperatively depending on the procedure performed. Antibiotic therapy is a common measure to prevent infection resulting from contamination of the abdominal cavity with gastric contents.*
- Resume oral food and fluids as ordered. Initial feedings may be clear fluids, progressing to free fluids and then frequent small feedings of regular foods. Monitor bowel sounds and for abdominal distension frequently during this period. *Oral feedings are reintroduced slowly, minimising abdominal distension and trauma to the suture lines.*
- Begin discharge planning and teaching. Consult with a nutritionist for instructions and menu planning, reinforce teaching. Advise about potential postoperative complications *such as abdominal abscess or bowel obstruction, their preventive measures and clinical manifestations.*

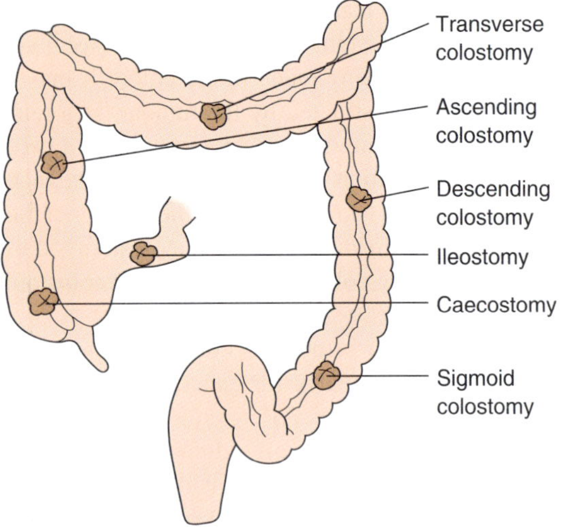

FIGURE 23.15 ***Various ostomy levels and sites***

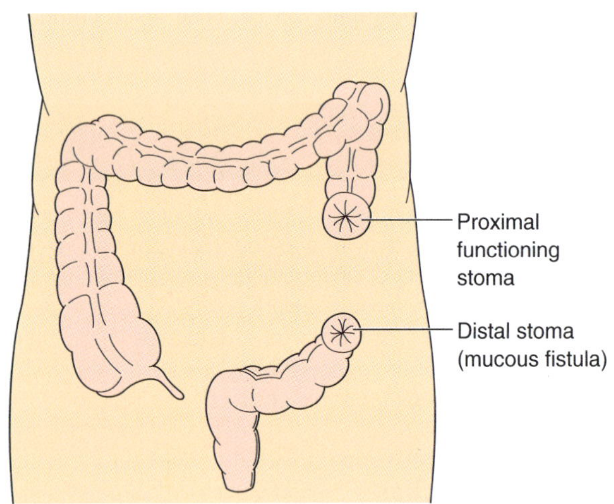

FIGURE 23.16 ***A double-barrel colostomy. The proximal stoma is the functioning stoma; the distal stoma expels mucus from the distal colon***

removed but bypassed. The proximal stoma, which is functional, diverts faeces to the abdominal wall. The distal stoma, also called the mucous fistula, expels mucus from the distal colon. It may be pouched or dressed with a 4 × 4 lint-free gauze dressing. A double-barrel colostomy may be created for cases of trauma, tumour or inflammation, and may be temporary or permanent.

An emergency procedure used to relieve an intestinal obstruction or perforation is called a *transverse loop colostomy*. During this procedure, a loop of the transverse colon is brought out from the abdominal wall and suspended over a plastic rod or bridge, preventing the loop from slipping back into the abdominal cavity. The loop stoma may be opened at the time of surgery or a few days later at the person's bedside. The bridge may be removed in 1 to 2 weeks. Transverse loop colostomies are generally temporary.

In a *Hartmann procedure*, a common temporary colostomy procedure, the distal portion of the colon is left in place and is over-sewn for closure. A temporary colostomy may be done to allow bowel rest or healing, such as following tumour resection or inflammation of the bowel. It may also be created following traumatic injury to the colon, such as a gunshot wound. Anastomosis of the severed portions of the colon is delayed because bacterial colonisation of the colon prevents proper healing of the anastomosis. About 3 to 6 months after a temporary colostomy, the colostomy is closed and the colon is reconnected. A person with a temporary colostomy requires the same care as an individual with permanent colostomy. See the 'Nursing care of the person with a colostomy' box.

Radiation therapy

Although radiation therapy is not used as a primary treatment for colon cancer, it is used with surgical resection for treating rectal tumours. Small rectal cancers may be treated with intracavitary, external or implantation radiation. Rectal cancer has a high rate of regional recurrence following complete surgical resection, particularly when the tumour has invaded tissues outside the bowel wall or regional lymph nodes. Pre- or postoperative radiation therapy reduces the recurrence of pelvic tumours, although the effect of radiation therapy on long-term survival is less clear. Radiation therapy is also used preoperatively to shrink large rectal tumours enough to permit their surgical removal. Further discussion about radiation therapy and nursing implications is included in the chapter 'Nursing care of people with cancer'.

Chemotherapy

Chemotherapeutical agents, such as intravenous fluorouracil (5-FU) and folinic acid (leucovorin), are also used postoperatively as adjunctive therapy for colorectal cancer. When combined with radiation therapy, chemotherapy reduces the rate of tumour recurrence and prolongs survival in people with stage II and stage III rectal tumours. The benefit for colon cancers is less clear, but chemotherapy may be used to reduce its spread to the liver and prevent recurrence. Irinotecan (CPT-11) or oxaliplatin may also be used in chemotherapy regimens for colorectal cancer. See the chapter 'Nursing care of people with cancer'.

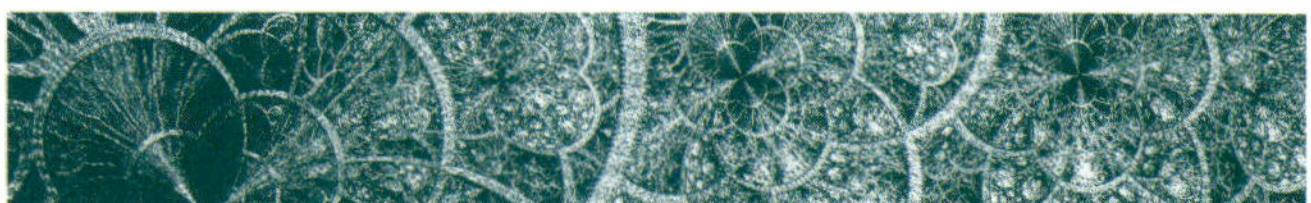

Nursing care

Health promotion

Primary prevention of colorectal cancer is a significant nursing care issue. Discuss the dietary recommendations provided by the Cancer Council (2022) for the prevention of colorectal cancer, including decreasing the amount of fat, refined sugar and red meats in the diet while increasing intake of dietary fibre. Foods containing high amounts of fibre include raw fruit and vegetables, legumes and wholegrain products.

NURSING CARE OF THE PERSON **with a colostomy**

- Assess the location of the stoma and the type of colostomy performed. *Stoma location is an indicator of the section of bowel in which it is located and a predictor of the type of faecal drainage to expect.*
- Assess stoma appearance and surrounding skin condition frequently (see the box 'Nursing care of the person having an ileostomy'). *Assessment of stoma and skin condition is particularly important in the early postoperative period, when complications are most likely to occur and are most treatable.*
- Position a collection bag or drainable pouch over the stoma. Initial drainage may contain more mucus and serosanguineous fluid than faecal material. As the bowel resumes function, drainage becomes faecal in nature. *The consistency of drainage depends on the stoma location in the bowel.*
- If ordered, irrigate the colostomy, instilling water into the colon similar to an enema procedure. *The water stimulates the colon to empty.*
- When colostomy irrigation is ordered for a person with a double-barrel or loop colostomy, irrigate the proximal stoma. Digital assessment of the bowel direction from the stoma can assist in determining the proximal stoma. *The distal bowel carries no faecal contents and does not need irrigation. It may be irrigated for cleansing just prior to reanastomosis.*
- Empty a drainable pouch or replace the colostomy bag as needed or when it is no more than one-third full. *If the pouch is allowed to overfill, its weight may impair the seal, causing leakage.*
- Provide stomal and skin care for a person with a colostomy as for a person with an ileostomy (see the box 'Nursing care of the person having an ileostomy'). *Good skin and stoma care is important to maintain skin integrity and function as the first line of defence against infection.*
- Use caulking agents, such as Stomahesive or karaya paste and a skin barrier wafer, as needed to maintain a secure ostomy pouch. *This is particularly important for a person with a loop colostomy. The main challenge for a person with a transverse loop colostomy is to maintain a secure ostomy pouch over the plastic bridge.*
- If the pouch does not incorporate an air vent, a small needle hole high on the colostomy pouch allows flatus to escape. This hole may be closed with a Band-Aid, and opened when the person is in the bathroom, for odour control. *Ostomy bags may 'balloon' out, disrupting the skin seal, if excess gas collects.*

HEALTH EDUCATION FOR THE PERSON AND FAMILY

- Prior to discharge, provide written, verbal and psychomotor instruction on colostomy care, pouch management, skin care and irrigation to the person. Whether the colostomy is temporary or permanent, the person will be responsible for its management. *Good understanding of procedures and care enhances the ability to provide self care, as well as self esteem and control.*
- Allow ample time for the person (and their family, if necessary) to practise changing the pouch, either on the person or a model. *Practice of psychomotor skills improves learning and confidence.*
- If an abdominoperineal resection has been performed, emphasise the importance of using no rectal suppositories, rectal temperatures or enemas. Suggest the person carry medical identification or a MedicAlert® tag or bracelet. *These measures are important to prevent tissue trauma when the rectum has been removed.*
- The diet for a person with a colostomy is individualised and may require no alteration from that consumed preoperatively. Dietary teaching should, however, include information on foods causing stool odour and gas, and foods that thicken or loosen stools. *Foods causing these effects on ostomy output are listed below.*

Foods increasing stool odour

- Asparagus
- Beans
- Cabbage
- Eggs
- Fish
- Garlic
- Onions
- Some spices

Foods increasing intestinal gas

- Beer
- Broccoli
- Brussels sprouts
- Cabbage
- Carbonated drinks
- Cauliflower
- Corn
- Cucumbers
- Dairy products
- Dried beans
- Peas
- Radishes
- Spinach

Foods thickening stools

- Apple sauce
- Bananas
- Bread
- Cheese
- Pasta
- Pretzels
- Rice
- Smooth peanut paste
- Tapioca
- Yoghurt

Foods loosening stools

- Chocolate
- Dried beans
- Fried foods
- Greasy foods
- Highly spiced foods
- Leafy green vegetables
- Raw fruits and juices
- Raw vegetables

Foods colouring stools

- Beetroot
- Red and green jelly

Stress the importance of regular health examinations, including digital rectal exams. Discuss recommendations for regular haemoccult testing of stool after age 50. Include the importance of seeking medical treatment if blood is noted in or on the stool. Teach the warning signs for cancer, including those specific to bowel cancer, such as a change in bowel habits.

Assessment

- *Health history*: usual bowel patterns and any recent changes; weight loss, fatigue, decreased activity tolerance; presence of blood in the stool; pain with defecation, abdominal discomfort, perineal pain; usual diet; family history of colon cancer; other specific risk factors such as IBD or colon polyps.
- *Physical examination*: general appearance; weight; abdominal shape, contour; bowel sounds, abdominal tenderness; stool haemoccult or guaiac.

Nursing diagnoses and interventions

In planning and implementing care, consider both physical care needs and the person's psychological response to the diagnosis. The psychological recovery of a person who is diagnosed with colorectal cancer may be influenced by the possible permanent changes to their body image and lifestyle. When planning care, open and genuine communication enables nurses to understand the person's anxieties and personal, family and social needs (Le, 2018). As colorectal cancer is often advanced at the time of diagnosis, the prognosis, even with treatment, may be poor. Denial and anger are common. Extensive abdominal surgery and potentially a colostomy may be necessary and the effects of chemotherapy and radiation therapy can leave the person fatigued and discouraged. See the nursing care plan for a person with colorectal cancer.

Nursing care includes providing emotional support, teaching and direct care before and after diagnostic procedures and surgery and during adjunctive treatments. When developing nursing care plans, it is imperative to incorporate the person's cultural, religious and personal viewpoints into the plan of care. Priority nursing diagnoses include *Acute pain*, *Imbalanced nutrition* and *Anticipatory grieving*. *Risk of sexual dysfunction* should be considered as a priority diagnosis if a colostomy was created.

CONSIDERATION FOR PRACTICE

If an abdominoperineal resection (AP) resection was performed, alert all care personnel to avoid rectal temperatures, suppository use or other procedures that could damage sutures.

Acute pain

A person with colorectal cancer may experience pain related to preparatory procedures, diagnostic examinations and surgery. Following an AP, 'phantom' rectal pain related to the severing of nerves during the wide excision of the rectum may develop. Finally, the primary tumour itself and, potentially, metastatic tumours may impinge on nerves and other organs, causing pain. In the early postoperative period, an epidural infusion or PCA is often used to manage pain. PCA, routine administration of ordered analgesics or a continuous analgesia delivery (CAD) system may also be used for pain management when the tumour is far enough advanced to preclude surgical resection. See the chapter 'Nursing care of people in pain' for more information on caring for a person with pain, the chapter 'Nursing care of people with cancer' for discussion of pain associated with cancer and the chapter 'Nursing care of people experiencing loss, grief and death' for discussion of end-of-life care.

- Assess and monitor for adequate pain relief. Use subjective and objective information, including the location, intensity and character of the pain, as well as non-verbal signs such as grimacing, muscle tension, apparent dozing, changes in pulse or blood pressure, and rapid, shallow respirations. Response to pain varies between individuals and is influenced by culture, beliefs, pathophysiological factors and psychological factors such as previous pain events (Picot, 2021). A person may assume that pain is to be expected or tolerated or may fear becoming addicted to analgesic medications. *Careful questioning and a holistic assessment can provide accurate information about pain status, allowing better control of discomfort.*
- Ask the person to rate pain using a 0 to 10 pain scale. Document the level of pain. Pain is a subjective experience. *People perceive and respond to pain differently. Religion and ethnic background may affect the response to pain.*
- Monitor analgesic effectiveness 30 minutes after administration. Monitor for pain relief and adverse effects. *The method of delivery, dosage or medication itself may need to be adjusted to provide adequate pain relief.*
- Assess the incision for inflammation or swelling; assess drainage catheters and tubes for patency. *Poorly controlled pain, or pain that changes, may be related to organ distension from an obstructed nasogastric tube, urinary catheter or wound drain, or may indicate an infection.*
- Assess the abdomen for distension, tenderness and bowel sounds. *Intra-abdominal bleeding, peritonitis or paralytic ileus can cause pain that may be confused with incisional pain.*
- Administer analgesia prior to an activity or procedure. *Adequate pain relief reduces muscle tension, allowing for more comfortable participation in activities.*
- Assist with adjunctive comfort measures, such as positioning, diversional activities, management of environmental stimuli, guided imagery and teaching relaxation techniques. *These measures enhance the effects of analgesia by reducing muscle tension.*
- Splint incision with a pillow and teach the person how to self-splint when coughing and deep breathing *to prevent respiratory complications related to fear of pain.*

Imbalanced nutrition: less than body requirements

Bowel preparation for diagnostic procedures, surgery, radiation therapy and chemotherapy place the person with colorectal cancer at risk of nutritional deficiencies. Fluid and electrolyte replacement is provided following surgery, along with possible TPN (see the chapter 'Nursing care of people with nutritional disorders'). Adequate kilojoule and nutrient intake is necessary

NURSING CARE PLAN **A person with colorectal cancer**

Bill Cunningham is a 65-year-old retired railway employee, husband and father of three grown children. For the past 3 months, Mr Cunningham has noticed small amounts of blood and occasional mucus in his stools. He has a sensation of pressure in the rectum and noticed his stools are smaller in diameter, about the size of a pencil. After palpating a mass on digital examination of the rectum, the doctor orders a colonoscopy. A large sessile lesion is found in the rectum and biopsied. The pathology report shows the lesion to be adenocarcinoma. Mr Cunningham is scheduled for an abdominoperineal resection and sigmoid colostomy.

ASSESSMENT

Madonna Hart, RN, completes the admission assessment. Mr Cunningham states his bowel habits have recently changed but denies pain or other symptoms. Physical assessment findings include T 36.9°C, P 82, R 18 and BP 118/78. He is 178 cm tall and weighs 84 kg. Laboratory findings are normal except for the previous pathology report of adenocarcinoma of rectal lesion.

Mr Cunningham states, 'I really don't want a colostomy, but if that is what it takes to get rid of this, I'm ready to get it over with.'

DIAGNOSES

- *Altered comfort* related to acute pain secondary to surgical intervention.
- *Risk of impaired skin integrity (peristomal)* related to faecal drainage and pouch adhesive.
- *Risk of constipation/diarrhoea* related to effects of surgery on bowel function.
- *Disturbed body image* related to colostomy.
- *Risk of sexual dysfunction* related to wide rectal incision, radiation therapy and colostomy.

PLANNING

When planning nursing care with Mr Cunningham, it is vital to consider his preferences and religious and cultural beliefs for incorporation into his plan of care.

Expected outcomes

- Mr Cunningham will report pain within an acceptable range that allows ease of movement and ambulation.
- Mr Cunningham will perform colostomy care using correct technique.
- Mr Cunningham will demonstrate willingness to discuss changes in sexual function.
- Mr Cunningham will wear clothing to enhance physical and emotional self-esteem.

IMPLEMENTATION

- Provide Mr Cunningham with analgesia as ordered, evaluating its effectiveness and monitoring for adverse reactions.
- Provide for privacy when teaching and discussing concerns about ostomy.
- Discuss with Mr Cunningham foods that cause odour and gas.
- Teach Mr Cunningham how to care for his colostomy.
- Maintain consistent nursing personnel assignment to facilitate trust.
- Provide Mr Cunningham information about the Australian Stoma Appliance Scheme. It is subsidised by the Australian Government and provides stoma products (medicine and appliances) for people with a permanent or temporary stoma free of charge to members of one of the 22 approved volunteer stoma associations.
- Refer Mr Cunningham to the local Stoma Association.

EVALUATION

At discharge, Mr Cunningham is able to empty and rinse out his colostomy pouch. He is changing the pouch and caring for surrounding skin appropriately. RN Hart gave him verbal and written instructions on colostomy care. He verbalised understanding of phantom rectal pain and the importance of avoiding rectal suppositories. He expresses an understanding of the need to avoid heavy lifting and the importance of follow-up care. RN Hart refers Mr Cunningham to a home healthcare agency in his community if he has further questions and for his follow-up care.

CRITICAL THINKING IN THE NURSING PROCESS

1. Describe the cause of phantom rectal pain.
2. Outline why it is important to discuss dietary concerns with a person with a colostomy, especially odour- and gas-forming foods.
3. Outline a plan to teach Mr Cunningham how to irrigate a colostomy.
4. Develop a care plan for Mr Cunningham for the nursing diagnosis *Disturbed body image*.

REFLECTION ON THE NURSING PROCESS

1. Reflect on what you learned from completing this section. Outline how you will apply this knowledge to assist you in your clinical reasoning when next on clinical placement.
2. Describe nursing interventions you can incorporate into your clinical practice to assist a person to be independent in caring for their colostomy.

for healing after surgery. Additionally, if the tumour is advanced, metabolic needs may be increased and the appetite decreased.

- Assess nutritional status using data such as height and weight, [illegible] body mass index (BMI) calculation (see the chapter 'A person-centred approach to assessing the gastrointestinal system') and laboratory data including serum albumin level. Refer to nutritionist for dietary management. *A person malnourished before beginning aggressive cancer treatment requires more vigorous nutrition management to promote healing.*
- Assess readiness for resumption of oral intake after surgery or procedures using data such as statements of hunger, presence of bowel sounds, passage of flatus and minimal abdominal distension. *Manipulation of the bowel interrupts peristalsis of the GI tract. It is important to ensure that peristalsis has resumed prior to resumption of oral intake.*
- Monitor and document food and fluid intake. *Documentation helps identify the adequacy of kilojoule and other nutrient intake.*

- Weigh daily. *Weight fluctuation may indicate adequate or inadequate dietary intake.*
- Maintain TPN and central intravenous lines as ordered. *Parenteral nutrition prevents tissue catabolism and promotes healing when food intake is disrupted for more than 2 to 3 days.*
- When oral intake resumes, help the person develop a meal plan incorporating their food preferences and that considers their schedule and environment. *Consideration of likes, dislikes and circumstances in meal planning promotes adequate intake.*

Anticipatory grieving

When a bowel resection is performed for colorectal cancer, the person needs to adjust to the loss of a major body part as well as to the diagnosis of cancer. Even when the prognosis for recovery is good, many people perceive cancer as fatal. Supporting the person and their family during the initial stages of grieving can improve physical recovery as well as psychological coping and eventual adaptation. See the chapter 'Nursing care of people experiencing loss, grief and death' for discussion of nursing care of people experiencing loss and grief.

- Work to develop a trusting relationship with the person and their family. *This increases the nurse's effectiveness in helping them work through the grieving process.*
- Listen actively, encouraging the person and their family to express their fears and concerns. Assist to identify strengths, experiences and support systems.
- Demonstrate respect for cultural, spiritual and religious values and beliefs; encourage use of these resources to cope with losses.
- Encourage discussion of the potential impact of loss on individual family members, family structure and family function. Assist family members to share concerns with one another.
- Refer to cancer support groups, social services or counselling as appropriate. *These resources can be used throughout the grieving process.*

Risk of sexual dysfunction

Colorectal cancer and ostomy surgery increase the risk of sexual dysfunction, defined as a change in sexual function so that it becomes unsatisfying, unrewarding or inadequate). Physical factors leading to sexual dysfunction include disruption of nerves and blood vessels supplying the genitals, radiation therapy, chemotherapy and other medications prescribed after surgery.

Psychologically, an *ostomate* (person with an ostomy) experiences an altered body image and may develop low self-esteem. The person may feel undesirable and fear rejection. They may be concerned about odours or pouch leakage during sexual activity. This emotional stress can also contribute to sexual dysfunction.

- Provide opportunities for the person and their family to express feelings about the cancer diagnosis, stoma and effects of other treatments. *Encouraging verbalisation of feelings about the diagnosis, stoma and treatments provides an opportunity to validate that feelings of anger and depression are normal responses to the diagnosis and change in body function.*
- Provide consistent care. *An accepting attitude and consistent care by nurses, as well as securing the appliance and controlling odour and leakage, can increase the person's confidence and independence in caring for the appliance.*
- Encourage expression of sexual concerns. Provide privacy for discussions with a caregiver who has an established trust with the person and their partner. Sexuality is a private concern to most people. *The person and their partner are not likely to express their concerns openly unless trust has been established.*
- Reassure the person and their partner that the effect of physical illness and prescribed interventions on sexuality is usually temporary. *The person and their partner may misinterpret an initial decrease in libido as evidence sexual activity will not be possible or resume following recovery.*
- Refer the person and their partner to social services or a family counsellor for further interventions. A person is often discharged from acute care settings well before concerns about sexual activity surface. *Ongoing counselling provides a continuing resource.*
- Arrange for a visit from a member of the Stoma Association. *People living and coping with an ostomy can provide information and support, helping the new ostomate overcome feelings of isolation and rejection.*

Community-based care

During the diagnostic and preoperative periods, provide instruction about the following topics:

- tests to be performed and preparatory procedures, including dietary restrictions, laxatives, enemas and food and fluid restrictions just prior to the procedure
- recommended post-procedure care and potential adverse effects to report
- preoperative care, such as intestinal preparation and food and fluid restrictions.

If a colostomy is planned, refer to a stomal therapist for stoma placement and initial teaching.

Once treatment has been initiated, include the following topics (as appropriate) in teaching for home care:

- pain management
- skin care and management of potential adverse effects of radiation therapy and/or chemotherapy (Refer to the chapter 'Nursing care of people with cancer' for further discussion of teaching needs related to these therapies.)
- incision and stoma care
- recommended diet
- follow-up appointments and care.

If the tumour is inoperable or a cure is not anticipated, provide information about pain and symptom management. Discuss the hospice philosophy and available services. Provide a referral to a local hospice or home health department. See the chapter 'Nursing care of people experiencing loss, grief and death' for discussion of end-of-life care and the chapter 'Nursing care of people with cancer' for nursing care of a person with cancer.

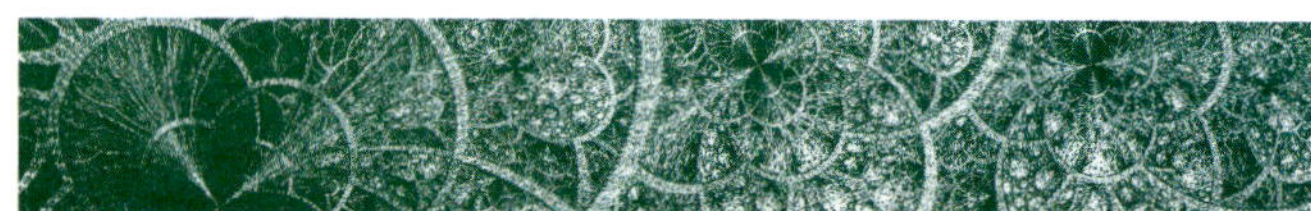

Structural and obstructive bowel disorders

Any portion of the intestines may be affected by a structural or obstructive disorder. When the structural defect is in the bowel wall, the intestine may be directly affected, as is the case with diverticula. Defects in the abdominal wall may allow intra-abdominal contents (such as loops of bowel) to protrude, indirectly affecting bowel function. Likewise, obstructions may result from disease of the bowel itself or from obstruction of the bowel lumen by an external force.

THE PERSON WITH A HERNIA

A hernia is a defect in the abdominal wall allowing abdominal contents to protrude out of the abdominal cavity. Trauma, surgery and increased intra-abdominal pressure caused by such conditions as pregnancy, obesity, weight lifting or tumours are risk factors for hernia formation.

Pathophysiology

Hernias are classified by location (see Figure 23.17) and are congenital or acquired. Most hernias occur in the groin (inguinal or femoral hernias). Inguinal hernias are often congenital, caused by improper closure of the tract developing as the testes descend into the scrotum during fetal development. Inguinal hernias may be acquired, resulting from weakness of fascia in a region called Hesselbach's area or from dilation of the femoral ring (e.g. during pregnancy and childbirth). Ventral or incisional hernias of the abdominal wall generally are acquired, caused by weakening of normal abdominal wall musculature. Umbilical hernias also are congenital and usually are detected in infancy. Hiatal hernias develop in the diaphragm (see the chapter 'Nursing care of people with upper gastrointestinal disorders').

Inguinal hernia

Inguinal hernias usually affect males and are classified as indirect or direct inguinal hernias. *Indirect inguinal hernias* are caused by improper closure of the tract developing as the testes descend into the scrotum before birth. A sac comprising abdominal contents protrudes through the internal inguinal ring into the inguinal canal. It often descends into the scrotum. Although indirect inguinal hernias are congenital defects, these often are not evident until adulthood, when increased intra-abdominal pressure and dilation of the inguinal ring allow abdominal contents to enter the channel.

Direct inguinal hernias are acquired defects resulting from weakness of the posterior inguinal wall. Direct inguinal hernias usually affect older adults. *Femoral hernias* are also acquired defects in which a peritoneal sac protrudes through the femoral ring. These hernias usually affect obese or pregnant women.

Inguinal hernias may produce no manifestations and are discovered during routine physical examination. These may cause a lump, swelling or bulge in the groin, particularly during lifting or straining. An inguinal hernia may cause sharp pain or a dull ache radiating into the scrotum. A palpable mass may be present in the groin, although it may be felt only with increased intra-abdominal pressure (as occurs during coughing) and invagination of the scrotum towards the inguinal ring.

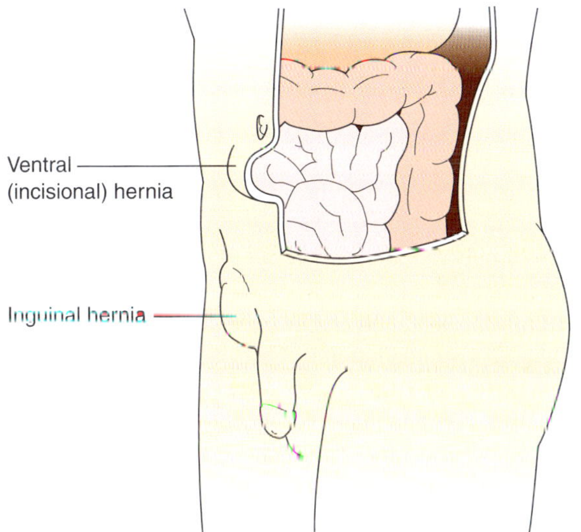

FIGURE 23.17 ***An abdominal wall (ventral or incisional) hernia and an inguinal hernia***

Umbilical hernia

Pregnancy and obesity contribute to the development of umbilical hernias in adults. *Umbilical hernias* may be congenital and evident during infancy, or acquired as the tissue closing the umbilical ring weakens, allowing protrusion of abdominal contents. These hernias are more common in women. Other predisposing factors include multiple pregnancies with prolonged labour, ascites and large intra-abdominal tumours.

Umbilical hernias tend to enlarge steadily and contain omentum, although these may also contain small or large bowel. These hernias may cause sharp pain on coughing or straining, or a dull, aching sensation. Strangulation is a common complication of umbilical hernias.

Incisional or ventral hernia

Incisional or *ventral hernias* occur at a previous surgical incision or following abdominal muscle tears. Inadequate healing of the incision or tear leads to hernia development. Contributing factors include poor wound closure, postoperative infection, age or debility, obesity, inadequate nutrition and excess incisional stress caused by vigorous coughing.

Ventral hernias are characterised by a bulge at the incisional site, often noted when the person pulls to a sitting position from a lying position. Ventral hernias often are asymptomatic and the risk of incarceration is low because of the size of the defect.

Manifestations

Abdominal contents (peritoneum, bowel and other abdominal organs) can protrude through the abdominal wall forming a sac covered by skin and subcutaneous tissues. In most cases, abdominal contents move into the sac when intra-abdominal pressure increases, then return to the abdominal cavity when pressure returns to normal or when manual pressure is placed on the bulging sac. This is known as a *reducible hernia*.

Complications

The risk of complications is low with a reducible hernia. If the contents of a hernia cannot be returned to the abdominal cavity, it is said to be *incarcerated*. Contents of an incarcerated hernia are trapped, usually by a narrow neck or opening to the hernia. Incarceration increases the risk of complications, including obstruction and strangulation. Obstruction occurs when the lumen of the bowel contained within the hernia becomes occluded, much like crimping of a hose. A *strangulated hernia* develops when blood supply to bowel and other tissues in the hernia sac is compromised, leading to necrosis. The affected bowel infarcts, leading to perforation and contamination of the peritoneal cavity. Clinical manifestations of a strangulated hernia include severe abdominal pain and distension, nausea, vomiting, tachycardia and fever.

INTERPROFESSIONAL CARE

The diagnosis of a hernia is made by a physical examination. The person is examined in a supine or standing position. A bulge may be seen or felt when the person coughs or bears down. No laboratory or diagnostic testing is usually required, unless bowel obstruction or strangulation is suspected.

Surgical repair, or *herniorrhaphy*, is the usual treatment of hernia. Surgery is generally well tolerated by people of all ages and carries a much lower risk than the complications of incarceration, obstruction and strangulation. Emergency surgery is indicated for hernias that are incarcerated, painful or tender. In a herniorrhaphy, the abdominal wall defect is closed by suturing or with wire or mesh over the defect. If incarceration occurs or strangulation is suspected, the abdominal cavity is explored during surgery and any infarcted bowel resected. Heavy lifting and heavy manual labour are restricted for approximately 3 weeks after surgery.

When surgery is contraindicated, a person can be taught to reduce their hernia by lying down and gently pushing against the mass. However, the person needs to be instructed if hernia incarceration is suspected, not to attempt to reduce their hernia and to seek medical assistance. A binder or truss may be worn to prevent or control the protrusion.

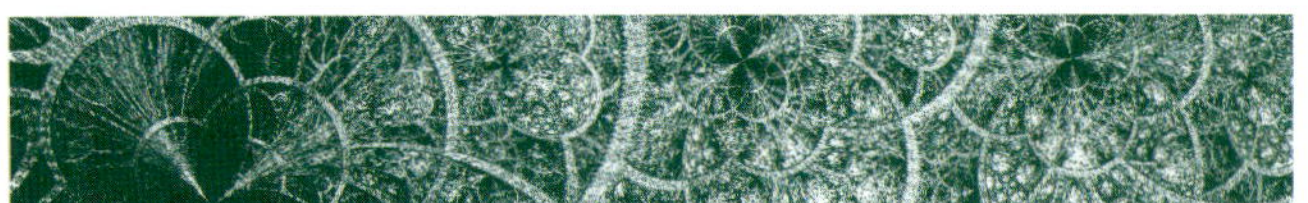

Nursing care

Assessment

- *Health history*: manifestations of hernia, such as bulging in the groin or of the abdominal wall when coughing, straining or moving from lying to standing; pain (abdominal, groin or scrotal); history of hernia or abdominal surgery.
- *Physical examination*: observe for bulging of the abdominal wall or around the umbilicus when raising head and shoulders from supine position; wearing gloves, palpate inguinal region for bulges when the person coughs or bears down (Valsalva manoeuvre) while standing.

Nursing diagnoses and interventions

Herniorrhaphy is generally an uncomplicated procedure, usually performed as day surgery. Preoperative assessment and teaching and immediate postoperative care are the primary nursing care needs. Care is similar to that provided for a person following an appendectomy.

Risk of decreased gastrointestinal tissue perfusion

When providing care for a person with a known hernia, the possibility of obstruction and strangulation must be considered throughout nursing assessments. Although nursing interventions may not be able to prevent these complications, rapid identification of the problem allows timely surgical treatment. Prompt treatment may prevent major complications related to infection and peritoneal contamination by bowel contents.

- Assess bowel sounds and abdominal distension at least every 8 hours. A change in bowel sounds—either cessation of sounds or an onset of hyperactive, high-pitched sounds—may indicate obstruction. *With obstruction, abdominal girth may increase.*

> **CONSIDERATION FOR PRACTICE**
>
> **Promptly report any acute increase in abdominal, groin, perineal or scrotal pain. An abrupt increase in the intensity of pain may indicate bowel ischaemia due to strangulation.**

- Notify medical staff if the hernia becomes painful or tender. *Pain and tenderness indicates incarceration and increased risk of strangulation.*
- If signs of possible obstruction or strangulation occur, notify the doctor. Place the person in a supine position with the hips elevated and knees slightly bent. Withhold all food and fluids (NBM) and begin preparations for surgery. *This position helps relax abdominal muscles and may facilitate reduction of the hernia. Strangulation or obstruction requires immediate surgical intervention.*

Community-based care

Include the following topics when teaching a person about hernias and home care:

- rationale for examining the groin and abdomen for bulges
- the nature of hernia, risk factors and manifestations
- surgical intervention for hernia
- how to reduce a hernia if necessary
- the importance of seeking immediate medical intervention for signs of strangulation or obstruction
- the need to notify the doctor if upper respiratory infection and cough develop preoperatively (forceful coughing is not recommended postoperatively)
- postoperative pain management and activity restrictions.

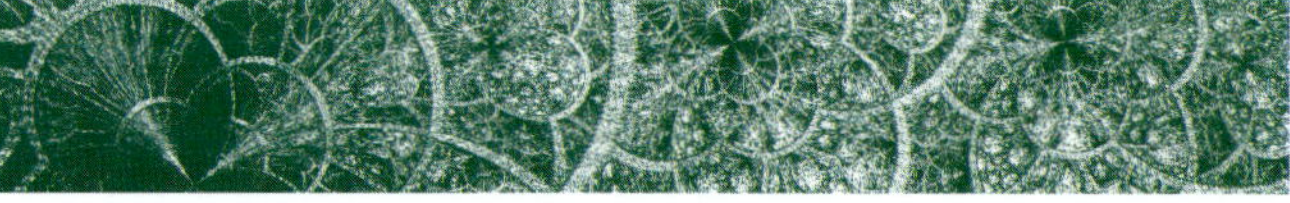

THE PERSON WITH INTESTINAL OBSTRUCTION

Intestinal obstruction is failure of intestinal contents to move through the bowel lumen. Intestinal obstructions affect either the large or small bowel. The small intestine is more commonly affected; however, bowel obstructions may also occur in the large intestine. Obstruction is the most common reason for small-bowel surgery.

Pathophysiology

Intestinal obstructions are either mechanical or functional in nature. *Mechanical* obstructions may be caused by: (1) problems outside the intestine, such as bands of scar tissue or hernias, (2) problems within the intestine—for example, tumours or IBD, or (3) obstruction of the intestinal lumen. Intestinal obstructions are partial or complete. *Functional* obstruction occurs when peristalsis fails to propel intestinal contents although there is no mechanical obstruction. *Adynamic ileus* (also known as **paralytic ileus** or simply *ileus*) is the most common functional obstruction after abdominal surgery and probably accounts for most intestinal obstructions (Marieb & Hoehn, 2019). Obstructions are further classified by the portion of intestine affected.

When the intestine is obstructed, gas and fluid accumulate proximal to and within the obstructed segment, distending the bowel. Swallowed air accounts for most of the gas. Ingested fluid, saliva, gastric juice and pancreatic secretions contribute to accumulated fluid. Water and sodium are drawn into the bowel lumen, contributing to fluid accumulation, distension and vascular fluid losses. Distension of the bowel lumen interferes with peristaltic movement, leading to atony and further distension. Significant distension of the bowel lumen comprises blood flow to mucosa, and eventually leads to necrosis. Gangrenous bowel may perforate resulting in peritonitis. Rapid bacterial growth in the obstructed bowel leads to sepsis and often death.

Significant bowel distension, vomiting and third spacing of fluids in the bowel and peritoneal cavity leads to massive loss of fluids and electrolytes with resulting hypovolaemia, hypokalaemia, renal insufficiency and shock.

Small-bowel obstruction

Adhesions or bands of scar tissue and hernias account for most mechanical small-bowel obstructions. In adults, adhesions develop following abdominal surgery or inflammatory processes. Adhesions usually produce a *simple obstruction* or single blockage in one portion of the intestine (see Figure 23.18A). The obstruction produced by an incarcerated hernia is a *closed-loop obstruction*, with two different portions of the bowel lumen obstructed (see Figure 23.18B).

Tumours, either intrinsic (of the bowel itself) or extrinsic (of another organ but affecting the bowel because of their size), can progressively occlude the bowel lumen and eventually obstruct it (see Figure 23.18C). Other, less common causes of bowel obstruction include intussusception (rare in adults) (see Figure 23.18D); volvulus, the rotation of loops of bowel about a fixed point (see Figure 23.18E); foreign bodies; stricture; and IBD.

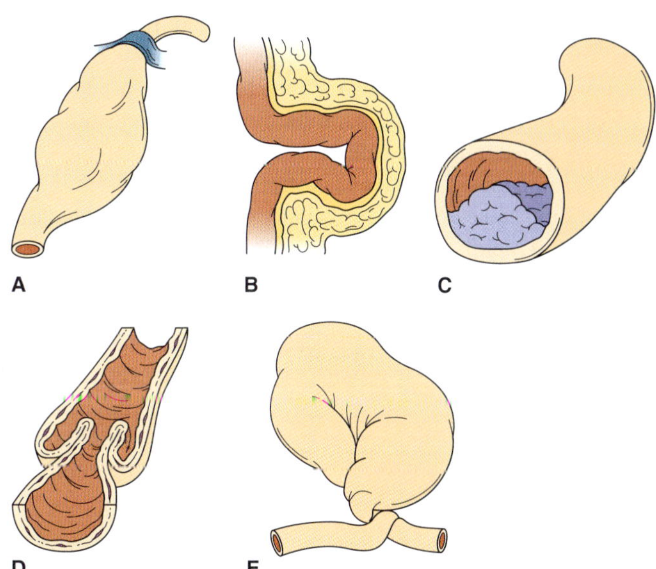

FIGURE 23.18 *Selected causes of mechanical obstruction. A, Adhesions; B, incarcerated hernia; C, tumour; D, intussusception; E, volvulus*

Both volvulus and an incarcerated hernia can cause a *strangulated obstruction*. In a strangulated obstruction, not only is the lumen of the bowel obstructed, but the blood supply to the affected portion is also compromised.

In a functional obstruction or adynamic ileus, peristalsis stops due to either neurogenic or muscular impairment. The bowel lumen remains patent; however, the contents are not propelled forward. Temporary ileus commonly follows gastrointestinal surgery. It may also result from tissue anoxia or peritoneal irritation due to haemorrhage, peritonitis or perforation of an organ. Other conditions precipitating paralytic ileus include renal colic, spinal cord injuries, uraemia and electrolyte imbalances, particularly hypokalaemia. Additionally, the effects of some narcotics, anticholinergic drugs and antidiarrhoeal medications such as diphenoxylate can produce a functional obstruction.

MANIFESTATIONS The manifestations of a small-bowel obstruction vary, depending on the level of obstruction and how rapidly it develops. Cramping or colic-like abdominal pain may be intermittent or increasing in intensity. Vomiting is common, particularly in high or proximal obstructions, because lumen distension stimulates the vomiting centre. As bacterial fermentation occurs, vomitus often contains faecal matter, particularly with a low or distal obstruction. Flatus and faeces already present in the lower bowel may be expelled early in the obstructive process. However, this expulsion ceases as the obstruction continues.

Early in the course of a mechanical obstruction, borborygmi and high-pitched tinkling bowel sounds are present, as the intestine attempts to propel contents past the obstruction. Visible peristaltic waves may be noted in the distended loops of bowel in thin people. In the later stages, the bowel becomes silent. With a paralytic ileus, bowel sounds are greatly diminished or absent throughout the process. Abdominal distension is minimal with proximal obstructions but may be pronounced with distal obstruction and paralytic ileus. The abdomen may be tender to palpation as well.

In addition to abdominal and gastrointestinal manifestations, signs of fluid and electrolyte imbalance develop. Hypovolaemia can develop rapidly as extracellular fluid is sequestered in the bowel and vomiting occurs. Although early vital signs may be normal, changes are noted as dehydration and hypovolaemia develop. The person becomes tachycardic and tachypnoeic and blood pressure falls. Temperature may be elevated. Urine output decreases and clinical manifestations of hypovolaemic shock may be seen. The clinical manifestations of mechanical small-bowel obstruction with their accompanying pathophysiological process are outlined in Table 23.13.

COMPLICATIONS Hypovolaemia and hypovolaemic shock with multiple-organ dysfunction is a significant complication of bowel obstruction and can lead to death. Renal insufficiency from hypovolaemia leads to acute kidney injury or dysfunction. Pulmonary ventilation may be impaired because abdominal distension elevates the diaphragm, impeding respiratory processes.

Strangulation associated with incarcerated hernia or volvulus impairs the blood supply to the bowel. Gangrene may rapidly result, causing bleeding into the bowel lumen and peritoneal cavity and eventual perforation. With perforation, bacteria and toxins from the strangulated intestine enter the peritoneum and, potentially, the circulation, resulting in peritonitis and possible septic shock. Strangulation greatly increases the risk of mortality.

Large-bowel obstruction

Obstruction of the large intestine occurs much less frequently than small-bowel obstruction. Although any portion of the colon may be affected, obstruction usually occurs in the sigmoid segment. Bowel cancer is the most common cause; other causes include volvulus, diverticular disease, inflammatory disorders and faecal impaction.

MANIFESTATIONS Constipation and colic-like abdominal pain are usual manifestations of large-bowel obstruction. The pain is often deep and cramping; severe continuous pain signals bowel ischaemia and possible perforation. Vomiting is a late sign, if it occurs at all. The abdomen is distended, with high-pitched, tinkling bowel sounds with rushes and gurgles. On palpation, localised tenderness or a mass may be noted.

COMPLICATIONS If the ileocaecal valve between the small and large intestines is competent, distension proximal to the obstruction is limited to the colon itself. This is known as a *closed-loop obstruction*. It leads to massive colon dilation as the ileum continues to empty gas and fluid into the colon. Increasing pressure within the obstructed colon impairs circulation to the bowel wall. Gangrene and perforation are potential complications.

INTERPROFESSIONAL CARE

The management of a bowel obstruction focuses on relieving the pressure and obstruction and providing supportive care. The intestine is decompressed and fluid and electrolyte balance is restored. Surgery may be necessary to relieve a mechanical obstruction or if strangulation is suspected.

Diagnosis

Radiological studies (x-rays and CT scan) are used to confirm the diagnosis of bowel obstruction. Laboratory testing is used to evaluate for the presence of infection and fluid and electrolyte imbalances.

An abdominal x-ray often shows distended loops of intestine with fluid and gas in a small-bowel obstruction. Free air under the diaphragm indicates a perforation. X-ray or CT scan with contrast media may be required to confirm a mechanical obstruction and assess the completeness of the obstruction. Meglumine diatrizoate (Gastrografin) is often used to provide contrast, rather than barium, when a bowel

TABLE 23.13 Clinical manifestations and pathophysiological processes of mechanical small-bowel obstruction

MANIFESTATION	PATHOPHYSIOLOGY
Abdominal pain: intermittent mid-abdominal, colicky; intensity may initially decrease, then become severe and steady	Peristaltic waves attempt to propel bowel contents past the obstruction. As the bowel becomes increasingly distended, peristalsis is inhibited and pain may decrease in intensity. If unrelieved, distension of bowel lumen impairs mucosal blood supply, leading to ischaemia and necrosis. Bowel infarction or perforation may occur, leading to chemical and bacterial peritonitis.
Bowel sounds: initially loud, possibly high pitched; may correspond with waves of abdominal pain; later infrequent or absent	Initial distension of the bowel proximal to the obstruction stimulates peristalsis as the bowel attempts to propel contents past the obstruction. With further distension and resulting electrolyte imbalances, peristalsis is inhibited and bowel sounds become less frequent to inaudible.
Vomiting	Distension of the bowel stimulates the vomiting centre of the brain, which, in turn, stimulates the vomiting reflex.
Abdominal distension	Fluid (saliva, gastric juice, bile, pancreatic secretions) and air are trapped in the bowel proximal to the obstruction.
Hypovolaemia, electrolyte imbalance	Normal movement of water and sodium from the bowel lumen to the interstitial and intravascular spaces is initially inhibited. Fluids and electrolytes are lost through vomiting. With continued obstruction and bowel distension, sodium and water move from the vascular system into the bowel lumen, further distending it. Intestinal venous return is inhibited, leading to tissue oedema and accumulation of fluid and electrolytes within the peritoneal cavity.

obstruction is suspected. Barium enema may be used to confirm the diagnosis of large-bowel obstruction and determine its location, unless perforation is suspected.

Laboratory tests include WBC, serum amylase, serum osmolality, electrolytes and arterial blood gases. These tests will show the following results with a bowel obstruction:

- *WBC* often shows mild leucocytosis due to an inflammatory response to changes within the obstructed bowel lumen. With strangulation, leucocytosis is marked.
- *Serum amylase levels* may be elevated, particularly when strangulation is present.
- *Serum osmolality* and *electrolyte levels* are affected by fluid and electrolyte losses from vomiting and fluid sequestering in the bowel lumen. With hypovolaemia, the serum osmolality and urine specific gravity increase. Potassium and chloride are lost through vomiting, leading to hypokalaemia and hypochloraemia.
- *ABGs* may reveal metabolic alkalosis (pH > 7.45, bicarbonate > 26 mmol/L, PCO_2 > 45 mmHg) with small-bowel obstruction due to loss of hydrochloric acid from the stomach.

Gastrointestinal decompression

Most partial small-bowel obstructions are successfully treated with gastrointestinal decompression using a nasogastric or long intestinal tube. Functional obstructions respond to treatment with bowel rest and intestinal decompression as well. Intestinal tubes (see Figure 23.5) may be inserted through the nares or via gastrostomy. A balloon or weighted tip draws the tube from the stomach into the intestine and to the area of obstruction. Collected fluid and gas are removed using low suction until peristalsis resumes or the obstruction is relieved. Sharma (2018) outlined the current clinical guidelines for low-pressure gastric suctioning, including regularly checking that suction reaches the specified pressure level—gastric contents move back down the tube towards the person when the suction is off and rise towards the container when the suction is on. If the fluid fails to move, the Salem sump may be blocked or the suction container is positioned too low or high relative to the height of the person's stomach. In a few hours, a person can lose more than 1,500 mL containing electrolytes and hydrogen ions when low-pressure suction is used (Sharma, 2018). It is important to closely assess the person's fluid, electrolyte and acid–base balance.

Surgery

Surgical intervention is required for complete mechanical obstructions as well as for strangulated or incarcerated obstructions of the small intestine. A person with incomplete mechanical obstruction may also require surgery if the obstruction persists.

Prior to surgery, a nasogastric tube is inserted to relieve vomiting and abdominal distension and to prevent aspiration of intestinal contents. Fluid and electrolyte balance must be restored before surgery. Isotonic intravenous fluids, such as normal (physiological) saline, Hartmann's solution or other balanced electrolyte solutions are used. Additional electrolytes may be added to the solution to correct low levels. It is particularly important to correct hypokalaemia prior to surgery. Acid–base imbalances are also addressed, often using intravenous acidifiers or alkalinising agents. If strangulation has occurred, the person may require plasma or blood replacement. Intravenous broad-spectrum antibiotics are administered prophylactically (see the section on peritonitis).

A laparotomy usually is performed to allow inspection of the small intestine and removal of infarcted or gangrenous tissue. If the obstruction was caused by adhesions, these are removed or lysed. Obstructing tumours are resected and foreign bodies are removed. Any bowel appearing gangrenous is resected, usually followed by an end-to-end anastomosis of remaining intestine. If a large tumour mass or dense adhesions are found, the area of obstruction may be bypassed by anastomosis of proximal small bowel to small or large intestine distal to the obstruction. See the box 'Nursing care of the person requiring bowel surgery'.

Obstructions of the large intestine usually necessitate surgery. The primary goal is to relieve colonic distension and prevent perforation. The secondary goal is to remove the obstructing lesion. In some cases, colonoscopy may be used to relieve the distension. If the person's condition prohibits major surgery or the obstructing tumour is advanced, laser photocoagulation may be used to enlarge the bowel lumen. Removal of the obstructing lesion is the preferred treatment. The proximal and distal bowel segments may be anastomosed or a permanent colostomy or ileostomy may be required.

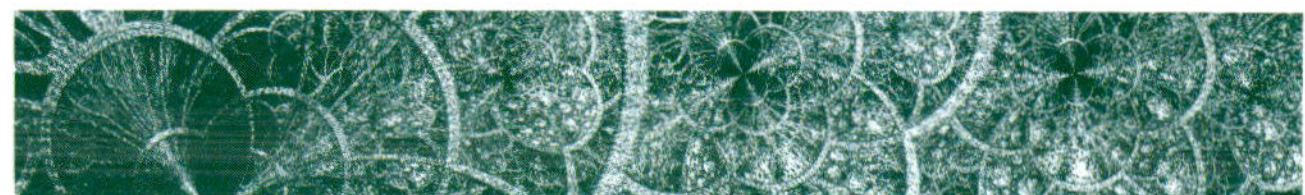

Nursing care

Health promotion

Advise the person, particularly older adults, regarding health promotion activities, such as increasing dietary fibre intake, maintaining a generous fluid intake and exercising daily to help prevent constipation and possible large-bowel obstruction. Stress the importance of maintaining dietary restrictions (such as avoiding popcorn) for a person experiencing repeated small-bowel obstructions.

Assessment

Nurses may be instrumental in the early identification of intestinal obstructions in older adults, the homebound or the institutionalised individual. Early identification and intervention significantly reduce morbidity from bowel obstruction.

- *Health history*: complaints of abdominal pain and bloating, constipation; previous history of bowel obstruction or risk factors such as hernia, IBD, diverticulosis or previous abdominal surgery; current medications.
- *Physical examination*: vital signs including orthostatic blood pressure, temperature; skin colour, temperature, texture and turgor; colour and moisture of mucous membranes; abdominal shape, contour, bowel sounds, presence of tenderness or masses on palpation.

Nursing diagnoses and interventions

In a person with suspected or confirmed bowel obstruction, frequent assessment for complications such as fluid and electrolyte imbalance, acid–base imbalances, hypovolaemic shock, perforation and peritonitis is necessary.

Deficient fluid volume

Because of the large collection of fluid in the bowel proximal to an obstruction, and the accompanying vomiting and nasogastric suction, a person with an intestinal obstruction often has a fluid volume deficit. If not corrected promptly, hypovolaemic shock, acute kidney injury and multiple-organ system dysfunction from poor tissue perfusion may result.

- Monitor vital signs, peripheral perfusion (skin temperature, peripheral pulses and capillary refill); pulmonary artery pressures, cardiac output (CO) (if Swan–Ganz catheter in situ) and central venous pressure (CVP) hourly (if able). *A decrease in blood pressure, tachycardia, tachypnoea and a decrease in peripheral perfusion may indicate hypovolaemia. Although invasive, haemodynamic parameters such as pulmonary artery pressures, CO and CVP allow accurate assessment of fluid volume status.*
- Measure urinary output hourly and nasogastric drainage every 2 to 4 hours. *A urinary output of 0.5 mL/kg/hr or more usually indicates an adequate glomerular filtration rate (GFR). Nasogastric output provides a tool for evaluating fluid replacement needs.*

CONSIDERATION FOR PRACTICE

Report promptly urine output of less than 0.5 mL/kg/hr for 2 consecutive hours. This often indicates hypovolaemia and an increased risk of shock and acute kidney injury or dysfunction.

- Maintain intravenous fluids and blood volume expanders as ordered. *The amount of fluid administered is calculated to meet ongoing fluid needs and replace previous and current losses. Restoration and maintenance of blood volume are necessary to maintain cardiac output and tissue and organ perfusion.*
- Measure abdominal girth every 4 to 8 hours. Mark the level of measurement on the abdomen. *A reference mark allows consistent, accurate measurements. An increase in abdominal girth indicates increasing intestinal distension.*
- Notify the doctor of changes in status. *Changes in vital signs, pain and signs of increasing distension can indicate the need for immediate surgical intervention.*

Ineffective tissue perfusion: gastrointestinal

Perfusion of the intestinal wall and mucosa may be impaired by the obstructive process itself (e.g. strangulation or volvulus) or by significant intestinal distension. The goal is to maintain tissue perfusion and promote normal peristalsis and bowel elimination.

- Monitor vital signs hourly. Assess peripheral pulses, skin colour, temperature and capillary refill. *Cardiovascular assessment is vital to detect early signs of hypovolaemic shock resulting from sequestering large volumes of fluid in the intestines. Hypovolaemia and shock can convert mild bowel ischaemia to infarction as the blood supply to the tissue falls.*
- Monitor urine output hourly. Report output of less than 0.5 mL/kg/hr. *Urine output is a good indicator of the GFR and tissue perfusion. The urine output often falls before vital sign changes are apparent in hypovolaemia.*
- Monitor temperature at least every 4 hours. *An elevated temperature may be an early indication of sepsis from bowel perforation as a result of gangrene.*
- Frequently assess pain. *A change in the character of pain or a rapid increase in its intensity may signal bowel infarction or perforation.*
- Maintain NBM status until peristalsis resumes. *Enteral food or fluids may increase distension and bowel ischaemia. These also are restricted until the possibility of perforation is eliminated.*

Ineffective breathing pattern

Significant abdominal distension from a bowel obstruction can cause the diaphragm to flatten, impairing pulmonary ventilation. Following surgery, splinting of abdominal muscles to avoid pain can lead to shallow respirations. These factors, plus the risk of aspiration of gastrointestinal contents during vomiting, place a person at high risk of respiratory complications, particularly with a small-bowel obstruction.

- Assess respiratory rate, pattern, pulse oximetry and lung sounds at least every 2 to 4 hours. *Tachypnoea, shortness of breath or apparent dyspnoea are early signs of respiratory compromise. Diminished breath sounds, particularly in the bases of the lungs, or crackles indicate poor lung expansion and possible impaired ventilation.*
- Monitor ABG results for possible effects of altered respiratory status. *Tachypnoea may lead to respiratory alkalosis as excess carbon dioxide is eliminated. Conversely, impaired chest expansion can lead to respiratory acidosis because of alveolar hypoventilation.*
- Elevate the head of the bed. *Elevating the head of the bed reduces the work of breathing and improves alveolar ventilation by reducing the pressure of abdominal distension on the diaphragm.*
- Provide a pillow or folded towel to use in splinting the abdomen while coughing postoperatively. *Splinting abdominal muscles and incisions improves the ease and effectiveness of coughing postoperatively.*
- Maintain nasogastric or intestinal tube patency. *Maintaining gastrointestinal suction helps reduce abdominal distension and prevent aspiration associated with vomiting.*

- Encourage use of incentive spirometer or other assistive device hourly. *These devices encourage deep breathing, opening distal airways and preventing atelectasis.*
- Contact physiotherapist as indicated. *The physiotherapist may suggest or perform additional measures to maintain effective pulmonary ventilation.*
- Provide good oral care 2 to 4 hourly. *Dehydration and nasogastric suction dry the mucous membranes of the mouth and throat, increasing the risk of bacterial growth. Many respiratory infections result from aspirated organisms.*

Community-based care

Include the following topics when teaching a person with intestinal obstruction in preparation for home care:

- wound care
- activity level, return to work and any other recommended restrictions
- recommended follow-up care
- care of temporary colostomy (if appropriate) and planned reanastomosis
- recurrent obstructions, their cause, early identification of manifestations and possible preventive measures.

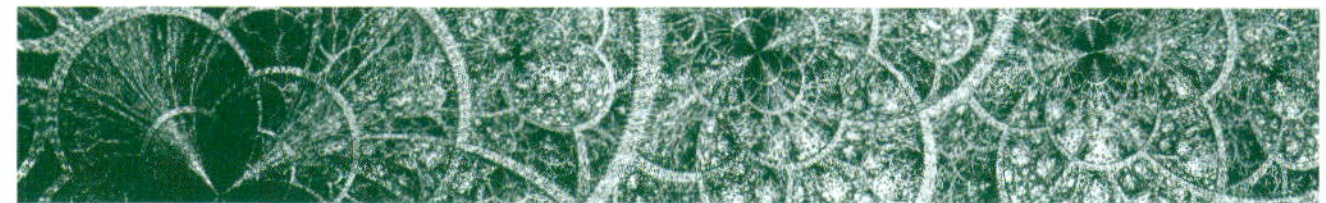

THE PERSON WITH DIVERTICULAR DISEASE

Diverticula are small (0.5 to 1.0 cm) outpouchings of the colon occurring in rows (see Figure 23.19). Diverticula may occur anywhere in the intestinal tract, excluding the rectum. The vast majority, however, affect the large intestine, with 85–95% occurring in the sigmoid colon (Loscalzo et al., 2022; Papadakis et al., 2022).

FAST FACTS

Diverticular disease

- People in Australia, the UK, France and the US have high and increasing incidence rates of diverticular disease. The incidence of diverticula increases with age, with 5–10% of the population older than 45 years of age and almost 80% of those older than 85 years of age experiencing it.
- Most people diagnosed with diverticular disease remain asymptomatic.
- Men and women are equally affected.

Cultural factors—diet, in particular—are thought to play an important role in the development of diverticula. A diet consisting of highly refined and fibre-deficient foods is believed to be a major contributor to the disease. Decreased activity levels and delaying defecation have also been suggested as contributing factors. The increasing incidence of diverticula with ageing suggests dietary factors (lack of fibre), a decrease in physical activity, poor bowel habits (neglecting the urge to defecate) and the effects of ageing contribute to development of the disease (Marieb & Hoehn, 2019).

Pathophysiology

Diverticula form when increased pressure within the bowel lumen causes bowel mucosa to herniate through defects in the colon wall. The circular and longitudinal muscles often thicken or hypertrophy in the area affected by diverticula. This narrows the bowel lumen, increasing intraluminal pressure. Deficient dietary fibre and a lack of faecal bulk contribute to muscle hypertrophy and narrowing of the bowel. Contraction of the muscles in response to normal stimuli such as meals may occlude the narrowed lumen, further increasing intraluminal pressure. The high pressure causes mucosa to herniate through

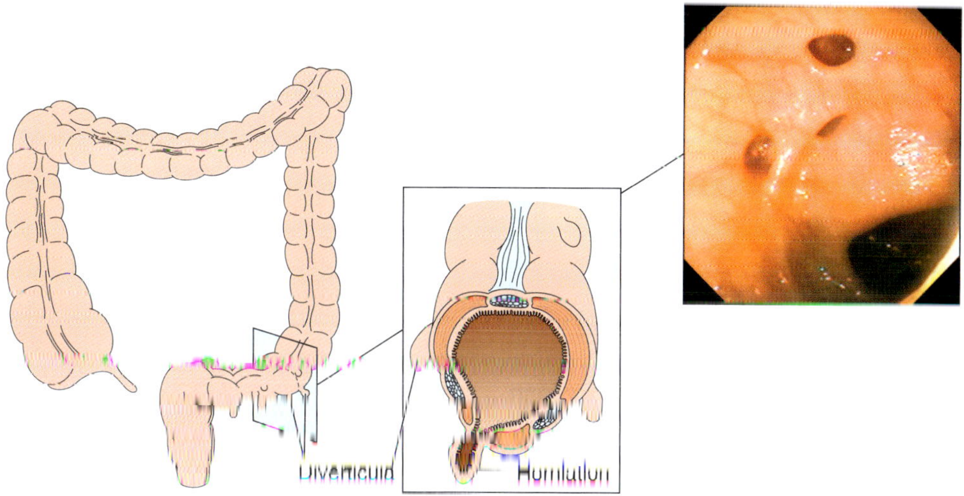

FIGURE 23.19 *Diverticula of the colon*

Source: Image © David M. Martin MD/Science Photo Library.

the muscle wall, forming a diverticulum. Areas where nutrient blood vessels penetrate the circular muscle layer are the most common sites for diverticula formation.

Diverticulosis

Diverticulosis indicates the presence of diverticula. More than two-thirds of people with diverticulosis are asymptomatic. When manifestations such as episodic pain (usually left-sided), constipation and diarrhoea occur, these often are attributed to IBS, commonly accompanying diverticular disease. As the disease progresses, abdominal cramping, narrow stools (decrease in calibre), increased constipation, bleeding in the stools, weakness and fatigue may develop.

Complications of diverticulosis include haemorrhage and diverticulitis. A diverticulum may bleed, whether it is inflamed or not, possibly due to erosion of an adjacent blood vessel by a faecalith (hard mass) in the diverticulum.

Diverticulitis

Diverticulitis is inflammation in and around the diverticular sac. It typically affects only one diverticulum, usually in the sigmoid colon. Undigested food and bacteria collect in the diverticula, forming a hard mass impairing the mucosal blood supply, allowing bacterial invasion. Mucosal ischaemia leads to perforation. With microscopic perforation, inflammation is localised. Gross perforation of a diverticulum results in more extensive bacterial contamination, leading to abscess formation or peritonitis.

MANIFESTATIONS Pain is a common clinical manifestation of diverticulitis. It is usually left-sided and may be mild to severe and either steady or cramping. The person may also experience either constipation or increased frequency of defecation. Depending on the location and severity of the inflammation, nausea, vomiting and a low-grade fever may occur. On examination, the abdomen may be distended, with tenderness and a palpable mass in the left lower quadrant resulting from the inflammatory response.

Older adults may have less specific manifestations, complaining of vague abdominal pain. A palpable mass and signs of a large-bowel obstruction may be present.

COMPLICATIONS Complications associated with diverticulitis (in addition to peritonitis and abscess formation) include bowel obstruction, fistula formation and haemorrhage. Severe or repeated episodes of diverticulitis may lead to scarring and fibrosis of the bowel wall, further narrowing the bowel lumen. This increases the risk of obstruction of the large bowel. Acutely inflamed tissue adheres to the small bowel, increasing the potential for small-bowel obstruction as well. Fistulas may form, usually between the sigmoid colon and the bladder. Urinary tract infection is the usual sign of a colovesical fistula. Fistulas may also perforate into the small intestine, ureter, vagina, perineum or abdominal wall. Bleeding from perforation of a vessel wall can occur with diverticulitis. Although it may be significant, bleeding usually stops spontaneously.

INTERPROFESSIONAL CARE

Management of diverticular disease varies from no prescribed treatment to surgical resection of affected colon, depending on the severity of the disease and its complications.

Diagnosis

Diagnostic testing is used to identify diverticular disease when the disease is symptomatic or complications develop. In addition to illustrating diverticula, a barium enema and x-rays can reveal segmental spasm and muscular thickening with a narrowed bowel lumen. Flexible sigmoidoscopy or colonoscopy may be done to detect diverticulosis, assess for strictures or bleeding, and rule out tumour as the cause of the person's manifestations. Abdominal x-ray films may show free abdominal air associated with diverticulitis and perforation. CT scan may be done with or without contrast media to assess inflammation and detect an abscess or fistula.

Laboratory tests include haemoccult or guaiac testing of stool to identify the presence of occult blood, and a WBC count may show leucocytosis with a left shift (an increased number of immature WBCs) due to inflammation in diverticulitis.

Medications

Systemic broad-spectrum antibiotics effective against usual bowel flora are prescribed to treat acute diverticulitis. Oral antibiotics such as metronidazole (Flagyl) and ciprofloxacin (Cipro) or trimethoprim-sulfamethoxazole (Septra, Bactrim) may be prescribed if manifestations are mild. Rifixamin (Xifaxan) is a poorly absorbed antibiotic that may be used together with fibre to treat unmanaged diverticular disease. Severe, acute attacks often require hospitalisation and treatment with intravenous fluids and antibiotics effective against anaerobic and Gram-negative bacteria. Therapy may include a second-generation cephalosporin such as cefoxitin (Mefoxin) or another antibiotic such as piperacillin-tazobactam (Tazocin) or ticarcillin-clavulanate (Timentin). Antibiotics and their nursing implications are discussed in the chapter 'Nursing care of people with infections'.

Although a stool softener such as docusate sodium (Coloxyl) may be prescribed, it is important to note that laxatives (which can further increase intraluminal pressure in the colon) are avoided for a person with diverticular disease.

Nutrition

Dietary modification is central to the management of diverticular disease. Dietary changes appear to reduce the risk of complications of diverticulosis. A high-fibre diet is recommended; this increases stool bulk, decreases intraluminal pressures and may reduce spasm (see Table 23.14). Bran is a low-cost fibre supplement that can be added to cereal, soups, salads or other foods. Commercial bulk-forming products—for example, psyllium seed (Metamucil)—may be recommended. These products are discussed in the 'Medication administration' box on laxatives. The person should be advised to avoid foods with small seeds (such as caraway seeds, figs or berries), which could obstruct diverticula.

Bowel rest is prescribed during an acute episode of diverticulitis. Initially the person may be NBM with intravenous

TABLE 23.14 Foods recommended in a high-fibre, high-residue diet

FOOD GROUP	RECOMMENDED FOODS
Cereals and grains	Wheat or oat bran; cooked cereals, such as oatmeal; dry cereals, such as bran buds or flakes, cornflakes, shredded wheat; wholegrain breads or biscuits; brown rice; popcorn
Fruits	Unpeeled raw apples, peaches and pears; blackberries, raspberries, strawberries; oranges
Vegetables	Dried beans (navy, kidney, pinto), lima beans; broccoli; peas; corn; squash; raw vegetables, such as carrots, celery and tomatoes; potatoes (with skins)

fluids and occasionally TPN. Feeding is resumed gradually. Initially, a clear liquid diet is prescribed, with gradual advancement to a soft, low-roughage diet (i.e. a diet low in insoluble fibre) with daily added psyllium seed to soften stool and increase its bulk. Among foods a person should avoid are wheat and corn bran, vegetable and fruit skins, nuts and dry beans. The high-fibre diet is resumed following full recovery.

Surgery

A person with acute diverticulitis may require surgery, usually to treat generalised peritonitis or an abscess failing to respond to medical treatment. Haemorrhage that recurs or cannot be controlled may also necessitate surgery. Elective surgery may be performed for recurrent episodes of diverticulitis or persistent diverticulitis with continuing pain, tenderness and a palpable mass.

The affected bowel segment is resected and, if possible, an anastomosis of the proximal and distal portions is performed. When an acute infection and diverticulitis are present, a two-stage Hartmann's procedure is required. A temporary colostomy is created and anastomosis delayed until the inflammation has subsided. A second surgery is performed 2 to 3 months later to reconnect the bowel and close the temporary colostomy.

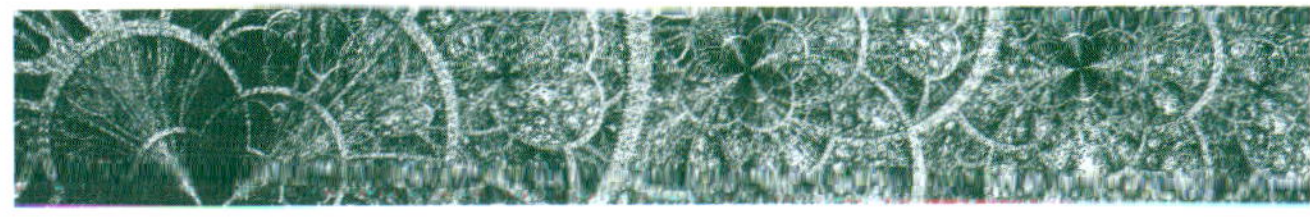

Nursing care

Health promotion

Advising a person about the benefits of a high-fibre diet is important primary prevention for diverticular disease. Nurses working with groups and individuals in the community should emphasise the importance of a high-fibre diet and its benefits in preventing diverticular disease and other disorders. In facilities such as residential settings, nurses can work with dietary staff and care providers to increase the amount of fibre in residents' diets, unless this is contraindicated by a pre-existing condition.

Assessment

Because most people with diverticular disease have few or no manifestations, nursing assessment focuses on manifestations of complications.

- *Health history*: abdominal pain or cramping, chronic constipation or irregular bowel habits; nausea and vomiting; history of diverticular disease or IBS.
- *Physical examination*: bowel sounds, presence of abdominal tenderness of masses and location; stool for occult blood.

Nursing diagnoses and interventions

A person with acute diverticulitis is acutely ill and has multiple nursing care needs. Priority nursing diagnoses include *Potential complication: perforation*, *Acute pain* and *Anxiety* related to the possibility of a significant complication or possible surgery.

Potential complication: perforation

During an acute attack of diverticulitis, inflammation and mucosal ischaemia the person is at risk of perforation and peritonitis. In addition to maintaining bowel rest to reduce the risk of perforation, nurses monitor for manifestations of perforation and possible sepsis.

- Monitor vital signs including temperature at least every 4 hours. *Tachycardia and tachypnoea may be early indications of increased inflammation and resulting fluid shift. Fever greater than 38.3°C may indicate increased inflammation or spread of inflammation. Note, however, that little temperature elevation may occur in older adults. A change in behaviour or increasing lethargy may be subtle indications of infection in the older adult.*
- Assess abdomen every 4 to 8 hours or more often as indicated, including measuring abdominal girth, auscultating bowel sounds and palpating for tenderness. Report promptly significant changes to the doctor. *Increasing abdominal distension, a decrease or change in the quality of bowel sounds, and/or increasing tenderness or guarding may indicate spread of the infectious process or peritonitis.*
- Assess for evidence of lower intestinal bleeding by visual examination and guaiac testing of stools for occult blood. *Perforation of a diverticulum may produce either intestinal or intra-abdominal bleeding and require immediate treatment such as surgery.*
- Maintain intravenous fluids, TPN and accurate intake and output records. *During acute diverticulitis, oral intake is usually prohibited or restricted. Intravenous fluids are given to maintain fluid and electrolyte balance; TPN is used to maintain nutritional status, facilitating healing and recovery.*

Acute pain

Pain is a common clinical manifestation of acute diverticulitis. It results from inflammation of the bowel and oedema of affected tissues. If surgery is required, postoperative pain is managed with narcotic analgesics.

- Ask the person to rate pain using a 0 to 10 pain scale. Document the level of pain and note any changes in location or character of pain. *The perception and response to pain is individual and is affected by past experiences, culture, ethnic background and other factors. A change in the character or intensity of the pain indicates a complication such as perforation or abscess formation.*
- Administer prescribed analgesic or maintain PCA as ordered. Assess analgesic effectiveness. Avoid administering morphine. Provide adjunctive medications as ordered and encourage use of adjunctive techniques, such as relaxation, positioning and distraction. Notify the doctor if pain management is inadequate. *If a person has not obtained adequate pain relief, further assessment and intervention are required.*
- Maintain bowel rest and total body rest (bed rest with limited activity). *Rest helps reduce inflammation and promotes healing, increasing comfort.*
- Reintroduce oral foods and fluids slowly, providing a soft, low-fibre diet with bulk-forming agents. *This allows continued healing of the affected bowel while promoting soft, easily expelled stools.*

Anxiety

A person with acute diverticulitis faces not only hospitalisation but also potential serious complications such as peritonitis and haemorrhage. Surgery and formation of a temporary colostomy may be necessary. Furthermore, episodes of acute diverticulitis are often recurrent and the person may fear future problems.

- Demonstrate empathy and awareness of the perceived health threat. *It is important to recognise and respect the person's feelings and perceptions as reality.*
- Assess level of understanding about disease and condition. *This allows misperceptions contributing to anxiety to be corrected.*
- Assess and document level of anxiety. *Severe anxiety or panic states interfere with the ability to respond to instructions and assist with care. Low to moderate anxiety levels enhance learning and compliance with prescribed interventions.*
- Assist the person to identify and use appropriate coping mechanisms. *Coping mechanisms provide immediate relief of anxiety while the person adapts to the situation.*
- Attend to physical care needs. *This provides reassurance these needs will be met and relieves concerns about them.*
- Spend as much time as possible with the person. *Presence of caring nurses helps relieve fears of abandonment or that help will not be available if needed. It also enhances trust and provides opportunity for expression of fears or concerns.*
- Encourage family and friends to remain with the person as much as possible. *This provides a supportive environment for the person and also distracts from physical concerns.*
- Involve the person and their family (as appropriate) in care decisions. *This increases a person's sense of control over the situation.*

Community-based care

A person with diverticular disease is responsible for self-care. Discuss the following topics for home care:

- prescribed high-fibre diet and the need to maintain the diet for life to reduce the incidence of complications, including ways to increase dietary fibre
- complications and their manifestations of diverticular disease
- provide a referral to a nutritionist for teaching as indicated.

Prior to discharge of a person with acute diverticulitis, discuss the following:

- food and fluid limitations, including recommendations for a low-residue diet during the initial period of healing
- colostomy management (if a temporary colostomy has been created), including where to obtain supplies and dietary management
- planned procedure to reanastomose the colon and revise the colostomy. Refer to community healthcare organisations as indicated.

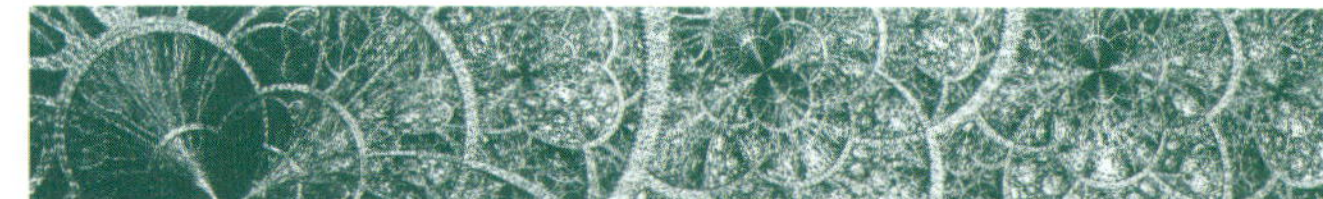

Anorectal disorders

Anorectal lesions include haemorrhoids, anal fissure, anorectal abscess, anorectal fistula and pilonidal disease.

THE PERSON WITH HAEMORRHOIDS

The anus and anal canal contain two superficial venous plexuses with the haemorrhoidal veins. When pressure on these veins is increased or venous return impeded, they can develop varices or varicosities, becoming weak and distended. This condition is commonly known as **haemorrhoids** or 'piles'. When asymptomatic, haemorrhoids are considered to be a normal condition found in all adults.

Pathophysiology and manifestations

Haemorrhoids develop when venous return from the anal canal is impaired. Straining to defecate increases venous pressure and is the most common cause of distended haemorrhoids. Pregnancy increases intra-abdominal pressure, raising venous pressure, and is another cause of haemorrhoids. Other factors that may contribute to symptomatic haemorrhoids include prolonged sitting, obesity, chronic constipation and a low-fibre diet.

Haemorrhoids are classed as either internal or external. *Internal haemorrhoids* affect the venous plexus above the mucocutaneous junction of the anus (see Figure 23.20).

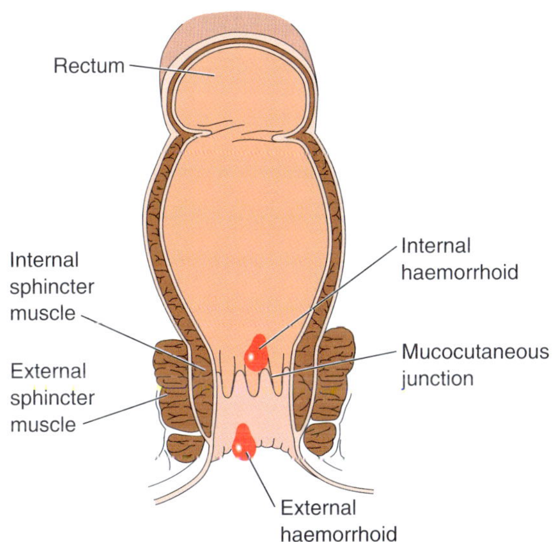

FIGURE 23.20 ***The location of internal and external haemorrhoids***

Internal haemorrhoids rarely cause pain, usually presenting with bleeding. Bleeding from internal haemorrhoids is bright red and unmixed with the stool. It varies in quantity from streaks on toilet tissue to enough to colour the water in the toilet. Recurrent bleeding of internal haemorrhoids may be sufficient to cause anaemia. Mucus discharge and a feeling of incomplete evacuation of stool may also be manifestations of internal haemorrhoids.

External haemorrhoids affect the inferior haemorrhoidal plexus below the mucocutaneous junction. Bleeding is rare with external haemorrhoids. Anal irritation, a feeling of pressure and difficulty cleaning the anal region may be manifestations of external haemorrhoids.

As these enlarge, haemorrhoids may prolapse or protrude through the anus. Initially, prolapse occurs only with defecation and the haemorrhoids spontaneously regress back into the anal canal. Eventually, a person may need to manually replace internal haemorrhoids after defecation or these may become permanently prolapsed, in which case replacement is not possible. Manifestations of permanently prolapsed haemorrhoids include mucus discharge and clothing soilage.

'Normal' haemorrhoids are not painful. Prolapsed haemorrhoids may become strangulated as a result of congestion and oedema, leading to thrombosis. Haemorrhoidal thrombosis causes extreme pain and may lead to infarction of skin and mucosa overlying the haemorrhoid. Internal haemorrhoids associated with portal hypertension in liver disease may bleed profusely if ruptured. (See the chapter 'Nursing care of people with gallbladder, liver and pancreatic disorders' for further discussion of portal hypertension.)

A *thrombosed external haemorrhoid* is a thrombosis of the subcutaneous external haemorrhoidal veins of the anal canal, rather than a true haemorrhoid. It appears as a painful bluish haematoma beneath the skin and typically occurs following a sudden increase in venous pressure (e.g. heavy lifting, coughing or straining). Pain is significant at onset; however, it gradually subsides. Spontaneous rupture with bleeding may occur. Thrombosed external haemorrhoids resolve without intervention.

INTERPROFESSIONAL CARE

Because haemorrhoids are a normal condition, management is conservative unless complications such as permanent prolapse or thrombosis occur.

Diagnosis

Haemorrhoids are diagnosed by the person's history and by examination of the anorectal area. External haemorrhoids can be seen on visual inspection, especially if thrombosed. The person is asked to strain (Valsalva manoeuvre) during the examination to detect prolapse. Internal haemorrhoids are usually not palpable or tender on digital examination of the rectum. *Anoscopic* examination is used to detect and evaluate internal haemorrhoids. For this exam, a speculum or endoscope is introduced into the anus to provide visual inspection of the tissues. Additional diagnostic examinations include testing of stool for occult blood and sigmoidoscopy, performed to rule out colon or rectal cancer, which may aggravate haemorrhoidal manifestations or produce similar manifestations. If liver disease with portal hypertension is suspected, liver function studies are ordered.

Medications

Bulk-forming laxatives such as psyllium seed (Metamucil) or stool softeners such as docusate sodium (Coloxyl) may be prescribed to relieve constipation as well as reducing discomfort. Suppositories and local ointments such as Preparation H or Nupercaine have an anaesthetic and astringent effect, reducing discomfort and irritation of surrounding tissues. These medications have little or no effect on the haemorrhoid itself. Warm sitz baths, bed rest and local astringent compresses may be recommended to reduce the swelling of oedematous prolapsed haemorrhoids after digital reduction.

Nutrition

Haemorrhoids that are not permanently prolapsed or acutely thrombosed generally are treated conservatively. A high-fibre diet and increased water intake to increase stool bulk, improve its softness and reduce straining are effective for most people with internal or external haemorrhoids.

Sclerotherapy

Haemorrhoids that are permanently prolapsed, are thrombosed or produce significant manifestations are treated more aggressively. *Sclerotherapy* involves injecting a chemical irritant into tissues surrounding the haemorrhoid to induce inflammation and eventual fibrosis and scarring. It is used to treat recurrent bleeding and early prolapse of internal haemorrhoids. The treatment produces minimal pain. Enlarged or prolapsing haemorrhoids may also be treated with rubber band ligation. A rubber band is placed snugly around the haemorrhoidal plexus and surrounding mucosa, causing the tissue to necrose and slough within 7 to 10 days. Treatment is limited to one haemorrhoidal complex at a time, so repeat treatments may be necessary. Pain should be minimal if the band is placed appropriately; persistent pain following band ligation may signal an infection. Bleeding can occur as the haemorrhoid sloughs. Other procedures used to treat haemorrhoids include cryosurgery (in which haemorrhoids are necrosed by freezing with a cryoprobe), infrared photocoagulation or electrocoagulation.

Haemorrhoidectomy

A person with chronic manifestations, permanent prolapse, chronic bleeding with associated anaemia or painful thrombosed haemorrhoids may be treated surgically with a *haemorrhoidectomy*. In this procedure, haemorrhoids are surgically excised, leaving normal skin and surrounding tissues. This procedure may use conventional techniques or a laser to remove both internal and external haemorrhoids. Few complications are associated with haemorrhoidectomy.

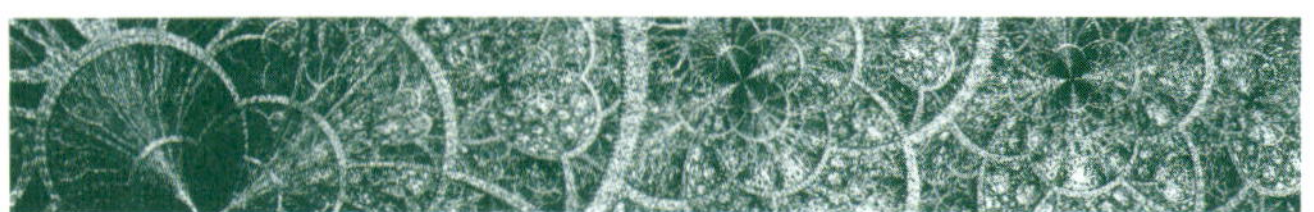

Nursing care

Primary prevention of symptomatic haemorrhoids involves education of people of all ages. Stress the importance of maintaining an adequate intake of dietary fibre, a liberal fluid intake and regular exercise to maintain stool bulk, softness and regularity. Discuss the need to respond to the urge to defecate rather than postponing defecation. Teach appropriate constipation management, including the use of bulk-forming laxatives.

Most people with haemorrhoids are treated in community settings where the primary nursing focus is educational. Discuss the appropriate use of over-the-counter preparations and sitz baths for the relief of minor haemorrhoidal manifestations. If necessary, teach the person how to reduce prolapsed haemorrhoids digitally.

Advise the person about possible complications, such as chronic bleeding, prolapse and thrombosis. Stress the need to seek medical evaluation if manifestations persist. Discuss the link between manifestations of haemorrhoids and colorectal cancer and urge the person to seek medical intervention for persistent, unresolved or progressive manifestations.

When a haemorrhoidectomy is performed, a person requires more direct nursing intervention. Postoperative care of a person with perianal surgery is outlined in Box 23.4. Anal packing may be in place for the first 24 hours following the procedure. When removed, observe the person closely for bleeding. Pain is a common postoperative problem. Although the operative procedure is minor, postoperative discomfort can be significant because the anal region is richly innervated and muscle spasms may occur. In addition to systemic analgesics, sitz baths usually are ordered. These not only help promote relaxation and reduce discomfort but also clean the anal area. Use of a rubber ring or doughnut device minimises pressure on the surgical site while the person sits in the bath.

BOX 23.4 Perianal postoperative care

Assessment

- Monitor vital signs every 4 hours for 24 hours.
- Inspect rectal dressing every 2 to 3 hours for 24 hours.
- Monitor fluid balance—urinary output.

Pain control

- Assist to position of comfort, usually side lying.
- Provide analgesics as prescribed.
- Keep fresh ice packs over the rectal dressing as ordered.
- Assist with sitz bath water sprays three to four times per day.
- Provide a flotation pad for use when sitting.

Elimination

- Give stool softeners as prescribed.
- Give an analgesic before the first postoperative bowel movement if possible.
- When tolerated, encourage fluid intake of at least 2,000 mL per day.

Individual and family teaching

- Take sitz bath or water spray after each bowel movement for 1 to 2 weeks after surgery.
- Drink at least 2,000 mL of fluid per day.
- Eat adequate dietary fibre and exercise moderately.
- Take stool softeners as prescribed.
- Report to the doctor the following symptoms: rectal bleeding, continued pain on defecation, fever greater than 38.3 °C, purulent rectal drainage.

A person may remain hospitalised until after the first postoperative bowel movement. Stool softeners, adequate fluids and analgesia before defecation aid in reducing anxiety and discomfort. Adequate cleaning following defecation, usually with a sitz bath, is vital.

Whether caring for a person with haemorrhoids or following a haemorrhoidectomy, consider the following nursing diagnoses:

- *Altered comfort* related to acute or chronic pain secondary to inflamed anal tissues.
- *Constipation* related to dietary habits and/or delay of defecation.
- *Risk of infection* related to disruption of anal tissue.

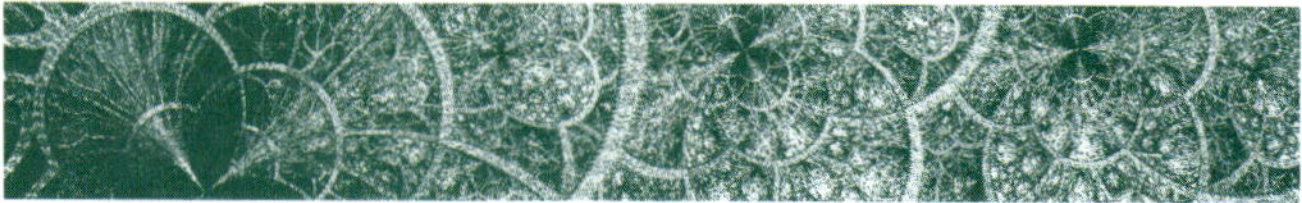

THE PERSON WITH AN ANORECTAL LESION

Unlike the rectum, which is relatively insensitive to pain, the anal canal is richly supplied with sensory nerves and is highly sensitive to painful stimuli. Lesions of the anorectal area may cause significant pain, particularly with defecation. Infection is a potential complication of anorectal lesions because of contamination by faecal bacteria. The superior boundary of the anal canal (the anorectal juncture or pectinate line) contains

8 to 12 anal crypts where anorectal abscesses or fistulas can form. Lesions of the anorectal area include fissures, abscesses, fistulas and pilonidal disease.

Anal fissure

Anal fissures or ulcers occur when the epithelium of the anal canal over the internal sphincter becomes denuded or abraded. Irritating diarrhoeal stools and tightening of the anal canal with increased sphincter tension are frequent causes of anal fissures. Other factors contributing to their development include childbirth trauma, habitual purgative use, laceration by a foreign body and anal intercourse. Chronic inflammation and infection of surrounding tissues accompanies an anal fissure.

A person with an anal fissure typically has periods of exacerbation and remission. Because these occur below the mucocutaneous line, anal fissures are painful. Pain occurring with defecation is described as tearing, burning or cutting. Bright red bleeding is noted with a bowel movement. Bleeding is typically minor and noted on toilet paper. Because of fear of defecation, the person may develop constipation, further disrupting normal bowel habits and aggravating manifestations.

The diagnosis of anal fissure is made by gentle digital examination of the anal canal and anoscopy using a small anoscope. Treatment is usually conservative, involving dietary changes to increase fibre intake and stool bulk, increased fluid intake and use of bulk-forming laxatives. A topical agent such as hydrocortisone cream may be prescribed. Surgical intervention with an internal sphincterotomy, an incision into the internal sphincter to increase its diameter, is considered when the fissure does not heal with medical intervention.

Anorectal abscess

Invasion of the pararectal spaces by pathogenic bacteria can lead to an *anorectal abscess*. Commonly caused by infection extending from the anal crypt into a pararectal space, the abscess may appear small but often contains a large amount of pus. Multiple pathogens may be present, including *E. coli*, *Proteus*, streptococci and staphylococci. Other factors contributing to the development of an anorectal abscess include infection of a hair follicle, sebaceous gland or sweat gland, and abrasions, fissures or anal trauma. The incidence of anorectal abscess is higher in men.

Pain is the primary manifestation of an anorectal abscess. Sitting or walking may aggravate the pain, but it is unrelated to defecation. External swelling, redness, heat and tenderness are apparent on examination. With a deeper abscess, swelling may not be visible, but the abscess is palpable on digital examination.

If the abscess either does not drain spontaneously or is not drained surgically, adjacent anatomical spaces are affected. Systemic sepsis is also a potential complication.

Incision and drainage is the treatment of choice for an anorectal abscess because it rarely resolves with antibiotic therapy alone. This treatment often leads to a persistent fistula, which is surgically closed after the infection has cleared.

Anorectal fistula

A fistula is a tunnel or tube-like tract with openings at each end. *Anorectal fistulas* have one opening in the anal canal, with the other usually found in perianal skin. Most occur spontaneously or as a result of anorectal abscess drainage. Crohn's disease is also a predisposing factor to fistula development.

The primary manifestation of an anorectal fistula is intermittent or constant drainage or purulent discharge. This may be accompanied by local itching, tenderness and pain associated with defecation.

Anoscopic and digital examination with gentle probing of the fistula tract are used to establish the diagnosis. Although some fistulas may heal spontaneously, the treatment of choice is a fistulotomy. The primary opening of the fistula is removed and the tract is opened to allow it to heal by secondary intention, from the inside outward. If the sphincter is involved, a two-stage operation may be done to preserve the muscle and prevent faecal incontinence.

Pilonidal disease

A person with *pilonidal disease* has an acute abscess or chronic draining sinus in the sacrococcygeal area. Underlying the abscess or sinus is a cyst with granulation tissue, fibrosis and, often, hair tufts. This disease usually affects young hirsute (hairy) males and is probably due to hair entrapment in deep tissues of the sacrococcygeal area. Some researchers, however, believe it is a congenital disorder.

The lesion of pilonidal disease is generally asymptomatic unless it becomes acutely infected. Manifestations of acute inflammation accompany infection, including pain, tenderness, redness, heat and swelling of the affected area. Purulent discharge may be noted from one or more sinuses or openings in the midline.

The preferred treatment option for pilonidal disease is incision and drainage. The sinus tract and underlying cyst are excised and closed by either primary- or secondary-intention healing. The person may be instructed to remove hair from the area routinely by shaving or using a depilatory to prevent further hair entrapment and recurrence of the problem.

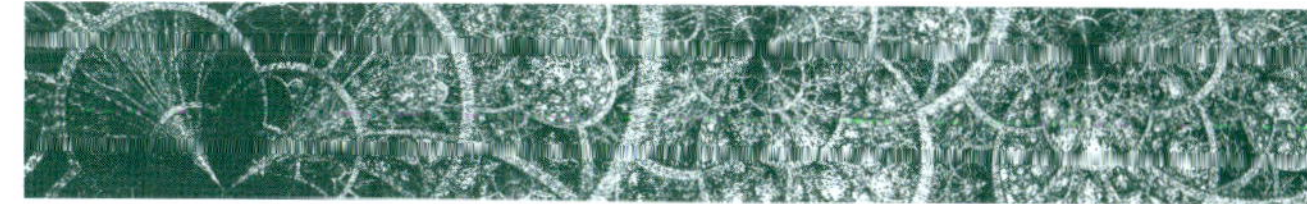

Nursing care

People with anorectal disorders are often treated in the community and the primary nursing responsibility is education. Highlight the importance of maintaining a high-fibre diet and liberal fluid intake to increase stool bulk and softness, thereby decreasing discomfort with defecation. Stress the importance of responding to the urge to defecate to prevent constipation.

Following surgical treatment of any of these disorders, inform the person to keep the perianal region clean and dry. If a dressing is in place, instruct to avoid soiling it with urine or faeces during elimination. Following removal of the dressing, teach to clean the area gently with soap and water following a bowel movement. Discuss the use of sitz baths for cleaning and comfort. Sitz baths are often recommended conservative management pre- and postoperatively for anorectal disorders. A systematic review by Sivapuram (2020) found no strong evidence to support the use of the sitz bath for pain relief or to accelerate fissure or wound healing among adult people with anorectal disorders. However, people with anorectal disorders were more satisfied when using interventions such as sitz baths and water sprays. Sivapuram (2020) highlighted that a person may find the use of the water spray method more convenient and an appropriate alternative to the sitz bath. The use of sitz baths is a personal choice.

Suggest taking an analgesic, if necessary, prior to defecation. However, caution that some analgesics promote constipation. Teach clinical manifestations of infection or other possible complications to report to the doctor. If an antibiotic has been prescribed, provide written and verbal instructions about its use, its desired and possible adverse effects, and their management.

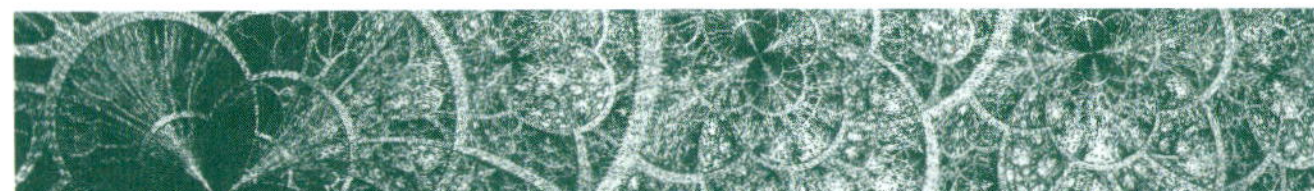

CHAPTER HIGHLIGHTS

- Disorders of intestinal motility include diarrhoea, constipation, irritable bowel syndrome and faecal incontinence. Diarrhoea is a manifestation of many other bowel disorders, including lactose intolerance, infections with bacteria and inflammatory diseases of the bowel. Constipation may be a primary problem (especially for the older adult) or a manifestation of another disorder. Irritable bowel syndrome (IBS) is a functional disorder without any identifiable organic cause. Faecal incontinence is usually considered to be the manifestation of a disorder, rather than a disorder itself.
- Appendicitis is an acute inflammation of the vermiform appendix, manifested by abdominal pain that localises in the right lower quadrant of the abdomen. On palpation, localised and rebound tenderness is present at McBurney's point. It is treated most often with an appendectomy.
- Peritonitis (inflammation of the peritoneum from infection or chemical irritant) is a serious complication of a wide variety of acute abdominal disorders, including perforated ulcer, ruptured appendix, abdominal trauma or surgery, or necrotic bowel. Complications may be life threatening; without prompt and effective treatment, septicaemia and septic shock may occur.
- Gastroenteritis may result from bacterial or viral infections, parasites or toxins, and is often the result of consuming contaminated water or food. Manifestations include nausea and vomiting, diarrhoea and abdominal discomfort.
- Nurses provide education to help prevent protozoal infections (e.g. giardiasis, amoebiasis) and helminthic infestations (by roundworms or tapeworms). Both are treated with medications.
- Chronic inflammatory bowel disease (IBD) includes two separate but closely related conditions: ulcerative colitis and Crohn's disease. Ulcerative colitis affects the mucosa and submucosa of the colon and rectum. Crohn's disease can affect any part of the GI tract, but usually involves the terminal ilium and ascending colon. Diarrhoea is common to both disorders. A colectomy (removal of the large colon) may be performed to treat ulcerative colitis; an ileostomy (artificial opening from the abdomen to the ileum) may be performed to treat Crohn's disease.
- Malabsorption syndromes, in which the intestinal mucosa ineffectively absorbs nutrients, are caused by a wide variety of diseases. However, three common malabsorption disorders in adults are coeliac disease (non-tropical and tropical), lactose intolerance of milk and milk products (resulting from a lactase deficiency) and short-bowel syndrome (a condition developing following resection of the small bowel).
- Malignant tumours of the lower bowel are the third leading cause of death from cancer in Australia. The risk of colon cancer may be reduced through health-related screenings and a diet high in fruits, vegetables, folic acid and calcium. Rectal bleeding is the most common initial manifestation but may not occur until the cancer is well advanced. Surgical treatment is through surgical resection of the bowel, accompanied by a colostomy for diversion of faecal contents.
- A hernia is a defect in the abdominal wall allowing intra-abdominal contents to protrude out of the abdominal cavity. Hernias may follow trauma, surgery and increased intra-abdominal pressure (as from pregnancy or obesity). Hernias may be congenital or acquired and may be inguinal, umbilical, incisional or ventral.
- Intestinal obstructions occur when intestinal contents cannot move through the lumen of the bowel. These may occur in either the large or small intestine, may be partial or complete, and are caused by many factors, ranging from surgical ileus following abdominal surgery to adhesions or tumours.
- Diverticula are sac-like projections of mucosa through the muscular layer of the colon. When these sacs become inflamed, the condition is labelled diverticulitis. A diet high in fibre is recommended for self-care.
- Anorectal disorders include haemorrhoids, anorectal lesions (fissures, abscess and fistula) and pilonidal disease. These disorders are painful and pose a risk of bleeding and infection.

CONCEPT CHECK

1 Mr William Brown presents at the urgent care clinic with complaints of diarrhoea for the past week. The RN should first:
1. advise Mr Brown to abstain from all food intake until the diarrhoea subsides
2. ask Mr Brown to describe the number and character of daily stools
3. question Mr Brown about possible exposure to an enterotoxin or protozoal infection
4. recommend an over-the-counter antidiarrhoeal preparation such as Kaomagma with Pectin Suspension

2 RN Sandra Smith, who is caring for Ms Wong admitted with possible appendicitis, appropriately plans which of the following?
1. Initiate bowel preparation for a barium enema.
2. Restrict intake to clear liquids.
3. Prepare for possible immediate appendectomy.
4. Insert saline lock for intravenous antibiotic therapy.

3 RN David Smith is teaching Mrs Doris Bishop with inflammatory bowel disease about prescribed sulfasalazine. RN Smith instructs Mrs Bishop to:
1 use a sunscreen while taking the drug
2 take the drug on an empty stomach
3 limit fluid intake to 1,500 mL per day or less
4 take vitamin C while on this drug

4 Mr Adam Jones reports frequent large, fatty, foul-smelling stools. RN Brown recognises this as:
1 haematochezia, a manifestation of GI bleeding
2 characteristic of inflammatory bowel disease
3 a common early manifestation of colorectal cancer
4 steatorrhoea, a manifestation of malabsorption

5 Mr Stanley Green tells RN Davis that his father and grandfather died of colon cancer and he is worried that he is going to die from 'the same horrible disease'. Which of the following does RN Davis include in his recommendations?
1 There is no genetic link seen in colon cancer, so his risk is equal to that of people with no family history of the disease.
2 He should plan for annual digital rectal exams and periodic colonoscopy for early identification of possible tumours.
3 He should have annual CEA levels drawn to screen for early tumour development.
4 It is imperative that he change his diet immediately, significantly increasing his intake of dietary fibre.

6 Mrs Phyllis Jones is a 75-year-old with a nasogastric tube in place to maintain gastric decompression. Which nursing actions are important in monitoring responses to *Deficient fluid volume* when caring for Mrs Jones? (Select all that apply.)
1 Low suction is used to decompress the stomach.
2 Give her as much water as she wants to drink.
3 Listen to bowel sounds prior to checking the placement of the NG tube.
4 Document the amount and colour of NG tube drainage every shift.
5 Keep an accurate record of intake and output every 2 to 4 hours.
6 Listen to bowel sounds after palpating the stomach for tenderness.
7 Measure abdominal girth every 4 to 8 hours.

7 Ms Stella Black developed a paralytic ileus following a recent abdominal surgery. What is the most important nursing consideration when caring for Ms Black?
1 Ensure Ms Black is able to eat a clear liquid diet.
2 Maintain Ms Black on strict bed rest.
3 Monitor Ms Black's bowel sounds every hour.
4 Ensure Ms Black's nasogastric tube is functioning.

8 Mrs Jones has a history of diverticulosis and has been having abdominal pain recently. When advising Mrs Jones about her diet prior to discharge from the hospital, what type of foods should Mrs Jones exclude from her diet?
1 wholemeal bread
2 popcorn
3 soup
4 apples

9 Mr Allen, an 85-year-old, was admitted with a diagnosis of constipation. Which of the following is important for you to incorporate in Mr Allen's discharge education? (Select all that apply.)
1 Eat plenty of fresh fruits and vegetables daily.
2 Take bisacodyl (Durolax) daily.
3 Drink 6 to 8 glasses of non-alcoholic fluid daily.
4 Take docusate (Coloxyl) at night time only.
5 Eat wholemeal bread instead of white bread.
6 Eat a bran cereal for breakfast.

10 A small-bowel obstruction can occur due to:
1 eating extra fibre in the diet
2 abdominal adhesions
3 drinking too much water
4 a nasogastric tube

BIBLIOGRAPHY

Aginga, L. (2021). *Inflammatory bowel syndrome: Acupuncture*. Joanna Briggs Institute. Retrieved from https://www.joannabriggs.edu.au

Alkalay, M. J. (2021). Nutrition in patients with lactose malabsorption, celiac disease, and related disorders. *Nutrients*, *14*(1), 2. https://doi.org/10.3390/nu14010002

Australian Institute of Health and Welfare (AIHW) (2018). *Colorectal and other digestive-tract cancers*. Retrieved from https://www.aihw.gov.au/

Australian Institute of Health and Welfare (AIHW) (2021). *Cancer in Australia 2021*. Canberra: AIHW.

Beeching, N. & Beadsworth, M. (2018). Gastrointestinal presentations. In N. Beeching & G. Gill (eds), *Tropical medicine lecture notes* (8th ed., pp. 1–10). Oxford, UK: Wiley Blackwell.

Hellmann, S. (2022). *Constipation management (older person): Pharmacological interventions*. Joanna Briggs Institute. Retrieved from https://www.joannabriggs.edu.au

Bourque, D. L., Neumayr, A., Libman, M. & Chen, L. H. (2022). Treatment strategies for nitroimidazole-refractory giardiasis: A systematic review. *Journal of Travel Medicine*, 29(1). https://doi.org/10.1093/jtm/taab120

Braun, L. & Cohen, M. (2015). *Herbs and natural supplements: An evidence-based guide* (4th ed.). Marrickville, NSW: Churchill Livingstone.

Brown, S. (2007). *Health and illness in older adults*. Frenchs Forest, NSW: Pearson Australia.

Bullock, S. & Manias, E. (2014). *Fundamentals of pharmacology* (7th ed.). Frenchs Forest, NSW: Pearson Australia.

Bullock, S. & Manias, E. (2022). *Fundamentals of pharmacology* (9th ed.). Frenchs Forest, NSW: Pearson Australia.

Cancer Council (2022). *Bowel cancer*. Retrieved from https://www.cancer.org.au/

Chey, W. D., Kurlander, J. & Eswaran, S. (2015). Irritable bowel syndrome: A clinical review. *JAMA*, *313*(9), 949–958. doi: 10.1001/jama.2015.0954

Coeliac Australia (n.d.). *Coeliac disease*. Retrieved from https://www.coeliac.org.au/

Communicable Diseases Network Australia – National Notifiable Diseases Surveillance System (CDNA–NNDSS) (2018). Retrieved from https://www.health.gov.au/

Continence Foundation of Australia (CFA) (2022). *Faecal incontinence*. Retrieved from https://www.continence.org.au/

Crohn's & Colitis Australia (CCA) (2022). *About Crohn's disease*. Retrieved from https://www.ccfa.org/

Crohn's & Colitis Foundation of America (CCFA) (2022). *About Crohn's disease*. Retrieved from https://www.ccfa.org/

Devuni, D. (2014). Toxic megacolon. *Medscape*. Retrieved from http://emedicine.medscape.com/

Fong, E. (2022). *Constipation in hospitalized patients: Management*. Adelaide: Joanna Briggs Institute.

Forssman, B., Manne, T., Musto, J. et al. (2007). *Vibrio cholerae* O1 El Tor cluster in Sydney linked to imported whitebait. *Medical Journal of Australia*, *187*(6), 345–347.

Gastroenterological Society of Australia (GSA) (2022). *Bowel polyps*. Retrieved from www.gesa.org.au/

Hanieh, S., Mahanty, S., Gurruwiwi, G. et al. (2021). Enteric pathogen infection and consequences for child growth in young Aboriginal Australian children: A cross-sectional study. *BMC Infectious Diseases*, 21(9). doi.org/10.1186/s12879-020-05005-1

Hanson, J. P. (2005). Tropical sprue in Far North Queensland. *Medical Journal of Australia*, 182(10) 536–537. Retrieved from https://www.mja.com.au

Kee, J. (2018). *Handbook of laboratory and diagnostic tests with nursing implications* (10th ed.). Upper Saddle River, NJ: Prentice Hall.

Kelly, P. (2014). Intestinal protozoa. In J. Farrar, P. Hotez, T. Junghanss, G. Kang, D. Lalloo & N. J. White (eds), *Manson's tropical diseases* (23rd ed., pp. 664–675). St Louis, MO: Elsevier.

Le, L. K. (2018). *Constipation management (older person)*. Joanna Briggs Institute. Retrieved from https://www.joannabriggs.edu.au

Lee, G. & Bishop, P. (2016). *Microbiology and infection control for health professionals* (6th ed.). Frenchs Forest, NSW: Pearson Australia.

Leggett, B. A. & Hewett, D. G. (2015). Colorectal cancer screening. *Internal Medicine Journal, 45*(1), 6–15. doi: 10.1111/imj.12636

Lizarondo, L. (2021). *Irritable bowel syndrome: Psychological therapies*. Joanna Briggs Institute. Retrieved from https://www.joannabriggs.edu.au

Lizarondo, L. (2022). *Faecal incontinence: Conservative management*. Joanna Briggs Institute. Retrieved from https://www.joannabriggs.edu.au

Loscalzo, J., Fauci, A. S., Kasper, D. L., Hauser, S. L. & Longo, D. (2022). *Harrison's principles of internal medicine* (21st ed.). New York: McGraw Hill Medical.

Magtoto, L. (2022). *Faecal incontinence: Assessment*. Joanna Briggs Institute. Retrieved from https://www.joannabriggs.edu.au

Manning, L. P., Tuck, C. J. & Biesiekierski, J. R. (2022). The lived experience of irritable bowel syndrome: A focus on dietary management. *Australian Journal of General Practice, 51*(6), 395–400. doi: 10.31128/AJGP-07-21-6080

Manuel, B. (2021). *Irritable bowel syndrome: Probiotics*. Joanna Briggs Institute. Retrieved from https://www.joannabriggs.edu.au

Marieb, E. N. & Hoehn, K. (2019). *Human anatomy and physiology* (11th ed.). International edition. San Francisco: Pearson.

Marin, T. (2021). *Irritable bowel syndrome: FODMAP diet*. Joanna Briggs Institute. Retrieved from https://www.joannabriggs.edu.au

Marin, T. (2022). *Irritable bowel syndrome: Peppermint oil*. Joanna Briggs Institute. Retrieved from https://www.joannabriggs.edu.au

Martin, T. D., Chan, S. S. & Hart, A. R. (2014). Environmental factors in the relapse and recurrence of inflammatory bowel disease: A review of the literature. *Digestive Diseases and Sciences, 60*(5), 1396–1405. doi: 10.1007/s10620-014-3437-3

Middleton, B. F., Danchin, M., Quinn, H., Ralph, A. P., Pingault, N., Jones, M., Estcourt, M. & Snelling, T. (2020). Retrospective case-control study of 2017 G2P[4] rotavirus epidemic in rural and remote Australia. *Pathogens (Basel), 9*(10), 790. https://doi.org/10.3390/pathogens9100790

Nepogodiev, D., Matthews, J. H., Morley, G. L. et al. (2020). Evaluation of appendicitis risk prediction models in adults with suspected appendicitis. *British Journal of Surgery, 107*(1), 73–86. https://doi.org/10.1002/bjs.11440

O'Dempsey, T. & Beeching, N. (2018a). Giardiasis and other intestinal protozoal infections. In N. Beeching & G. Gill (eds), *Tropical medicine lecture notes* (7th ed., pp. 218–221). Oxford, UK: Wiley Blackwell.

O'Dempsey, T. & Beeching, N. (2018b). Hydatid disease. In N. Beeching & G. Gill (eds), *Tropical medicine lecture notes* (7th ed., pp. 218–221). Oxford, UK: Wiley Blackwell.

Odhiambo, M. (2022). *Enteral nutrition: Infection control*. The Joanna Briggs Institute. Retrieved from https://www.joannabriggs.edu.au

Papadakis, M., McPhee, S. & Rabow, M. (2022). *Current medical diagnosis and treatment* (61st ed.). New York: McGraw-Hill Education.

Picot, E. (2021). *Administration of PRN analgesia. Evidence summary*. Joanna Briggs Institute. Retrieved from https://www.joannabriggs.edu.au

Porritt, K. (2020). *Enema: Administration (older person)*. Joanna Briggs Institute. Retrieved from https://www.joannabriggs.edu.au

Principi, M. & De Censi, A. (2015). Prevention of colorectal adenomas. *Colorectal Disease, 17*, 20–24. doi: 10.1111/codi.12817

Queensland Health (2017). *Hydatid disease*. Retrieved from http://conditions.health.qld.gov.au/

Queensland Health (2019). *Rotavirus fact sheet*. Retrieved from http://conditions.health.qld.gov.au/

Sharma, L. (2018). *Nasogastric suction: Clinician information. Evidence summary*. Joanna Briggs Institute. Retrieved from https://www.joannabriggs.edu.au

Shussman, N. & Wexner, S. D. (2014). Colorectal polyps and polyposis syndromes. *Gastroenterology Report, 2*(1), 1–15. doi: 10.1093/gastro/got041

Sivapuram, M. S. (2020). *Anorectal disorders: Sitz baths*. Joanna Briggs Institute. Retrieved from https://www.joannabriggs.edu.au

Slade, S. (2021). *Fecal incontinence (adult): Biofeedback and/or sphincter exercises*. Joanna Briggs Institute. Retrieved from https://www.joannabriggs.edu.au

Sperber, A. D., Bangdiwala, S. I., Drossman, D. et al. (2021). Worldwide prevalence and burden of functional gastrointestinal disorders, results of Rome Foundation Global Study. *Gastroenterology, 60*(1), 99–114.e3. doi: 10.1053/j.gastro.2020.04.014

Stewart, M., Biddle, M. & Thomas, T. (2017). Evaluation of current feeding practices in the critically ill: A retrospective chart review. *Intensive and Critical Care Nursing, 38*, 24–30. doi: 10.1016./j.iccn.2016.05.004

Tiziani, A. (2021). *Harvard's nursing guide to drugs* (11th ed.). Chatswood, NSW: Mosby.

World Health Organization (WHO) (2015). *Rotavirus*. Retrieved from Retrieved from http://www.who.int

World Health Organization (WHO) (2017a). *Diarrhoeal disease*. Retrieved from http://www.who.int

World Health Organization (WHO) (2017b). *Food safety*. Retrieved from http://www.who.int

World Health Organization (WHO) (2018). *Salmonella (non-typhoidal)*. Retrieved from http://www.who.int

World Health Organization (WHO) (2020). *Soil-transmitted helminthiasis*. Retrieved from http://www.who.int

World Health Organization (WHO) (2022). *Cholera*. Retrieved from http://www.who.int

CHAPTER 24

Nursing care of people with gallbladder, liver and pancreatic disorders

Jane Medved

Key terms

alcoholic (Laënnec's) cirrhosis 789
ascites 783
balloon tamponade 797
biliary colic 776
cholecystitis 777
cholelithiasis 776
chronic hepatitis 786
cirrhosis 789
fulminant hepatitis 786
hepatitis 784
hepatorenal syndrome 783
jaundice 783
laparoscopic cholecystectomy 778
liver transplantation 798
oesophageal varices 790
pancreatitis 805
paracentesis 796
portal hypertension 783
portal systemic encephalopathy 783
transjugular intrahepatic portosystemic shunt (TIPS) 797

Learning outcomes

- Discuss the pathophysiology, manifestations and associated nursing care of the person suffering from a disorder of the gallbladder.
- Compare and contrast the pathophysiology, manifestations and complications of hepatitis, cirrhosis, trauma and cancer of the liver.
- Discuss pathophysiology, manifestations and interprofessional care of a person with pancreatitis or cancer of the pancreas.

Clinical competencies

- Assess functional health status of people with gallbladder, liver or pancreatic disease.
- Monitor for, document and report expected and unexpected manifestations in people with gallbladder, liver or pancreatic disease.
- Prepare people for, and understand the purpose and significance of, diagnostic tests for gallbladder, liver and pancreatic disorders.
- Integrate appropriate dietary, pharmacological and other interprofessional measures into nursing care and teaching of the person with a gallbladder, liver or pancreatic disorder.
- Provide appropriate nursing care for the person who has surgery of the gallbladder, liver or pancreas.
- Integrate psychosocial, cultural and spiritual considerations into the plan of care for a person with a gallbladder, liver or pancreatic disorder.
- Use evidence-based practice to develop, implement, evaluate and, as needed, revise the plan of care for people with disorders of the gallbladder, liver or pancreas.
- Provide appropriate person and family health education to promote, maintain and restore functional health status for people with gallbladder, liver and pancreatic disorders.

Gallbladder, liver and exocrine pancreatic disorders may occur as primary disorders or develop secondarily to other disease processes. One organ's functioning frequently affects that of another. Duct inflammation or obstruction and changes in the multiple functions of these organs can cause significant health effects.

People with a gallbladder, liver or pancreatic disorder may experience pain, multiple metabolic and nutritional disturbances, and altered body image. Nursing care addresses the physiological and psychosocial needs of the person and family.

Gallbladder disorders

Altered bile flow through the hepatic, cystic or common bile duct is a common problem. It often leads to inflammation and other complications. Gallstones are the most common cause of obstructed flow. Tumours and abscesses also can obstruct bile flow.

THE PERSON WITH GALLSTONES

Cholelithiasis is the formation of stones (*calculi*, or *gallstones*) within the gallbladder or biliary duct system. Gallstones are common with ageing, with prevalence up to 15% in people aged 50 years or older (Gastroenterological Society of Australia, 2021). Box 24.1 lists risk factors for gallstones. The incidence of gallstones varies among people of different ethnic backgrounds.

Physiology review

Normally bile is formed by the liver and stored in the gallbladder. Bile contains bile salts, bilirubin, water, electrolytes, cholesterol, fatty acids and lecithin. In the gallbladder, some of the water and electrolytes are absorbed, further concentrating the bile. Food entering the intestine stimulates the gallbladder to contract and release bile through the common bile duct and sphincter of Oddi into the intestine. The bile salts in bile increase the solubility and absorption of dietary fats.

Pathophysiology and manifestations

Cholelithiasis

Gallstones form when several factors interact: abnormal bile composition, biliary stasis and inflammation of the gallbladder. Most gallstones (80%) consist primarily of cholesterol; the rest contain a mixture of bile components. Excess cholesterol in bile is associated with obesity; a high-kilojoule, high-cholesterol diet; and drugs that lower serum cholesterol levels. When bile is supersaturated with cholesterol, it can precipitate out to form stones. Biliary stasis, or slowed emptying of the gallbladder, contributes to cholelithiasis. Stones do not form when the gallbladder empties completely in response to hormonal stimulation. Slowed or incomplete emptying allows cholesterol to concentrate and increases the risk of stone formation. Finally, inflammation of the gallbladder allows excess water and bile salt reabsorption, increasing the risk of lithiasis.

BOX 24.1 Risk factors for gallstones

- Age
- Family history of gallstones
- Race or ethnicity
- Obesity, hyperlipidaemia
- Rapid weight loss
- Female gender; use of oral contraceptives
- Biliary stasis: pregnancy, fasting, prolonged parenteral nutrition
- Diseases or conditions: cirrhosis; ileal disease or resection; sickle cell anaemia; glucose intolerance

CONSIDERATION FOR PRACTICE

Certain very-low-kilojoule diets are associated with a high risk of cholelithiasis. Increased cholesterol concentration in the bile and decreased gallbladder contractions associated with fasting increase the risk of gallstone formation.

Most gallstones are formed in the gallbladder. They then may migrate into the ducts (see Figure 24.1), leading to *cholangitis* (duct inflammation). Although some people with cholelithiasis are asymptomatic, many develop manifestations. Early manifestations of gallstones may be vague: epigastric fullness or mild gastric distress after eating a large or fatty meal. Stones that obstruct the cystic duct or common bile duct lead to distension and increased pressure behind the stone. This causes **biliary colic**, a severe, steady pain in the epigastric region or right upper quadrant of the abdomen. The pain may radiate to the back, right scapula or shoulder. The pain often begins suddenly following a meal and may last as long as 5 hours. It often is accompanied by nausea and vomiting.

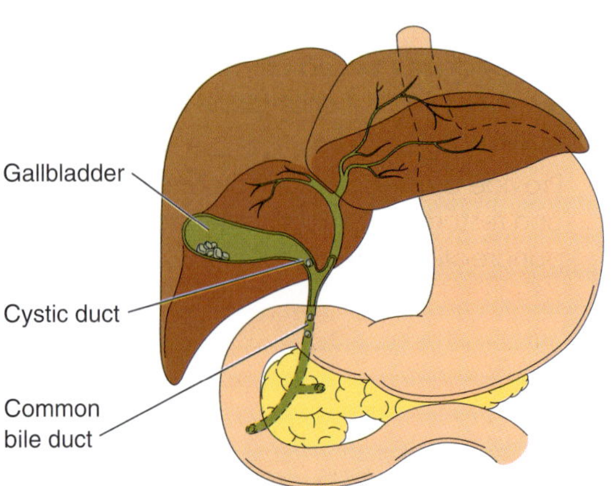

FIGURE 24.1 *Common locations of gallstones*

TABLE 24.1 Manifestations and complications of cholelithiasis and cholecystitis

MANIFESTATIONS	CHOLELITHIASIS	CHOLECYSTITIS
Pain	• Abrupt onset • Severe, steady • Localised to epigastrium and RUQ of abdomen • May radiate to back, right scapula and shoulder • Lasts 30 minutes to 5 hours	• Abrupt onset • Severe, steady • Generalised in RUQ of abdomen • May radiate to back, right scapula and shoulder • Lasts 12 to 18 hours • Aggravated by movement, breathing
Associated symptoms	• Nausea, vomiting	• Anorexia, nausea, vomiting • RUQ tenderness and guarding • Rigors and fever
Complications	• Cholecystitis • Common bile duct obstruction with possible jaundice and liver damage • Common duct obstruction with pancreatitis	• Gangrene and perforation with peritonitis • Chronic cholecystitis • Empyema • Fistula formation • Gallstone ileus

Obstruction of the common bile duct may cause bile reflux into the liver, leading to jaundice, pain and possible liver damage. If the common duct is obstructed, pancreatic enzymes will be unable to enter the small intestine and pancreatitis (discussed later in this chapter) becomes a potential complication.

Cholecystitis

Cholecystitis is inflammation of the gallbladder. *Acute cholecystitis* usually follows obstruction of the cystic duct by a stone. The obstruction increases pressure within the gallbladder, leading to ischaemia of the gallbladder wall and mucosa. Chemical and bacterial inflammation often follows. The ischaemia can lead to necrosis and perforation of the gall bladder wall.

Acute cholecystitis usually begins with an attack of biliary colic. The pain involves the entire right upper quadrant (RUQ) and may radiate to the back, right scapula or shoulder. Movement or deep breathing may aggravate the pain. The pain usually lasts longer than biliary colic, continuing for 12 to 18 hours. Anorexia, nausea and vomiting are common. Fever often is present and may be accompanied by rigors. The RUQ is tender to palpation.

Chronic cholecystitis may result from repeated bouts of acute cholecystitis or from persistent irritation of the gallbladder wall by stones. Bacteria may be present in the bile as well. Chronic cholecystitis is often asymptomatic.

Complications of cholecystitis include *empyema*, a collection of infected fluid within the gallbladder; gangrene and perforation with resulting peritonitis or abscess formation; formation of a fistula into an adjacent organ (such as the duodenum, colon or stomach); or obstruction of the small intestine by a large gallstone (*gallstone ileus*). Table 24.1 compares the manifestations and complications of acute cholelithiasis with those of cholecystitis.

INTERPROFESSIONAL CARE

Treatment of the person with cholelithiasis or cholecystitis depends on the acuity of the condition and the person's overall health status. When gallstones are present but asymptomatic and the person has a low risk of complications, conservative treatment is indicated. However, when the person experiences frequent symptoms, has acute cholecystitis or has very large stones, the gallbladder and stones are usually surgically removed.

Diagnosis

Diagnostic tests are ordered to identify the presence and location of stones, identify possible complications and help differentiate gallbladder disease from other disorders.

- *Serum bilirubin* is measured. Elevated direct (conjugated) bilirubin may indicate obstructed bile flow in the biliary duct system (see Box 24.2).

BOX 24.2 Total, direct and indirect bilirubin levels

When serum bilirubin levels are measured, the results usually are reported as the total bilirubin, direct bilirubin and indirect bilirubin levels. Most bilirubin is formed from haemoglobin, as ageing or abnormal red blood cells (RBCs) are removed from circulation and destroyed. It is then bound to protein and transported to the liver. This protein-bound bilirubin is called *indirect* or *unconjugated* bilirubin. Once in the liver, bilirubin is separated from the protein and converted to a soluble form, *direct* or *conjugated* bilirubin. Conjugated bilirubin is then excreted in the bile.

- *Total* (serum) *bilirubin*, the total bilirubin in the blood, includes both indirect and direct forms. In adults, the normal total bilirubin is < 20 micromol/L. Total bilirubin levels increase when more is being produced (e.g. RBC haemolysis) or when its metabolism or excretion is impaired (e.g. liver disease or biliary obstruction).
- *Direct* (conjugated) *bilirubin* levels, normally < 7 micromol/L adults, rise when its excretion is impaired by obstruction within the liver (e.g. in cirrhosis, hepatitis, exposure to hepatotoxins) or in the biliary system.
- *Indirect* (unconjugated) *bilirubin* levels, 3.4–12 micromol/L in adults, rise in RBC haemolysis (e.g. sickle cell disease or transfusion reaction).

- *Full blood count (FBC)* may indicate infection and inflammation if the white blood cell (WBC) count is elevated.
- *Serum amylase* and *lipase* are measured to identify possible pancreatitis related to common duct obstruction.
- *Abdominal x-ray* may show gallstones that have high calcium content.
- *Ultrasonography of the gallbladder* is a non-invasive exam that can accurately diagnose cholelithiasis. It also can be used to assess emptying of the gallbladder.
- *Oral cholecystogram* is performed using a dye administered orally to assess the gallbladder's ability to concentrate and excrete bile.
- *Gallbladder scans* use an intravenous radioactive solution that is rapidly extracted from the blood and excreted into the biliary tree to diagnose cystic duct obstruction and acute or chronic cholecystitis.

See the chapter 'A person-centred approach to assessing the gastrointestinal system' for more information about these diagnostic tests and their nursing implications.

The primary disadvantages of pharmacological treatment for gallstones include its cost, long duration (2 years or more) and the high incidence of recurrent stone formation when treatment is discontinued. If infection is suspected, antibiotics may be ordered to cure the infection and reduce associated inflammation and oedema. People with pruritus (itching) due to severe obstructive jaundice and an accumulation of bile salts on the skin may be given cholestyramine (Questran Lite). This medication binds with bile salts to promote their excretion in the faeces. An opioid analgesic such as morphine may be required for pain relief during an acute attack of cholecystitis.

Treatments

SURGERY **Laparoscopic cholecystectomy** (removal of the gallbladder) is the treatment of choice for symptomatic cholelithiasis or cholecystitis. This minimally invasive procedure has a low risk of complications and generally requires a hospital stay of less than 24 hours. Not all people are candidates for laparoscopic cholecystectomy and there is a risk that a laparoscopic cholecystectomy may be converted to a *laparotomy* (surgical opening into the abdomen) during the procedure. The 'Translation to practice' box discusses evidence-based practice for managing pain in people undergoing laparoscopic cholecystectomy.

TRANSLATION TO PRACTICE Evidence-based practice: a person undergoing laparoscopic cholecystectomy

There are several advantages of laparoscopic cholecystectomy, including minimally invasive procedure, reduced postoperative pain and shorter hospitalisation. Most people are discharged home the day after surgery. The most significant challenge to date remains postoperative pain management. Poor management of pain post laparoscopic cholecystectomy puts the person at risk of prolonged immobility, thromboembolism and respiratory complications such as pneumonia. Long term, people may experience chronic local pain syndrome. Studies have shown that the most common types of pain after laparoscopic cholecystectomy are visceral pain caused by organ damage during surgery and surgical incision pain. These require a multimodal analgesia response. Most people respond to analgesia regimens comprising oral opioids and NSAIDs or wound-infiltrating local anaesthetics. However, these may still cause complications such as altered respiratory function, hypotension, intestinal obstruction, nausea and vomiting, urinary retention and pruritis.

Singh et al. (2013) studied the effects of pre-emptive intravenous (IV) ketamine infusion for analgesia in the first 24 hours post surgery to manage surgical pain. There was a marked reduction in pain score compared to those who did not receive IV ketamine. The purpose of pre-emptive analgesia administration is to reduce the central sensitisation from a variety of noxious stimuli, with the benefits being better postoperative pain management, reduced use of analgesia and improved patient outcomes. Zhu and Sun (2023) completed a systematic review and meta-analysis on the analgesic effects of local anaesthetic ropivacaine with alpha-2 adrenergic agonist dexmedetomidine (DEX) via transversus abdominis plane block. They concluded that using this combination therapy reduced pain as well as the frequency for analgesia with fewer side effects.

IMPLICATIONS FOR NURSING

Effective pain relief is known to promote healing and immune function following surgery. The above studies are an example of the continuing need to explore effective multimodal options for short-stay surgical patients. Effective postoperative pain management requires a combination of good preoperative education, discharge planning related to the person's expectations of pain and postoperative pain management. Local surgical centre policies need to be reviewed to ensure the appropriate training of staff and monitoring of people prescribed with this type of postoperative analgesia.

CRITICAL THINKING IN PERSON-CENTRED CARE

1 One of the side effects of ketamine is hallucinations. How can the nurse ensure appropriate patient safety while promoting effective postoperative pain management? What teaching could you provide to help people manage adverse effects of the prescribed drug?
2 Nausea and vomiting are common yet easily preventable side effects of laparoscopic cholecystectomy. How will the incidence of nausea and vomiting impact on the pain management of a person undergoing laparoscopic cholecystectomy?

Source: Zhu & Sun (2023). Analgesic effects of ropivacaine combined with dexmedetomidine in transversus abdominis plane block in patients undergoing laparoscopic cholecystectomy: A systematic review and meta-analysis. *Journal of PeriAnesthesia Nursing*. doi: https://doi.org/10.1016/j.jopan.2022.09.003.

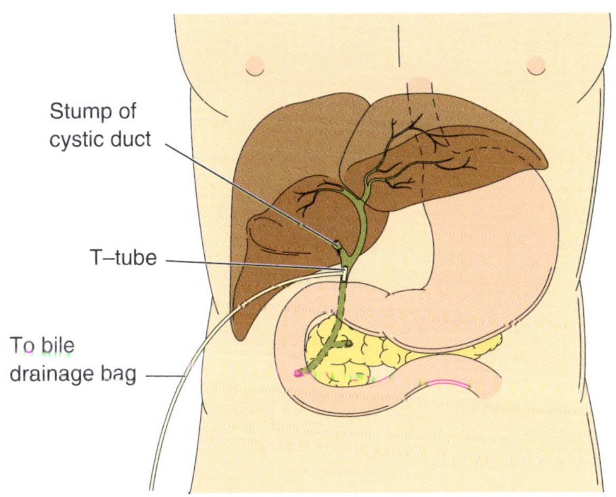

FIGURE 24.2 ***T-tube placement in the common bile duct. Bile fluid flows with gravity into a drainage collection device below the level of the common bile duct***

When stones are lodged within the ducts, a cholecystectomy with common bile duct exploration may be done. A T-tube (see Figure 24.2) is inserted to maintain patency of the duct and promote bile passage while the oedema decreases. Excess bile is collected in a drainage bag secured below the surgical site. If it is suspected that a stone has been retained following surgery, a postoperative cholangiogram via the T-tube or direct visualisation of the duct with an endoscope may be performed. See the accompanying box for nursing care for a person with a T-tube.

Some people who are poor surgical risks and for whom laparoscopic cholecystectomy is inappropriate may have either a *cholecystostomy* to drain the gallbladder or a *choledochostomy* to remove stones and position a T-tube in the common bile duct.

NUTRITION Food intake may be eliminated during an acute attack of cholecystitis and a nasogastric tube inserted to relieve nausea and vomiting. Dietary fat intake may be limited, especially if the person is obese. If bile flow is obstructed, fat-soluble vitamins (A, D, E and K) and bile salts may need to be administered.

OTHER THERAPIES In some cases, shock wave lithotripsy may be used with drug therapy to dissolve large gallstones. In extracorporeal shock wave lithotripsy, ultrasound is used to align the stones with the source of shock waves and the computerised lithotripter. Positioning is of prime importance throughout the procedure, which usually takes an hour. Mild sedation may be given during the procedure. Nursing care after the procedure includes monitoring for biliary colic, which can result from the gallbladder contracting to remove stone fragments; nausea; and transient haematuria. *Percutaneous cholecystostomy*, ultrasound-guided drainage of the gallbladder, may be done in high-risk people to postpone or even eliminate the need for surgery.

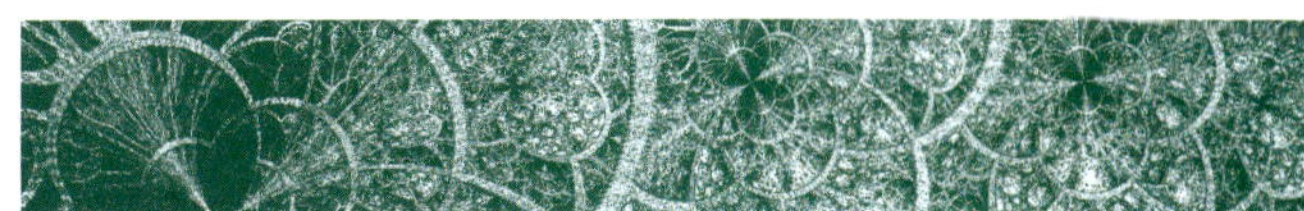

Nursing care

In addition to the nursing care discussed in this section, see the accompanying nursing care plan for a person with cholelithiasis.

Health promotion

Although most risk factors for cholelithiasis cannot be controlled or modified, several can. Modifiable risk factors include obesity, hyperlipidaemia, extremely low-kilojoule diets and diets high in cholesterol. Encourage people who are obese to increase their activity level and follow a low-carbohydrate, low-fat, low-cholesterol diet to promote weight loss and reduce their risk of developing gallstones. Discuss the dangers of 'yo-yo' dieting, with cycles of weight loss followed by weight gain, and of extremely low-kilojoule diets. Encourage people with high serum cholesterol levels to talk with their primary care provider about using cholesterol-lowering drugs.

NURSING CARE OF THE PERSON **with a T-tube**

- Ensure that the T-tube is properly connected to a sterile container; keep the tube below the level of the surgical wound. *This position promotes the flow of bile and prevents backflow or seepage of caustic bile on to the skin. The tube itself decreases biliary tree pressure.*
- Monitor drainage from the T-tube for colour and consistency; record as output. Normally, the tube may drain up to 500 mL in the first 24 hours after surgery; drainage decreases to less than 200 mL in 2 to 3 days and is minimal thereafter. Drainage may be blood tinged initially, changing to green–brown. Report excessive drainage immediately. (After 48 hours, drainage greater than 500 mL is considered excessive.) *Stones or oedema and inflammation can obstruct ducts below the tube, requiring treatment.*
- Place in Fowler's position. *This promotes gravity drainage of bile.*
- Assess skin for bile leakage during dressing changes. *Bile irritates the skin; it may be necessary to apply skin protection with a barrier product.*
- Teach the person how to manage the tube when turning, ambulating and performing activities of daily living. *Direct pulling or traction on the tube must be avoided.*
- If indicated, teach care of the T-tube, how to clamp it, signs of infection and when to report these symptoms to clinicians. People may be discharged home with the tube in place. *Reporting early signs of infection facilitates prompt treatment.*

NURSING CARE OF THE PERSON having a laparoscopic cholecystectomy

PREOPERATIVE CARE

- Provide routine preoperative care as ordered (see the chapter 'Nursing care of people having surgery').
- Reinforce teaching about the procedure and postoperative expectations, including pain management, deep breathing and mobilisation. *Preoperative teaching reduces anxiety and promotes rapid postoperative recovery.*

POSTOPERATIVE CARE

- Provide routine postoperative recovery care as outlined in the chapter 'Nursing care of people having surgery'.
- Assist to chair at bedside as allowed. *Early mobilisation promotes lung ventilation and circulation, reducing the potential for postoperative complications.*
- Advance oral intake from ice chips to regular diet as tolerated. *Oral intake can be rapidly resumed due to minimal disruption of the gastrointestinal tract during surgery.*
- Provide and reinforce teaching: pain management, incision care, activity level and postoperative follow-up appointments. *With early discharge, the person and family assume responsibility for the majority of postoperative care. A clear understanding of this care and expected needs reduces anxiety and the risk of postoperative complications.*
- Initiate follow-up contact 24 to 48 hours after discharge to evaluate adequacy of pain control, incision management and discharge understanding. *Contact following discharge provides an opportunity to evaluate care and reinforce teaching.*

Assessment

Assessment data related to cholelithiasis and cholecystitis include the following:

- *Health history*: current manifestations, including RUQ pain, its character and relationship to meals, duration and radiation, nausea and vomiting or other symptoms; duration of symptoms; risk factors or previous history of symptoms; chronic diseases such as diabetes, cirrhosis or inflammatory bowel disease; current diet; use of oral contraceptives or possibility of pregnancy.
- *Physical assessment*: current weight; colour of skin and sclera; abdominal assessment including light palpation for tenderness; colour of urine and stool.
- *Diagnostic tests*: monitor results of WBC count, serum bilirubin, liver enzymes and pancreatic enzymes (amylase and lipase).

Nursing diagnoses and interventions

Priority nursing diagnoses for the person with cholelithiasis or cholecystitis often include pain related to biliary colic or surgery, imbalanced nutrition related to the effects of altered bile flow and to nausea and anorexia, and risk of infection related to potential rupture of an acutely inflamed gallbladder. Nursing interventions for the person who has undergone a laparoscopic or open cholecystectomy are similar to those for other people having abdominal surgery (see the chapter 'Nursing care of people having surgery').

Pain

The pain associated with cholelithiasis can be severe. Sometimes a combination of interventions is indicated.

- Discuss the relationship between fat intake and the pain. Teach ways to reduce fat intake. *Fat entering the duodenum initiates gallbladder contractions, causing pain when gallstones are present in the ducts.*
- Withhold oral food and fluids during episodes of acute pain. Insert nasogastric tube and connect to low suction if ordered. *Emptying the stomach reduces both the amount of chyme entering the duodenum and the stimulus for gallbladder contractions, thus reducing pain.*
- For severe pain, administer morphine or other opioid analgesia as ordered. *Recent research indicates that morphine is not likely to cause spasms of the sphincter of Oddi.*
- Place in Fowler's position. *Fowler's position decreases pressure on the inflamed gallbladder.*
- Monitor vital signs, including temperature, at least every 4 hours. *Bacterial infection often is present in acute cholecystitis and may cause an elevated temperature and respiratory rate.*

Imbalanced nutrition: less than body requirements

The person with severe gallbladder disease may develop nutritional imbalances related to anorexia, pain and nausea following meals and impaired bile flow that alters absorption of fat and fat-soluble vitamins (A, D, E and K) from the gut.

- Assess nutritional status, including diet history, height and weight, and skinfold measurements (see the chapters 'A person-centred approach to assessing the gastrointestinal system' and 'Nursing care of people with nutritional disorders'). *Although often obese, people with gallbladder disease may have an imbalanced diet or may have specific vitamin deficiencies, particularly of the fat-soluble vitamins.*
- Evaluate laboratory results, including serum bilirubin, albumin, glucose and cholesterol levels. Report abnormal results to the doctor. *Elevated serum bilirubin may indicate impaired bilirubin excretion due to obstructed bile flow. A low serum albumin may indicate poor nutritional status. Glucose intolerance and hypercholesterolaemia are risk factors for cholelithiasis.*

NURSING CARE PLAN A person with cholelithiasis

Joyce Wing is a 44-year-old married mother of three children. She works full time as a cook at a local restaurant. Recently Mrs Wing has noticed a dull pain in her upper abdomen that gets worse after eating fatty foods; nausea and sometimes vomiting accompany the pain. She had a similar pain after the birth of her last child. She is diagnosed with cholelithiasis and is admitted for a laparoscopic cholecystectomy.

ASSESSMENT

David Corbin, RN, takes Mrs Wing's admission history. It includes intolerance to fatty foods and intermittent 'stabbing' abdominal pain that radiates to her back. Her usual diet includes regular takeaway meals due to her busy lifestyle. She reports 'not wanting to eat much of anything lately'. She states she has never had surgery before and hopes 'everything goes well'. Physical assessment includes T 37.7°C, P 88, R 20 and BP 130/84. She has had a recent 3 kg weight loss, currently weighing 59 kg. She is 160 cm tall. Abdominal examination elicits tenderness in the right upper abdominal quadrant. She has no jaundice, rigors or evidence of complications.

DIAGNOSES

- *Risk of imbalanced nutrition: less than body requirements* related to anorexia and manifested by recent weight loss.
- *Risk of pain* related to inflamed gallbladder and surgical incisions manifested by increased heart rate and blood pressure and decreased inspiratory volume.
- *Risk of infection* related to potential bacterial contamination of abdominal cavity, manifested by increased white cell count, temperature, heart and respiratory rate and decreased blood pressure.
- *Risk of anxiety* related to lack of information about perioperative experience and manifested by restlessness, increased heart rate and blood pressure.

PLANNING

- Teach about the gallbladder and the function of bile.
- Discuss pre- and postoperative care, including self-care following discharge.
- Teach home care of incisions and recognition of signs of infection.

Expected outcomes

- Maintain present weight within 2 kg over the next 3 weeks.
- Resume regular diet, decreasing intake of foods high in fat.
- Verbalise adequate pain control after surgery and with activity resumption.
- Remain free of infection.
- Verbalise a decrease in anxiety before surgery.

IMPLEMENTATION

- Promote mobility as soon as allowed after surgery.
- Review specific high-fat foods to avoid and ways to maintain her weight. Consultation with a dietitian if available would be beneficial.
- Provide analgesia as needed postoperatively. Teach appropriate analgesic use after discharge.

EVALUATION

Mrs Wing is discharged the morning after her surgery. She is afebrile, has no signs of infection and is able to appropriately care for her incisions. She identifies signs of infection and talks about ways to reduce her fat intake while keeping her weight stable. She verbalises understanding of initial activity restrictions and resumption of normal activities. Mrs Wing states, 'It wasn't as bad as I thought it would be at first.' She has an appointment to see her surgeon in 1 week.

CRITICAL THINKING IN THE NURSING PROCESS

1. What is the rationale for a low-fat diet with cholelithiasis? Discuss nutritional practices as they relate to the medical problem and Mrs Wing's lifestyle.
2. How would your discharge teaching for Mrs Wing differ if she had had an open cholecystectomy instead of a laparoscopic cholecystectomy?

REFLECTION ON THE NURSING PROCESS

1. Develop a care plan for Mrs Wing for the nursing diagnosis *Risk of infection*.
2. Discuss strategies you can use to encourage Mrs Wing's postoperative mobilisation.

- Refer to a dietitian or nutritionist for diet counselling to promote healthy weight loss and reduce pain episodes. *A low-carbohydrate, low-fat, higher-protein diet reduces symptoms of cholecystitis. While fasting and very low kilojoule diets are contraindicated, a moderate reduction in kilojoule intake and increased activity levels promote weight loss.*
- Administer vitamin supplements as ordered. *People who do not absorb fat well due to obstructed bile flow may require supplements of the fat-soluble vitamins.*

Risk of infection

An acutely inflamed gallbladder may become necrotic and rupture, releasing its contents into the abdominal cavity. While the resulting infection often remains localised, peritonitis can result from chemical irritation and bacterial contamination of the peritoneal cavity.

CONSIDERATION FOR PRACTICE

Rupture of an acutely inflamed gallbladder may be heralded by abrupt but transient pain relief as contents are released from the distended gallbladder into the abdomen. Promptly report this change to the doctor.

Following open cholecystectomy (*laparotomy*), the risk of pulmonary infection is significant due to the high abdominal incision.

- Monitor vital signs, including temperature, every 4 hours. Promptly report vital sign changes or temperature elevation. *Tachycardia, increased respiratory rate or an elevated temperature may indicate an infectious process.*

- Assess abdomen every 4 hours and as indicated (e.g. when pain level changes abruptly). *Increasing abdominal tenderness or a rigid, board-like abdomen may indicate rupture of the gallbladder with peritonitis.*
- Assist to cough and deep breathe or use an incentive spirometer every 1 to 2 hours while awake. Splint abdominal incision with a blanket or pillow during coughing. *The high abdominal incision of an open cholecystectomy interferes with effective coughing and deep breathing, increasing the risk of atelectasis and respiratory infections such as pneumonia.*
- Place in Fowler's position and encourage ambulation as allowed. *Fowler's position and ambulation promote lung expansion and airway clearance, reducing the risk of respiratory infections.*
- Administer antibiotics as ordered. *Antibiotics may be given preoperatively to reduce the risk of infection from infected gallbladder contents and may be continued postoperatively to prevent infection.*

Community-based care

Teaching varies, depending on the choice of treatment options for cholelithiasis and cholecystitis. If surgery is not an option, teach about maintaining a low-fat, low-carbohydrate diet if indicated. Include an explanation about the role of bile and the function of the gallbladder in terms that the person and family can understand.

Provide appropriate preoperative teaching for the planned procedure. Discuss the possibility of open cholecystectomy even when a laparoscopic procedure is planned. Teach postoperative self-care measures to manage pain and prevent complications. If the person will be discharged with a T-tube, provide instructions about its care (see the 'Nursing care' box). Discuss manifestations of complications to report to the doctor. Stress the importance of follow-up appointments.

Following cholecystectomy, a low-fat diet may be initially recommended. Refer the person and food preparer to a dietitian to review low-fat foods. (See Box 24.3 for examples of high-fat foods to avoid.) Higher-fat foods may be gradually added to the diet as tolerated.

BOX 24.3 Examples of high-fat foods

- Whole-milk products (e.g. cream, ice-cream, cheese)
- Doughnuts, deep-fried
- Sausage, bacon, hot dogs
- Sauces with fat, cream
- Most nuts (e.g. pecans, cashews)
- Corn chips and potato chips
- Butter and cooking oils
- Fried foods (e.g. hamburgers, hot chips)
- Peanut butter
- Chocolate

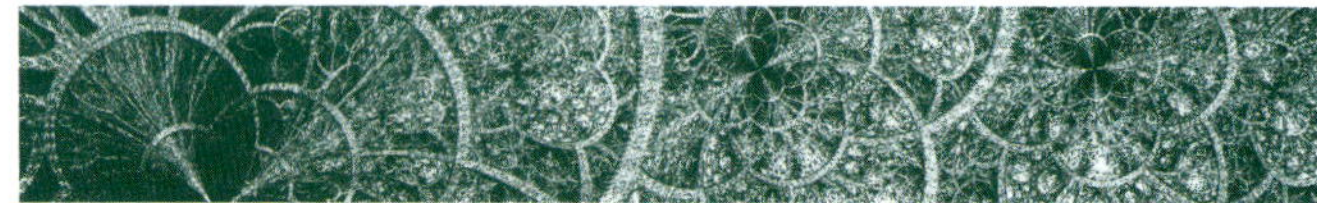

THE PERSON WITH CANCER OF THE GALLBLADDER

Gallbladder, or bile duct, cancer is a very rare form of cancer, with about 3–4 cases per 100,000 annually in Australia (Cancer Council, 2020). The survival rate is 20% after 5 years (GI Cancer, 2022). More than 85% of gallbladder cancer types are adenocarcinomas that start in the gland cells lining the gallbladder. Due to the cancer being asymptomatic, most people present with advanced, incurable disease. Clinical manifestations include:

- intense pain and a palpable mass in the RUQ of the abdomen
- unexplained nausea and vomiting
- unexplained weakness
- unexplained loss of appetite and weight loss
- fevers and chills
- pain in the right side of the abdomen
- darkened urine
- pale bowel movements
- itchy skin (GI Cancer, 2022).

Gallbladder cancers spread by direct extension to the liver and metastasise via the blood and lymph system.

Nursing care is palliative, focusing on maintaining comfort and independence to the extent possible.

Liver disorders

The liver is a complex organ with multiple metabolic and regulatory functions. Optimal liver function is essential to health. Because of the significant amount of blood in the liver at all times, it is exposed to the effects of pathogens, drugs, toxins and possibly malignant cells. As a result, liver cells may become inflamed or damaged, or cancerous tumours may develop. Malignancy of the liver or intrahepatic bile ducts, and diseases of the liver such as cirrhosis were ranked in the top 20 causes of Australian deaths in 2020 (Australian Bureau of Statistics (ABS), 2020). Aboriginal and Torres Strait Islander people were three times more likely to die from liver disease than the rest of the population. Non-alcoholic fatty liver disease is now the most common cause of liver disease in the industrialised world, with a projected increase of 25% from 5,551,000 cases in 2019 to over 7 million cases by 2030 in Australia alone (Adams et al., 2020).

Physiology review

The essential functions of the liver include the metabolism of proteins, carbohydrates and fats. It also is responsible for the metabolism of steroid hormones and most drugs. It synthesises essential blood proteins, including albumin and clotting factors in particular. The liver detoxifies alcohol and other toxic substances. Ammonia, a toxic by-product of protein metabolism, is converted to urea in the liver for elimination by the kidneys. The liver produces bile, an essential substance for absorbing fats and eliminating bilirubin from the body. Minerals and fat-soluble vitamins are stored in the liver, as is glycogen (stored carbohydrate for energy reserves). The Kupffer cells that line the sinusoids phagocytise foreign cells and damaged blood cells. See the chapter 'A person-centred approach to assessing the gastrointestinal system' for more information about the liver.

Common manifestations of liver disorders

Although many different disorders can disrupt liver function, their manifestations relate to three primary effects: disrupted liver cell function, impaired bilirubin conversion and excretion leading to jaundice and disrupted blood flow through the liver, with resulting portal hypertension.

Hepatocellular failure

The liver is vital to the digestion and metabolism of nutrients; the production of plasma proteins, including those involved in clotting; and the metabolism and excretion of compounds such as bilirubin, steroid hormones and ammonia, as well as toxins (such as alcohol) and drugs. Impaired function of liver cells has multiple effects, including:

- Impaired protein metabolism with decreased production of albumin and clotting factors. Low albumin levels contribute to oedema in peripheral tissues and **ascites** (accumulation of fluid in the abdomen) as plasma oncotic pressure is reduced. Impaired clotting factor production increases the risk of bleeding.
- Disrupted glucose metabolism and storage with resulting alterations in blood glucose levels (either hyperglycaemia or hypoglycaemia).
- Reduced bile production that impairs the absorption of lipids and fat-soluble vitamins. Inadequate vitamin K, a fat-soluble vitamin, affects the production of clotting factors, leading to a bleeding tendency.
- Impaired metabolism of steroid hormones (including oestrogen and testosterone) leads to feminisation in men and irregular menses in women.

Jaundice

Disrupted metabolism and excretion of bilirubin allows it to accumulate in tissues, leading to **jaundice** (yellow staining of tissues). Jaundice (also called *icterus*) often is first noticeable in the sclera of the eyes, then the skin.

When RBCs are destroyed (due to cell ageing or disease), haemoglobin is released. The haemoglobin molecule breaks up into globin, a protein, and haem, the iron-containing portion of the molecule. In this process, biliverdin, later converted to fat-soluble bilirubin (*unconjugated bilirubin*), is released. The bilirubin binds with albumin to be transported to the liver. In the liver, it is converted to a water-soluble form (*conjugated bilirubin*) to be excreted in the bile. See Box 24.2 for more information about bilirubin metabolism.

Jaundice can result from disruptions at any point in the production and metabolism of bilirubin:

- *Haemolytic jaundice* develops when excess RBC destruction (haemolysis) releases more bilirubin into circulation than the liver is able to process. High blood levels of unconjugated bilirubin are seen.
- *Hepatic jaundice* occurs when impaired liver cell (*hepatocyte*) function disrupts the conversion and excretion of bilirubin. Blood levels of both conjugated and unconjugated bilirubin may be elevated. Stools may appear normal or clay coloured and urine is dark because the conjugated bilirubin is excreted by the kidneys.
- Obstruction of bile flow within the biliary system (the gallbladder and bile ducts) impairs bilirubin excretion, leading to *obstructive jaundice*. Levels of conjugated bilirubin are elevated. Stools are light or clay coloured due to lack of bile pigment, and urine is dark because the kidneys excrete bilirubin.

Portal hypertension

Impaired blood flow through the liver increases pressure in the portal venous system that drains the gastrointestinal tract, the spleen and surface veins of the abdomen. **Portal hypertension**, increased pressure in the portal system, has several effects when it is prolonged:

- Dilation of veins in the gastrointestinal tract and the abdominal wall. This congestion tends to suppress the appetite and lead to the formation of collateral vessels in the distal oesophagus, stomach and rectum. The dilated, congested vessels in the oesophagus are known as
- *oesophageal varices*; in the rectum, they lead to the development of haemorrhoids. In advanced liver failure, superficial varices may develop around the umbilicus, a feature known as *caput medusae*.
- Splenomegaly or enlargement of the spleen.
- Ascites (accumulation of fluid in the peritoneal cavity). Increased hydrostatic pressure in abdominal vessels forces fluid out of the vessels and into the peritoneal cavity. Low serum albumin levels (*hypoalbuminaemia*) contribute to fluid accumulation by reducing the osmotic draw of fluid back into vessels.
- **Portal systemic encephalopathy** (or hepatic encephalopathy), impaired consciousness and mental status due to the accumulation of toxic waste products in the blood (ammonia, in particular) as blood bypasses the congested liver. It appears that factors other than elevated ammonia levels contribute, including toxic fatty acids, altered neurotransmitters and an imbalance of plasma amino acid ratios. Cerebral oedema develops late in the course of liver failure, resulting from both the accumulation of toxins and vascular mechanisms. As cerebral oedema progresses, intracranial pressure increases, cerebral perfusion decreases and brain cells become hypoxic.
- **Hepatorenal syndrome** is acute renal failure due to disrupted blood flow to the kidneys. See the chapter 'Nursing care of people with kidney disorders' for more information about renal failure.

See the section of this chapter on cirrhosis for more information about the effects and complications associated with portal hypertension.

THE PERSON WITH HEPATITIS

Hepatitis is inflammation of the liver. It is usually caused by a virus, although it may result from exposure to alcohol, drugs and toxins, or other pathogens. Hepatitis may be acute or chronic in nature. Cirrhosis, discussed in the next section, is a potential consequence of severe hepatocellular damage. Chronic hepatitis also increases the risk of developing liver cancer.

Pathophysiology and manifestations

The inflammatory process of hepatitis, whether caused by a virus, a toxin or another mechanism, damages hepatic cells and disrupts liver function. Cell-mediated immune responses damage hepatocytes and Kupffer cells, leading to hyperplasia, necrosis and cellular regeneration. The flow of bile through bile canaliculi and into the biliary system can be impaired by the inflammatory process, leading to jaundice. When the inflammatory process is mild (e.g., hepatitis A), the liver parenchyma is not significantly damaged. The inflammatory processes associated with hepatitis B and hepatitis C, however, can lead to severe liver damage. The metabolism of nutrients, drugs, alcohol and toxins and the process of bile elimination are disrupted by the inflammation of hepatitis. See the chapter 'A person-centred approach to assessing the gastrointestinal system' for more information about the liver and the preceding section for more information about the effects of disrupted liver function.

Viral hepatitis

At least five viruses are known to cause hepatitis: hepatitis A virus (HAV), hepatitis B virus (HBV), hepatitis C virus (HCV), the hepatitis-B-associated delta virus (HDV) and hepatitis E virus (HEV). With the exception of HBV, all of the hepatitis viruses are RNA viruses; HBV is a DNA virus. The viruses differ from one another in mode of transmission, incubation period, the severity and type of liver damage they cause, and their ability to become chronic or develop a carrier (asymptomatic) state. The illnesses they cause, however, are clinically very similar. Table 24.2 identifies unique features of the primary hepatitis viruses.

Hepatitis viruses replicate in the liver, damaging liver cells (hepatocytes). The viruses provoke an immune response that causes inflammation and necrosis of hepatocytes as well. Although the extent of damage and the immune response vary among the different hepatitis viruses, the disease itself usually follows a predictable pattern.

No manifestations are present during the incubation period after exposure to the virus. The *prodromal* or *pre-icteric* (before jaundice) *phase* may begin abruptly or insidiously, with general malaise, anorexia, fatigue and muscle and body aches. These manifestations often are mistaken for the flu. Nausea, vomiting, diarrhoea or constipation may develop, as well as mild RUQ abdominal pain. Rigors and fever may be present.

The *icteric* (jaundiced) *phase* usually begins 5 to 10 days after the onset of symptoms. It is heralded by jaundice of the sclera, skin and mucous membranes. Inflammation of the liver and bile ducts prevents bilirubin from being excreted into the small intestine. As a result, the serum bilirubin levels are elevated, causing yellowing of the skin and mucous membranes. Pruritus may develop due to deposition of bile salts on the skin. The stools are light brown or clay coloured because bile pigment is not excreted through the normal faecal pathway. Instead, the pigment is excreted by the kidneys, causing the urine to turn brown. Whereas people with acute hepatitis A or B are likely to develop jaundice, many people with hepatitis C do not develop jaundice. As a result, the infection may go undiagnosed for an extended period of time.

During the icteric phase, the initial prodromal manifestations usually diminish even though the serum bilirubin increases. The appetite increases and the temperature returns to normal. When uncomplicated, spontaneous recovery usually begins within 2 weeks of the onset of jaundice.

The *convalescent phase* follows jaundice and lasts several weeks. During this time, manifestations gradually improve: serum enzymes decrease, liver pain decreases and gastrointestinal symptoms and weakness subside. See the 'Manifestations' box for the manifestations of each phase of hepatitis.

TABLE 24.2 Comparison of types of viral hepatitis

VIRUS	HEPATITIS A (HAV)	HEPATITIS B (HBV)	HEPATITIS C (HCV)	HEPATITIS D (HDV)	HEPATITIS E (HEV)
Mode of transmission	Faecal-oral	Blood and body fluids; perinatal	Blood and body fluids	Blood and body fluids; perinatal	Faecal-oral
Incubation (in weeks)	2-6	6-24	5-12	3-13	3-6
Onset	Abrupt	Slow	Slow	Abrupt	Abrupt
Carrier state	No	Yes	Yes	Yes	Yes
Possible complications	Rare	Chronic hepatitis Cirrhosis	Chronic hepatitis Cirrhosis	Chronic hepatitis Cirrhosis	May be severe in pregnant women
		Liver cancer	Liver cancer	Fulminant hepatitis	
Laboratory findings	Anti-HAV antibodies present	Positive HBsAg (HBV surface antigen); anti-HBV antibodies present	Anti-HCV antibodies present	Positive HDVAg (delta antigen) early; anti-HDV antibodies later	Anti-HEV antibodies present

MANIFESTATIONS Acute hepatitis

PRE-ICTERIC PHASE
- 'Flu-like' symptoms: malaise, fatigue, fever
- Gastrointestinal: anorexia, nausea, vomiting, diarrhoea, constipation
- Muscle aches, polyarthritis
- Mild right upper abdominal pain and tenderness

ICTERIC PHASE
- Jaundice
- Pruritus
- Clay-coloured stools
- Brown urine
- Decrease in pre-icteric phase symptoms (e.g. appetite improves; no fever)

POST-ICTERIC/CONVALESCENT PHASE
- Serum bilirubin and enzymes return to normal levels
- Energy level increases
- Pain subsides
- Appetite returns

HEPATITIS A Hepatitis A (HepA), or infectious hepatitis, is a highly contagious disease caused by the hepatitis A virus (HAV) causing inflammation of the liver. HAV lasts on unwashed hands for several hours and longer in room temperature food, and is resistant to heat and freezing. HepA is transmitted by the faecal–oral route via contact with faecal-contaminated food, liquid, eating utensils, water, clothing, nappies, linen and towels, used condoms and direct (including sexual) contact with an infected person. HepA illness may last from a few weeks to several months; however, it usually does not cause the same long-term damage as other types of hepatitis. Symptoms present 2–4 weeks after exposure to HAV. The infectious period is from 2 weeks before onset of symptoms until all symptoms are resolved.

Symptoms include abdominal pain (mostly right side), fever, nausea, vomiting, loss of appetite, malaise, joint pain, dark urine, pale faeces and jaundice. Diagnosis is confirmed with medical and travel history and a blood test. Treatment is based on symptoms and is primarily fluid replacement and avoiding contact with others. Alcohol consumption should also be avoided to protect the liver. Prevention of transmission includes good hand hygiene, correct food handling, not sharing eating utensils, not drinking contaminated water and food (in developing countries and disaster areas) and vaccination. In Australia, the HepA vaccine is available for all people 2 years and older and has proven to be effective in preventing infection in about 95% of people.

FAST FACTS

- HepA is the most common cause of food poising outbreaks worldwide.
- In Australia, HepA is a nationally notifiable disease
- The infection rate for HAV, HBV and HCV is higher in people participating in high-risk sexual activity and intravenous drug users.
- Injection drug use accounted for 50% of new cases of HBV infection; heterosexual sex accounted for another 18%.
- Untreated HBV is a major cause of liver cancer.

HEPATITIS B Hepatitis B virus (HBV) causes hepatitis B (HepB) and is the most common cause of liver disease worldwide, with more than 220,000 Australians living with the disease. It is estimated that 2 billion people globally have been infected with HBV, with approximately 1.5 million new cases annually, of which only 10% are diagnosed. Almost 300 million people are chronically infected with HBV (Hepatitis B Foundation, 2022).

HBV can cause acute hepatitis, chronic hepatitis, *fulminant* (rapidly progressive) hepatitis or a carrier state. In a *carrier state*, the person harbours the active virus and is capable of spreading it to others, even though there are no discernible manifestations of the disease. This virus is spread through contact with infected blood and body fluids.

Healthcare workers are at risk through exposure to blood and body fluids, and needle-stick injuries. Other high-risk groups for HBV include people frequently receiving blood products (such as people on haemodialysis).

The exact mechanism of liver injury by HBV is unclear: however, it is known that liver cells are damaged by the immune response to this antigen. The liver shows evidence of injury and scarring, regeneration and proliferation of inflammatory cells. Damage may affect only portions of the liver or the majority of the liver. During the prodromal period, people with HepB may experience nausea, vomiting, fatigue, malaise, muscle and joint pains, headache, photophobia and flu-like symptoms 1 to 2 weeks prior to the onset of jaundice.

HEPATITIS C Hepatitis C (HepC) is a blood-borne virus caused by vepatitis C virus (HCV). HCV was first discovered in 1988 as a cause for 'non-A, non-B hepatitis', with testing in Australia developed in 1990. The World Health Organization (WHO) (2019) estimates that 58 million people globally have chronic HepC, with approximately 1.5 million acute infections annually. The WHO estimates that almost 300,000 people die from HepC each year, mostly from liver cirrhosis or hepatocellular carcinoma (WHO, 2019). In Australia, over 115,000 live with HepC. While there is no effective vaccine for HepC, antiviral medications are 95% effective against HCV. As HepC is a blood-borne virus, the most common modes of transmission are via:

- reuse of healthcare equipment such as syringes and needles
- inadequate processing and sterilisation of healthcare equipment including tattoo and body piercing equipment
- transfusion of unscreened blood products
- intravenous drug users sharing injecting equipment
- sharing toothbrushes, razors or nail files.

HepC may also be transmitted from mother to fetus (5% chance) and via sexual contact, especially in people who have multiple partners or in male to male sex (Hepatitis Australia,

2022). At-risk populations include people with haemophilia treated with clotting factors prior to 1987 and people requiring haemodialysis.

The incubation period for HCV is from 2 weeks to 6 months. Acute HepC usually is asymptomatic and occurs in 25% of cases. If symptoms do develop, they often are mild and non-specific and do not cause life-threatening disease. Symptoms of HepC include fever, fatigue, nausea and vomiting, abdominal pain, dark urine, pale faeces, joint pain, dry eyes and oral mucosa and jaundice (WHO, 2019). The WHO estimates that 30% of people infected with HCV spontaneously clear the virus within 6 months of infection and with no treatment. The remaining 55–85% will develop chronic HCV infection, with a 15–30% chance of developing cirrhosis within 20 years. Diagnosis is with serological testing for anti-HCV antibodies. Further testing for HCV ribonucleic acid is required to confirm chronic HepC infection. Early diagnosis in high-risk populations (IV drug users, sex workers, renal dialysis patients) assists with prevention of further illness and, most importantly, prevention of transmission.

HEPATITIS DELTA Hepatitis delta virus (HDV) is the least common form of viral hepatitis. HDV requires HBV for its replication, so infection with hepatitis D (HepD) only occur with co-infection of both HBV and HDV, or via superinfection (the person is already infected with HBV). As with HBV, HDV is transmitted via blood and body fluids. Five per cent of people with chronic HepB also carry HDV. HDV–HBV co-infection is considered the most severe form of viral hepatitis due to its rapid progression to hepatocellular carcinoma and liver-related mortality. Populations most at risk include Aboriginal and Torres Strait Islander peoples, people receiving haemodialysis, men who have sex with men, IV drug users and sex workers. HepD treatment success rates are low; however, HDV infection is prevented with HBV vaccine.

HEPATITIS E Hepatitis E virus (HEV) is a is a major cause of mortality and morbidity in pregnant women, people with chronic liver disease and the immunocompromised. In Australia, people at highest risk are those who eat undercooked pork products, particularly pork livers. HEV is a nationally notifiable disease in Australia. Hepatitis E is rare in Australia, with approximately 10 to 30 cases diagnosed and reported each year. HEV rates are highest in areas of poor sanitation and contamination of water supplies such as South-East Asia, Africa and Central America. It is transmitted by faecal–oral route. The chance of developing a chronic illness is very low (1–4%) except in pregnant women (20% mortality).

Chronic hepatitis

Chronic hepatitis is chronic infection of the liver. Although it may cause few symptoms, it is the primary cause of liver damage leading to cirrhosis, liver cancer and liver transplantation. Three of the known hepatitis viruses cause chronic hepatitis: HBV, HCV and HDV. Manifestations of chronic hepatitis include malaise, fatigue and hepatomegaly. Occasional icteric (jaundiced) periods may occur. Liver enzymes, particularly serum aminotransferase levels, typically are elevated.

In *chronic active hepatitis*, inflammation extends to involve entire hepatic lobules. Chronic active hepatitis usually leads to cirrhosis and end-stage liver failure.

Fulminant hepatitis

Fulminant hepatitis is a rapidly progressive disease, with liver failure developing within 2 to 3 weeks after the onset of symptoms. Although uncommon, it is usually related to HBV with concurrent HDV infection.

Toxic hepatitis

Many substances, including alcohol, certain drugs and other toxins, can directly damage liver cells. Alcoholic hepatitis can result from chronic alcohol abuse or from an acute toxic reaction to alcohol. Alcoholic hepatitis causes necrosis of hepatocytes and inflammation of the liver parenchyma (functional tissue). Unless alcohol intake is avoided, progression to cirrhosis is common.

Other potential hepatotoxins include paracetamol, benzene, carbon tetrachloride, halothane, chloroform and poisonous mushrooms. These substances directly damage liver cells, leading to necrosis. The degree of damage often depends on age and the extent of exposure to (dose of) the hepatotoxin. Paracetamol overdose is a common cause of hepatocellular damage.

Hepatobiliary hepatitis

Hepatobiliary hepatitis is due to cholestasis, the interruption of the normal flow of bile. Cholestasis may result from obstruction of the hepatic duct with stones or inflammation secondary to cholelithiasis. Other agents, such as oral contraceptives and allopurinol (a drug used to lower uric acid levels), also can cause cholestasis. When bile flow is disrupted, the liver parenchyma may become inflamed. Re-establishing bile flow by removing the stone or other causative agent is the treatment for hepatobiliary hepatitis.

INTERPROFESSIONAL CARE

Management of hepatitis focuses on determining its cause, providing appropriate treatment and support, and teaching strategies to prevent further liver damage. Effective management begins with thorough assessment of diagnostic and laboratory data.

Diagnosis

Liver function tests, such as blood levels of bilirubin and enzymes commonly released when liver cells are damaged, are obtained. These include the following:

- *Alanine aminotransferase (ALT)* is an enzyme contained within each liver cell. When liver cells are damaged, ALT is released into the blood. Levels may exceed 1,000 U/L or more in acute hepatitis.
- *Aspartate aminotransferase (AST)* is an enzyme found predominantly in heart and liver cells. AST levels rise when liver cells are damaged; with severe damage, blood levels may be 20 to 100 times normal values.

- *Alkaline phosphatase (ALP)* is an enzyme present in liver cells and bone. Serum ALP levels often are elevated in hepatitis.
- *Gamma-glutamyltransferase (GGT)* is an enzyme present in cell membranes. Its blood levels rise in hepatitis and obstructive biliary disease and remain elevated until function is restored.
- *Lactic dehydrogenase (LDH)*, an enzyme present in many body tissues, is a non-specific indicator of tissue damage. Its isoenzyme, LDH5, is a specific indicator of liver damage.
- *Serum bilirubin* levels, including *conjugated* and *unconjugated*, are elevated in viral hepatitis due to impaired bilirubin metabolism and obstruction of the hepatobiliary ducts by inflammation and oedema. The bilirubin level decreases as inflammation and oedema subside.
- Laboratory tests for viral antigens and their specific antibodies may be done to identify the infecting virus and its state of activity.
- A *liver biopsy* may be done to detect and evaluate chronic hepatitis. (Nursing implications for this test are outlined in the 'Diagnostic tests' box in the chapter 'A person-centred approach to assessing the gastrointestinal system'.)

Medications

PREVENTION HAV and HBV are preventable diseases. Vaccines are available, as are preparations to prevent the disease following known or suspected exposure.

Vaccines Hepatitis A vaccine provides long-term protection against HAV infection. It is an inactivated whole-virus vaccine available in paediatric and adult formulations. Although more than 95% of adults achieve immunity after one dose of the vaccine, two doses are recommended for full protection. (See Table 24.3.)

Three doses of hepatitis B vaccine provide immunity to HBV infection in 90% of healthy adults. Because the hepatitis delta virus requires the presence of HBV, hepatitis B vaccine also protects against HDV. Hepatitis B vaccine is a recombinant vaccine. Vaccines produced by different manufacturers may be used interchangeably, although their dosages differ. Older adults are less likely to achieve immunity than younger adults. People on haemodialysis and people who are immunocompromised may need larger or more doses of the vaccine to achieve adequate protection. Serological testing for immunity is recommended on completion of the series for people in these high-risk groups.

A combined hepatitis A and hepatitis B vaccine is available for use. It is recommended for the same high-risk populations as the single vaccines. Three doses are given: the initial dose, followed by doses no sooner than 4 weeks and 6 months later.

Post-exposure prophylaxis Post-exposure prophylaxis may be recommended for household or sexual contacts of people with HAV or HBV and other people who are known to have been exposed to these viruses. It may also be necessary for health professionals who are not immunised

TABLE 24.3 Recommendations for hepatitis prevention in adults

DISEASE/STRATEGY	IMMUNISATION	ADVERSE REACTIONS	POPULATION RECOMMENDATIONS
Hepatitis A			
Prevention	Hepatitis A vaccine (Havrix; VAQTA Adult), 2 doses (initial dose with booster in 6–12 months) given IM into deltoid muscle Combined hepatitis A and hepatitis B vaccine (Twinrix), 3 doses (initial dose followed by doses 1 and 6 months later) given IM into deltoid muscle	Pain at injection site	• All travellers to, and all expatriates living in, moderately to highly endemic areas • Indigenous Australian children residing in the Northern Territory, Queensland, South Australia and Western Australia • Those whose lifestyle may put them at risk of acquiring HVA • People with occupational risk
Post-exposure prophylaxis	Standard immune globulin IM into large muscle mass within 2 weeks of exposure	Rare; risk of anaphylaxis in people with IgA deficiency	• Close contacts of people with known HVA • People potentially exposed to hepatitis A at childcare centre or restaurant with infected food handler
Hepatitis B			
Prevention	Recombinant hepatitis B vaccine (Engerix-B Adult), 3 doses (initial dose followed by doses at 1 and 6 months later) given IM into deltoid muscle Combined hepatitis A and hepatitis B vaccine (Twinrix), 3 doses (initial dose followed by doses 4 weeks and 6 months later) given IM into deltoid muscle	Pain at injection site; fever, nausea, dizziness, malaise, myalgia and arthralgia	• Infants and adolescents • Household contacts of acute and chronic HBV carriers • Men who have sex with men • Haemodialysis patients, HIV-positive individuals and other adults with impaired immunity • Prostitutes; heterosexuals with multiple sexual partners • People with an STD • Intravenous drug users Long-term male prisoners • Healthcare workers
Post-exposure prophylaxis	Hepatitis B immune globulin (HBIG) given IM into large muscle mass within 72 hours of exposure.	Infrequent; muscle stiffness, pain, fever, nausea, dizziness, malaise, myalgia and arthralgia	• Infants born to women with HBV infection • Percutaneous or permucosal exposure to HBV when unvaccinated or antibody response is negative or unknown

Source: Based on Australian Technical Advisory Group on Immunisation (ATAGI) (2022). *Australian immunisation handbook*. Canberra: Australian Government Department of Health and Aged Care. Retrieved from https://immunisationhandbook.health.gov.au.

against HBV post needle-stick injury. It is not necessary if the exposed person has been vaccinated and is known to be immune.

Hepatitis A prophylaxis is provided by a single dose of immune globulin (IG) given within 2 weeks after exposure. IG is recommended for all people with household or sexual contact with a person known to be infected with HAV. See Table 21.3 for further recommendations.

Hepatitis B post-exposure prophylaxis is indicated for people exposed to HBV. Hepatitis B immune globulin (HBIG) is given to provide short-term immunity. Hepatitis B vaccine may be given concurrently. Candidates for post-exposure prophylaxis include those with known or suspected percutaneous or permucosal contact with infected blood, sexual partners of people with acute HBV or who are HBV carriers, and household contacts of people with acute HBV infection (Department of Health and Aged Care, 2022).

Treatments

In most cases of acute viral hepatitis, pharmacological treatment of the infection is not indicated. However, acute HCV generally is treated with interferon alpha, and direct-acting antiviral (DAA) agent, to reduce the risk of chronic HCV. The Hepatitis C Virus Infection Consensus Statement Working Group (2020) recommends DAA agents as these target numerous stages in the HCV replication life cycle. These medications are highly effective and safe, with a short treatment duration. Virtually all people with HCV are suitable for DAA therapy, including those previously intolerant of or ineligible for interferon therapy. In Australia, the Therapeutic Goods Administration has approved multiple DAAs including NS3 protease inhibitors (glecaprevir, grazoprevir and voxilaprevir), NS5B nucleotide inhibitor (sofosbuvir) and NS5A inhibitors (velpatasvir, pibrentasvir, elbasvir and ledipasvir). Additionally, several interferon-free regimens combining these DAAs are available to treat people with HCV infection, including people with compensated and decompensated liver disease (Hepatitis C Virus Infection Consensus Statement Working Group, 2020).

Interferon alpha is used to treat both chronic HBV and chronic HCV. Interferon alpha interferes with viral replication, reducing the viral load. It is given by intramuscular or subcutaneous injection. Virtually all people treated with interferon alpha develop a flu-like syndrome with fever, fatigue, muscle aches, headache and chills. Paracetamol helps alleviate some of these adverse effects. Depression also is a common adverse effect of this drug.

An alternative treatment for chronic HBV is lamivudine (3TC, Zeffix), an antiviral drug that can reduce liver inflammation and fibrosis. Although it has minimal side effects, people may become resistant to the beneficial effects of lamivudine.

Treatment of acute hepatitis also includes as-needed bed rest, adequate nutrition as tolerated and avoidance of strenuous activity, alcohol and agents that are toxic to the liver. In most cases, clinical recovery takes 3 to 16 weeks.

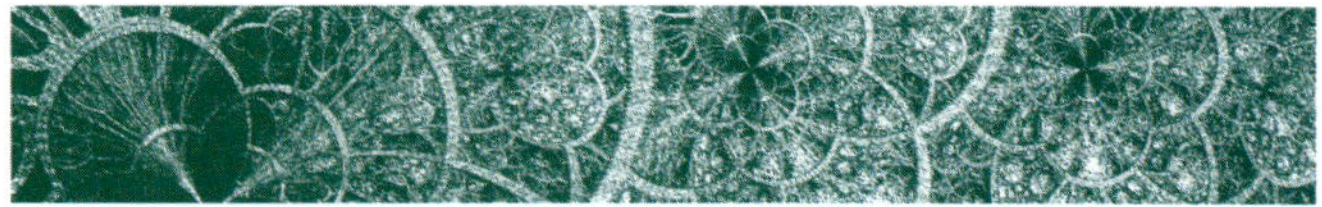

Nursing care

Health promotion

Nurses play an instrumental role in preventing the spread of hepatitis. Stress the importance of hygiene measures such as handwashing after toileting and before all food handling. Discuss the dangers of intravenous drug use and, with drug users, of sharing needles or other equipment. Encourage all sexually active people to use safer sexual practices such as mutual monogamy and barrier protection (such as male or female condoms).

Discuss recommendations for hepatitis A and hepatitis B vaccine with people in high- or moderate-risk groups for these infections. Ensure that nurses and other healthcare workers at risk of exposure to blood and body fluids are effectively vaccinated against hepatitis A and B. Encourage all people with known or probable exposure to HAV or HBV to obtain post-exposure prophylaxis.

Assessment

Collect assessment data related to hepatitis, such as the following:

- *Health history*: current manifestations, including anorexia, nausea, vomiting, abdominal discomfort, changes in bowel elimination or colour of stools; muscle or joint pain, fatigue; changes in colour of skin or sclera; duration of symptoms; known exposure to hepatitis; travel history; high-risk behaviours such as intravenous drug use or multiple sexual partners; previous history of liver disorders; current medications, prescription and over the counter.
- *Physical assessment*: vital signs including temperature; colour of sclera and mucous membranes; skin colour and condition; abdominal contour and tenderness; colour of stool and urine.
- *Diagnostic tests*: serum bilirubin, liver function tests, serological antibody–antigen levels.

Nursing diagnoses and interventions

People with acute or chronic hepatitis usually are treated in community settings; rarely is hospitalisation required. Nursing care focuses on preventing spread of the infection to others and promoting the person's comfort and ability to provide self-care.

Risk of infection (transmission)

An important goal when caring for people with acute viral hepatitis is preventing spread of the infection.

- Use standard precautions. Practise meticulous handwashing. The hepatitis viruses are spread by direct contact with faeces or blood and body fluids. *Standard precautions and good handwashing protect both healthcare workers and other people from exposure to the virus.*
- For people with HAV or HEV, use standard precautions and contact isolation if faecal incontinence is present. *The faecal–oral route is the primary mode of transmission of these viruses. Other hepatitis viruses are transmitted through blood and other body fluids.*

- Encourage prophylactic treatment of all members of household and intimate sexual contacts. *Prophylactic treatment of others in close contact with the person decreases their risk of contracting the disease or, if already infected, the severity of the disease.*

> **CONSIDERATION FOR PRACTICE**
>
> If the person diagnosed with HAV is employed as a food handler or childcare worker, contact the local health department to report possible exposure of patrons. Maintain confidentiality. Prophylactic treatment of people who have possibly been exposed to the virus can prevent a local epidemic of the disease.

Fatigue

Fatigue and possible weakness are common in acute hepatitis. Although bed rest is rarely indicated, adequate rest periods and limitation of activities may be necessary. Many people with acute hepatitis may be unable to resume normal activity levels for 4 or more weeks.

- Encourage planned rest periods throughout the day. *Adequate rest is necessary for optimal immune function.*
- Assist to identify essential activities and those that can be deferred or delegated to others. *Identifying essential and non-essential activities promotes the person's sense of control.*
- Suggest using level of fatigue to determine activity level, with gradual resumption of activities as fatigue and sense of wellbeing improves. *Fatigue associated with activity is an indicator of appropriate and inappropriate activity levels. As recovery progresses, increasing activity levels are tolerated with less fatigue.*

Imbalanced nutrition: less than body requirements

Adequate nutrition is important for immune function and healing in people with acute or chronic hepatitis.

- Help plan a diet of appealing foods that provides a high-kilojoule intake of approximately 65 carbohydrate kilojoules per kilogram of ideal body weight. *Sufficient energy is required for healing; adequate carbohydrate intake can spare protein.*
- Encourage planning food intake according to symptoms of the disease. Discuss eating smaller meals and using between-meal snacks to maintain nutrient and kilojoule intake. *People with acute hepatitis often are more anorexic and nauseated in the afternoon and evening; planning the majority of kilojoule intake for in the morning helps maintain adequate intake. Limiting fat intake and the size of meals may reduce the incidence of nausea.*
- Instruct to avoid alcohol intake and diet drinks. *Alcohol avoidance is vital to prevent further liver damage and promote healing. Diet drinks (e.g. diet soft drinks or juice drinks) provide few kilojoules when an increased kilojoule intake is needed for healing.*
- Encourage use of nutritional supplements such as Ensure or instant breakfast drinks to maintain kilojoule and nutrient intake. *Nutritional supplement drinks are an additional source of concentrated kilojoules and nutrients.*

Disturbed body image

Jaundice and associated rashes and itching can affect the person's body image. Nursing measures to prevent skin breakdown and address body image are discussed in the following section on cirrhosis.

Community-based care

Provide discharge teaching to people and their families for home care. Include the following topics:

- recommended prophylactic treatment
- infection control measures such as frequent handwashing, not sharing eating utensils, avoiding food handling or preparation activities by the person with hepatitis A; abstaining from sexual relations during acute infection and using barrier protection if a carrier or for chronic infection
- managing fatigue and limited activity
- managing pruritus and maintaining skin integrity: use warm, not hot, water when bathing, use mild or no soap, limit duration of baths and showers; pat dry, do not rub, apply an alcohol-free lotion soon after bathing to retain skin moisture; wear loose cotton garments that allow moisture to evaporate from skin; reduce room temperature, especially at night, to prevent overheating; keep fingernails short and wear cotton mittens or gloves as needed to prevent scratching during sleep
- promoting nutrient intake
- avoiding hepatic toxins such as alcohol, paracetamol and selected other drugs; encourage to alert all care providers to presence of infection
- recommended follow up.

If chronic HBV or HCV is being treated with medications, teach how to administer the medication, its dosing schedule, precautions and management of adverse effects. Stress the importance of keeping follow-up appointments, including recommended laboratory testing.

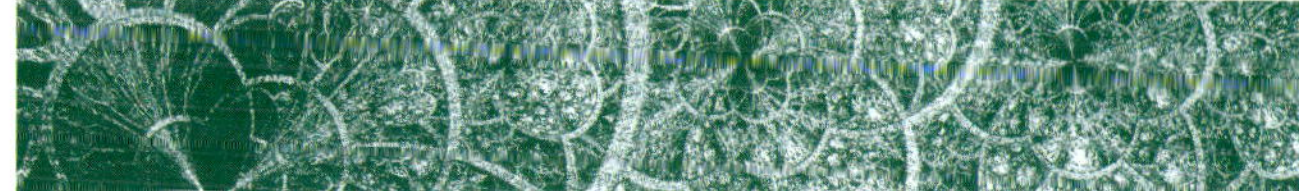

THE PERSON WITH CIRRHOSIS

Cirrhosis is the end-stage of chronic liver disease. It is a progressive, irreversible disorder, eventually leading to liver failure.

Alcoholic, or **Laënnec's**, **cirrhosis** is the most frequent cause of death related to long-term, high-risk alcohol consumption. Excessive alcohol consumption is one of the leading causes of morbidity and mortality in Australia (Selvanathan, Selvanathan & Jayasinghe, 2020). Cirrhosis also may result from chronic HBV or HCV; prolonged obstruction of the biliary (bile drainage) system; long-term, severe right heart failure and other uncommon liver disorders. The incidence of and mortality attributable to cirrhosis and chronic liver disease vary significantly among populations.

Pathophysiology

In cirrhosis, functional liver tissue is gradually destroyed and replaced by fibrous scar tissue. As hepatocytes and liver lobules are destroyed, the metabolic functions of the liver are lost.

Structurally abnormal nodules encircled by connective tissue form. This fibrous connective tissue forms constrictive bands that disrupt blood and bile flow within liver lobules. Blood no longer flows freely through the liver to the inferior vena cava. This restricted blood flow leads to portal hypertension (increased pressure in the portal venous system).

FAST FACTS

- Alcoholic liver disease is the most common cause of alcohol-related deaths in Australia. In 2015, chronic liver disease was the nineth leading cause of death in Australia.
- In 2017, an estimated two-thirds of alcohol-induced deaths were due to alcoholic liver disease, with males over the age of 60 at highest risk.
- The rate of alcoholic liver disease mortality is approximately five times higher for Aboriginal and Torres Strait Islander people than other groups in Australia (ABS, 2020).

Laënnec's, or portal, cirrhosis was first described by Rene Laënnec in 1819. It is the final stage of alcoholic liver disease. Its development is directly related to alcohol consumption: total amount of alcohol consumed, number of years of excessive alcohol consumption and blood alcohol levels. Cirrhosis mortality is prevalent in men due to men generally consuming more alcohol than women and the percentage of men consuming large amounts of alcohol.

Alcohol causes metabolic changes in the liver: triglyceride and fatty acid synthesis increases and the formation and release of lipoproteins decrease, leading to fatty infiltration of hepatocytes (fatty liver). At this stage, abstinence from alcohol can allow the liver to heal. With continued alcohol abuse, the disease progresses. Inflammatory cells infiltrate the liver (alcoholic hepatitis), causing necrosis, fibrosis and destruction of functional liver tissue. In the final stage of alcoholic cirrhosis, regenerative nodules form and the liver shrinks and develops a nodular appearance. Malnutrition commonly accompanies alcoholic cirrhosis. See 'Pathophysiology illustrated: cirrhosis and portal hypertension'.

Biliary cirrhosis

When bile flow is obstructed within the liver or in the biliary system, retained bile damages and destroys liver cells close to the interlobular bile ducts. This leads to inflammation, fibrosis and formation of regenerative nodules.

Post-hepatic cirrhosis

Advanced progressive liver disease resulting from chronic hepatitis B or C or from an unknown cause is known as post-hepatic or post-necrotic cirrhosis. The liver is shrunken and nodular, with extensive liver cell loss and fibrosis.

Manifestations and complications

Early in the course of cirrhosis, few manifestations may be present. The liver usually is enlarged and may be tender. Symptoms may be vague such as a dull, aching pain in the RUQ along with fever, nausea, vomiting, diarrhoea, anorexia and malaise (Craft et al., 2018).

As the disease progresses, manifestations related to complications of liver cell failure and portal hypertension develop including ascites, oedema, gastrointestinal haemorrhage, jaundice or encephalopathy. Men may have decreased body hair, gynaecomastia and testicular atrophy; women may have dysmenorrhoea or amenorrhoea. Laboratory tests may show anaemia from chronic gastrointestinal bleeding, hypersplenism or nutritional deficiencies, total serum bilirubin may be elevated with advanced cirrhosis, clotting factors are prolonged and liver enzymes elevated (Craft et al., 2018). See 'Multisystem effects of cirrhosis'.

See the 'Manifestations' box for selected manifestations of cirrhosis and their underlying pathophysiology.

PORTAL HYPERTENSION Portal hypertension causes blood to be rerouted to adjoining lower-pressure vessels. This *shunting* of blood involves collateral vessels. Affected veins, which become engorged and congested, are located in the oesophagus, rectum and abdomen. Portal hypertension increases the hydrostatic pressure in vessels of the portal system. Increased hydrostatic pressure in the capillaries pushes fluid out, contributing to ascites formation.

SPLENOMEGALY The spleen enlarges (splenomegaly) because portal hypertension causes blood to be shunted into the splenic vein. Splenomegaly increases the rate at which red and white blood cells and platelets are removed from circulation and destroyed. This increased blood cell destruction leads to anaemia, leucopenia and thrombocytopenia (Craft et al., 2018).

ASCITES Ascites is the accumulation of plasma-rich fluid in the abdominal cavity. Although portal hypertension is the primary cause of ascites, decreased serum proteins and increased aldosterone also contribute to the fluid accumulation. *Hypoalbuminaemia*, low serum albumin, decreases the colloidal osmotic pressure of plasma. This pressure normally holds fluid in the intravascular compartment; when plasma colloidal osmotic pressure decreases, fluid escapes into extravascular compartments. *Hyperaldosteronism*, an increase in aldosterone, causes sodium and water retention, contributing to ascites and generalised oedema.

OESOPHAGEAL VARICES **Oesophageal varices** are enlarged, thin-walled veins that form in the submucosa of the oesophagus. These collateral vessels form when blood is shunted from the portal system due to portal hypertension. The thin-walled varices may rupture, causing massive haemorrhage; even eating high-roughage foods can precipitate bleeding. Thrombocytopenia, platelet deficiency and impaired production of clotting factors by the liver contribute to the risk of haemorrhage.

PORTAL SYSTEMIC ENCEPHALOPATHY Portal systemic encephalopathy (*hepatic encephalopathy*) results from accumulation of neurotoxins in the blood and cerebral oedema. Ammonia, a by-product of protein metabolism, contributes to hepatic encephalopathy. Ammonium ion is produced as proteins and amino acids are broken down by bacteria in the intestinal tract. Normally, the ammonia produced is then converted by the liver to urea before entering the general

MANIFESTATIONS **Cirrhosis with underlying cause**

MANIFESTATION	UNDERLYING PATHOPHYSIOLOGY
Oedema, ascites	Impaired plasma protein synthesis (hypoalbuminaemia) Disrupted hormone balance and fluid retention Increased pressure in portal venous system
Bleeding, bruising	Decreased clotting factor synthesis Increased platelet destruction by enlarged spleen Impaired vitamin K absorption and storage
Oesophageal varices, haemorrhoids	Increased pressure in portal venous system with collateral vessel development
Gastritis, anorexia, diarrhoea	Engorged veins in gastrointestinal system Alcohol ingestion Impaired bile synthesis and fat absorption
Abdominal wall vein distension (caput medusae)	Portal hypertension
Jaundice	Impaired bilirubin metabolism and excretion
Malnutrition, muscle wasting	Impaired nutrient metabolism Impaired fat absorption Impaired hormone metabolism
Anaemia, leucopenia, increased risk of infection	Bleeding Increased blood cell destruction by spleen
Asterixis, encephalopathy	Accumulated metabolic toxins Impaired ammonia metabolism and excretion
Gynaecomastia, infertility, impotence	Altered sex hormone metabolism

circulation. As functional liver tissue is destroyed, ammonia can no longer be converted to urea and it accumulates in the blood. Other nervous system depressants, such as narcotics and tranquillisers, also can contribute to hepatic encephalopathy. Box 24.4 lists selected precipitating factors for hepatic encephalopathy. Accumulation of other metabolic toxins is thought to contribute as well.

Asterixis (liver flap), a muscle tremor that interferes with the ability to maintain a fixed position of the extremities and causes involuntary jerking movements, is an early sign of portal systemic encephalopathy. Asterixis primarily affects the upper extremities, but also may affect the tongue and feet. Asterixis is elicited by instructing the person to extend the arms and dorsiflex the wrists. If present, asterixis causes a downward flapping of the hands (see Figure 24.3). Changes in personality and mentation develop; agitation, restlessness, impaired judgment and slurred speech also are early manifestations of hepatic encephalopathy. As it progresses, confusion, disorientation and incoherence develop. Cerebral oedema that leads to increased intracranial pressure and cerebral hypoxia is the leading cause of death in people with portal systemic encephalopathy and liver failure.

BOX 24.4 Precipitating factors for hepatic encephalopathy

- High serum ammonia level
- Constipation
- Blood transfusions
- Gastrointestinal bleeding
- Medications: sedatives, tranquillisers, narcotic analgesics, anaesthetics
- Hypoxia
- High-protein diet
- Severe infection
- Surgery

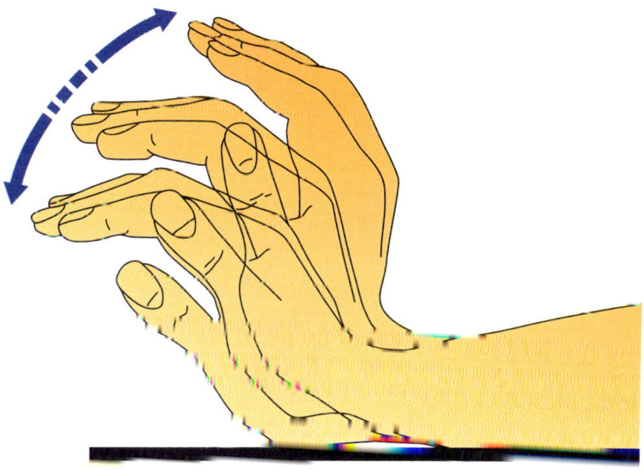

FIGURE 24.3 *Asterixis. Note the downward tremor of the hand on dorsiflexion of the wrist*

Cirrhosis and portal hypertension

Normal liver

The liver contains multiple lobules made up of plates of hepatocytes, the functional cells of the liver, surrounded by small capillaries called sinusoids. These sinusoids receive a mixture of venous and arterial blood from branches of the portal vein and hepatic artery. Blood from the sinusoids drains into the central vein of the lobule. Hepatocytes produce bile, which drains outward to bile ducts.

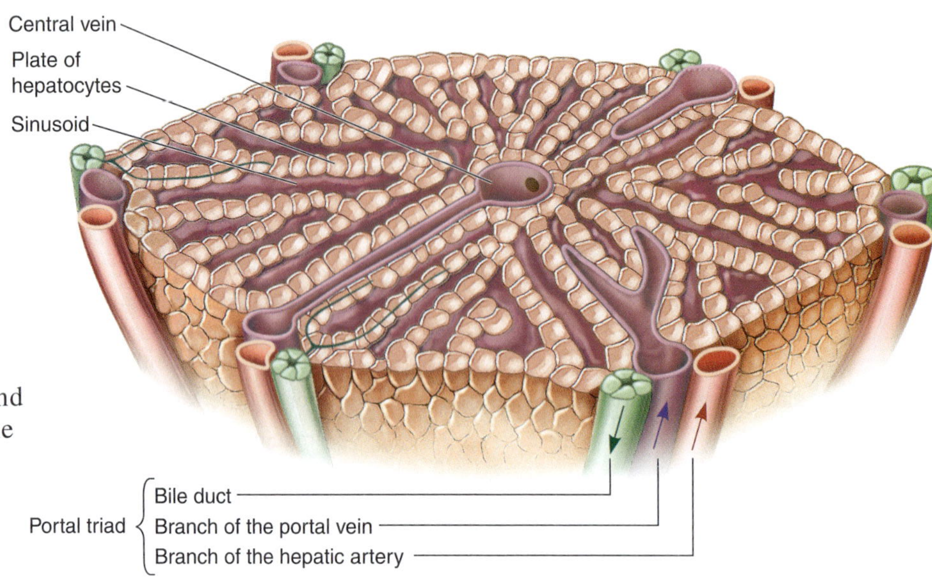

Fatty liver

Ingested alcohol is primarily metabolised in the liver. Acetaldehyde, formed when alcohol is metabolised, damages hepatocytes and impairs the oxidation of fatty acids. As a result, fat accumulates within hepatocytes and liver lobules. Other alcohol metabolism by-products, including oxygen free radicals, promote inflammation and may stimulate autoantibody production.

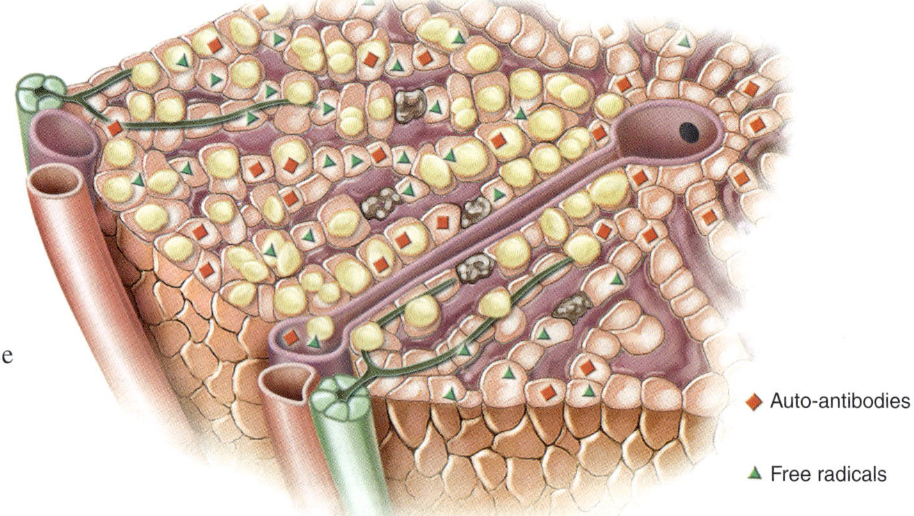

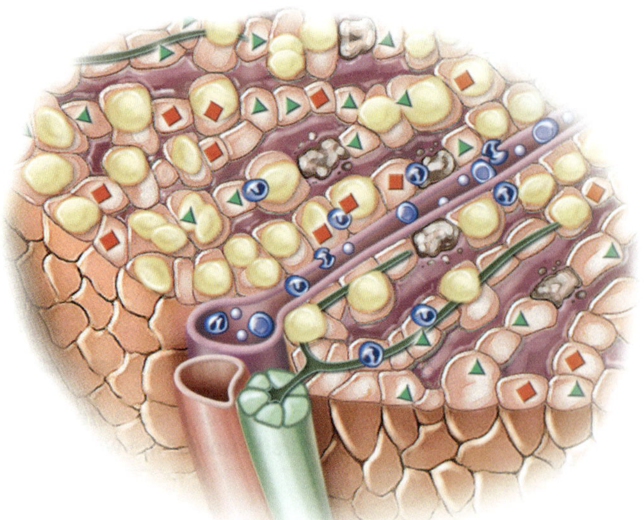

Alcoholic hepatitis

With continued alcohol intake, liver cells degenerate and spotty cellular necrosis occurs. Inflammatory cells such as polymorphonuclear leucocytes and lymphocytes infiltrate the lobule.

Alcoholic cirrhosis

Cellular necrosis and inflammation transform some liver cells into fibroblasts that produce and deposit collagen. Web-like bands of connective tissue develop around the portal triads and central vein, eventually connecting with one another. Small islands of liver cells continue to regenerate, forming nodules. Hepatocyte destruction outpaces regeneration. As a result of cell loss, fibrosis and scarring, the liver shrinks and becomes hard and nodular.

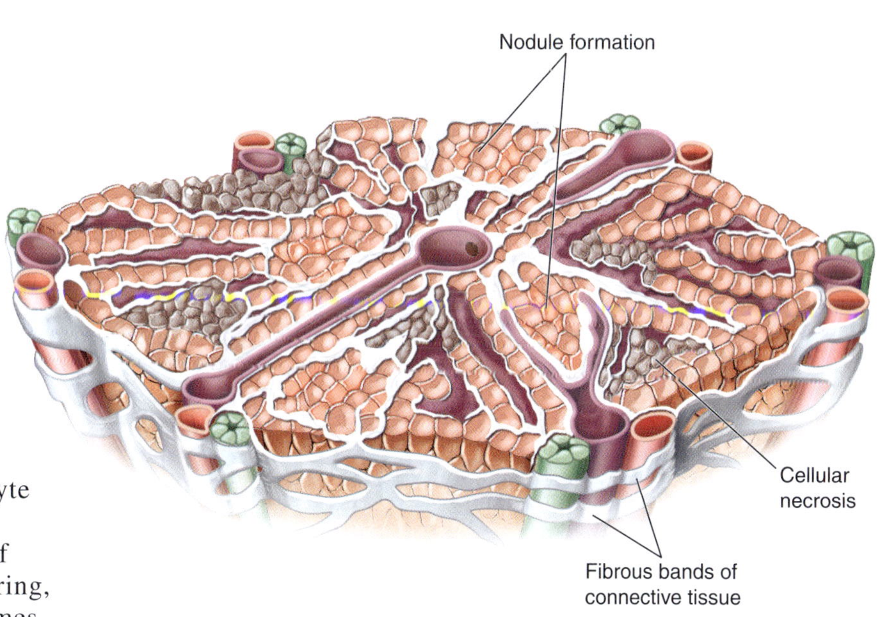

Portal hypertension

Bands of fibrotic scar tissue obstruct the sinusoids and blood flow from the portal vein to the hepatic vein. Pressure in the portal venous system, which drains the gastrointestinal tract, pancreas and spleen, increases. This increased pressure opens collateral vessels in the oesophagus, anterior abdominal wall and rectum, allowing blood to bypass the obstructed portal vessels. Prolonged portal hypertension leads to the development of (1) varices (fragile, distended veins) in the lower oesophagus, stomach and rectum; (2) splenomegaly (an enlarged spleen); (3) ascites (accumulation of fluid in the abdomen); and (4) hepatic encephalopathy (disrupted CNS function with altered consciousness).

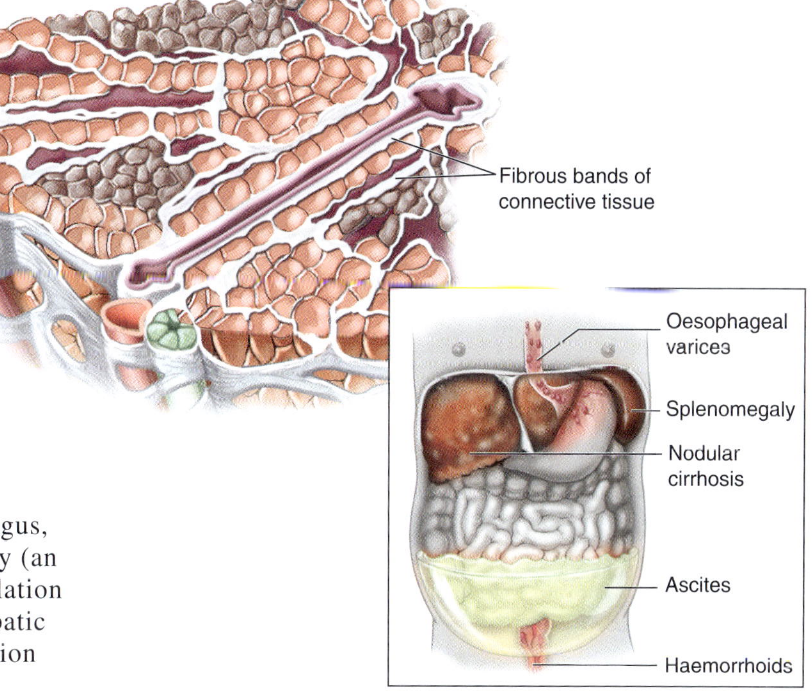

Multisystem effects of cirrhosis

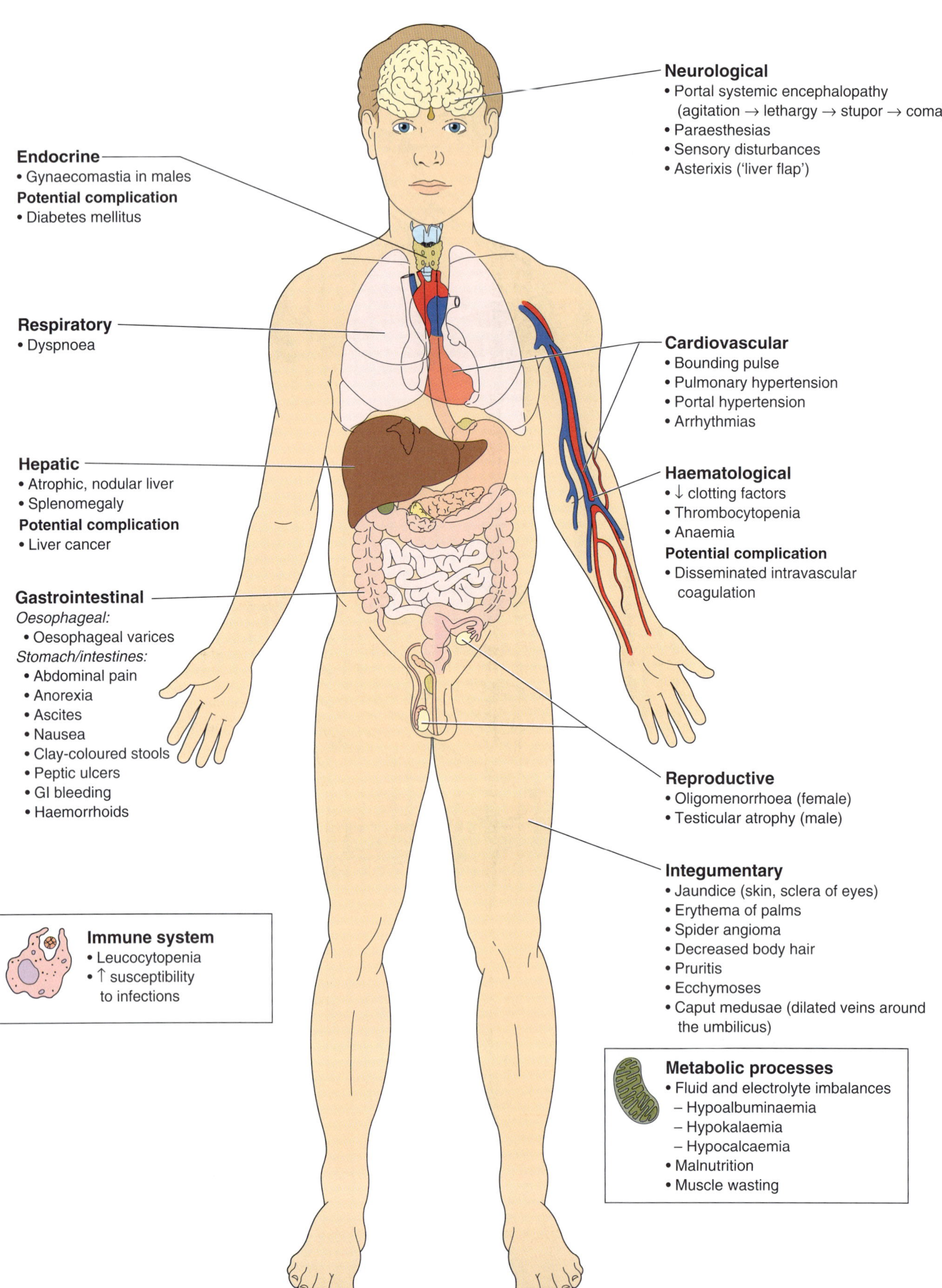

HEPATORENAL SYNDROME Although the cause is unclear, renal failure with azotaemia (excess nitrogenous waste products in the blood), sodium retention, oliguria and hypotension may develop in people with advanced cirrhosis and ascites. Hepatorenal syndrome appears to be the result of imbalanced blood flow, leading to constriction of vessels leading to and within the kidneys. The syndrome may be precipitated by gastrointestinal bleeding, aggressive diuretic therapy or by an unknown cause.

SPONTANEOUS BACTERIAL PERITONITIS People with cirrhosis and ascites may develop bacterial peritonitis, even in the absence of known contamination of the peritoneal cavity or other specific risk factors (e.g. paracentesis). The inflammatory response to peritonitis worsens ascites by increasing the permeability of capillaries in the mesentery. The manifestations of spontaneous bacterial peritonitis may be subtle, with increased abdominal discomfort or pain, fever, increasing ascites, worsening encephalopathy and an overall decline in condition.

INTERPROFESSIONAL CARE

Care for the person with cirrhosis is holistic, addressing physiological, psychosocial and spiritual needs. The importance of including the family in the plan of care cannot be overemphasised, particularly if alcohol abuse is identified as the cause. Abstinence from alcohol is the cornerstone of treatment for alcoholic liver cirrhosis (Arun, Ilangovan & Rajma, 2020). Other treatment includes medications to help regulate protein metabolism, maintenance of fluid and electrolyte balance, and supportive therapies, including treatment of underlying problems such as malnutrition, anaemia, bleeding, encephalopathy, renal failure and infections.

Diagnosis

Studies to confirm the diagnosis of cirrhosis and identify its cause and effects are performed. Diagnostic tests may include the following:

- *Liver function studies* include *ALT*, *AST*, *ALP* and *GGT*. All may be elevated in cirrhosis, but usually not as severely as in acute hepatitis. Elevations in these enzymes may not correlate well with the extent of liver damage in cirrhosis.
- *FBC with platelets* is done. A low RBC count, haemoglobin and haematocrit demonstrate anaemia related to bone marrow suppression, increased RBC destruction, bleeding and deficiencies of folic acid and vitamin B_{12}. Platelets are low, related to increased destruction by the spleen. Leucopenia (low WBC count) also relates to splenomegaly.
- *Coagulation studies* show a prolonged prothrombin time due to impaired production of coagulation proteins and lack of vitamin K.
- *Serum electrolytes* are measured. Hyponatraemia is common, due to haemodilution. Hypokalaemia, hypophosphataemia and hypomagnesaemia also are frequently seen, related to malnutrition and altered renal excretion of these electrolytes.
- *Bilirubin* levels are usually elevated in severe cirrhosis, including both direct (conjugated) and indirect (unconjugated) bilirubin.
- *Serum albumin* levels show hypoalbuminaemia due to impaired liver production.
- *Serum ammonia* levels are elevated because the liver fails to effectively convert ammonia to urea for renal excretion.
- *Serum glucose* and *cholesterol* levels frequently are abnormal in people with cirrhosis.
- *Abdominal ultrasound* is performed to evaluate liver size, detect ascites and identify liver nodules. Liver biopsy under ultrasound is useful to aid diagnosis; however, this is contraindicated in people who are still drinking alcohol. Biopsy may be deferred if the bleeding time is prolonged (such as a prothrombin time (PT) greater than 3 seconds over the control). See the 'Diagnostic tests' box in the chapter 'A person-centred approach to assessing the gastrointestinal system' for nursing implications for a person having a liver biopsy. Figure 20.8 shows the site and position for liver biopsy.
- Endoscopy may be done to determine the presence of oesophageal varices.

More information about the above diagnostic tests and their nursing implications can be found in the chapter 'A person-centred approach to assessing the gastrointestinal system'.

Medications

Medications are used to treat the complications and effects of cirrhosis; they do not reverse or slow the process of cirrhosis itself. Known hepatotoxic drugs and alcohol are avoided, as are drugs metabolised by the liver (e.g. barbiturates, sedatives, hypnotics and paracetamol). Several groups of drugs are commonly prescribed. See the 'Medication administration' box for nursing responsibilities and teaching for commonly used drugs for people with cirrhosis.

- Diuretics reduce fluid retention and ascites. Spironolactone is frequently the drug of first choice because it addresses one of the causes of ascites —increased aldosterone levels. If additional diuresis is necessary, a loop diuretic such as frusemide may be added to the regimen.
- Medications to reduce the nitrogenous load and lower serum ammonia levels are added when manifestations of hepatic encephalopathy develop. Two commonly administered medications are lactulose and neomycin. Both exert their effects locally, in the bowel. Lactulose reduces the number of ammonia-forming organisms in the bowel and increases the acidity of colon contents, converting ammonia into ammonium ion. Ammonium ion is not absorbable and is excreted in the faeces. Neomycin sulfate is a locally acting antibiotic that also reduces the number of ammonia-forming bacteria in the bowel.
- Ferrous sulfate and folic acid are given as indicated to treat anaemia. Vitamin K may be ordered to reduce the risk of bleeding. When bleeding is acute, packed RBCs, fresh frozen plasma or platelets may be administered to restore blood components and promote haemostasis.

MEDICATION ADMINISTRATION The person with cirrhosis

DIURETICS

Spironolactone

Frusemide

Spironolactone is a potassium-sparing diuretic that competes with aldosterone. It reduces ascites by increasing renal excretion of fluid and decreasing aldosterone levels. Frusemide is a loop diuretic that promotes the excretion of potassium. Drugs may be given in combination if serum potassium level permits.

Nursing responsibilities

- Monitor ECG, serum potassium, BUN, creatinine levels and hydration status.
- Weigh daily.
- Carefully monitor intake and output.
- Monitor for signs of hyperkalaemia if taking spironolactone alone: bradycardia; widening QRS, spiking T waves or ST segment depression on ECG; diarrhoea; and muscle twitching.
- Assess for hyponatraemia: confusion, lethargy, apprehension.

Health education for the person and family

- Maintain diet and fluid restrictions as prescribed.
- Report increases in weight or oedema.
- Immediately report signs of hyponatraemia, hyperkalaemia or hypokalaemia (see the chapter 'Nursing care of people with altered fluid, electrolyte and acid–base balance').
- Expect increased urinary output; take medications in morning hours to avoid nocturia.

LAXATIVES

Lactulose

Lactulose is a disaccharide laxative that is not absorbed by the gastrointestinal tract. It reduces the number of ammonia-producing bacteria and lowers the pH in the colon. The lower pH (increased acidity) converts ammonia to ammonium ion, a non-absorbable form that is excreted in the faeces. Lactulose also pulls water into the bowel lumen, increasing the number of daily stools.

Nursing responsibilities

- Assess bowel sounds and abdominal girth.
- Maintain accurate stool chart.
- Adjust dose to achieve two to four soft stools per day.
- Monitor electrolytes and hydration.

Health education for the person and family

- Drink adequate fluids.
- Report diarrhoea; if present, decrease dose. You should have an average of two to four stools per day.
- Lactulose may cause nausea. Continue taking lactulose; taking it with water crackers or a soft drink may reduce nausea.

ANTI-INFECTIVE AGENTS

Neomycin sulfate

Neomycin sulfate is a non-systemic aminoglycoside antibiotic that reduces intestinal bacteria and decreases ammonia production in the bowel lumen. The drug may be administered as an oral or rectal preparation.

Nursing responsibilities

- Monitor hearing, renal and neurological functions. Neomycin is ototoxic, nephrotoxic and neurotoxic.
- Prior to administration, check for previous hypersensitivity reaction.
- Monitor intake and output.
- Monitor BUN and creatinine levels.
- If the person is taking digitalis, monitor levels; oral neomycin interferes with its absorption.

Health education for the person and family

- Report dizziness, tinnitus (ringing in ears), hearing loss, headaches, tremors or vision changes immediately.
- Keep follow-up appointments.
- Maintain fluids, avoid dehydration. (Teach signs of dehydration.)

- Antacids are prescribed as indicated. A drug regimen to treat *H. pylori* infection may also be effective (see the chapter 'Nursing care of people with upper gastrointestinal disorders').
- Oxazepam a benzodiazepine anti-anxiety/sedative drug, is not metabolised by the liver and may be used to treat acute agitation.

Treatments

Treatment of cirrhosis is supportive, directed at slowing the progression to liver failure and reducing complications.

NUTRITION Dietary support is an essential part of care for the person with cirrhosis. Dietary needs change as hepatic function fluctuates.

- Sodium intake is restricted to under 2 g/day and fluids are restricted as necessary to reduce ascites and generalised oedema. Fluids are often limited to 1,500 mL/day. Fluid needs are calculated based on response to diuretic therapy, urine output and serum electrolyte values.
- Unless serum ammonia levels are high, a palatable diet with adequate kilojoules and protein is recommended. Previously protein was discouraged in people with encephalopathy; however, the negative impact of that restriction on overall nutrition is thought to outweigh the benefit (Merli, 2020). The diet is high in kilojoules and includes moderate fat intake to promote healing. Parenteral nutrition is used as needed to maintain nutritional status when food intake is limited.
- Vitamin and mineral supplements are ordered based on laboratory values. Deficiencies in the B-complex vitamins, particularly thiamine, folate and B_{12}, and the fat-soluble vitamins A, D and E are common. These vitamins may need to be administered in a water-soluble form. People with alcohol-induced cirrhosis are at high risk of magnesium deficiency, which needs to be replaced.

COMPLICATION MANAGEMENT **Paracentesis**, aspiration of fluid from the peritoneal cavity, may be a diagnostic or a therapeutic procedure. It may be done therapeutically to relieve severe ascites that does not respond to diuretic therapy. The goal of paracentesis is to relieve respiratory distress caused by excess fluid in the abdomen. Ascites fluid may be withdrawn in moderate amounts of 500 mL to 1 L daily to reduce the risk of fluid and electrolyte imbalances. Large-volume paracentesis, withdrawal of 4 to 6 L of fluid at one time, may be used. Albumin is often administered intravenously during large-volume paracentesis to maintain intravascular volume as the pressure of the ascites fluid in the abdomen is relieved. Nursing implications for the person undergoing paracentesis are listed in Box 24.5. Figure 24.4 shows insertion sites and positioning during paracentesis.

Bleeding oesophageal varices are life threatening and require critical care management. Restoration of haemodynamic stability is the first priority. A central line is inserted and central venous and pulmonary artery pressures are monitored (see the chapter 'Nursing care of people with cardiac disorders'). Blood is given to restore blood volume, and fresh frozen plasma may be administered to restore clotting factors. Octreotide, a drug that constricts blood vessels in the gut, is given intravenously to reduce blood flow in the portal venous system. Vasopressin, a drug that produces generalised vasoconstriction, may also be used.

When the blood pressure and cardiac output have stabilised, upper endoscopy is performed to evaluate and treat the varices. During endoscopy, the varices may be banded or sclerosed to reduce the risk of recurrent bleeding. In *banding* (*variceal ligation*), small rubber bands are placed on varices to occlude blood flow. *Endoscopic sclerosis* involves injecting a sclerosing agent directly into the varices to induce inflammation and clotting. See the chapter 'A person-centred approach to assessing the gastrointestinal system' for the nursing implications of endoscopic investigation.

Balloon tamponade of bleeding varices may be used if bleeding cannot be controlled through vasoconstriction or if endoscopy is unavailable. A multiple-lumen nasogastric (NG) tube (such as a Sengstaken–Blakemore tube or a Minnesota tube) is inserted and the gastric and oesophageal balloons are inflated to apply direct pressure on the bleeding varices (see Figure 24.5). Tension is applied to the tube to further compress the varices. Balloon tamponade carries a number of risks, including aspiration, airway obstruction and tissue ischaemia and necrosis. An endotracheal tube is inserted prior to nasogastric intubation to support the airway and reduce the risk of aspiration. This short-term measure is used only until more definitive treatment can be done.

Transjugular intrahepatic portosystemic shunt (TIPS) is used to relieve portal hypertension and its complications of oesophageal varices and ascites. A channel is created through the liver tissue using a needle inserted transcutaneously (see Figure 24.6). An expandable metal stent is inserted into this channel to allow blood to flow directly from the portal vein

BOX 24.5 Nursing implications for abdominal paracentesis

Preparation of the person

- Verify presence of an informed consent.
- Weigh prior to paracentesis.
- Assess vital signs for baseline.
- Have person void immediately prior to the test to avoid bladder puncture.
- Position seated, either on the side of the bed or in a chair, with feet supported.

Health education for the person and family

- Describe what to expect during and following paracentesis. Blood pressure is monitored during the procedure.
- The doctor will clean abdomen with Betadine and insert local anaesthesia. A small incision may be made and a needle or catheter is inserted to withdraw fluid. The needle is connected to tubing and a collection bottle; specimens may be sent to laboratory.
- A small dressing is placed over the puncture site after the needle is withdrawn. There may be some fluid leakage from the site.
- Salt-poor albumin may be given after the procedure to replace lost protein.

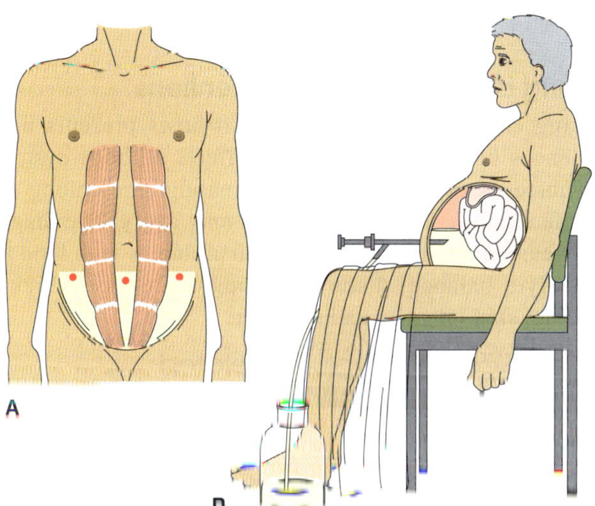

FIGURE 24.4 *Sites and position for paracentesis. A, Potential sites of needle or trocar insertion to avoid abdominal organ damage. B, The person sits comfortably; in this position, the intestines float back and away from the insertion site*

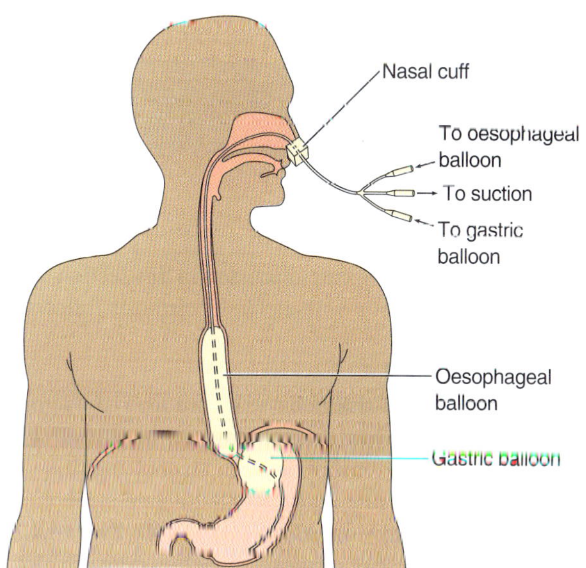

FIGURE 24.5 *Triple-lumen nasogastric tube (Sengstaken–Blakemore) used to control bleeding oesophageal varices*

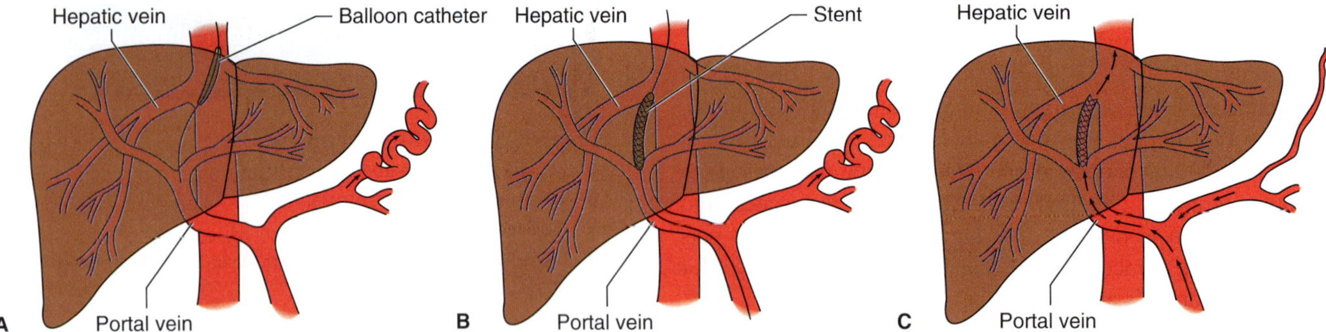

FIGURE 24.6 *Transjugular intrahepatic portosystemic shunt (TIPS). A, Guided by angiography, a balloon catheter inserted via the jugular vein is advanced to the hepatic veins and through the substance of the liver to create a portacaval (portal vein to vena cava) channel. B, A metal stent is positioned into the channel and expanded by inflating the balloon. C, The stent remains in place after the catheter is removed, creating a shunt for blood to flow directly from the portal vein into the hepatic vein*

into the hepatic vein, bypassing the cirrhotic liver. The shunt relieves pressure in oesophageal varices and allows better control of fluid retention with diuretic therapy. Stenosis and occlusion of the shunt are frequent complications. TIPS also increases the risk of developing hepatic encephalopathy (due to decreased perfusion of the liver and impaired ammonia metabolism) and may reduce long-term survival. It generally is used as a short-term measure until a liver transplant is performed.

SURGERY **Liver transplantation** is indicated for some people with irreversible, progressive cirrhosis. A decline in functional status, increasing bilirubin levels, falling albumin levels and increasing problems with complications that respond poorly to treatment are indications for liver transplantation. Malignancy, active alcohol or drug abuse, and poor surgical risk are contraindications for the surgery. See the accompanying box for nursing care of the person undergoing a liver transplant.

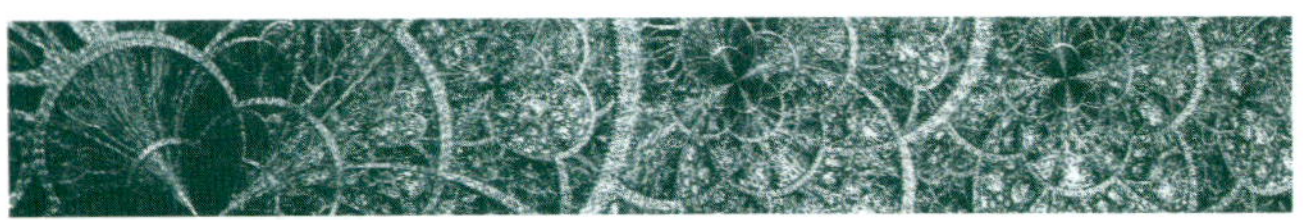

Nursing care

In addition to the nursing care discussed in this section, a nursing care plan for a person with alcoholic cirrhosis follows.

Health promotion

For most people, high-risk behaviours are the risk factors for cirrhosis. With all people (including children and young adults), stress the relationship between alcohol and drug abuse and liver disorders. While many people tolerate alcohol use in moderation with no adverse effects on the liver, excess alcohol use is the leading cause of cirrhosis. Injection drug use also is a significant risk factor, increasing the risk of contracting blood-borne hepatitis (B, C or D). These types of viral hepatitis can lead to chronic hepatitis and, ultimately, to cirrhosis. Discuss abstinence or safer sex practices as another measure to prevent viral hepatitis and potential liver damage.

Assessment

Assessment data related to cirrhosis include the following:

- *Health history*: current manifestations, including abdominal pain or discomfort, recent weight loss, weakness and anorexia; altered bowel elimination; excess bleeding or bruising; abdominal distension; jaundice, pruritus; altered libido or impotence; duration of symptoms; history of liver or gallbladder disease; pattern and extent of alcohol or injection drug use; use of other prescription and non-prescription drugs.
- *Physical assessment*: vital signs; mental status; colour and condition of skin and mucous membranes; peripheral pulses and presence of peripheral oedema; abdominal assessment including appearance, shape and contour, bowel sounds, abdominal girth, percussion for liver borders and palpation for tenderness and liver size.

Nursing diagnoses and interventions

Nursing care of the person with cirrhosis presents many challenges because liver function affects all body systems. The nurse is responsible for coordinating care among care providers. Many nursing diagnoses may apply. The diagnoses discussed in this section focus on problems with fluid and electrolyte balance, disturbed thought processes, risk of bleeding, skin integrity and nutrition.

Risk of excess fluid volume related to portal hypertension

Cirrhosis affects water and salt regulation due to portal hypertension, hypoalbuminaemia and hyperaldosteronism. Signs of fluid volume overload and portal hypertension may develop: ascites, peripheral oedema, internal haemorrhoids and varices, and prominent abdominal wall veins. Careful monitoring is necessary, because treatment measures can lead to further fluid and electrolyte imbalances.

- Weigh daily. Assess for jugular vein distension, measure abdominal girth daily and check for peripheral oedema. Monitor intake and output. *Careful assessment is important to detect fluid shifts.*
- Assess urine specific gravity. *Specific gravity measures the concentration of urine, an indicator of hydration.*
- Provide a low-sodium diet (500 to 2,000 mg/day) and restrict fluids as ordered. *Excess sodium leads to water retention and can increase fluid volume, ascites and portal hypertension.*

CONSIDERATION FOR PRACTICE

Monitor the person with cirrhosis for signs of impaired renal function, such as oliguria, a fixed urine specific gravity of about 1.012, central oedema (around the eyes and of the face) and increasing serum creatinine and BUN levels. Such signs may indicate hepatorenal syndrome or acute renal failure from another cause.

Risk of disturbed thought processes due to hepatic encephalopathy

Accumulated nitrogenous waste products and other metabolites affect mental status and thought processes. Effects of

NURSING CARE OF THE PERSON undergoing liver transplantation

PREOPERATIVE CARE

- Obtain a complete nursing history and physical examination. *A complete preoperative nursing assessment provides baseline data for comparison after surgery.*
- Provide routine preoperative care as ordered (see the chapter 'Nursing care of people having surgery'). *Preoperative care is similar to that provided for other people undergoing major surgery.*
- Discuss preoperative and postoperative expectations with the person and family. Introduce to the intensive care unit and discuss anticipated drainage tubes and supportive measures in the immediate postoperative period. Provide information about visiting policies and family accommodation (if available). *Preoperative teaching helps relieve anxiety in the person and family members. After a transplant people return from surgery to an intensive care or specialised care unit. Restrictions on the number of visitors and the time they may spend with the person are common.*
- Once a donor liver is located, check for evidence of infection; if no infection is present, begin preoperative antibiotics as ordered. *An acute or chronic infection may contraindicate liver transplantation as drugs given postoperatively to suppress rejection of the transplanted organ also impair the ability to fight infection.*

POSTOPERATIVE CARE

- Maintain airway and ventilatory support until awake and alert. *Until the new liver clears the anaesthesia, the person requires measures to support respirations and ventilation.*
- Monitor temperature and implement rewarming measures (such as warming blankets, heating lamps and head covers) as indicated. *The person often is hypothermic after liver transplant, necessitating careful rewarming while maintaining haemodynamic stability.*
- Frequently monitor haemodynamic pressures, including arterial blood pressure, central venous pressure and pulmonary artery pressures. *Postoperative fluid volume status may be difficult to determine without careful pressure measurements. The rate and type of fluids administered are determined by haemodynamic status.*
- Monitor urine output hourly; maintain careful intake and output records. Weigh daily. *Urine output and weight provide additional information about fluid volume status. In addition, renal function may be altered after liver transplant; acute renal failure is a significant risk. See the chapter 'Nursing care of people with kidney disorders' for more information about acute renal failure.*
- Monitor for signs of active bleeding, including excess drainage, increasing abdominal girth, bloody nasogastric drainage, black tarry stools, tachypnoea, tachycardia, diminished peripheral pulses or pallor. Report immediately. *Altered coagulation in the early postoperative period increases the risk of bleeding. Blood products to replace volume and clotting factors may be necessary.*
- Monitor serum electrolytes and laboratory values related to blood coagulation, liver function and renal function. Report abnormal results or significant changes immediately. *Electrolyte imbalances are common postoperatively. Altered liver or renal function tests may indicate rejection of the transplanted liver or acute renal failure. Other early signs of transplant rejection include fever, a drop in bile output or a change in bile colour and viscosity (Urden, Stacy & Lough, 2021).*
- Monitor neurological status. *With good function of the transplanted organ, mental status should clear within days of the transplant.*

HEALTH EDUCATION FOR THE PERSON AND FAMILY

- Teach how to reduce risk of infection and signs of infection to report.
- Instruct to recognise and report signs of organ rejection.
- Discuss all medications, including their purpose, schedule, adverse effects and potential long-term effects. Stress the importance of complying with all prescribed medications and postoperative precautions for the remainder of the person's life.
- Discuss possible changes in body image and psychological responses to receiving a transplanted organ. Refer to a social worker or support group as indicated.
- Refer for home health services for continued assessment and teaching.
- Stress importance of continued follow-up with transplant team and general practitioner.

NURSING CARE PLAN A person with alcoholic cirrhosis

Richard Wright is a 48-year-old divorced father of two teenagers. Mr Wright has been admitted to hospital with ascites and malnutrition. He has had three previous hospital stays for cirrhosis, the most recent 6 months ago.

ASSESSMENT

Mr Wright is lethargic but responds appropriately to verbal stimuli. He complains of 'spitting up blood the past week or so' and says, 'I'm just not hungry'. He has lost 9 kg since his previous admission. He is jaundiced and has petechiae and bruising on his arms and legs. Liz Mowdi, Mr Wright's nurse, notes pitting pre-tibial oedema. Abdominal assessment reveals a tight, protuberant abdomen with caput medusae. The liver margin is not palpable; the spleen is enlarged. Vital signs are T 37.7°C, P 110, R 24 and BP 110/70.

Abnormal laboratory results include WBC 3,700/L (normal 3.4–9.6 billion cells/L); RBC 4.0/L (male normal 4.35 to 5.65/L); platelets 75,000/mm^3 (male normal 135–317/L); serum ammonia (normal < 50micromol/L); total bilirubin 40 micromol/L (normal 3–20 micromol/L); and serum sodium 150 mEq/L (normal 135 to 145 mEq/L). Potassium, haemoglobin, haematocrit, total protein and albumin levels are markedly decreased. Liver enzymes are elevated. Blood urea nitrogen and creatinine levels are marginally elevated. Oxygen saturation (O_2 sat) is 88% (RA) (normal range: 96% to 100%) per pulse oximetry.

Endoscopy shows bleeding from gastric ulcer and the diagnosis of alcoholic cirrhosis with gastritis is made. Mr Wright is started on spironolactone, 25 mg PO q8h; lactulose, 30 mL prn until onset of diarrhoea, then 15 mL tds; and low-sodium diet; fluid restriction of 1,500 mL/day.

DIAGNOSES

- *Risk of impaired gas exchange* related to pressure of ascites fluid on the diaphragm as manifested by tachypnoea and decreased oxygen saturation.
- *Risk of excess fluid volume* related to electrolyte imbalance and hypoalbuminaemia as manifested by ascites and peripheral oedema.
- *Risk of imbalanced nutrition: less than body requirements* related to anorexia and possible alcohol abuse as manifested by weight loss and low serum protein levels.
- *Risk of disturbed thought processes* related to effects of high ammonia levels as manifested by lethargy.
- *Risk of ineffective protection* related to impaired platelet formation and malnutrition.

PLANNING

- Teach the importance of activity, turning, coughing and deep breathing prior to the procedure.
- Encourage Mr Wright's family to visit at mealtimes to encourage oral intake.
- Ensure buzzer is kept by bedside at all times and encourage Mr Wright to alert nursing staff immediately if he experiences any signs of bleeding such as haematemesis or dizziness.
- Arrange for social work review for referral to community support services.

Expected outcomes

- Respiratory rate and SpO_2 will be within normal limits.
- Abdominal girth will decrease by 1 to 2 cm per day; peripheral oedema will decrease.
- Will gain 0.5 kg per week without evidence of increased fluid retention. Serum albumin levels will return to normal range.
- Will be alert and oriented; serum ammonia levels are within normal range.
- Will demonstrate no further evidence of active bleeding.
- Will verbalise willingness to join a community support group.

IMPLEMENTATION

- Weigh daily.
- Provide high-kilojoule, low-salt, low-protein diet with between-meal snacks.
- Maintain stool chart.
- Assign same nurses to care as much as possible to facilitate evaluation of mental status. Promptly report changes in status or laboratory values.
- Measure abdominal girth every 8 hours, marking level of measurement.
- Institute bleeding precautions.
- Elevate head of bed; assist to chair with legs elevated as tolerated. When resting in bed encourage to turn, cough and deep breathe every 2 to 4 hours.
- Include significant others in care and teaching.

EVALUATION

A week after admission, Mr Wright's ascites has decreased and no further active bleeding is noted. His serum protein levels have increased and his laboratory values are improving. No further bruising is noted during hospitalisation. Although he shows a 2 kg weight loss as excess water is eliminated, he is consuming 100% of his diet. His serum ammonia levels have returned to normal. On discharge, SpO_2 is 96%; respirations are 18. Lactulose will be continued on discharge.

Ms Mowdi provides both written and verbal information about the medication and cirrhosis, including measures to prevent complications. Mr Wright and his children express interest in Alcoholics Anonymous and are referred to this agency. Prior to discharge, follow-up appointments are made with a mental health team, social worker and a general practitioner.

CRITICAL THINKING IN THE NURSING PROCESS

1. Describe the relationship between portal hypertension, liver dysfunction and ascites.
2. What is the pathophysiological basis for hepatic encephalopathy? What are the nursing responsibilities related to lactulose and neomycin?
3. Design a nursing care plan for Mr Wright for the diagnosis *Ineffective coping*.

REFLECTION ON THE NURSING PROCESS

1. Outline what you have learned from this case study that you will apply to your future practice.
2. Mr Wright confides to you that he is worried about whether he will be able to completely abstain from alcohol. Reflect on how you would respond.

hepatic encephalopathy can range from mild confusion to agitation to coma.

- Assess neurological status, including level of consciousness and mental status. Observe for signs of early encephalopathy: changes in handwriting, speech and asterixis. *Early identification of evidence of encephalopathy allows prompt intervention—subtle changes in neurological functioning are important!*
- Avoid factors that may precipitate hepatic encephalopathy. Avoid hepatotoxic medications and CNS-depressant drugs. *Cautious use of medications and close monitoring can eliminate iatrogenic causes of encephalopathy.*
- If possible, plan for consistent nursing care assignments. *Consistent care providers facilitate early identification of subtle neurological changes indicative of hepatic encephalopathy.*
- Administer medications or enemas as ordered to reduce nitrogenous products. Monitor bowel function and provide measures to promote regular elimination and prevent constipation. *Oral or rectally administered medications are ordered to reduce intestinal bacteria and the ammonia they produce. Regular bowel elimination promotes protein and ammonia elimination in the faeces.*
- Orientate to surroundings, person and place; provide simple explanations and reassurance. *Modification of verbal interactions to level of understanding and mental status may reduce anxiety and agitation.*

CONSIDERATION FOR PRACTICE

Closely monitor people who have experienced gastrointestinal bleeding for signs of hepatic encephalopathy. Blood in the intestinal tract is digested as a protein, increasing serum ammonia levels and the risk of hepatic encephalopathy.

Ineffective protection

Impaired coagulation, oesophageal varices and possible acute gastritis place the person with cirrhosis at significant risk of haemorrhage. Clotting is altered by vitamin K deficiency; impaired manufacture of coagulation factors II, VII, IX and X; and increased platelet destruction due to splenomegaly.

- Monitor vital signs; report tachycardia or hypotension. *Increased pulse and decreasing blood pressure may indicate hypovolaemia due to haemorrhage.*
- Institute bleeding precautions (see Box 24.6). *Preventive measures can decrease the risk of active bleeding.*
- Monitor coagulation studies and platelet count. *Report abnormal results. Coagulation studies help determine the risk of bleeding and the need for treatment.*
- Carefully monitor the person who has had bleeding oesophageal varices for evidence of rebleeding: haematemesis, haematochezia (bright blood in the stool) or tarry stools, signs of hypovolaemia or shock. *Rebleeding is common following variceal haemorrhage, especially within the first week.*

BOX 24.6 Bleeding precautions

- **Prevent constipation.**
- **Avoid rectal temperatures or enemas.**
- **Avoid injections; if needed, use small-gauge needle and apply gentle pressure.**
- **Monitor platelet count, PT and APTT.**
- **Assess for bruised areas and areas of purpura.**
- **Apply pressure to bleeding sites. After venepuncture, apply direct pressure for at least 5 minutes.**
- **Use only a soft toothbrush.**
- **Avoid blowing nose.**
- **Assess oral cavity for bleeding gums.**

Impaired skin integrity

Severe jaundice with bile salt deposits on the skin may cause pruritus. Scratching related to the pruritus damages the skin and impairs its integrity. Malnutrition, particularly protein deficiency, and oedema also increase the risk of tissue breakdown and impaired skin integrity.

- Use warm water rather than hot water when bathing. *Hot water increases pruritus.*
- Use measures to prevent dry skin: apply an emollient or lubricant as needed to keep skin moist, avoid soap or preparations with alcohol, and do not rub the skin. *Dry skin contributes to pruritus.*
- If indicated, apply gloves to prevent scratching. *People with encephalopathy may not understand the need to refrain from scratching.*
- Institute measures to prevent skin and tissue breakdown: turn at least every 2 hours, use an alternating-pressure mattress and frequently assess skin condition. *Frequent position changes relieve pressure and promote circulation and tissue oxygenation.*
- Administer prescribed antihistamine (to relieve pruritus) cautiously. *Decreased liver function increases the risk of altered drug responses.*

Imbalanced nutrition: less than body requirements

The person with cirrhosis is at risk of malnutrition for a number of reasons: possible chronic alcohol use, anorexia, impaired vitamin and mineral absorption, and impaired protein metabolism. In addition, salt restrictions may make the diet less palatable and appealing to the person.

- Weigh daily. Instruct to weigh at least weekly at home. Weight is a good indicator of both nutritional status and fluid balance. *Short-term weight fluctuations tend to reflect fluid balance, while longer-term changes in weight are more reflective of nutritional status.*

- Provide small meals with between-meal snacks. *A small meal is more appealing for an anorexic person. Between-meal snacks help to maintain adequate kilojoule and nutrient intake.*
- Unless protein is restricted due to impending hepatic encephalopathy, promote protein and nutrient intake by providing nutritional supplements such as Ensure or instant breakfasts. *The sodium and protein content of all meals and snacks must be calculated when maintaining restrictions of these nutrients.*
- Arrange for consultation with a dietitian for diet planning while hospitalised and at home. *The dietitian can provide detailed instructions, sample menus and suggestions for improving the palatability of the diet and promoting intake.*

Community-based care

Cirrhosis is a chronic, progressive disease. As such, the person and family assume major roles in managing the disease and its manifestations, and in preventing complications. Teaching topics for home care include:

- The absolute necessity of avoiding alcohol and other hepatotoxic drugs. Suggest inpatient or community-based alcohol treatment programs and Alcoholics Anonymous as indicated.
- Diet and fluid intake restrictions and recommendations. Include suggestions to promote nutritional intake and increase the flavour of food when sodium is restricted.
- Prescribed medications—their timing, intended and adverse effects and manifestations to report to the primary care provider.
- Bleeding precautions (see Box 24.6).
- Manifestations of potential complications to be reported to the primary care provider. Stress the importance of promptly reporting evidence of gastrointestinal bleeding for prompt intervention for potential haemorrhage.
- Skin care techniques to reduce pruritus and the risk of damage.
- Ways to manage fatigue and conserve energy.

Provide referrals for home health services, dietary consultation, social services and counselling as needed by the person and family. Suggest local support groups where available. If appropriate, suggest hospice services for the person with end-stage liver disease.

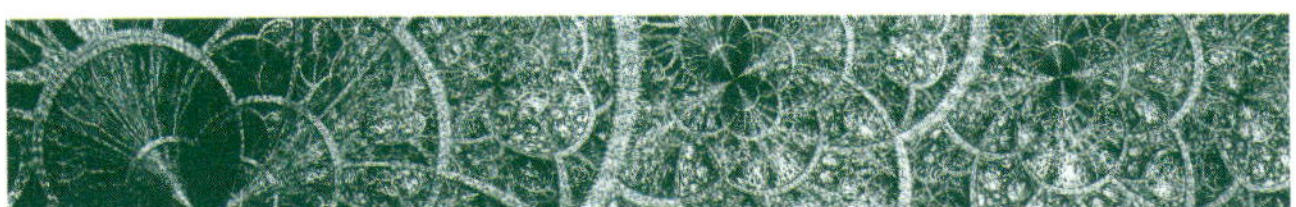

THE PERSON WITH CANCER OF THE LIVER

In 2022, 2,905 new cases of hepatocellular or liver cancer were diagnosed, with over 2,000 cases being male. This is estimated at almost 2% of the total new cases of cancer diagnosed in 2022. There is an estimated 22% survival rate after 5 years, which has improved almost four times the survival rates in the 1990s. Liver cancer accounts for approximately 5% of all cancer deaths, making it the seventh-highest cause of cancer-related deaths in Australia (ABS, 2020). Metastasis to the liver from primary tumours of the lung, breast and gastrointestinal tract is relatively common.

Pathophysiology

About 80–90% of primary hepatic cancers arise from the liver's parenchymal cells (hepatocellular carcinoma); the remainder form in the bile ducts (cholangiocarcinoma). Regardless of the origin, the progress of the disease is similar. Several aetiological factors have been identified (see Box 24.7). Most primary liver cancer in Australia is related to alcoholic cirrhosis, HBV or HCV.

The underlying pathophysiology of primary liver cancer is damage to hepatocellular DNA. This damage may be caused by integration of HBV or HCV into the DNA or by repeated cycles of cell necrosis and regeneration that facilitate DNA mutations. HBV and aflatoxins damage a specific tumour suppressor gene, p53. Tumours may be limited to one specific area, may occur as nodules throughout the liver or may develop as surface infiltrates. The tumour interferes with normal hepatic function, leading to biliary obstruction and jaundice, portal hypertension and metabolic disruptions (hypoalbuminaemia, hypoglycaemia and bleeding disorders). It also may secrete bile products and produce hormones (paraneoplastic syndrome) that may lead to polycythaemia, hypoglycaemia and hypercalcaemia. Tumours usually grow rapidly and metastasise early.

Manifestations

Initial manifestations of liver cancer develop insidiously and often are masked by the presence of cirrhosis or chronic hepatitis. See the 'Manifestations' box for manifestations of primary liver cancer. Ascites and jaundice may be present at diagnosis. Signs of liver failure with portal hypertension, splenomegaly and altered metabolism develop as the tumour progresses.

BOX 24.7 Suspected causes of primary liver cancer

- Chronic hepatitis C infection
- Chronic hepatitis B infection
- Cirrhosis, regardless of type
- Chronic aflatoxin (a toxin produced by *Aspergillus* moulds) exposure
- Arsenic-contaminated water
- Carcinogens in food
- Possible hormonal factors (e.g. long-term use of androgens)

MANIFESTATIONS Primary liver cancer

- Malaise
- Anorexia
- Lethargy
- Weight loss
- Fever of unknown origin
- Jaundice
- Feeling of abdominal fullness
- Painful right upper quadrant mass
- Manifestations of liver failure

INTERPROFESSIONAL CARE

Liver tumours are identified by CT scans and MRI. A liver biopsy may be done to confirm the diagnosis and identify the tumour type or origin. See the 'Diagnostic tests' box in the chapter 'A person-centred approach to assessing the gastrointestinal system' for the nursing implications of liver biopsy. Serum alpha-fetoprotein (AFP) levels, normally low in non-pregnant adults, rise in most people with hepatocellular cancer.

Small, localised tumours may be surgically resected, offering the only viable chance for cure. Most tumours, however, have spread extensively or have distant metastasis at the time of diagnosis, so this is frequently not an option. Liver transplantation may be done; however, the tumour may recur in the transplanted organ.

Radiation therapy is used to shrink the tumour, decreasing pressure on surrounding organs and reducing pain. Chemotherapy may be used as primary treatment or adjunctive therapy. Direct continuous hepatic arterial infusion with an implanted pump has shown promise in prolonging survival rates. See the chapter 'Nursing care of people with cancer' for nursing care for people receiving radiation therapy or chemotherapy.

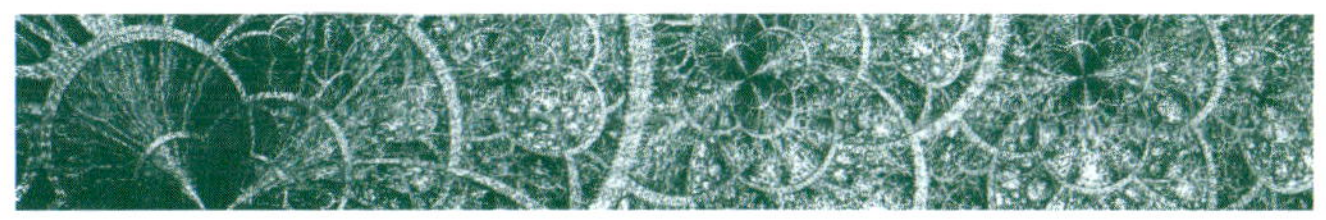

Nursing care

Encourage people with risk factors for primary liver cancer to avoid alcohol and other substances that may further damage the liver. Urge them to discuss regular screening for liver tumours (such as serum AFP levels) with their general practitioner.

Both the person and the family need extensive nursing support. Controlling pain is a priority. Because of the poor prognosis, early referral for hospice services may be appropriate.

Nursing diagnoses, interventions and teaching for the person with liver cancer are similar to those for people with cirrhosis; see above.

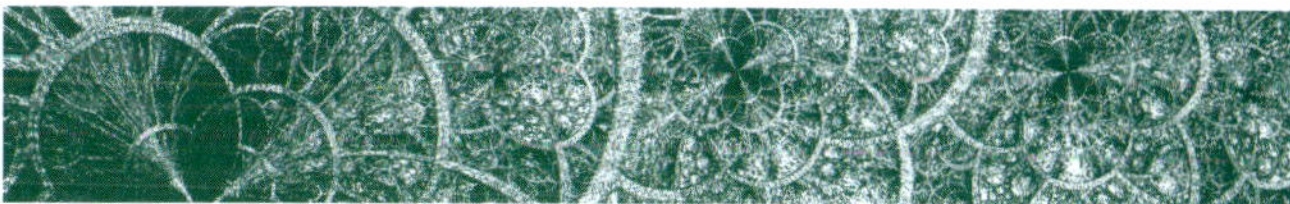

THE PERSON WITH LIVER TRAUMA

Blunt or penetrating trauma to the abdomen can damage the liver. Liver trauma is frequently seen in combination with injuries to other abdominal organs. Motor vehicle crashes, stab or gunshot wounds, and iatrogenic sources such as liver biopsy are among the causes of these injuries.

Pathophysiology and manifestations

Liver trauma generally causes bleeding due to the vascularity of the organ. Liver injury may cause a surface haematoma, a haematoma within the liver parenchyma, laceration of liver tissue or disruption of vessels leading to or from the liver. Severe bleeding can rapidly disrupt haemodynamic stability and lead to shock.

CONSIDERATION FOR PRACTICE

Bleeding due to liver trauma may not be immediately apparent. Instruct the person with apparent or potential liver trauma to immediately report light-headedness, rapid heart rate, shortness of breath, thirst or increasing abdominal pain.

INTERPROFESSIONAL CARE

Diagnostic peritoneal lavage (DPL) may be used along with CT scan to diagnose liver trauma. The procedure is performed by making a small abdominal incision into the peritoneum (after the bladder has been emptied) and inserting a small catheter into the peritoneal cavity. If blood is immediately detected, the person is taken directly to surgery for abdominal exploration or transferred to a trauma facility where this surgery can occur. If frank bleeding is not apparent, a litre of isotonic fluid is instilled into the abdomen, then drained and sent for laboratory analysis.

A *FAST (focused abdominal sonography in trauma)* scan is more frequently used to identify free intraperitoneal fluid associated with liver injuries from blunt trauma. Unlike DPL, FAST scans are non-invasive, quick, and pose no risk to the person. DPL carries a 1–9.5% risk to the person, including perforation of a viscus, vascular laceration and wound complications (Lee et al., 2019). Intravenous fluids, fresh frozen plasma, platelets and other clotting factors are administered to restore blood volume and promote haemostasis. Haemodynamic status is closely monitored; continued instability may indicate a need for surgical intervention to control haemorrhage. Postoperative nursing care focuses on preventing pulmonary complications, such as atelectasis, and detecting and preventing infection.

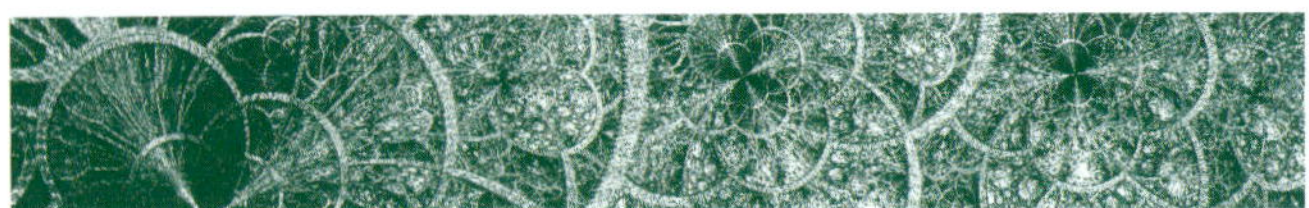

Nursing care

Nursing care of the person with liver trauma focuses on fluid management and other supportive care related to shock. Keeping family members informed is an important aspect of care, especially during the period of haemodynamic instability. Diagnoses include the following:

- *Deficient fluid volume* related to haemorrhage.
- *Risk of infection* related to wound or abdominal contamination.
- *Ineffective protection* related to impaired coagulation.

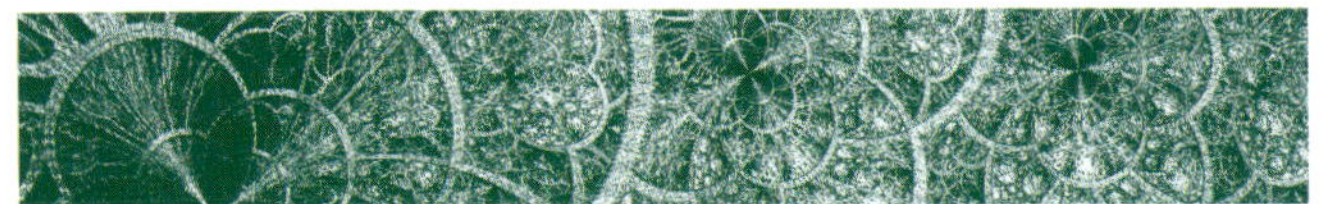

THE PERSON WITH LIVER ABSCESS

Liver abscesses usually are bacterial or amoebic (protozoal) in origin. Bacterial abscesses may follow trauma or surgical procedures, including biopsy. Multiple or single abscesses occur most commonly in the right lobe. Amoebic abscesses most frequently occur following infestation of the liver by *Entamoeba histolytica*. Amoebic infestation is associated with poor hygiene, unsafe sexual practices or travel in areas where drinking water is contaminated.

Pathophysiology and manifestations

Following bacterial or amoebic invasion of the liver, healthy tissue is destroyed, leaving an area of necrosis, inflammatory exudate and blood. This damaged region becomes walled off from the healthy liver tissue. Pyogenic (bacterial) liver abscess may be caused by cholangitis or distant or intra-abdominal infections, such as peritonitis or diverticulitis. *Escherichia coli* is the most frequently identified causative organism. The onset of pyogenic abscess is usually sudden, causing acute symptoms such as fever, malaise, vomiting, hyperbilirubinaemia and pain in the right upper abdomen.

The infection pathway for amoebic hepatic abscesses usually is the portal venous circulation from the right colon. Generally, the onset of amoebic abscess is insidious.

INTERPROFESSIONAL CARE

Hepatic abscess is diagnosed through biopsy, hepatic aspirate, blood and faecal cultures, and CT scan and ultrasound studies. Therapy is based on identifying the causative organism through laboratory cultures. Pyogenic abscesses are treated with antibiotics to which the causative organism is sensitive.

Pharmacological agents used for amoebic hepatic abscess are the same as those used for intestinal amoebic infestation (see the chapter 'Nursing care of people with bowel disorders'); combination therapy is commonly used. Two commonly used drugs for treating amoebic liver abscesses are metronidazole and iodoquinol. Both medications can cause gastrointestinal symptoms. Bone marrow suppression is a risk with metronidazole.

If the abscess does not respond to antibiotic therapy, percutaneous aspiration or surgical drainage may be done. In these procedures, a *percutaneous closed-catheter drain* is placed in the abscess to promote drainage of purulent material.

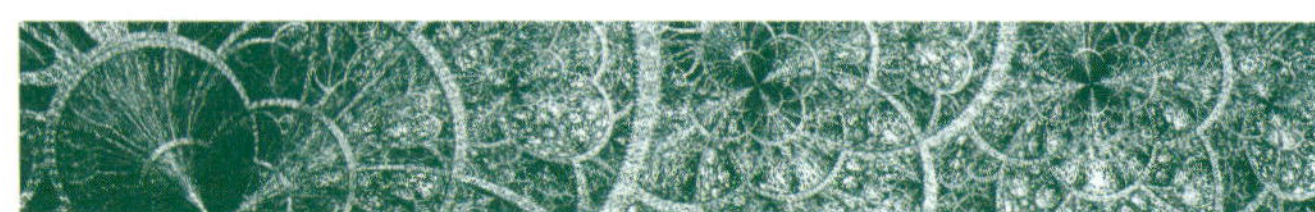

Nursing care

A major aspect of nursing care is prevention; teaching people to avoid contaminated water and foods is especially important. Nursing interventions include teaching hikers to treat water and food handlers to wash hands thoroughly.

People who have a liver abscess require supportive care to prevent dehydration from the accompanying fever, nausea, vomiting and anorexia. Careful monitoring of fluid and electrolyte status is indicated, as are comfort measures for abdominal pain. Possible nursing diagnoses include the following:

- *Risk of deficient fluid volume* related to effects of prolonged fever and vomiting.
- *Deficient knowledge* related to transmission of amoebic abscess.
- *Activity intolerance* related to pain and weakness.

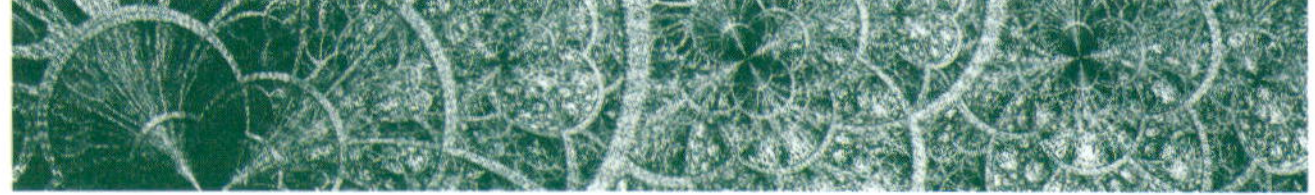

Exocrine pancreas disorders

The pancreas is both an exocrine and an endocrine gland. It is made up of two basic cell types, each having different functions. The exocrine cells produce enzymes that empty through ducts into the small intestine, whereas the endocrine cells produce hormones that enter the bloodstream directly. Disorders of the exocrine pancreas affect the secretion and glandular control of digestive enzymes, whereas disorders of the endocrine pancreas affect the production of hormones necessary for normal carbohydrate, protein and fat metabolism. Disorders of the exocrine pancreas are discussed in this section of the chapter; diabetes mellitus, a disorder of the endocrine pancreas, is discussed in the chapter 'Nursing care of people with diabetes mellitus'.

THE PERSON WITH PANCREATITIS

Pancreatitis, or inflammation of the pancreas, is characterised by release of pancreatic enzymes into the tissue of the pancreas itself, leading to haemorrhage and necrosis. Pancreatitis may be either acute or chronic.

Gallstones and chronic alcohol abuse account for 80% of acute pancreatitis causes. The incidence of acute pancreatitis varies in different countries depending on the cause. In Australia, the estimated incidence is around 70 cases per 1,00,000 people.

The incidence of chronic pancreatitis is less clear, because many people with chronic pancreatitis do not have classic manifestations of the disease. People with pancreatitis may have long-term effects of the disease, with chronic changes in enzyme and hormone production.

Physiology review

Knowledge of the normal structure and functions of the exocrine pancreas is important to understand how inflammation affects it and the person. The exocrine pancreas consists of lobules of acinar cells. The acinar cells secrete digestive enzymes and fluids (pancreatic juices) into ducts that empty into the main pancreatic duct (the duct of Wirsung). The pancreatic duct joins the common bile duct and empties into the duodenum through the ampulla of Vater. (In some people, the main pancreatic duct empties directly into the duodenum.) The epithelial lining of the pancreatic ducts secretes water and bicarbonate to modify the composition of the pancreatic secretions. Pancreatic enzymes are secreted primarily in an inactive form and are activated in the intestine, a modification that prevents digestion of pancreatic tissue by its own enzymes (Norris, 2018). The pancreatic enzymes, with related functions, are as follows:

- proteolytic enzymes, including trypsin, chymotrypsin, carboxypolypeptidase, ribonuclease and deoxyribonuclease, which break down dietary proteins
- pancreatic amylase, which breaks down starch
- lipase, which breaks down fats into glycerol and fatty acids.

Pathophysiology

Acute pancreatitis

Acute pancreatitis is an inflammatory disorder that involves self-destruction of the pancreas by its own enzymes through autodigestion. The milder form of acute pancreatitis, *interstitial oedematous pancreatitis*, leads to inflammation and oedema of pancreatic tissue. It often is self-limiting. The more severe form, *necrotising pancreatitis*, is characterised by inflammation, haemorrhage and, ultimately, necrosis of pancreatic tissue.

Acute pancreatitis incidence is higher in men than in women. Acute pancreatitis is usually associated with gallstones in women and with alcoholism in men. Some people recover completely, others experience recurring attacks and still others develop chronic pancreatitis. The mortality and symptoms depend on the severity and type of pancreatitis: with mild pancreatic oedema, mortality is low; with severe necrotic pancreatitis, the mortality rate is high (Craft et al., 2018).

Although the exact cause of pancreatitis is not known, the following factors may activate pancreatic enzymes within the pancreas, leading to autodigestion, inflammation, oedema and/or necrosis.

- Gallstones may obstruct the pancreatic duct or cause bile reflux, activating pancreatic enzymes in the pancreatic duct system.
- Alcohol causes duodenal oedema and may increase pressure and spasm in the sphincter of Oddi, obstructing pancreatic outflow. It also stimulates pancreatic enzyme production, thus raising pressure within the pancreas.

Other factors associated with acute pancreatitis include tissue ischaemia or anoxia, trauma or surgery, pancreatic tumours, third-trimester pregnancy, infectious agents (viral, bacterial or parasitic), elevated calcium levels and hyperlipidaemia. Some medications have been linked with this disorder, including thiazide diuretics, oestrogen, steroids, salicylates and NSAIDs.

Regardless of the precipitating factor, the pathophysiological process begins with the release of activated pancreatic enzymes into pancreatic tissue. Activated proteolytic enzymes—trypsin, in particular—digest pancreatic tissue and activate other enzymes such as phospholipase A, which digests cell membrane phospholipids, and elastase, which digests the elastic tissue of blood vessel walls. This leads to proteolysis, oedema, vascular damage and haemorrhage, and necrosis of parenchymal cells. Cellular damage and necrosis release activated enzymes and vasoactive substances that produce vasodilation, increase vascular permeability and cause oedema. A large volume of fluid may shift from circulating blood into the retroperitoneal space, the peripancreatic spaces and the abdominal cavity.

MANIFESTATIONS Acute pancreatitis develops suddenly, with an abrupt onset of continuous severe epigastric and abdominal pain. This pain commonly radiates to the back and is relieved somewhat by sitting up and leaning forward. The pain often is initiated by a fatty meal or excessive alcohol intake.

Other manifestations include nausea and vomiting, abdominal distension and rigidity, decreased bowel sounds, tachycardia, hypotension, elevated temperature, and cold, clammy skin. Within 24 hours, mild jaundice may appear. Retroperitoneal bleeding may occur 3 to 6 days after the onset of acute pancreatitis; signs of bleeding include bruising in the flanks (Turner's sign) or around the umbilicus (Cullen's sign). See the 'Manifestations' box.

COMPLICATIONS Systemic complications of acute pancreatitis include intravascular volume depletion with acute tubular necrosis and renal failure (see the chapter 'Nursing care of people with kidney disorders' for more information about acute renal failure) and acute respiratory distress syndrome (ARDS). Acute renal failure usually develops within 24 hours

MANIFESTATIONS **Acute and chronic pancreatitis**

ACUTE PANCREATITIS

- Abrupt onset of severe epigastric and left upper quadrant pain; may radiate to back
- Nausea, vomiting; fever
- Decreased bowel sounds; abdominal distension and rigidity
- Tachycardia, hypotension; cold, clammy skin
- Possible jaundice
- Positive Turner's sign (flank bruising) or Cullen's sign (periumbilical bruising)

CHRONIC PANCREATITIS

- Recurrent epigastric and LUQ pain; radiates to back
- Anorexia, nausea and vomiting, weight loss
- Flatulence, constipation
- Steatorrhoea

after the onset of acute pancreatitis. Manifestations of ARDS may be seen 3 to 7 days after its onset, particularly in people who have experienced severe volume depletion. See the chapter 'Nursing care of people with gas exchange disorders' for more information about ARDS.

Localised complications include pancreatic necrosis, abscess, pseudocysts and pancreatic ascites. Pancreatic necrosis causes an inflammatory mass that may be infected. It may lead to shock and multiple organ failure. A pancreatic abscess may form late in the course of the disease (6 or more weeks after its onset), causing an epigastric mass and tenderness (Papadakis, McPhee & Rabow, 2022). Pancreatic pseudocysts, encapsulated collections of fluid, may develop both within the pancreas itself and in the abdominal cavity. They may impinge on other structures or may rupture, causing generalised peritonitis. Rupture of a pseudocyst or of the pancreatic duct can lead to pancreatic ascites. Pancreatic ascites is recognised by gradually increasing abdominal girth and persistent elevation of the serum amylase level without abdominal pain.

Chronic pancreatitis

Chronic pancreatitis is characterised by gradual destruction of functional pancreatic tissue. In contrast to acute pancreatitis, which may completely resolve with no long-term effects, chronic pancreatitis is an irreversible process that eventually leads to pancreatic insufficiency. Alcoholism is the primary risk factor for chronic pancreatitis in Australia. Malnutrition is a major worldwide risk factor. About 10–20% of chronic pancreatitis is idiopathic, with no identified cause. A genetic mutation on a gene associated with cystic fibrosis may play a role in these cases. Children or young adults with cystic fibrosis may develop chronic pancreatitis as well.

In chronic pancreatitis related to alcoholism, pancreatic secretions have an increased concentration of insoluble proteins. These proteins calcify, forming plugs that block pancreatic ducts and the flow of pancreatic juices. This blockage leads to inflammation and fibrosis of pancreatic tissue. In other cases, a stricture or stone may block pancreatic outflow, causing chronic obstructive pancreatitis. In chronic pancreatitis, recurrent episodes of inflammation eventually lead to fibrotic changes in the parenchyma of the pancreas, with loss of exocrine function. This leads to malabsorption from pancreatic insufficiency. If endocrine function is disrupted as well, clinical diabetes mellitus may develop.

MANIFESTATIONS Chronic pancreatitis typically causes recurrent episodes of epigastric and left upper abdominal pain that radiates to the back. This pain may last for days to weeks. As the disease progresses, the interval between episodes of pain becomes shorter. Other manifestations include anorexia, nausea and vomiting, weight loss, flatulence, constipation and steatorrhoea (fatty, frothy, foul-smelling stools caused by a decrease in pancreatic enzyme secretion).

COMPLICATIONS Chronic pancreatitis complications include malabsorption, malnutrition and possible peptic ulcer disease. Pancreatic pseudocysts or abscesses may form or stricture of the common bile duct may develop. Diabetes mellitus may develop and there is an increased risk of pancreatic cancer. Opioid tolerance related to frequent, severe pain episodes is common.

INTERPROFESSIONAL CARE

Acute pancreatitis often is a mild, self-limiting disease. Treatment focuses on reducing pancreatic secretions and providing supportive care. Treatment to eliminate the causative factor is begun after the acute inflammatory process resolves. Severe necrotising pancreatitis may require intensive care management. Treatment for chronic pancreatitis often focuses on managing pain and treating malabsorption and malnutrition.

Diagnosis

The laboratory tests that may be ordered when pancreatitis is suspected are summarised in Table 24.4. Diagnostic studies include the following:

- *Ultrasonography* can identify gallstones, a pancreatic mass or pseudocyst.
- *CT scan* may be ordered to identify pancreatic enlargement, fluid collections in or around the pancreas, and perfusion deficits in areas of necrosis.
- *Endoscopic retrograde cholangiopancreatography (ERCP)* may be performed to diagnose chronic pancreatitis and to differentiate inflammation and fibrosis from carcinoma.
- *Magnetic endoscopic retrograde cholangiopancreatography (MRCP)* is a non-invasive procedure that does not use contrast media and is safer for people with known contrast adverse reactions.
- *Endoscopic ultrasonography* can detect changes indicative of chronic pancreatitis in the pancreatic duct and parenchyma.
- *Percutaneous fine-needle aspiration biopsy* may be performed to differentiate chronic pancreatitis from cancer of the pancreas; the cells that are aspirated are examined for malignancy.

TABLE 24.4 Laboratory tests in exocrine pancreatic disorders

TEST	NORMAL VALUE	SIGNIFICANCE
Serum amylase	0–130 U/L (U = units)	Rises within 2 to 12 hours of onset of acute pancreatitis to three times normal. Returns to normal in 3 to 4 days.
Serum lipase	0–160 U/L	Levels rise to three times normal in acute pancreatitis; remain elevated for 7 to 14 days.
Serum trypsinogen	< 80 microgram/L	Elevated in acute pancreatitis; may be decreased in chronic pancreatitis.
Urine amylase	4–37 U/L/2 h	Urine amylase levels rise in acute pancreatitis.
Serum glucose	70–110 mmol/L	May be transient elevation in acute pancreatitis.
Serum bilirubin	< 20 micromol/L	Compression of the common duct may increase bilirubin levels in acute pancreatitis.
Serum alkaline phosphatase	30–110 U/L	Compression of the common duct may increase levels in acute pancreatitis.
Serum calcium	2.10–2.60 mmol/L	Hypocalcaemia develops in up to 25% of people with acute pancreatitis.
White blood cells	$4.0–11.0 \times 10^9$/L	Leucocytosis indicates inflammation and is usually present in acute pancreatitis.

More information about these tests and their nursing implications can be found in the chapter 'A person-centred approach to assessing the gastrointestinal system'.

Medications

The treatment of acute pancreatitis is largely supportive. Early, aggressive fluid replacement with intravenous crystalloid fluids is recommended for mild to severe pancreatitis diagnoses. In addition, the person should be kept nil by mouth until nausea, vomiting and pain dissipates. Narcotic analgesics such as morphine sulfate are used to control pain. Antibiotics may be prescribed to treat infection.

People with chronic pancreatitis also require analgesics but are closely monitored to prevent drug dependence. Narcotics are avoided when possible. Pancreatic enzyme supplements are given to reduce steatorrhoea (see the 'Medication administration' box). People with chronic pancreatitis may need to remain on pancreatic enzyme supplements for life. H_2 blockers such as cimetidine and ranitidine and proton pump inhibitors such as omeprazole may be given to neutralise or decrease gastric secretions. Octreotide, a synthetic hormone, suppresses pancreatic enzyme secretion and may be used to relieve pain in chronic pancreatitis.

Treatments

NUTRITION Oral food and fluids are withheld during acute episodes of pancreatitis to reduce pancreatic secretions and promote rest of the organ. A nasogastric tube may be inserted and connected to suction. Intravenous fluids are administered for 48–72 hours to maintain vascular volume. If there is no improvement, enteral feeding will be commenced via either a nasogastric or a nasojejunal tube. Enteral feeding is preferable to total parenteral nutrition (TPN) as it maintains gut barrier integrity, which reduces bacteria translocation risk, and is more physiological than TPN (Chandran & Mammen, 2020). Oral food and fluids are begun once the serum amylase levels have returned to normal, bowel sounds are present and pain disappears. A low-fat diet is ordered and alcohol intake is strictly prohibited.

SURGERY If the pancreatitis is the result of a gallstone lodged in the sphincter of Oddi, an *endoscopic transduodenal sphincterotomy* may be performed to remove the stone. When cholelithiasis is identified as a causative factor, a cholecystectomy is performed once the acute pancreatitis has resolved. Surgical procedures to promote drainage of pancreatic enzymes into the duodenum or resection of all or part of the pancreas

MEDICATION ADMINISTRATION The person with chronic pancreatitis

PANCREATIC ENZYME REPLACEMENT

Pancrelipase

Pancrelipase enhances the digestion of starches and fats in the gastrointestinal tract by supplying an exogenous source of the enzymes protease, amylase and lipase. The drug promotes nutrition and decreases the number of bowel movements.

Nursing responsibilities

- Assess for allergy to pork protein.
- Monitor frequency and consistency of stools.
- Weigh every other day and record.
- Give with meals; if not enteric coated, H_2 antagonists or antacids may be given concurrently to prevent destruction of the enzymes by hydrochloric acid.
- Monitor for side effects: rash, hives, respiratory difficulty, haematuria, hyperuricaemia or joint pain.

Health education for the person and family

- Take with meals or snacks.
- If medicine is enteric coated, do not crush, chew or mix with alkaline foods (e.g. milk, ice-cream).
- Be sure to follow prescribed diet.
- Continue taking this drug until or unless advised by the doctor that it is no longer necessary.

may be done to provide pain relief in people with chronic pancreatitis. Large pancreatic pseudocysts may be drained endoscopically or surgically.

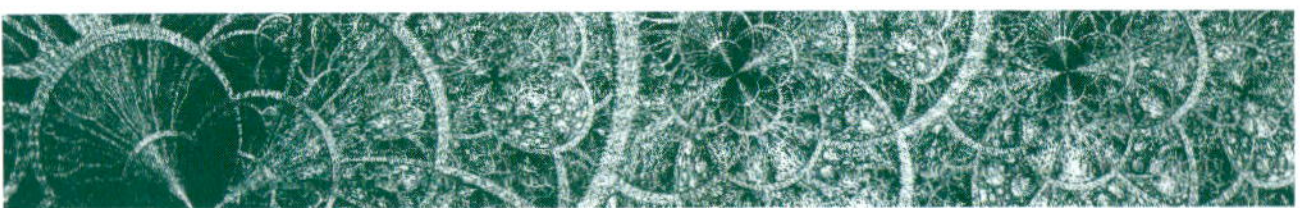

Nursing care

In addition to the nursing care discussed in this section, see the accompanying nursing care plan for a person with acute pancreatitis.

Health promotion

Teach people who abuse alcohol about the risk of developing pancreatitis. Advise abstinence to reduce this risk and refer to an alcohol treatment program or Alcoholics Anonymous.

Assessment

Assessment data related to acute or chronic pancreatitis include the following:

- *Health history*: current manifestations; abdominal pain (location, nature, onset and duration, identified precipitating factors); anorexia, nausea or vomiting; flatulence, diarrhoea, constipation or stool changes; recent weight loss; history of previous episodes or gallstones; alcohol use (extent and duration); current medications.
- *Physical assessment*: vital signs including orthostatic vitals and peripheral pulses; temperature; skin temperature and colour, presence of any flank or periumbilical ecchymoses; abdominal assessment including bowel sounds, presence of distension, tenderness or guarding.

Nursing diagnoses and interventions

Nursing care for the person with acute pancreatitis focuses on managing pain, nutrition and maintaining fluid balance.

Pain

Obstruction of pancreatic ducts and inflammation, oedema and swelling of the pancreas caused by pancreatic autodigestion cause severe epigastric, left upper abdominal or mid-scapular back pain. The pain often is accompanied by nausea and vomiting, abdominal tenderness and muscle guarding.

- Using a standard pain scale (see the chapter 'Nursing care of people in pain'), assess pain, including location, radiation, duration and character. Note non-verbal cues of pain: restlessness or remaining rigidly still; tense facial features; clenched fists; rapid, shallow respirations; tachycardia; and diaphoresis. Administer analgesics on a regular schedule. *Pain assessment before and after analgesic administration measures its effectiveness. Administering analgesics on a regular schedule prevents pain from becoming established, severe and difficult to control. Unrelieved pain has negative consequences; for example, pain, anxiety and restlessness may increase pancreatic enzyme secretion.*
- Maintain NBM status and nasogastric tube patency as ordered. *Gastric secretions stimulate hormones that stimulate pancreatic secretion, aggravating pain. Eliminating oral intake and maintaining gastric suction reduce gastric secretions. Nasogastric suction also decreases nausea, vomiting and intestinal distension.*
- Maintain bed rest in a calm, quiet environment. Encourage use of non-pharmacological pain management techniques such as meditation and guided imagery. *Decreasing physical movement and mental stimulation decreases metabolic rate, gastrointestinal secretion, pancreatic secretions and resulting pain. Adjunctive pain relief measures enhance the effectiveness of analgesics (see the chapter 'Nursing care of people in pain').*
- Assist to a comfortable position, such as a side-lying position with knees flexed and head elevated 45 degrees. *Sitting up, leaning forward or lying in a fetal position tends to decrease pain caused by stretching of the peritoneum by oedema and swelling.*
- Remind family and visitors to avoid bringing food into the person's room. *The sight or smell of food may stimulate secretory activity of the pancreas through the cephalic phase of digestion.*

> **CONSIDERATION FOR PRACTICE**
>
> **Regularly assess respiratory status (at least every 4 to 8 hours), including respiratory rate, depth and pattern; breath sounds; oxygen saturation and arterial blood gas results. Report tachypnoea, adventitious or absent breath sounds, oxygen saturation levels below 92%, $PaO_2 > 70$ mmHg or $PaCO_2 < 45$ mmHg. Severe abdominal pain causes shallow respirations and hypoventilation, and suppresses cough effectiveness, which can lead to pooling of secretions, atelectasis and pneumonia.**

Imbalanced nutrition: less than body requirements

The effects of pancreatitis and its treatment may result in malnutrition. Inflammation increases metabolic demand and frequently causes nausea, vomiting and diarrhoea. At a time of increased metabolic demand, NBM status and gastric suction further decrease available nutrients. In the person with chronic pancreatitis, loss of digestive enzymes affects the digestion and use of nutrients.

- Monitor laboratory values: serum albumin, serum transferrin, haemoglobin and haematocrit. *Serum albumin, serum transferrin (which transports iron in the blood), haemoglobin and haematocrit levels are decreased in malnutrition. Decreased pancreatic enzymes affect protein catabolism and absorption; decreased transferrin affects iron absorption and transport, thereby decreasing haematocrit and haemoglobin levels.*
- Weigh daily or every other day. *Short-term weight changes (over hours to days) accurately reflect fluid balance, whereas weight changes over days to weeks reflect nutritional status.*
- Maintain stool chart; note frequency, colour, odour and consistency of stools. *Protein and fat metabolism are impaired in pancreatitis; undigested fats are excreted in the stool. Steatorrhoea indicates impaired digestion and, possibly, an increase in the severity of pancreatitis.*

NURSING CARE PLAN A person with acute pancreatitis

Rose Schliefer is a 59-year-old wife, mother of three and grandmother of four. She has been hospitalised for the past 6 weeks for acute haemorrhagic pancreatitis and pseudocyst. The pancreatitis was caused by gallstones. Mrs Schliefer spent 3 weeks in intensive care and then underwent surgery to remove the gallstones and to insert drains into the pseudocyst. Prior to discharge, she had progressed to a soft, high-carbohydrate, low-fat diet; had all drains removed; and was able to walk in the hall. Mrs Schliefer was referred to the community nurses in her home town for continued follow up.

ASSESSMENT

Lee Quinn, the community health nurse, assesses Mrs Schliefer at home after discharge. Mrs Schliefer is thin and appears anxious and tired. She states that she lost 13 kg in the hospital and now weighs only 46 kg. She is 168 cm tall. Her vital signs are within normal limits. Mrs Schliefer has a well-healed upper abdominal scar and two small wounds (from drains) on each side of her abdomen. The wounds are closed but still have scabs. Her skin is cool and dry and turgor is poor. She is alert and oriented and responds appropriately to questions. Blood glucose levels are normal. Mrs Schliefer states that her main problems are lack of energy and lack of appetite for the low-fat diet that has been ordered. Mrs Schliefer's husband and daughters express concern about their ability to provide care. Although they have been taught all about the disease and how to provide care, they still are not sure they know exactly what should be done now that Mrs Schliefer is at home.

DIAGNOSES

- *Fatigue* related to decreased metabolic energy production.
- *Imbalanced nutrition: less than body requirements* related to prolonged hospitalisation, dietary restrictions and impaired digestion.
- *Bathing/hygiene self-care deficit* (Level II: requires help of another person, supervision and teaching) related to decreased strength and endurance.
- *Risk of caregiver role strain* related to inexperience with care-giving tasks.

PLANNING

- Develop activity goals, incorporating small, incremental steps towards achieving goals. Instruct Mrs Schliefer to:
  a. Rest in bed each day from 1 pm to 3 pm.
  b. Eat six small meals a day with family members or friends.
  c. Sit and rest quietly for 15 minutes before eating.
- Arrange for regular family discussions of concerns about future and goal setting and acknowledge family strengths.

Expected outcomes

- Set priorities for daily and weekly activities and incorporate a rest period into daily activity.
- Gain 0.5–1 kg per week.
- Bathe and maintain personal hygiene without assistance.
- Family members will verbalise comfort with providing necessary care.

IMPLEMENTATION

- Explain causes of fatigue. Review effects of pancreatitis, surgery and acute illness on energy levels.
- Mrs Schliefer indicates that she wants to cook a meal for the whole family. To reach this goal, she will:
  a. Schedule the meal when her energy level is highest.
  b. List actions necessary to prepare the meal and delegate difficult tasks to family members.
  c. Ask her daughters to reorganise the kitchen to avoid unnecessary steps.
  d. Plan the meal no sooner than the third week after being home.
- Discuss dietary restrictions and how to adapt them to usual diet.
- Advise to use shower chair and develop self-care goals for bathing and hygiene in small steps. Add self-care tasks gradually as tolerated.
- Discuss division of responsibilities for physical care, home maintenance and medical care with family members.

EVALUATION

One month after discharge, Mrs Schliefer and her family have established new routines based on her energy levels. Mrs Schliefer now makes lunch because she feels best around midday. She and her husband share this time together without interruption. Mrs Schliefer still rests during the day but can now provide self-care. She has gained only 1 kg, but states that she is getting used to the new diet and that 'things are even starting to taste good without butter'. She also says that sitting quietly before meals is helpful and that she prefers eating six small meals a day. Mr and Mrs Schliefer and their daughters agree that their initial worries about Mrs Schliefer's care have been resolved now they all know what they must do and the future looks much brighter.

CRITICAL THINKING IN THE NURSING PROCESS

1 You are caring for a person who has acute pancreatitis and is also an alcoholic. Describe assessments that indicate the beginnings of withdrawal.
2 Discuss the pathophysiological basis of hypovolaemic shock in acute necrotic pancreatitis.
3 Outline a teaching plan that includes specific foods to omit and to include in a high-carbohydrate, low-protein, low-fat diet.
4 Develop a plan of care for the nursing diagnosis of *Impaired home maintenance*.

REFLECTION ON THE NURSING PROCESS

1 Outline what you have learned from this case study that you will apply to your future practice.
2 Reflect on Mrs Schliefer's discharge process from hospital. What could have been done differently to avoid her loss of appetite and fatigue at home?

- Monitor bowel sounds. *The return of bowel sounds indicates return of peristalsis; nasogastric suction usually is discontinued within 24 to 48 hours thereafter.*
- Administer prescribed intravenous fluids and/or enteral feeds. *Intravenous fluids are given to maintain hydration. Enteral feeds are used to provide fluids, electrolytes and kilojoules when fasting is prolonged (more than 2 to 3 days).*
- Provide oral and nasal care every 1 to 2 hours. *Fasting and nasogastric suction increase the risk of mucous membrane irritation and breakdown.*
- When oral intake resumes, offer small, frequent feedings. Provide oral hygiene before and after meals. *Oral hygiene decreases oral microorganisms that can cause foul odour and taste, decreasing appetite. Small, frequent feedings reduce pancreatic enzyme secretion and are more easily digested and absorbed.*

Risk of deficient fluid volume

Acute pancreatitis can lead to a fluid shift from the intravascular space into the abdominal cavity (third spacing). Third spacing of fluid may cause hypovolaemic shock, affecting cardiovascular function, respiratory function, renal function and mental status.

- Assess cardiovascular status every 4 hours or as indicated, including vital signs, cardiac rhythm, haemodynamic parameters (central venous and pulmonary artery pressures); peripheral pulses and capillary refill; skin colour, temperature, moisture and turgor. *These measurements are indicative of fluid volume status and are used to monitor response to treatment. Stable values are as follows: heart rate less than 100; blood pressure within 10 mmHg of baseline; central venous pressure 0–8 mmHg; pulmonary wedge pressure 8–12 mmHg; cardiac output approximately 5 L/min; and skin warm, dry, with good turgor and colour. (See the chapter 'Nursing care of people experiencing trauma and shock' for a full discussion of hypovolaemic shock.)*
- Monitor renal function. Obtain hourly urine output; report if less than 0.5 mL/kg/hour. Weigh daily. *Urine output of less than 0.5 mL/kg/hour indicates decreased renal perfusion or acute renal failure, a major complication of acute pancreatitis. Weight changes are an effective indicator of fluid volume status.*
- Monitor neurological function, including mental status, level of consciousness and behaviour. *Hypotension and hypoxaemia may decrease cerebral perfusion, causing changes in mental status, decreased level of consciousness and changes in behaviour. In addition, alcohol withdrawal is a risk in the person with acute pancreatitis.*

Community-based care

The person with pancreatitis is often acutely ill and, along with family members, needs information about both hospital procedures and self-care at home following discharge. During the acute stage, keep explanations brief and simple.

Prior to discharge, teach the person and family about the disease and how to prevent further attacks of inflammation. Include the following topics as appropriate:

- Alcohol can cause stones to form, blocking pancreatic ducts and the outflow of pancreatic juice. Continued alcohol intake is likely to cause further inflammation and destruction of the pancreas. Avoid alcohol entirely.
- Smoking and stress stimulate the pancreas and should be avoided.
- If pancreatic function has been severely impaired, discuss appropriate use of pancreatic enzymes, including timing, dose, potential side effects and monitoring of effectiveness.
- A low-fat diet is recommended. Provide a list of high-fat foods to avoid. Crash dieting and binge eating also should be avoided as they may sometimes precipitate attacks. Spicy foods, coffee, tea or colas, and gas-forming foods stimulate gastric and pancreatic secretions and may precipitate pain. Avoid them if this occurs.
- Report symptoms of infection (fever of 38.5°C or more, pain, rapid pulse, malaise) because a pancreatic abscess can develop after initial recovery.

Refer to a dietitian or nutritionist for diet teaching as needed. If appropriate, refer to community agencies, such as Alcoholics Anonymous, or to an alcohol treatment program. Provide referrals to community or home health agencies, as needed, for continued monitoring and teaching at home.

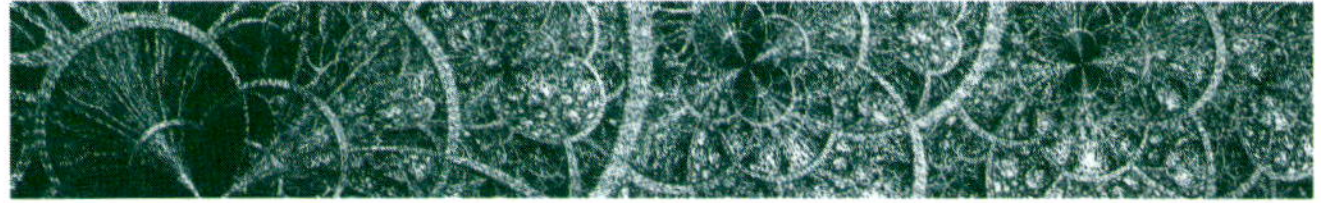

THE PERSON WITH PANCREATIC CANCER

Pancreatic cancer accounts for about one-sixth of all deaths associated with cancers in Australia. It has a 5-year survival rate of less than 6%. Complete resection is the best hope for cure if the cancer is in the head of the pancreas. However, by the time of initial presentation most people already have advanced disease. Only about 30% of these people can be offered curative resection. If the cancer is in the body or tail of the pancreas, only about 10% of these people can be offered curative resection (Cancer Council, 2022).

FAST FACTS

Identified risk factors for pancreatic cancer include:

- Cigarette smoking—the incidence is twice as high in smokers as in non-smokers
- Exposure to industrial chemicals or environmental toxins
- Chronic pancreatitis
- Diabetes mellitus
- Obesity; high-fat diet.

In contrast to acute and chronic pancreatitis, alcohol abuse and gallstones are not identified risk factors for pancreatic cancer.

Pathophysiology and manifestations

Most cancers of the pancreas occur in the exocrine pancreas, are adenocarcinomas and cause death within 1 to 3 years after diagnosis.

Cancer of the pancreas has a slow onset, with manifestations of anorexia, nausea, weight loss, flatulence and dull epigastric pain. The pain increases in severity as the tumour grows. Other manifestations depend on the location of the tumour. Cancer of the head of the pancreas, which is the most common site, often obstructs bile flow through the common bile duct and the ampulla of Vater, resulting in jaundice, clay-coloured stools, dark urine and pruritus. Cancer of the body of the pancreas presses on the coeliac ganglion, causing pain that increases when the person eats or lies supine. Cancer of the tail of the pancreas often causes no symptoms until it has metastasised. Other late manifestations include a palpable abdominal mass and ascites. Because the manifestations are non-specific, up to 85% of people with cancer of the pancreas do not seek healthcare until the cancer becomes too far advanced for a cure.

INTERPROFESSIONAL CARE

Early cancers of the head of the pancreas may be resectable. A pancreatoduodenectomy (commonly called Whipple's procedure) is performed to remove the head of the pancreas, the entire duodenum, the distal third of the stomach, a portion of the jejunum and the lower half of the common bile duct. The common bile duct is then sutured to the end of the jejunum and the remaining pancreas and stomach are sutured to the side of the jejunum (see Figure 24.7). Radiation and chemotherapy are often used in addition to surgery.

Postoperative nursing care of the person undergoing Whipple's procedure is outlined in the accompanying nursing care box. Immediate postoperative care is often provided in the intensive care unit.

The person with pancreatic cancer has multiple problems requiring nursing care. The chapter 'Nursing care of people with cancer' provides a discussion of care of the person with cancer. The nursing diagnoses and interventions discussed for the person with pancreatitis are also appropriate for the person with pancreatic cancer.

NURSING CARE OF THE PERSON undergoing Whipple's procedure

PREOPERATIVE CARE

- Provide routine preoperative nursing care as outlined in the chapter 'Nursing care of people having surgery'.
- Clarify teaching and learning as needed. Provide psychological support for person and family. *The person and family faced with a diagnosis of pancreatic cancer may require reinforcement of teaching as anxiety, fear and possible denial can interfere with learning.*

POSTOPERATIVE CARE

- Provide postoperative care as outlined in the chapter 'Nursing care of people having surgery'.
- Maintain in semi-Fowler's position. *Semi-Fowler's position facilitates lung expansion and reduces stress on the anastomosis and suture line.*
- Maintain low gastrointestinal suction. If drainage is not adequate, obtain an order to irrigate, using minimal pressure. Do not reposition nasogastric tube. *Pressure within the operative area from retained secretions increases intraluminal pressure and places stress on the suture line. Forceful irrigations and repositioning of the nasogastric tube may disrupt the suture line.*
- Maintain pain control using analgesics as prescribed (PCA, infusion or given on a regular basis). Assess effectiveness of pain management. *Doses higher than normal may be required if narcotic analgesics have been used prior to surgery to manage pain.*
- *Increased pain may indicate complications such as disruption of suture line, leakage from anastomosis or peritonitis. Adequate pain management increases resistance to stress, facilitates healing and increases the ability to cough, deep breathe and change position.*
- Assist with coughing, deep breathing and changing position every 1 to 2 hours. Splint incision during coughing and deep breathing. *The location of the incision makes coughing and deep breathing more painful. The prolonged surgical procedure, anaesthesia, location of incision and immobility increase the risk of retained secretions, atelectasis and pneumonia. Changing position facilitates drainage of secretions; effective coughing and deep breathing remove secretions and open distal alveoli.*
- Monitor for complications:
  a. Take vital signs every 2 to 4 hours or as indicated; immediately report changes (such as elevated temperature; hypotension; weak, thready pulse; increased or difficult respirations).
  b. Assess skin colour, temperature, moisture and turgor.
  c. Measure urinary output, gastrointestinal output and drainage from any other tubes; monitor amount and type of wound drainage.
  d. Assess level of consciousness.
  e. Monitor results of laboratory tests, especially arterial blood gases, haemoglobin and haematocrit.

The main potential complications following Whipple's procedure are haemorrhage, hypovolaemic shock and hepatorenal failure. *The assessments listed provide information about the person's status and alert the nurse to abnormal findings that signal the onset of these complications.*

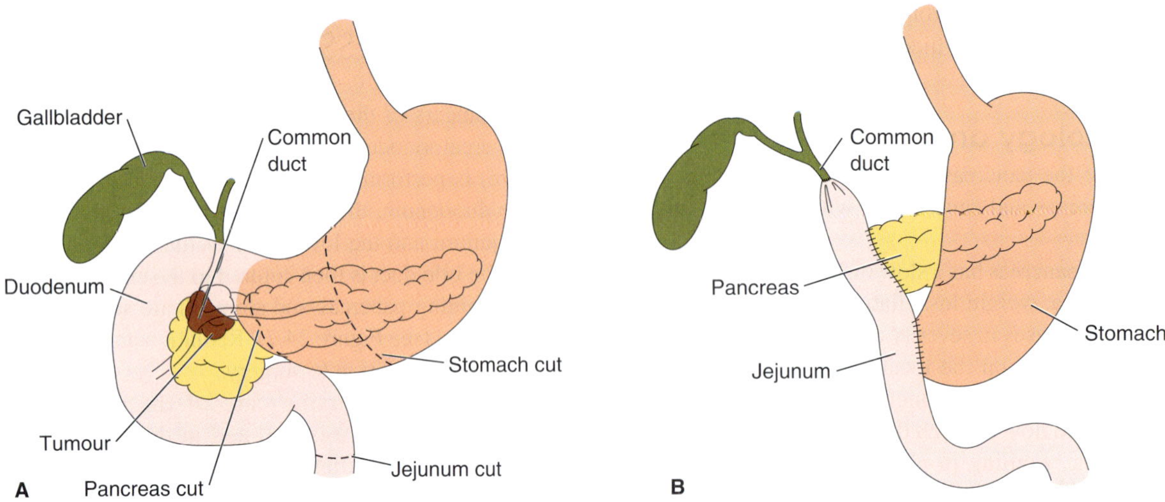

FIGURE 24.7 *Pancreatoduodenectomy (Whipple's procedure). A, areas of resection; B, appearance following resection*

CHAPTER HIGHLIGHTS

- Gallstones (cholelithiasis) are common and often unrecognised until the person develops manifestations of biliary colic or acute cholecystitis. Laparoscopic cholecystectomy is the treatment of choice for symptomatic gallbladder disease.
- Hepatitis, inflammation of functional liver tissue, is usually a viral disease and therefore cannot be cured at this time. Preventing the spread of hepatitis through use of standard and body substance precautions is an important nursing responsibility.
- Hepatitis A, commonly transmitted via the faecal–oral route, is generally a self-limiting disease with few long-term sequelae. Some types of viral hepatitis, most notably hepatitis B and C, can become chronic and ultimately lead to liver failure and an increased risk of liver cancer. Hepatitis B and C can result in a carrier state in which the infected person has no symptoms of the disease but can spread it to others.
- Alcohol abuse is a significant risk factor for liver and pancreatic disorders. Prevention, early identification and treatment of alcohol abuse reduce the risk of these disorders. Absolute abstinence from alcohol is an important part of the treatment plan for people with liver and pancreatic disorders.
- Cirrhosis leads to portal hypertension and liver failure, which, in turn, account for most of the manifestations and complications of the disorder. Complications, such as ascites, splenomegaly, oesophageal varices and hepatic encephalopathy, affect multiple body systems and significantly contribute to mortality and morbidity associated with cirrhosis.
- Bleeding from oesophageal varices may be massive, resulting in a medical emergency and requiring prompt control to maintain cardiac output.
- Acute pancreatitis often develops as a complication of gallstones. Acute pancreatitis often resolves with no long-term consequences. Chronic pancreatitis is more frequently related to alcohol abuse and can lead to continuing pain and digestive disruptions.

CONCEPT CHECK

1 When assessing the person admitted for a laparoscopic cholecystectomy, the nurse would expect to find:

1 a history of intermittent episodes of right upper quadrant pain
2 significant jaundice of the sclera and skin
3 complaints of recurrent heartburn and acid reflux
4 ascites and peripheral oedema

2 Which of the following does the nurse include in her teaching for a person with acute cholecystitis? (Select all that apply.)

1 Avoid consumption of foods high in fat, such as sauces and peanut butter.
2 Limit your intake to dry cracker biscuits and clear liquids during episodes of acute pain.
3 A low-carbohydrate diet such as the Atkins diet is recommended for weight loss.
4 Call your doctor if you develop severe abdominal pain and a temperature.
5 Surgery for gallstones is optional; they pose little risk when fat intake is minimal.

3 During an outbreak of hepatitis A traced to a food handler at a local restaurant, the nurse teaches staff at the restaurant that the most cost-effective means of protecting customers from further outbreaks is to:

1 insist that all food handlers be immunised against hepatitis A
2 test all new employees for hepatitis A antigen
3 wash hands thoroughly before handling food and after using the bathroom
4 use gloves for handling food if any cuts or scrapes are on hands

4 The nurse would evaluate teaching as effective when a person with chronic hepatitis C states which of the following?

1 'I will reduce my alcohol intake and use only paracetamol for pain relief.'

2 'I understand that I must return to the doctor every year for a follow-up liver biopsy.'
3 'Even though no treatment is available for this disease, I plan to live a long life.'
4 'I will avoid donating blood and will use barrier protection during sex.'

5 When evaluating for people possibly exposed to hepatitis A by a recently diagnosed person, the nurse inquires about:
1 sexual partners within the past 6 months
2 close household contacts within the past 4 weeks
3 food preparation activities since the development of jaundice
4 immunisation status of the person

6 A person hospitalised with cirrhosis, ascites and mild hepatic encephalopathy suddenly vomits 200 mL of bright red blood. Which of the following should the nurse do first?
1 Insert a nasogastric tube.
2 Place in Fowler's position.
3 Contact the doctor.
4 Check stool for occult blood.

7 The nurse caring for a person scheduled for an abdominal paracentesis instructs the person to:
1 avoid eating or drinking fluid for 6 hours prior to the procedure
2 scrub the abdomen with antiseptic soap before the procedure
3 empty the bladder before the procedure
4 report excess flatus following the procedure to the doctor

8 A person hospitalised with severe ascites due to cirrhosis develops a fever and confusion. The nurse should:
1 auscultate bowel sounds and palpate for abdominal tenderness
2 enquire about headache and check for nuchal rigidity
3 observe for neck vein distension and auscultate lung sounds
4 measure abdominal girth and percuss for shifting dullness

9 A 54-year-old woman admitted with acute pancreatitis says, 'I don't understand how I got this disease. I thought alcoholics got pancreatitis—I never drink.' Which of the following is the most appropriate response by the nurse?
1 'Was there a time in your life that you did drink heavily?'
2 'It also is prevalent in smokers; do you smoke cigarettes?'
3 'Gallstones also are a risk factor. We'll evaluate for them.'
4 'Intravenous drug use is a risk factor. Do you use drugs by injection?'

10 The nurse caring for a person returning to the unit following Whipple's procedure identifies which of the following as of highest priority in the plan of care?
1 referral to a smoking cessation program
2 frequent turning, coughing and deep breathing exercises
3 early mobilisation including ambulation as tolerated
4 maintaining patency of the nasogastric tube

BIBLIOGRAPHY

Adams, L. A., Roberts, S. K., Strasser, S. I. et al. (2020). Nonalcoholic fatty liver disease burden: Australia, 2019–2030. *Journal of Gastroenterology and Hepatology*, *35*(9), 1628–1635.

Arun, A. C., Ilangovan, N. & Rajma, J. (2020). Risk factors for alcohol use relapse after abstinence in patients with alcoholic liver disease. *Journal of Family Medicine and Primary Care*, *9*(12), 5995–5999. doi: 10.4103/jfmpc.jfmpc_1401_20

Australian Bureau of Statistics (ABS) (2020). *Causes of death, Australia 2020. Statistics on the number of deaths, by sex, selected age groups, and cause of death classified to the International Classification of Diseases (ICD) reference period 2020.* Retrieved from https://www.abs.gov.au/

Australian Technical Advisory Group on Immunisation (ATAGI) (2022). *Australian immunisation handbook.* Canberra: Australian Government Department of Health and Aged Care. Retrieved from https://immunisationhandbook.health.gov.au

Cancer Council (2020). *Understanding gall bladder cancer.* Retrieved from https://www.cancer.org.au/

Cancer Council (2022). *Understanding pancreatic cancer.* Retrieved from https://www.cancer.org.au/

Chandran, K. & Mammen, S. C. (2020). Effects of early feeding on recovery profile in mild acute pancreatitis. *International Surgery Journal*, *7*(6), 1964–1967. http://dx.doi.org/10.18203/2349-2902.isj20202414

Craft, J., Gordon, C., Huether, S., McCance, K. & Brashers, V. (2018). *Understanding pathophysiology* (ANZ 3rd ed.). Chatswood, NSW: Elsevier.

Department of Health and Aged Care (2022). *National immunisation program.* Canberra: Australian Government. Retrieved from https://www.health.gov.au/

Gastroenterological Society of Australia (2021). *Gallstones.* Retrieved from https://www.gesa.org.au/

GI Cancer (2022). *Gallbladder and bile duct cancer: Symptoms and risk factors.* Retrieved from https://gicancer.org.au/

Hepatitis Australia (2022). *Stopping the spread of hepatitis C.* Retrieved from https://www.hepatitisaustralia.com

Hepatitis B Foundation (2022). *What is hepatitis B?* Retrieved from https://www.hepb.org

Hepatitis C Virus Infection Consensus Statement Working Group (2020). *Australian recommendations for the management of hepatitis C virus infection: A consensus statement* (June 2020). Melbourne: Gastroenterological Society of Australia.

Lee, C., Balk, D., Schafer, J. et al. (2019). Accuracy of focused assessment with sonography for trauma (FAST) in disaster settings: A meta-analysis and systematic review. *Disaster Medicine and Public Health Preparedness*, *13*(5–6), 1059–1064.

Merli, M. (2020). Nutrition in cirrhosis: Dos and don'ts. *Journal of Hepatology*, *73*(6), 1563–1565. https://doi.org/10.1016/j.jhep.2020.07.010

Norris, T. L. (2018). *Porth's pathophysiology: Concepts of altered health states* (10th ed.). Philadelphia: Lippincott Williams & Wilkins.

Papadakis, M., McPhee, S. & Rabow, M. (2022). *Current medical diagnosis and treatment* (61st ed.). New York: McGraw-Hill Education.

Selvanathan, E. A., Selvanathan, S. & Jayasinghe, M. (2020). Nexus between drinking patterns, gender and life satisfaction: Some evidence from Indigenous Australians. *The Australian Journal of Social Issues*, *55*(4), 396–417. https://doi.org/10.1002/ajs4.109

Singh, H., Kundra, S., Singh, R. M., Grewal, A., Kaul, T. K. & Sood, D. (2013). Preemptive analgesia with ketamine for laparoscopic cholecystectomy. *Journal of Anaesthesiology, Clinical Pharmacology*, *29*(4), 478–484.

Urden, L. D., Stacy, K. M. & Lough, M. E. (2021). *Critical care nursing: Diagnosis and management* (9th ed.). St Louis, MO: Elsevier.

World Health Organization (2019). *Hepatitis C fact sheet.* Retrieved from http://www.who.int/

Zhu, M. & Sun, W. (2023). Analgesic effects of ropivacaine combined with dexmedetomidine in transversus abdominis plane block in patients undergoing laparoscopic cholecystectomy: A systematic review and meta-analysis. *Journal of PeriAnesthesia Nursing*. doi: https://doi.org/10.1016/j.jopan.2022.09.003

UNIT 6 BUILDING CLINICAL COMPETENCE

Responses to altered gastrointestinal function

Clinical scenario

You have been assigned to work with the following four people for the 0700 shift. Significant data obtained during report are as follows:

- Thomas Jones, aged 56, was transferred to your unit yesterday after treatment in the critical care unit for oesophageal varices. Significant history includes alcohol consumption (6 to 12 beers daily for several years) and smoking (2 packets per day for the past 30 years). Current vital signs are T 37.7°C, P 96, R 28, BP 150/90. He complains of abdominal tenderness and dyspnoea. He appears anxious and irritable.
- Ruth Green, aged 35, was admitted with right upper quadrant pain radiating to the left shoulder and a feeling of abdominal fullness. She has a history of cholelithiasis and cholecystitis. Her assessment reveals T 37.2°C, P 90, R 24, BP 140/84, with pallor, diaphoresis and complaints of nausea. She is scheduled for a cholecystectomy at 9 am.
- Tanya Cooper, aged 21, was admitted with dehydration, weakness and fainting. Her weight is 40.9 kg and height is 165 cm. Her vital signs are T 36.1°C, P 70, R 26, BP 90/56 mmHg with orthostatic BP 70/48 mmHg. She has a 3-year history of anorexia nervosa and laxative abuse. She has an IV of 0.9% NaCl with 20 mmol KCl infusing. She is to be monitored for food intake and watched for 1 hour after meals. She is ringing her call light to get up to the bathroom.
- Grace Freeman is a 36-year-old who had a temporary colostomy formed 5 days ago following an abdominal injury from a motor vehicle crash. Vital signs at 0400 were T 36.8°C, P 78, R 14, BP 112/78. She buzzed for assistance because her colostomy bag is full and she needs help emptying it.

Critical-thinking questions

1 In what order would you visit these people after report?

1. ______________________________
2. ______________________________
3. ______________________________
4. ______________________________

2 What top two priority nursing diagnoses would you choose for each of the people presented above? Can you explain, if asked, the rationale for your choices?

	Priority Nursing Diagnosis #1	Priority Nursing Diagnosis #2
Thomas Jones		
Ruth Green		
Tanya Cooper		
Grace Freeman		

3 You need to complete preoperative preparation on Mrs Green. Which of the following do you need to do?

1. Complete preoperative checklist, witness signed consent and administer preoperative medication when requested.
2. Explain the procedure, obtain informed consent and complete the preoperative checklist.
3. Sign the operative consent, explain complications of the procedure and take vital signs on call.
4. Obtain signed consent, discuss with the family the surgical procedure and have the person void prior to going to the OR.

4 Mrs Green understands the postoperative teaching done by the nurse when she states:

1. 'I wlll be on bed rest for two days after surgery.'
2. 'I will need to cough and deep breathe while splinting my incision.'
3. 'I will be able to begin eating when I return from surgery.'
4. 'I will be medicated for pain without having to request it.'

5 The nurse explains a diet of low-fat foods to Mrs Green. She understands this diet when she picks which meal plan?

1. eggs, sausage and toast
2. chicken, mashed potatoes and gravy and corn
3. grilled fish, tossed salad, peaches
4. hamburger with lettuce and tomato, chips

6 To prepare Mr Jones for an oesophagoscopy, the nurse institutes the following interventions:

1. Explain that it is not a painful procedure but he will be medicated for pain.
2. Keep Mr Jones NBM for 12 hours prior to the procedure.
3. Remove dentures and provide mouth care.
4. Place in a supine position with the head slightly hyperextended.

7 Which discharge instructions will the RN advise Mrs Freeman regarding how to take care of the colostomy?

1. 'The types of foods you eat will not affect the colostomy output.'
2. 'Empty the colostomy pouch or replace the bag when it is half full.'
3. 'Irrigate the colostomy with water to stimulate the colon to empty.'
4. 'Cleanse the area around the stoma with deodorant soap to decrease odour.'

8 Which of the following is the most common initial manifestation of malignant tumours of the lower bowel?

1. rectal bleeding
2. diarrhoea
3. rectal pain
4. constipation

9 A person with severe diarrhoea may develop metabolic acidosis. Which arterial blood gases indicates metabolic acidosis?

1. pH 7.45, $PaCO_2$ 40 mmHg, bicarbonate 25 mEq/L
2. pH 7.28, $PaCO_2$ 30 mmHg, bicarbonate 19 mEq/L
3. pH 7.55, $PaCO_2$ 50 mmHg, bicarbonate 30 mEq/L
4. pH 7.33, $PaCO_2$ 36 mmHg, bicarbonate 24 mEq/L

10 Teaching appropriate constipation management includes which actions? (Select all that apply.)

1. Decrease dietary fibre.
2. Increase fluid intake.
3. Increase exercise activity.
4. Use bulk-forming laxatives.
5. Use enemas daily.

11 With Ms Cooper's history of anorexia for 3 years, which is a priority nursing intervention in the plan of care for her?

1. Monitor for cardiac arrhythmias due to electrolyte imbalances.
2. Monitor weight for loss or gain to determine effectiveness of nursing care.

3. Maintain close observation for at least 1 hour after meals.
4. Serve small, frequent meals, increasing serving size gradually.

12 In planning discharge for Ms Cooper, the family and person participate in teaching and diet counselling sessions. Which is the priority item for the family and Ms Cooper to follow after discharge?

1. Monitor weight regularly to determine further weight loss.
2. Use rewards for food and kilojoule intake rather than weight gain.
3. Gradually increase the amount of food taken at meals.
4. Attend support groups for people with eating disorders.

Case study

Lewis Haches, an 82-year-old white male, has a history of hypertension, degenerative arthritis and angina pectoris for which he takes frusemide, atenolol, extra-strength aspirin and glyceryl trinitrate. He states that his blood pressure is controlled when he takes his medications as prescribed. Lately, he has been having some financial difficulties and does not take his medications as often as he should. He lives with his 80-year-old wife, who also has health problems. He does the cooking and grocery shopping. He has a son who lives nearby who looks in on them every couple of days.

Mr Haches feels that he cooked some outdated food that made him ill. He states he has been trying to stretch their grocery budget by reducing their serving sizes and shopping less frequently. He says he has had nausea and loose, dark stools for the past 2 days. This morning, he is weak and dizzy and states he nearly fainted in the shower. He also states he has not been able to take his medications for the past 2 days and feels that his heart is beating too fast. His son brought him to the hospital because he was weak, confused and very pale when he checked on him prior to going to work in the morning.

Based on Mr Haches' medical diagnosis and treatment plan, *Imbalanced nutrition: less than body requirements* is identified as the priority nursing diagnosis at this time.

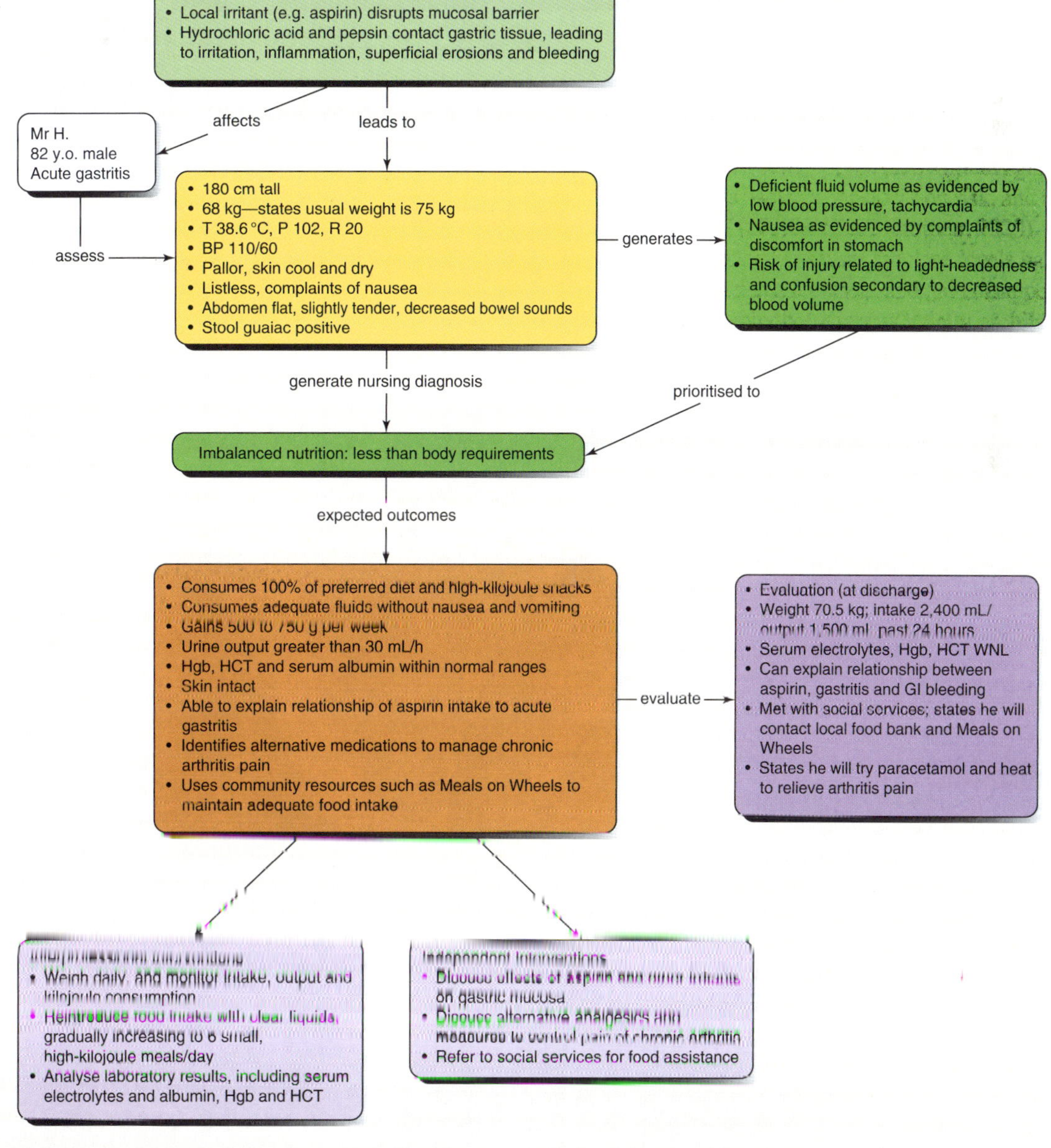

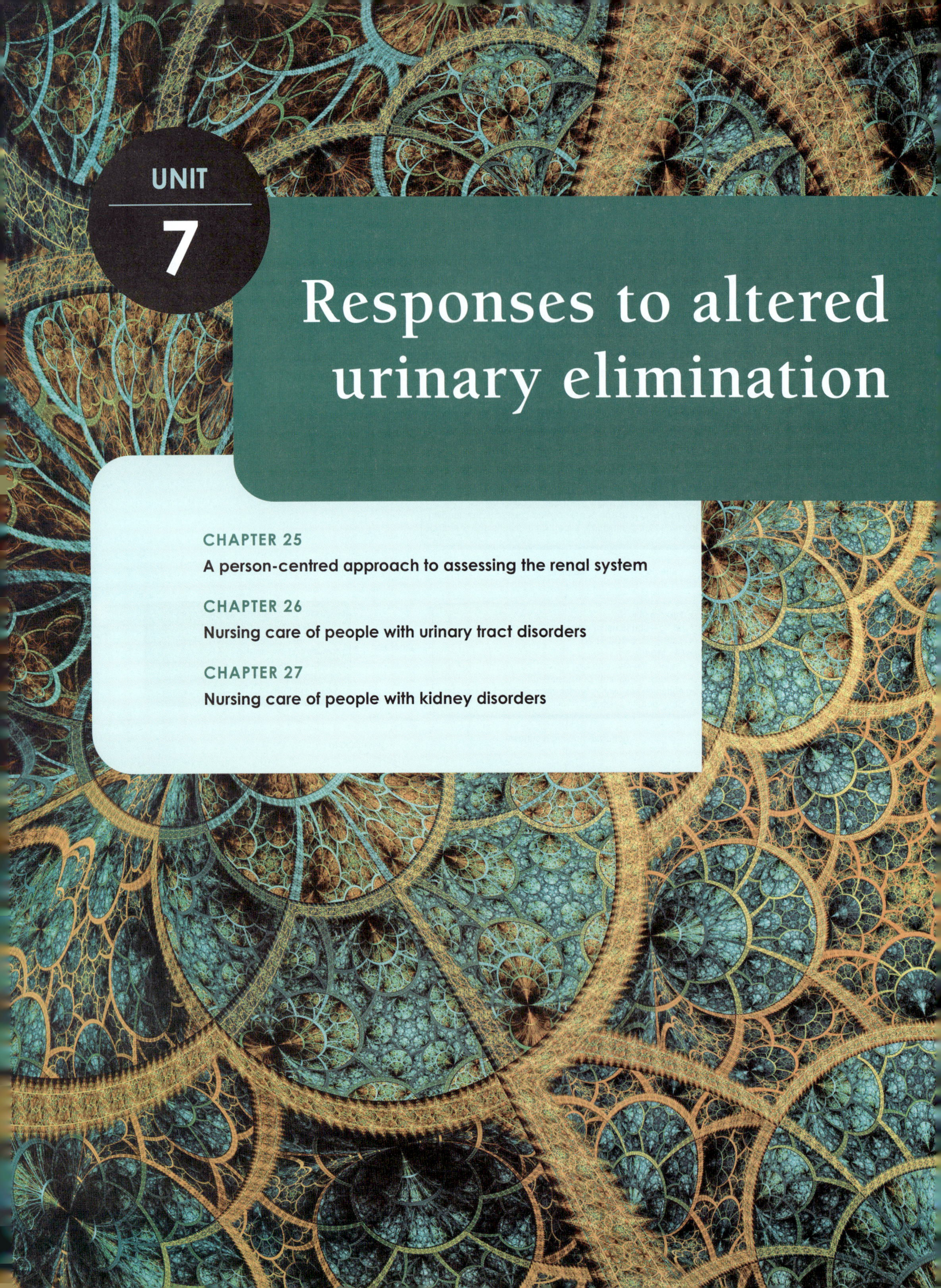

UNIT

7

Responses to altered urinary elimination

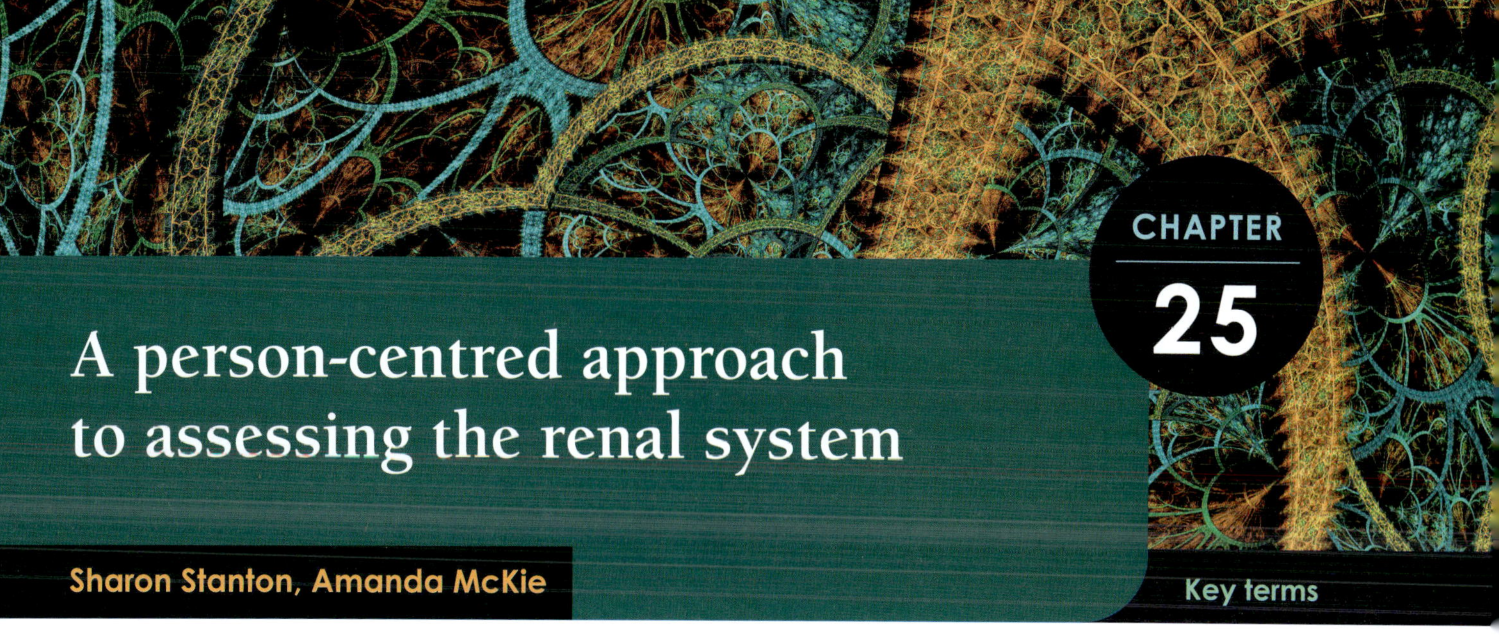

CHAPTER 25

A person-centred approach to assessing the renal system

Sharon Stanton, Amanda McKie

Key terms

albuminuria 829
calculi 828
chronic kidney disease (CKD) 821
creatinine 823
dysuria 824
glomerular filtration rate (GFR) 820
haematuria 824
micturition 824
nocturia 824
oliguria 824
polyuria 824
pyuria 825
urea 823

Learning outcomes

- Describe the anatomy, physiology and functions of the renal system.
- Examine investigations, techniques and observations important for assessing a person's renal system function.
- Demonstrate accurate interpretation of normal and aberrant data obtained from assessment of a person's renal system.

Clinical competencies

- Conduct and document a health history for people who have or are at risk of alterations in urinary elimination.
- Conduct and document a physical assessment of the renal system.
- Monitor the results of diagnostic tests and report abnormal findings.

Equipment needed

- Urine specimen cup
- Disposable gloves

The functions of the renal system (also called the urinary system or kidney structure) are to regulate and maintain body fluids and electrolyte balance, to filter metabolic wastes from the bloodstream, to reabsorb needed substances and water into the bloodstream and to eliminate metabolic wastes and water as urine. The renal system also indirectly maintains the body's the blood pressure, acid–base balance and an endocrine function. Any alteration in the structure or function of the renal system affects the whole body. In turn, healthy renal system function depends on the health of other body systems, especially the circulatory, endocrine and nervous systems.

Anatomy, physiology and functions of the renal system

The organs of the renal system are the paired kidneys (produce urine), the paired ureters (transport urine to the bladder), the urinary bladder (collects the urine) and the urethra (transports urine to outside the body) (see Figure 25.1). There are three major functions of the renal system:

1. *excretion*, the removal of wastes from body fluids
2. *elimination*, the elimination of these wastes from the body
3. *homeostatic regulation* of the volume and solute concentration of the plasma in the blood (Martini, Nath & Bartholomew, 2017).

Each structure is essential to the total functioning of the renal system.

THE KIDNEYS

The two kidneys are located outside the peritoneal cavity and on either side of the vertebral column at the levels of T_{12} to L_3. The left kidney is slightly superior to the right kidney. These highly vascular, bean-shaped organs are approximately 11.5 cm long, 5–7.5 cm wide, 2.5 cm thick and weigh about 150 g. The lateral surface of the kidney is convex; the medial surface is

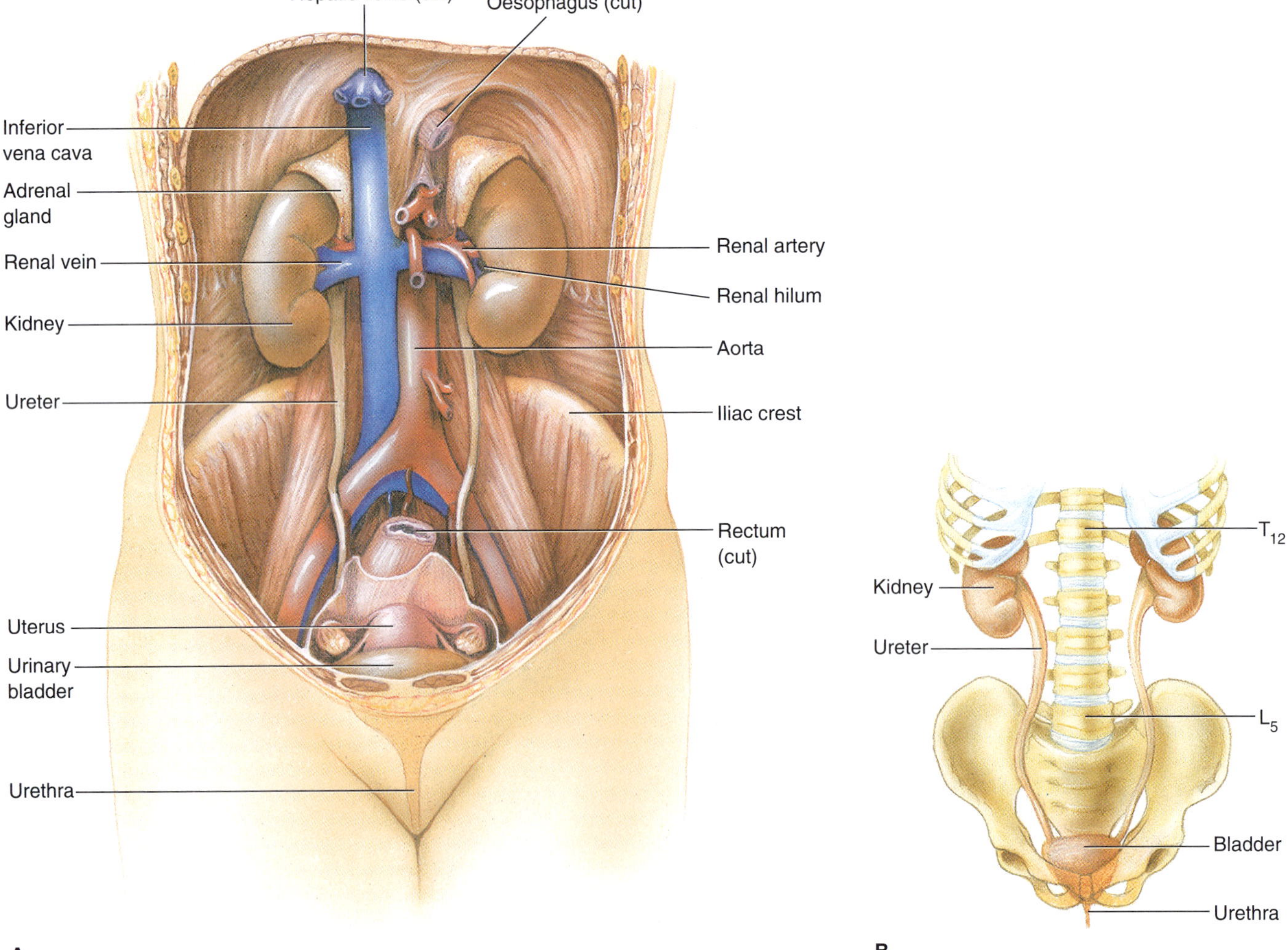

FIGURE 25.1 ***The renal/kidney/urinary system. A, Anterior view of the renal system in a female. B, The kidneys are shown in relation to the vertebrae and ribs***

concave and forms a vertical cleft, the hilum. The ureter, renal artery, renal vein, lymphatic vessels and nerves enter or exit the kidney at the level of the hilum.

The kidney is supported by three layers of connective tissue: the outer renal fascia, the middle adipose capsule and the inner renal capsule. The renal fascia, made up of dense connective tissue, surrounds the kidney (and the adrenal gland, a discrete organ that sits on top of each kidney) and anchors it to surrounding structures. The middle adipose capsule is a fatty mass that holds the kidney in place and also cushions it against trauma. The inner renal capsule provides a barrier against infection and helps protect the kidney from trauma.

Internally, each kidney has three distinct regions: the cortex, medulla and pelvis. The outer region, or renal cortex, is light in colour and has a granular appearance (see Figure 25.2). This region of the kidney contains the glomeruli, small clusters of capillaries. The glomeruli bring blood to and carry waste products from the nephrons, the functional units of the kidney.

The renal medulla, just below the cortex, contains cone-shaped tissue masses called renal pyramids, formed almost entirely of bundles of collecting tubules. Areas of lighter-coloured tissue called renal columns are extensions of the cortex and serve to separate the pyramids. The collecting tubules that make up the pyramids channel urine into the innermost region, the renal pelvis.

The renal pelvis is continuous with the ureter as it leaves the hilum. Branches of the pelvis known as the major and minor calyces extend towards the medulla and serve to collect urine and empty it into the pelvis. From the pelvis, urine is channelled through the ureter and into the bladder for storage. The walls of the calyces, the renal pelvis and the ureter contain smooth muscle that moves urine along by peristalsis.

Each kidney contains approximately 1 million nephrons, which process the blood to make urine (see Figure 25.3). Each nephron consists of a renal corpuscle and a renal tubule (Martini et al., 2017). The renal corpuscle contains a tuft of capillaries called the glomerulus, which is completely surrounded by the glomerular capsule (or Bowman's space). The renal tubule is a

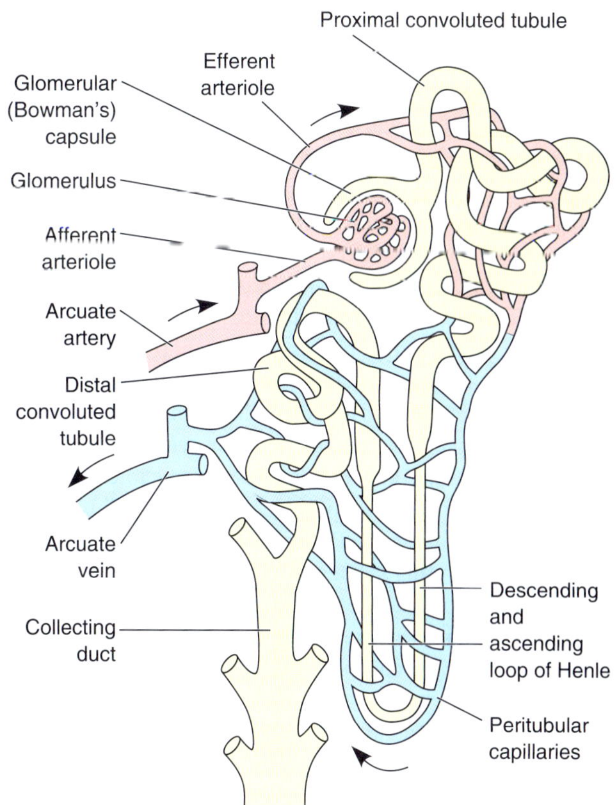

FIGURE 25.3 ***The structure of a nephron, showing the glomerulus within the glomerular capsule***

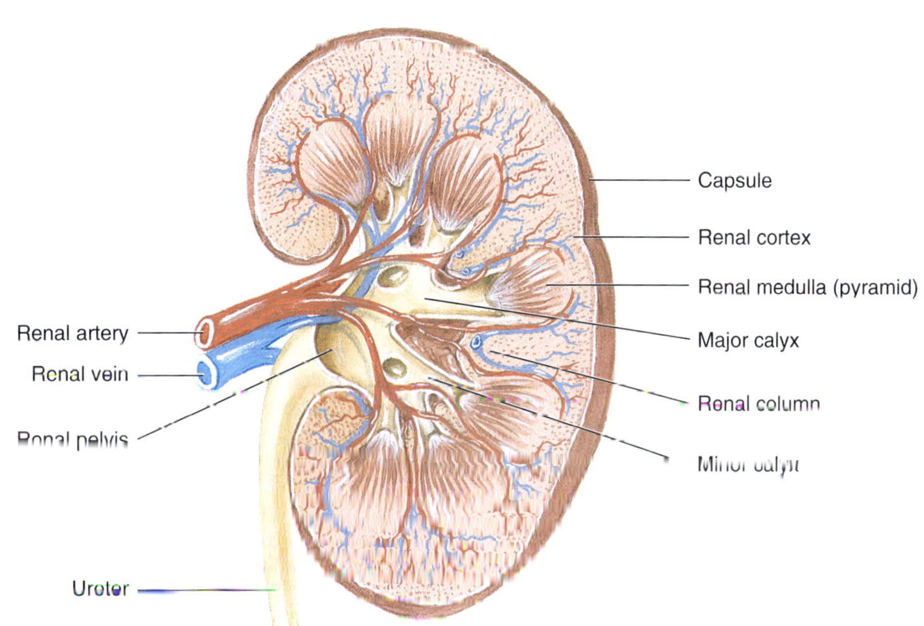

FIGURE 25.2 ***Internal anatomy of the kidney***

tubular passageway that may be up to 50 mm in length (Martini et al., 2017).

The endothelium of the glomerulus allows capillaries to be extremely porous. Thus, large amounts of solute-rich fluid pass from the capillaries into the capsule. This fluid, called the filtrate, is the raw material of urine. Filtrate leaves the capsule and is channelled into the renal tubule, which consists of two convoluted (twisted or coiled) segments: the proximal convoluted tubule (PCT) and the distal convoluted tubule (DCT) (Martini et al., 2017). In the PCT of the nephron, microvilli on the tubular cells increase the surface area for reabsorption of substances from the filtrate into plasma in the peritubular capillaries. Substances moved by active transport include glucose, sodium, potassium, amino acids, proteins and vitamins. About 70% of the water in the filtrate, as well as chloride and bicarbonate, is reabsorbed by passive transport.

The filtrate then moves into the U-shaped loop of Henle, where it is concentrated. The descending limb of the U is relatively thin and freely permeable to water, whereas the ascending segment is thick and thereby less permeable. The DCT receives filtrate from the loop of Henle. Although this segment is structurally similar to the PCT, it lacks microvilli and is more involved with secreting solutes into the filtrate than in reabsorbing substances from it. The collecting duct receives the newly formed urine from many nephrons and channels urine through the minor and major calyces of the renal pelvis and into the ureter.

The functions of the kidney are to:

- form urine
- balance solute and water transport
- excrete metabolic waste products
- conserve nutrients
- regulate acid–base balance
- secrete hormones to help regulate blood pressure, erythrocyte production and calcium metabolism.

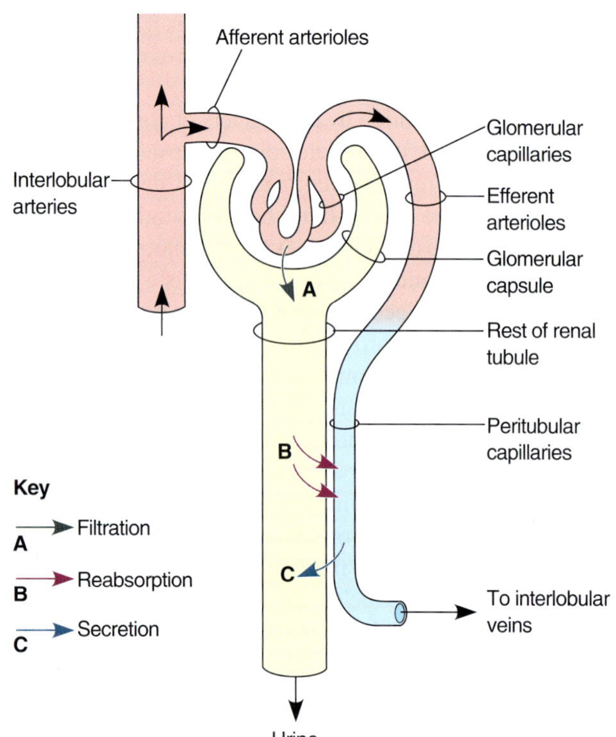

FIGURE 25.4 ***Schematic view of the three major mechanisms by which the kidneys adjust to the composition of plasma: A, glomerular filtration; B, tubular reabsorption; and C, tubular secretion***

Formation of urine

The complex structures of the kidneys process about 180 L of blood-derived fluid each day. Of this amount, only 1% is excreted as urine; the rest is returned to the circulation. Performing a urinalysis is a quick way to early identify infections and some diseases to ensure appropriate management (Chukwu et al., 2022). Normal and abnormal findings of urine on laboratory analysis are listed in Table 25.1. Urine formation is accomplished entirely by the nephron through three processes: glomerular filtration, tubular reabsorption and tubular secretion (see Figure 25.4).

Glomerular filtration

Glomerular filtration is a passive, non-selective process in which hydrostatic pressure forces fluid and solutes through a membrane. The amount of fluid filtered from the blood into the capsule per minute is called the **glomerular filtration rate (GFR)**. Three factors influence this rate: the total surface area available for filtration, the permeability of the filtration membrane and the net filtration pressure.

The glomerulus is a far more efficient filter than most capillary beds because the filtration membrane of the glomerulus is much more permeable to water and solutes than are other capillary membranes. In addition, the glomerular blood pressure is much higher, resulting in higher net filtration pressure.

Net filtration pressure is responsible for the formation of filtrate and is determined by two forces: hydrostatic pressure ('push') and osmotic pressure ('pull'). The glomerular hydrostatic pressure pushes water and solutes across the membrane. This pressure is opposed by the osmotic pressure in the glomerulus (primarily the colloid osmotic pressure of plasma proteins in the glomerular blood) and the capsular hydrostatic pressure exerted by fluids within the glomerular capsule. The difference between these forces determines the net filtration pressure, which is directly proportional to the GFR.

The normal GFR in both kidneys is 120 to 125 mL/min in adults, or about 10% of the blood delivered to the glomeruli (Martini et al., 2017). This rate is held constant under normal conditions by intrinsic controls (or renal autoregulation). The myogenic mechanism, which responds to pressure changes in the renal blood vessels, controls the diameter of the afferent arterioles, thereby achieving autoregulation. An increase in systemic blood pressure causes the renal vessels to constrict, whereas a decline in blood pressure causes the afferent arterioles to dilate. These changes adjust the glomerular hydrostatic pressure and, indirectly, maintain the GFR. The GFR is difficult to measure, so an estimated GFR (eGFR) is calculated from the serum creatinine (Kidney Health Australia (KHA), 2020a). The eGFR is discussed in greater depth in the chapter 'Nursing care of people with kidney disorders'. The normal eGFR in the healthy adult

TABLE 25.1 **Normal and abnormal findings: urinalysis**

CHARACTERISTIC OR COMPONENT	NORMAL RESULTS	ABNORMAL FINDING WITH POSSIBLE CAUSE
Colour	Light straw to deep amber-yellow	• Red, dark, smoky colour may be the result of blood in the urine (haematuria or menstrual blood). • Colourless urine indicates very dilute urine, such as in overhydration, kidney disease, alcohol ingestion or diabetes insipidus. • Dark yellow urine indicates dehydration and/or fever. • Red or red-brown urine may be caused by medications such as phenytoin (Dilantin), chlorpromazine (Largactil) and phenolphthalein (Probanthine), and by beetroot, carrots, rhubarb or food colouring. • Purple urine may be caused by eating beetroot or can occur in people with permanent bladder catheters who have *Escherichia coli* infections; called 'purple bag syndrome'. • Orange urine may be caused by fever, urobilin, nitrofurantoin (Macrodantin), sulfonamides and foods such as carrots or food colouring. • Blue or green urine may be caused by *Pseudomonas* urinary tract infection, ingested substances such as amitriptyline (Endep), methylene blue, cimetidine (Tagamet), propofol (Diprivan) infusion and yeast concentrate. • Brown or black urine may be caused by Lysol poisoning, melanin, bilirubin, methaemoglobin, herbal medicines such as cascara and injectable iron.
Appearance	Clear	• Hazy or cloudy urine indicates bacteria, pus, RBCs, WBCs, phosphates, prostatic fluid spermatozoa or urates. • Milky urine is the result of fats or pyuria. • Yellow foam results from bilirubin, bile or severe cirrhosis of the liver. • Frothy urine may signify protein. • A dark yellow to brownish colour is seen with deficient fluid volume.
Odour	Aromatic	• Ammonia smell increases as urine stands outside the body. • Urinary tract infection (UTI) causes a foul or unpleasant odour, depending on the causative organism. • Asparagus causes a distinctive odour. • Mousy odours result from phenylketonuria. • Sweet or fruity odours occur in starvation and diabetic ketoacidosis.
pH	5-8.0	• $<$ 4.5: metabolic acidosis, respiratory acidosis, diet high in protein or cranberries, ammonium chloride and mandelic acid. • $>$ 8.0: bacteriuria, UTI, antibiotics (neomycin, kanamycin), sulfonamides, sodium bicarbonate, acetazolamide (Diamox), potassium citrate, vegetarian diet, low-carbohydrate diet and ingestion of citrus fruits.
Specific gravity	1.005-1.030	• $<$ 1.005: diabetes insipidus, overhydration, renal disease, severe potassium deficit. • $>$ 1.030: dehydration, fever, diabetes mellitus, vomiting, diarrhoea, contrast media.
Protein	2-8 mg/dL	• $>$ 8 mg/dL: proteinuria, exercise, fever, stress, acute infection, kidney disease, lupus erythematosus, leukaemia, multiple myeloma, cardiac disease, toxaemia of pregnancy, sexual intercourse (in men), septicaemia, lead, mercury, neomycin, barbiturates, sulfonamides.
Glucose	Negative	• $>$ 15 mg/dL: or +4: diabetes mellitus, stroke, Cushing's syndrome, anaesthesia, glucose infusions, severe stress, infections, ascorbic acid, aspirin, cephalosporins and adrenaline.
Ketones	Negative	• +1 to +3: ketoacidosis, starvation, high-protein diet, severe exercise, exposure to cold, loss of carbohydrates.
RBCs	Rare	• $>$ 2 per low-power field: kidney trauma, kidney diseases, renal calculi, cystitis, excess aspirin, anticoagulants, sulfonamides, menstrual contamination. *Note:* high false-positive rate of haematuria with 'dipstick testing'.
WBCs	3-4	• $>$ 4 per low-power field: UTI, fever, strenuous exercise, kidney diseases.
Bilirubin	Negative	• Liver disease, biliary obstruction.
Urobilinogen	Low concentrations	• Liver disease such as hepatitis or cirrhosis, or haemolytic conditions.
Casts	Occasional hyaline	• Fever, kidney diseases, heart failure.

is equal to or greater than 90 mL/min/1.73 m^2. However, an eGFR $<$ 60 mL/min/1.73m^2 is common in older people and should not be labelled as age appropriate as this could be predictive of increased risks of adverse outcomes (KHA, 2020a). Two aspects of the kidney are used to determine kidney function: eGFR and the presence of albuminuria (KHA, 2020a).

Chronic kidney disease (CKD) is defined as the presence of impaired or reduced kidney function that lasts longer than 3 months (Australian Institute of Health and Welfare, 2020). There are difficulties with the terminology as chronic renal failure, kidney impairment, insufficiency and dysfunction have been used interchangeably to describe CKD. Approved nomenclature for kidney function and disease indicates the use of 'CKD' or 'kidney failure' to describe impairment of kidney function that has endured more than 3 months (Levey et al., 2020).

Another intrinsic control of the GFR results from the renin–angiotensin mechanism at work in the kidneys. Special cells known as the juxtaglomerular apparatus are located in the distal tubules and respond to slow filtrate flow by releasing chemicals that cause intense vasodilation of the afferent arterioles. Conversely, an increase in the flow of filtrate promotes vasoconstriction, decreasing the GFR. A drop in systemic blood pressure often triggers the juxtaglomerular cells to release renin. Renin acts on a plasma globulin, angiotensinogen, to release angiotensin I, which is in turn converted to angiotensin II. As a vasoconstrictor, angiotensin II activates vascular smooth muscle throughout the body, causing systemic blood pressure to rise. Thus, the renin–angiotensin mechanism is a factor in renal autoregulation, even though its main purpose is the control of systemic blood pressure.

Glomerular filtration is also under an extrinsic control mechanism through the sympathetic nervous system. During periods of extreme stress or emergency, sympathetic nervous system stimulation causes strong constriction of the afferent arterioles and inhibits filtrate formation. The sympathetic nervous system also stimulates the juxtaglomerular cells to release renin, increasing systemic blood pressure.

Tubular reabsorption

Tubular reabsorption is a transepithelial process that begins as the filtrate enters the proximal tubules. In healthy kidneys, virtually all organic nutrients such as glucose and amino acids are reabsorbed. However, the tubules constantly regulate and adjust the rate and degree of water and ion reabsorption in response to hormonal signals. Reabsorption may be active or passive. Substances reclaimed through active tubular reabsorption are usually moving against electrical and/or chemical gradients. These substances, including glucose, amino acids, lactate, vitamins and most ions, require an ATP-dependent carrier to be transported into the interstitial space. In passive tubular reabsorption, which includes diffusion and osmosis, substances move along their gradient without expenditure of energy.

Tubular secretion

The final process in urine formation is tubular secretion, which is essentially reabsorption in reverse. Substances such as hydrogen and potassium ions, creatinine, ammonia and organic acids move from the blood of the peritubular capillaries into the tubules themselves as filtrate. Thus, urine consists of both filtered and secreted substances. Tubular secretion is important for disposing of substances not already in the filtrate, such as medications. This process eliminates undesirable substances that have been reabsorbed by passive processes and rids the body of excessive potassium ions. It is also a vital force in the regulation of blood pH.

Maintaining normal composition and volume of urine

Maintaining the normal composition and volume of urine involves a countercurrent exchange system. In this system, fluid flows in opposite directions through the parallel tubes of the loop of Henle and the vasa recta, tiny capillaries that run along the loop of Henle. Fluid is exchanged across these parallel membranes in response to a concentration gradient (see Figure 25.5). When the filtrate enters the proximal convoluted tubule, its osmolality (300 mOsm/kg) is the same as plasma and

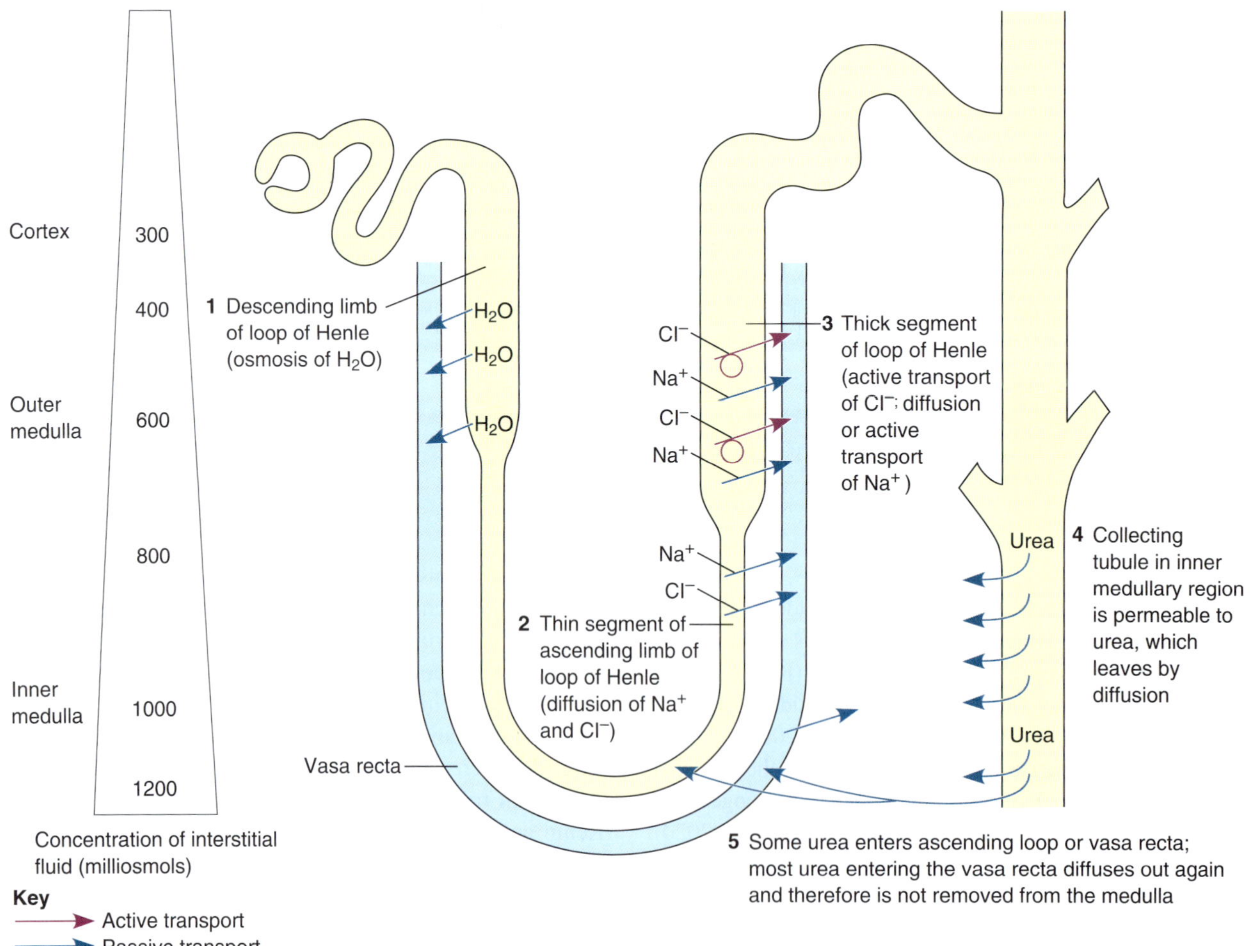

FIGURE 25.5 ***The countercurrent exchange system is responsible for establishing and maintaining an osmotic gradient necessary to the composition, volume and pH of urine***

the interstitial fluid of the renal cortex. Note the following steps in the process:

1. The descending loop of Henle is highly permeable to water and allows chloride and sodium to enter the loop through diffusion. The hyperosmotic interstitium causes water to move out of the descending loop, so remaining filtrate becomes increasingly concentrated.
2. The lumen of the ascending loop of Henle is impermeable to water but allows chloride and sodium to move out into the interstitium of the medulla. As a result, the filtrate in the ascending loop becomes hypoosmotic and the medullary interstitium becomes hyperosmotic.
3. As the filtrate progresses through the ascending limb of the loop of Henle and enters the distal convoluted tubule, sodium and chloride are removed and water is retained. Thus, the filtrate becomes more dilute.
4. As the filtrate passes through the deep medullary regions, urea (an end product of protein metabolism and, along with water, the main constituent of urine) begins to diffuse out from the collecting tubules into the interstitial space and establishes a concentration gradient to facilitate water movement.
5. Some urea enters the ascending loop of Henle. Urea entering the vasa recta typically diffuses out again.

The dilution or concentration of urine is largely determined by the action of antidiuretic hormone (ADH), which is secreted by the posterior pituitary gland. ADH causes the pores of the collecting tubules to enlarge, so that increased amounts of water move into the interstitial space. As the end result, water is reabsorbed and urine is more highly concentrated. When ADH is not secreted, the filtrate passes through the system without further water reabsorption, so that the urine is more dilute.

Urine is composed, by volume, of about 95% water and 5% solutes. The largest component of urine by weight is urea. Other solutes normally excreted in the urine include sodium, potassium, phosphate, sulfate, creatinine, uric acid, calcium, magnesium and bicarbonate.

Clearing waste products

The kidneys excrete water-soluble waste products and other chemicals or substances from the body. This process is called renal plasma clearance, which refers to the ability of the kidneys to clear (cleanse) a given amount of plasma of a particular substance in a given time (usually 1 minute). The kidneys clear 25 to 30 g of **urea** (a nitrogenous waste product formed in the liver from the breakdown of amino acids) each day. They also clear **creatinine** (an end product of creatine phosphate, found in skeletal muscle), uric acid (a metabolite of nucleic acid metabolism) and ammonia, as well as bacterial toxins and water-soluble drugs. Tests of renal clearance are often used to determine the GFR and glomerular damage.

Renal hormones

Hormones that are either activated or synthesised by the kidneys include the active form of vitamin D, erythropoietin and natriuretic hormone.

Vitamin D is necessary for the absorption of calcium and phosphate by the small intestine. In an inactive form, vitamin D enters the body either by dietary intake or through the action of ultraviolet rays on cholesterol in the skin. Activation occurs in two steps, the first in the liver and the second in the kidneys. The renal step is stimulated by parathyroid hormone, which in turn responds to a decreased plasma calcium level. High calcium and phosphate levels may lead to calcium deposits in the small capillaries in the eyes, lungs and heart. Calcium deposits increase the risk of cardiovascular disease over time (KHA, 2020b).

Erythropoietin (EPO) stimulates the bone marrow to produce red blood cells in response to tissue hypoxia. The stimulus to produce erythropoietin by the kidneys is decreased oxygen delivery to kidney cells.

The right atria of the heart releases natriuretic hormone in response to increased volume and stretch, as occurs in increased extracellular volume. This hormone inhibits ADH secretion, so that the collecting tubules are less porous and a large amount of dilute urine is produced.

THE URETERS

The ureters are bilateral tubes approximately 25 to 30 cm long. They transport urine from the kidney to the bladder through peristaltic waves originating in the renal pelvis. The wall of the ureter has three layers: an inner epithelial mucosa, a middle layer of smooth muscle and an outer layer of fibrous connective tissue.

THE URINARY BLADDER

The urinary bladder is posterior to the pubic symphysis and serves as a storage site for urine. In males, the bladder lies immediately in front of the rectum; in females, the bladder lies in front of the vagina and the uterus. Openings for the ureters and the urethra are inside the bladder: the trigone is the smooth triangular portion of the base of the bladder outlined by these three openings (see Figure 25.6).

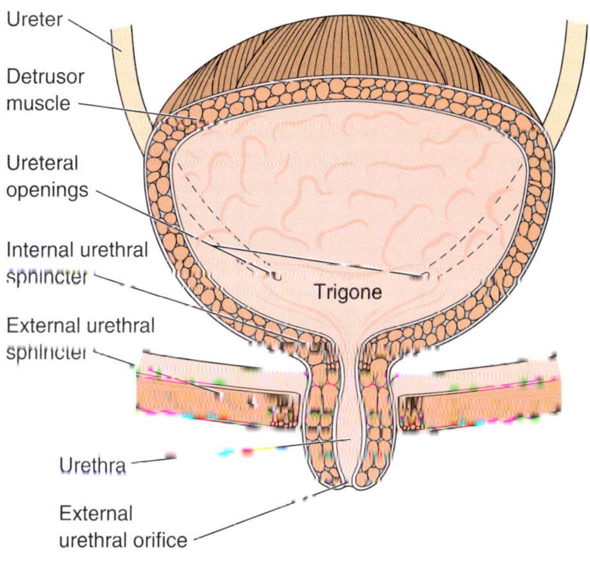

FIGURE 25.6 ***Internal view of the urinary bladder and trigone***

The layers of the bladder wall (from internal to external) are the epithelial mucosa lining the inside, the connective tissue submucosa, the smooth muscle layer and the fibrous outer layer. The muscle layer, called the detrusor muscle, consists of fibres arranged in inner and outer longitudinal layers and in a middle circular layer. This arrangement allows the bladder to expand or contract according to the amount of urine it holds.

The size of the bladder varies with the amount of urine it contains. In healthy adults, the bladder holds about 300 to 500 mL of urine before internal pressure rises and signals the need to empty the bladder through **micturition** (also called urination or voiding). However, the bladder can hold more than twice that amount if necessary. The bladder has an internal urethral sphincter that relaxes in response to a full bladder and signals the need to urinate. A second external urethral sphincter is formed by skeletal muscle and is under voluntary control.

THE URETHRA

The urethra is a thin-walled muscular tube that channels urine to the outside of the body. It extends from the base of the bladder to the external urinary meatus. In females, the urethra is approximately 3 to 5 cm long and the urinary meatus is anterior to the vaginal orifice. In males, the urethra is approximately 20 cm long and serves as a channel for semen as well as urine. The prostate gland encircles the urethra at the base of the bladder in males. The male urinary meatus is located at the end of the glans penis.

HEALTH ASSESSMENT, DIAGNOSTICS AND DOCUMENTATION

Renal system function is assessed by findings from a health assessment interview to collect subjective data, a physical assessment to collect objective data and diagnostic tests. Sample documentation of an assessment of renal system function is included in the 'Sample documentation' box.

Health assessment interview

A health assessment interview to determine problems with urinary structure and function may be conducted during a health screening, may focus on a chief complaint (such as burning on urination or difficulty starting the stream when urinating) or may be part of a total health assessment. As with alterations in bowel function, people with problems with renal system function may be embarrassed to talk about urinary elimination patterns. It is often helpful to discuss less personal information first.

Current urinary status should include the following data:

- colour, odour and amount of urine
- difficulty initiating a stream of urine
- frequency of urination
- painful urination (**dysuria**)
- excessive urination at night (**nocturia**)
- blood in the urine (**haematuria**)
- voiding scant amounts of urine (**oliguria**)
- voiding excessive amounts of urine (**polyuria**)
- discharge
- flank pain.

If you identify a problem with urinary elimination, analyse its onset, characteristics and course, severity, precipitating and relieving factors, and any associated symptoms, noting the timing and circumstances. For example, you may ask the following questions:

- Have you noticed any burning when you pass urine?
- Do you have difficulty starting to urinate?
- When did you first notice that you were unable to control the loss of urine from your bladder?

Further explore any abnormalities in the person's current renal status. Focus questions on changes in patterns of urination, changes in the urine and pain.

SAMPLE DOCUMENTATION

Assessment of renal system function

10/7/2023 NURS 1030 hrs — Home visit made to 66-year-old woman with end-stage chronic kidney disease. Skin pale and oral mucous membranes dry. 4+ oedema in ankles and feet. Eyelids swollen. Skin tight and shiny over abdomen and bilateral lower extremities. Abdomen distended and tender on light palpation; further palpation deferred. Urinary bladder not palpable. Urine output for past 24 hours is 15 mL.__________ A Lam

(APRIL LAM, RN)

Links to National Patient Safety Standards

NSQHS: Partnering with Consumers Standard

In line with the intent of the NSQHS Partnering with Consumers Standard (Australian Commission on Safety and Quality in Health Care (ACSQHC), 2021) and creating a consumer-centred approach, nurses when conducting renal assessment and obtaining a history should include patients in the decision-making processes. People experiencing incontinence may be reluctant to discuss or disclose information, potentially impacting on healthcare decisions. Here, the nurse must consider and be respectful of the individual's concerns when collecting health information to ensure plans developed incorporate their concerns.

Identify opportunities for open communication such as conducting assessments in a private environment, discussing less personal information first, regular communication checks during healthcare team rounds and establishing an agreed communication process (written and verbal).

Source: ACSQHC (2021). *National Safety and Quality Health Service Standards* (2nd ed.). Sydney: ACSQHC. © Australian Commission on Safety and Quality in Health Care. https://www.safetyandquality.gov.au/standards/nsqhs-standards/partnering-consumers-standard

Assess changes in patterns of urination by asking the person: How many times a day do you urinate? Do you feel that you empty your bladder each time? How many times do you get up at night to urinate? Do you experience a very strong desire to urinate and feel that you just cannot wait? Have you noticed that you urinate small amounts of dark, strong-smelling urine?

Changes in the urine that should be explored include the presence of blood or a cloudy appearance of the urine. If the person has noticed blood, explore the use of medications (such as anticoagulants or dye-containing drugs) and other bleeding problems. Women may not understand that blood in the toilet or on toilet tissue after urination is normal during menstruation. Cloudy, foul-smelling urine often indicates infection (**pyuria**); ask the person about temperature elevations, chills and general malaise. Cloudy urine in men may result from retrograde ejaculation (when semen is discharged into the bladder instead of from the penis) during ejaculation.

If the person reports pain, explore its location, duration and intensity. Kidney pain is experienced in the back and the costovertebral angle (the angle between the lower ribs and adjacent vertebrae) and may spread towards the umbilicus. Renal colic (pain in response to renal calculi moving through the ureter) is severe, sharp, stabbing and excruciating; often it is felt in the flank, bladder, urethra, testes or ovaries. Bladder and urethral pain is usually dull and continuous but may be experienced as spasms. The person with a distended bladder experiences constant pain increased by any pressure over the bladder.

Information about surgeries or other treatment of previous urinary problems is essential to the health history, as is a family history of altered structure or function. A family history of kidney problems may be the first clue to abnormalities in the person's kidney function. Explore information regarding family occurrence of end-stage renal disease, renal calculi and frequent infections, as well as related problems such as hypertension and diabetes mellitus.

Questions about cultural background, lifestyle, diet and work history should explore cigarette smoking and/or exposure to toxic chemicals (to identify risks for cancer), usual fluid intake, type of fluid intake and self-care measures to replace fluids lost during work or physical activity in hot temperatures.

Interview questions categorised by functional health patterns are listed in the 'Functional health pattern interview' box.

PATIENT SAFETY COMPETENCY FRAMEWORK

3 Cultural competence

The Patient Safety Competency Framework indicates that nursing students should demonstrate cultural competence by respecting each person's cultural values, beliefs, life experiences and health practices (Levett-Jones et al., 2017).

FUNCTIONAL HEALTH PATTERN INTERVIEW Renal system

FUNCTIONAL HEALTH PATTERN	INTERVIEW QUESTIONS AND LEADING STATEMENTS
Health perception–Health management	■ Have you ever had a bladder or kidney disease, injury or surgery? Describe.
	■ If so, how was the problem treated?
	■ Describe your usual intake of fluids for a 24-hour period. What type of fluids do you drink?
	■ Have you ever smoked? If so, how many cigarettes per day?
	■ Describe the problem you are having with your kidneys or bladder.
	■ Are you taking medications for this or any other health problem? If so, what do you take and how often?
	■ *For women.* Describe how you care for yourself when you urinate (e.g. direction of wiping with tissue).
	■ If you have a surgical diversion of urine, describe how you care for yourself. (What skin and appliance care do you use? How often do you empty the bag?)
	■ Do you wear or have you ever worn an external catheter, indwelling catheter or incontinence briefs? Explain.
	■ Have you ever done self-catheterisation? If so, why and how often?
Nutritional–Metabolic	■ How much coffee, tea or alcohol do you drink in a 24-hour period?
	■ Have you ever limited your fluid intake? Explain.
	■ Do you limit the amount of salt you eat? Explain.
	■ Do you have swelling in your ankles? If so, what do you do?
Elimination	■ How many times a day do you urinate? Do you have to get up at night to urinate? Has there been a change in your usual pattern of urination?

(continued)

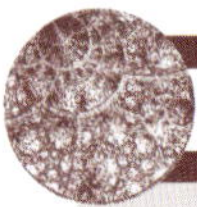

FUNCTIONAL HEALTH PATTERN INTERVIEW **Renal system (continued)**

FUNCTIONAL HEALTH PATTERN	INTERVIEW QUESTIONS AND LEADING STATEMENTS
	■ Do you experience a sudden urge to urinate?
	■ Has there been a change in your urine, such as a change in amount, colour or odour? Have you ever noticed blood in your urine or on the tissue after you wipe?
	■ Is it difficult for you to begin or end your flow of urine?
	■ Have you ever had problems controlling your urine when you laugh, sneeze or cough?
	■ Do you have any discharge from your urethra? Explain.
Activity–Exercise	■ Do your urinary problems interfere with your activities of daily living? Explain.
	■ Describe your usual energy level. Has there been a change? Explain.
	■ Have you ever been taught to do Kegel exercises to help you control your urination? If so, how often do you practise these?
Sleep–Rest	■ Does a problem with urination interfere with your ability to sleep and rest? Explain.
	■ Has there been a change in the number of times you wake up at night to urinate? Explain.
Cognitive–Perceptual	■ Do you have any pain or burning when you urinate?
	■ Have you experienced any tenderness or pain over the lower sides of your back or severe pain that spreads over your lower abdomen? If so, describe its location, intensity, aggravating factors and duration.
Self-perception–Self-concept	■ How does having this condition make you feel about yourself?
Role–Relationships	■ How does having this condition affect your relationships with others?
Sexuality–Reproductive	■ Has this condition interfered with your usual sexual activity?
Coping–Stress–Tolerance	■ Has having this condition created stress for you?
	■ Have you experienced any kind of stress that makes this condition worse? Explain.
	■ Describe what you do when you feel stressed.
Value–Belief	■ Describe how specific relationships or activities help you cope with this problem.
	■ Describe specific cultural beliefs or practices that affect how you care for and feel about this problem.
	■ Are there any specific treatments that you would not use to treat this condition?

Physical assessment

The structure and function of the renal system is assessed by examination of the skin, abdomen, kidneys, bladder and urinary meatus. Guidelines for abdominal assessment are outlined in the chapter 'A person-centred approach to assessing the gastrointestinal system'. Normal age-related changes in the kidney are summarised in Tables 25.2 and 27.2. These changes are similar to changes seen with chronic kidney disease (CKD).

Physical assessment of the renal system may be performed as part of a total health assessment, as part of an abdominal assessment or as part of a back examination (for the kidneys). The techniques of inspection, auscultation, palpation and percussion are used.

Before beginning the assessment, ask the person to provide a clean urine specimen. Assess the specimen for colour, odour and clarity before sending to the laboratory.

Prior to the examination, collect all necessary equipment and explain the techniques to the person to decrease anxiety. Because the examination involves exposure of the genital area, give the person a gown and drape them appropriately to minimise exposure.

Guidelines for percussion and palpation of the kidneys are outlined in Box 25.1. This is an advanced assessment skill and should not be performed without an understanding of the patient's history or underlying disease processes.

CONSIDERATION FOR PRACTICE

Auscultate immediately after inspection, because percussion or palpation may increase bowel motility and interfere with sound transmission during auscultation.

TABLE 25.2 Age-related renal system changes

AGE-RELATED CHANGE	SIGNIFICANCE
Kidneys: ↓ loss of renal mass, ↓ cortical volume, ↓ medullary volume, ↓ growth of renal tissue, atherosclerosis and constriction, all of which may result in atrophy of the kidneys (Rowland et al., 2018).	• ↓ renal blood flow. • ↓ GFR by about 50% between ages 20 and 90. eGFR of < 60 mL/min/1.73 m^2 is very common in older people (KHA, 2020a).
Renal tubules: ↓ number and length of proximal tubules, diverticular and cysts of distal tubules, ↓ function, with less effective exchange of substances, water and sodium conservation, and plasma renin and aldosterone levels; ↑ vasoconstrictive response to stimuli (e.g. volume depletion) (Rowland et al., 2018).	• Risk of dehydration, hyponatraemia, hyperkalaemia and nocturia. • Effects of medications may be altered (with decreased filtration). • ↓ reabsorption of glucose may result in proteinuria and glycosuria, which are not of major clinical significance.
Bladder: • Muscles weaken and bladder capacity decreases. • More difficult to empty bladder. • Delayed micturition reflex. • Prostatic gland enlargement compresses the urethra (Martini et al., 2017).	• Urinary frequency, urgency and nocturia are more common with ageing. • Larger amounts of residual urine present after voiding. • Some stress incontinence may occur, especially in women who have had several children. • Urinary incontinence is not a normal outcome of ageing. • Urinary retention is more common.

BOX 25.1 Guidelines for physical assessment of the kidneys

Percussion of the kidneys

Percussion of the kidneys helps assess pain or tenderness. Assist the person to a sitting position and stand behind them. For indirect percussion, place the palm of your non-dominant hand over the costovertebral angle (see Figure A). Strike this area with the ulnar surface of your dominant hand, curled into a fist (see Figure B). For direct percussion, also strike the area over the costovertebral angle with the ulnar surface of your dominant hand, curled into a fist. Repeat the technique for the other kidney. Kidneys should be percussed with just enough pressure that the person feels a gentle thud; fingertip pressure may be enough to elicit tenderness (Bilal et al., 2017). Percussion is usually done at the end of the assessment.

Palpation of the kidneys

Although the technique of palpation of the kidneys is outlined here, this technique is best performed by an advanced practitioner because it involves deep palpation. In addition, the kidneys are difficult to palpate.

Assist the person to the supine position and stand at their right side. To palpate the left kidney, reach across the person and place your left hand under their left flank with your palm upward. Elevate the left flank with your fingers, displacing the kidney upward. Ask the person to take a deep breath and use the palmar surface of your right hand to palpate the kidney (see Figure C) (Bilal et al., 2017). Repeat the technique for the right kidney, which may be more anterior and should be distinguished from the liver, which feels sharper.

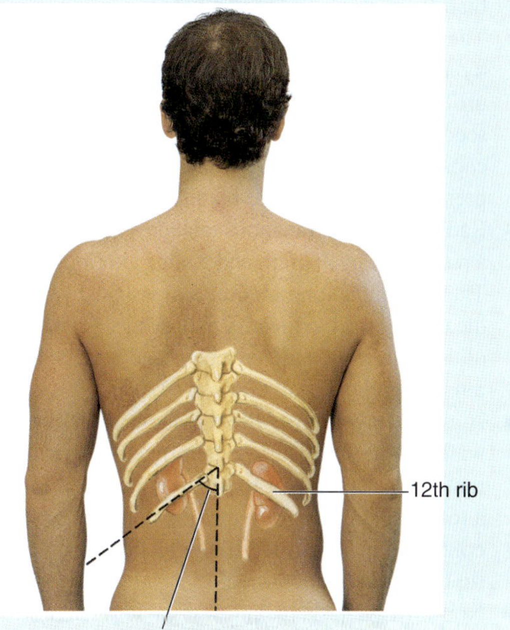

***A** Location of the kidneys and the costovertebral angle*

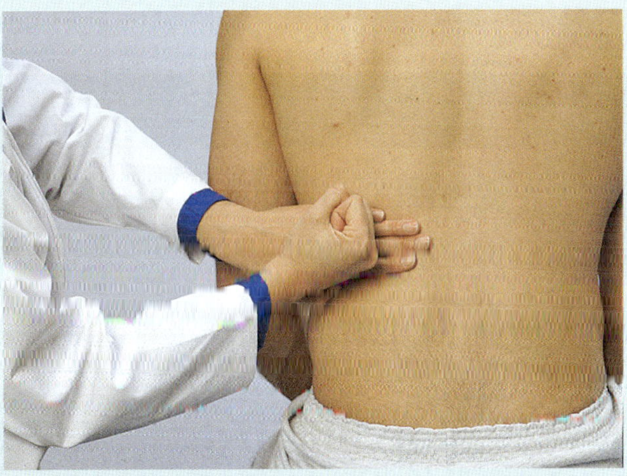

***B** Percussing the kidney*

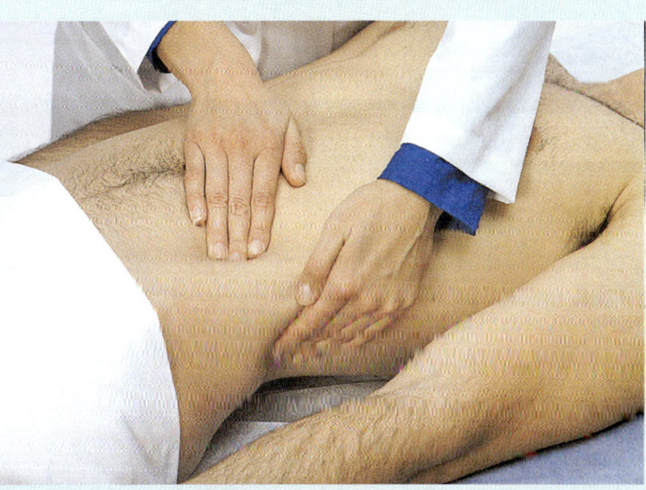

***C** Palpating the left kidney*

Diagnostic tests

The results of diagnostic tests of renal system function are used to support the diagnosis of a specific disease, to provide information to identify or modify the appropriate medication or therapy, and to monitor the person's responses to treatment and nursing care interventions. Diagnostic tests used to assess the structures and functions of the renal system are described in the 'Diagnostic tests' box and summarised in the bulleted list that follows. More information is included in the discussion of specific disorders in the chapters 'Nursing care of people with urinary tract disorders' and 'Nursing care of people with kidney disorders'.

- Urine may be tested through routine analysis, a urine culture, a post-voiding residual urine and a 24-hour collection for creatinine. Results of these tests include findings to serve as baseline data, to support diagnosis of various health problems, to evaluate the ability to empty the bladder of urine and to evaluate kidney function.
- The ability to empty the bladder of urine may be evaluated by a portable bladder scan to evaluate for residual urine, uroflowmetry to measure the volume of urine voided per second and a cystometrogram (CMG) to evaluate bladder capacity, neuromuscular functions of the bladder, urethral pressures and causes of bladder dysfunction.
- Radiological examinations include an intravenous pyelogram, a retrograde pyelogram and a renal arteriogram or angiogram. These examinations are useful in visualising (via x-ray film) the urinary tract to identify abnormal size, shape and function of the kidneys, the kidney pelvis and ureters; and to detect renal **calculi** (stones), tumours or cysts.
- A cystoscopy allows direct visualisation of the bladder wall and urethra. During the procedure small stones can be removed, a sample of tissue may be taken for biopsy and a retrograde pyelogram may be done at the same time. If a contrast dye is instilled in the bladder, fistulas, tumours or ruptures can be identified.
- Non-invasive tests include a renal ultrasound, computed tomography (CT) scan, magnetic resonance imaging (MRI) and renal scan. These tests are used to identify and evaluate kidney size and structure, as well as renal or perirenal masses and obstructions. In addition, a renal scan may be used to evaluate kidney blood flow, perfusion and urine production.
- A kidney biopsy is done to obtain tissue to diagnose or monitor kidney disease.

The nurse should explain the procedure and required preparation, assess medication use that may affect the outcome of the tests, support the person during the examination as necessary and document and monitor the results of the tests.

Genetic considerations

When conducting a health assessment interview and physical assessment, consider the genetic influences on adult health (see the 'Genetic considerations' box). Ask if family members have health problems affecting kidney function such as polycystic disease or diabetes mellitus. If data are found to indicate genetic risk factors or alterations, ask about genetic testing and refer for appropriate genetic counselling and evaluation. The chapter 'Genetic implications of adult health nursing' provides further information about genetics in medical–surgical nursing.

GENETIC CONSIDERATIONS Renal system

- Autosomal dominant polycystic kidney disease (ADPKD), or adult polycystic kidney disease, is an inherited disease characterised by large cysts in one or both kidneys. It is the most commonly inherited kidney disease, with rates of 1:500 to 1:4,000 in Australia. Because of its inheritance pattern, there is a 50% chance that the children of people with PKD will inherit the disorder. Hypertension is an early finding in ADPKD, affecting 60% of people, more commonly in males (KHA, 2020c).
- CKD may be a complication of type 1 and type 2 diabetes mellitus (DM), but is seen more often in people with type 1 DM. Type 1 and type 2 DM are classified as multifactorial inheritance disorders because both genetic and environmental factors are necessary for onset of the disorder.

DIAGNOSTIC TESTS Renal system disorders

NAME OF TEST Serum urea

PURPOSE AND DESCRIPTION This blood test measures urea, the end product of protein metabolism. Increased levels may result from dehydration, vomiting, diarrhoea, GI bleeding, renal impairment, excessive protein catabolism or congestive cardiac failure. It may be decreased with protein deficiency in diet, dieresis and pregnancy.

Normal values:
3.0–8.0 mmol/L

RELATED NURSING CARE No special preparation is needed. If values are increased in a person who is dehydrated, they should return to normal with hydration. If not, this is an indicator of renal impairment.

DIAGNOSTIC TESTS Renal system disorders (continued)

NAME OF TEST Serum creatinine

PURPOSE AND DESCRIPTION This blood test is used to diagnose renal impairment. Creatinine is a by-product of the breakdown of muscle and is excreted by the kidneys. Serum creatinine levels may rise when 50% or more nephrons are destroyed or there is acute muscle wasting. Levels may fall with chronic muscle wastage (such as muscular dystrophy, muscle sclerosis).

Normal values:
Serum (adult female): 0.05–0.11. Serum (adult male): 0.06–0.12 mmol/L. (Creatinine varies with size and muscle mass. Older adults may have decreased values due to decreased muscle mass.)

RELATED NURSING CARE No special preparation is needed. Values may be increased by antibiotics, ascorbic acid, L-dopa, methyldopa and lithium carbonate. Values are not affected by hydration status. Three to four hours after eating meat the plasma creatinine can double, so fasting prior to measurements may be recommended.

NAME OF TEST Estimated glomerular filtration rate (eGFR)

PURPOSE AND DESCRIPTION GFR is the best measurement of kidney function; the eGFR can estimate the GFR.

Normal values:
GFR < 60 mL/min/1.73 m^2 for 3 months. Normal findings and abnormal findings with causes are outlined in Table 25.1.

RELATED NURSING CARE eGFR may be unreliable if diet is vegetarian, high in protein or includes creatine supplements; in people with large muscle mass and amputees; in children under 18 years; and in those with severe liver disease.

NAME OF TEST Routine urinalysis (UA) (dipstick or ward urinalysis)

PURPOSE AND DESCRIPTION An examination of the constituents of a sample of urine to establish a baseline, to provide data for diagnosis or to monitor results of treatment. Normal findings and abnormal findings with causes are outlined in Table 25.1.

RELATED NURSING CARE Provide a clean specimen cup for a sample of urine. Note if the person is menstruating. Assess medications, fluid status and foods that might affect urinalysis results.

NAME OF TEST Urine culture (microscopy urine (MSU), clean-catch)

PURPOSE AND DESCRIPTION A culture of a urine sample to identify the causative organism of a urinary tract infection (UTI).

Normal value:
< 10,000 organisms/mL (urine is sterile but urethra contains bacteria and a few WBCs).

Values of > 100,000 organisms/mL indicate UTI.

RELATED NURSING CARE Provide the person with sterile container. Ask women to separate labia with one hand and clean labia with other hand, using sterile cotton sponges saturated with a cleansing solution (may be 0.9% sodium chloride) and wiping three times front to back. Ask men to retract the foreskin and cleanse glans with three cotton sponges saturated with a cleansing solution, using a circular motion. After cleaning, ask the person to begin voiding and then collect specimen in the container (initial voiding will contain urethral contaminants). If the person is unable to void, it may be necessary to obtain a specimen with a urinary catheterisation.

NAME OF TEST Urinary albumin:creatinine ratio (ACR)

PURPOSE AND DESCRIPTION Used to detect albumin (a protein) in the urine. A marker of kidney damage is excessive amounts of albumin in the urine (**albuminuria**). The presence of albuminuria is determined by the albumin-to-creatinine ratio (ACR). Low levels of albumin in the urine are normal; however, levels increase with age, reaching the highest levels after the age of 70 (Barzilay et al., 2020). Other causes of transient elevations in urinary ACR include UTIs, diurnal variations in urinary excretion, non-steroidal anti-inflammatory drugs (NSAIDs), fluid overload and acute febrile illness (AACB, 2022). Elevated ACR may occur when kidney damage is present.

Normal value:
< 30 mg albumin/g creatinine (RCPA, 2022)

Microalbuminuria: 30 to 300 mg albumin/g creatinine (RCPA, 2022)

Macroalbuminuria: > 300 mg albumin/g creatinine (RCPA, 2022)

(continued)

DIAGNOSTIC TESTS **Renal system disorders (continued)**

Evaluations of significance can include an increased excretion of albumin (> 30 mg/g creatinine) of insufficient degree to be detected by urinalysis. This may be an early sign of diabetic nephropathy. Further, microalbuminuria (30–300 mg/g creatinine) may be considered an early marker of renal damage. This could be progressive if risk factors are not adequately treated (RCPA, 2022). Vigorous exercise should be avoided 24 hours prior to testing (RCPA, 2022).

RELATED NURSING CARE This should be a first-void spot specimen. Albuminuria is said to be present if two out of three ACR results are positive (National Kidney Foundation, 2022). A routine 'dipstick' for protein in the urine is not recommended to investigate for CKD.

NAME OF TEST Portable ultrasonic bladder scan

PURPOSE AND DESCRIPTION Used to obtain information about bladder volume or residual urine left in the bladder after voiding. Where possible, place the person in a supine position. Warm ultrasound gel and apply over the lower abdomen. The ultrasound probe is placed just above the pubic bone. Select 'male' on the machine if the person has had a hysterectomy. The scanner shows an outline of the bladder and displays the amount of urine in the bladder in millilitres. Obtain several readings and use the largest (the most accurate). Print the information, place it on the person's chart and document the residual urine amount.

RELATED NURSING CARE No special preparation is needed, but the test is usually not used for pregnant women. Remember, the machine will measure any fluid collection in the suprapubic region such as ascites, haematoma or lymphocele. Report and monitor a residual of more than 100 mL or if the residual is greater than the amount voided. A urinary catheter may have to be inserted if the volume is greater than 600 mL, or if the person has not voided for 5 to 6 hours or is uncomfortable.

NAME OF TEST Creatinine clearance

PURPOSE AND DESCRIPTION A 24-hour urine test and a blood sample (collected at either the end or beginning of the 24-hour urine collection) are used to identify renal dysfunction and to monitor renal function.

Normal value:

90–125 mL/min

Calculation of estimated glomerular function rate (eGFR), using a single blood sample, is another straightforward method of estimating kidney function.

RELATED NURSING CARE Assess medications: drugs that may decrease the creatinine clearance measurement are steroids, aminoglycosides, thiazides, cimetidine, cisplatin and cephalosporins. Ascorbic acid, steroids, methyldopa (Aldomet), cefoxitin and diuretics can increase the result. Levels of creatinine are elevated in hypothyroidism, hypertension, pregnancy and exercise.

Obtain appropriate specimen container. Ask person to void and discard first voiding. Instruct the person, family and staff to then save all urine for a clearly designated 24-hour period, keeping the specimen in the fridge. If the person misses a sample, the test is invalid.

NAME OF TEST Uroflowmetry

PURPOSE AND DESCRIPTION This test measures the volume passed per second, maximum and average flow rate, and voiding time.

RELATED NURSING CARE Ask the person to increase fluid intake and refrain from voiding for several hours before the test to ensure a full bladder and a strong urge to void during testing. Tell the person they will be asked to urinate into a funnel. Residual urine may be measured following the test.

NAME OF TEST Micturating cysto-urethrogram (cystometrogram (CMG))

PURPOSE AND DESCRIPTION Conducted to evaluate bladder capacity and neuromuscular functions of the bladder, urethral pressures and causes of bladder dysfunction. A measured quantity of fluid (contrast media) is instilled into the bladder (via urethral catheter) and the filling capacity and voiding pressures are measured. The catheter is removed and a series of x-ray pictures are taken as the person micturates. A catheter may also be placed in the rectum during the test.

RELATED NURSING CARE Tell the person that the bladder will be filled and during filling they will be asked to describe the first urge to void and the sensation of being unable to delay urination any longer.

DIAGNOSTIC TESTS Renal system disorders (continued)

NAME OF TEST Intravenous pyelogram (IVP)

PURPOSE AND DESCRIPTION This radiological examination is done to visualise the entire urinary tract to identify abnormal size, shape and function of the kidneys, or to detect renal calculi (stones), tumours or cysts. A urinary catheter is placed into the bladder and a radiopaque substance is injected intravenously and a series of x-rays taken.

PERSON PREPARATION

- Assess knowledge and understanding of procedure, clarifying information as needed. The person may have to fast (from food); clear fluids allowed up to 2 hours prior to the procedure.
- Schedule IVP prior to any ordered barium test or gallbladder studies using contrast material.
- Assess if the person has any form of reaction to x-ray contrast dye, or an iodine or seafood allergy, or if they are asthmatic.
- Verify the presence of a signed consent for the procedure.
- Assess renal and fluid status, including serum osmolality, creatinine and urea results. Notify the doctor of any abnormal values.
- Instruct the person to follow preparation protocol. This may include pre-test bowel preparation and fasting for 3 hours prior to the procedure.
- Obtain baseline vital signs and record.

AFTER THE TEST

- Monitor vital signs and urine output.
- Report manifestations of delayed reaction to the contrast media such as dyspnoea, tachycardia, itching, hives or flushing.

HEALTH EDUCATION FOR THE PERSON AND FAMILY

- X-rays and a dye that is rapidly excreted in the urine are used to show the structures of the kidney, ureters and bladder. The test takes about 30 minutes.
- As the dye is injected, you may feel a transient warm flushing sensation along with possible nausea and a metallic taste.
- A wide band may be placed around your waist at some stage and tightened for a few minutes to stop the contrast from draining to the bladder through the ureters (the tubes joining the kidneys to the bladder).
- Notify your doctor immediately if you develop a rash, difficulty breathing, rapid heart rate or hives during or after the test.
- Increase fluid intake after the test is completed.

NAME OF TEST Retrograde pyelogram

PURPOSE AND DESCRIPTION This radiological test is done to evaluate the structures of the ureters and kidney pelvis. It may be performed alone or in conjunction with a cystoscopy. A contrast dye is injected through a catheter into the ureters and kidney pelvis and x-rays are taken.

RELATED NURSING CARE Nursing care for the person having a retrograde pyelogram is the same as that for people having an IVP.

NAME OF TEST Renal arteriogram or angiogram

PURPOSE AND DESCRIPTION This radiological test is done to visualise renal blood vessels in order to detect renal artery stenosis, renal thrombosis or embolism, tumours, cysts or aneurysm; to determine the causative factor for hypertension; and to evaluate renal circulation. A contrast medium is injected into the femoral artery.

RELATED NURSING CARE Assess for allergy to iodine, seafood or other contrast dye from other x ray procedures. A laxative or cleansing enema may be required the night before and the person should be fasted for 8–12 hours prior to the test. Results may be affected by faeces, gas and barium sulfate. Anticoagulants should be discontinued.

After the test, pressure will be applied to the insertion site for up to 20 minutes to prevent bleeding. Continue to monitor for bleeding from the femoral artery, restrict activity for a day, assess peripheral pulses and monitor urine output.

NAME OF TEST Cystoscopy (cystogram), cystography

PURPOSE AND DESCRIPTION Direct visualisation of the bladder wall and urethra is accomplished by using a cystoscope. During the procedure small renal calculi can be removed from the ureter, bladder or urethra and tissue biopsy can be done. It also permits determination of the cause of haematuria or UTI. A stent may be inserted during the procedure to facilitate urinary drainage past an obstruction. A retrograde pyelogram may be done during the cystoscopy. By instilling a contrast dye into the bladder (*cystography*), neurogenic bladder, fistulas, tumours or ruptures can be identified.

(*continued*)

DIAGNOSTIC TESTS Renal system disorders (continued)

PERSON PREPARATION

- Assess knowledge and understanding of the procedure, clarifying information as needed.
- Verify the presence of a signed consent for the procedure.
- Instruct in pre-test preparation as ordered, which may include prescribed antibiotics, laxatives the evening prior to the test or food or fluid restrictions.
- Administer sedation and other medications as ordered prior to the test.
- Cystoscopy is performed using either a local or general anaesthetic. The person may feel some pressure or a need to urinate as the scope is inserted through the urethra into the bladder. The procedure takes approximately 15 to 30 minutes.

HEALTH EDUCATION FOR THE PERSON AND FAMILY

- Burning on urination or more frequent urination for a day or two after the procedure is to be expected.
- Notify the doctor if your urine remains bloody for more than three voidings after the procedure or if you develop bright bleeding, low urine output, abdominal or flank pain, chills or fever.
- Warm baths may help; however, the doctor may ask you to avoid baths.
- Analgesic agents and antispasmodic medications may relieve discomfort after the procedure.
- Increasing fluid intake will flush the bladder, decrease irritation and difficulty voiding, and reduce the risk of infection.

NAME OF TEST Renal ultrasound

PURPOSE AND DESCRIPTION This non-invasive test is conducted to detect renal or perirenal masses, identify obstructions and diagnose renal cysts and solid masses. It is done by applying a conductive gel to the skin and placing a small external ultrasound probe on the person's skin. Sound waves are recorded on a computer as they are reflected off tissues.

RELATED NURSING CARE No special preparation is indicated.

NAME OF TEST CT scan of kidneys

PURPOSE AND DESCRIPTION The CT scan allows evaluation of kidney size, tumours, abscesses, suprarenal masses and obstructions. A contrast dye is injected intravenously, allowing increased visualisation of the density of renal tissue and masses in comparison to an ultrasound.

RELATED NURSING CARE Assess the person for allergies to iodine, x-ray contrast dye and seafood. Tell the person to fast for 4 hours prior to the test and that laxatives or enemas may be ordered to remove gas or faecal material from the bowel.

NAME OF TEST MRI of the kidneys

PURPOSE AND DESCRIPTION An MRI is used to visualise the kidneys by assessing computer-generated films of radiofrequency waves and changes in magnetic fields.

RELATED NURSING CARE Ask the person to remove all metal objects. Assess for metal implants. (Test may not be conducted if present.)

NAME OF TEST Renal scan

PURPOSE AND DESCRIPTION This test is done to evaluate kidney blood flow, location, size and shape; and to assess kidney perfusion and urine production. Radioactive isotopes are injected intravenously and radiation detector probes are placed over the kidneys to monitor activity in the kidneys. Radioisotope distribution in the kidneys is scanned and graphed. Non-functioning tissue, such as in tumours and cysts, appears as cold spots.

RELATED NURSING CARE Ask the person to drink several glasses of water prior to the test. Obtain weight and have the person void. After the procedure, increase fluid intake.

DIAGNOSTIC TESTS Renal system disorders (continued)

NAME OF TEST Renal biopsy

PURPOSE AND DESCRIPTION A renal biopsy is done to obtain tissue to diagnose or monitor kidney disease. The test is usually done by inserting a needle through the skin into the lower lobe of the kidney. It can also be done with CT, fluoroscopy or ultrasound guidance.

PERSON PREPARATION

- Informed consent is required for a kidney biopsy. Answer questions and provide additional information as needed.
- May be asked to fast for 4 to 6 hours prior to the procedure.
- As ordered, stop blood thinning medications (anticoagulants), aspirin and NSAIDs, or certain dietary supplements (omega-3 fatty acids).
- Note haemoglobin, haematocrit and coagulation profile prior to the procedure.
- If the procedure is to be performed at the bedside, obtain biopsy tray and other necessary supplies.
- May need to rest in bed for 12 to 24 hours post biopsy.
- Monitor closely for bleeding during the first 24 hours after the procedure:
  a. Check vital signs frequently. Notify the doctor of tachycardia, hypotension or other signs of bleeding or shock.
  b. Monitor biopsy site for bleeding.
  c. Check haemoglobin and haematocrit, comparing with pre-procedure values.
  d. Observe for and report complaints of flank or back pain, shoulder pain (caused by diaphragmatic irritation if haemorrhage occurs), pallor, light-headedness.
  e. Monitor urine output for quantity and haematuria. Initial haematuria should clear within 24 hours.
- Monitor for other potential complications such as inadvertent penetration of the liver or bowel. Report abdominal pain, guarding and decreased bowel sounds.
- Encourage fluids during the initial post-procedure period.

HEALTH EDUCATION FOR THE PERSON AND FAMILY

- Local anaesthesia is used at the injection site. The procedure may be uncomfortable but should not be painful.
- When the needle is inserted, you will be instructed not to breathe to prevent kidney motion.
- The entire procedure takes approximately 10 minutes.
- Avoid coughing during the first 24 hours after the procedure. Strenuous activity such as heavy lifting may be prohibited for approximately 2 weeks after the procedure.
- Report any manifestations of complications, such as haemorrhage or urinary tract infection, to the doctor.

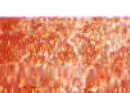

RENAL/KIDNEY ASSESSMENTS

Technique/normal findings	Abnormal findings
Skin assessment	
Inspect the skin and mucous membranes, noting colour, turgor and excretions. *The colour of skin and mucous membranes should be even and appropriate to the person's age and race; skin should be dry with no visible excretions.*	■ Pallor of the skin and mucous membranes may indicate kidney disease with resultant anaemia. ■ Decreased turgor of the skin may indicate dehydration. ■ Oedema (generalised or in the lower extremities) may indicate fluid volume excess. (Changes in skin turgor may indicate renal insufficiency with either excess fluid loss or retention.) ■ An accumulation of uric acid crystals, called uraemic frost, may be seen on the skin of the person with late-stage kidney disease.
Abdominal assessment	
Inspect the abdomen, noting size, symmetry, masses or lumps, swelling, distension, glistening or skin tightness. *The abdomen should be slightly concave, symmetric, without distension or masses.*	■ Enlargements or asymmetry may indicate a hernia or superficial mass. ■ If the urinary bladder is distended, it rises above the pubic symphysis as a rounded mass. ■ Distension, glistening or skin tightness may be associated with fluid retention. ■ Ascites is an accumulation of fluid in the peritoneal cavity.

(continued)

RENAL/KIDNEY ASSESSMENTS (continued)

Technique/normal findings	Abnormal findings
Urinary meatus assessment This technique is not part of a routine assessment, but it is an important component in caring for people with health problems of the renal system. Further discussion is included in the chapter 'A person-centred approach to assessing the male and female reproductive systems'. *For the male:* With the person in a sitting or standing position, compress the tip of the glans penis with your gloved hand to open the urinary meatus (see Figure 25.7). *For the female:* With the person in the dorsal lithotomy position, spread the labia with your gloved hand to expose the urinary meatus. *The urinary meatus should be midline and free of redness, lesions or discharge.*	■ Increased redness, swelling or discharge from the urinary meatus may indicate infection or sexually transmitted infection. ■ Ulceration of the urinary meatus may indicate a sexually transmitted infection. ■ Hypospadias is displacement of the urinary meatus to the ventral surface of the penis. ■ Epispadias is displacement of the urinary meatus to the dorsal surface of the penis. 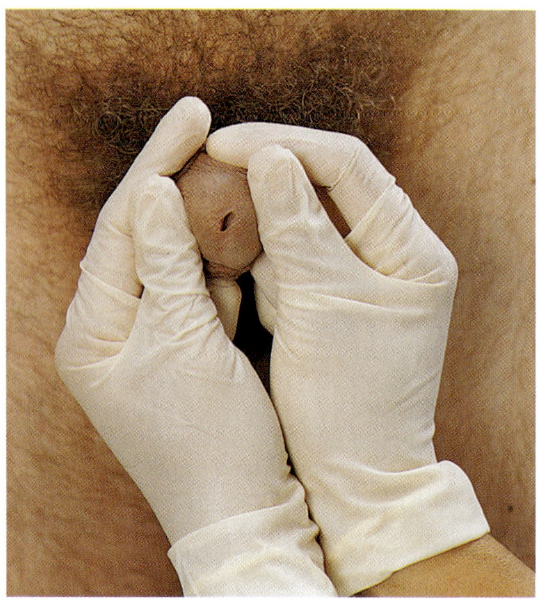 **FIGURE 25.7** ***Inspecting the urinary meatus of the male***
Kidney assessment See Box 25.1 for assessment guidelines for percussion and palpation of the kidneys. Auscultate the renal arteries by placing the bell of the stethoscope lightly in the areas of the renal arteries, located in the left and right upper abdominal quadrants. *Bruits are not normally heard over the renal arteries.*	■ Systolic bruits ('whooshing' sounds) may indicate renal artery stenosis.
Percuss the kidneys for tenderness or pain. *No tenderness or pain should be elicited.*	■ Tenderness and pain on percussion of the costovertebral angle suggest glomerulonephritis or glomerulonephrosis.
Palpate the kidneys. The lower pole of the right kidney may be palpable with deep palpation; the remaining right kidney and the left kidney are normally not palpable. *If palpable, they should be non-tender, bilaterally of appropriate size and density, without palpable masses. Note: Deep palpation should not be attempted by the novice practitioner.*	■ A mass or lump may indicate a tumour or cyst. ■ Tenderness or pain on palpation may suggest an inflammatory process. ■ A soft kidney that feels spongy may indicate chronic renal disease. ■ Bilaterally enlarged kidneys may suggest polycystic kidney disease. ■ Unequal kidney size may indicate hydronephrosis.
Bladder assessment Percuss the bladder for tone and position. *The bladder should be midline without dullness.*	■ Dull percussion tone over the bladder of a person who has just urinated may indicate urinary retention.
Palpate the bladder (over the pubic symphysis and abdomen) for distension. *The bladder is normally not palpable.*	■ Distended bladder may be palpated at any point from the pubic symphysis to the umbilicus and is felt as a firm, rounded organ. It indicates urinary retention.

CONCEPT CHECK

1 What part of the kidney processes the blood to make urine?
1 ureter
2 medulla
3 pyramids
4 nephrons

2 A person has been vomiting for 4 hours. What hormone is increased as a result?
1 thyroxine
2 renin
3 aldosterone
4 ADH

3 What diagnostic test can be used to determine GFR as well as glomerular damage?
1 routine urinalysis
2 renal scan
3 creatinine clearance
4 renal biopsy

4 What gland encircles the male urethra at the base of the bladder?
1 spleen
2 pancreas
3 prostate
4 adrenal

5 The person tells you they are getting up to void several times a night. You record this finding as:
1 polyuria
2 nocturia
3 dysuria
4 haematuria

6 Which question would you ask a person prior to an IVP?
1 'Are you allergic to shellfish?'
2 'Do you have burning on urination?'
3 'Have you ever had kidney stones?'
4 'Why are you having this test?'

7 Before beginning the physical assessment of the renal system, you should ask the person to:
1 empty the bladder
2 take several deep breaths
3 provide a urine specimen
4 drink several glasses of water

8 Following surgery, an older adult has not voided for 12 hours. What assessment should you make?
1 Palpate for bladder distension.
2 Auscultate for bowel sounds.
3 Inspect for oedema of the urethra.
4 Percuss for gastric tympany.

9 Of the following health problems an older woman may have, which is not normally a part of ageing of the renal system?
1 increased risk of haematuria
2 decreased risk of infection
3 urine that is darker in colour
4 urinary incontinence

10 What assessment would you use to assess hydration status of a person?
1 auscultation of renal arteries
2 palpation for skin turgor
3 percussion for dullness over bladder
4 palpation of both kidneys

BIBLIOGRAPHY

Australasian Association for Clinical Biochemistry and Laboratory Medicine (AACB) (2022). Albumin/creatinine ratio urine. *Pathology Tests Explained*. Retrieved from https://pathologytestsexplained.org.au/

Australian Commission on Safety and Quality in Health Care (ACSQHC) (2021). *National Safety and Quality Health Service Standards* (2nd ed.). Sydney: ACSQHC.

Australian Institute of Health and Welfare (2020). *Chronic kidney disease*. Retrieved from https://www.aihw.gov.au/

Barzilay, J. I., Buzkova, P., Shlipak, M. G., Bansal, N., Garimella, P. & Mukamal, K. J. (2020). Hospitalization rates in older adults with albuminuria: The Cardiovascular Health Study. *The Journals of Gerontology. Series A, Biological Sciences and Medical Sciences, 75*(12), 2426–2433. doi: 10.1093/gerona/[illegible]

Bilal, M., Voin, V., Topale, N., Iwanaga, J., Loukas, M. & [illegible] (2017). The clinical anatomy of the physical examination of the abdomen: A comprehensive review. *Clinical Anatomy, 30*, 352–356. doi: 10.1002/ca.22832

Chukwu, C. A., Rao, A., Kalra, P. A. & Middleton, R. (2022). Managing recurrent urinary tract infections in kidney transplant recipients using smartphone assisted urinalysis test. *Journal of Renal Care, 24*(2), 119–127.

Kidney Health Australia (KHA) (2020a). *Estimated glomerular filtration rate (eGFR) fact sheet*. Retrieved from www.kidney.org.au

Kidney Health Australia (KHA) (2020b). *Chronic kidney disease management in primary care* (4th ed.). Retrieved from www.kidney.org.au

Kidney Health Australia (KHA) (2020c). *Polycystic kidney disease—Diagnosis and monitoring*. Primary Care Education Workshop. Retrieved from https://www.kidney.org.au/

Levett-Jones, T., Dwyer, T., Reid-Searl, K., Heaton, L., Flenady, T., Applegarth, J., Guinea, S. & Andersen, P. (2017). *Patient Safety Competency Framework (PSCF) for Nursing Students*. Sydney. Retrieved from http://psframework.wpengine.com/

Levey, A. S. et al. (2020). Nomenclature for kidney function and disease: Report of a kidney disease: Improving global outcomes (KDIGO consensus conference). *Kidney International, 97*, 1117–1129.

Martini, F., Nath, J. & Bartholomew, E. (eds) (2017). *Fundamentals of anatomy and physiology* (11th ed.). San Francisco: Pearson Education, Inc.

National Kidney Foundation Inc. (2022). *Albuminuria*. Retrieved from https://www.kidney.org/

Rowland, J., Akbarov, A., Akhlaq, M., Eales, J. & Dormer, J. (2018). Tick tock chimes the kidney clock—From biology of renal ageing to clinical applications. *Kidney and Blood Pressure Research, 43*(1), 55–67.

The Royal College of Pathologists of Australasia (RCPA) (2022). *Albumin urine*. Retrieved from https://www.rcpa.edu.au/

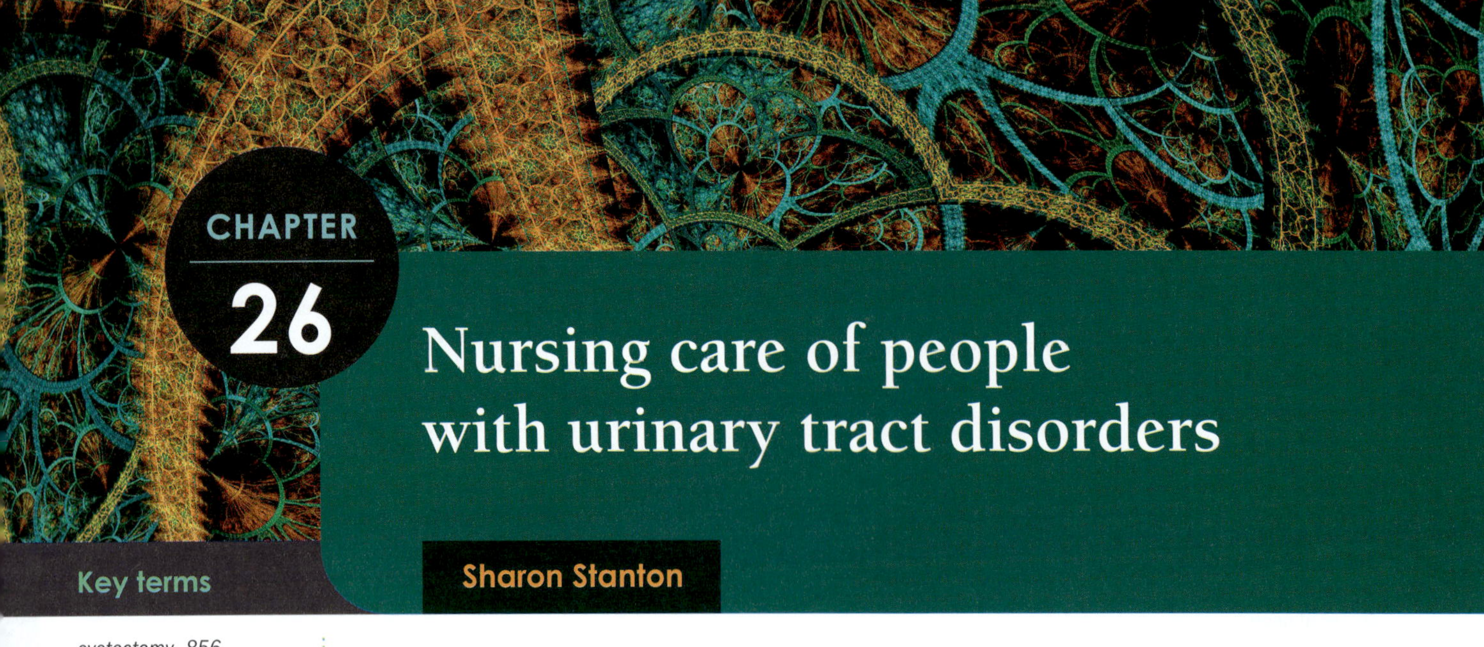

CHAPTER 26

Nursing care of people with urinary tract disorders

Sharon Stanton

Key terms

cystectomy 856
cystitis 838
dysuria 838
extracorporeal shock wave lithotripsy (ESWL) 850
haematuria 839
healthcare-associated infection 838
hydronephrosis 848
lithiasis 846
lithotripsy 850
neurogenic bladder 863
nocturia 838
pyelonephritis 839
reflux 838
renal colic 847
ureteral (or ureteric) stent 842
ureteroplasty 842
urgency 838
urinary calculi 846
urinary diversion 856
urinary drainage system 837
urinary incontinence (UI) 865
urinary retention 861

Learning outcomes

- Evaluate the interprofessional care and health management implications for a person with urinary tract infection to the pathophysiology of the condition.
- Explain the risk factors, course, pathophysiology and interventions required to competently care for a person with an obstruction of the urinary tract.
- Describe the interprofessional care and health management when caring for individuals experiencing various urinary flow disorders.

Clinical competencies

- Assess the functional health status of people with urinary tract disorders.
- Identify, report and document abnormal or unexpected assessment findings and their effect on personal status.
- Use evidence-based research to plan and implement nursing care for people with urinary tract disorders, integrating interprofessional care and health management plans.
- Knowledgeably and safely administer prescribed medications and treatments for people with urinary tract disorders.
- Provide effective nursing care for people undergoing surgery of the urinary tract.
- Plan and provide appropriate teaching for prevention and self-care of urinary tract disorders.
- Evaluate personal responses, revising plan of care as needed to promote, maintain or restore functional health of individuals with urinary tract disorders.

The urinary system includes the kidneys, ureters, urinary bladder and urethra. This organ system can be affected by a variety of disorders, including congenital malformations, infections, obstructions, trauma, tumours and neurological conditions. Any portion of the system—from the kidney through to the urethra—can be affected, with serious or even life-threatening consequences unless the problem is appropriately diagnosed and treated. Kidney disorders that can affect urine production and waste elimination directly are discussed in the next chapter. Disorders of the **urinary drainage system** may obstruct urine flow or may affect the kidneys and urine production and elimination. The anatomy, physiology and nursing assessment related to the urinary tract are presented in the chapter 'A person-centred approach to assessing the renal system'.

When caring for people with urinary tract disorders, it is important to consider their modesty with respect to voiding, possible difficulty in discussing the genitals, embarrassment over exposure during examination and testing, and fear of changes in body image or function. These psychosocial issues may interfere with willingness to seek help, discuss treatment and learn about preventive measures.

Nursing interventions for people with urinary tract disorders are directed towards primary prevention, early detection and management of disorders through nursing care and health education.

THE PERSON WITH URINARY TRACT INFECTION

In Australia in 2020, there were 4,019 deaths from diseases of the kidney and urinary tract, with these being the ninth leading cause of death (Australian Bureau of Statistics (ABS), 2021). Untreated or poorly managed urinary tract infections (UTIs) may result in significant morbidity, including kidney damage, and are the cause of 17.2% of all nosocomial infections (Sihra et al., 2018). People who are diabetic or have nephritis or hypertensive vascular disease have an increased risk of developing kidney failure or chronic kidney disease (CKD). Indigenous Australians have an even greater risk than non-Indigenous Australians, with a three times higher death rate from the disease (ABS, 2021).

UTIs are common community-acquired bacterial infections and comprise 1.2% of all Australian general practice consultations (Australian Commission on Safety and Quality in Health Care, 2021). Community-acquired UTIs are more common in women than males, are unusual in men under the age of 50 and may be symptomatic or asymptomatic.

Most community-acquired UTIs (80%) are caused by *Escherichia coli* (Matsui et al., 2020), a common Gram-negative enteral bacteria. About 5–10% of symptomatic UTIs are caused by *Staphylococcus saprophyticus*, a Gram-positive organism. Catheter-associated UTIs often involve other Gram-negative bacteria such as *Proteus*, *Klebsiella*, *Serratia* and *Pseudomonas*.

Risk factors

A variety of factors can predispose to UTI (see Box 26.1). Some factors cannot be changed (e.g. ageing and the short urethra of the female); others may be a result of individual behaviour—for example, poor fluid intake or delaying going to the toilet, especially in the elderly.

BOX 26.1 Risk factors for UTI

Female
- Short, straight urethra
- Proximity of urinary meatus to vagina and anus
- Sexual intercourse
- Use of diaphragm and spermicidal compounds for birth control
- Pregnancy

Male
- Uncircumcised
- Prostatic hypertrophy
- Unprotected anal intercourse

Both
- Ageing
- Urinary tract obstruction
- Neurogenic bladder dysfunction
- Vesicoureteral reflux
- Genetic factors
- Catheterisation

In women, poor perineal hygiene or cleansing techniques after micturition or defecation may result in bacterial deposition close to the external urethral orifice. Sexual activity also increases the risk of UTI because bacteria can be introduced into the bladder via the urethra during sexual intercourse. Use of spermicidal compounds with a diaphragm, cervical cap or condom alters the normal bacterial flora of the vagina and perineal tissues and further increases the risk of UTI. Some females lack a normally protective mucosal enzyme and have decreased levels of cervicovaginal antibodies to enterobacteria, further increasing their risk. Prostatic hypertrophy and bacterial prostatitis are risk factors among males, as is unprotected anal intercourse, although circumcision appears to have a protective effect. Congenital or acquired factors contributing to the risk of infection include urinary tract obstruction by tumours or calculi, structural abnormalities such as strictures, impaired bladder innervation, bowel incontinence and chronic diseases such as diabetes mellitus.

Instrumentation of the urinary tract (e.g. catheterisation or cystoscopy) is a major risk factor for UTI. The placement of the catheter prevents the flushing action of voiding and bacteria may ascend to the bladder either through the catheter lumen or via exudate between the urethral mucosa and the catheter. Even when performed under strict aseptic conditions, catheterisation can result in bladder infection. Research indicates that the risk of catheter associated UTI is reduced when anaesthetic lubricating gels are inserted into the urethra prior to catheter insertion (Payne & Kerrigan, 2020). Prophylactic antibiotics are not recommended at insertion or replacement of an indwelling urinary catheter unless otherwise recommended. Use of a local anaesthetic minimises the discomfort experienced by the patient (Payne & Kerrigan, 2020).

Older individuals have an increased incidence of UTI. The greatest degree of increase is seen in men, as the ratio of female-to-male UTI in older adults changes from 50:1 to less than 5:1. An increased risk of urinary stasis, chronic disease states such as diabetes mellitus and an impaired immune response contribute to the higher incidence of UTI in the older adult. In men, the prostate typically hypertrophies with ageing, potentially resulting in urinary retention as the urethra narrows. Prostatic secretions are lessened, diminishing their protective, antibacterial effect. In older women, loss of tissue elasticity and weakening of perineal muscles often contribute to the development of a cystocele or rectocele. Resulting changes in bladder and urethral position increase the risk of incomplete bladder emptying.

FAST FACTS

- For females, there is a 50–60% lifetime incidence of UTI (Medina & Castillo-Pino, 2019).
- In healthy adult men, however, UTIs are unusual and may prompt additional diagnostic testing.

Physiology review

The urinary tract is normally sterile above the urethra. Adequate urine volume, a free flow from the kidneys through the urinary meatus and complete bladder emptying are the most important mechanisms in maintaining sterility. Any pathogens that enter and contaminate the distal urethra are then washed out during voiding. Other defences for maintaining sterile urine include its normal acidity and the bacteriostatic properties of the bladder and urethral cells. The peristaltic activity of the ureters and a competent vesicoureteral junction help maintain sterility of the upper urinary tract. As the ureter enters the bladder, its distal portion tunnels between the mucosa and muscle layers of the bladder wall (see Figure 26.1). During voiding, increased *intravesicular* (within the bladder) pressure compresses the ureter, preventing **reflux**, or backflow of urine towards the kidneys. In males, a long urethra and the antibacterial effect of zinc in prostatic fluid also help prevent contamination of this normally sterile environment.

Pathophysiology and manifestations

Pathogens usually enter the urinary tract by ascending from the mucous membranes of the perineal area into the lower urinary tract. Bacteria that have colonised the urethra, vagina or perineal tissues are the usual source of infection and are most often *E. coli*, which are linked to higher incidents of recurrence (Cai, 2021). From the bladder, bacteria may continue to ascend the urinary tract, eventually infecting the *parenchyma* (functional tissue) of the kidneys (Loscalzo et al., 2022). Haematogenous spread of infection to the urinary tract is rare. Infections introduced in this manner are usually associated with previous damage or scarring of the urinary tract. Bacteria introduced into the urinary tract may cause asymptomatic bacteriuria or an inflammatory response with manifestations of UTI.

Urinary tract infections can be categorised in several ways. Anatomically, UTIs may affect the lower or the upper urinary tract. Lower urinary tract infections include *urethritis*, inflammation of the urethra; *prostatitis*, inflammation of the prostate gland (discussed in the chapter 'Nursing care of men with reproductive system and breast disorders'); and cystitis, inflammation of the urinary bladder. The most common upper urinary tract infection is pyelonephritis, inflammation of the kidney and renal pelvis. The infection may involve superficial tissues such as the bladder mucosa or may invade other tissues such as prostate or renal tissues. Epidemiologically, UTIs are identified as community-acquired infections or **healthcare-associated infections** associated with catheterisation.

Cystitis

Cystitis, inflammation of the urinary bladder, is the most common UTI. The infection tends to remain superficial, involving the bladder mucosa. The mucosa becomes hyperaemic (red) and may haemorrhage (see Figure 26.2). The inflammatory response results in pus formation, causing the classic manifestations associated with cystitis. Typical presenting symptoms of cystitis include **dysuria** (painful or difficult urination), urinary frequency and **urgency** (a sudden, compelling need to urinate), and **nocturia** (voiding two or more times at night). In addition, the urine may be foul smelling and cloudy (*pyuria*) or bloody

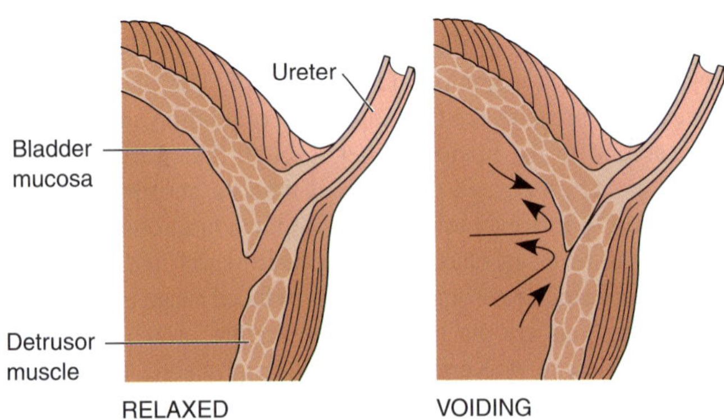

FIGURE 26.1 *A competent vesicoureteral junction. Note how increased intravesicular pressure during voiding occludes the distal portion of the ureter, preventing reflux*

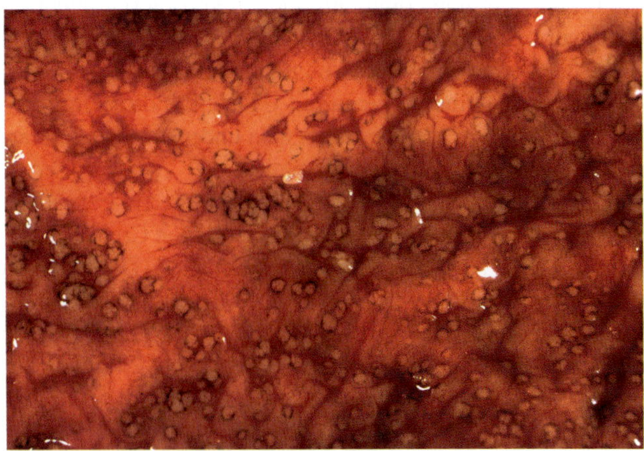

FIGURE 26.2 *Appearance of the bladder wall affected by cystitis*

Source: © CNRI/Science Photo Library.

MANIFESTATIONS Cystitis

- Dysuria
- Pyuria
- Frequency
- Haematuria
- Urgency
- Suprapubic discomfort
- Nocturia

(**haematuria**) because of mucus, excess white cells in the urine and bleeding of the inflamed bladder wall. Suprapubic pain and tenderness also may be present. See the 'Manifestations' box for manifestations of cystitis.

Cystitis occurs most frequently in adult females, usually because of colonisation of the bladder by bacteria normally found in the lower gastrointestinal tract. These bacteria gain entry by ascending the short, straight female urethra. In addition to the risk factors listed above, personal hygiene practices and voluntary urinary retention can contribute to the risk of UTI in women.

Older people may not experience the classic symptoms of cystitis. Instead, they often present with non-specific manifestations such as nocturia, incontinence, confusion, behaviour change, lethargy, anorexia or 'just not feeling right'. Fever and hypothermia may also be present.

Although the bacteriostatic effect of prostatic fluid and a longer urethra provide an effective barrier to bladder infection for adult males, the prostatic hypertrophy commonly associated with ageing increases the risk of cystitis in elderly males. An enlarged prostate can impede urine flow, leading to incomplete bladder emptying and urinary stasis. Bacteria are not completely flushed with voiding, allowing colonisation of the bladder.

Cystitis is usually uncomplicated and readily responds to treatment. Severe or prolonged infection may lead to sloughing of bladder mucosa and ulcer formation; when left untreated, the infection can ascend to involve the kidneys. Chronic cystitis can also lead to bladder stones (discussed later in this chapter).

Catheter-associated UTI

Up to 70% of hospitalised patients and 95% of those in ICU will develop a UTI, with the length of time of catheterisation one of the most influential factors (Khan, Tabassum & Kim, 2020). Bacteria, including *E. coli*, *Proteus*, *Pseudomonas* and *Klebsiella*, reach the bladder either by migrating through the column of urine within the catheter or by moving up the mucous sheath of the urethra outside the catheter (Loscalzo et al., 2022). Bacteria enter the catheter system at the connection between the catheter and drainage system or through the emptying tube of the drainage bag. Colonisation of perineal skin by bowel flora is a common source of infection in catheterised women.

Catheter-associated UTIs are often asymptomatic. Gram-negative bacteraemia is the most significant complication associated with these. Most catheter-associated UTIs resolve quickly when the catheter is removed and a short course of antibiotics is given. Intermittent catheterisation carries a lower risk of infection than does an indwelling catheter and is preferred for those who are unable to empty their bladder by normal voiding.

Pyelonephritis

Pyelonephritis is inflammation of the renal pelvis and parenchyma, the functional kidney tissue. *Acute pyelonephritis* is a bacterial infection of the kidney; *chronic pyelonephritis* is associated with repeated non-bacterial infections and inflammatory processes that may be metabolic, chemical or immunological in origin.

ACUTE PYELONEPHRITIS Acute pyelonephritis usually results from an infection that ascends to the kidney from the lower urinary tract. Asymptomatic bacteriuria or cystitis can lead to acute pyelonephritis. Risk factors include pregnancy (because of slowed ureteral peristalsis), urinary tract obstruction and congenital malformation. Urinary tract trauma, scarring, calculi (stones), kidney disorders such as polycystic or hypertensive kidney disease, and chronic diseases such as diabetes may also contribute to pyelonephritis. *Vesicoureteral reflux*, a condition in which urine moves from the bladder back towards the kidney, is a common risk factor in children who develop pyelonephritis and is also seen in adults when bladder outflow is obstructed.

The infection spreads from the renal pelvis to the renal cortex. The pelvis, calyces and medulla of the kidney are primarily affected, with white blood cell (WBC) infiltration and inflammation. The kidney becomes grossly oedematous. Localised abscesses may develop on the cortical surface of the kidney. As with cystitis, *E. coli* is the organism responsible for 80% (Matsui et al., 2020) of the cases of acute pyelonephritis. Other organisms commonly found include *Proteus* and *Klebsiella*, bacteria that normally inhabit the intestinal tract.

The onset of acute pyelonephritis is typically rapid, with chills and fever, malaise, vomiting, flank pain, costovertebral tenderness, urinary frequency and dysuria (see the 'Manifestations' box). Symptoms of cystitis also may be present. The older adult may present with a change in behaviour, acute confusion, incontinence or a general deterioration in condition.

CHRONIC PYELONEPHRITIS Chronic pyelonephritis involves chronic inflammation and scarring of the tubules and interstitial tissues of the kidney and is a common cause of chronic renal failure. It may develop as a result of ascending UTIs or other conditions that damage the kidneys, such as hypertension, vascular conditions, severe vesicoureteral reflux or obstruction of the urinary tract.

The person with chronic pyelonephritis may be asymptomatic or have mild manifestations such as urinary frequency, dysuria and flank pain. Hypertension can develop as kidney tissue is destroyed.

MANIFESTATIONS Acute pyelonephritis

URINARY

- Urinary frequency
- Dysuria
- Pyuria
- Haematuria
- Flank pain
- Costovertebral tenderness

SYSTEMIC

- Vomiting
- Diarrhoea
- Acute fever
- Shaking chills
- Malaise

FAST FACT

The most common route of entry for a urinary tract infection is ascending, from colonisation of the perineal tissues by faecal bacteria (usually *E. coli*), through the urethra, into the bladder (cystitis) and possibly kidney tissue (pyelonephritis).

INTERPROFESSIONAL CARE

Treatment of UTI focuses on eliminating the causative organism, preventing relapse or reinfection, and identifying and correcting any contributing factors. Drug treatment with antibiotics and urinary anti-infectives is commonly used. In some cases, surgery may be indicated to correct contributing factors.

Diagnosis

Laboratory testing for UTI includes:

- *Urinalysis*, to assess for pyuria, bacteria and blood cells in the urine. A bacteria count greater than 10×10^6/L suggests infection. Rapid tests for bacteria in the urine include using a *nitrite dipstick* (which turns pink in the presence of bacteria) and the *leucocyte esterase test*, which is positive in the presence of WBCs (neutrophils), indicating infection or inflammation.

  Urine should be a midstream clean-catch specimen in a sterile container. If necessary, catheterisation or 'mini-cath', with aseptic technique, may be used. However, catheterisation should be avoided if possible to reduce the risk of further infection. (A 'Diagnostic tests' box for nursing care related to collecting a urinalysis specimen is included in the chapter 'A person-centred approach to assessing the renal system'.)
- *Gram stain of the urine* may be done to identify the infecting organism by shape and characteristic (Gram-positive or Gram-negative).
- *Urine culture and sensitivity* tests may be ordered to identify the infecting organism and the most effective antibiotic. Culture requires 24 to 72 hours, so treatment to eliminate the most common organisms may be initiated without culture followed by antibiotic therapy according to sensitivity results.
- *WBC with differential* may be done to detect typical changes associated with infection, such as *leucocytosis* (elevated WBC) and increased numbers of neutrophils.

In men and in adult women with recurrent infections or persistent bacteriuria, additional diagnostic testing may be ordered to evaluate for structural abnormalities and other contributing factors:

- *Intravenous pyelography (IVP)* is used to evaluate the structure and excretory function of the kidneys, ureters and bladder. As the kidneys clear an intravenously injected contrast medium from the blood, the size and shape of the kidneys, their calyces and pelvises, the ureters and the bladder can be identified and structural or functional abnormalities, such as vesicoureteral reflux, may be detected.
- *Antegrade pyelogram* is used when an IVP fails to identify an obstruction in the ureters or bladder. Contrast medium is injected into the collecting system of the kidney and renal flow is monitored by radiology.
- *Computed tomography (CT scan)* may be used in preference to IVP for identifying renal calculi. It uses a radiation beam to build a three-dimensional picture of the renal system.
- *Ultrasound* is a non-invasive technique that utilises sound waves to visualise soft tissue masses, obstructions, some renal calculi and renal blood flow.
- *Micturating cystogram (MCU)* is a procedure conducted on infants or children, and involves instilling contrast medium into the bladder, then using x-rays to assess the bladder and urethra when filled and during voiding. This study can detect structural or functional abnormalities of the bladder and urethral strictures. This test has a lower risk of allergic response to the contrast dye than IVP.
- *Cystoscopy*, direct visualisation of the urethra and bladder through a cystoscope, may be used to diagnose conditions such as prostatic hypertrophy, urethral strictures, bladder calculi, tumours, polyps or diverticula, and congenital abnormalities. A tissue biopsy may be obtained during the procedure and other interventions performed (e.g. stone removal or stricture dilation).
- *Manual pelvic* or prostate examinations are performed to assess for structural changes of the genitourinary tract, such as prostatic enlargement, cystocele or rectocele.

Nursing implications for these diagnostic procedures are presented in the chapter 'A person-centred approach to assessing the renal system'.

Medications

Most uncomplicated infections of the lower urinary tract can be treated with a short course of antibiotic therapy. Upper urinary tract infections, in contrast, usually require longer treatment (2 or more weeks) to eradicate the infecting organism.

Short-course therapy (either a single antibiotic dose or a 3-day course of treatment) reduces treatment cost, increases compliance and has a lower rate of side effects. Single-dose therapy is associated with a higher rate of recurrent infection and continued vaginal colonisation with *E. coli*, making a 3-day course of treatment the preferred option for uncomplicated cystitis. Oral trimethoprim (TMP) or cephalexin as a first choice may be ordered (Jarvis et al., 2014), although formal culture and susceptibility testing should be performed to ensure correct antimicrobial therapy to minimise the growing incidence of antibiotic resistance. This is particularly true in high-risk groups and events of recurrence.

Men and women with pyelonephritis, urinary tract abnormalities, stones or a history of previous infections with antibiotic-resistant infections may be prescribed a variety of drugs including cephalexin, amoxicillin/clavulanic acid, trimethoprim or ciprofloxacin as a 7- to 10-day course. Those with severe illness may need hospitalisation for initial parenteral treatment, changing to oral therapy when there is clinical improvement. Drugs used for severe illness or sepsis associated with UTI include ciprofloxacin, gentamicin or ceftriaxone, or amoxicillin/ampicillin. (See the chapter 'Nursing care of people with infections' for the nursing implications for antibiotic therapy.)

The outcome of treatment for UTI is determined by follow-up urinalysis and culture. *Cure*, as evidenced by no pathogens present in the urine, is the desired outcome. When therapy fails to eradicate bacteria in the urine, it is known as unresolved bacteriuria. *Persistent bacteriuria* or *relapse* occurs when a persistent source of infection causes repeated infection after initial cure. *Reinfection* is the development of a new infection with a different pathogen following previous successful UTI treatment (Papadakis, McPhee & Rabow, 2022).

> **CONSIDERATION FOR PRACTICE**
>
> **Follow-up urine culture should be performed 10 days to 2 weeks following completion of antibiotic therapy for UTI to ensure bacterial eradication from the urinary tract.**

Individuals experiencing frequent symptomatic UTIs may be treated with prophylactic antibiotic therapy with a drug such as TMP or nitrofurantoin). TMP and nitrofurantoin do not achieve effective plasma concentrations at recommended doses but do reach effective concentrations in the urine. Nitrofurantoin also may be used to treat UTI in pregnant women. Nursing implications for these urinary anti-infectives are outlined in the 'Medication administration' box.

Antibiotics and urinary anti-infectives are not generally recommended to treat asymptomatic bacteriuria in catheterised people. The recommended treatment for catheter-associated UTI is removal (or replacement if required) of the indwelling catheter followed by a 10- to 14-day course of antibiotic therapy to eliminate the infection.

Surgery

Surgery may be indicated for recurrent UTI if diagnostic testing indicates calculi, structural anomalies or strictures that contribute to the risk of infection. Table 26.1 lists major causes of urinary tract obstruction that may contribute to UTI.

Stones or *calculi* in the renal pelvis or in the bladder are an irritant and provide a matrix for bacterial colonisation. Treatment may include surgical removal of a large calculus from the renal pelvis or cystoscopic removal of bladder calculi. *Percutaneous ultrasonic pyelolithotomy* or *extracorporeal shock wave lithotripsy* (described in the next section) may be used instead of surgery to crush and remove stones. (See the 'Diagnostic tests'

MEDICATION ADMINISTRATION Urinary anti-infectives

URINARY ANTI-INFECTIVES
Nitrofurantoin (Furadantin, Macrodantin)
Trimethoprim (Bactrim, Triprim)

Urinary anti-infectives are usually used prophylactically to prevent recurrence of UTI in those with frequent symptomatic infections. Nitrofurantoin may be used to treat UTI in pregnant women but only if medically essential.

Nursing responsibilities

- Ensure adequate fluid intake (1,500 to 2,000 mL/day) to maintain a urine output of at least 1,500 mL of urine per 24 hours (unless contraindicated). Do not overhydrate.
- Administer with meals to minimise GI side effects, such as nausea, gastric upset and abdominal cramping.
- Trimethoprim is contraindicated for use in people with renal or hepatic impairment; nitrofurantoin is contraindicated for those with impaired renal function. Report abnormal laboratory values such as elevated creatinine or BUN, decreased eGFR, bilirubin, alanine aminotransferase (ALT), aspartate aminotransferase (AST) and lactic dehydrogenase (LDH).
- Monitor for skin irritations, rash, nausea, vomiting and fever. If bruising or unusual bleeding occurs, discontinue the drug and notify the doctor.
- Use with caution in older or chronically ill people. Monitor closely for adverse effects.
- Do not administer trimethoprim to pregnant women unless essential because of possible adverse effects on the fetus.
- Monitor the person taking nitrofurantoin for an acute or chronic pulmonary reaction with manifestations of dyspnoea, cough, chills, fever and chest pain. Discontinue the drug and notify the doctor.
- Nitrofurantoin may cause peripheral neuropathy, especially in older individuals and adult diabetics. Notify the doctor if symptoms develop.
- Nitrofurantoin oral suspension may stain the teeth; therefore, instruct the person to rinse the mouth thoroughly after administering.
- Monitor for signs of phenytoin toxicity (sedation, ataxia and increased blood levels) if trimethoprim is given concurrently. Phenytoin doses may need to be reduced.

Health education for the person and family

- These drugs are used with good hygiene practices to prevent UTI recurrence. Take as directed even when no symptoms are present, until the course is completed.
- Drink six to eight glasses of water a day (2,500–3,500 mL) while taking these drugs.
- Take the drug with meals or food to reduce gastric effects; however, avoid milk products because they may interfere with absorption.
- Trimethoprim should not be taken during pregnancy. Contact your doctor before attempting to become pregnant.
- Contact your doctor if you develop any of the following: chest pain, difficulty breathing, cough, chills and fever; numbness and tingling or weakness of the extremities; rash or pruritus (itching), bruising or bleeding.
- If you are taking an oral suspension of nitrofurantoin, rinse your mouth thoroughly after each dose to avoid staining the teeth.
- Nitrofurantoin turns the urine brown. This is not harmful and disappears when the drug is discontinued.
- If you are taking trimethoprim along with phenytoin (Dilantin) or a related anticonvulsant, contact your doctor if you become sedated or begin to stagger.

TABLE 26.1 Major causes of urinary tract obstruction by location

LOCATION	OBSTRUCTIVE PROCESS
Kidney pelvis	Calculi (stones) Polycystic kidney disease Infection and scarring
Ureters	Calculi Scarring and stricture Congenital defects or strictures External processes such as pregnancy, tumours, lymph node enlargement
Bladder	Neurogenic bladder Tumours Calculi and other foreign bodies
Urethra	Benign prostatic hypertrophy Tumours Scarring and stricture Trauma

box in the chapter 'A person-centred approach to assessing the renal system' for nursing care related to cystoscopy.)

Ureteroplasty, surgical repair of a ureter, may be indicated for structural abnormality or stricture of a ureter. This may be combined with a ureteral reimplantation if vesicoureteral reflux is present. The person returns from these surgeries with an indwelling urinary catheter (Foley or suprapubic) and a **ureteral** (or **ureteric**) stent (a thin catheter inserted into the ureter to provide for urine flow and ureteral support) which remains in place for 3 to 5 days. Ureteral stents can remain in place for several months if required. However, they are a risk for calculi build up which may lead to other complications. Care of those with a ureteral stent is outlined in the 'Nursing care of the person' box.

Complementary therapies

Complementary therapies such as aromatherapy or herbal preparations, particularly cranberry juice, have been advocated

NURSING CARE OF THE PERSON with a ureteral stent

Ureteral stents are used to maintain patency and promote healing of the ureters (see figure). A stent may be temporary, used during and after a surgical procedure, or it may be used for longer periods in individuals with ureteral obstruction due to tumours, strictures or other causes.

Stents may be positioned during surgery or cystoscopy. They are made of a non-toxic material such as silicone or polyurethane, with side drainage holes placed along the length of the stent. Stents are radiopaque for easy radiographic identification and one or both ends of the stent may be pigtail or J shaped to prevent migration or dislodgement.

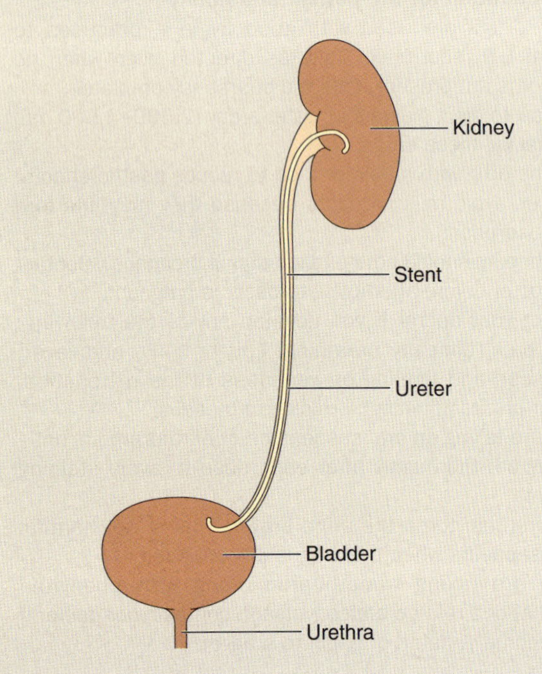

- If the stent has been brought to the surface, secure it and maintain its position. The stent is usually placed in the renal pelvis. *It is important to secure it well to prevent trauma to the kidney, inadvertent removal of the stent and ureter obstruction.*
- Label all drainage tubes, including stents, for easy identification. Attach each catheter and stent to a separate closed drainage system. *Careful labelling allows close monitoring of output from all sources and reservoirs. Separate drainage systems minimise the risk of infection.*
- Monitor urine output, including colour, consistency and odour. Monitor for signs of infection, bleeding, fever, tachycardia, pain, haematuria and cloudy or foul-smelling urine. *The stent facilitates urine flow but may become obstructed because of bleeding, calculi or sediment. Obstruction may result in hydronephrosis and kidney damage. The stent itself is a foreign body in the urinary tract and can increase the risk of UTI.*
- Maintain fluid intake, encouraging the use of fluids that acidify urine, such as low-sugar apple, cranberry and blueberry juice. *The stent can precipitate calculus formation as well as UTI. Increasing fluid intake (unless contraindicated) and acidifying the urine may assist in preventing these complications.*
- For an indwelling stent, stress the need for regular follow-up to monitor for and prevent complications such as UTI and calculi. *The person with an indwelling stent may tend to forget that the stent is in place and become lax in compliance with follow-up and preventive measures.*
- Some indwelling stents are associated with discomfort and pain. Offer reassurance and support, and stress follow-up to ensure no complications. *Pain and discomfort can be distressing to a person, particularly when they are not 'sick'. Some evidence reports limited effect of analgesia, but the use of alfuzosin or tamsulosin is showing promise. Discomfort may be related to spasm in the ureteral smooth muscle (Sali & Joshi, 2020).*

for use in conjunction with antibiotics to treat UTI. However, despite being recommended for prevention and treatment of UTI, cranberry juice and capsule studies have been inconclusive as to their effectiveness. While some studies have shown there may be benefits from cranberry juice, in controlled studies cranberry juice does not prevent UTIs (Gbinigie et al., 2021). There are also risks of interaction between cranberry juice and other drugs—for example, warfarin. People who wish to take herbal supplements or alternative/complementary therapies should consult their doctor due to potential drug interaction risks.

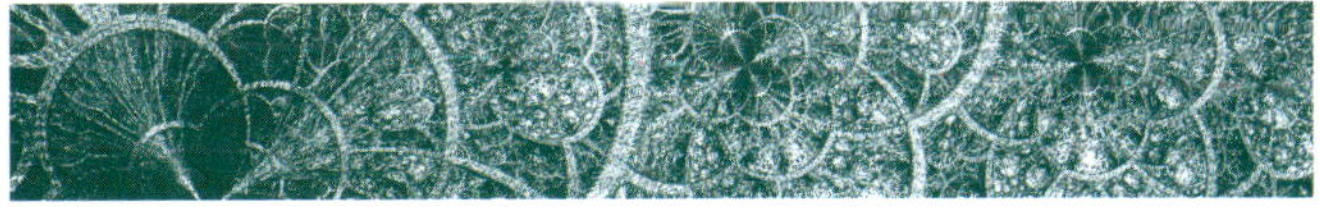

Nursing care

Health promotion

Teach measures to prevent UTI to all sexually active women, particularly younger women. Encourage the maintenance of a generous fluid intake of 2,000–2,500 mL per day, increasing intake during hot weather or strenuous activity, if not contraindicated. Discuss the need to avoid voluntary urinary retention, emptying the bladder every 3 to 4 hours. Instruct women to cleanse the perineal area from front to back after voiding and defecating. Teach to void before and after sexual intercourse to flush out bacteria introduced into the urethra and bladder. Teach measures to maintain the integrity of perineal tissues: avoid bubble baths, feminine hygiene sprays and vaginal douches; wear cotton briefs, avoid synthetic materials as they may irritate the perineal area.

Assessment

Focused assessment data for the person with a UTI include the following:

- *Health history*: current symptoms, including frequency, urgency, burning on urination, number of voidings per night; colour, clarity and odour of urine; other manifestations such as lower abdominal, back or flank pain, nausea or vomiting, fever; duration of symptoms and any treatment attempted; history of previous UTIs and their frequency; possibility of pregnancy and type of birth control used; chronic diseases such as diabetes; current medications and any known allergies.
- *Physical examination*: general health; vital signs including temperature; abdominal shape, contour, tenderness to palpation (especially suprapubic); percuss for costovertebral tenderness (see Box 25.1).

See the Chapter 'A person-centred approach to assessing the renal system' for complete nursing assessment of the urinary system.

Nursing diagnoses and interventions

General health, abilities for self-care and risk factors that may contribute to UTI are considered when planning and implementing nursing care for the person with a UTI. Priority nursing diagnoses focus on comfort, urinary elimination and teaching/learning needs. See the 'Nursing care plan' box for the person with cystitis.

Pain

Pain is a common manifestation of both lower and upper UTI. Urinary tract pain is caused primarily by distension and increased pressure within the tract. The severity of the pain is related to the rate at which inflammation and distension develop.

In cystitis, inflammation causes a sensation of fullness; dull, constant suprapubic pain; and possibly lower back pain. The inflamed bladder wall and urethra cause dysuria, pain and burning on urination. Bladder spasms may develop, causing periodic severe, stabbing discomfort. Pain associated with pyelonephritis is often steady and dull, but may include severe, stabbing spasms, localised to the outer abdomen or flank region. Urological disorders rarely cause central abdominal pain.

- Assess pain: timing, quality, intensity, location, duration and aggravating and alleviating factors. *A change in the nature, location or intensity of the pain could indicate an extension of the infection or a related but separate problem.*
- Teach or provide comfort measures such as warm baths, warm packs or heating pads, and balanced rest and activity. Systemic analgesics, urinary analgesics or antispasmodic medication may be used as ordered. *Warmth relaxes muscles, relieves spasms and increases local blood supply. Because pain can stimulate a stress response and delay healing, it should be relieved when possible.*
- Increase fluid intake unless contraindicated. *Increased fluid dilutes urine, reducing irritation of the inflamed bladder and urethral mucosa.*
- Instruct to notify primary care provider if pain and discomfort continue or intensify after therapy is initiated. *Pain and discomfort in voiding typically are relieved within 24 hours of the initiation of antibiotic therapy. Continued discomfort may indicate a complicated UTI or other urinary tract disorder.*

> **CONSIDERATION FOR PRACTICE**
>
> **The older adult with a UTI may not complain of dysuria with a UTI. Be alert for other manifestations of UTI such as incontinence or cloudy or foul-smelling urine, as well as cognitive decline or confusion. Inflammatory and immune responses tend to diminish with ageing, reducing the irritative effects of UTI symptoms.**

Impaired urinary elimination

Inflammation of the bladder and urethral mucosa affects the normal process and patterns of voiding, causing frequency, urgency and burning on urination, as well as nocturia. Urine may be tinged with blood, cloudy and foul smelling. The person with short or long-term urinary retention requires

NURSING CARE PLAN A person with cystitis

Alana Stanton is a 22-year-old second-year university student. She is single and lives in a share house with three other students near the university she attends. Alana has never been pregnant and uses a Mirina® for birth control, as well as condoms for protection from STDs, although she admits only 'most' times. She presents to the university GP clinic complaining of lower back pain, frequency, urgency and burning on urination that began the day before.

ASSESSMENT

The RN admits Alana to the clinic and completes an assessment. Alana denies having had similar symptoms in the past or ever having been diagnosed with a urinary tract infection. The data collected show a constant dull ache that does not change with movement. Alana feels the need to urinate almost constantly, but experiences difficulty in starting her stream, with a burning pain and cramping when voiding. She reports getting up four times the night before to urinate. She denies painful intercourse and states that her last menstrual period began 2 weeks previously. A physical examination reveals: BP 112/68; P 90 and regular, T afebrile. Suprapubic tenderness was noted but no flank or costovertebral angle tenderness. A clean-catch urine specimen shows haematuria, multiple WBCs and a bacteria count greater than 10^6/L.

After assessing for allergies and diabetes, Alana was prescribed trimethoprim (TMP) 160/800 mg PO bd for 3 days and paracetamol 1 g PO every 4 hours as needed for pain; with a maximum of 4 g per day. She was also advised to increase her fluid intake to at least 3,000 mL every day to flush out the urinary system.

Alana is instructed to return to the clinic in 7 days for a follow-up urine culture or sooner if her symptoms do not improve or become worse.

DIAGNOSES

- *Pain* related to infection and inflammatory process in the urinary tract.
- *Impaired urinary elimination* related to inflammation as evidenced by frequency, urgency, nocturia and dysuria.
- *Deficient knowledge* related to lack of information about risk factors for UTI.

PLANNING

- Plan for effective pain management.
- Plan for elimination of burning on urination.
- Plan for effective psychological care.
- Plan to monitor for fluid balance.
- Plan for incorporating health prevention activities into daily routine.

Expected outcomes

- Relief of lower back pain and burning on urination.
- Regains a normal voiding pattern without frequency, urgency, nocturia and abnormal urine characteristics.
- Verbalises understanding of the disease process, related risk factors, follow-up instructions and symptoms of any recurrence indicating the need for medical attention.

IMPLEMENTATION

- Teach comfort measures: warm baths (avoiding the use of any additives such as bubble bath, perfumes or oils), a heating pad on low heat applied to her lower back or abdomen, rest, increased fluid intake, avoiding caffeinated beverages and taking paracetamol as ordered.
- Advise to avoid the use of antacids when taking trimethoprim-sulfamethoxazole and to take the medication on an empty stomach.
- Advise to stop taking the medication and return to doctor if rash and/or skin irritation occurs, which may signify allergic response to medication.
- Advise to refrain from sexual intercourse until infection and inflammation have cleared to avoid further irritation of inflamed tissues.
- Discuss dietary and hygiene practices to prevent UTI, including voiding post coitus, and symptoms which may indicate the need for further intervention and the risks of under treatment.
- Suggest how strategies designed to prevent further attacks of UTI can be incorporated into daily activities.
- Ensure details of Alana's history, diagnosis, treatment and response are recorded on the appropriate documents.

EVALUATION

On her follow-up visit, Alana reports that her symptoms and urine cleared within about a day after starting the antibiotic and she has had no further problems. She has increased her intake of fluid and vitamin C, and no longer puts off urinating until she 'has time to go'.

CRITICAL THINKING IN THE NURSING PROCESS

1. Which physiological and psychosocial factors put Alana at risk of developing a UTI?
2. Why is it necessary to ascertain whether or not Alana had allergies or diabetes? What would be the implications of these for the prescribed treatment?
3. Why was it appropriate to use short-course therapy for Alana? What was the importance of advising her to return if the symptoms did not clear?

REFLECTION ON THE NURSING PROCESS

1. Compare and contrast the benefits and disadvantages to short-course therapy versus conventional therapy for UTI in this case.
2. What are the potential dangers of repeated attacks of UTIs and why is it important to prevent these?
3. What lessons from this scenario could be used in health education programs to promote awareness of UTI and its treatment?

additional measures in assessing for and preventing UTI. (See the section on urinary retention later in this chapter.)

- Monitor (or give instructions to monitor) colour, clarity and odour of urine. *Urine should return to clear yellow within 48 hours, unless drug therapy causes a change in the colour of urine. If clarity does not return, further investigation may be necessary.*

> **CONSIDERATION FOR PRACTICE**
>
> Provide for close, easy access to a bedpan, urinal, commode or bathroom. Make sure that lighting is adequate and that pathways are free of obstacles. Frequency, urgency and nocturia increase the risk of urinary incontinence and, importantly, of injury due to falls, particularly in the older or debilitated individual.

- Instruct to avoid caffeinated drinks, including coffee, tea and cola; citrus juices; drinks containing artificial sweeteners; and alcoholic beverages. *Caffeine, citrus juices and artificial sweeteners irritate bladder mucosa and the detrusor muscle, and can increase urgency and bladder spasms.*
- Use strict aseptic non-touch technique (ANTT) and a closed urinary drainage system when inserting a straight or indwelling urinary catheter. Insert indwelling catheters to the full recommended length (5–6 cm in women and 15–25 cm in men) until urine flows before inflating the balloon. Never inflate the balloon until urine flows freely and stop if pain is felt. *Bacteria colonising the perineal tissues or on the nurse's hands can be introduced into the bladder during catheterisation. ANTT reduces this risk. Inflation of the balloon while in the urethra damages urethral tissues and can cause significant discomfort. See the 'Translation to practice' box for evidence-based practice for catheterisation.*

> **CONSIDERATION FOR PRACTICE**
>
> In males, fully insert the catheter to the 'Y' connection; in females, 2.5 cm beyond the point of urine flow (Society of Urological Nurses Association, 2014).

- When possible, use intermittent straight catheterisation to relieve urinary retention. Remove indwelling urinary catheters as soon as possible. *Using intermittent straight catheterisation allows the bladder to fill and completely empty in a more normal manner, maintaining physiological function. The risk of infection associated with an indwelling catheter is about 3–5% per day of catheterisation (Loscalzo et al., 2022).*

TRANSLATION TO PRACTICE Evidence-based practice: catheterisation

Insertion of an indwelling (retention) catheter is performed in hospitals and long-term care facilities. The location of the female urethral meatus presents a challenge to maintaining catheter sterility during insertion, whereas the anatomy of the male urethra presents a different set of challenges. Best practice guidelines for inserting the catheter in females is to insert the catheter until urine flows, then advance the catheter a further 2–4 cm to ensure the balloon is clear of the urethra; for males insert the catheter until resistance is felt at the first sphincter, then continue to the Y bifurcation. Ensure the retention balloon is well within the urinary bladder prior to its inflation (ANZUNS, 2013). Insertion to any lesser distance is inadequate to ensure safe balloon inflation without potential damage to the urethra.

IMPLICATIONS FOR NURSING

Nursing fundamentals and skills texts recommend inserting the catheter from 15.25 cm into the male urethra until urine flows. To ensure safe practice and reduce the risk of injury and discomfort, insert a retention catheter to the bifurcation before inflating the balloon.

SAFETY ALERT

Maintain the closed urinary drainage system and use aseptic technique when emptying the catheter drainage bag. Maintain gravity flow, preventing reflux of urine into the bladder from the drainage system. Bacteria can enter the drainage system when its integrity is interrupted as, for example, when disconnecting the catheter from the drainage system or during emptying of the drainage bag. Bacteria can ascend the column of urine to the bladder, causing UTI.

- Provide perineal care on a regular basis and following defecation. Use antiseptic preparations only as ordered. Regular cleansing of perineal tissues reduces the risk of colonisation by bacteria from the bowel or other sources. *While antiseptic solutions may be ordered for catheter care, they can dry perineal tissues and reduce normal flora, increasing the risk of colonisation by pathogens, and therefore should not be routinely used.*

CRITICAL THINKING IN PERSON-CENTRED CARE

1. Why is insertion of a urinary catheter frequently a more uncomfortable and difficult procedure for a male than a female? What nursing measures or techniques can be used to reduce this discomfort?
2. Sterile technique is generally used when catheterising people in acute care settings. However, those who require intermittent catheterisation to empty their bladder typically use clean technique. Would clean technique be appropriate in an acute or long-term care setting? Why or why not?

Source: ANZUNS (2013). *Catheterisation guideline working party*. Retrieved from https://www.anzuns.org/

Promoting health maintenance

The person with a urinary tract infection is at an increased risk of future UTI and needs to understand the disease process, risk factors, measures needed to prevent recurrent infection, diagnostic procedures required and appropriate home care. In addition, once the symptoms of UTI are relieved, individual motivation to continue the treatment plan declines. Failure to complete the full course of therapy and recommended follow-up can lead to continued bacteriuria and recurrent infections.

- Teach how to obtain a midstream clean-catch urine specimen. *Ninety per cent of urethral bacteria are cleared in the first 10 mL of voided urine; a midstream specimen is representative of urine in the bladder. Cleansing of the urinary meatus and perineal area reduces contamination of the specimen by external cells and bacteria.*
- Assess knowledge about the disease process, risk factors and preventive measures. *The individual may have little understanding of UTI, its causes and contributing factors.*
- Discuss the prescribed treatment plan and the importance of taking all prescribed antibiotics.
- Help the person develop a plan for taking medications, such as taking them with meals or on an empty stomach (unless contraindicated) or setting out all doses for the day in the morning. Discuss other over-the-counter medications or alternative therapies and assess understanding of interactions. *Missed doses of antibiotic can result in lowered therapeutic blood levels and reduced effectiveness. Taking medication in association with meals helps with remembering doses.*

CONSIDERATION FOR PRACTICE

Symptoms are largely relieved within 24 to 48 hours of starting antibiotic therapy; however, bacteria may remain in the urinary tract. Completing the prescribed regimen is important to prevent recurrent infections and resistant bacteria.

- Instruct to keep appointments for follow-up and urine culture. *Follow-up urine culture, often scheduled 7 to 14 days after completion of antibiotic therapy, is vital to ensure complete eradication of bacteria and prevention of relapse or recurrence.*
- Teach measures to prevent future UTI (see the preceding 'Health promotion' section). *Keep urine dilute and acidic and void regularly to flush bacteria out of the bladder and urethra. The proximity of the female urethral meatus to the vagina and anus increases the risk of bacterial contamination, especially during intercourse. Bubble baths, feminine hygiene sprays, synthetic fibres and douches may dry and irritate perineal tissues, promoting bacterial growth. Maintain adequate fluid intake to ensure renal function and production of urine.*

Community-based care

Because both upper and lower urinary tract infections are usually managed in the community, health education is the most important nursing intervention. Provide instruction on the following topics:

- Risk factors for UTI and how to minimise or eliminate these factors through increased fluid intake, regular elimination and personal hygiene measures.
- Early manifestations of UTI and the importance of seeking medical intervention promptly.
- Maintaining optimal immune system function by attending to contributory physical and psychosocial stressors, such as lack of adequate rest, poor nutrition and high levels of emotional stress.
- The importance of completing the prescribed treatment and keeping follow-up appointments.
- Minimising the risk of UTI when an indwelling urinary catheter is necessary:
  a. Use alternatives to an indwelling catheter when possible. For urinary incontinence, try scheduled toileting, incontinence pads or external catheters if possible. For urinary retention, teach the person or a family member to perform straight catheterisation every 3 to 4 hours using clean technique.
  b. Teach care measures such as perineal care, managing and emptying the collection chamber, maintaining a closed system and bladder irrigation or flushing if ordered when an indwelling catheter is necessary.

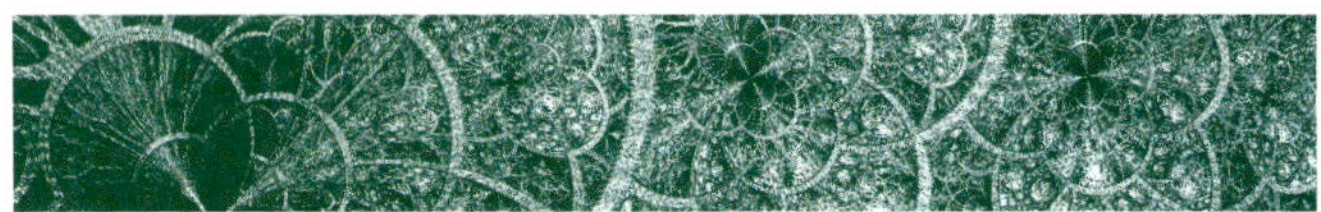

THE PERSON WITH URINARY CALCULI

Urinary calculi, stones in the urinary tract, are the most common cause of upper urinary tract obstruction (Wilson, Farrow & Holden, 2022). The term **lithiasis** means 'stone formation'; when the stones form in the kidney, it is known as *nephrolithiasis*; when they form elsewhere in the urinary tract (e.g. the bladder), it is called *urolithiasis*. Stones may form and obstruct the urinary tract at any point (see Figure 26.3). In Australia, the US and other industrialised countries, renal or kidney stones are the most common.

Incidence and risk factors

Urolithiasis is the third most common urological condition. It affects more males (1:10) than females (1:35) and, in Australia, the Indigenous population is at greater risk than non-Indigenous Australians. The incidence may vary according to geographical areas. Most people affected are in young or middle adulthood.

Although the majority of stones are idiopathic (having no demonstrable cause), a number of risk factors have been identified. The greatest risk factor for stone formation is a prior personal or family history of urinary calculi. A genetic predisposition towards the accumulation of certain mineral substances in the urine or a congenital lack of protective factors may explain the familial link. Other identified risk factors include dehydration with resultant increased urine concentration, immobility and excess dietary intake of calcium, oxalate or proteins. Gout, hyperparathyroidism and urinary stasis or repeated infections also contribute to calculus formation.

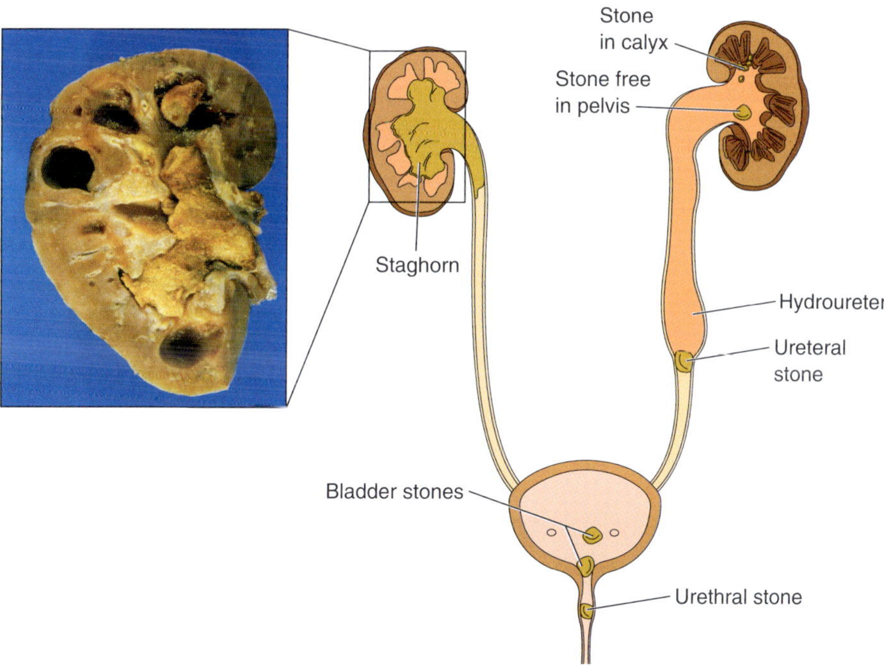

FIGURE 26.3 ***Development and location of calculi within the urinary tract***

Source: Image © Dr E. Walker/Science Photo.

Physiology review

Normally, a balance exists in the kidneys between the need to conserve water and to eliminate poorly soluble materials such as calcium salts. This balance is affected by factors such as diet, environmental temperature and activity. Protective inorganic and organic substances in the urine, such as pyrophosphate, citrate and glycoproteins, normally inhibit stone formation.

Pathophysiology

Three factors contribute to urolithiasis: supersaturation, nucleation and lack of inhibitory substances in the urine.

When the concentration of an insoluble salt in the urine is very high (supersaturated), crystals may form. Usually, these crystals disperse and are eliminated because the chemical bonds holding them together are weak. However, a nucleus of crystals may develop stable bonds to form a stone with crystals forming around an organic matrix or mucoprotein nucleus. The stimulus required to initiate crystallisation in supersaturated urine may be minimal. Ingesting a meal high in insoluble salt, or decreased fluid intake as occurs during sleep, allows the concentration to increase to the point where salt precipitation occurs, and stones are formed and grow. When fluid intake is adequate, no stone growth occurs. The acidity or alkalinity of the urine and the presence or absence of calculus-inhibiting compounds also affect lithiasis.

Most (75–80%) kidney stones are calcium stones composed of calcium oxalate and/or calcium phosphate. These stones are generally associated with high concentrations of calcium in the blood or urine. *Uric acid stones* develop when the urine concentration of uric acid is high. They are more common in men and may be associated with gout. Genetic factors contribute to the development of uric acid stones and calcium stones. *Struvite stones* are associated with UTI caused by urease-producing bacteria such as *Proteus*. These stones can become very large, filling the renal pelvis and calyces, and are often called *staghorn stones* because of their shape. *Cystine stones* are rare and are associated with a genetic amino acid metabolic defect. The types of renal calculi, contributing factors and recommended dietary modifications are listed in Table 26.2. Manifestations develop as a result of obstructed urine flow with resulting distension, and tissue trauma caused by passage of the rough-edged, crystalline stone.

Manifestations

The symptoms caused by urinary calculi vary with their size and location (see the 'Manifestations' box).

> **FAST FACTS**
>
> - Most urinary stones form in the renal pelvis and are composed primarily of calcium salts.
> - Loss of calcium from the bones (e.g. due to immobility, osteoporosis) and dehydration are major risk factors for urinary stones.

Calculi affecting the kidney calyces and pelvis may cause few symptoms. If the stone has gradually or partially obstructed urinary flow, dull, aching flank pain may be present, but renal calculi may be silent, without symptoms. Bladder calculi may cause few symptoms other than dull suprapubic pain on exercise or after voiding.

Renal colic—acute, severe flank pain on the affected side—develops when a stone obstructs the ureter, causing ureteral spasm. The pain of renal colic may radiate to the suprapubic

TABLE 26.2 Risk factors and interventions for renal calculi

STONE TYPE AND INCIDENCE	RISK FACTORS	MANAGEMENT
Calcium phosphate and/or oxalate 75–80%	Hypercalciuria and hypercalcaemia: hyperparathyroidism, immobility, bone disease, vitamin D intoxication, multiple myeloma, renal tubular acidosis, prolonged steroid intake, alkaline urine, dehydration, inflammatory bowel disease	Pharmacology: thiazide diuretics, phosphates, calcium-binding agents Dietary: limit foods high in calcium and oxalate, increase foods that acidify urine Other: increase hydration, exercise
Struvite 15–20%	UTIs, especially *Proteus* infections	Pharmacology: antibiotic therapy for UTI Other: surgical intervention or lithotripsy to remove stone
Uric acid 5–10%	Gout, increased purine intake, acid urine	Pharmacology: potassium citrate, allopurinol Dietary: low-purine diet Other: increase hydration
Cystine (uncommon)	Genetic defect, acid urine	Pharmacology: penicillamine, sodium bicarbonate Dietary: sodium restriction Other: increase hydration

MANIFESTATIONS Urinary calculi

KIDNEY STONES
- Often asymptomatic
- Dull, aching flank pain
- Microscopic haematuria
- Manifestations of UTI

URETERAL STONES
- Renal colic
- Acute, severe flank pain on affected side
- Often radiates to suprapubic region, groin and external genitals
- Nausea, vomiting, pallor and cool, clammy skin

BLADDER STONES
- May be asymptomatic
- Dull suprapubic pain, possibly associated with exercise or voiding
- Gross or microscopic haematuria
- Manifestations of UTI

region, groin and external genitals (the scrotum or labia). The severity of the pain often causes a sympathetic response with associated nausea, vomiting, pallor and cool, clammy skin.

Manifestations of UTI, including chills and fever, frequency, urgency and dysuria, may accompany urinary calculi at any level. Trauma to the urinary tract by the calculi may cause gross or microscopic haematuria. Gross haematuria may also be the only sign of bladder stones.

Complications

Urinary stones may obstruct urine flow at any point of the urinary tract, leading to complications such as hydronephrosis and urinary stasis with subsequent infection.

Obstruction

Stones can obstruct the urinary tract at any point from the calyces of the kidney to the distal urethra, impeding the outflow of urine. If the obstruction develops slowly, there may be few or no symptoms, whereas sudden obstruction (e.g. blockage of a ureter by a passing stone) may cause severe manifestations. Urinary tract obstruction can ultimately lead to renal failure. The degree of obstruction, its location and the duration of impaired urine flow determine the effect on renal function.

HYDRONEPHROSIS The kidneys continue to produce urine, causing increased pressure and distension of the urinary tract behind the obstruction. **Hydronephrosis**, distension of the renal pelvis and calyces, and *hydroureter*, distension of the ureter, are possible results. If the pressure is unrelieved, the collecting tubules, proximal tubules and glomeruli of the kidney are damaged, causing a gradual loss of renal function.

Acute hydronephrosis typically causes colicky pain on the affected side. The pain may radiate into the groin. Chronic hydronephrosis develops slowly and may have few manifestations other than dull, aching back or flank pain. When hydronephrosis is significant, a palpable mass may be felt in the flank region. Haematuria and signs of UTI such as pyuria, fever and discomfort may occur. Gastrointestinal symptoms such as nausea, vomiting and abdominal pain may accompany hydronephrosis (see the 'Manifestations' box). In severe cases, shock caused by pain may develop and urgent treatment may be necessary.

INFECTION The urinary stasis associated with partial or complete obstruction increases the risk of urinary infection in the upper or lower urinary tract.

MANIFESTATIONS Acute and chronic hydronephrosis

ACUTE
- Acute, colicky pain; may radiate into groin
- Haematuria, pyuria
- Fever
- Nausea, vomiting, abdominal pain

CHRONIC
- Dull, aching flank pain
- Haematuria, pyuria
- Fever
- Palpable flank mass

INTERPROFESSIONAL CARE

Management of urinary calculi focuses on relieving acute symptoms, destroying or removing stones, and preventing further stone formation. Asymptomatic stones (those not causing pain, infection or obstruction) are treated conservatively.

Diagnosis

Laboratory and diagnostic tests that may be ordered when urinary calculi are suspected include the following:

- *Urinalysis* to assess for haematuria and the possible presence of WBCs and crystal fragments. The urine pH is helpful in identifying the type of stone.
- *Chemical analysis* of any stones passed in the urine determines the type of stone and suggests measures to prevent further stone formation. Retrieving stones or teaching the person to do so is a nursing responsibility. All urine is strained and may be saved. Any visible stones or sediment is sent for analysis.
- *Urine calcium, uric acid* and *oxalate* levels measure the amount of these substances excreted over a 24-hour period and may be assessed to help identify possible causes of lithiasis. Elevated calcium levels occur in hyperparathyroidism, Cushing's syndrome and osteoporosis, all of which may contribute to lithiasis. Uric acid levels may be elevated in people with gout and those at risk of forming uric acid calculi. Urine oxalate excretion may help to differentiate calcium oxalate from calcium phosphate stones.
- *Serum calcium, phosphorus* and *uric acid* levels may be obtained to help identify factors contributing to calculus formation.
- *X-ray* (kidneys, ureters and bladder) of the lower abdomen that requires no special preparation. Calculi may be identified as opacities in the kidneys, ureters and bladder.
- *Renal ultrasound* is a non-invasive test that uses reflected sound waves to detect stones and evaluate the kidneys for possible hydronephrosis.
- *Computed tomography (CT) scan* of the kidney, with or without contrast medium, directed at the kidney from many angles to provide a computer-generated photograph that shows calculi, ureteral obstruction and other renal disorders.
- *IVP* may be done to visualise the kidneys, ureters and bladder after injection of a contrast medium. IVP may be done when x-rays, renal ultrasonography and CT scan fail to demonstrate clear evidence of urinary calculi. (See 'Diagnostic tests, intravenous pyelogram (IVP)' in the chapter 'A person-centred approach to assessing the renal system'.)
- *Cystoscopy* is used to visualise and possibly remove calculi from the urinary bladder and distal ureters.

Nursing implications and care for people undergoing these tests and procedures are outlined in the chapter 'A person-centred approach to assessing the renal system'.

Medications

An acute episode of renal colic is treated with analgesia and hydration. A narcotic analgesic such as morphine sulfate is given, often intravenously, to relieve pain and reduce ureteral spasm. Indomethacin, a non-steroidal anti-inflammatory drug (NSAID), given as a suppository, may reduce the amount of narcotic analgesia required for acute renal colic. Oral or intravenous fluids reduce the risk of further stone formation and promote urine output.

After analysis of the calculus, various medications may be ordered to inhibit or prevent further lithiasis. A thiazide diuretic, frequently prescribed for calcium calculi, acts to reduce urinary calcium excretion and is very effective in preventing further stones. Potassium citrate alkalinises urine by raising the pH and is often prescribed to prevent stones that tend to form in acidic urine (uric acid, cystine and some forms of calcium stones). See Table 26.2 for other preparations related to types of stones. Nursing responsibilities focus on teaching the person about the prescribed medication, its importance in preventing further stone formation and potential adverse effects.

Nutrition and fluid management

Diet modifications are often prescribed to change the character of the urine and prevent further lithiasis.

Increased fluid intake of 2,500 to 3,000 mL per day is recommended, unless contraindicated, regardless of stone composition. A fluid intake to ensure the production of approximately 2,000 to 2,500 mL of urine a day prevents the stone-forming salts from becoming concentrated enough to precipitate. Fluid intake should be spaced throughout the day and evening. Recommended dietary changes may include reduced intake of the primary substance forming the calculi. For calcium stones, dietary calcium and vitamin-D-enriched foods are limited. Limiting vitamin D inhibits the absorption of calcium from the GI tract. Calcium stones may be a calcium phosphate salt, calcium oxalate or a combination of both; therefore, phosphorus and/or oxalate may also be limited in the diet.

The person with uric acid stones requires a diet low in purines. Organ meats, sardines and other high-purine foods may be limited.

In addition to limiting certain foods, the diet may be modified to maintain a urinary pH that does not promote lithiasis. Uric acid and cystine stones tend to form in acid urine. Foods that tend to alkalinise the urine may be recommended. Because alkaline urine promotes formation of calcium stones and urinary tract infections, the diet may be modified to lower the pH of the urine. Foods that affect urinary pH and foods high in various stone components are summarised in Table 26.3.

TABLE 26.3 Teaching people with urolithiasis: possible food and fluid modifications

Foods high in calcium	Beans and lentils, chocolate and cocoa, dried fruits, canned or smoked fish except tuna, flour, milk and milk products
Foods high in oxalate	Asparagus, beer and colas, beetroot, cabbage, celery, chocolate and cocoa, fruits, green beans, nuts, tea, tomatoes
Purine-rich foods	Goose, organ meats, sardines and herring, venison; moderate in beef, chicken, crab, pork, salmon, veal
Acidifying foods	Cheese, cranberries, eggs, grapes, meat and poultry, plums and prunes, tomatoes, whole grains
Alkalinising foods	Green vegetables, fruit (except as noted previously), legumes, milk and milk products, rhubarb

Surgery

Treatment of existing calculi depends on the location of the stones, the extent of obstruction, renal function, the presence or absence of UTI, and the individual's general state of health. In general, a stone is removed if it is causing severe obstruction, infection, unrelieved pain or serious bleeding (Loscalzo et al., 2022).

Lithotripsy, using sound or shock waves to crush a stone, is the preferred treatment for urinary calculi. Several techniques are available. **Extracorporeal shock wave lithotripsy (ESWL)** is a non-invasive technique for fragmenting kidney stones using shock waves generated outside the body. Acoustic shock waves are aimed under fluoroscopic guidance at the stone (see Figure 26.4). These shock waves travel through soft tissue without causing damage but shatter the stone as its greater density stops their progress. Repeated shock waves pulverise the stone into fragments small enough to be eliminated in the urine. The procedure may require 30 minutes to 2 hours to complete. Intravenous sedation generally is adequate to maintain comfort during the procedure (Reesink et al., 2018). See the nursing care box.

Lithotripsy also may be performed using a percutaneous ultrasonic or laser technique. *Percutaneous ultrasonic lithotripsy* uses a nephroscope inserted into the kidney pelvis through a small flank incision (see Figure 26.5). The stone is fragmented using a small ultrasonic transducer and the fragments are removed through the nephroscope. *Laser lithotripsy* is an alternative to ultrasonic lithotripsy. Laser beams are used to disintegrate the stone, without damaging soft tissue. A nephroscope or a ureteroscope (passed up the ureter from the bladder during cystoscopy) is used to guide the laser probe into direct contact with the stone.

A double J stent (ureteric stent) may be inserted into the affected ureter to maintain its patency following ESWL or other lithotripsy procedures. (See the 'Nursing care of the person having lithotripsy' box.)

On rare occasions, surgical intervention is necessary to remove a calculus in the renal pelvis or ureter. *Ureterolithotomy* is an incision in the affected ureter to remove a calculus. *Pyelolithotomy* is an incision into and removal of a stone from the kidney pelvis. A staghorn calculus that invades the calyces and renal parenchyma may require a *nephrolithotomy* for removal. See the chapter 'Nursing care of people having surgery' for care of the person having surgery.

Bladder stones may be removed using an instrument passed through a cystoscope to crush the stones. The remaining stone fragments are then irrigated out of the bladder using an acid solution to counteract the alkalinity that precipitated stone formation.

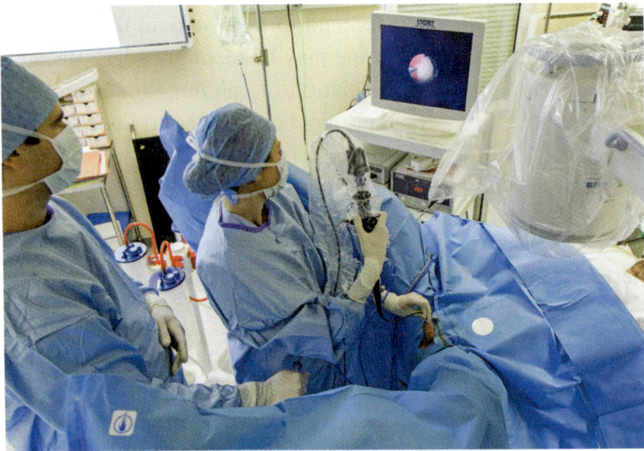

FIGURE 26.4 ***Extracorporeal shock wave lithotripsy. Acoustic shock waves generated by the shock wave generator travel through soft tissue to shatter the urinary stone into fragments, which are then eliminated in the urine***

Source: GARO/PHANIE/Alamy Stock Photo.

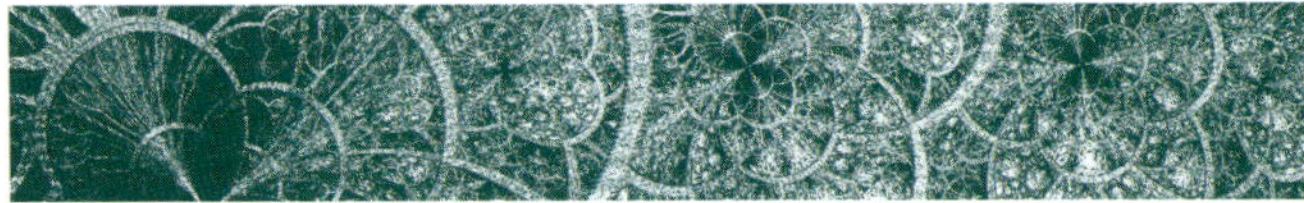

Nursing care

Nursing care for the person with urolithiasis is directed at providing for comfort during acute renal colic, assisting with diagnostic procedures, ensuring adequate urinary output and teaching information necessary to prevent future stone formation.

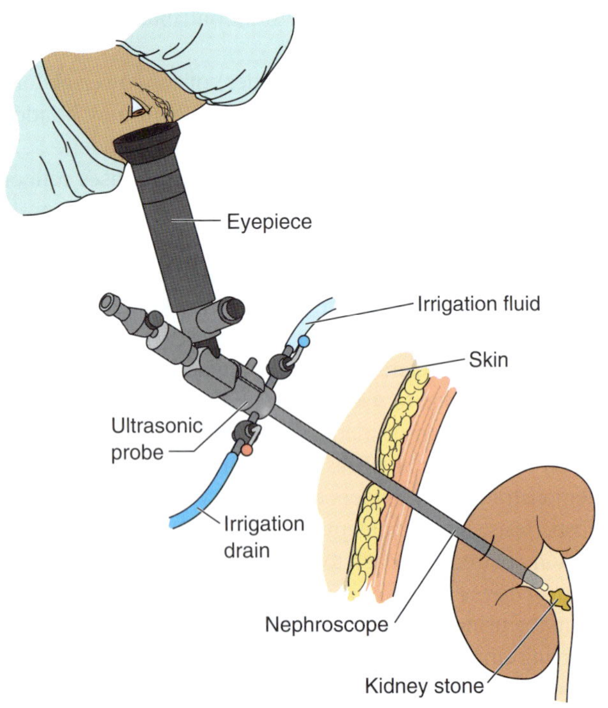

FIGURE 26.5 ***Percutaneous ultrasonic lithotripsy. A nephroscope is inserted into the renal pelvis and ultrasonic waves are used to fragment the stone. The fragments are then removed through the nephroscope.***

NURSING CARE OF THE PERSON having lithotripsy

PREOPERATIVE CARE

- Assess knowledge and understanding of the procedure, providing information as needed. *Anxiety is reduced and recovery is enhanced and hastened when the individual is fully prepared for surgery.*
- Follow directions from the radiology department, doctor or anaesthetist for withholding food and fluids and for bowel preparation prior to surgery. Conscious sedation, general anaesthesia or spinal anaesthesia may be required, depending on the procedure. *Faecal material in the bowel may impede fluoroscopic visualisation of the kidney and stone.*

POSTOPERATIVE CARE

- In the initial period, monitor vital signs frequently. *The kidney is highly vascular; therefore, haemorrhage and resulting shock are potential complications of lithotripsy. Bleeding may be internal or retroperitoneal and difficult to detect.*
- Monitor amount, colour and clarity of urine output. *Urine is often bright red initially, but bleeding should diminish within 48 to 72 hours. Cloudy urine may indicate the presence of an infection.*
- Maintain placement and patency of urinary catheters. Anchor ureteral catheters or nephrostomy tubes securely. Label all lines and ensure separate drainage systems for all drainage tubes. Irrigate gently if ordered. *A kinked or plugged catheter may result in hydroureter, hydronephrosis and kidney damage. Decreased urinary output and flank pain are possible symptoms of obstructed urine flow. Excessive force in irrigation may cause trauma and bleeding and should not be attempted without education and/or support from suitably experienced staff.*
- Ensure fluid intake of at least 3 L per day to promote urine production and to flush the renal system, unless contraindicated.

HEALTH EDUCATION FOR THE PERSON AND FAMILY

- Prepare for discharge by teaching care of the indwelling catheter, urine-collection device and incision site (if present). Teach signs and symptoms to report: urine leakage from incision for more than 4 days, symptoms of infection, pain, bright haematuria. *If discharged with dressings and catheters in place, the individual and family need necessary information to provide self-care. Assessment of patient and/or family understanding may lead to further referral to specialised services (i.e Community Health or Hospital in the Home).*
- Teach measures to reduce the risk of further lithiasis. Prevention of stone formation is important to preserve renal function, as many people *have repeated episodes of lithiasis and renal colic. Dietary advice may be required.*

Health promotion

Discuss the importance of maintaining an adequate fluid intake with all people. Stress the need to increase fluid intake during warm weather and strenuous exercise or physical labour.

Discuss the relationship between weight-bearing activity and retention of calcium in the bones. Encourage the maintenance of physical activity as much as possible to prevent bone resorption (loss) and possible hypercalciuria.

Instruct people with known gout to maintain a generous fluid intake so as to produce at least 2,000 mL of urine every day, unless contraindicated. Discuss the risk of lithiasis with individuals who have frequent UTIs and teach measures to reduce the incidence of UTI and the risk of lithiasis.

Assessment

Obtain subjective and objective assessment data specific to urolithiasis:

- *Health history*: complaints of flank, back or abdominal pain, radiation, characteristics and timing, aggravating or relieving factors, other symptoms such as nausea and vomiting; possible contributing factors such as dehydration; previous or family history of kidney stones; current or previous treatment measures.
- *Physical examination*: general appearance including position, vital signs; skin colour, temperature, moisture, turgor; abdominal, flank or costovertebral tenderness; amount, colour and characteristics of urine (presence of haematuria, bacteria, pyuria, pH).

Nursing diagnoses and interventions

See the nursing care plan that follows this section for additional nursing diagnoses and interventions.

Acute pain

Pain is the primary outward manifestation of urolithiasis, particularly when a stone lodges within a ureter causing acute obstruction and distension. Invasive and non-invasive procedures to remove or crush stones also may be painful. People undergoing surgery also experience incisional pain.

CONSIDERATION FOR PRACTICE

The intensity of renal colic pain can cause a vasovagal response with resulting hypotension and syncope. Always provide for the person's personal safety and ensure they are not at risk from shock in this situation.

- Assess pain using a standard pain scale and its characteristics. Administer analgesia as ordered and monitor its effectiveness. *The intensity, type of pain and its responsiveness to analgesia provide valuable clues as to its cause. Regular administration of prescribed analgesics controls pain more effectively than waiting until pain becomes intolerable. Administering an ordered NSAID on a routine schedule may significantly reduce the need for narcotic analgesia for those with renal colic.*
- Unless contraindicated, encourage fluid intake and ambulation for people with renal colic. *Increased fluids and ambulation encourage urinary output, thereby facilitating movement of the calculus through the ureter and decreasing pain.*
- Use non-pharmacological measures such as positioning, moist heat, relaxation techniques, guided imagery and diversion as adjunctive therapy for pain relief. *Adjunctive pain relief measures can enhance the effectiveness of analgesics and other prescribed treatment.*
- If surgery has been performed, monitor urinary output, catheters, incision and wound drainage. *Pain may be a symptom of proximal distension due to a blocked catheter. Infection or haematoma at the surgical site can significantly increase pain.*

Impaired urinary elimination

Obstruction of the urinary tract is the primary problem associated with urolithiasis. Obstruction can ultimately lead to stasis, infection or irreversible renal damage.

- Monitor amount and character of urine output. If catheterised, measure output hourly. Document any haematuria, dysuria, frequency, urgency and pyuria. Strain all urine for stones, saving any recovered stones for laboratory analysis. *The amount of urine output helps determine possible urinary tract obstruction and adequacy of hydration. Gross or microscopic haematuria is often associated with calculi and with procedures used to remove stones, such as cystoscopy or lithotripsy. A change in the amount of haematuria may indicate stone passage or a complication. Dysuria, frequency, urgency and cloudy urine are symptoms of UTI, often associated with urolithiasis. Antibiotic therapy may be required. Analysis of stones recovered from the urine can direct measures to prevent further lithiasis.*

> **CONSIDERATION FOR PRACTICE**
>
> **A stone that completely obstructs the ureter can lead to hydronephrosis and kidney damage on the affected side. Report symptoms of hydronephrosis such as dull flank pain or aching and changes in renal function studies (blood urea nitrogen (BUN) and serum creatinine). As the other kidney continues to function, urine output may not fall significantly with obstruction of one ureter. A rising BUN and serum creatinine may be early signs of renal failure.**

- Maintain patency and integrity of all catheter systems. Secure catheters well, label as indicated and use sterile technique for all ordered irrigations or other procedures. *A kinked or plugged catheter, particularly a ureteral catheter or nephrostomy tube, may damage the urinary system. Labelling catheters can prevent mistakes such as inappropriate irrigation or clamping. Any catheter increases the risk of infection; aseptic technique in all procedures reduces this risk.*

Deficient knowledge

The person with urolithiasis has multiple learning needs. These include information about the disease and its possible consequences, any diagnostic or therapeutic procedures performed and strategies to prevent future lithiasis.

- Assess understanding and previous learning. *Relating information to previously learned material enhances retention and understanding.*
- Present all information in a manner appropriate to knowledge base, developmental and educational level, and current needs. *Learning is an active process that requires the individual's participation. Tailoring teaching to the individual increases involvement.*
- Educate about all diagnostic and treatment procedures. *Knowing what to expect reduces anxiety, enhances compliance and hastens recovery.*
- If the person will be managed in the community, educate to:
  a. Collect and strain all urine, saving any stones.
  b. Report stone passage to the doctor and deliver the stone for analysis.
  c. Report any changes in the amount or character of urine output to doctor.

  When pain can be managed with oral analgesics, urinary stones are managed in the community. The individual needs to know how and why to collect the calculus and indicators of complications, such as reduced urine output, cloudy or bloody urine or marked increase in pain.
- Teach measures to prevent further urolithiasis:
  a. Increase fluid intake to 2,500 to 3,500 mL per day (unless contraindicated).
  b. Follow recommended dietary guidelines.
  c. Maintain activity level to prevent urinary stasis and bone resorption.
  d. Take medications as prescribed.
  e. Obtain prompt treatment for any further urinary infections.
  f. Reduce/minimise tea and coffee and reduce salt in the diet. Restrict carbonated drinks such as cola and beer as these contain phosphoric acid, a precursor to calculi formation.

  The risk of recurrent lithiasis is approximately 50%; however, this risk can be reduced by measures to prevent conditions favouring stone formation.
- Teach about the relationship between urinary calculi and UTI, emphasising preventive measures and the importance of prompt treatment. *Urinary tract infection promotes urolithiasis and thus requires prompt treatment to reduce this risk.*

Community-based care

The person with urinary calculi will need to know how to manage existing stones and what to do to reduce the risk of future stone formation. Discuss the following topics to prepare the person and family for home care:

- importance of maintaining a fluid intake adequate to produce 2,000 to 2,500 mL of urine per day, unless contraindicated
- prescribed medications, their management and potential adverse effects
- dietary recommendations
- prevention, recognition and management of UTI
- any further diagnostic or treatment measures planned.

If the person is to be discharged with dressings, a nephrostomy tube or a catheter, educate the individual and family about the following:

- how to change dressings, maintaining aseptic technique
- assessment of the wound and skin for healing and possible complications such as infection or skin breakdown
- how to manage drainage systems and maintain their patency with aseptic considerations
- emptying drainage bags and assessing urine output
- recommendations for follow-up care and when to contact the doctor.

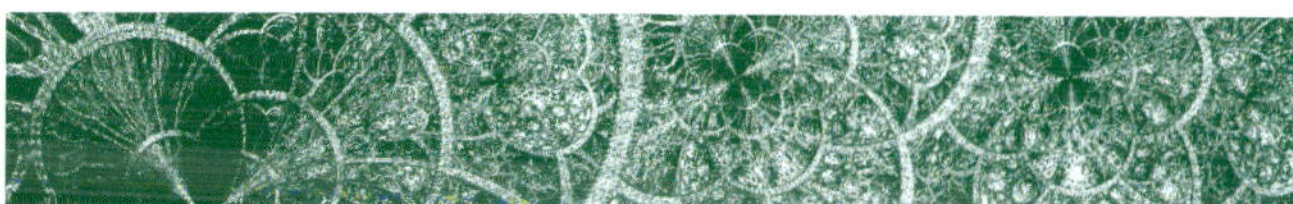

NURSING CARE PLAN **A person with urinary calculi**

Richard Leton, aged 44, owns a small business. He is admitted to the medical unit from the emergency department after awakening at 4 am with severe right-sided pain. His FBC is normal and urinalysis reveals microscopic haematuria, but no protein or bacteria. A renal ultrasound shows a 4–5 mm stone partially obstructing the right ureter.

The admitting nurse notes that Mr Leton is pale, diaphoretic and very anxious. He complains of nausea and asks for an emesis basin. Mr Leton received 4 mg of intravenous morphine sulfate approximately 2.5 hours ago. He denies pain at this time but says, 'I'm scared to death that it'll come back. I couldn't even move, it hurt so bad.'

ASSESSMENT

Mr Leton's history reveals no previous episodes of renal calculi. He felt well until the pain awakened him during the night. He admits that he has been working under a deadline to complete a construction project and that he probably has not been drinking enough fluids, 'considering how hot it's been'. Physical assessment findings include T 38.05°C, P 98, R 24 and BP 160/86. Colour is pale to ashen, skin cool and moist. His abdomen is firm with moderate tenderness in the right upper outer quadrant. The doctor orders an IV of 5% dextrose in normal saline at 200 mL/h until nausea is relieved, then PO fluids of at least 3,000 mL/24 h; morphine sulfate 2 to 10 mg IV prn for pain; indomethacin (Indocid) 50 mg per rectal suppository q8h; ondansetron (Zofran) 4 mg wafer PRN for nausea; activity to tolerance; and strain all urine, sending recovered stones for analysis.

DIAGNOSES

- *Anxiety* related to anticipation of recurrent severe pain.
- *Risk of imbalanced nutrition: less than body requirements* related to nausea.
- *Acute pain* related to partial obstruction of right ureter by calculus.
- *Impaired urinary elimination* related to partial obstruction of ureter by calculus.
- *Deficient knowledge* related to lack of information about disease process, contributing factors and management.

PLANNING

- Plan interventions to reduce pain and anxiety.
- Plan interventions to reduce nausea and facilitate adherence to increased fluid intake.
- Develop collaboratively a nutrition and fluid education program.

Expected outcomes

- Demonstrate reduced anxiety by relaxed facial expression, vital signs within his normal range and ability to rest when not disturbed.
- Consume at least 50% of diet and 100% of ordered fluids without nausea or vomiting.
- Request analgesia as needed at onset of pain; report effective pain relief.
- Maintain urine output of 2,500 mL/24 h with no signs of infection or obstruction (such as increased pain, dysuria, pyuria or haematuria).
- Demonstrate an understanding of the process of urolithiasis and contributing factors.
- Verbalise knowledge of dietary, fluid intake and other measures required to reduce risk of future stone formation.

IMPLEMENTATION

- Reassure that measures to prevent further episodes of renal colic are being implemented and that medication is available to relieve pain promptly.
- Assess the effectiveness of analgesia and its adverse effects, especially nausea.
- Maintain IV as ordered until oral fluid intake exceeds 200 mL of fluid per hour while awake.
- Measure and strain all urine. Assess urine for colour, clarity and odour.
- Teach about urolithiasis and its risk factors, especially as they relate to Mr Leton.
- Teach the importance of maintaining a high fluid intake, especially when working outdoors in hot weather; recommended dietary modifications and their rationale; ordered medications and their effects; how to identify and prevent UTI; and symptoms that should be reported to the doctor.

EVALUATION

Mr Leton passed the obstructing stone the evening after admission and is discharged the following day. On discharge, he states he has no pain or nausea, his urine is clear and pale yellow, and urinalysis is normal. Laboratory analysis shows that the calculus was calcium. Mr Leton is able to affirm the importance of continuing a high fluid intake. He confirms that he will

(continued)

NURSING CARE PLAN A person with urinary calculi (countinued)

reduce his intake of calcium-rich foods, such as milk and milk products, and that he will increase his intake of foods to acidify his urine. He is able to list foods to include in his diet and comments: 'You can be sure I'll follow my diet, drink my water and make sure I don't get an infection. I hope to never feel pain like that again!'

CRITICAL THINKING IN THE NURSING PROCESS

1 What factors contributed to the onset and timing of Mr Leton's ureteral colic?
2 What is the rationale for administering indomethacin, an NSAID, to a person with ureteral colic?
3 Why did the nurse include a nursing intervention to assess for a relationship between Mr Leton's nausea, his pain and the ordered analgesic agent?

REFLECTION ON THE NURSING PROCESS

1 Reflect on the educational strategies offered to Mr Leton and consider how you could incorporate these into your workday to prevent a reoccurrence for people at risk.
2 Considering the case study above, identify what new knowledge you have gained that will enhance how you deliver care to a person with ureteral colic.

THE PERSON WITH A URINARY TRACT TUMOUR

A malignancy can develop in any part of the urinary tract; however, 90% develop in the bladder, about 8% develop in the renal pelvis and only 2% develop in the ureter or urethra (Loscalzo et al., 2022). Overall prognosis for bladder cancer is dependent on the type of carcinoma present. In Australia, the 5-year survival rate for bladder cancer is 53.3% (Australian Institute of Health and Welfare, 2017).

Incidence and risk factors

The incidence of bladder cancer is higher in people who smoke or are over the age of 65, and is three times higher in men than in women. Women experience poorer outcomes and survival (Krimprove et al., 2019).

Two main factors are implicated in the development of bladder cancer: the presence of carcinogens in the urine and chronic inflammation or infection of bladder mucosa. Cigarette smoking is the primary risk factor for bladder cancer. Bladder cancer accounts for 3% of cancer diagnoses worldwide and 50–65% of all cases are linked to tobacco smoking, which is the strongest risk factor (Saginala et al., 2020). The chemicals and dyes used in the plastics, rubber and cable industries; substances in the work environment of textile workers, leather finishers, spray painters and petroleum workers; and the chronic use of phenacetin-containing analgesic agents also are associated with a higher risk. Additional risk factors for bladder cancer include residence in an urban area, chronic UTIs and bladder calculi. The parasite *Schistosoma haematobium*, endemic to Egypt and the Sudan, also increases the risk of bladder cancer (Saginala et al., 2020). The risk of bladder cancer appears to be reduced by changes in diet, fluid intake and exercise (Saginala et al., 2020).

FAST FACTS

The main risk factors for bladder cancer are:

- Male gender, age > 55, residence in urban area
- Cigarette smoking
- Occupational exposure to dyes or solvents
- Chronic UTI or bladder calculi
- Long-term use of cyclophosphamide

Pathophysiology

Most urinary tract malignancies arise from epithelial tissue. Transitional epithelium lines the entire tract from the renal pelvis through to the urethra. Carcinogenic products of nicotine metabolism and cigarette smoke are stored in the bladder then excreted in urine. It is possible the presence of carcinogens in bladder urine may cause abnormal bladder cell development. Squamous cell carcinoma of the urinary tract occurs less frequently than transitional epithelial cell tumours.

Urinary tract tumours begin as non-specific cellular alterations that develop into either flat or papillary lesions.

These lesions may be either superficial or invasive. About 75% of bladder tumours are papillary lesions (*papillomas*), a polyp-like structure attached by a stalk to the bladder mucosa (see Figure 26.6). Papillomas are generally superficial, non-invasive tumours that bleed easily and frequently recur (Loscalzo et al., 2022). They rarely progress to become invasive and the prognosis for recovery is good.

Carcinoma in situ (CIS), which occurs less frequently, is a poorly differentiated flat tumour that invades directly and is associated with a poorer prognosis. Bladder tumours are rated by their cell type and grade. Grade I tumours are highly differentiated and rarely progress to become invasive,

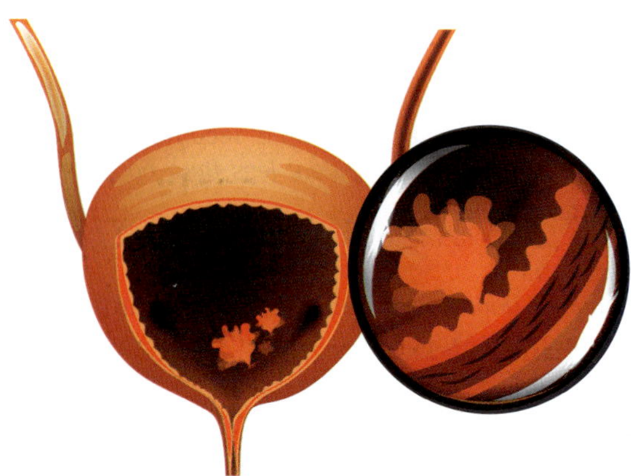

FIGURE 26.6 ***Papillary transitional cell carcinoma of the urinary bladder***

Source: Viktoriya Kabanova/Alamy Stock Vector.

TABLE 26.4 Bladder tumour staging

DEPTH OF INVOLVEMENT	TNM (TUMOUR, NODE, METASTASIS) STAGE	TUMOUR INVOLVEMENT
Superficial	T_a	Limited to the bladder mucosa
	T_1	Involvement of the bladder mucosa and submucosal layers
Invasive	T_2	Invasion of superficial muscle of bladder wall
	T_{3a}	Deep muscle invasion
	T_{3b}	Involvement of perivesicular fat
	$T_{3-4}N_+$	Regional (pelvic) lymph node involvement
	$T_{3-4}M_1$	Metastasis to distant lymph nodes or organs

whereas grade III tumours are poorly differentiated and usually progress (Loscalzo et al., 2022). The staging of bladder tumours is outlined in Table 26.4. See the chapter 'Nursing care of people with cancer' for more information about tumour grading and staging. When metastasis occurs, the pelvic lymph nodes, lungs, bones and liver are most commonly involved.

Manifestations

Painless haematuria is the presenting sign in 75% of urinary tract tumours. Haematuria may be gross or microscopic and is often intermittent, causing delay in seeking treatment (Saginala et al., 2020). Inflammation surrounding the tumour occasionally causes manifestations of a urinary tract infection, including frequency, urgency and dysuria. Ureteral tumours may cause colicky pain from obstruction. Tumours of the urinary tract typically cause few outward signs and may not be discovered until obstructed urine flow causes flank pain or renal failure.

CONSIDERATION FOR PRACTICE

Intermittent painless haematuria is the most common presenting symptom of bladder cancer. Instruct all people with painless haematuria to contact their doctor for follow-up testing.

INTERPROFESSIONAL CARE

Treatment of the person with a tumour of the urinary tract focuses on removing or destroying the cancerous tissue, preventing further invasion or metastasis and maintaining renal and urinary function.

Diagnosis

When a urinary tract tumour is suspected, the following diagnostic tests may be ordered:

- *Urinalysis* is done to evaluate for haematuria. Gross or microscopic haematuria is often the first indicator of a neoplasm in the urinary tract.
- *Urine cytology*, microscopic examination of cells in the urine, is performed to identify abnormal cells (tumour or pre-tumour cells). Periodic urine cytology is recommended for those at high risk of bladder cancer or its recurrence due to carcinogen exposure.
- *Ultrasound of the bladder* is a non-invasive test to detect bladder tumours. No dye is required and there is no exposure to radiation.
- *Intravenous pyelography* is used to evaluate the structure and function of the kidneys, ureters and bladder. IVP may reveal a rigid deformity of the bladder wall, obstruction of urine flow at the point of the tumour, or bladder filling or emptying defects.
- *Cystoscopy* and *ureteroscopy* allow direct visualisation, assessment and biopsy of lesions of the urethra, bladder or ureters using a lighted scope inserted through the urethra. Cystoscopy or ureteroscopy with biopsy allows definitive diagnosis of urinary tract tumours.
- *CT scan* or *MRI* is primarily used to evaluate tumour invasion or metastasis if suspected.
- See the chapter 'A person-centred approach to assessing the renal system' for nursing care related to these diagnostic tests.

Medications

Immunological or chemotherapeutic agents administered by intravesical instillation (into the bladder) may be used either as the primary treatment for bladder cancer when multiple early lesions are present or to prevent recurrence following endoscopic tumour removal. Bacillus Calmette-Guérin (BCG; BCGLive, TheraCys) is a suspension of attenuated *Mycobacterium bovis* used to treat carcinoma in situ (CIS) and recurrent bladder tumours. Instillation into the bladder causes a local inflammatory reaction that eliminates or reduces superficial tumours. Systemic mycobacterial infection is a rare complication of intravesical BCG therapy that may require antitubercular treatment (Papadakis et al., 2022). Other chemotherapeutic agents also may be administered intravesically, including doxorubicin, mitomycin C and interferon. Bladder irritation, frequency, dysuria and contact dermatitis are possible adverse reactions to intravesical chemotherapy. Suppression of bone marrow function also can occur as a result of intravesical treatment.

Radiation therapy

Radiation is an adjunctive therapy used in the treatment of urinary tumours. Although radiation alone is not curative, it can reduce tumour size prior to surgery and is used as palliative treatment for inoperable tumours and those who cannot tolerate surgery. Radiation therapy also is used in combination with systemic chemotherapy to improve local and distant relapse rates (Papadakis et al., 2022) (see the chapter 'Nursing care of people with cancer').

Surgery

A number of surgical procedures, ranging from simple resection of non-invasive tumours to removal of the bladder and surrounding structures, are used to treat urinary tract tumours. Indications for each procedure and specific nursing implications are outlined in Table 26.5.

TABLE 26.5 Surgical procedures to treat bladder tumours

PROCEDURE	INDICATIONS	NURSING IMPLICATIONS
Transurethral resection of bladder tumour	Diagnose and treat superficial bladder tumours having low rate of recurrence; control bleeding	Maintain continuous bladder irrigation postoperatively; monitor for excessive bleeding; ensure catheter patency. Increase fluids to 2,500–3,000 mL/day if not contraindicated. Give stool softeners to prevent straining.
Partial cystectomy	Resect solitary, isolated tumour at stage T_2 or T_3 not involving trigone	Maintain patency of urethral and/or suprapubic catheter to make sure suture lines are free of pressure; monitor for excess bleeding.
Complete or radical cystectomy	Remove large, invasive tumours; involvement of trigone	Permanent urinary diversion is required. Maintain patency and position of stents; urethral catheter may be in place to drain pelvic cavity.

Transurethral tumour resection may be performed by excision, *fulguration* (destruction of tissue using electric sparks generated by high-frequency current) or *laser photocoagulation* (use of light energy to destroy abnormal tissue). Laser surgery carries the lowest risk of bleeding and perforation of the bladder wall. Following cystoscopic tumour resection, individuals are followed at 3-month intervals for tumour recurrence. Recurrences may develop anywhere in the urinary tract, including the renal pelvis, ureter or urethra (Loscalzo et al., 2022).

Cystectomy, surgical removal of the bladder, is necessary to treat invasive cancers. Partial cystectomy may be done to remove a solitary lesion; however, radical cystectomy is the standard treatment for invasive tumours. The bladder and adjacent muscles and tissues are removed. In men, the prostate and seminal vessels are also removed, resulting in significant side effects such as erectile dysfunction. In women, a total hysterectomy and bilateral salpingo-oophorectomy (removal of the uterus, fallopian tubes and ovaries) accompanies the procedure. At the time of surgery, a **urinary diversion** is created to provide for urine collection and drainage. Either an *ileal conduit* (see Figure 26.7A) or a *continent urinary diversion* (see Figure 26.7B) is created to collect and drain urine. Table 26.6 describes the most frequently used urinary diversion techniques. Surgical procedures to remove tumours involving other portions of the urinary tract vary according to the site and stage of the tumour. When the distal ureter is involved, the tumour may be resected and the ureter implanted into the opposite ureter to provide for drainage. A proximal ureteral tumour necessitates removal of the ureter and kidney on the affected side.

See the 'Nursing care of the person having a cystectomy and urinary diversion' box.

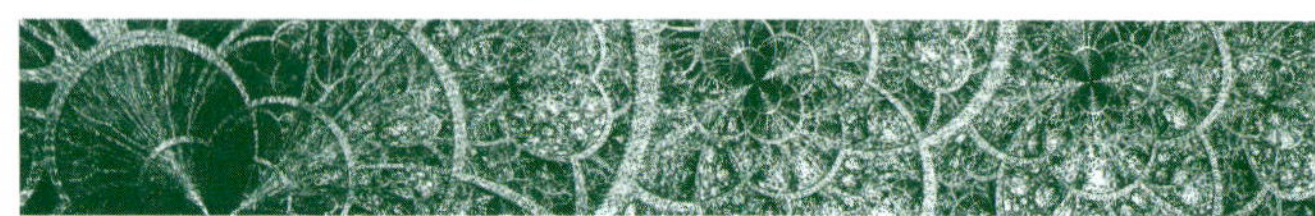

Nursing care

The person who undergoes treatment for a tumour of the urinary tract has many nursing care needs because of alterations in the functional health patterns of elimination, health perception–health management, cognitive–perceptual, self-perception–self-concept, role–relationships and coping–stress–tolerance.

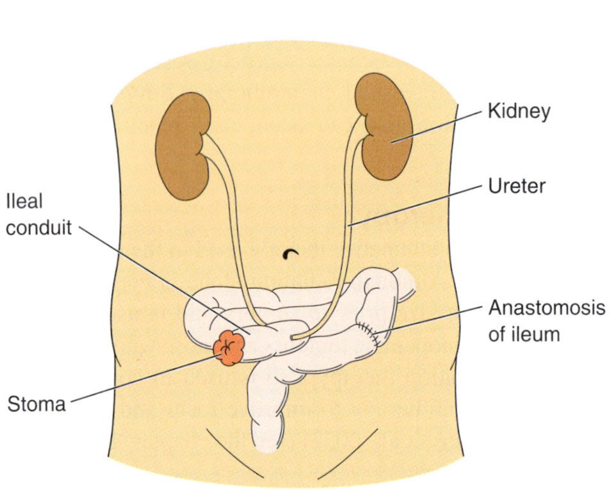

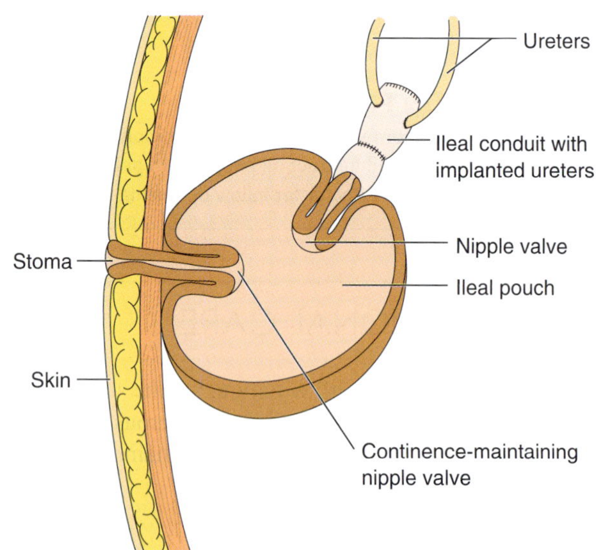

FIGURE 26.7 *Common urinary diversion procedures. A, Ileal conduit. A segment of ileum is separated from the small intestine and formed into a tubular pouch with the open end brought to the skin surface to form a stoma. The ureters are connected to the pouch. B, A continent urinary diversion. A segment of ileum is separated from the small intestine and formed into a pouch. Nipple valves are formed at each end of the pouch by intussuscepting tissue backwards into the reservoir to prevent leakage*

TABLE 26.6 Urinary diversion procedures

PROCEDURE	DESCRIPTION	NURSING CONSIDERATIONS
Ileal conduit	Portion of ileum is isolated from small intestine, leaving vascular, lymphatic and neural connections intact; ileum is formed into pouch with open end brought to surface to form a stoma; ureters are inserted into pouch.	Most common urinary diversion. Continuous urine drainage necessitates appliance. Postoperative oedema may interfere with urine output. Risk of infection is less than for cutaneous ureterostomy, but potential for reflux is high. Good skin care vital because of constant contact with urine.
Continent internal ileal reservoir or continent ileal bladder conduit (Kock pouch)	Pouch is created as for ileal conduit but nipple valves are formed by intussuscepting tissue backwards into a reservoir to connect pouch to the skin and ureters to the pouch; filling pressure closes valves, preventing leakage and reflux.	Drainage collection device not necessary. The person must be willing and able to perform clean intermittent self-catheterisation every 2 to 4 hours. Continence valve mechanism may fail, requiring surgery for revision.
Indiana pouch (continent diversion)	A portion of the terminal ileum, ascending colon and caecum is isolated from the bowel with vascular and neural connections intact. Reservoir is formed from colon and caecum; portion of the ileum is brought to the surface to form nipple valve and stoma or is attached to urethral stump.	As for Kock pouch. The person must be able and motivated to manage self-catheterisation. Reservoir may absorb urea and electrolytes, resulting in imbalances. Significant portion of bowel is required to form pouch and stoma.
Ileocystoplasty	Section of the ileum is isolated and formed into U shape. Ureters are implanted in upper portion of the Urethra. Urethra is anastomosed to central section.	Appropriate for men only because urethra is removed with cystectomy in women. Allows the person to void by relaxing pelvic muscles and using Valsalva manoeuvre.

Health promotion

Encourage all individuals not to smoke. Provide referral to smoking cessation programs or clinics for those who wish to give up smoking. Encourage people at high risk of developing bladder cancer (see above) to have periodic examinations, including urinalysis and urine cytology.

Assessment

Nursing assessment related to urinary tract cancer includes both subjective and objective information:

- *Health history*: risk factors; history of haematuria or manifestations of UTI (dysuria, frequency, urgency, pyuria); lower abdominal discomfort or flank pain.
- *Physical examination*: general health; abdominal tenderness; urine for analysis.

Nursing diagnoses and interventions

Maintaining urinary output is the priority nursing care focus for the person with a bladder tumour. For additional potential nursing diagnoses and interventions for those with a bladder tumour, see the nursing care plan.

Impaired urinary elimination

Whether the person has undergone transurethral resection of a bladder tumour or radical cystectomy with urinary diversion, urinary elimination is altered at least temporarily.

- Monitor urine output from all catheters, stents and tubes for amount, colour and clarity hourly for the first 24 hours postoperatively, then every 4 to 8 hours dependent on patient status. *Decreased urine output may indicate impaired catheter or drainage system patency. Prompt intervention is necessary to prevent hydronephrosis. A change in colour or clarity may indicate a complication such as haemorrhage or infection.*
- Label all catheters, stents and their drainage containers. Maintain separate closed gravity drainage systems for each. *Clear identification of each tube can prevent errors in irrigating and calculating outputs. Separate closed systems minimise the risk and extent of potential bacterial contamination and resultant infection.*

CONSIDERATION FOR PRACTICE

Promptly report low urine output. This may indicate low vascular volume or renal insufficiency. Prompt intervention is vital to restore cardiac output and prevent acute kidney injury (previously known as acute renal failure).

- Secure ureteral catheters and stents with tape; prevent kinking or occlusion; and maintain gravity flow by keeping drainage bag below the level of the kidneys. *Impaired urine flow can lead to urinary retention and distension of the bladder, a newly created reservoir or the renal pelvis (hydronephrosis).*

CONSIDERATION FOR PRACTICE

Using aseptic techniques, strictly follow guidelines for irrigating catheters. Catheters placed in the kidney pelvis are irrigated using gentle pressure and small amounts of fluid (10 to 15 mL) to avoid damaging renal tissues.

- Encourage fluid intake of 3,000 mL per day, unless contraindicated. Increased fluid intake maintains a high urinary output, reducing the risk of infection. *Dilute urine is less irritating to the skin surrounding the stoma site. Electrolyte reabsorption from reservoirs may increase risk of calculi; high fluid intake and urine output reduce this risk.*
- Encourage activity to tolerance. *Ambulation promotes drainage of urine from reservoirs and helps prevent calcium loss from bones, which could precipitate calculus formation.*

CONSIDERATION FOR PRACTICE

Monitor urine output closely for first 24 hours after stents or ureteral catheters are removed. Oedema or stricture of ureters may impede output, leading to hydronephrosis and kidney damage.

Risk of impaired skin integrity

The skin surrounding the stoma site of an ileal conduit is at risk of irritation and breakdown. Because urine is acidic and contains high concentrations of electrolytes, it has a corrosive effect on skin. In addition, adhesives and sealants used to prevent pouch leakage may irritate the skin.

- Assess peristomal skin for redness, excoriation or signs of breakdown. Assess for urine leakage from catheters, stents or drains. Keep the skin clean and dry. Change wet dressings. *Intact skin is the first line of defence against infection. Impaired skin integrity may lead to local or systemic infection and impaired healing.*
- Ensure gravity drainage of urine collection device or empty bag every 2 hours. *Overfilling of the collection bag may damage the seal, allowing leakage and contact of urine with skin.*
- Change urine collection appliance as needed, removing any mucus from stoma. See Box 26.2 for care of a urinary stoma. *Meticulous care and protection of skin surrounding stoma can maintain integrity and prevent breakdown.*

Disturbed body image

A radical cystectomy and urinary diversion affect the person's body image. In most cases, an abdominal stoma is created, requiring either a drainage appliance or regular catheterisation of the stoma to drain urine. Removal of the prostate and seminal vesicles or the uterus and ovaries leaves the person infertile. If radiation or chemotherapy is planned as adjunctive therapy, the individual may experience hair loss, stomatitis, nausea and vomiting, or other disturbing side effects of therapy.

- Use therapeutic communication techniques to help the person deal with the situation by actively listening and responding to the individual's and the family's concerns. *People must know that their feelings and concerns are respected and valued. Grief is a common process for the person's disordered body and normal for those undergoing a significant change in body image.*
- Recognise and accept behaviours that indicate use of coping mechanisms, encouraging adaptive mechanisms. *The person may initially use defensive coping mechanisms such as denial, minimisation and dissociation from the immediate situation to reduce anxiety and maintain psychological integrity. Adaptive mechanisms include learning as much as possible about the surgery and its effects, practising procedures, setting realistic goals and rehearsing various alternative outcomes.*
- Encourage looking at, touching and caring for the stoma and appliance as soon as possible. Allow the person to proceed gradually, providing support and encouragement. *Accepting the stoma as part of the self is vital to adapting to the changed body image and is indicated by a willingness to begin self-care.*
- Discuss concerns about returning to usual activities, perceived relationship changes and resumption of sexual relations. Provide referral to the support group or provide for contact with someone who has successfully adjusted to a urinary diversion. *Individuals and families may be reluctant to discuss topics of concern. An atmosphere of openness and acceptance facilitates expression of concerns and anxieties related to the changed body image.*

PATIENT SAFETY COMPETENCY FRAMEWORK

2 Therapeutic communication

The Patient Safety Competency Framework indicates that nursing students should demonstrate the ability to use verbal and non-verbal communication to convey respect and empathy and be able to develop therapeutic relationships while maintaining professional boundaries (Levett-Jones et al., 2017).

BOX 26.2 Urinary stoma care

- Ensure your own knowledge of policy/procedures of the facility related to the task.
- Gather all supplies: a clean, disposable pouch; liquid skin barrier or barrier ring; 4 × 4 gauze squares; stoma guide; adhesive solvent; clean gloves; and a clean washcloth.
- Assess knowledge, learning needs and ability and willingness to assist with procedure. Explain the procedure as needed.
- Use standard precautions.
- Remove old pouch, pulling gently away from skin. Warm water or adhesive solvent may be used to loosen the seal if necessary.
- Assess stoma. Normally the stoma is bright red and appears moist. Report a dark purple, black or very pale stoma to the doctor. Slight bleeding with cleansing is normal, especially in the immediate postoperative period.
- Prevent urine flow during cleaning by placing a rolled gauze square or tampon over the stoma opening.
- Cleanse skin around the stoma with soap and water; rinse and pat or air dry.
- Use the stoma guide to determine correct size for the bag opening and/or protective ring seal. Trim the bag or seal as needed.
- Apply skin barrier; allow to dry.
- Apply the bag with an opening no more than 1 to 2 mm wider than outside of stoma. Allow no wrinkles or creases where the bag contacts the skin. Smooth side edges and lower edges first to ensure smooth fit.
- Connect bag to the urine-collection device. Dispose of old pouch, used supplies and gloves appropriately. Wash hands.
- Chart procedure, including stoma appearance and response of the person.

NURSING CARE OF THE PERSON having a cystectomy and urinary diversion

PREOPERATIVE CARE

- Provide routine preoperative care as outlined in the chapter 'Nursing care of people having surgery'.
- Assess knowledge of the proposed surgery and its long-term implications, clarifying misunderstandings and discussing concerns. *Those having surgery for cancer of the urinary tract are trying to cope with a diagnosis of cancer and may not fully understand the surgery and its potential effects. Open discussion can reduce the need for postoperative analgesia and facilitate postoperative recovery and adjustment.*
- Begin teaching about postoperative tubes and drains, self-care of stoma and control of drainage and odour. *Postoperative physiological and psychological stressors may interfere with learning. A basic understanding of what to expect in the way of tubes, drains and procedures reduces stress in the immediate postoperative period. Preoperative teaching can enhance recall and postoperative learning.*
- Refer to the Continence Nurse Advisor (or appropriate alternative; i.e. Stomal Therapy Nurse) to help prepare the person physically and psychologically for the outcomes of surgery and changed body image.
- Assist in identifying a stoma site, avoiding folds of skin, bones, scar tissue and the waistline or belt area. The site should be visible and accessible for manipulation. Be sure to consider the person's occupation and style of clothing. *Stoma placement is a vital component of adjustment and self-care. Care is taken to place the stoma away from areas of constant irritation by clothing or movement. It should be located so that the person can cover and disguise the collecting device, maintain the seal to prevent leakage and effectively cleanse and maintain the site.*
- Perform bowel-preparation activities as ordered. *Bowel preparation is done to prevent faecal contamination of the peritoneal cavity and to decompress the bowel during surgery.*

PATIENT SAFETY COMPETENCY FRAMEWORK

4 Teamwork and collaborative practice

The Patient Safety Competency Framework indicates that nursing students must demonstrate the ability to collaborate and communicate effectively with all members of the healthcare team by engaging in shared goal setting and decision making when planning person-centred care (Levett-Jones et al., 2017).

POSTOPERATIVE CARE

- Provide routine postoperative care (see the chapter 'Nursing care of people having surgery').
- Monitor intake and output carefully, assessing urine output every hour for the first 24 hours, then every 4 hours or as ordered. Call the doctor if urine output is reduced. *Tissue oedema and bleeding may interfere with urinary output from stoma, catheters or drains. Maintenance of urine outflow is vital to prevent hydronephrosis and possible renal damage. An adequate urine output is necessary for effective renal function.*
- Assess colour and consistency of urine. Expect pink or bright red urine fading to pink and then clearing by the third postoperative day. Urine may be cloudy due to mucus production by bowel mucosa. *Bright red blood in the urine from a urinary diversion may indicate haemorrhage, necessitating further surgery. Excessive cloudiness or foul-smelling urine may indicate infection.*
- Assess size, colour and condition of the stoma and surrounding skin every 2 hours for the first 24 hours, then every 4 hours for 48 to 72 hours. Expect the stoma to initially appear bright red and slightly oedematous. Slight bleeding during cleansing is normal. *Compromised circulation causes the stoma to appear pale, grey or cyanotic, or to blanch when touched. Other complications, such as infection or impaired healing, may be evidenced by a change in the appearance of the stoma or incision.*
- Irrigate the ileal diversion catheter with 30 to 60 mL of normal saline every 4 hours or as ordered. *Mucus produced by the bowel wall may accumulate in the newly devised reservoir or obstruct catheters.*
- Monitor serum electrolyte values, acid–base balance and renal function tests such as BUN and serum creatinine. *Reabsorption of electrolytes from reservoirs created by portions of bowel may result in electrolyte imbalance and metabolic acidosis. Optimal renal function is necessary to maintain a normal state of homeostasis.*

HEALTH EDUCATION FOR THE PERSON AND FAMILY

- Teach the person and family about stoma and urinary diversion care, including odour management, skin care, increased fluid intake, pouch application and leakage prevention, self-catheterisation for those with continent reservoirs and signs of infection and other complications. *The ability to provide self-care is a significant factor in the adjustment to a changed body image. Teaching family members facilitates acceptance and adjustment. The family also needs this knowledge in case illness or disability interferes with the self-care capacity.*
- Ensure the Continence Nurse Advisor is available for counselling, guidance and support for the person and family in the postoperative period.

NURSING CARE PLAN A person with a bladder tumour

Ben Hussain is a 61-year-old car salesman. He is married and has five children, all of whom are grown and living away from home. A week ago Mr Hussain became alarmed when his urine was bright red. He called his doctor, who ordered urinalysis and urine cytology which revealed gross haematuria and poorly differentiated abnormal cells. Cystoscopy and tissue biopsy confirmed a tumour involving the bladder trigone area. Mr Hussain was admitted for a radical cystectomy and continent urinary diversion.

ASSESSMENT

Mr Hussain's admission history, obtained by the Registered Nurse, indicated that he had lost 4–7 kg during the last few months. He smoked two to three packets of cigarettes a day for 40 years but cut back to a packet a day about a year ago, saying he could not quit smoking entirely. He drinks five to six cups of coffee daily and consumes a moderate amount of alcohol, averaging three to four drinks a day. Mr Hussain says that he is 'a little nervous about surgery and what they're going to find'. The nurse notes that he fidgets and talks rapidly throughout their interview. Mr Hussain also expresses concern about how he will handle the pain after surgery, because he had never been hospitalised before his cystoscopy, and voices concerns related to sexual function postoperatively. Physical assessment findings include T 36.7°C, P 84, R 18 and BP 154/86. Examinations of the skin, neuromuscular and cardiac systems show no abnormalities. Auscultation of lung fields showed scattered expiratory crackles. Bowel sounds were very active; Mr Hussain explained that he began taking his bowel-preparation laxative the day before admission. Slight tenderness was noted in the suprapubic region and Mr Hussain's urine was clear and bright pink. CBC and chemistry screening results were within normal limits. Surgery was planned for 9 am the following day.

DIAGNOSES

- *Anxiety* related to undetermined extent of disease, fear of pain and unknown outcomes of erectile/sexual dysfunction.
- *Deficient knowledge* related to care and management of continent urinary diversion.
- *Impaired urinary elimination* related to cystectomy and urinary diversion.
- *Risk of impaired gas exchange* related to smoking history and effects of anaesthesia.

PLANNING

- Plan education to reduce anxiety and concerns around surgery.
- Plan to include family in education sessions.
- Plan adequate pain reduction interventions.
- Plan collaborative quit smoking and alcohol-reduction intervention programs.

Expected outcomes

- Verbalise decreased feelings of anxiety.
- Demonstrate appropriate postoperative pain relief through subjective reports of pain severity and objective findings.
- Be able to care for urinary diversion and surrounding skin prior to discharge.
- Demonstrate self-catheterisation of stoma using appropriate technique prior to discharge.
- Maintain normal urine output with acceptable colour and clarity and no signs of infection.
- Maintain adequate gas exchange as evidenced by good skin colour, O_2 saturation greater than 95% and clear lung sounds on auscultation.

IMPLEMENTATION

- Spend as much time as possible with Mr Hussain and his family preoperatively, answering questions fully and encouraging expression of fears and anxieties.
- Reinforce teaching given by the Continence Nurse Advisor and ensure that Mr Hussain understands his condition, the surgery and his postoperative plan of care.
- Provide verbal explanations supported by printed material and application examples when appropriate.
- Administer postoperative analgesia on a regular basis for the first 48 to 72 hours. Monitor for objective signs of unrelieved pain.
- Explain all procedures related to stoma and diversion care as they are being performed.
- Encourage Mr Hussain to look at the stoma and touch it when ready.
- Teach stoma and skin care, as well as self-catheterisation, emphasising measures to prevent skin irritation and urinary tract infection.
- Monitor urine output, colour, clarity and consistency every hour for first 24 hours, then every 4 hours for 24 hours, then every 8 hours. Report output of less than 30 mL per hour, bright bleeding, excessively cloudy or foul-smelling urine.
- Assist with use of incentive spirometer to promote respiratory function every hour while awake. Ambulate as soon as possible. Assess lung sounds every 4 hours, reporting increased crackles or diminished breath sounds.
- Refer Mr and Mrs Hussain to a local stoma group on discharge.

EVALUATION

On discharge, Mr Hussain has performed self-catheterisation and stoma and skin care several times. His wife also is able to catheterise the stoma and demonstrate skin care. His urine is pale yellow and slightly cloudy. Mr Hussain is ambulating independently and using oxycodone twice a day for pain relief. His lungs are clear and he is very proud of having 'survived' 7 days without a cigarette. He says, 'Now I'm going to try for 7 weeks, then 7 months, then 7 years without a cigarette!' A community care referral is made to continue supporting Mr Hussain in caring for his diversion and appliance at home. Information related to support groups is supplied.

CRITICAL THINKING IN THE NURSING PROCESS

1. How does cigarette smoking contribute to the increased risk of urinary tract tumours?
2. Suppose Mr Hussain had become confused, disoriented and tremorous, and had begun to experience visual hallucinations 2 to 3 days postoperatively. What would you suspect the cause to be? What would be the appropriate response?
3. Develop a plan of care for Mr Hussain for the nursing diagnosis *Risk of sexual dysfunction*.

REFLECTION ON THE NURSING PROCESS

1. Reflect on how Mr Hussain's attitudes towards smoking, alcohol and caffeine intake may have influenced his adherence and contribution to planned education programs.
2. How has involvement of the family in education programs influenced Mr Hussain's adherence to the programs?

Risk of infection

Diagnostic instrumentation procedures, surgical manipulation and disruption of normal urinary tract defence mechanisms increase the risk of ascending urinary tract infection. When an ileal conduit or artificial bladder is created using bowel tissue, the normal bacteriostatic activity of bladder mucosa is lost. In addition, the peristaltic action of the ureters may be disrupted and the vesicoureteral junction no longer prevents urine reflux. Adjunctive chemotherapy or radiation treatments may impair normal immune function and further increase the risk of infection.

- Maintain separate closed drainage systems, keeping drainage bags lower than the kidney, and prevent loops or kinks in drainage tubing, which impede urine flow. *Although urine is sterile when it leaves the kidney, bacteria grow rapidly in it. Therefore, prevention of urine reflux is essential to preventing UTI.*
- Monitor for signs of infection: elevated temperature, cloudy or foul-smelling urine, haematuria, general malaise, back or abdominal pain, and nausea and vomiting. *Infection undermines the healing process. Early detection and treatment help prevent long-term consequences such as chronic pyelonephritis.*

> **CONSIDERATION FOR PRACTICE**
>
> **Impaired immune capability (due to ageing or the effects of chemotherapy) and urine cloudiness (related to the effects of urine on ileal mucosa) can mask signs of UTI such as fever and altered urine clarity. Be alert for more generalised manifestations, such as increased fatigue and malaise.**

- Teach signs and symptoms of infection and self-care measures to prevent UTI. The person with a cystectomy and ileal diversion, urostomy or continent reservoir is at risk of UTI for life because of impaired urinary defence mechanisms. *Using clean or aseptic technique in providing care, increasing fluid intake and using measures to acidify urine minimise this risk, but does not eliminate it.*

> **PATIENT SAFETY COMPETENCY FRAMEWORK**
>
> **8 Infection prevention and control**
>
> The Patient Safety Competency Framework indicates that nursing students must demonstrate infection prevention and control strategies, such as employing strict aseptic technique, to reduce the risk of introducing infectious organisms when immune responses are impaired (Levett-Jones et al., 2017)

Community-based care

The need for individual and family teaching for the person who has had surgery to treat a urinary tract tumour is significant. For many, surgery means a lifelong change in urinary elimination. Even the individual who has undergone transurethral excision of bladder tumours requires follow-up cystoscopy on a regular basis and needs to be alert for signs of tumour recurrence.

The person who has had a urinary diversion needs teaching about care of the stoma and surrounding skin, prevention of urine reflux and infection, signs and symptoms of UTI and renal calculi, and, in some cases, self-catheterisation using clean technique. Referral to community health services will be an important aid to the individual and family in adapting to their changed situation and the impact on their lifestyles.

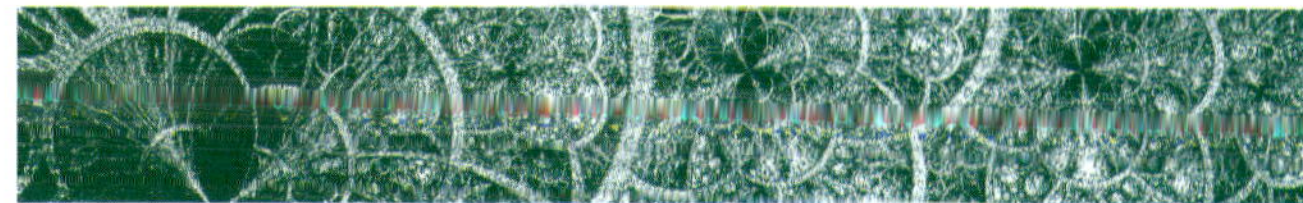

THE PERSON WITH URINARY RETENTION

Urinary retention, incomplete emptying of the bladder, can lead to overdistension of the bladder, poor detrusor muscle contractility and inability to urinate. If the problem persists, hydroureter and hydronephrosis can result. In addition, the person is at higher risk for infection and potential for urinary stones.

Physiology review

Normally, bladder emptying is controlled by the interaction of muscle tone and the autonomic nervous system. The sympathetic nervous system (SNS) relaxes the detrusor muscle, allowing the bladder to fill with urine. The internal sphincter, a continuation of the detrusor muscle, remains closed during filling. Pressures within the bladder remain low during filling, in contrast to high sphincter and urethral pressures. Voluntary muscles of the external sphincter and pelvic floor help maintain these high pressures. When the bladder contains 150 to 300 mL of urine, signals from stretch receptors in the bladder wall are transmitted to the spinal cord and cerebral cortex. Reflexive bladder emptying can be consciously inhibited. During *micturition* (bladder emptying), parasympathetic stimulation causes the detrusor muscle of the bladder fundus to contract, opening the internal sphincter. The external sphincter then relaxes, allowing urine to flow out.

Pathophysiology

Either mechanical obstruction of the bladder outlet or a functional problem can cause urinary retention. Benign prostatic hypertrophy (BPH) is a common cause; difficulty initiating and maintaining urine flow is often the presenting complaint in men with BPH. Acute inflammation associated with infection or trauma of the bladder, urethra or perineal tissues may also interfere with micturition. Scarring due to repeated urinary tract infection can lead to urethral stricture and a mechanical obstruction. Bladder calculi may also obstruct the urethral opening from the bladder.

Surgery, particularly abdominal or pelvic surgery, may disrupt detrusor muscle function, leading to urine retention. Drugs also may interfere with its function. Anticholinergic medications such as atropine, glycopyrrolate, propantheline bromide, hyoscine and others can lead to acute urinary retention and bladder distension. Other drugs with anticholinergic side effects may also cause urinary retention. Among these are anti-anxiety agents such as diazepam, antidepressant and tricyclic drugs such as imipramine, antiparkinsonian drugs, antipsychotic agents and some sedative/hypnotic drugs. In addition, antihistamines common in over-the-counter cough, cold, allergy and sleep-promoting drugs have anticholinergic effects which may interfere with bladder emptying. Diphenhydramine is an example of a non-prescription antihistamine.

Voluntary urinary retention (particularly common among nurses!) may lead to overfilling of the bladder and a loss of detrusor muscle tone.

Manifestations

The person with urinary retention is unable to empty the bladder completely. Overflow voiding or incontinence may occur, with 25 to 50 mL of urine eliminated at frequent intervals. Assessment reveals a firm, distended bladder that may be displaced to one side of midline. Percussion of the lower abdomen reveals a dull tone, reflective of fluid in the bladder.

Severe urinary retention with resulting bladder distension impairs the ability of the vesicoureteral junction to prevent backflow of urine into the ureters (see Figure 26.1 earlier in the chapter). Reflux of urine from the distended bladder distends the ureters (hydroureter) and kidneys (hydronephrosis). Hydronephrosis impairs renal function and acute kidney injury can result. See the chapter 'Nursing care of people with kidney disorders' for more information about acute kidney injury (previously known as acute renal failure).

INTERPROFESSIONAL CARE

Urinary retention is confirmed using a bladder scan or by inserting a urinary catheter (if possible, depending on the reason for retention—BPH creating almost total occlusion) and measuring the urine output. Use of a bladder scan is preferred to reduce the risk of UTI (Brackmann et al., 2020).

An indwelling urinary catheter or intermittent straight catheterisation can prevent urinary retention and overdistension of the bladder. Cholinergic medications such as bethanechol chloride, which promote detrusor muscle contraction and bladder emptying, may be used. A medication with no anticholinergic side effects may be substituted when urinary retention is related to drug therapy.

Mechanical obstructions are treated by removing or repairing the obstruction when possible. Resection of the prostate gland may be done for urinary retention related to BPH. Bladder calculi are removed and measures to prevent their formation are instituted.

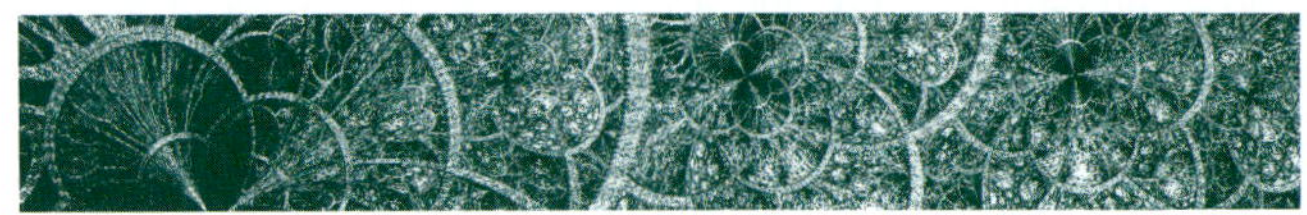

Nursing care

Health promotion measures to prevent urinary retention include monitoring urine output in at-risk individuals and evaluating drug regimens for medications known to interfere with detrusor muscle function. Pay particular attention to elimination when these drugs are ordered for (or used by) those with BPH or if there is known mechanical obstruction of urine flow.

Nursing diagnoses and interventions

Impaired urinary elimination

Nursing measures to promote urination include placing the individual in normal voiding position and providing for privacy. Additional measures include running water, placing the person's hands in warm water, pouring warm water over the perineum or warm showering.

In acute urinary retention, catheterisation may be necessary to relieve bladder distension and prevent hydronephrosis. Use a relatively small catheter (14 Fr. for a man, 12 Fr. for a woman). A coudé-tipped catheter is passed more easily in the older man with an enlarged prostate. Using 2% lignocaine gel (10 mL injected into the male urethra or 6 mL injected into the female urethra) reduces discomfort during catheterisation and the risk of catheter-associated infection and promotes pelvic muscle relaxation (Payne & Kerrigan, 2020). Carefully observe the person as the distended bladder drains for signs of discomfort or shock. Home care for the person with urinary retention varies, depending on the cause. Some people may be taught intermittent self-catheterisation. Instruct all those who have experienced urinary retention to avoid over-the-counter drugs that affect micturition, especially those with an anticholinergic effect (allergy and cold medications, and many non-prescription sleep aids). Other home care measures include double-voiding (urinate, remain on the toilet for 2 to 5 minutes, then urinate again), scheduled voiding, or, when other measures fail, an indwelling catheter. When an indwelling catheter is necessary, teach the person and family to use clean technique when changing from overnight bag to leg bag and to promptly report signs of UTI to the primary care provider.

CONSIDERATION FOR PRACTICE

Some people may experience a vasovagal response, becoming pale, sweaty and hypotensive if the bladder is rapidly drained (decompression). Draining urine in 500 mL increments and clamping the catheter for 5 to 10 minutes between increments may prevent this response. Haematuria also may occur with rapid bladder decompression. Promptly notify the doctor if haematuria develops.

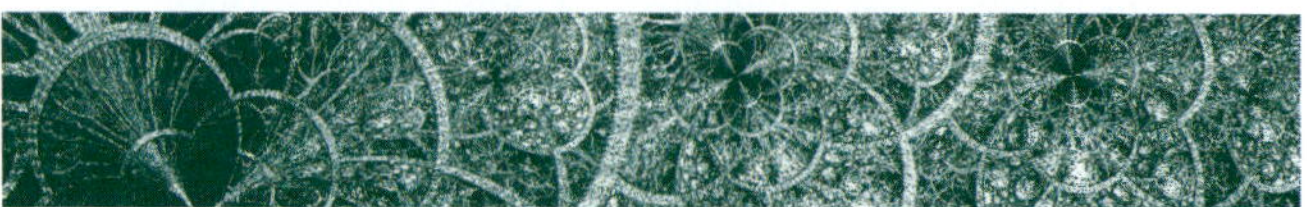

THE PERSON WITH A NEUROGENIC BLADDER

The neurological connections influencing bladder filling, the perception of fullness and the need to void, and bladder emptying are complex. Disruption of the central or peripheral nervous systems may interfere with normal mechanisms, causing **neurogenic bladder**.

Pathophysiology

As noted in the physiology section on urinary retention, bladder filling and emptying are controlled by the central nervous system (CNS). This neurological control can be disrupted at any level: the cerebral cortex (voluntary impulses), the micturition centre of the midbrain, the spinal cord tracts or the peripheral nerves of the bladder itself.

Spastic bladder dysfunction

A simple reflex arc exists between the bladder and the spinal cord at levels S_2 to S_4. The stimulus of more than 400 mL of urine in the bladder causes reflex contraction of the detrusor muscle and bladder emptying unless voluntary control (cerebral input) is used to suppress it. Disruption of CNS transmission above the sacral spinal cord segment typically leads to *spastic neurogenic bladder*. Both sensory and voluntary control of urination is interrupted partially or totally, while the sacral reflex arc remains intact. The stimuli generated by bladder filling causes frequent spontaneous detrusor muscle contraction and involuntary bladder emptying. Spinal cord injury above the sacral segment is the most common cause of a spastic bladder. Other causes include stroke, multiple sclerosis and other CNS lesions (Lee, 2021).

Flaccid bladder dysfunction

Damage to the sacral spinal cord at the level of the reflex arc, the cauda equina or the sacral nerve roots causes loss of detrusor muscle tone and a *flaccid neurogenic bladder*. The perception of bladder fullness is lost and the bladder becomes overdistended, with weak and ineffective detrusor muscle contractions. Flaccid neurogenic bladder is seen with myelo-meningocele and during the spinal shock phase of a spinal cord injury above the sacral region. During the spinal shock phase, all reflex activity below the level of spinal cord injury is suppressed.

Peripheral neuropathies may also cause bladder atony and overfilling. Either sensory or motor pathways (or both) may be disrupted, leading to incomplete bladder emptying and large residual volumes after voiding (Wittig et al., 2019). Diabetes mellitus is the most common cause of peripheral bladder neuropathy. Other causes include multiple sclerosis, chronic alcoholism and prolonged overdistension of the bladder.

INTERPROFESSIONAL CARE

Management of a neurogenic bladder focuses on maintaining continence and avoiding complications associated with overfilling or incomplete emptying of the bladder. Because self-care is the goal, teaching is a primary intervention for the healthcare team.

Diagnosis

The following diagnostic tests may be ordered for the person with a neurogenic bladder:

- *Urine culture* to detect possible urinary tract infection related to impaired bladder function.
- *Urinalysis* and *serum creatinine* and *BUN* to evaluate renal function. See the diagnostic tests table in the chapter 'A person-centred approach to assessing the renal system' for normal BUN and creatinine levels. Ascending infection or hydronephrosis resulting from bladder overfilling and vesicoureteral reflux can damage the kidneys. Impaired renal function may lead to blood cells or protein in the urine and elevated BUN and creatinine levels.
- *Post-void bladder scan* and/or *catheterisation* to measure residual urine. Amounts greater than 50 mL may indicate ineffective detrusor muscle contractions, common in a neurogenic bladder.
- *Cystometrography* to evaluate bladder filling and the detrusor muscle tone and function. See the chapter 'A person-centred approach to assessing the renal system' for nursing care of the person undergoing cystometrography.

Medications

Medications may be prescribed to increase or decrease the contractility of the detrusor muscle, to increase or decrease the tone of the internal sphincter, or to relax the external urethral sphincter.

Bethanechol, a cholinergic drug, stimulates detrusor muscle contraction in a flaccid neurogenic bladder. It is generally used to manage short-term urinary retention (e.g. following surgery or childbirth). It may be used in combination with bladder-training techniques to promote complete emptying of a neurogenic bladder. Anticholinesterase drugs such as neostigmine also may be used to increase detrusor muscle tone.

Anticholinergic drugs (parasympathetic blockers) relax the detrusor muscle and contract the internal sphincter, increasing bladder capacity in people with spastic bladder dysfunction. Oxybutynin and tolterodine inhibit the muscarinic effects of acetylcholine on smooth muscle, reducing detrusor muscle spasticity and promoting bladder filling. Other anticholinergic drugs also may be used, including propantheline or flavoxate. Dry mouth, blurred vision and constipation are potential adverse effects of anticholinergic medications. See the 'Medication administration' box for drugs used to modify detrusor muscle activity.

Nutrition

Dietary measures to reduce the risk of UTI and urinary calculi may be suggested for the person with a neurogenic bladder. A moderate to high fluid intake and a diet that acidifies the urine are helpful. Cranberry juice may be recommended to maintain urine acidity. See Table 26.3 for additional foods to include or avoid in the diet to help prevent UTI and urolithiasis. The timing of fluid intake may be regulated to promote continence.

Bladder retraining

Individuals with a spastic neurogenic bladder may use measures to stimulate reflex voiding, allowing scheduled toileting. Techniques include using trigger points—for example, stroking or pinching the abdomen, inner thigh or glans penis. Pulling pubic hairs, tapping the suprapubic region or inserting a gloved

MEDICATION ADMINISTRATION The person with a neurogenic bladder

ANTICHOLINERGIC DRUGS TO TREAT SPASTIC BLADDER

Oxybutynin (Ditropan)
Tolterodine (Detrusitol)
Propantheline bromide (Pro-Banthine)
Flavoxate hydrochloride (Urispas)

Anticholinergic drugs inhibit the response to acetylcholine, relaxing the detrusor muscle and increasing internal sphincter tone. The combination of detrusor relaxation and internal sphincter contraction increases the bladder capacity of those with spastic or hyper-reflexive neurogenic bladder. Of these medications, tolterodine has the most specific effects on the detrusor muscle with fewer anticholinergic side effects.

Nursing responsibilities

- Assess for contraindications, such as glaucoma, gastrointestinal or urinary tract obstruction, severe ulcerative colitis or toxic megacolon, unstable cardiovascular status or myasthenia gravis.
- Observe for the desired effect of increased bladder capacity with decreased incontinence and spasm.
- Monitor for possible interaction with other drugs such as narcotic analgesics, antiarrhythmic medications, antihistamines, antidepressants or psychoactive drugs.
- Monitor vital signs, particularly heart rate and blood pressure, especially when given to people with known cardiovascular disease.
- Assess for adverse effects such as urinary hesitancy or retention, arrhythmias, mental status changes and gastrointestinal disturbances.

Health education for the person and family

- Promptly report eye pain, rapid heartbeat, difficulty breathing, rash or hives, or changes in mental function to your primary care provider.
- These drugs may cause drowsiness or blurred vision. Use caution when driving, operating machinery or performing other tasks requiring mental acuity.
- Boiled sugar-free sweets or gum may assist relieve dry mouth associated with these drugs.
- Do not use alcohol or non-prescription antihistamines while taking these drugs.

CHOLINERGIC DRUGS TO STIMULATE MICTURITION

Bethanechol chloride (Urocarb)

Bethanechol stimulates the parasympathetic nervous system, increasing detrusor muscle tone and producing a contraction strong enough to initiate micturition. It is used primarily to treat acute postoperative and postnatal urinary retention.

Nursing responsibilities

- Assess for contraindications, including hypersensitivity, hyperthyroidism, peptic ulcer disease, asthma, significant bradycardia or hypotension, coronary heart disease, epilepsy and parkinsonism.
- Do not give to individuals who have had recent gastrointestinal or bladder surgery, or those with possible gastrointestinal or urinary tract obstruction.
- Give oral forms on an empty stomach to reduce the risk of nausea and vomiting.
- Administer parenteral bethanechol (Urocarb) subcutaneously. Keep atropine, the antidote for bethanechol overdose or toxicity, available.
- Observe for desired effect within 30 to 60 minutes after oral administration, 5 to 15 minutes after injection.
- Assess for adverse effects such as malaise, headache, abdominal cramping, nausea, hypotension with reflex tachycardia, wheezing and dyspnoea.

Health education for the person and family

- Take the medication 1 hour before or 2 hours after meals.
- Use caution when rising from a recumbent or sitting position; you may feel dizzy or light-headed.

finger into the rectum and gently stretching the anal sphincter can also stimulate urination.

Credé's method (applying pressure to the suprapubic region with the fingers of one or both hands), manual pressure on the abdomen and the Valsalva manoeuvre (bearing down while holding the breath) promote bladder emptying for the person with a spastic or flaccid bladder.

CONSIDERATION FOR PRACTICE

Increasing lower abdominal and bladder pressure with Credé's method can stimulate autonomic dysreflexia in some people with spinal cord injuries. Autonomic dysreflexia is a medical emergency in which the blood pressure rises rapidly due to SNS stimulation.

See the chapter 'Nursing care of people with cerebrovascular and spinal cord disorders' for a discussion of autonomic dysreflexia.

The person with a flaccid bladder may require catheterisation to completely empty the bladder. An indwelling catheter may be used initially, but intermittent catheterisation is preferred. Clean intermittent self-catheterisation is performed every 3 to 4 hours to prevent overdistension of the bladder (see Procedure 42.1).

Surgery

Surgery may be required when urination cannot be effectively managed using more conservative measures. *Rhizotomy*, or destruction of the nerve supply to the detrusor muscle or the external sphincter, may be used for those with hyperreflexia or spasticity. Urinary diversion is another surgical technique used when conservative management fails. Implantation of an artificial sphincter may be useful for some people with neurogenic bladder. See Table 26.6 for urinary diversion techniques.

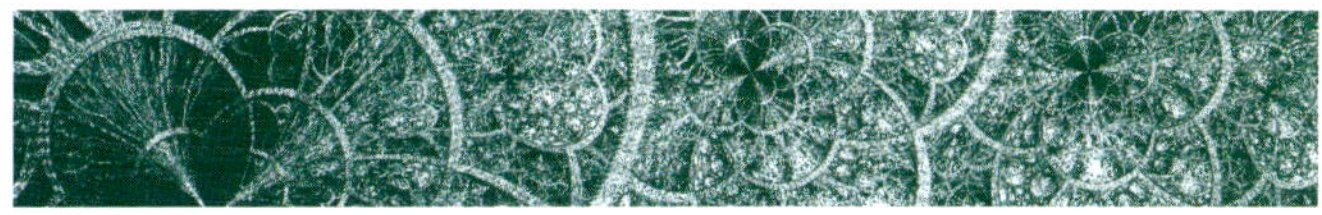

Nursing care

Nursing care of the person with a neurogenic bladder is directed towards promoting urinary drainage and continence, preventing complications, and teaching the person and family self-care techniques.

Assessment

Nursing assessment for neurogenic bladder includes obtaining a complete nursing history, focusing on information related to CNS or spinal cord injury or disease as well as disorders that affect the peripheral nervous system (e.g. diabetes). Ask about measures used to stimulate or control urination. Inspect and palpate the lower abdomen and suprapubic region for tenderness or bladder distension. Percuss the suprapubic region for a dull percussion tone indicative of a full bladder. Assess urine for colour, clarity and odour. Collect a specimen for analysis as indicated.

Nursing diagnoses and interventions

Although each person has individual nursing care needs, examples of nursing diagnoses appropriate for those with a neurogenic bladder include the following:

- *Impaired urinary elimination* related to impaired bladder innervation.
- *Self-care deficit: toileting* related to neurological injury.
- *Risk of impaired skin integrity* related to urinary incontinence.
- *Risk of infection* related to impaired urination reflex.

Community-based care

Include the following in teaching for the person with a neurogenic bladder and family members:

- measures to stimulate reflex voiding and promote bladder emptying
- use of prescribed medications, including desired and adverse effects and interactions with other drugs
- manifestations of UTI or urolithiasis and measures to reduce the risk of these complications.

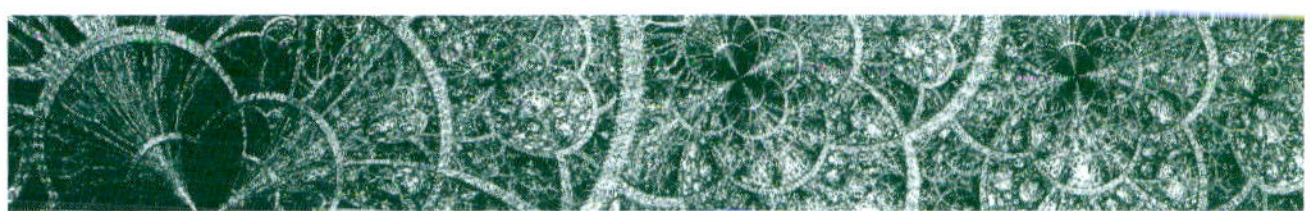

THE PERSON WITH URINARY INCONTINENCE

The most common manifestation of impaired bladder control is **urinary incontinence (UI)**, or involuntary urination. UI can have a significant impact on individuals, leading to physical problems such as skin breakdown, maceration, infection and rashes. Psychosocial consequences include embarrassment, isolation and withdrawal, feelings of worthlessness and helplessness, and depression.

Incidence and prevalence

According to the Continence Foundation of Australia (CFA) (2021), approximately 38% of Australian women and 10% of Australian men are affected by urinary incontinence. An estimated 65% of women and 30% of men visiting their general practitioner reported UI, but only 31% reported seeking assistance from a healthcare professional (CFA, 2021). The actual prevalence of urinary incontinence is nearly impossible to determine. Embarrassment and the availability of products to protect clothing and prevent detection contribute to people not seeking evaluation of and treatment for incontinence.

Pathophysiology

Urinary continence requires a bladder be able to expand and contract, and sphincters that can maintain a urethral pressure higher than that in the bladder. Incontinence results when the pressure within the urinary bladder exceeds urethral resistance, allowing urine to escape. Any condition causing higher than normal bladder pressures or reduced urethral resistance can potentially result in incontinence. Relaxation of the pelvic musculature, disruption of cerebral and nervous system control, and disturbances of the bladder and its musculature are common contributing factors.

Incontinence may be an acute, self-limited disorder or it may be chronic. The causes may be congenital or acquired, reversible or irreversible. Congenital disorders associated with incontinence include *epispadias* (absence of the upper wall of the urethra) and *meningomyelocele* (a neural tube defect in which a portion of the spinal cord and its surrounding meninges protrude through the vertebral column). CNS or spinal cord trauma, stroke and chronic neurological disorders such as multiple sclerosis and Parkinson's disease are examples of acquired, irreversible causes of incontinence. Reversible causes include acute confusion, medications such as diuretics or sedatives, prostatic enlargement, vaginal and urethral atrophy, UTI and faecal impaction.

> **FAST FACTS**
>
> - Urinary incontinence is especially common among older individuals. Although the prevalence of UI increases in older adults, it is *not* a normal consequence of ageing and it can be treated.
> - Over 70% of women suffer from UI as a result of childbirth and menopause.
> - The incidence of UI in males increases with age, especially in the 80+ age group.

Incontinence is commonly categorised as stress incontinence, urge incontinence (also known as overactive bladder), overflow incontinence and functional incontinence. Table 26.7 summarises each type with its physiological cause and associated factors. *Mixed incontinence*, with elements of both stress and urge incontinence, is common. *Total incontinence* is loss of all voluntary control over urination, with urine loss occurring without stimulus and in all positions.

Incontinence is associated with an increased risk of falls, fractures, pressure ulcers, urinary tract infection and depression. It contributes to the stress of caregivers and may be a factor in institutionalising the affected person.

TABLE 26.7 Types of urinary incontinence

	DESCRIPTION	PATHOPHYSIOLOGY	CONTRIBUTING FACTORS
Stress	Loss of urine associated with increased intra-abdominal pressure during sneezing, coughing, lifting. Quantity of urine lost is usually small	Relaxation of pelvic musculature and weakness of urethra and surrounding muscles and tissues leads to decreased urethral resistance	• Multiple pregnancies • Decreased oestrogen levels • Short urethra, change in angle between bladder and urethra • Abdominal wall weakness • Prostate surgery • Increased intra-abdominal pressure due to tumour, ascites, obesity
Urge	Involuntary loss of urine associated with a strong urge to void	Hypertonic or overactive detrusor muscle leads to increased pressure within bladder and inability to inhibit voiding	• Neurological disorders such as stroke, Parkinson's disease, multiple sclerosis; peripheral nervous system disorders • Detrusor muscle overactivity associated with bladder outlet obstruction, ageing or disorders such as diabetes
Overflow	Inability to empty bladder, resulting in overdistension and frequent loss of small amounts of urine	Outlet obstruction or lack of normal detrusor activity leads to overfilling of bladder and increased pressure	• Spinal cord injuries below S_2 • Diabetic neuropathy • Prostatic hypertrophy • Faecal impaction • Drugs, especially those with anticholinergic effect
Functional	Incontinence resulting from physical, environmental or psychosocial causes	Ability to respond to the need to urinate is impaired	• Confusion or dementia • Physical disability or impaired mobility • Therapy or sedation • Depression • Regression

NURSING CARE OF THE OLDER ADULT Minimising the risk of UTI and UI

Older adults have a higher incidence of two common urinary tract disorders: urinary tract infection and urinary incontinence.

URINARY TRACT INFECTION

Ageing affects the normal protective mechanisms which prevent UTI. The pH of urine increases with ageing, allowing bacteria to grow and multiply more readily. Glucosuria, more common in older adults due to the higher incidence of diabetes, facilitates bacterial growth. Incomplete bladder emptying and urinary retention are more common due to problems such as prostatic hypertrophy in men, bladder prolapse in women and neurogenic bladder in both sexes. Changes in vaginal pH in women post menopause and decreased prostatic secretions in men may also contribute to an increased incidence of UTI.

While many UTIs in older adults are asymptomatic and self-limited, infections can lead to bacteraemia, sepsis and shock. Manifestations of UTI in the elderly include dysuria, urgency, frequency, incontinence, occasional haematuria and increased confusion. Symptoms such as fever, chills and flank pain and tenderness may be absent. Dementia may make diagnosis more difficult.

URINARY INCONTINENCE

Urinary incontinence, the involuntary loss of urine, is a common problem in older adults. While incontinence should never be considered a *normal* consequence of ageing, age-related changes contribute to its development. Bladder capacity tends to decline with age and involuntary bladder muscle contractions are more common. In women, decreased oestrogen levels and pelvic muscle relaxation decrease bladder outlet and urethral resistance pressures. Decreased oestrogen also causes atrophic vaginitis and urethritis, with manifestations of dysuria and urgency. Other risk factors for UI in older adults include impaired mobility and chronic degenerative diseases, impaired cognition, medications, low fluid intake, diabetes and stroke.

ASSESSING FOR HOME CARE

Assessment for urinary problems in the older adult focuses on risk factors, the extent and manifestations of the disorder, and contributing factors. Using clear language, ask about problems with urine loss, its frequency and any contributing factors. Enquire about frequency, urgency and burning on urination. Identify current medications and the time of day each is taken. Assess patterns of fluid intake and output. Assess the abdomen for evidence of bladder distension or tenderness. Perform a mental status examination if indicated.

Assess the home environment (whether in the community or a residential living facility) for possible barriers to urinary elimination:

- inadequate lighting, particularly at night
- narrow doorways that may interfere with access to the toilet
- inadequate toilet facilities
- physical placement of toilet facilities resulting in long walks for disabled or incapacitated individuals
- the need for mobility aids such as safety bars, a raised toilet seat or a bedside commode.

TEACHING FOR HOME CARE

Discuss the following points to help prevent UTI and UI in the older adult:

- Maintain a generous fluid intake (unless contraindicated). Reduce or eliminate fluid intake after 7 pm in the evening to reduce nocturia.
- Wear comfortable clothing that is easy to remove for toileting.
- Maintain good hygiene, but do not bathe more often than necessary. Frequent bathing and feminine hygiene sprays or douches may dry perineal tissues, increasing the risk of UTI or UI.
- Perform pelvic muscle exercises (Kegel exercises) several times a day to increase perineal muscle tone.

NURSING CARE OF THE OLDER ADULT Minimising the risk of UTI and UI (continued)

- Reduce consumption of caffeine-containing beverages (coffee, tea, colas), citrus juices and artificially sweetened beverages containing aspartame.
- Use behavioural techniques such as scheduled toileting, habit training and bladder training to reduce the frequency of incontinence. *Scheduled toileting* is toileting at regular intervals (e.g. every 2 to 4 hours). *Habit training* is toileting the person on a schedule that corresponds with the normal pattern. *Bladder training* gradually increases the bladder capacity by increasing the intervals between voidings and resisting the urge to void.
- See your primary care provider regularly for a pelvic or prostate examination to assess for physical abnormalities.
- For women, discuss possible benefits and risks of hormone replacement therapy, physical therapy, incontinence aids or surgery to treat incontinence.
- Report a change in urine colour, odour or clarity, or symptoms such as burning, frequency or urgency, to your primary care provider.

RESOURCES

Continence Foundation of Australia (National Office)
AMA House, 293 Royal Parade
Parkville Vic 3052
Telephone: 03 9347 2522
Fax: 03 9347 2533
E-mail: info@incontinence.or.au
National Continence Helpline: 1800 330 066
Website: https://www.continence.org.au
(State offices' contact details can be obtained from the national office.)
The organisation provides a wide range of services, from professional advice to referrals to continence clinics and education resources.

Community health services

Blue Care Services
Telephone: 07 3377 3377
Website: https://www.bluecare.org.au
Provides care to all members of the community. Keep in mind this service may have a cost associated, may require ACAT assessments and may attract NDIS funding.

Continence Management Advice Services
Telephone: 1300 787 055
Website: https://www.silverchain.org.au/wa/health-care/continence-management/
Gives professional advice and may be able to provide access to products at a reduced cost.

INTERPROFESSIONAL CARE

Urinary incontinence management is directed at identifying and correcting the cause if possible. If the underlying disorder cannot be corrected, techniques to manage urine output can often be taught.

Evaluation for incontinence begins with a complete history, including the duration, frequency, volume and associated circumstances of urine loss. A voiding diary (see Figure 26.8) is often used to collect detailed information. The history also includes information about chronic or acute illnesses, previous surgeries (childbirth in women) and current medication use, both prescription and over the counter.

Physical assessment includes abdominal, rectal and pelvic assessment, as well as evaluation of mental and neurological status, mobility and dexterity. Findings often associated with incontinence in women include weak abdominal and pelvic muscle tone, cystocele or urethrocele, and atrophic vaginitis. In men, an enlarged prostate gland is the physical finding most commonly associated with incontinence.

See the 'Translation to practice' box on evidence-based practice for diagnosing urge incontinence using specific personal assessment data.

Diagnosis

- *Urinalysis* and *urine culture* using a clean-catch specimen are done to rule out infection and other acute causes of incontinence.
- *Post-voiding residual (PVR) volume* is measured to determine how completely the bladder empties with voiding. Less than 50 mL PVR is expected; when 100 mL or more is obtained, further testing is indicated.
- *Cystometrography* is used to assess neuromuscular function of the bladder by evaluating detrusor muscle function, pressure within the bladder and the filling pattern of the bladder. The person describes sensations and any urge to void as sterile water or saline is instilled into the bladder. Normally, the urge to void is perceived at 150 to 450 mL and the bladder feels full at 300 to 500 mL. Bladder pressure and volume are recorded on a graph. When the bladder is full, the individual voids and intravesical pressure is noted during voiding.
- *Uroflowmetry* is a non-invasive test used to evaluate voiding patterns. The uroflowmeter, contained in a funnel, measures the rate of urine flow, the continuous flow time and the total voiding time.
- *IVP* may be ordered to evaluate structure and function of the upper and lower urinary tract.
- *Cystoscopy* or *ultrasonography* may be ordered to identify structural disorders contributing to incontinence, such as an enlarged prostate or a tumour.

Nursing implications for the specialised studies for urinary incontinence are outlined in the chapter 'A person-centred approach to assessing the renal system'.

Medications

Both stress and urge incontinence may improve with drug treatment.

When incontinence is associated with postmenopausal atrophic vaginitis, oestrogen therapy may be effective. Both systemic oestrogens and local creams are used.

People with urge incontinence may be treated with preparations that increase bladder capacity. The primary drugs used to

Your Daily Voiding Diary Date ____________

This diary will help you and your healthcare team identify factors causing bladder control problems. Choose a 24-hour period when you can record your fluid intake (type and amount), urine output and episodes of urine leakage, any strong urge to void just prior to leaking, and your activity when leak episodes occur. The line below illustrates how to use your diary.

Time 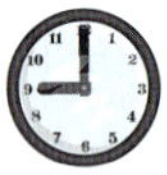	Fluid Intake 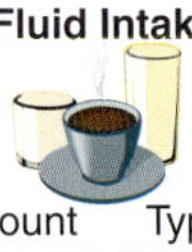 Amount	Fluid Intake Type	Urine Output 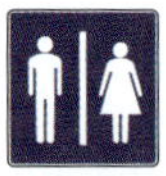	Leaks 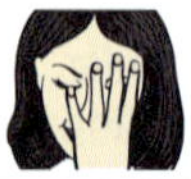	Urge 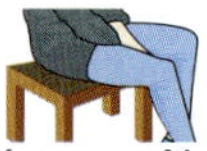 Yes No	Activity 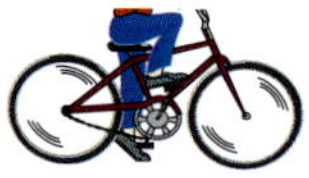
7 am	2 cups	coffee	sm (med) lg	(sm) med lg	Yes	walking
			sm med lg	sm med lg		
			sm med lg	sm med lg		
			sm med lg	sm med lg		
			sm med lg	sm med lg		
			sm med lg	sm med lg		
			sm med lg	sm med lg		
			sm med lg	sm med lg		
			sm med lg	sm med lg		
			sm med lg	sm med lg		
			sm med lg	sm med lg		
			sm med lg	sm med lg		
			sm med lg	sm med lg		
			sm med lg	sm med lg		
			sm med lg	sm med lg		
			sm med lg	sm med lg		
			sm med lg	sm med lg		
			sm med lg	sm med lg		

I used___pads today. I used___nappies today.

Questions to ask my healthcare team: ____________

FIGURE 26.8 ***A sample voiding diary***

Source: Adapted from *Your daily bladder diary*, National Kidney and Urologic Diseases Information Center, National Institute of Diabetes and Digestive and Kidney Disease (NIDDK), National Institutes of Health.

inhibit detrusor muscle contractions and increase bladder capacity include oxybutynin, an anticholinergic drug, and tolterodine, a more specific antimuscarinic agent. These drugs can be taken once or twice a day and have fewer side effects than less specific anticholinergic drugs. Drugs with anticholinergic effects are contraindicated for the person with acute glaucoma. Urinary retention is a potential side effect that must be considered when these drugs are used (see the 'Medication administration: the person with a neurogenic bladder' box).

Surgery

Surgery may be used to treat stress incontinence associated with cystocele or urethrocele and overflow incontinence associated with an enlarged prostate gland.

Suspension of the bladder neck, a technique that brings the angle between the bladder and urethra closer to normal, is effective in treating stress incontinence associated with urethrocele in 80–95% of individuals. A laparoscopic, vaginal or abdominal approach may be used to perform this surgery. Care of the person with a bladder neck suspension is outlined in the 'Nursing care of the person' box.

Transurethral resection of the prostate (TURP), or prostatectomy, is indicated for the person who is experiencing overflow incontinence as a result of an enlarged prostate gland and urethral obstruction. Care of the person with a prostatectomy is outlined in the chapter 'Nursing care of men with reproductive system and breast disorders'.

Other surgical procedures of potential benefit in the treatment of incontinence include implantation of an artificial sphincter, formation of a urethral sling to elevate and compress the urethra, and augmentation of the bladder with bowel segments to increase bladder capacity.

Complementary therapies

Biofeedback and relaxation techniques may help reduce episodes of urinary incontinence. Biofeedback uses electronic monitors to teach conscious control over physiological responses of which the individual is not normally aware. Developing awareness of perceptible information allows the person to gain voluntary control over urination. Biofeedback is widely used to manage urinary incontinence.

TRANSLATION TO PRACTICE Evidence-based practice: urinary incontinence

While an accurate diagnosis of stress urinary incontinence often is made based on clinical data, motor urge incontinence has been more difficult to diagnose accurately without urodynamic investigations. This presents difficulty for nurses and nurse practitioners planning care for incontinent individuals when urological testing is not feasible or readily available. A model developed by Gray et al. (2001) may be useful to address this problem in cognitively intact adults. By comparing personal data with urodynamic testing results, this team of researchers identified factors predictive of motor urge incontinence. These factors included age, gender and three key symptoms: diurnal frequency (urinating more often than every 2 hours while awake), nocturia (awakening with urge to urinate more than once per night if under age 65, twice per night if over age 65) and urge incontinence (urine loss associated with a strong desire to urinate). The presence of all three symptoms was more than 92% predictive of motor urge incontinence in study participants of all ages (range 18 to 89; median 61) and both genders.

IMPLICATIONS FOR NURSING

Asking specific questions about urinary tract symptoms can facilitate accurate identification of the nursing diagnosis *Urinary incontinence: urge*. Accurate diagnosis is vital to planning and implementing appropriate care measures and achieving the desired outcome of continence. Successful treatment promotes self-esteem and provides positive reinforcement for continuing planned strategies.

CRITICAL THINKING IN PERSON-CENTRED CARE

1 What nursing care measures and person-centred teaching will you provide for the person with stress incontinence that may not be appropriate or necessary for the person with urge incontinence but not stress incontinence?
2 Identify circumstances in which it may not be possible or feasible to have the person undergo urodynamic testing to differentiate stress, urge or mixed (stress and urge) incontinence.
3 The individuals in this study lived independently in the community and were cognitively intact. Can the data in this study be generalised to people residing in a long-term care facility? Can the results be applied to all types of incontinence? Why or why not?

Source: Gray et al. (2001). A model for predicting motor urge urinary incontinence. *Nursing Research, 50*(2), 116–122.

NURSING CARE OF THE PERSON having a bladder neck suspension

PREOPERATIVE CARE

- Provide routine preoperative care and teaching as outlined in the chapter 'Nursing care of people having surgery'.
- Discuss the need to avoid straining and the Valsalva manoeuvre postoperatively. Suggest measures such as increasing fluid and fibre intake and using a stool softener to prevent postoperative constipation. *Straining and increased abdominal pressure during the Valsalva manoeuvre may place excessive stress on suture lines and interfere with healing.*

POSTOPERATIVE CARE

- Provide routine postoperative care as outlined in the chapter 'Nursing care of people having surgery'.
- Monitor urine output, including quantity, colour and clarity. Expect urine to be pink initially, gradually clearing. *Bright red urine, excessive vaginal drainage or incisional bleeding may indicate haemorrhage. Instrumentation of the urinary tract increases the potential for UTI; cloudy urine may be an early sign.*
- Maintain stability and patency of suprapubic and/or urethral catheters. Secure catheters in position. *Maintaining bladder decompression eliminates pressure on suture lines. Preventing movement or pulling of catheters reduces the risk of resultant pressure on surgical incisions.*
- Carefully monitor urine output after catheter removal. *Difficulty voiding is common following catheter removal. Early intervention to prevent bladder distension is important to prevent pressure on suture lines.*
- If the urethral or suprapubic catheter will remain in place on discharge, teach proper care to the person and family members as needed. *Appropriate self-care and early recognition of problems reduce the risk of significant complications.*

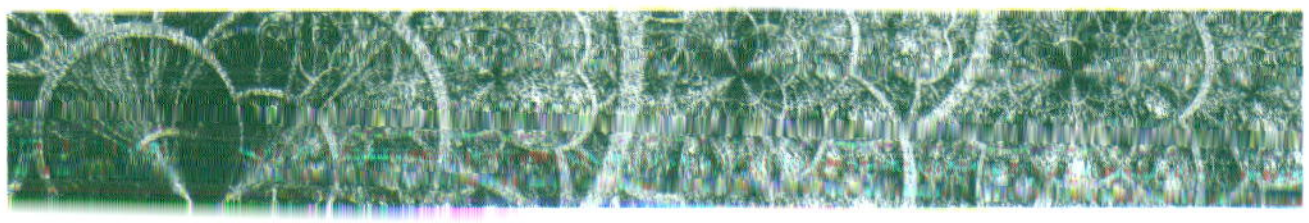

Nursing care

Health promotion

Although urinary incontinence rarely causes serious physical effects, it frequently has significant psychosocial effects and can lead to lowered self-esteem, social isolation and even institutionalisation (Mohammed et al., 2021). Inform all people that UI is not a normal consequence of ageing and that treatments are available. To reduce the incidence of UI, teach everyone to perform pelvic floor muscle (Kegel) exercises (see Box 26.3) to improve perineal muscle tone. Advise women to seek advice from their women's healthcare or primary care practitioner about using topical or systemic hormone therapy during menopause to maintain perineal tissue integrity. Advise older men to have routine prostate

BOX 26.3 Pelvic floor muscle (Kegel) exercises

Kegel exercises are particularly important for postnatal, menopausal or post-vaginal hysterectomy women

- Identify the pelvic muscles with these techniques:
  a. Stop the flow of urine during voiding and hold for a few seconds.
  b. Tighten the muscles at the vaginal entrance around a gloved finger or tampon.
  c. Tighten the muscles around the anus as though resisting defecation.
- Perform exercises by tightening pelvic muscles, holding for 10 seconds and relaxing for 10 to 15 seconds. Continue the sequence (tighten, hold, relax) for 10 repetitions.
- Keep abdominal muscles and breathing relaxed while performing exercises.
- Initially, exercises should be performed twice per day, working up to four times a day.
- Encourage exercising at a specific time each day or in conjunction with another daily activity (such as bathing or watching the news). Establish a routine as these exercises should be continued for life.
- This process is the same for men, particularly post prostatectomy, with a slightly different technique used to identify the correct muscle groups.

examinations to prevent urethral obstruction and overflow incontinence.

Assessment

Nursing assessment for the person with urinary incontinence includes both subjective and objective data:

- *Health history*: voiding diary; frequency of incontinent episodes, amount of urine loss and activities associated with incontinence; methods used to deal with incontinence; use of Kegel exercises or medications; any chronic diseases, related surgeries; effects of incontinence on usual activities, including social activities.
- *Physical examination*: physical and mental status, including any physical limitations or impaired cognition; inspect, palpate and percuss abdomen for bladder distension; inspect perineal tissues for redness, irritation or tissue breakdown; observe for bulging of bladder into vagina when bearing down; assess pelvic muscle tone as indicated.

Nursing diagnoses and interventions

In planning nursing care, consider the person's mental status, mobility and motivation. Behavioural techniques can be effective, but they require long-term commitment and the physical and mental capability to use them.

Nursing care and modification of routines can restore continence fully or partially even in the institutionalised person. Scheduled toileting, bladder training and prompted voiding, combined with positive reinforcement such as praise, can reduce the need for incontinence pads and/or catheterisation.

See the nursing care plan for additional nursing diagnoses and interventions for the person with urinary incontinence.

Urinary incontinence: stress and/or urge

Exercises to strengthen pelvic floor muscles, dietary modifications and bladder training programs often are effective to restore and maintain continence.

- Instruct to keep a voiding diary, recording the time and amount of all fluid intake and urinary output, status at the time of voiding (dry or wet) and on arising from sleep and activities. *Voiding diaries provide valuable information for identifying the type of incontinence and possible measures to reduce or eliminate incontinent episodes.*
- Teach pelvic floor muscle exercises (see Box 26.3). Instruct to consciously tighten pelvic muscles when the need to void is perceived and to relax the abdomen while walking to the bathroom. *Improved pelvic muscle strength helps retain urine and prevent stress incontinence by increasing urethral pressure. Exercises also decrease abnormal detrusor muscle contractions, decreasing pressure within the bladder.*

CONSIDERATION FOR PRACTICE

Do not advise people who have difficulty emptying the bladder completely to stop urine flow while voiding to identify pelvic floor muscles. Repeated interruption of micturition can interfere with complete bladder emptying and increase the risk of UTI.

- Using the person's voiding diary, suggest dietary and fluid intake modifications to reduce stress and urge incontinence. Include limiting caffeine, alcohol, citrus juice and artificial sweetener consumption; limiting fluid intake to no less than 1.5 to 2.0 L per day; and limiting evening fluid intake. *Caffeine, alcohol and citrus juices are bladder irritants and tend to promote detrusor instability, increasing the risk of urge incontinence. Artificial sweeteners may also irritate the bladder. Fluid intake of 1.5 to 2.0 L per day is adequate to maintain health for most people; excess fluid may increase stress incontinence if bathroom facilities are not readily available.*

CONSIDERATION FOR PRACTICE

Limiting total fluid intake to less than 1.5 to 2.0 L per day is not recommended for those with urinary incontinence. Inadequate fluid increases urine concentration, leading to bladder wall irritation and possibly increasing problems of urge incontinence.

Self-care deficit: toileting

Functional incontinence may be the predominant problem in an institutionalised older adult. Limited mobility, impaired vision, dementia, lack of access to facilities and privacy, and tight staffing patterns increase the risk of incontinence in previously continent residents. The primary problem in functional incontinence is an outside factor that interferes with the ability to respond normally to the urge to void. An immobilised person may wet the bed if a call light is not within reach; a person with Alzheimer's disease may perceive the urge to void but be unable to interpret its meaning or respond by seeking a bathroom. For these people, self-care deficit in toileting is a primary problem.

- Assess physical and mental abilities and limitations, usual voiding pattern and ability to assist with toileting. *A thorough assessment allows planned interventions to address specific needs and promote independence.*
- Provide assistive devices as needed to facilitate independence, such as raised toilet seats, grab bars, a bedside commode or night-lights. *Fostering independence in toileting bolsters self-concept and maintains a positive body image.*
- Plan a toileting schedule based on the person's normal elimination patterns to achieve approximately 300 mL of urine output with each voiding. *Allowing the bladder to fill to a point at which the urge to void is experienced and then emptying it completely helps maintain normal bladder capacity and bacteriostatic functions.*
- Position for ease of voiding and provide privacy. *Normal positioning, usual toileting facilities and privacy enhance the ability to void on schedule and empty the bladder completely.*
- Adjust fluid intake so that the majority of fluids are consumed during times of the day when the person is most able to remain continent. Unless fluids are to be restricted, maintain a fluid intake of at least 1.5 to 2.0 L per day. *An adequate fluid intake is vital to promote hydration and urinary function. Overly concentrated urine can irritate the bladder, increasing incontinence.*
- Assist with clothing that is easily removed (e.g. elastic-waist pants or loose dresses). Velcro and may be easier than snaps and buttons. *Clothing that is difficult to remove can increase the risk of incontinence for those with mobility problems or impaired dexterity.*

Social isolation

Urinary incontinence increases the risk of social isolation due to embarrassment, fear of not having ready access to a bathroom, body odour or other factors. Social isolation can, in turn, increase problems of incontinence because normal cues and relationships are lost and the need to remain dry is less strongly felt.

- Assess reasons for and extent of social isolation. Verify the degree of social isolation with the person or significant other. Do not assume that social isolation is only related to urinary incontinence. *Other problems frequently associated with ageing (such as a hearing deficit) may be primary or contributing factors.*
- Refer the person for urological examination and incontinence evaluation. *People who assume that urinary incontinence is a normal part of the ageing process may not be aware of treatment options.*
- Explore alternative coping strategies with the person, significant other, staff and other healthcare team members. *Protective pads or shields, good perineal hygiene, scheduled voiding and clothing that does not interfere with toileting can enhance continence.*

Community-based care

Because urinary incontinence is a contributing factor in the institutionalisation of many older people, person-centred teaching and family teaching can have a significant impact on maintaining independence and residence in the community. Address possible causes of incontinence and appropriate treatment measures. Refer for urological examination if not already completed. Discuss fluid intake management, perineal care and products for clothing protection.

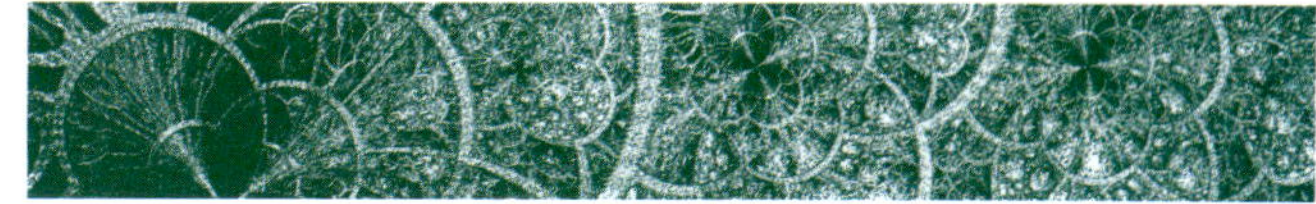

NURSING CARE PLAN A person with urinary incontinence

Anna Giovanni, a 76-year-old retired teacher, has been widowed for 10 years and lives alone. Mrs Giovanni's eldest daughter expresses concern that her mother seems increasingly reluctant to leave her apartment to visit friends and family. She reports a strong odour of urine throughout her mother's apartment and that her mother's bed is often wet. She is worried about needing to place her mother in an aged care facility if she cannot continue to live independently.

ASSESSMENT

The community nurse visits Mrs Giovanni to assess her situation. Mrs Giovanni admits that she has problems with urine leakage when laughing and coughing and has a strong urge to void on hearing the sound of running water. At night, her urge to void is so strong that she often cannot reach the bathroom in time. Mrs Giovanni does not have a history of UTIs, neurological disorders or difficulty with her bowels. She had a hysterectomy at age 52 and was on hormone replacement therapy for about 10 years afterwards. She is taking digoxin 0.125 mg daily, frusemide 40 mg twice daily and potassium chloride 20 mEq three times daily for mild heart failure.

Physical assessment reveals a moderate cystourethrocele and atrophy of vaginal and vulvar tissues. Moderate perineal dermatitis is also noted and her pelvic floor strength is weak. Urinalysis is within normal limits and post-voiding residual urine is 5 mL.

Analysis of Mrs Giovanni's voiding diary shows moderate consumption of tea and juices throughout the day, nine day time voidings and four night voidings with an average volume of about 250 mL per void. She notices urine leakage most often in the late afternoon and at night. The community nurse identifies stress incontinence with an urgency component and decides to try a conservative approach before referring Mrs Giovanni for further testing and possible doctor referral for

(continued)

NURSING CARE PLAN A person with urinary incontinence (continued)

cystourethrocele repair. Oestrogen cream, tolterodine and a barrier cream to treat Mrs Giovanni's vulvitis are prescribed.

DIAGNOSES

- *Stress urinary incontinence* related to weak pelvic floor musculature and tissue atrophy.
- *Urge urinary incontinence* related to excess intake of caffeine and citrus juices.
- *Impaired skin integrity* related to constant contact of urine with perineal tissues.
- *Ineffective coping* related to inability to control urine leakage.

PLANNING

- Plan interventions to facilitate a return of normal bladder function.
- Plan interventions that foster a resumption of previous levels of social activity.

Expected outcomes

- Remain dry between voidings and at night.
- Demonstrate improved perineal muscle strength.
- Regain and maintain perineal skin integrity.
- Return to her previous level of social activity.

IMPLEMENTATION

- Teach how to identify pelvic floor muscles and how to perform Kegel exercises.
- Suggest drinking decaffeinated tea and non-citrus fruit juices (grape, apple and cranberry).
- Encourage to minimise fluid intake after evening meal.
- Change evening dose of frusemide from 9 pm to 3 pm.
- Instruct to void by the clock, gradually increasing intervals from every 45 to 60 minutes to every 2 to 2.5 hours. Advise to maintain shorter voiding intervals for 2 to 3 hours after frusemide doses.
- Teach to how to cleanse perineal area, wiping front to back after each voiding or incident of urine leakage.
- Introduce commercial products available for clothing and furniture protection, encouraging experimentation to identify the most helpful product(s).
- Provide a commode for bedside at night and adequate lighting to prevent injury.
- Schedule follow-up visits and evaluations to reinforce teaching.

EVALUATION

Three months after her initial visit, Mrs Giovanni states that she is doing very well, experiencing only occasional leakage of small amounts of urine, primarily when sneezing, coughing or laughing. She finds a minipad adequate for protection and is often able to remain dry all day. She has had no further problems with enuresis since changing her evening frusemide dose to late afternoon and limiting her fluids after dinner. She can make it to the bathroom and no longer needs the bedside commode. Her perineal tissue is intact and she demonstrates improved muscle strength. Anna's daughter says her mother is beginning to resume her normal social activities and that she is no longer worried about her mother's ability to care for herself independently.

CRITICAL THINKING IN THE NURSING PROCESS

1. What factors in Mrs Giovanni's medical history and current medication regimen contributed to her night-time incontinence?
2. What is the rationale for including an intervention to teach Mrs Giovanni about perineal cleansing as part of her care plan?

REFLECTION ON THE NURSING PROCESS

1. Outline what you have learned from Mrs Giovanni's situation that you could apply to your future practice.
2. What educational strategies would you give Mrs Giovanni's family to prevent her developing social isolation related to the urinary incontinence?

CHAPTER HIGHLIGHTS

- **Urinary tract infections are very common and are a leading complication among hospitalised individuals. Short-course antibiotic therapy is appropriate for uncomplicated infections of the lower urinary tract that are not associated with the presence of an indwelling urinary catheter.**
- **Teach people about perineal hygiene and the importance of maintaining adequate fluid intake as measures to help prevent UTI.**
- **Urinary calculi can obstruct the urinary tract at any level and cause significant pain as they move from the kidney through the ureter. Instruct those who have had a renal stone to maintain a generous fluid intake particularly during exercise and warm weather, to reduce the risk of further stone formation.**
- **The risk of bladder cancer is greater among men than women, although women have poorer outcomes, and cigarette smoking is the most significant risk factor for bladder cancer. Most tumours can be resected transurethrally if diagnosed early, before spreading to deeper layers of the bladder wall, the lymph nodes and adjacent tissue.**
- **When resection of the urinary bladder is necessary, a urinary diversion is created to collect urine. A collection appliance must be worn constantly on an ileal conduit; when a continent urinary diversion is created, the pouch is emptied by intermittent catheterisation of the stoma.**
- **Urinary retention may occur as a result of some medications, neurological damage or disease, or obstruction (e.g. an enlarged prostate gland). If the underlying condition cannot be treated, medications or intermittent catheterisation are used to promote bladder emptying.**
- **Older adults, in particular, are at risk of urinary incontinence, a treatable condition. A health history, voiding diary and diagnostic testing are used to establish the type of urinary incontinence and direct treatments such as surgery, pelvic floor muscle exercises, medications and scheduled toileting.**

CONCEPT CHECK

1 A 30-year-old male presents to the urgency clinic complaining of concentrated bright yellow urine and of discomfort in his lower back area. The assessment reveals no significant nursing history. Additional questions the nurse should ask include:
1 'Have you had any injury to your abdominal area?'
2 'When did you first notice your urine's colour?'
3 'How often do you void?'
4 'How much fluid do you drink each day?'

2 The man volunteers the information that he has just started cycling, has been following a strict high-level exercise program and has a high-protein diet. His fluid intake is about 1 L per day. The nurse should then ask:
1 'Do you take any prescribed medications?'
2 'How much exercise do you have each day?'
3 'How long have you been on this exercise program?'
4 'Do you take any additional supplements; e.g. vitamins?' (Multivitamins will colour urine orange.)

3 After an assessment and a nursing history nothing of significance is noted except mild tenderness over the lower back area. The man admits he has been taking multivitamins because he wanted to improve his physical performance. The nurse recommends the man:
1 reduces the amount of exercise he does on a daily basis
2 applies a warm pack to his lower back when he rests
3 stops taking the multivitamin medication until his urine returns to a normal colour
4 increases his fluid intake to at least 3 L per day

4 A 58-year-old woman presents at her doctor with symptoms of frequency, urgency, nocturia, dysuria and cloudy, rust-coloured urine for the third time in the past 2 years. The nurse should plan to include which of the following in her teaching for this woman? (Select all that apply.)
1 return to the office in 10 days for follow-up culture
2 preprocedure instruction for an IVP
3 the potential benefits of oestrogen vaginal cream
4 recommendations for perineal cleansing
5 recommendations for screening cystoscopy

5 Recognising the risk of urolithiasis in the immobilised person, the nurse appropriately plans to:
1 administer a calcium supplement
2 regularly monitor urine pH
3 maintain an indwelling urinary catheter
4 increase fluid intake to 3,000 mL per day

6 A person admitted with possible kidney stones develops sudden complaints of acute crampy pain on the left side that radiates into the groin. He is nauseated and vomits clear fluid. On voiding, his urine is pink. The nurse should:
1 obtain a bladder scan to assess for residual urine
2 administer the prescribed narcotic analgesic
3 notify the doctor
4 strain all urine

7 The nurse teaching a group of community members about wellness and disease prevention includes which of the following as a measure to reduce the risk of bladder cancer?
1 Do not start smoking. If you smoke, stop.
2 Avoid using hair dyes and pesticides in the home.
3 Limit your intake of coffee and other caffeinated beverages.
4 Empty your bladder every 2 hours.

8 A person remarks to the nurse that his urine occasionally appears pink. He wonders if this is anything to be concerned about. The nurse should:
1 instruct the man to notify his doctor if he develops pain or difficulty voiding
2 advise the man to make an appointment to see his doctor
3 instruct the man to record if the urine is pink following exercise
4 tell the man to increase his fluid intake to 4 L per day

9 The nurse caring for a person in the spinal shock phase following spinal cord injury appropriately plans to:
1 insert a Foley catheter to accurately measure output
2 stimulate voiding using Credé's method
3 assess for urinary retention following each voiding
4 catheterise with a straight catheter every 3 to 4 hours

10 The nurse implements a nursing care necessary for this individual with a Foley catheter in place to:
1 maintain the closed system of drainage tubing and collection bag to prevent ascending infection
2 irrigate the person with 1% neosporin solution three times a daily
3 clamp the catheter for 1 hour every 4 hours to maintain the bladder's elasticity
4 maintain the drainage tubing and collection bag below bladder level to facilitate drainage by gravity

BIBLIOGRAPHY

Australian & New Zealand Urological Nurses Society (ANZUNS) (2013). *Catheterisation guideline working party*. Retrieved from https://www.anzuns.org/

Australian Bureau of Statistics (ABS) (2021). *Causes of death, Australia, 2020*. Retrieved from http://www.abs.gov.au/

Australian Commission on Safety and Quality in Health Care (ACSQHC) (2021). *The Fourth Atlas of Healthcare Variation 2021—2.4 Kidney infections and urinary tract infections*. Developed by the Australian Commission on Safety and Quality in Health Care (ACSQHC). ACSQHC: Sydney. Retrieved from https://www.safetyandquality.gov.au/

Australian Institute of Health and Welfare (AIHW) (2017). *Cancer in Australia 2017*. Cancer series no. 101. Cat. no. CAN 100. Canberra: AIHW.

Brackman, M., Carballo, E., Uppal, S., Torski, J., Reynolds, R. K. & McLean, K. (2020). Implementation of a standardized voiding management protocol to reduce unnecessary re-catheterization—A quality improvement project. *Gynecologic Oncology*, *157*, 487–493. https://doi.org/10.1016/j.ygyno.2020.01.036

Cai, T. (2021). Recurrent uncomplicated urinary tract infections: Definitions and risk factors. *Urogenital Infections and Inflammations*, *9*, 1–5. doi. 10.3205/id000072

Continence Foundation of Australia (CFA) (2021). *Key statistics on incontinence*. Retrieved from https://www.continence.org.au/

Gbinigie, O. A., Spencer, E. A., Heneghan, C. J., Lee, J. J. & Butler, C. C. (2021). Cranberry extract for symptoms of acute, uncomplicated urinary tract infection: A systematic review. *Antibiotics*, *10*(1), 1–14. https://doi.org/10.3390/antibiotics10010012

Gray, M., McClain, R., Peruggia, M. et al. (2001). A model for predicting motor urge urinary incontinence. *Nursing Research*, *50*(2), 116–122.

Jarvis, T., Chan, L. & Gottlieb, T. (2014). Assessment and management of lower urinary tract infection in adults. *Australian Prescriber*, *37*, 7–9. https://doi.org/10.1016/j.urology.2018.10.010

Khan, F., [illegible], N. & Kim, Y. M. (2020). A strategy to control colonization of pathogens: Embedding of lactic acid bacteria on the surface of urinary catheter. *Applied Microbiology and Biotechnology*, *104*, [illegible]. https://doi.org/10.1007/s00253-020-10903-0

Krimphove, M. J., Szymaniak, J., Marchese, M. et al. (2019). Sex-specific differences in the quality of treatment of muscle-invasive bladder cancer do not explain the overall survival discrepancy. *European Urology Focus*, 7, 124–131. https://doi.org/10.1016/j.euf.2019.06.001

Lee, J. K. (2021). Neurogenic bladder management. *Radiologic Technology*, *92*(3), 281–295.

Levett-Jones, T., Dwyer, T., Reid-Searl, K., Heaton, L., Flenady, T., Applegarth, J., Guinea, S. & Andersen, P. (2017). *Patient Safety Competency Framework (PSCF) for Nursing Students*. Sydney. Retrieved from http://psframework.wpengine.com/

Loscalzo, J., Fauci, A. S., Kasper, D. L., Hauser, S. L. & Longo, D. (2022). *Harrison's principles of internal medicine* (21st ed.). New York: McGraw Hill Medical.

Matsui, Y., Hu, Y., Rubin, J., Souza de Assis, R., Suh, J. & Riley, L. W. (2020). Multilocus sequence typing of *Escherichia coli* isolates from urinary tract infection patients and from fecal samples of healthy subjects in a college community. *Microbiology Open*, 9, e1032. https://doi.org/ 10.1002/mbo3.1032

Medina, M. & Castillo-Pino, E. (2019) An introduction to the epidemiology and burden of urinary tract infections. *Therapeutic Advances in Urology*, *11*, 3–7. doi: 10.1177/1756287219832172

Mohammed, R. F., Taha, S. H., Abd-Elaziz, N. M. & Abd-Elziz Omar, E. (2021). Effect of selective behavioural therapy on stress urinary incontinence and self-esteem among institutionalized elderly women. *Assiut Scientific Journal*, 9(25.0), 45–55. doi: 10.21608/asnj.2021.80932.1199

Papadakis, M., McPhee, S. & Rabow, M. (2022). *Current medical diagnosis and treatment* (61st ed.). New York: McGraw-Hill Education.

Payne, D. & Kerrigan, P. (2020). One Trust's rationale for choosing a lubrication gel for use in catheterisation. *British Journal of Nursing*, *29*(18), S38–S43. https://doi.org/10.12968/bjon.2020.29.18.S38

Reesink, D. J., Scheltema, J. M. W., Barendrecht, M. M., Boeken Kruger, A. E., Jansonius, A., Wiltink, J. & van der Windt, F. (2018). Extracorporeal shock wave lithotripsy under intravenous sedation for treatment of urolithiasis. *Scandinavian Journal of Urology*, *52*(5–6), 453–458. doi: 10.1080/21681805.2018.1524398

Saginala, K., Barsouk, A., Aluru, J. S., Rawla, P., Padala, S. A. & Barsouk, A. (2020). Epidemiology of bladder cancer. *Medical Sciences*, *8*(1), 15–27. https://dx.doi.org/10.3390/medsci8010015

Sali, G. M. & Joshi, H. B. (2020). Ureteric stents: Overview of current clinical applications and economic implications. *International Journal of Urology*, *27*, 7–15. doi: 10.1111/iju.14119

Sihra, N., Goodman, A., Zakri, R., Sahai, A. & Malde, S. (2018). Nonantibiotic prevention and management of recurrent urinary tract infection. *Nature Reviews Urology*, *15*, 750–776. https://doi.org/10.1038/s41585-018-0106-x

Society of Urological Nurses Association (2014). *Streamlined evidence-based RN tool: Catheter associated urinary tract infection (CAUTI) prevention*. Retrieved from http://nursingworld.org/

Wilson, J., Farrow, E. & Holden, C. (2022). Urinary tract obstruction. *InnovAiT*, *15*(5), 265–271. https://doi.org/10.1177/17557380221080781

Wittig, L., Carlson, K. V., Andrews, J. M., Trafford Crump, R. & Baverstock, R. J. (2019). Diabetic bladder dysfunction: A review. *Urology*, *123*, 1–6. https://doi.org/10.1016/j.urology.2018.10.010

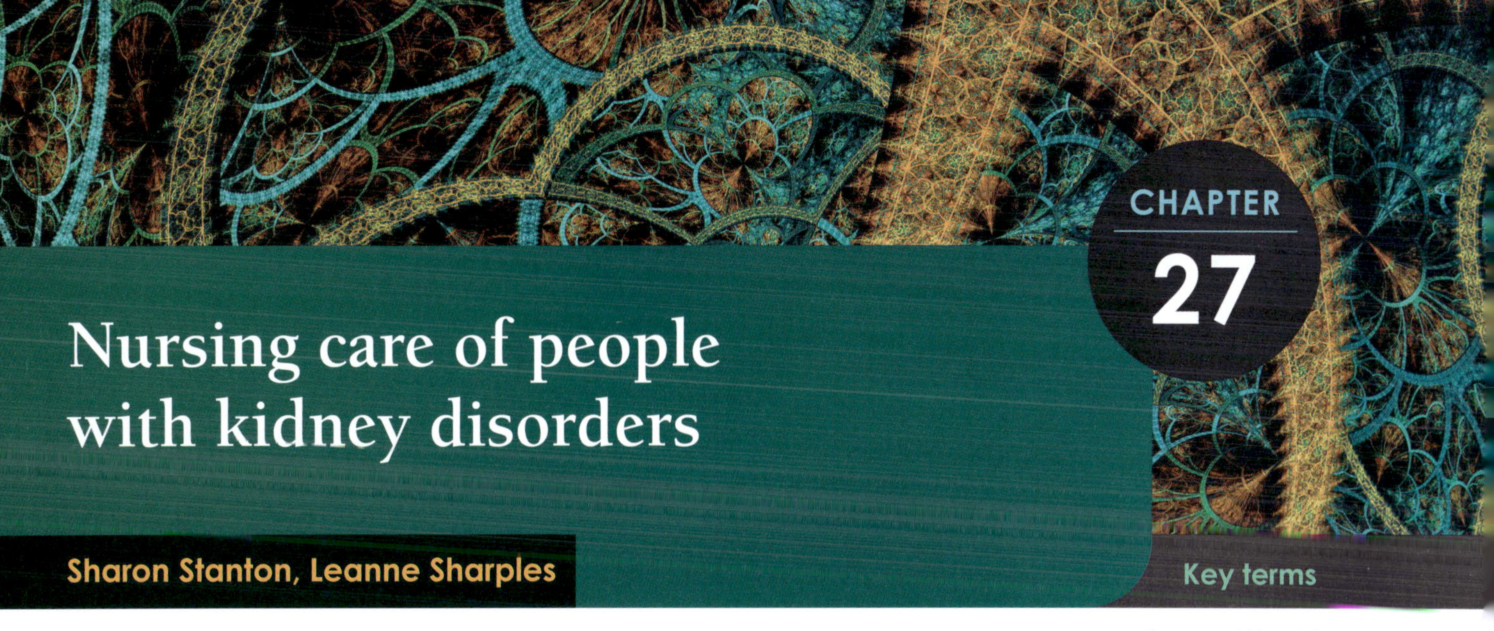

CHAPTER 27

Nursing care of people with kidney disorders

Sharon Stanton, Leanne Sharples

Learning outcomes

- Discuss the course, implications and health management options for a person with acute kidney injury.
- Relate the pathophysiology, clinical manifestations and possible interventions required for a person with chronic kidney disease to the pathophysiology of the condition.
- Discuss the risk factors, implications and health management and treatment options for a person who has end-stage kidney disease (kidney failure).

Clinical competencies

- Assess the functional health status of people with kidney disease.
- Monitor, document and report unexpected or abnormal manifestations in people with kidney disease.
- Provide appropriate and effective nursing care for people undergoing dialysis, surgery involving the kidneys or kidney transplant.
- Based on assessment data, determine priority nursing diagnoses and interventions for people with kidney disease.
- Plan and implement evidence-based nursing care for people with kidney disease using research and best practices.
- Collaborate with the person and other members of the interprofessional team to prioritise and implement care.
- Provide teaching appropriate to both people with kidney disease and their personal circumstances.
- Evaluate responses to care, revising the plan of care as needed to promote, maintain or restore functional health status for people with kidney disease.

Key terms

The internal environment of the body normally remains in a relatively constant or *homeostatic* state. One of the easiest ways to reflect on the nursing roles necessary when looking after a person with renal insufficiency is to recall the functions of the kidney (see Table 27.1) and then consider how we support the loss of those functions.

RENAL INSUFFICIENCY: TOWARDS A NEW UNDERSTANDING

Renal insufficiency is a broad term that describes any condition in which the kidneys are unable to remove accumulated metabolites from the blood, leading to altered fluid, electrolyte and acid–base balance. The cause may be an acute insult or a primary kidney disorder, or may be secondary to a systemic disease or urological defects.

Before we continue to explore the many facets of renal insufficiency, it is important to understand the disease trajectory of any kidney-related disorder and the meanings of the terms used to describe them. One point to note when reviewing the renal literature is that there has been a change in the past few years as to how we describe renal insufficiency. You may note that some literature uses the term 'chronic renal failure' or 'acute renal failure', whereas more modern texts use the terms 'chronic kidney disease' and 'acute kidney injury or dysfunction', respectively. These changes in terminology reflect the changes in our understanding of both the illness trajectory and the pathophysiology of renal insufficiency and that in fact, more often than not, there is a disease process occurring and not merely 'renal failure'.

The sub-types of renal insufficiency are described as either acute, chronic or end-stage. **Acute kidney injury (AKI)** is characterised by a rapid onset of symptoms that are potentially reversible with prompt intervention that addresses the initial cause of the injury. Chronic kidney disease (CKD), by contrast, is a largely silent disease that presents as an insidious irreversible decline in renal function. A more detailed definition of CKD will be discussed later in this chapter. People with CKD are also at high risk of acute episodes, which is referred to as 'acute on chronic kidney disease'. As the phrase suggests, an acute injury is superimposed on a background of CKD. For example, a person with a history of CKD may become dehydrated and experience a rapid decline in renal function which may be reversible with adequate rehydration.

There is often some confusion in the literature when the terms 'chronic kidney disease' (CKD) and 'end-stage kidney disease' (ESKD) are used interchangeably. This use is incorrect, as the final stage of chronic kidney disease, when the glomerular filtration rate falls below 15 mL/min, sees its description change to 'end-stage kidney disease' (ESKD) or 'kidney failure' to denote the terminal phase of the disease trajectory. ESKD is not synonymous with active treatment and it is at this stage that the person may choose to undergo a kidney replacement therapy (KRT) or to withdraw from active treatment.

TABLE 27.1 Functions of the kidney

EXCRETORY	REGULATORY	HORMONAL/ METABOLIC
Removal of metabolic waste products	Maintain fluid and electrolyte balance Maintain acid-base balance Regulate blood pressure	Activation of vitamin D Erythropoietin production Renin production

FAST FACTS

- Acute kidney injury has a sudden onset and is often reversible with prompt treatment.
- Chronic kidney disease is a slowly progressive and often silent disease that is irreversible.
- End-stage kidney disease, or kidney failure, is the final stage of the CKD continuum.
- Diagnosis/staging of disease is multifaceted and not based on glomerular filtration rate (GFR) alone.

AGE-RELATED CHANGES IN KIDNEY FUNCTION

Structural and functional changes occur in the ageing kidney. Structurally, the number of nephrons decreases. Glomeruli in the renal cortex (see the chapter 'A person-centred approach to assessing the renal system' for a review of normal kidney structure and function) are lost with ageing, reducing kidney mass. Because of the large functional reserve of the kidneys, however, renal function remains adequate unless additional stressors affect the renal system. Any additional stressors such as hypotension, exposure to nephrotoxic drugs or an inflammatory process such as glomerulonephritis may precipitate an acute episode in the older adult. The **glomerular filtration rate (GFR)**, the amount of filtrate made by the kidneys per minute, declines due to age-related factors affecting the renovascular system (such as arteriosclerosis, decreased renal vascularity and decreased cardiac output). By age 80, the GFR may be less than half of what it was at age 30. Serum creatinine levels may rise slowly. Because older adults have less muscle mass, they produce less creatinine. Likewise, the urea may remain within normal limits.

Age-related changes in renal function have significant implications. The kidneys are less able to concentrate urine and compensate for increased or decreased salt intake. When combined with the diminished effectiveness of antidiuretic hormone (ADH) and a reduced thirst response, both common in ageing, this decreased ability to concentrate urine increases the risk of dehydration. Potassium excretion may be decreased because of lower aldosterone levels. As a result, fluid and electrolyte imbalances are more common and potentially critical in older people.

Decreased GFR in the older adult also reduces the clearance of drugs excreted through the kidneys. This reduced clearance prolongs the half-life of drugs and may necessitate lower drug doses and longer dosing intervals. Common medications affected by decreased GFR include:

- cardiac drugs: digoxin
- antibiotics: aminoglycosides, tetracyclines, cephalosporins
- histamine H_2 antagonists: cimetidine
- hypoglycaemic agents: metformin.

TABLE 27.2 Nursing implications of age-related changes in kidney function

FUNCTIONAL CHANGE	EFFECT	IMPLICATIONS
Decreased GFR	Decreased clearance of drugs excreted primarily through the kidneys increases drug half-life and blood levels and risk of drug toxicity.	Monitor carefully for signs of toxicity, especially when administering contrast media, amphotericin B, digoxin, aminoglycoside antibiotics, tetracyclines, vancomycin, cimetidine and cephalosporin antibiotics.
Decreased number of functional nephrons; lower levels of aldosterone; increased resistance to ADH	Decreased ability to conserve water and sodium; impaired potassium excretion; and decreased hydrogen ion excretion, resulting in reduced ability to compensate for acidosis.	Monitor for dehydration and hyponatraemia; maintain fluid intake of 1,500 to 2,500 mL/day unless contraindicated; monitor for hyperkalaemia, especially if taking a potassium-sparing diuretic, heparin, ACE inhibitor, beta-blocker or NSAID; increased risk of acidosis.
Reduced numbers of functional nephrons	Decreased renal reserve with increased risk of acute injury.	Avoid giving nephrotoxic drugs if possible; monitor urine output and blood chemistries for early signs of renal failure.

When caring for older adults or any person at risk of chronic kidney disease due to reduced GFR, it is especially important to monitor drugs that are toxic to the renal tubules. Age-related changes in renal function and related nursing implications are summarised in Table 27.2.

THE PERSON WITH ACUTE KIDNEY INJURY

The use of the term 'AKI' suggests some form of structural injury to the renal parenchyma, yet classifications of AKI that were proposed by the Kidney Disease: Improving Global Outcomes (KDIGO) group, which merges the earlier RIFLE (Risk, Injury, Failure, Loss, End-stage kidney disease) and the Acute Kidney Injury Network (AKIN) criteria (see Table 27.3), define AKI in terms of functional decreases. In basic terms, AKI manifests as a rapid decline in renal function with uraemic symptoms and fluid and electrolyte imbalances. The deterioration in renal function sees an increase in serum creatinine levels. However, what is important in terms of outcomes for people experiencing AKI is the context and environment in which the insult to the kidney occurs as this is directly associated with mortality and morbidity.

AKI is a broad clinical syndrome, which includes both direct injury to the kidney and the acute impairment of function.

TABLE 27.3 Staging of AKI

STAGE	SERUM CREATININE	URINE OUTPUT
1	1.5–1.9 times baseline OR ≥ 0.3 mg/dL (≥ 26.5 µmol/L) increase	< 0.5 mL/kg/h for 6–12 hours
2	2.0–2.9 times baseline	< 0.5 mL/kg/h for ≥ 12 hours
3	3.0 times baseline OR Increase in serum creatinine to ≥ 4.0 mg/dL (≥ 353.6 µmol/L) OR Initiation of renal replacement therapy OR, in patients < 18 years, [illegible] in eGFR to < [illegible] mL/min per 1.73 m²	< 0.3 mL/kg/h for ≥ 24 hours OR Anuria for ≥ 12 hours

Source: Kidney Disease: Improving Global Outcomes (KDIGO) Acute Kidney Injury Workgroup (2012). KDIGO clinical practice guideline for acute kidney injury. *Kidney International Supplements*, 2, 1–138. See also Levey et al. (2020). Nomenclature for kidney function and disease: Report of a Kidney Disease: Improving Global Outcomes (KDIGO) Consensus Conference. *Kidneys International*, 97, 1117–1129. https://doi.org/10.1016/j.kint.2020.02.010.

Incidence and risk factors

Approximately 5–7% of all people hospitalised develop AKI and the incidence jumps to as high as 30% in critical care units, with an associated mortality rate exceeding 50% (Khan, Deepak & Kumar, 2017). While research indicates that mortality rates associated with AKI are steadily declining, 53 Australians die from kidney-related diseases every day (Kidney Health Australia, 2018).

Major trauma or surgery, infection, haemorrhage, severe heart failure, severe liver disease and lower urinary tract obstruction are risk factors for AKI. Drugs and radiological contrast media that are toxic to the kidney (*nephrotoxic*) also increase the risk of AKI. Older adults develop AKI more frequently due to a higher incidence of serious illness, hypotension, major surgeries, diagnostic procedures and treatment with nephrotoxic drugs. The older adult also may have some degree of pre-existing renal insufficiency associated with ageing (O'Sullivan, Hughes & Ferenbach, 2017).

The most common causes of AKI are ischaemia and exposure to nephrotoxic agents. The kidney is particularly vulnerable to both due to the amount of blood that passes through it. A fall in blood pressure or volume can result in ischaemic injury to the kidney tissues. Alternatively, nephrotoxins in the blood damage kidney tissue directly.

Physiology review

The functional unit of the kidneys, the nephron (see Figure 25.3), produces urine through three processes: glomerular filtration, tubular reabsorption and tubular secretion. In the *glomerulus*, a filtrate of water and small solutes is formed. The solute concentration of this filtrate is equal to that of plasma, with the exception of large molecules such as plasma proteins and blood cells. The GFR is affected by blood volume and pressure, the autonomic nervous system and other factors. From the glomerulus, the filtrate flows into the *tubules*, where its composition is changed by the processes of *tubular reabsorption* and *tubular secretion*. Most water and many filtered solutes such as electrolytes and glucose are reabsorbed. Metabolic waste products such as urea, hydrogen ion, ammonia and some creatinine are secreted into the tubule for elimination. By the time urine [illegible] the collecting [illegible] renal pelvis, 99% of the filtrate [illegible].

Pathophysiology

Acute kidney injury is categorised as being pre-renal, intrinsic or post-renal. In *pre-renal AKI*, hypoperfusion leads to kidney dysfunction without directly affecting the integrity of kidney

TABLE 27.4 Causes of acute kidney injury

	CAUSE	EXAMPLES
Pre-renal	Hypovolaemia	Haemorrhage, dehydration, excess fluid loss from GI tract, burns, wounds, sepsis
	Decreased cardiac output	Heart failure, cardiogenic shock
	Altered vascular resistance	Sepsis, anaphylaxis, vasoactive drugs
	Renovascular obstruction	Renal artery stenosis, aneurysm, trauma, emboli, thrombi
Intra-renal	Glomerular/microvascular injury	Glomerulonephritis, disseminated intravascular coagulation, vasculitis, hypertension, toxaemia of pregnancy, haemolytic uraemic syndrome
	Acute tubular necrosis	Ischaemia due to conditions associated with pre-renal failure; toxins such as drugs, heavy metals; haemolysis, rhabdomyolysis (muscle cell breakdown)
	Interstitial nephritis	Acute pyelonephritis, toxins, metabolic imbalances, idiopathic
Post-renal	Ureteral/urethral obstruction	Calculi, carcinoma, external compression, stricture, prostatic hypertrophy, blood clot, neuropathy

tissues. *Intrinsic* (or *intra-renal*) *AKI* is due to direct damage to functional kidney tissue. Causes include medications, radiographic contrast agents, hypercalcaemia and poisonous substances (Alscher, Erley & Kuhlmann, 2019). *Post-renal AKI* is related to urinary obstruction, with prostatic hypoplasia a major cause. Renal function can somewhat recover after the occurrence of obstruction has been resolved (Alscher et al., 2019). Table 27.4 summarises the causes of AKI. See also 'Pathophysiology illustrated: acute kidney injury'.

Pre-renal AKI

Pre-renal AKI results from any condition that decreases renal blood flow, causing subsequent hypoperfusion of the kidney; as a result, it is also termed 'volume responsive AKI'. Renal blood flow can be decreased though renovascular obstruction (e.g. renal artery stenosis), during surgical procedures or as a result of any condition that significantly decreases vascular volume, cardiac output or systemic vascular resistance. The kidney's natural response is to use its own autoregulatory system in an attempt to restore renal blood flow. The afferent and efferent arterioles dilate and constrict, respectively, while the enzyme angiotensinogenase (more commonly known as renin) is simultaneously released to activate the renin–angiotensin system to stimulate the production of the potent vasoconstrictor angiotensin II. Angiotensin II has multiple functions, including the constriction of the efferent arterioles, which increases the pressure within the glomeruli. It also facilitates the release of aldosterone from the adrenal cortex to increase sodium and chloride reabsorption. The ensuing increase in plasma sodium stimulates the secretion of ADH from the posterior pituitary gland, which increases water reabsorption and assists peripheral vasoconstriction. The sum effect of these autoregulatory features of the kidney is a decrease in urine production and an increase in circulating blood volume, which collectively increase blood pressure. The unfortunate by-product of this autoregulation is that urea reabsorption also occurs, which sees a corresponding elevation in serum urea levels. If these autoregulatory mechanisms are unsuccessful and renal perfusion is not restored, the continuing ischaemia can lead to acute tubular necrosis.

FAST FACTS

- Pre-renal AKI is common, particularly in trauma, surgical and critically ill people.
- Restoration of blood pressure and blood flow to the kidneys rapidly reverses pre-renal AKI.
- If not promptly identified and treated, pre-renal AKI leads to ischaemic acute tubular necrosis and intrinsic AKI.

Intrinsic (intra-renal) AKI

Intrinsic or intra-renal failure is characterised by acute damage to the renal parenchyma and nephrons. The major structures of the kidney that may be affected are the blood vessels, the glomerulus, the tubules and the interstitium. Intra-renal causes include diseases of the kidney itself, such as acute glomerulonephritis and **acute tubular necrosis (ATN)**, the most common intrinsic cause of AKI.

Acute glomerulonephritis

Acute **glomerulonephritis** can be caused by a number of different factors; however, the key feature is inflammation of the glomerulus, which can decrease renal blood flow and cause AKI. Acute glomerulonephritis can result from infection, immunological abnormalities, drugs, toxins and systemic diseases such as lupus erythematosus. Acute post-streptococcal glomerulonephritis (also known as acute proliferative glomerulonephritis) is a common cause of glomerulonephritis. Infection of the pharynx or skin with group A beta-haemolytic *Streptococcus* is the usual initiating event for this disorder. Staphylococcal or viral infections, such as hepatitis B, mumps or varicella (chickenpox), can lead to a similar post-infectious acute glomerulonephritis (McCance & Huether, 2019). See 'Pathophysiology illustrated: acute glomerulonephritis'.

MANIFESTATIONS AND COMPLICATIONS Post-infectious acute glomerulonephritis is characterised by an abrupt onset of **haematuria**, **proteinuria**, salt and water retention and evidence of uraemic symptomology occurring 10 to 14 days after the initial infection. The urine often appears brown or cola-coloured. Salt and water retention

Acute kidney injury

The initial kidney injury is usually associated with an acute condition such as sepsis, trauma and hypotension, or the result of treatment for an acute condition with a nephrotoxic medication. Injury to the kidney can occur because of glomerular injury, vasoconstriction of capillaries or tubular injury. All consequences of injury lead to decreased glomerular filtration and oliguria.

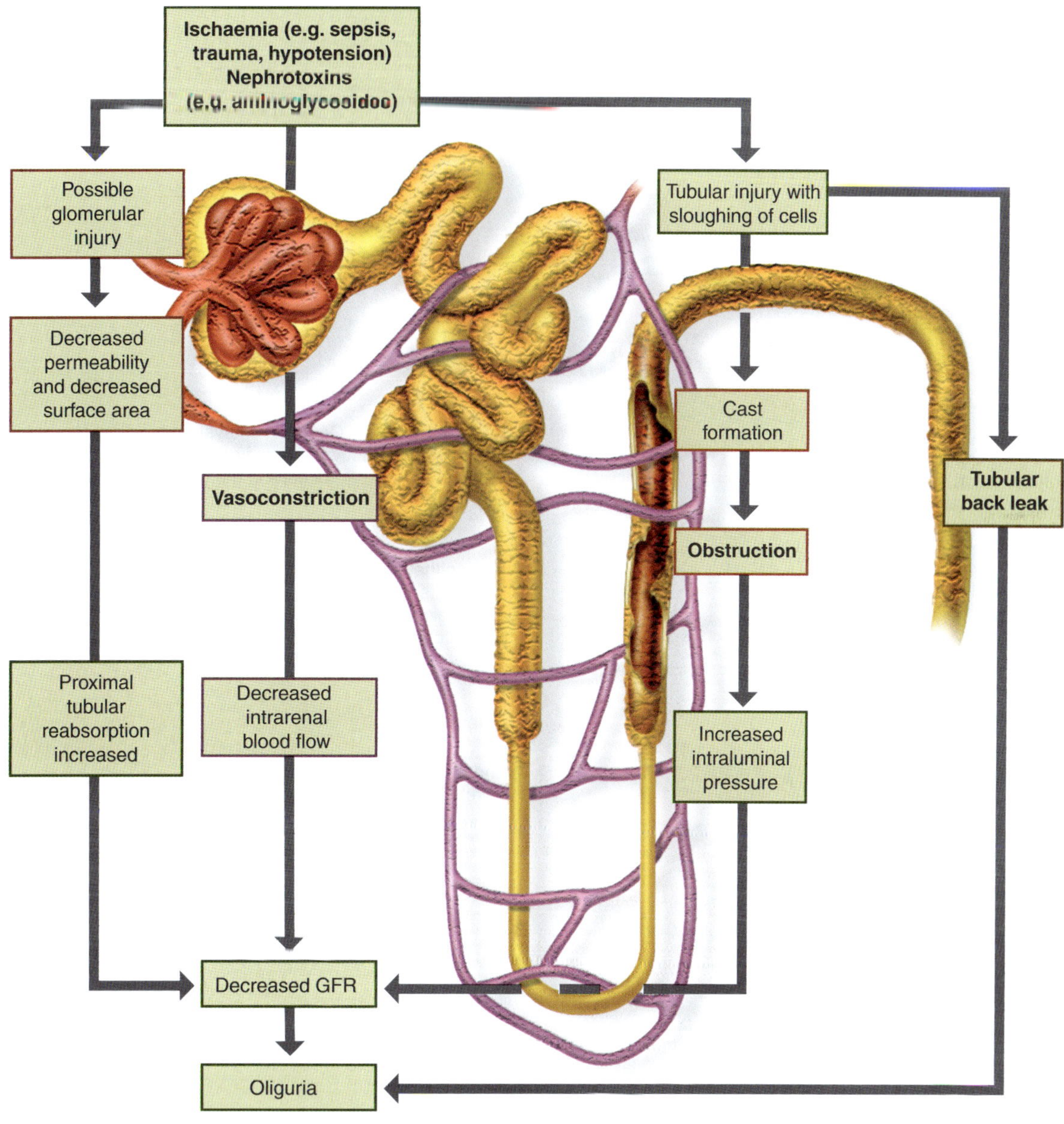

increase extracellular fluid volume, leading to hypertension and oedema. The oedema is primarily noted in the face, particularly around the eyes (*periorbital* oedema). Dependent oedema, affecting the hands and upper extremities in particular, may also be noted. Other manifestations may include fatigue, anorexia, nausea and vomiting, and headache. See the 'Manifestations' box.

The older adult may have fewer apparent symptoms. Nausea, malaise, arthralgias and proteinuria are common manifestations; hypertension and oedema are seen less often. Pulmonary infiltrates may occur early in the disorder, often due to worsening of a pre-existing condition such as heart failure.

MANIFESTATIONS Acute glomerulonephritis

- Haematuria, cola-coloured urine
- Proteinuria
- Salt and water retention
- Oedema, periorbital and facial, dependent oedema
- Hypertension
- Uraemia
- Fatigue
- Anorexia, nausea and vomiting
- Headache

Acute glomerulonephritis

Infection from group A beta-haemolytic *Streptococcus* causes an immune response that causes inflammation and damage to the glomeruli. Protein and red blood cells are allowed to pass through the glomeruli. Blood flow to the glomeruli is reduced due to obstruction with damaged cells and renal insufficiency results, leading to the retention of sodium, water and waste.

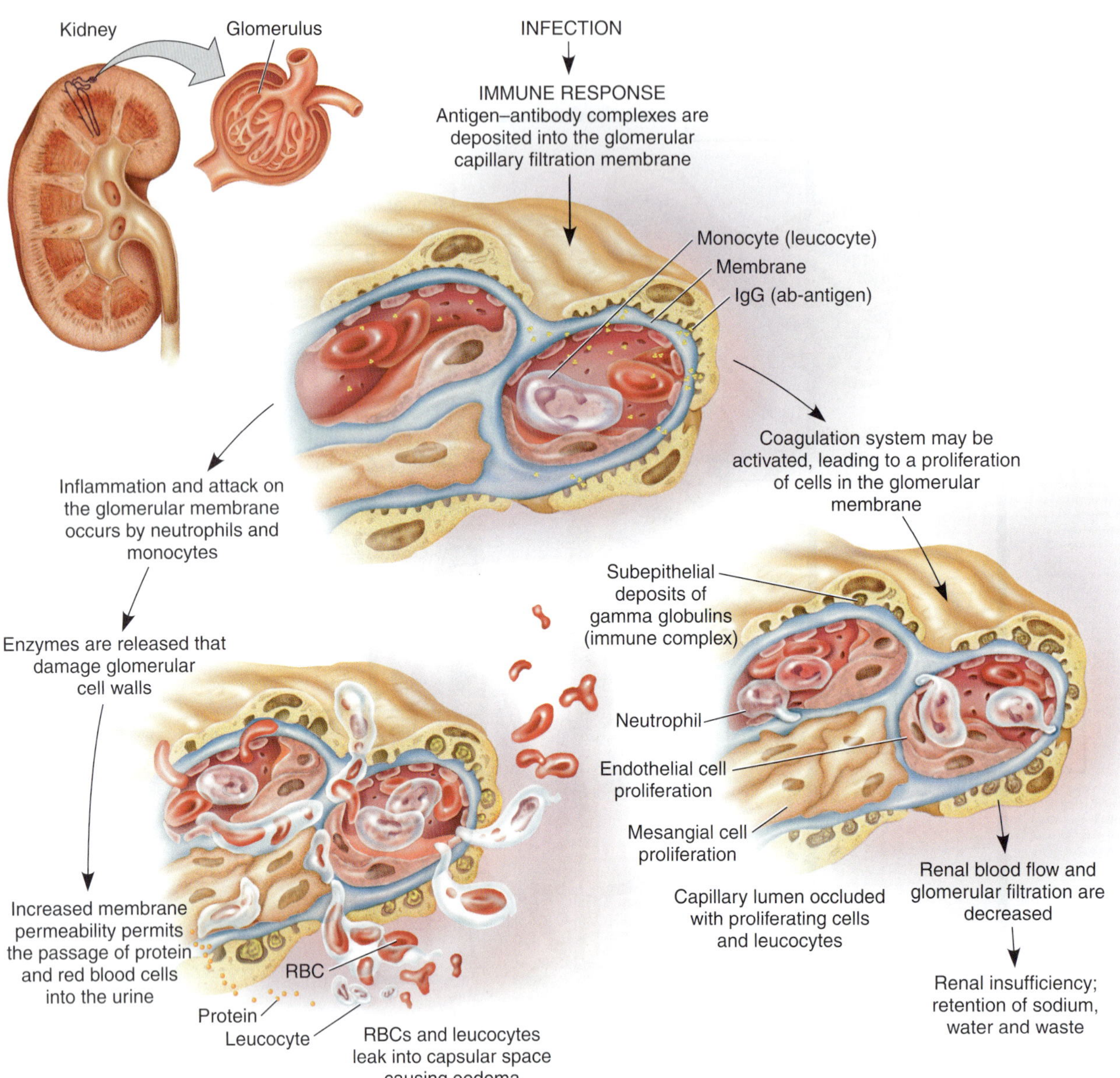

The prognosis for adults with acute post-infectious glomerulonephritis is less favourable than it is for children. The symptoms usually resolve spontaneously within 10 to 14 days in up to 95% of patients, with the GFR returning to normal over 1 to 3 months. Full recovery is usual in children, whereas approximately only 60% of adults recover completely, decreasing to 25% in the older population (Balasubramanian & Marks, 2017).

ACUTE TUBULAR NECROSIS ATN is characterised pathologically by structural damage to the tubular epithelial cells and cell death if the insult is not reversed promptly. Nephrons are particularly susceptible to injury from ischaemia or exposure to nephrotoxic agents. Prolonged ischaemia is the primary cause of ATN. When ischaemia and nephrotoxin exposure occur concurrently, the risk of ATN and tubular dysfunction increases. See Figure 27.1 for the pathogenesis of acute kidney injury due to ATN. Risk factors for ischaemic ATN include major surgery, severe hypovolaemia, sepsis, trauma and burns. The impact of ischaemia resulting from vasodilation and fluid loss in sepsis, trauma and burns is often compounded by toxins and inflammatory markers released by bacteria or from damaged tissue (Chakraborty & Burns, 2022).

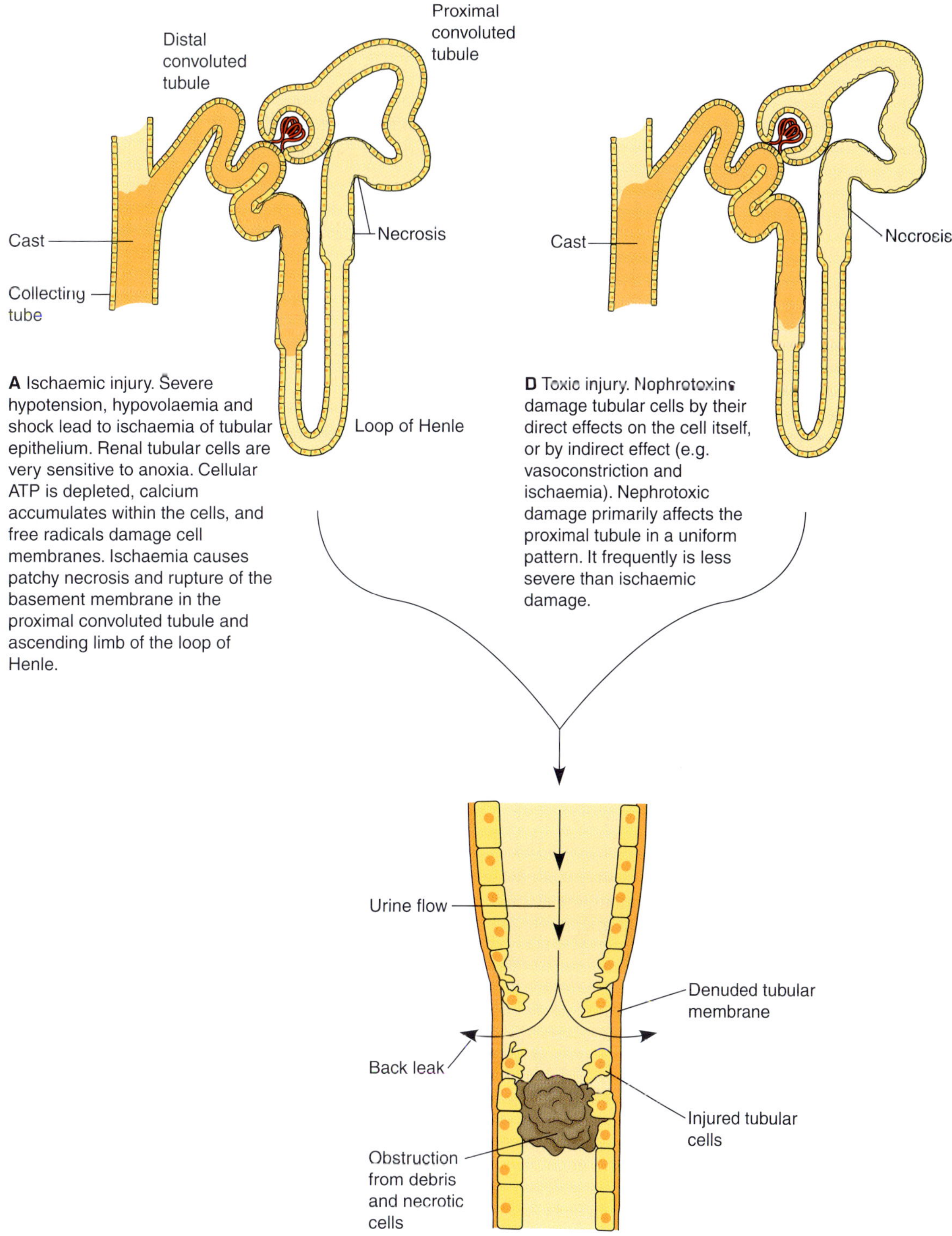

C Injured tubular cells release intracellular debris, which combines with proteins within the tubules to form casts. These casts, together with sloughed necrotic cells, occlude the tubular lumen, increasing tubular pressure and disrupting the flow of glomerular filtrate. Glomerular filtration slows. The increased pressure pushes filtrate out of the damaged tubule into interstitial tissues (back leak). Renal blood flow and glomerular filtration may be further reduced by intrarenal angiotension II release and vasoconstriction.

FIGURE 27.1 Acute tubular necrosis. *In ATN, tubular epithelial cells are destroyed by either ischaemic or toxic injury*

Ischaemia lasting more than 2 hours causes severe and irreversible damage to kidney tubules with patchy cellular necrosis and sloughing. The GFR is significantly reduced as a result of: (1) ischaemia, (2) activation of the renin–angiotensin system, and (3) tubular obstruction by cellular debris, which raises the pressure in the glomerular capsule.

Common nephrotoxic agents associated with ATN include the aminoglycoside antibiotics and radiological contrast media. Research has demonstrated AKI to be a common problem in the hospitalised and ambulatory population and the term contrast-induced AKI (CI-AKI) is proposed for people who develop AKI following intravenous radiological contrast media. Many other drugs (e.g. NSAIDs, antineoplastics and some immunosuppressants), heavy metals such as mercury and gold, and some common chemicals such as ethylene glycol (antifreeze) are also potentially toxic to the renal tubule. The risk of ATN is higher when nephrotoxic drugs are given to older people or those with pre-existing renal insufficiency and when used concomitantly with other nephrotoxic agents. Dehydration also increases the risk by increasing the toxin concentration in nephrons (Yang, We & Li, 2020).

Nephrotoxins destroy tubular cells by both direct and indirect effects. As tubular cells are damaged and lost through necrosis and sloughing, the tubule becomes more permeable. This increased permeability results in filtrate reabsorption, further reducing the ability of the nephron to eliminate wastes.

Rhabdomyolysis is a pathological syndrome that is characterised by damage to skeletal muscle fibres, which causes the release of excess myoglobin. Myoglobin is a protein that acts as the oxygen reservoir for muscle fibres, much as haemoglobin does for the blood. Muscle trauma and other factors can precipitate rhabdomyolysis. The myoglobin obstructs renal tubules, causing ischaemic injury, and contains an iron pigment that directly damages the tubules. Common causes of rhabdomyolysis include crush injuries, strenuous exercise, drug overdose and infection. Although no epidemiological data exists in Australia, 15–33% of people experiencing rhabdomyolysis will develop AKI (Kidney Health Australia, 2018). Renal injury occurs secondary to the myoglobin-induced tubule obstruction, renal hypoperfusion and intratubular cast formation. Prompt intervention with fluid resuscitation and urinary alkalinisation will minimise the impact of AKI and contribute to positive outcomes.

FAST FACTS

Clues for identifying pre-existing CKD in people with suspected AKI:

- Review biochemistry history: does the person currently have an elevated parathyroid hormone or is there a record of elevated serum creatinine levels anywhere in their patient history?
- Renal ultrasound revealing small kidneys with decreased cortical width is consistent with a history of CKD.
- Does the person have a long-standing history of uraemic symptoms?

Post-renal AKI

Obstructive causes of acute kidney injury are classified as post-renal. Any condition that prevents urine excretion can lead to post-renal AKI. Benign prostatic hypertrophy is the most common precipitating factor. Others include renal or urinary tract calculi and tumours. See the chapter 'Nursing care of people with urinary tract disorders' for further discussion of urinary tract obstruction.

Clinical course and manifestations of acute kidney injury

Not all people with AKI experience an identical clinical course; however, more often than not it progresses as a continuum through four phases: initiation, maintenance, diuretic and recovery.

Initiation phase

The *initiation phase* may last hours to days. It begins with the initiating event (e.g. haemorrhage) and ends when tubular injury occurs. If AKI is recognised and the initiating event is effectively treated during this phase, the prognosis is good. The initiation phase of AKI has few manifestations; in fact, it is often identified only when manifestations of the maintenance phase develop.

Maintenance phase

The *maintenance phase* of AKI is characterised by a significant fall in GFR and tubular necrosis. **Oliguria** may develop, although many people continue to produce normal or near-normal amounts of urine (non-oliguric AKI). Even though urine may be produced, the kidney cannot efficiently eliminate metabolic wastes, water, electrolytes and acids from the body during the maintenance phase of AKI. Uraemic symptoms, fluid retention, electrolyte imbalances and metabolic acidosis develop. These abnormalities are more severe in oliguric AKI than non-oliguric AKI. Up to 50% of AKI is non-oliguric, which generally reflects a less severe insult and is associated with a more favourable prognosis than in people with oliguric AKI.

During the maintenance phase, salt and water retention cause oedema, increasing the risk of heart failure and pulmonary oedema. Impaired potassium excretion leads to hyperkalaemia. When the serum potassium level is greater than 6.0 to 6.5 mmol/L, manifestations of its effect on neuromuscular function develop. These include muscle weakness, nausea and diarrhoea, electrocardiographic changes, arrhythmias and possible cardiac arrest. Other electrolyte imbalances include hyperphosphataemia and hypocalcaemia. Metabolic acidosis results from impaired hydrogen ion elimination by the kidneys.

Anaemia develops after several days of AKI due to suppressed erythropoietin secretion by the kidneys. Immune function is often impaired, increasing the risk of infection, and is one of the leading causes of mortality in AKI. Other manifestations of the maintenance phase include:

- oedema and hypertension due to salt and water retention
- confusion, disorientation, agitation or lethargy, hyperreflexia and possible seizures or coma due to uraemic toxicity and electrolyte and acid–base imbalances
- anorexia, nausea, vomiting and decreased or absent bowel sounds
- uraemic syndrome if AKI is prolonged (see the section on chronic kidney disease that follows).

Diuretic phase

The diuretic phase, if it occurs, can last up to 1 to 2 weeks. An increase in diuresis occurs because patency within the renal tubules is re-established. Nephrons have not recovered functionally and still cannot concentrate urine; and the solutes previously retained, such as urea and sodium, promote an osmotic effect, thus increasing urine output. It is crucial during this phase that the nurse ensures that fluid intake matches urine output so that renal perfusion is maintained. As the diuretic phase ends, urea and creatinine levels begin to decrease and electrolyte imbalances begin to resolve, and the kidneys start to regain their ability to regulate hydrogen and bicarbonate ion exchange. This sees the commencement of the recovery phase.

Recovery phase

The recovery phase of AKI is characterised by the fibrous scar tissue laid down within the glomerular basement membrane during the initial insult being replaced with a more contractile scar tissue. This process of tubular cell regeneration and repair sees a gradual return of the GFR to normal or pre-AKI levels. Serum creatinine, urea, potassium and phosphate levels remain high and may continue to rise in spite of increasing urine output. Renal function improves rapidly during the first 5 to 25 days of the recovery phase and continues to improve for up to a year.

> **FAST FACTS**
>
> The classification of urine output:
> - Anuria: no urine output
> - Oliguria: less than 400 mL/day
> - Polyuria: greater than 2,500 mL/day

Diagnostics

Diagnostic tests are used to identify the cause of acute kidney injury and monitor its effects on homeostasis:

- *Urinalysis* often shows the following abnormal findings in acute kidney injury:
  a. Urine-specific gravity is typically higher in pre-renal AKI as the kidney attempts to conserve water, and lower in intrinsic AKI as the tubules are unable to concentrate the filtrate. However, urine osmolality provides a more accurate measurement.
  b. Proteinuria if glomerular damage is the cause of AKI.
  c. The presence of RBCs (due to glomerular dysfunction), WBCs (related to inflammation) and renal tubular epithelial cells (indicating ATN).
  d. Cell casts, which are protein and cellular debris moulded in the shape of the tubular lumen. (In AKI, RBCs, WBCs and renal tubular epithelial casts may be present. Brownish pigmented urine and positive tests for occult blood indicate haemoglobinuria or myoglobinuria.)
- *Serum creatinine* and *urea* are used to evaluate renal function. In AKI, serum creatinine levels increase rapidly, within 24 to 48 hours of the onset. Creatinine levels generally peak within 5 to 10 days. Creatinine and urea levels tend to increase more slowly when urine output is maintained. The onset of recovery is marked by a halt in the rise of the serum creatinine and urea. eGFR is an inaccurate marker to evaluate kidney function in AKI as the formula used to determine GFR relies on a steady-state creatinine level and does not account for fluctuating or rapid changes in creatinine levels. It is also important to note that eGFR has not been validated in children or the Indigenous population.
- *Serum electrolytes* are monitored to evaluate the fluid and electrolyte status. The serum potassium rises at a moderate rate and is often used to indicate the need for dialysis. Hyponatraemia is common, due to the water excess associated with AKI.
- *Arterial blood gases* often show a metabolic acidosis due to the kidneys' inability to adequately eliminate metabolic wastes and hydrogen ions (see the chapter 'Nursing care of people with altered fluid, electrolyte and acid–base balance').
- *FBC* shows reduced RBCs, moderate anaemia and a low haematocrit. AKI affects erythropoietin secretion and RBC production. Iron and folate absorption may also be impaired, further contributing to anaemia.

INTERPROFESSIONAL CARE

Identifying people at risk and preventing acute kidney injury should be a goal for health professionals, especially for people in high-risk groups. Treatment goals for acute kidney injury are to: (1) identify and correct the underlying cause, (2) prevent additional kidney damage, (3) restore the urine output and kidney function, and (4) compensate for renal impairment until kidney function is restored.

Maintaining an adequate vascular volume, cardiac output and blood pressure is vital to preserve kidney perfusion. The nursing team is ideally placed to facilitate the coordination of interprofessional care and is able to notify the treating team of any changes in status and to identify the need for timely referral to other members of the healthcare team. AKI is a serious life-threatening illness that requires multidisciplinary collaboration, agreed guidelines and implementation to deliver high-quality care (Kashani et al., 2019).

Medications

The primary focus in drug management for acute kidney injury is to restore and maintain renal perfusion and volume homeostasis, correct biochemical imbalances and eliminate nephrotoxic agents from the treatment regimen.

Intravenous fluids and blood volume expanders are given as needed to restore renal perfusion. Low or 'renal' dose dopamine has been historically administered via intravenous infusion to increase renal blood flow. Dopamine is a sympathetic neurotransmitter that improves cardiac output and dilates blood vessels of the mesentery and kidneys when given in low therapeutic doses. However, research has shown that low-dose dopamine may worsen renal perfusion in critically ill people and it has fallen out of favour (Lauschke et al., 2006; Schnuelle, Benck & Yard, 2018).

If restoration of renal blood flow does not improve urinary output, a loop diuretic such as frusemide may be given with intravenous fluids. The purpose is twofold. First, if nephrotoxins are present, the combination of fluids and potent diuretics may, in effect, 'wash out' the nephrons, reducing toxin concentration. Second, re-establishing urine output may prevent oliguria and reduce the degree of uraemic toxin accumulation and fluid and electrolyte imbalances. Frusemide also may be used to manage salt and water retention associated with AKI.

Aggressive hypertension management limits renal injury when AKI is associated with disorders such as toxaemia and pregnancy-induced hypertension. ACE inhibitors or other antihypertensive medications are used to control arterial pressures.

All drugs that are either directly nephrotoxic or that may interfere with renal perfusion may be discontinued. NSAIDs, nephrotoxic antibiotics and other potentially harmful drugs are avoided throughout the course of acute kidney injury. When a nephrotoxic drug or substance must be used, the risk of AKI can be reduced by using the minimum effective dose, maintaining hydration and eliminating other known nephrotoxins from the medication regimen.

People with kidney injury are at an increased risk of GI bleeding; this is related to the stress response and impaired platelet function. The cause is likely due to the combined effect of uraemic toxins, medications like warfarin or heparin, or coexisting GI tract pathologies. Histamine H_2-receptor antagonists or proton pump inhibitors are used to prevent GI haemorrhage. These drug classes protect the gastric mucosa by profoundly reducing gastric acid secretion. Antacids are used infrequently due to the inconvenience of dosing, whereas the other drug classes afford more convenient administration routes and less dosing intervals. Hyperkalaemia may require active intervention in combination with the restriction of dietary potassium intake. Serum levels of greater than 6.0–6.5 mmol/L are treated to prevent cardiac effects of hyperkalaemia. With significant hyperkalaemia, calcium chloride, sodium bicarbonate or insulin and glucose may be given intravenously to reduce serum potassium levels by moving potassium into the cells. A potassium-binding exchange resin such as calcium resonium may be given orally or by enema. This agent removes potassium from the body by exchanging sodium for potassium, primarily in the large intestine. When given orally, it is often co-administered with an aperient to prevent constipation. Rectally, it is instilled as a retention enema, allowed to remain in the bowel for approximately 30 to 60 minutes and then irrigated out using a tap-water enema.

Hyperphosphataemia is generally managed conservatively in AKI unless it is severe and there is a clinically significant reduction in serum calcium. Generally, it is only when the episode of AKI is protracted that oral phosphate binders are initiated (see the CKD section on medications later in this chapter for a more comprehensive review of phosphate binders).

Because many drugs are eliminated from the body by the kidney, drug dosages may need to be adjusted. Doses within the usual range can lead to potentially toxic blood levels, because their elimination is slowed and half-life prolonged. Nursing implications for medications commonly prescribed for the person with AKI are summarised in the 'Medication administration' box.

Fluid management

Once vascular volume and renal perfusion is restored, fluid intake is usually restricted. The allowed daily fluid intake is calculated by allowing 500–700 mL for insensible losses (respiration, perspiration, bowel losses) and adding the amount excreted as urine (or lost in vomitus) during the previous 24 hours. For example, if a person with AKI excretes 325 mL of urine in 24 hours, they are allowed a fluid intake allowance (including oral and intravenous fluids) of 825 mL for the next 24 hours. Fluid balance is carefully monitored, using accurate weight measurements and strict fluid balance charts as the primary indicators.

Nutrition

Nutritional management is critical in supporting the person with AKI. AKI is associated with the accumulation of electrolytes and fluids and the accelerated breakdown of body proteins (*catabolism*), which creates a negative nitrogen balance. Poor nutritional status is associated with increased mortality and morbidity; people with malnutrition are at higher risk of sepsis and haemorrhage. Managing nutritional intake remains a challenge in which the determinants of treatment requirements are based not on the degree of renal insufficiency, but on the cause of the AKI and the degree of catabolism experienced. People in hypercatabolic states experience multiple metabolic sequelae, including insulin resistance, hormonal alterations and metabolic acidosis. The goal of nutritional management is to maintain lean body mass through the provision of adequate kilojoule and nutritional intake, and to restore immunocompetence and an anabolic state (Wiesen & Preiser, 2014). Early referral to the dietitian is essential in order to provide comprehensive and timely management of the individual's nutritional status. Nutritional requirements are highly individualised and are influenced by the cause and treatment of the AKI. Due to the well-established association of malnutrition with morbidity and mortality, protein restriction is not recommended. Dietary proteins should be of high biological value (rich in essential amino acids). Carbohydrates are increased to maintain adequate kilojoule intake and provide a protein-sparing effect. Where possible, oral diet should be the initial route of nutrition (Ostermann, Macedo & Oudemans-van Straaten, 2019).

Parenteral nutrition providing amino acids, concentrated carbohydrates and fats may be instituted when the individual with AKI cannot tolerate enteral nutrition or consume an adequate diet (e.g. due to impaired gut function, nausea, vomiting or underlying critical illness) (Ostermann et al., 2019). The disadvantages of parenteral nutrition in these instances are the high volume of fluid required and the risk of infection through the central venous access.

MEDICATION ADMINISTRATION **The person with acute kidney injury**

LOOP DIURETICS

Frusemide

Ethacrynic acid

The loop diuretics, named for their primary site of action in the loop of Henle, are *high-ceiling diuretics*: the response increases with increasing doses. These are highly effective diuretics used in early AKI to re-establish urine flow and convert oliguric renal failure to non-oliguric renal failure. In ATN secondary to exposure to a nephrotoxic agent, loop diuretics are often used to clear the toxin from the nephrons more rapidly. Loop diuretics cause potassium wasting, which is generally not a concern in AKI because renal dysfunction impairs normal potassium elimination.

Nursing responsibilities

- Assess weight and vital signs for baseline data.
- Monitor intake and output, daily weight (or more frequently as ordered), vital signs, skin turgor and other indicators of fluid volume status frequently.
- Assess for postural hypotension because these potent diuretics can lead to hypovolaemia.
- Monitor laboratory results, especially serum electrolyte, glucose, urea and creatinine levels.
- Administer by mouth or, if ordered, by intravenous injection:
  a. Frusemide undiluted at a rate of no more than 20 mg per minute
  b. Ethacrynic acid 50 mg diluted with 50 mL of normal saline at a rate of no more than 10 mg per minute
- Assess response. Urine output typically increases within 10 minutes after intravenous administration.
- Monitor hearing and for complaints such as tinnitus. High doses of loop diuretics increase the risk of ototoxicity, especially with ethacrynic acid. These effects may be reversible if detected early and the drug is discontinued.
- Avoid administering concurrently with other ototoxic agents, such as aminoglycoside antibiotics and cisplatin.

Health education for the person and family

- Unless contraindicated, maintain a fluid intake that is equal to the previous day's urine output plus 500–700 mL to allow for insensible losses.
- Rise slowly from lying or sitting positions because a fall in blood pressure may cause light-headedness.
- Administer in the morning and at lunchtime if ordered twice a day, to avoid sleep disturbance.
- Take with food or milk to prevent gastric distress.
- NSAIDs interfere with the effectiveness of loop diuretics and should be avoided.

ELECTROLYTES AND ELECTROLYTE MODIFIERS

Calcium chloride

Calcium gluconate

Sodium bicarbonate

Calcium polystyrene sulfonate

Calcium chloride or gluconate and sodium bicarbonate are administered intravenously in the initial management of hyperkalaemia. Calcium can also be administered to correct hypocalcaemia and reduce hyperphosphatemia. (Calcium and phosphate have a reciprocal relationship in the body, as the level of one rises, the level of the other falls.) Sodium bicarbonate helps to correct acidosis and move potassium back into the intracellular space. Calcium polystyrene sulfonate is used to remove excess potassium from the body by exchanging calcium ions for potassium in the large intestine.

Nursing responsibilities

- Assess serum electrolyte levels prior to and during therapy. Report rapid shifts or adverse responses to the treating team.
- Administer as appropriate:
  a. Intravenous calcium chloride at less than 1 mL per minute; intravenous calcium gluconate at 0.5 mL per minute. Inject into a large vein through a small-bore needle; avoid infiltration because extravasation of intravenous solution will cause tissue necrosis.
  b. Intravenous sodium bicarbonate infusion over 4 to 8 hours; oral tablets as prescribed.
  c. Calcium polystyrene sulfonate as an oral solution can be taken with a laxative to prevent constipation or as a retention enema mixed with warm water. Leave in the bowel for 30 to 60 minutes; irrigate using a small tap-water enema.
- Monitor for adverse reactions, such as arrhythmias, electrolyte imbalances and metabolic alkalosis.

Health education for the person and family

- Intravenous calcium may make you light-headed; remain in bed for at least 30 minutes after administration.
- Do not take sodium bicarbonate tablets with milk.
- Retain the calcium polystyrene sulfonate enema as long as possible.

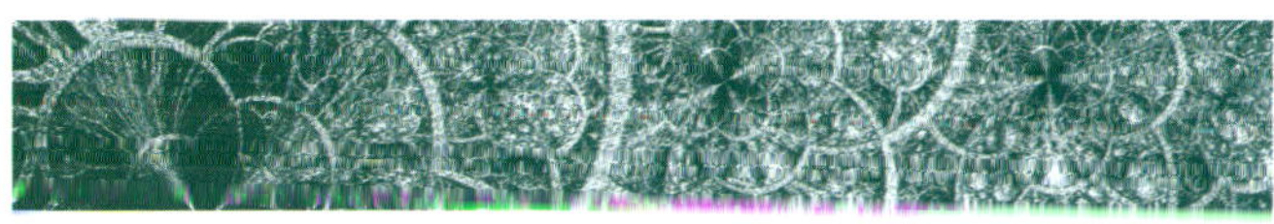

Nursing care

Health promotion

Acute kidney injury often can be prevented by measures that maintain fluid volume and cardiac output and reduce the risk of exposure to nephrotoxins.

- Carefully monitor critically ill, postoperative and other people who are at high risk of early signs of hypovolaemia (low urine output, altered mental status or changes in vital signs, skin colour or temperature).
- Report significant decreases in urine output and other evidence of decreased cardiac output.
- Maintain intravenous fluids as ordered.
- Alert the treating team if you note that the individual is receiving more than one nephrotoxic drug or if a nephrotoxic drug is ordered for a person who is dehydrated.

- Closely observe people receiving blood or blood cells for early signs of transfusion reaction and intervene appropriately.

Assessment

Both subjective and objective data are useful when assessing the person with acute kidney injury:

- *Health history*: complaints of anorexia, nausea, weight gain or oedema; recent exposure to a nephrotoxin such as an aminoglycoside antibiotic or radiological procedure using an injected contrast medium; previous transfusion reaction; chronic diseases such as diabetes, heart failure or kidney disease.
- *Physical examination*: vital signs, including temperature; urine output (amount, colour, clarity, specific gravity, presence of blood cells or protein); weight; skin colour, peripheral pulses; presence of oedema (periorbital or dependent); lung sounds, heart sounds and bowel tones.

Nursing diagnoses and interventions

In line with the National Safety and Quality Health Service (NSQHS) Recognising and Responding to Acute Deterioration Standard (Australian Commission on Safety and Quality in Health Care (ACSQHC), 2021), nurses must consider the nursing care required in relation to the renal dysfunction and also to the underlying condition that precipitated it. Priority nursing care needs relate to fluid volume alterations, appetite and nutrition, and teaching/learning. For additional nursing diagnoses and interventions, see the nursing care plan.

Excess fluid volume

In AKI, the kidneys often cannot excrete adequate urine to maintain a normal extracellular fluid balance. Fluid retention is greater in oliguric renal failure than in non-oliguric failure. Rapid weight gain and oedema indicate fluid retention. In addition, heart failure and pulmonary oedema may develop.

- Maintain hourly intake and output records. *Accurate intake and output records help guide therapy, especially fluid restrictions.*
- Weigh daily. Use standard technique (same scale, time, clothing or coverings) to ensure accuracy. *Rapid weight changes are an accurate indicator of fluid volume status, particularly in the oliguric person.*
- Assess vital signs at least every 4 hours. *Hypertension, tachycardia and tachypnoea may indicate excess fluid volume.*

> **CONSIDERATION FOR PRACTICE**
>
> **Frequently assess breath and heart sounds, neck veins for distension and back and extremities for oedema. Report abnormal findings. Adventitious breath sounds (crackles), abnormal heart sounds such as an S_3 or S_4 gallop, distended neck veins and peripheral oedema may indicate hypervolaemia, heart failure or pulmonary oedema.**

- If not contraindicated, place in semi-Fowler's position *to enhance cardiac and respiratory function.*
- Report abnormal serum electrolyte values and manifestations of electrolyte imbalance. People with AKI are at particular risk of the following electrolyte imbalances:
  a. *Hyperkalaemia* due to impaired potassium excretion. Manifestations include irritability, nausea, diarrhoea, abdominal cramping, muscle weakness, cardiac arrhythmias and ECG changes.
  b. *Hyponatraemia* due to water retention. Manifestations include nausea, vomiting and headache, with possible central nervous system (CNS) manifestations of lethargy, confusion, seizures and coma. The body's natural physiological response post surgery is to retain sodium and water.
  c. *Hyperphosphataemia* due to decreased phosphate excretion. Manifestations include hyperreflexia, paraesthesias and possible tetany secondary to hypocalcaemia.

  AKI impairs electrolyte and water excretion, causing multiple electrolyte imbalances.
- Restrict fluids as ordered. Provide frequent mouth care and strategies to decrease thirst drive (chewing gum, boiled lollies). If ice chips are allowed, include the water content (approximately one-half of the total volume) as intake. *Fluids are restricted to minimise fluid retention and complications of fluid volume excess.*
- Administer medications with meals if not contraindicated. *Giving oral medications with meals minimises ingestion of excess fluids.*
- Turn frequently and provide good skin care. *Oedema decreases tissue perfusion and increases the risk of skin breakdown.*

Imbalanced nutrition: less than body requirements

Anorexia and nausea associated with any form of renal insufficiency often interfere with oral intake and nutrition. In addition, the disease process leading to AKI may contribute to increased nutritional needs for healing and decreased food intake.

- Monitor and record food intake, including the amount and type of food consumed. *A detailed intake record helps guide decisions about nutritional status and necessary supplements.*
- Weigh daily. Weight changes over time (days to weeks) reflect nutritional status, while rapid weight changes are more reflective of fluid volume status. *In AKI, weight may remain stable or increase due to fluid retention even though tissue mass is being lost.*
- Arrange for dietary consultation to plan meals within prescribed limitations that consider individual food preferences. *Diets restricted in protein, salt and potassium can be unpalatable; intake and appetite improve when preferred foods are included as allowed.*
- Engage in planning daily menus in line with dietary allowances. *Participation in meal planning increases the individual's sense of control and autonomy.*
- Allow family members to prepare meals within dietary restrictions. Encourage family members to eat with the

person. *Familiar foods and social interaction encourage eating and increase enjoyment of meals.*

- Provide frequent, small meals or between-meal snacks. *These measures promote food intake in people who are fatigued or anorexic.*
- Administer anti-emetics as ordered and provide mouth care prior to meals. *Nausea and a metallic taste in the mouth, common manifestations of uraemia, can decrease food intake.*
- Administer parenteral nutrition as ordered if the person is unable to eat or tolerate enteral nutrition. *Preventing or slowing tissue catabolism is important for people with AKI.*

> **CONSIDERATION FOR PRACTICE**
>
> **Intravenous lines and parenteral nutrition solutions can increase the risk of infection. Monitor sites carefully for signs of infection or inflammation and adhere to local policy for line replacement.**

Deficient knowledge

The person with AKI has multiple learning needs. These include information about AKI, diagnostic and laboratory studies, management strategies and implications for the recovery period.

- Assess anxiety level and ability to comprehend instruction. Tailor information and presentation to developmental level and physical, mental and emotional status. *The person with AKI may be critically ill or have uraemic effects that hinder learning. During the initial stages of AKI it may be necessary to limit information to immediate concerns.*
- Assess knowledge and understanding. *To enhance understanding and retention, relate information presented to previous learning.*
- Teach about diagnostic tests and therapeutic procedures. *Teaching reduces anxiety and improves understanding and cooperation.*
- Discuss dietary and fluid restrictions. *These measures may be continued after discharge.*
- If discharge is planned prior to the recovery phase of AKI, teach the signs and symptoms of complications, such as fluid volume excess or deficit, heart failure and electrolyte imbalances. *As kidney function returns, urine output increases, but the concentrating ability of the nephrons and electrolyte excretion remain impaired. This impaired function increases the risk of excess fluid loss, possible dehydration, postural hypotension and electrolyte imbalance.*
- Teach how to monitor weight, blood pressure and pulse. *These are important means of assessing fluid status.*
- Instruct to avoid nephrotoxic agents for up to 1 year following an episode of AKI. *During recovery, nephrons remain vulnerable to damage by nephrotoxins such as NSAIDs, some antibiotics, radiological contrast media and heavy metals. Because alcohol can increase the nephrotoxicity of some materials, discourage alcohol intake.*

Community-based care

Quite often people develop AKI when they are critically ill. Critical illness and the resulting state of personal and family crisis can impair learning and retention of information. Include family members in teaching during the initial stages to promote understanding of what is happening and the reasons for specific treatment measures. Inclusion of the family reduces their anxiety and provides a valuable resource for reinforcing key health education points about care after discharge.

Teaching needs for home care include:

- avoiding exposure to nephrotoxins, particularly those in over-the-counter products
- preventing infection and other major stressors that can slow healing
- monitoring weight, blood pressure and pulse
- manifestations of relapse
- continuing dietary restrictions
- knowing when to contact the GP or present to the local emergency department.

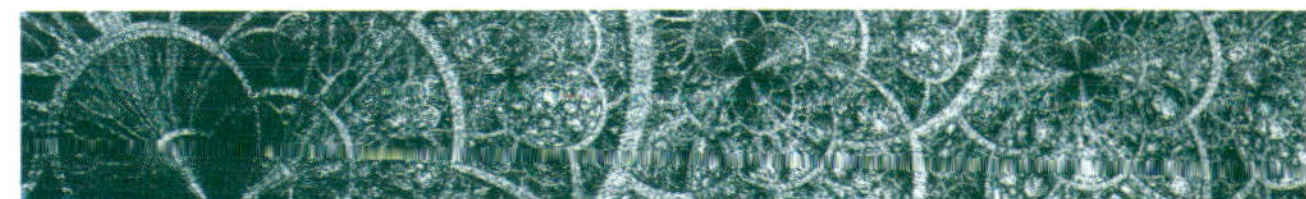

NURSING CARE PLAN A person with acute kidney injury

Sharon Jones is driving home late one evening when she loses control of her car trying to avoid hitting a kangaroo on the road. Her car strikes a tree and rolls into a deep ditch beside the road, out of sight of passing cars. The wreck is not discovered until 8 hours later. On arrival at the accident scene, the paramedics find Ms Jones hypotensive: BP 90/60, P 120, R 24 and GCS 11/15. She appears disorientated and in severe pain, with a [illegible] right femur and multiple facial fractures. 1 L of crystalloid is infused, analgesia administered and oxygen applied. After immobilising Ms Jones' neck and back and extricating her from the car, they apply a traction splint to her leg and transport her to the local hospital.

ASSESSMENT

Upon arriving at the high-dependency unit Ms Jones is more responsive, her pain score is 4/10 and GCS is 14/15. Lexi Ballinger, RN, obtains a nursing history on Ms Jones' admission and notes no significant medical history and nil known allergies. Ms Jones is not currently taking prescription or non-prescription drugs. Physical assessment findings on admission to the unit include T [illegible]°C, P 100, R 10 and BP [illegible]. Skin pale, cool and dry, with multiple scrapes and [illegible] on her face and extremities. A linear bruise is noted on her chest and abdomen from the seat belt. Lung sounds clear, heart tones normal and abdomen tender but soft to palpation. Right leg alignment

(continued)

NURSING CARE PLAN **A person with acute kidney injury (continued)**

maintained with skeletal traction. One unit of whole blood was infused in the emergency department. An indwelling urinary catheter and nasogastric tube were in situ.

During the first few hours after admission, Ms Ballinger notes that Ms Jones' hourly output has dropped from 55 mL to 45 mL to 28 mL of clear yellow urine. The resident medical officer is notified and orders a 500 mL intravenous fluid challenge, 40 mg frusemide IV, urinalysis, serum urea, creatinine and electrolytes. The fluid challenge and frusemide produces only a slight increase in urine output. Urinalysis results show a specific gravity of 1.010 and the presence of WBCs, red and white cell casts, and tubular epithelial cells in the sediment. Ms Jones' blood results reveal: urea 10 mmol/L; creatinine 133 μmol/L and potassium 5.9 mmol/L. The resident medical officer diagnoses probable acute kidney injury and orders sodium polystyrene sulfonate 15 g TDS. In addition, the physician orders aluminium hydroxide, 10 mL every 2 hours per nasogastric tube and ranitidine 50 mg intravenously every 8 hours.

DIAGNOSES

- *Acute pain* related to injuries sustained in accident.
- *Anxiety* related to admission to the high-dependency unit.
- *Risk of excess fluid volume* related to impaired renal function.
- *Impaired physical mobility* related to skeletal traction.
- *Ineffective protection* related to injuries and invasive procedures.

PLANNING

- Plan for effective pain management.
- Plan for effective psychological care.
- Plan to monitor for bleeding, fluid balance and respiratory distress.
- Plan for skin care, pressure ulcer prevention and to prevent infection.

Expected outcomes

- Report adequate pain control.
- Verbalise reduced anxiety.
- Maintain stable weight and vital signs within normal range.
- Maintain skin integrity.
- Use the trapeze appropriately to adjust position in bed while maintaining body alignment.
- Remain free of infection, bleeding or respiratory distress.

IMPLEMENTATION

- Maintain PCA.
- Assess frequently for pain control and response to analgesia.
- Encourage expression of thoughts, feelings and fears about condition and placement in the critical care unit.
- Document vital signs and heart and lung sounds at least every 4 hours.
- Weigh daily as tolerated by pain.
- Document hourly intake and output.
- Restrict fluids as ordered, including diluents for all intravenous medications as intake.
- Assist with mouth care every 3 to 4 hours; allow frequent rinsing of mouth, and ice chips as allowed.
- Assist with position changes at least every 2 hours; teach use of the overhead trapeze.
- Monitor frequently for signs of infection, bleeding or respiratory distress.

EVALUATION

After just over 3 days of oliguria, Ms Jones' urine output increases. By the end of the fourth day she is excreting 60 to 80 mL/h of urine. Although her urea and creatinine levels remain slightly elevated, they never reach a critical point and dialysis is not required. She is transferred from the high-dependency unit on the fourth day after admission. When Ms Jones is able to begin eating, she is placed on a low-potassium diet, restricted to 60 g of protein. Her renal function gradually improves. By discharge, the results of her renal function studies, including urea and serum creatinine, are nearly normal. Ms Jones verbalises an understanding of the need to avoid nephrotoxic agents such as NSAIDs in order to prevent another insult to her kidneys and agrees to be followed up by her GP in 2 weeks.

CRITICAL THINKING IN THE NURSING PROCESS

1. What was the most likely specific precipitating factor for Ms Jones' acute kidney injury? Did anything else contribute to her risk?
2. Why did the physician prescribe aluminium hydroxide and ranitidine? Consider both the acute kidney injury and Ms Jones' placement in the high-dependency unit.
3. Ms Jones is at risk of respiratory distress related to potential fluid volume excess. How does her fractured femur further contribute to risk of respiratory distress?
4. Develop a care plan for Ms Jones for the nursing diagnosis of *Deficient diversional activity*.

REFLECTION ON THE NURSING PROCESS

1. Consider the case study above and identify what new knowledge you have gained that will enhance the care you deliver to a person with AKI.
2. Reflect on a time you have provided education in the clinical setting. What are some of the key factors you would need to consider when educating Ms Jones about avoiding nephrotoxic agents?

THE PERSON WITH KIDNEY TRAUMA

Despite the kidneys being relatively well protected by the rib cage and back muscles, kidney trauma due to blunt force accounts for 80–90% of urological trauma (Singh & Sookraj, 2022). The majority of kidney trauma is managed successfully without surgery, but prompt diagnosis and treatment is essential and can be lifesaving in the event of major damage.

Pathophysiology and manifestations

Blunt force is the most common cause of kidney injury. Falls, motor vehicle accidents and sports injuries can damage the kidney. The injury may be minor, resulting in a contusion or small haematoma, or more serious, resulting in laceration or other damage. The kidney may fragment or 'shatter', causing significant blood loss and urine extravasation. Tearing of the renal artery or vein may cause rapid haemorrhage, with shock and possible death.

Gunshot wounds, knife wounds, impalement injuries and fractured ribs are more likely to require surgical intervention including nephrectomy (Singh & Sookraj, 2022). Minor penetrating injuries may lacerate the capsule or renal cortex. Major injuries include laceration or destruction of renal parenchyma or the vascular supply.

The primary manifestations of kidney trauma are haematuria (gross or microscopic), flank or abdominal pain, and oliguria or anuria. There may be localised swelling, tenderness or ecchymoses in the flank region. Retroperitoneal bleeding from the kidney may cause Turner's sign, a bluish discolouration of the flank. Signs of shock may be present, including hypotension, tachycardia, tachypnoea, cool and pale skin, and an altered level of consciousness.

INTERPROFESSIONAL CARE

The radiology team plays a crucial role in differentiating between cases that require immediate surgical intervention or conservative management. In blunt force trauma, renal imaging is indicated if there is suspected trauma (e.g. following a blunt injury or falling from a height) associated with either gross haematuria or microhaematuria with concurrent shock. Renal imaging is used immediately in penetrating trauma unless severe haemodynamic instability warrants urgent surgical intervention (Singh & Sookraj, 2022). Haemoglobin and haematocrit levels fall in significant renal injury with haemorrhage. Haematuria is typically noted on urinalysis and aspartate transaminase (AST) levels rise within 12 hours of significant renal trauma. Renal ultrasound is used to diagnose bleeding and kidney damage. It is non-invasive but lacks the resolution afforded by a CT scan. An abdominal CT scan with contrast medium may be done to visualise renal structures to establish a definitive diagnosis (Singh & Sookraj, 2022).

Treatment of minor kidney injuries is generally conservative, including bed rest, regular observation of vital signs, abdominal symptomology and full blood count. In these injuries, bleeding is typically minor and self-limiting, as opposed to major or critical trauma where immediate treatment focuses on controlling haemorrhage and treating or preventing shock. Major lacerations may require surgical repair or partial or total **nephrectomy** (removal of the affected kidney) (Singh & Sookraj, 2022).

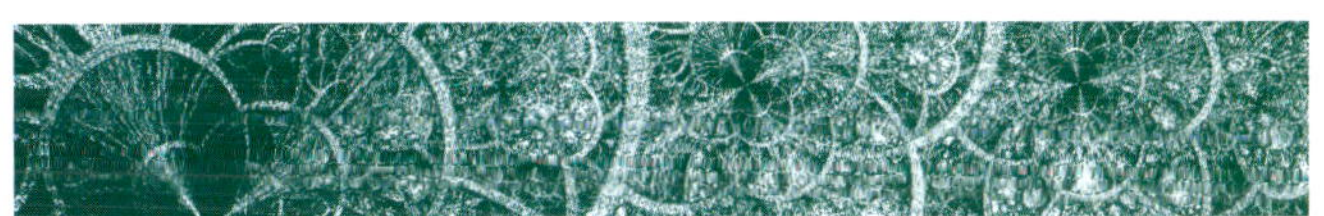

Nursing care

Nursing care for people who have experienced renal trauma focuses on timely and accurate assessment and appropriate intervention to preserve life and prevent complications. A urine specimen for analysis should be obtained when kidney trauma is suspected. Monitor level of consciousness, vital signs, skin colour and temperature, and urine output for possible signs of shock. See the chapter 'Nursing care of people experiencing trauma and shock' for additional nursing care measures for the person who has had a traumatic injury or who develops shock.

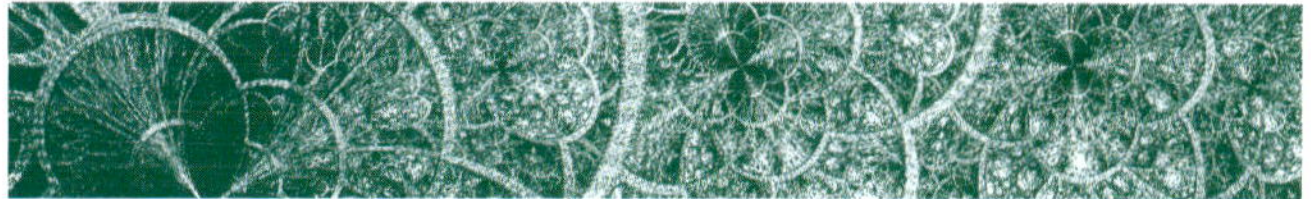

THE PERSON WITH A RENAL TUMOUR

Renal tumours are classified as benign or malignant, primary or metastatic. Benign renal tumours are infrequent and are often found only on autopsy. In 2011, renal cell carcinoma accounted for 2.4% of all adult cancers in Australia (Australian Institute of Health and Welfare (AIHW), 2022). Most primary renal tumours arise from renal cells; a primary tumour also may develop in the renal pelvis, although less frequently. Metastatic lesions to the kidney are associated with lung and breast cancer, melanoma and malignant lymphoma.

Males are affected by renal cancer more than females by a 2:1 ratio. The highest incidence is seen in people over the age of 55 years. Risk factors include smoking, obesity, prolonged time on dialysis, environmental exposure and genetic predisposition. The chronic irritation associated with renal calculi may also contribute (Kidney Health Australia, 2018).

Pathophysiology and manifestations

The most prevalent renal tumours are renal cell carcinomas, which develop in the renal cortex. The tumour, which can range in size up to several centimetres, has clearly defined margins and contains areas of ischaemia, necrosis and haemorrhage. Renal tumours tend to invade the renal vein and often have metastasised when first identified. Metastases tend to occur in the lungs, bone, lymph nodes, liver and brain (Loscalzo et al., 2022; Tran & Ornstein, 2021).

Renal tumours are often silent, with few manifestations. The classic triad of symptoms—gross haematuria, flank pain and a palpable abdominal mass—is seen in only about 10% of people with renal cell carcinoma. Haematuria, often microscopic, is the most consistent symptom. Systemic manifestations include fever without infection, fatigue and weight loss.

The tumour may produce hormones or hormone-like substances, including parathyroid hormone, prostaglandins, prolactin, renin, gonadotropins and glucocorticoids. These substances produce *paraneoplastic syndromes*, with additional manifestations such as hypercalcaemia, hypertension and hyperglycaemia. The progression of renal cell carcinomas varies from prolonged periods of stable disease to very aggressive. Table 27.5 outlines the staging and prognosis for renal cell cancers.

INTERPROFESSIONAL CARE

Haematuria is often the only initial manifestation of renal cancer, its presence indicates a need for further diagnostic studies. Commonly used imaging studies are discussed later in this chapter.

TABLE 27.5 Renal cell cancer staging

STAGE	EXTENT OF TUMOUR	PROGNOSIS
I	Confined to the kidney capsule	> 90% 5-year survival
II	Invasion through the capsule but confined to local fascia	85% 5-year survival
III	Renal vein or inferior vena cava involvement (IIIA), local lymph node (IIIB) and local lymph nodes and vessels (IIIC)	60% 5-year survival
IV	Spread to nearby organs or distant metastases	≤ 10% 5-year survival

Source: Adapted from Loscalzo et al. (2022). *Harrison's principles of internal medicine* (21st ed.). New York: McGraw Hill Medical.

MANIFESTATIONS Renal tumours

- Microscopic or gross haematuria
- Flank pain
- Palpable abdominal mass
- Fever
- Fatigue
- Weight loss
- Anaemia or polycythaemia

Radical nephrectomy is the treatment of choice for kidney tumours. In a radical nephrectomy, the adrenal gland, upper ureter, fat and fascia surrounding the kidney, as well as the entire kidney, are removed. Regional lymph nodes may also be resected. Although nephrectomy can be done using a laparoscopic approach, laparotomy primarily is used for radical nephrectomy. Nursing care for the person having a nephrectomy is summarised in the accompanying box.

No effective treatment is available for advanced renal carcinoma with metastases. Biological therapies such as interferon or interleukin-2 have been used, but rarely achieve a durable effect. No chemotherapy drug consistently causes tumour regression in more than 20% of individuals (Loscalzo et al., 2022), but research leading to new therapies is ongoing.

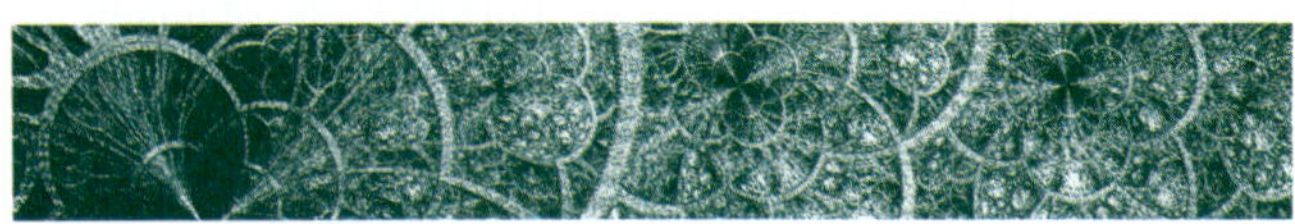

Nursing care

Nursing diagnoses and interventions

Nursing care focuses on needs related to the cancer diagnosis and to the surgical intervention. Postoperative pain may be significant and the risk of respiratory complications is high. The remaining kidney must be protected from damage to preserve renal function. Psychologically, the person may grieve the loss of a major organ and the diagnosis of cancer.

Pain

The size and location of the incision used for a radical nephrectomy (see Figure 27.2) make pain management a challenge. Intercostal blocks, patient-controlled analgesia (PCA) or routine analgesic administration can effectively relieve the discomfort. Nursing care focuses on assessing pain relief, providing supportive measures to enhance analgesia and ensuring that pain or the fear of pain does not lead to respiratory complications.

- Assess frequently for adequate pain relief. Use a standard pain scale and non-verbal signs such as grimacing, tense body position, apparent dozing, elevated pulse, change of blood pressure or rapid, shallow respirations. Notify the physician of inadequate pain relief. *The person may assume that pain is to be expected or may fear becoming addicted to analgesics. Careful questioning and assessment allow effective pain management. Responses to analgesics are individual and the prescribed dose may need to be adjusted.*
- Assess the incision for inflammation or swelling, and drainage catheters and tubes for patency. *An obstructed catheter can lead to hydronephrosis, haematoma or abscess, increasing incisional pain.*
- Use adjunctive pain relief measures such as positioning, diversional activities, management of environmental stimuli, guided imagery and relaxation techniques. *These can enhance the effects of analgesia.*

CONSIDERATION FOR PRACTICE

Assess for abdominal distension, tenderness and bowel sounds. Intra-abdominal bleeding, peritonitis or paralytic ileus can cause pain that may be confused with incisional pain.

Ineffective breathing pattern

The location of the incision combined with the respiratory depressant effects of narcotic analgesics increases the risk of respiratory complications in the person who has had a nephrectomy.

- Position to promote respiratory excursion, using semi-Fowler's position and side-lying positions as allowed and tolerated. *Lung expansion is improved in semi-Fowler's and Fowler's positions.*
- Change position frequently, ambulate as soon as possible. *These measures promote lung expansion and the movement of mucus out of airways.*
- Encourage frequent (every 1 to 2 hours) deep breathing, spirometer use and coughing. *Assist to splint the incision. These measures promote alveolar ventilation, gas exchange and airway clearance.*

CONSIDERATION FOR PRACTICE

Assess respiratory status frequently, including rate and depth, cough, breath sounds, oxygen saturation and temperature. Pneumothorax is not an uncommon complication during nephrectomy (Wu & Zhang, 2018). Early identification and intervention can prevent major respiratory complications.

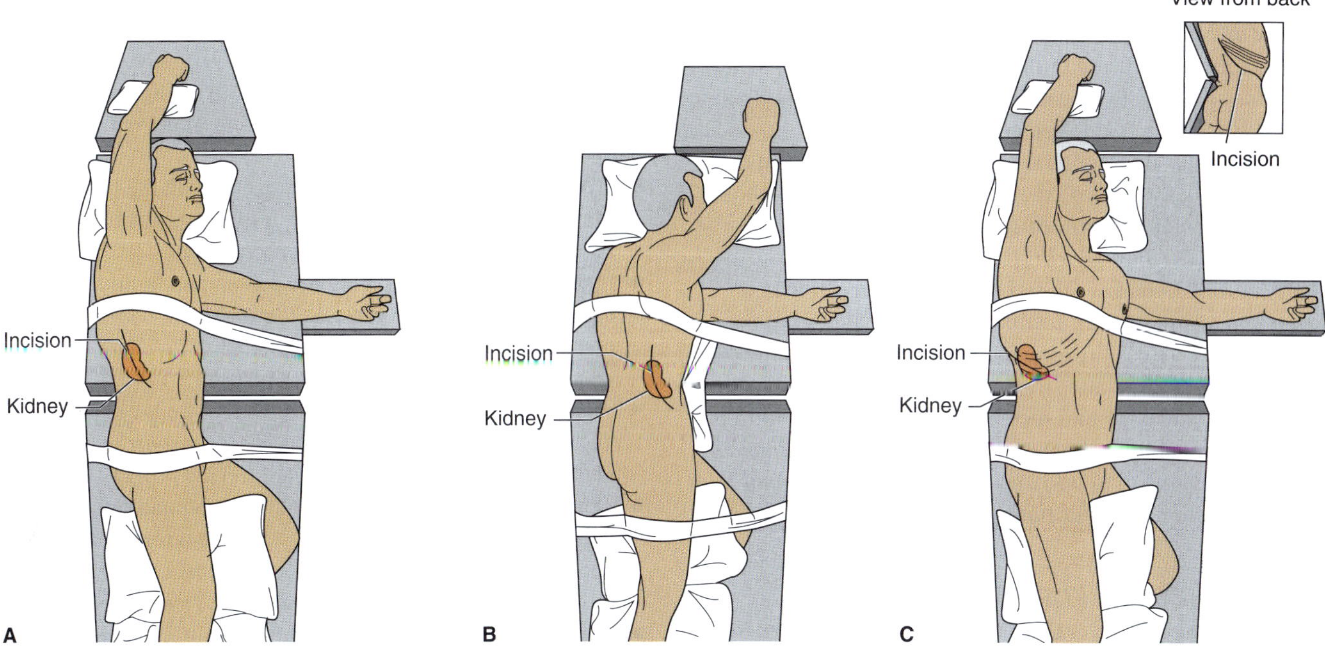

FIGURE 27.2 *Incisions used for kidney surgery: A, flank; B, lumbar; and C, thoracoabdominal*

NURSING CARE OF THE PERSON having a nephrectomy

PREOPERATIVE CARE

- Provide routine preoperative care as outlined in the chapter 'Nursing care of people having surgery'.
- Report abnormal laboratory values to the surgical team. *Bacteriuria, blood coagulation abnormalities or other significant abnormal values may affect surgery and postoperative care.*
- Discuss operative and postoperative expectations as indicated, including the location of the incision and anticipated tubes, stents and drains. *Preoperative teaching about postoperative expectations reduces anxiety for the person and family during the early postoperative period.*

POSTOPERATIVE CARE

- Provide routine postoperative care as described in the chapter 'Nursing care of people having surgery'.
- Frequently assess urine colour, amount and character, noting any haematuria, pyuria or sediment. Promptly report any significant decreases in urine output or changes in colour or clarity. *Preserving function of the remaining kidney is critical; frequent assessment allows early intervention for potential problems.*
- Note the placement, status and drainage from ureteral catheters, stents, nephrostomy tubes or drains. Label each clearly. Maintain gravity drainage; irrigate only as ordered. *Maintaining drainage tube patency is vital to prevent potential hydronephrosis. Bright bleeding or unexpected drainage may indicate a surgical complication.*
- Support the grieving process and adjustment to the loss of a kidney. Loss of a major organ leads to a body image change and grief response. *When renal cancer is the underlying diagnosis, the person may also grieve the loss of health and potential loss of life.*
- Provide the following home care instructions for the person and family:
  a. The importance of protecting the remaining kidney by preventing UTI, renal calculi and trauma. See the chapter 'Nursing care of people with urinary tract disorders' for measures to prevent UTI and calculi. *Damage to the remaining kidney by UTI, renal calculi or trauma can lead to renal failure.*
  b. Maintain a fluid intake of 2,000 to 2,500 mL per day unless contraindicated. *This important measure helps prevent dehydration and maintain good urine flow.*
  c. Gradually increase exercise to tolerance, avoiding heavy lifting for a year after surgery. Participation in contact sports is not recommended to reduce the risk of injury to the remaining kidney. Lifting is avoided to allow full tissue healing. *Trauma to the remaining kidney could seriously jeopardise renal function.*
  d. Care of the incision and any remaining drainage tubes, catheters or stents. *This routine postoperative instruction is vital to prepare the person for self-care and prevent complications.*
  e. Report abnormal signs and symptoms to the treating team, including manifestations of UTI (dysuria, frequency, urgency, nocturia, cloudy, malodorous urine) or systemic infection (fever, general malaise, fatigue), redness, swelling, pain or drainage from the incision or any catheter or drain tube site. *Prompt treatment of postoperative infection is vital to allow continued healing and prevent compromise of the remaining kidney.*

Risk of impaired urinary elimination

Surgery involving the urinary tract increases the risk of altered renal function and urine elimination. In addition, removal of one kidney dictates extra caution to maintain renal circulation, a sterile urinary tract and free urine flow.

- Monitor vital signs, central venous pressure (CVP) and urine output every 1 to 2 hours initially, then every 4 hours. *Hypovolaemia due to haemorrhage, diuresis or fluid sequestering (third spacing) reduces blood flow to the kidney and increases the risk of renal ischaemia with possible acute tubular necrosis and acute kidney injury.*
- Frequently assess the amount and nature of drainage on surgical dressings and from drainage tubes, stents and catheters. Measure and record output from each drain or catheter separately. *Frequent and accurate assessment of drainage helps to identify excess bleeding, abnormal fluid loss, infection or other potential surgical complications.*

CONSIDERATION FOR PRACTICE

Prevent kinking, twisting or tension on drains and tubes. Do not clamp. Ensure clear and consistent labelling of drains and that each drain is connected to a single, exclusive closed drainage system. Notify the surgical team immediately if any tube becomes dislodged. It is vital to maintain the patency of drains, particularly any affecting the remaining kidney, to prevent the excess pressure of hydronephrosis.

- Maintain fluid intake with intravenous fluids until oral intake is resumed. Encourage an intake of 2,000 to 2,500 mL per day if not contraindicated. *A liberal fluid intake prevents dehydration, helps to dilute any nephrotoxic substances and promotes good urinary output.*
- Use strict aseptic technique in caring for all urinary catheters, tubes, stents, drains and incisions. *Asepsis is vital to prevent infection and possible compromise of the remaining kidney.*
- Following catheter removal, assess frequently for urinary retention. Notify the physician if the person is unable to void within 4 to 6 hours or if manifestations of retention (distended bladder, discomfort, urinary dribbling) develop. *Maintenance of urine output is vital to prevent stasis and possible complications such as infection and hydronephrosis.*
- Monitor laboratory results, including urinalysis, serum urea, creatinine and electrolytes. Report abnormal findings to the treating team. *Abnormal values may indicate early acute kidney injury; prompt intervention is necessary to preserve renal function.*

Anticipatory grieving

The person having a radical nephrectomy for renal cancer not only loses a major organ but also has to adjust to the diagnosis of cancer. Although the prognosis for recovery may be good, there may be fears of recurrence. Without support and education, some people will perceive a cancer diagnosis as terminal. The NSQHS Standard Partnering with Consumers reminds clinicians to provide care that is respectful, supportive and encouraging (ACSQHC, 2021). Providing support during the initial stages of grieving can improve physical recovery, psychological coping and eventual adaptation.

- Work to develop a trusting relationship with the person and family. *Trust increases the nurse's effectiveness in helping them work through the process of grieving.*
- Listen actively, encouraging the person and family to express fears and concerns. *As they begin to express their concerns, person and family can begin to deal more effectively with them.*
- Assist the person and family to identify strengths, past experiences and support systems. *These resources can be employed in working through the grieving process.*
- Demonstrate respect for cultural, spiritual and religious values and beliefs; encourage use of these resources to cope with losses. *Value and belief systems can provide a structure and form for dealing with the grieving process.*
- Encourage discussion of the potential impact of loss on the person and the family structure and function. Assist family members to share concerns with one another. *Sharing of fears and concerns among family members promotes involvement and support of the entire family unit so that the individual is not left to cope alone.*
- Refer to cancer support groups, social services or counselling as appropriate. *Support groups and counselling services provide additional resources for coping.*

Community-based care

If renal cancer was detected at an early stage and cure is anticipated, teaching for home care focuses on protecting the remaining kidney. Include the following measures to prevent infection, renal calculi, hydronephrosis and trauma:

- Maintain a fluid intake of 2,000 to 2,500 mL per day, increasing the amount during hot weather or strenuous exercise, unless contraindicated.
- Urinate when the urge is perceived and before and after sexual intercourse.
- Properly clean the perineal area.
- Watch for symptoms of UTI and understand the importance of early and appropriate evaluation and intervention.
- If the person is an older adult male, he should watch for symptoms of prostatic hypertrophy, a major cause of urinary tract obstruction. Stress the importance of routine screening examinations.
- Avoid contact sports such as football or hockey; use measures to prevent injury which could damage the remaining kidney (i.e. motor vehicle accidents and falls).

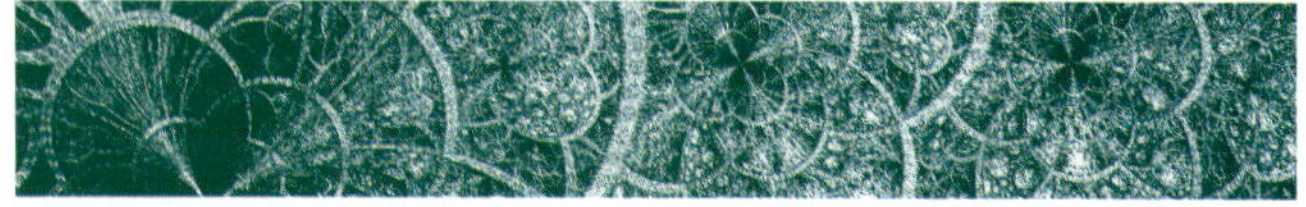

THE PERSON WITH A CONGENITAL KIDNEY MALFORMATION

Congenital kidney disorders can affect the form and/or function of the kidney. Functional congenital kidney disorders are usually identified in childhood or adolescence. If function is not affected, congenital malformations may be detected only coincidentally. Malformations include agenesis, hypoplasia, alterations in kidney position and fusion anomalies such as horseshoe kidney.

Agenesis, absence of the kidney, and *hypoplasia*, underdevelopment of the kidney, typically affect only one of these paired organs. Renal function remains normal unless the unaffected kidney is compromised. Abnormal kidney position affects the ureters and urine flow, potentially leading to urinary stasis, increased risk of UTI and lithiasis or stone formation (see the chapter 'Nursing care of people with urinary tract disorders').

One in every 400 to 600 people has *horseshoe kidney*, making it one of the most common renal malformations (Kirkpatrick & Leslie, 2022). Failure of the embryonic kidneys to ascend normally can result in a single, horseshoe-shaped organ. The two kidneys are fused at either the upper or lower pole (usually the lower). This malformation does not typically affect renal function; however, because the ureters cross the fused poles, there is an increased risk of *hydronephrosis* or distension of the renal pelvis and calyces with urine (see the chapter 'Nursing care of people with urinary tract disorders'). Recurrent UTI and renal calculi are also common in people with horseshoe kidney.

Renal ultrasound and intravenous pyelography are used to diagnose horseshoe kidney. Correction of the abnormality is rarely necessary, although surgical resection of the isthmus (connection between the kidneys) may be done to relieve ureteral obstruction or allow access to the abdominal aorta, which lies behind it.

Nursing care for people with horseshoe kidney or other congenital malformations is primarily educational. Because abnormal kidney shape or position increases the risk of infection and stone formation, teach the person to maintain a fluid intake of at least 2,500 mL per day unless contraindicated. Emphasise the importance of avoiding dehydration by increasing fluids during hot weather and strenuous exercise. Teach hygiene practices such as perineal cleansing and voiding before and after intercourse to help prevent UTI. Teach the early manifestations of UTI and instruct to seek treatment promptly to prevent infection of the kidney. See the chapter 'Nursing care of people with urinary tract disorders'.

THE PERSON WITH CHRONIC KIDNEY DISEASE

Although the kidneys usually recover from acute damage, some disease and injury can lead to permanent destruction of kidney tissue and loss of function. This process of **chronic kidney disease (CKD)** is often a slow, progressive deterioration that may occur over many years, with an absence of symptoms until the late stages. As nephron units are lost and kidney mass decreases, the functions of glomerular filtration, tubular secretion and tubular reabsorption fail. Kidney failure (CKD stage 5) is the final stage of CKD that occurs when the kidneys are no long able to adequately excrete metabolic waste or regulate fluid and electrolyte balance.

A person is described as having CKD if they have a GFR < 60 mL/min/1.73 m^2 for more than 3 months with or without evidence of kidney damage, *or* evidence of kidney damage (with or without decreased GFR) for more than 3 months including microalbuminuria, proteinuria, glomerular haematuria or any anatomical or pathological abnormality (KDIGO, 2013). There are five stages of CKD (see Figure 27.3). In Australia, 1 in 10 adults has indications of CKD including decreased GFR and microalbuminuria (AIHW, 2020).

Conditions causing CKD typically involve diffuse, bilateral disease of the kidneys with progressive scarring and destruction of the entire nephron. As indicated in Table 27.6, diabetic nephropathy continues to be the leading cause of ESKD in all population groups in Australia and New Zealand, and in fact in most of the Western world. Glomerulonephritis and hypertension follow as the next two leading causes of ESKD (ANZDATA Registry, 2021).

CKD is a public health concern in Australia, with the AIHW National Mortality Database reporting that CKD contributed to 18,600 deaths in Australia in 2018 (AIHW, 2020). In the period of 2017–2018, CKD accounted approximately

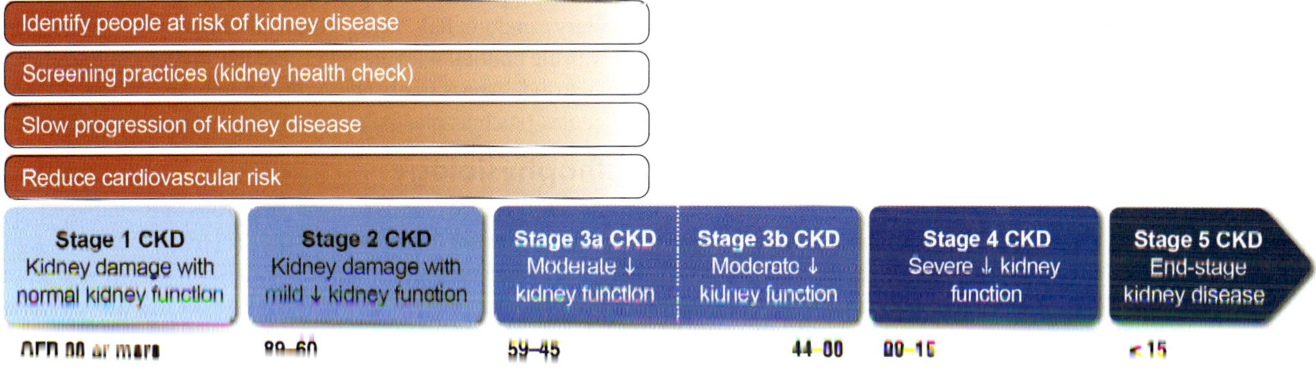

FIGURE 27.3 *Stages of chronic kidney disease*

Source: Nephrology Educators Network.

TABLE 27.6 Incidence of primary disease leading to kidney failure (CKD stage 5) in the Australian population, 2020

CAUSE (% OF PEOPLE)	EXAMPLES
Diabetic nephropathy (38%)	Multifactorial. Changes in the glomerular basement membrane lead to sclerosis of the glomerulus and gradual destruction of the nephron.
Glomerulonephritis (18%)	Bilateral inflammatory process of the glomeruli leads to ischaemia, nephron loss and shrinkage of the kidney.
Hypertension (12%)	Long-standing hypertension damages the vasculature supplying the kidneys and leads to renal arteriosclerosis and ischaemia, resulting in glomerular destruction and tubular atrophy.
Polycystic kidney disease (5%)	Multiple bilateral cysts gradually destroy normal renal tissue by compression.
Reflux nephropathy (2%)	Results from chronic infection (pyelonephritis) commonly associated with an obstructive or neurological process and vesicoureteral reflux. The end result is renal scarring, atrophy and dilated calyces.

Source: Data from ANZDATA Registry (2021). *44th annual report*. Adelaide: ANZDATA. Retrieved from https://www.anzdata.org.au.

1.8 million hospital admissions across Australia, this is 16% of all hospitalisations (AIHW, 2020). Many area health services have now put into action CKD management programs to identify and screen people at risk, implement risk reduction and prevention strategies, and prevent its progression while managing the comorbid associations of CKD.

The incidence of **end-stage kidney disease (ESKD)** is increasing, particularly in older adults. In 2020, 3,259 and 710 people in Australia and New Zealand respectively began receiving treatment for ESKD. That same year, in Australia, a total of 14,554 people with ESKD were treated with dialysis, and a further 13,130 people were living with functioning kidney transplants (ANZDATA Registry, 2021). The cumulative cost of treatment for ESKD from 2009 to 2020 was between $11.3 billion and $12.3 billion (Cass, Chadban & Gallagher, 2020). This cost excludes not only the financial costs incurred by people undertaking kidney replacement therapy, but also the immeasurable costs and burden placed on their lifestyle.

The burden of kidney disease on Aboriginal and Torres Strait Islander peoples

CKD exemplifies the differences in health equality between Aboriginal and Torres Strait Islander peoples and the non-Indigenous Australian population. Indigenous Australians are twice as likely to have biomedical markers of CKD and are five times more likely than the Australian population as a whole to progress to kidney failure (AIHW, 2020).

Aboriginal and Torres Islander people represent 3.3% of the general Australian population but 8.8% of the total Australian population with kidney failure requiring kidney replacement therapy (AIHW, 2021; ANZDATA Registry, 2021). Indigenous Australians living in very remote regions have an incidence of renal failure up to 20 times higher than non-Indigenous Australians (Kidney Health Australia, 2018). The rate of death associated with CKD is four times higher for Aboriginal and Torres Strait Islander people than for non-Indigenous Australians (AIHW, 2020).

Indigenous Australians have additional risk factors that predispose them to CKD, particularly in remote and very remote areas. These factors include low birth-weight; crowded housing (leading to increased infections); socioeconomic disadvantage including low levels of education; decreased access to preventive health and medical care; and increased rates of hypertension and diabetes (Dart, 2022; Hoy, Mott & McDonald, 2016).

The burden for Aboriginal and Torres Strait Islander peoples can be increased when they are required to leave their traditional lands for complex healthcare treatment in a distant Australian city. Indigenous Australians undertaking dialysis away from their traditional homeland, or Country, can experience overwhelming feelings of disempowerment related to their disconnection from cultural and social structures and networks, and dependence on health professionals and dialysis treatment (Conway et al., 2018). Thus, the prevention or identification of early-stage CKD in the Aboriginal and Torres Strait Islander population is critical to ensure people receive appropriate management to delay, minimise or halt disease progression.

Physiology review

The glomeruli are the filtering units of the kidney, with each glomerulus consisting of a tuft of capillaries surrounded by a thin, double-walled capsule (Bowman's capsule) (see Figure 25.3). About 20% of the resting cardiac output flows through the glomeruli of the kidneys, forming approximately 180 L of plasma ultrafiltrate each day. More than 99% of this filtrate is reabsorbed in the renal tubules. The glomerular filtration rate (GFR) is controlled by opposing forces: the pressure and amount of blood flowing through the glomeruli promote filtration, and the pressure in the Bowman's capsule and colloid osmotic (*oncotic*) pressure of the blood oppose it. The total surface area of glomerular capillaries also affects the GFR. The glomerular capillary membrane has three layers: the capillary endothelial layer, the basement membrane and the capsule epithelial layer. Water and the smallest solutes (such as electrolytes) pass freely across this membrane, whereas larger molecules (such as plasma proteins) are retained in the blood.

Pathophysiology

In the early stages of CKD, as nephrons are damaged the remaining functional nephrons hypertrophy. Glomerular capillary flow and pressure increase in these nephrons and more solute particles are filtered to compensate for lost kidney mass. This increased demand predisposes the remaining nephrons to glomerular sclerosis (scarring), resulting in their eventual destruction. This process of continued loss of nephron function may continue even after the initial disease process has resolved (Loscalzo et al., 2022).

Haematuria, microalbuminuria and proteinuria are manifestations of glomerular capillary membrane damage, which allows blood cells and proteins to escape from the blood into the glomerular filtrate. Haematuria may be either gross or microscopic. Microalbuminuria (30–300 mg/day), the precursor to proteinuria, may be detected early on in the disease process, but this is highly reliant on screening practices and the type of testing methodology utilised. The degree of albuminuria can be measured with a simple early morning spot urine test to determine the albumin:creatinine ratio (ACR). Proteinuria is measured similarly with a protein:creatinine ratio (PCR) and is considered an important indicator of glomerular injury, because it increases progressively with increased glomerular damage. Loss of plasma proteins leads to hypoalbuminaemia (low serum albumin levels), which in turn reduces the plasma oncotic pressure (osmotic pressure created by plasma proteins), leading to oedema.

As plasma proteins are lost, the forces opposing filtration diminish and the amount of filtrate increases. The increased flow of filtrate stimulates the renin–angiotensin–aldosterone mechanism (see the chapter 'A person-centred approach to assessing the renal system'), producing vasoconstriction and a fall in GFR. Increased aldosterone production causes salt and water retention, which further contributes to oedema. As the GFR falls, filtration and elimination of nitrogenous wastes, including urea, decrease. Oliguria, urine output of less than 400 mL in 24 hours, may result from the decreased GFR. Hypertension results from fluid retention and disruption of the renin–angiotensin system, a key regulator of blood pressure.

Table 27.6 outlines common pathological processes causing CKD that lead to ESKD in Australia.

The course of CKD is variable, progressing over a period of months to many years. In stage 1 the GFR remains essentially normal or slightly elevated as a result of a hyperperfusive state whereby unaffected nephrons compensate for the lost nephrons. As the disease progresses to stage 2 the GFR falls to between 89 and 60 mL/min and the individual remains asymptomatic. Any further insult to the kidneys at this stage (such as infection, dehydration, exposure to nephrotoxins or urinary tract obstruction) can further reduce function and precipitate the onset of an acute decline in kidney function. Stage 3 is characterised by a moderate decrease in renal function with a GFR of between 59 and 30 mL/min. The serum creatinine and urea may begin to rise and the person may begin to notice some feelings of tiredness, itchiness or loss of appetite, but it is not unusual to remain asymptomatic. Stage 4 sees a severe decrease in kidney function, with the GFR declining to between 28 and 15 mL/min. Symptomology of this decreased function, including increased tiredness, shortness of breath and general malaise, may be enough to prompt the individual to schedule a visit to their general practitioner if they have not already been diagnosed with CKD. In the final stage of CKD, kidney failure, the GFR is less than 15 mL/min and kidney replacement therapy is required to maintain life (see Figure 27.3).

Diabetic nephropathy

Diabetic nephropathy is one of the main microvascular complications of diabetes mellitus (DM) which sees the combination of haemodynamic, genetic and metabolic sequelae contribute to the development of increased vascular permeability at the glomerular basement membrane. Diabetic nephropathy is the leading cause of ESKD in Australia and New Zealand, with type 2 representing the majority of diabetic nephropathy cases requiring kidney replacement therapy (ANZDATA Registry, 2021).

The characteristic lesion of diabetic nephropathy is glomerulosclerosis and thickening of the glomerular basement membrane. Hyperglycaemia impairs the ability of afferent and efferent arterioles and glomerular capillaries to regulate glomerular pressure and respond to systemic changes in blood pressure. As the disease progresses, the glomerular capillary lumen narrows, reducing the surface area for glomerular filtration. Arteriosclerosis, a common feature of long-term diabetes and hypertension, contributes to the disease process, as do nephritis and tubular lesions. Pyelonephritis, inflammation of the kidney, is also implicated in the development of diabetic nephropathy. A further discussion is found in the chapter 'Nursing care of people with diabetes mellitus'.

Diabetic nephropathy progresses from a stage of hyperfiltration to early-stage glomerular damage signified by microalbuminuria, which is typically seen within 10 to 15 years after the onset of diabetes. If this damage is not detected early or is poorly controlled, it will lead to overt proteinuria (within 15 to 20 years of the initial diagnosis) and decreased GFR and may also see the concomitant development of hypertension. Eventually ESKD will develop and the individual will require kidney replacement therapy to sustain life.

Glomerulonephritis

Glomerulonephritis (GN) affects both the structure and function of the glomerulus, disrupting glomerular filtration, and is the second leading cause of ESKD in Australia (ANZDATA Registry, 2021). Histologically, glomerular involvement may be diffuse, involving all glomeruli, or focal, involving some glomeruli while others remain essentially normal. GN can present as either an acute or chronic condition and describes any disease that is mediated by either an inflammatory or immune mechanism that affects the glomerulus. Circulating antigen–antibody immune complexes formed during the initiating event become trapped in the glomerular membrane, leading to an inflammatory response. The complement system is activated and vasoactive substances and inflammatory mediators are released. Endothelial cells proliferate and the glomerular membrane swells and becomes permeable to plasma proteins and blood cells (see Figure 27.4). This increased permeability causes the manifestations common to glomerular disorders: haematuria, proteinuria and oedema.

The taxonomy of GN sometimes causes confusion as it attempts to classify the histopathological characteristics of the disease (e.g. focal segmental GN), the clinical presentation (e.g. nephrotic syndrome) or the aetiology of the disease (e.g. autoimmune) (Haas, 2017; Rosenberg & Kopp, 2017). From an immunological perspective, GN is described as either primary, where the disease is immunological or idiopathic in origin, or secondary, where it is associated with a multisystem disease or hereditary condition. Systemic lupus erythematosus (SLE) and Goodpasture's syndrome are frequently implicated in secondary glomerular disorders.

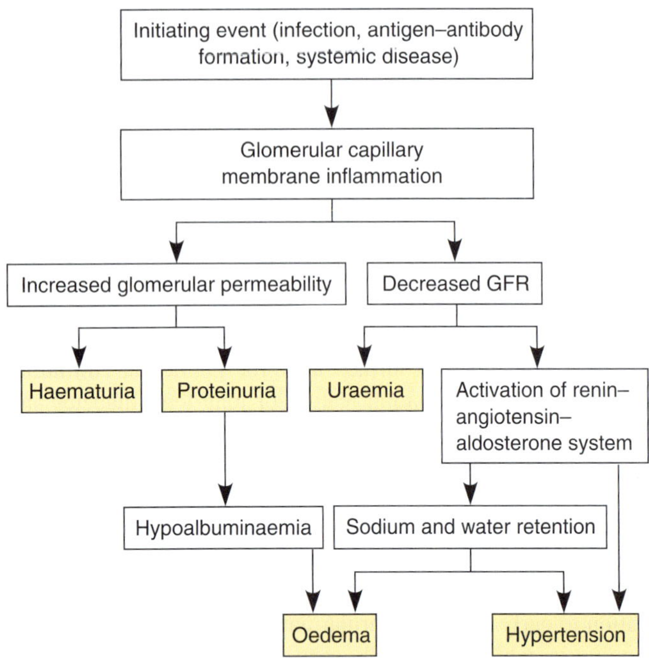

FIGURE 27.4 *The pathogenesis of glomerulonephritis*

FAST FACTS

- Glomerulonephritis is the second leading cause of kidney failure in Australia, with diabetes as the number one cause.
- Haematuria and microalbuminuria are early manifestations of kidney failure.
- IgA mesangioproliferative GN is the most common histologically proven form of glomerulonephritis in Australia, followed by focal sclerosing GN.

Primary glomerular disorders include IgA mesangioproliferative GN, rapidly progressive glomerulonephritis, focal sclerosing glomerulonephritis and nephrotic syndrome. Goodpasture's syndrome and lupus nephritis are the most common secondary forms of glomerular disease.

IgA MESANGIOPROLIFERATIVE GLOMERULONEPHRITIS

IgA mesangioproliferative glomerulonephritis, or IgA nephropathy (IgAN) as it is more commonly known, is characterised by the deposition of the antibody immunoglobulin A in the glomerular mesangium. IgAN has a highly variable course which can range from a benign condition to either a chronically slow or rapidly progressive disease. Children and young adults generally present with haematuria post respiratory tract infection or gastrointestinal illness; adults present later in the disease trajectory with proteinuria, haematuria and hypertension (KDIGO, 2021a). IgAN can only be diagnosed via renal biopsy; therefore, early biopsy is essential in order to implement appropriate treatment, with the goal of slowing the progression of the disease (KDIGO, 2021a).

RAPIDLY PROGRESSIVE GLOMERULONEPHRITIS

Rapidly progressive glomerulonephritis (RPGN) is characterised by manifestations of severe glomerular injury without a specific, identifiable cause. This type of glomerulonephritis often progresses to renal failure within months. It may be idiopathic (primary) or secondary to a systemic disorder such as SLE or Goodpasture's syndrome. It affects people of all ages.

In RPGN, glomerular cells proliferate and, together with macrophages, form crescent-shaped lesions that obliterate Bowman's space (Bagga & Menon, 2016). Glomerular damage is diffuse, leading to a rapid, progressive decline in renal function. Irreversible renal failure often develops over weeks to months (Loscalzo et al., 2022).

People with RPGN typically present with complaints of weakness, nausea and vomiting. Some may relate a history of flu-like illness preceding the onset of the glomerulonephritis. Other symptoms include oliguria and abdominal or flank pain. On urinalysis, haematuria and massive proteinuria are noted. People with RPGN are often treated with plasma exchange as an adjunct to immunosuppressive therapy (see Box 27.1).

Nephrotic syndrome

Nephrotic syndrome is a group of clinical findings as opposed to a specific disorder. It is characterised by massive proteinuria, hypoalbuminaemia, hyperlipidaemia and oedema. A number of disorders can affect the glomerular capillary membrane, changing its porosity and allowing plasma proteins to escape into the urine.

With plasma protein loss in the urine and resulting hypoalbuminaemia, the oncotic pressure of the plasma falls. Fluid shifts from the vascular compartment to interstitial spaces, causing the oedema characteristic of nephrotic syndrome. Salt and water retention, possibly due to activation of the renin–angiotensin system, contribute to the oedema. Oedema may be severe, affecting the face and periorbital area as well as dependent tissues (see Figure 27.5).

BOX 27.1 Therapeutic plasma exchange

Therapeutic plasma exchange (**plasmapheresis**) is a procedure performed by nurses with specialty training to remove disease-mediating antibodies from the plasma. It is used in conjunction with immunosuppressive therapy to treat RPGN and Goodpasture's syndrome. Blood is removed from the person via a large vein or central venous device and then the plasma containing the glomerular-damaging antibodies is separated and discarded using either centrifugal or membrane separation technologies. The RBCs are then returned to the person along with albumin or human plasma to replace the plasma removed. This procedure is usually done in a series of treatments. It is not without risk and informed consent is required. Procedural complications are mainly associated with the type of technology used to achieve plasma separation. The most common complications are transfusion reactions, citrate toxicity (with centrifugal methods), altered coagulation status, vascular access infection and hypotension secondary to fluid volume shifts.

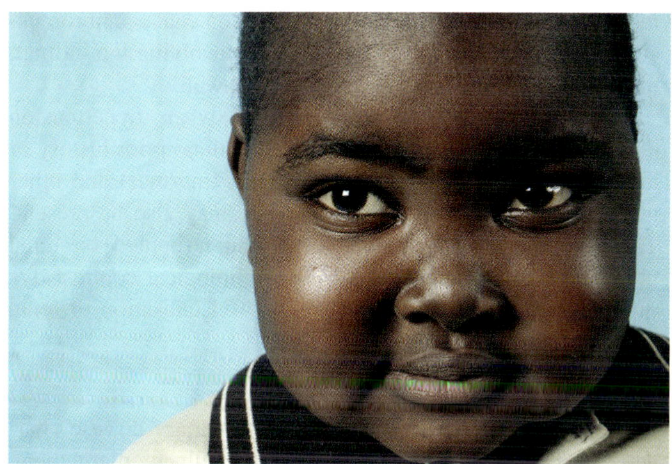

FIGURE 27.5 ***Severe oedema characteristic of nephrotic syndrome***

Source: © MedicImage/Alamy Stock Photo.

Loss of plasma proteins stimulates the liver to increase albumin production and lipoprotein synthesis. As a result, serum triglyceride and low-density lipoprotein (LDL) levels increase, as do urine lipids (*lipiduria*). Hyperlipidaemia increases the risk of atherosclerosis in people with nephrotic syndrome.

Thromboemboli (mobilised blood clots) are a relatively common complication of nephrotic syndrome. Loss of clotting and anti-clotting factors along with plasma proteins disrupts coagulation pathways and increases the risk of renal venous thrombosis, deep venous thrombosis and pulmonary embolism. Renal venous thrombosis can cause flank or groin pain on one or both sides, gross haematuria and a reduced GFR (McCance & Huether, 2019).

Nephrotic syndrome usually resolves without long-term effects in children. The prognosis for adults is less optimistic because the syndrome often occurs secondarily to another disorder. Many adults do not recover completely, experiencing persistent proteinuria and, potentially, progressive renal impairment.

Goodpasture's syndrome

Goodpasture's syndrome is a rare autoimmune disorder of unknown aetiology. It is characterised by formation of antibodies to the glomerular basement membrane. These antibodies may also bind to alveolar basement membranes, damaging alveoli and causing pulmonary haemorrhage. Goodpasture's syndrome usually affects young men aged between 18 and 35, although it can occur at any age and affect women as well.

Although the glomeruli may be nearly normal in appearance and function in Goodpasture's syndrome, extensive cell proliferation and crescent formation characteristic of rapidly progressive glomerulonephritis are more common. Renal manifestations include haematuria, proteinuria and oedema. Rapid progression through the CKD continuum may occur. Alveolar membrane damage can lead to mild or life threatening pulmonary haemorrhage. Cough, shortness of breath and haemoptysis (bloody sputum) are early respiratory manifestations.

Lupus nephritis

Systemic lupus erythematosus (SLE) is an inflammatory autoimmune disorder affecting the connective tissue of the body. Between 60% and 80% of people with SLE develop manifestations of nephritis (Loscalzo et al., 2022). Immune complexes that form within the glomerular capillary wall are the usual trigger for glomerular injury in SLE. Manifestations of lupus nephritis range from microscopic haematuria to massive proteinuria. Its progression may be slow and chronic or *fulminant*, with a sudden onset and the rapid development of renal disease. Most people with minimal or mild lesions survive for at least 10 years. Improved management of the underlying disease, immunotherapy, dialysis and renal transplantation have significantly improved the prognosis in recent years.

THE PERSON WITH A RENOVASCULAR DISORDER

Renal function is dependent on an adequate supply of blood. Blood supports renal cell metabolism and is vital to kidney function, the nephron in particular. The kidney can regulate fluid, electrolyte and acid–base balance, and serve as a major organ of excretion, only when its blood supply is sufficient. Vascular disorders, therefore, can have a significant impact on renal function.

Hypertension

Hypertension, sustained elevation of the systemic blood pressure, can result from or cause kidney disease. In 2020, it was the cause of 12% of all new cases of ESKD (kidney failure (CKD stage 5)) in Australia (ANZDATA Registry, 2021).

Prolonged hypertension damages the walls of arterioles and accelerates the process of atherosclerosis. This damage primarily affects the heart, brain, kidneys, eyes and major blood vessels. In the kidney, arteriosclerotic lesions develop in the *afferent* (leading into) and *efferent* (going out of) arterioles and the glomerular capillaries. GFR declines and tubular function is affected, resulting in proteinuria and microscopic haematuria.

Malignant hypertension is a rapidly progressive form of hypertension that can develop in people with untreated primary hypertension. Here, the diastolic pressure is in excess of 120 mmHg and may be as high as 150 to 170 mmHg. Malignant hypertension affects less than 1% of people with hypertension; it is more common in African Americans than in people of European ancestry. Untreated, malignant hypertension causes a rapid decline in renal function due to vessel changes, renal ischaemia and infarction.

Approximately 5–10% of hypertension is a manifestation of an underlying disease and is termed 'secondary hypertension'. Renal vascular disease and diseases of the renal parenchyma, such as diabetic nephropathy, are commonly associated with secondary hypertension. Ensuring blood pressure lies within normal limits is vital to prevent kidney damage. When hypertension is secondary to kidney disease, maintaining blood pressure control is an integral step in attempting to slow the decline in kidney function. Hypertension and its management are discussed in depth in the chapter 'Nursing care of people with vascular and lymphatic disorders'.

Renal artery occlusion

Renal arteries can be occluded by either a primary process affecting the renal vessels or by emboli, clots or other foreign material. Risk factors for acute renal artery thrombosis (formation of a blood clot in the renal artery) include severe abdominal trauma, vessel trauma from surgery or angiography, aortic or renal artery aneurysms, and severe aortic or renal artery atherosclerosis. Emboli from the left side of the heart can travel via the aorta to occlude the renal artery. Emboli may form as a result of atrial fibrillation (irregular and uncoordinated electrical activity of the atria), following myocardial infarction, as vegetative growths on heart valves associated with bacterial endocarditis or from fatty plaque in the aorta.

Renal arterial occlusion may be asymptomatic when the occlusion develops slowly and the affected vessels are small. Acute occlusion leading to ischaemia and infarction typically causes sudden, severe localised flank pain, nausea and vomiting, fever and hypertension. Haematuria and oliguria may occur. In the older person, the new onset of hypertension or worsening of previously controlled hypertension may signal renal artery thrombosis.

Laboratory studies reveal leucocytosis (elevated WBCs) and elevated renal enzyme levels, including aspartate transaminase (AST) and lactic dehydrogenase (LDH). These enzymes, normally present in renal cells, are released into the circulation when cells necrose and die. With bilateral arterial occlusion and infarction, renal function deteriorates rapidly, leading to acute kidney injury (Loscalzo et al., 2022).

Surgery to restore blood flow to the affected kidney may be indicated for acute occlusion. Management, where possible, is usually more conservative using anticoagulant therapy, hypertension control and supportive treatment.

Renal vein occlusion

A thrombus (clot) formed in a renal vein can occlude the vessel. The cause of the thrombus often is unclear. In adults, renal venous thrombosis usually occurs with nephrotic syndrome. Other predisposing factors include pregnancy, oral contraceptive use and certain malignancies.

Gradual or acute deterioration of renal function may be the only manifestation of renal vein occlusion. If the thrombus breaks loose, it can become a pulmonary embolism. The definitive diagnosis is made by visualising the thrombus through renal venography.

Thrombolytic drugs such as streptokinase or tissue plasminogen activator (tPA) may be given to dissolve or break up the thrombus. Anticoagulant therapy also is used to prevent further clotting and pulmonary emboli. Renal function often improves with treatment.

Renal artery stenosis

Renal artery stenosis is narrowing of the artery that supplies blood to the kidney; it can be unilateral or bilateral. Quite often a person can go through life with unilateral renal artery stenosis undetected; however, this is not always the case.

Atherosclerosis with gradual occlusion of the renal artery lumen by plaque is the primary cause of renal artery stenosis in men. In younger women, the most common cause is fibromuscular dysplasia, structural abnormalities involving the intimal, medial or adventitial layers of the arterial wall.

Renal artery stenosis is suspected when hypertension develops before age 30 or after age 50 with no prior history of high blood pressure. An epigastric bruit (murmur) and other manifestations of vascular insufficiency may also be present. The affected kidney appears small and atrophied on renal ultrasound. Renal angiography uses radiological contrast dye injected into the renal arteries to allow visualisation of renal blood vessels.

Polycystic kidney disease

Polycystic kidney disease (PKD), a hereditary disease characterised by cyst formation and massive kidney enlargement, affects both children and adults. This disease has two forms: the autosomal dominant form, which affects adults; and the autosomal recessive form, which is present at birth (McCance & Huether, 2019). Autosomal recessive PKD is rare. It usually is diagnosed prenatally or in infancy. Autosomal dominant PKD is relatively common. In 2020, PKD accounted for approximately 6% of people newly diagnosed with ESKD in Australia (ANZDATA Registry, 2021). This section focuses on autosomal dominant PKD, the more common adult form of the disorder.

Pathophysiology

Renal cysts are fluid-filled sacs affecting the nephron, the functional unit of the kidneys. The cysts may range in size from microscopic to several centimetres in diameter and affect the renal cortex and medulla of both kidneys. As the cysts fill, enlarge and multiply, the kidneys also enlarge. Renal blood vessels and nephrons are compressed and obstructed and functional tissue is destroyed (see Figure 27.6).

Although the name suggests the disease affects the kidneys, polycystic kidney disease is actually a systemic disease process and manifests with both renal and non-renal abnormalities. Often cysts develop elsewhere in the body, including the liver,

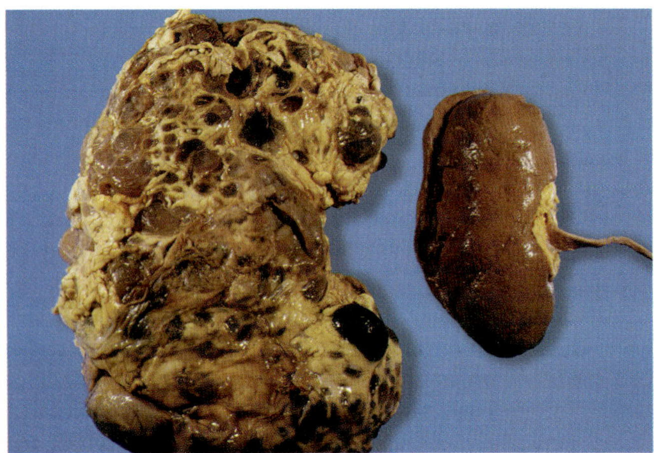

FIGURE 27.6 ***A polycystic kidney. The functional tissue of the kidneys is gradually destroyed and replaced with fluid-filled cysts***

Source: Arthur Glauberman/Science Source.

spleen, pancreas and other organs. Diverticular disease of the colon is common and may lead to perforation of the bowel (Loscalzo et al., 2022). Up to 10% of people affected experience subarachnoid haemorrhage from a type of congenital intracranial aneurysm.

Manifestations

Polycystic kidney disease is slowly progressive. Symptoms usually develop by age 40 to 50. Common manifestations include flank pain, microscopic or gross haematuria, proteinuria, and *polyuria* and *nocturia*, as the concentrating ability of the kidney is impaired. Urinary tract infection and renal calculi are common, as cysts interfere with normal urine drainage. Most people will develop hypertension from disruption of renal vessels. The kidneys become palpable, enlarged and knobby. Symptoms of renal insufficiency typically develop in approximately 60% of people by the age of 70. The progression to ESKD tends to occur more rapidly in men than in women.

GENETIC CONSIDERATIONS

Adult polycystic kidney disease

- Parents with autosomal dominant PKD will pass on the faulty gene to approximately 50% their offspring.
- Approximately 90% of cases are inherited as an autosomal dominant trait; the remaining 10% are due to spontaneous mutations.
- In autosomal recessive PKD, both parents must carry the defective gene and have a 25% chance of their child inheriting this disease.

MANIFESTATIONS AND COMPLICATIONS OF CKD

Uraemia

Uraemia, which literally means 'urine in the blood', refers to a group of symptoms associated with the decline in renal function generally in the final stages of the disease trajectory. In uraemia, fluid and electrolyte balance is altered, the regulatory and endocrine functions of the kidney are impaired, and accumulated metabolic waste products affect essentially every other organ system (Amerman, 2018; Loscalzo et al., 2022).

Early manifestations of uraemia include nausea, apathy, weakness and fatigue, symptoms that may be dismissed as a viral infection or just being run down. See 'Multisystem effects of uraemia'.

Fluid and electrolyte effects

Loss of kidney function impairs its ability to regulate fluid, electrolyte and acid–base balance. In the early stages of CKD, impaired filtration and reabsorption lead to proteinuria, haematuria and decreased urine-concentrating ability. Salt and water are poorly conserved and the risk of dehydration increases. Polyuria, nocturia and a fixed specific gravity of 1.008 to 1.012 are common (Amerman, 2018). As the GFR decreases and kidney function deteriorates further, sodium and water retention are common, necessitating salt and water restrictions.

Hyperkalaemia develops as kidney disease progresses. Manifestations of hyperkalaemia, such as muscle weakness, paraesthesias and ECG changes, are not usually seen until the GFR is less than 5–10 mL/min. Phosphate excretion is also impaired, leading to hyperphosphataemia and hypocalcaemia. Reduced calcium absorption due to impaired vitamin D activation also contributes to hypocalcaemia. Hypermagnesaemia develops with advancing kidney disease; magnesium-containing antacids are avoided for this reason.

As kidney disease advances, hydrogen-ion excretion and buffer production are impaired, leading to metabolic acidosis. Respiratory rate and depth increase (Kussmaul's respirations) to compensate for metabolic acidosis. Although metabolic acidosis is often asymptomatic, other possible manifestations include general malaise, weakness, headache, nausea and vomiting, and abdominal pain (see the chapter 'Nursing care of people with altered fluid, electrolyte and acid–base balance').

Cardiovascular effects

In 2020, cardiovascular causes were attributed as the second leading cause of deaths in dialysis-dependent people in Australia and New Zealand, behind only withdrawal from dialysis treatment (ANZDATA Registry, 2021). A combination of malnutrition, inflammatory processes, vascular calcification, hypertension, dyslipidaemia and glucose intolerance all contribute to the increased cardiovascular burden on people with kidney disease (Jankowski et al., 2021). Cerebral and peripheral vascular manifestations of atherosclerosis are also seen.

Systemic hypertension is a common complication of ESKD Hypertension results from excess fluid volume, increased renin–angiotensin activity, increased peripheral vascular resistance and decreased prostaglandins. Increased extracellular fluid volume also can lead to oedema and heart failure. Pulmonary oedema may result from heart failure and increased permeability of the alveolar capillary membrane.

Retained metabolic toxins can irritate the pericardial sac, causing an inflammatory response and signs of pericarditis. *Cardiac tamponade*, a potential complication of pericarditis, occurs when inflammatory fluid in the pericardial sac interferes with ventricular filling and cardiac output.

Haematological effects

Anaemia is a common sequela in CKD and its cause is multifactorial. The kidneys produce erythropoietin, a hormone that controls RBC production. In kidney disease, erythropoietin production declines. Retained metabolic toxins further suppress RBC production and contribute to a shortened RBC lifespan. Nutritional deficiencies (iron and folate) and increased risk of blood loss from the GI tract also contribute to anaemia. (See the chapter 'Nursing care of people with haematological disorders' for more information on anaemia.)

Anaemia contributes to symptoms such as fatigue, weakness, depression and impaired cognition. It also affects cardiovascular

Multisystem effects of uraemia

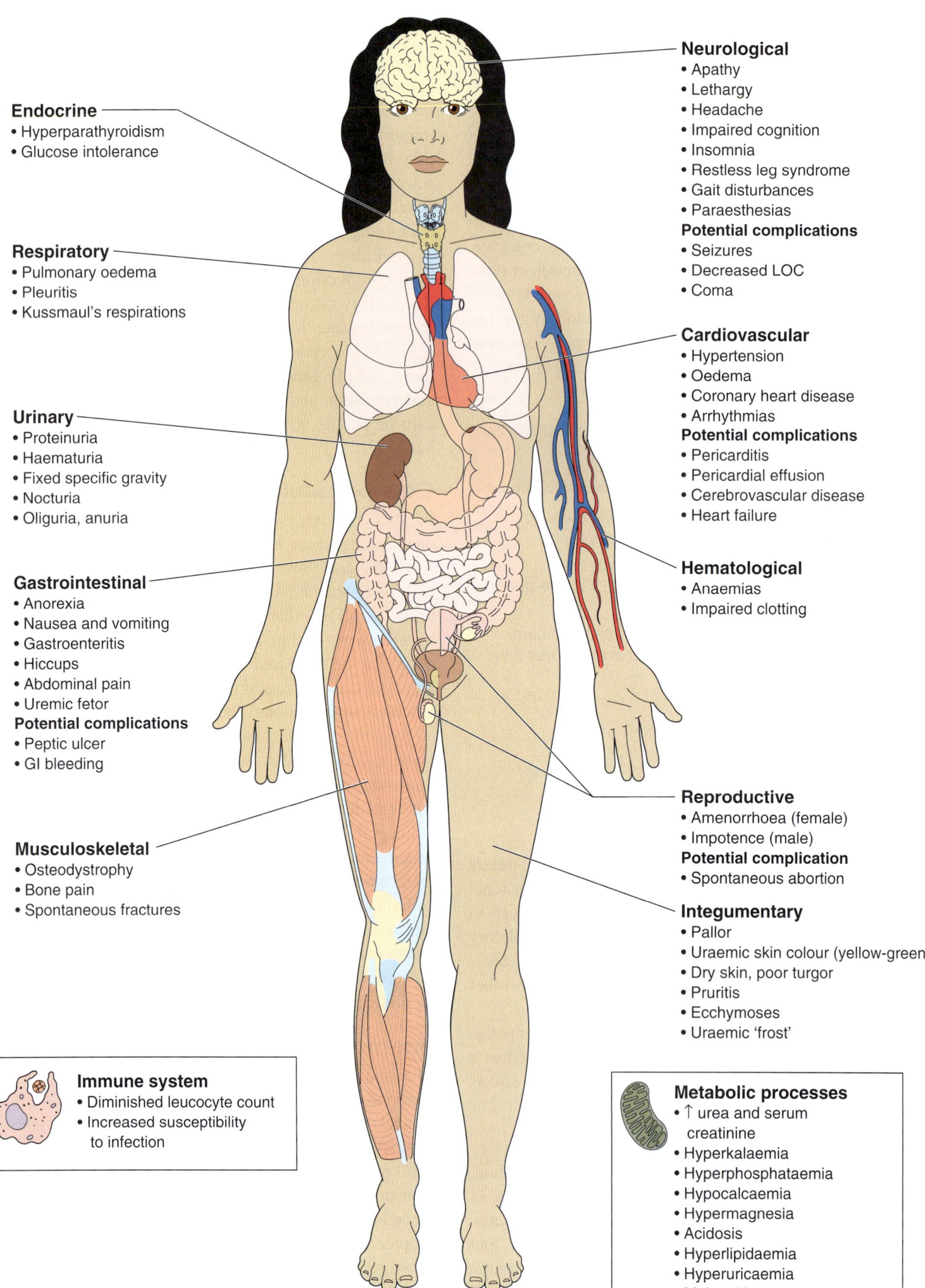

function, as the heart's natural response to anaemia is to increase cardiac output, which leads to increased cardiac remodelling and left ventricular hypertrophy. As such, anaemia is associated with an increased risk of cardiovascular disease.

People with kidney disease are at increased risk of bleeding disorders such as ecchymoses, epistaxis and GI bleeding. The combination of anaemia, platelet abnormalities, drug interactions, impaired platelet–vessel wall interaction and circulating uraemic toxins in the blood are all associated with this increased risk.

Immune system effects

Uraemia increases the risk of infection. High levels of urea and retained metabolic wastes impair all aspects of inflammation and immune function. The WBC declines, humoral and cell-mediated immunity are impaired and phagocyte function is defective. Both the acute inflammatory response and delayed hypersensitivity responses are affected (Amerman, 2018). Fever is suppressed, often delaying the diagnosis of infection.

Gastrointestinal effects

Anorexia, nausea and vomiting are the most common early symptoms of uraemia. Hiccups also are commonly experienced. Gastroenteritis is frequent. Ulcerations may affect any level of the GI tract and contribute to an increased risk of GI bleeding. Peptic ulcer disease is particularly common in people with uraemia. *Uraemic fetor*, a urine-like breath odour often associated with a metallic taste in the mouth, may develop. Uraemic fetor can further contribute to anorexia.

Neurological effects

Uraemia alters both central and peripheral nervous system function. CNS manifestations occur early and include changes in mentation, difficulty concentrating, fatigue and insomnia. Psychotic symptoms, seizures and coma are associated with advanced uraemic encephalopathy.

Peripheral neuropathy is also common in advanced uraemia. Both the sensory and motor tracts are involved. The lower limbs are initially affected. 'Restless leg syndrome', sensations of crawling or creeping, prickling or itching of the lower legs with frequent leg movement, increases during rest. Paraesthesias and sensory loss typically occur in a 'stocking-glove' pattern. As uraemia progresses, motor function is also impaired, causing muscle weakness, decreased deep tendon reflexes and gait disturbances.

Musculoskeletal effects

Hyperphosphataemia and hypocalcaemia associated with uraemia stimulate parathyroid hormone secretion. Parathyroid hormone causes increased calcium resorption from bone. In addition, osteoblast (bone-forming) and osteoclast (bone destructing) cell activity is affected. This bone resorption and remodelling combined with decreased vitamin D synthesis and decreased calcium absorption from the GI tract, lead to *renal osteodystrophy*. Osteodystrophy is characterised by *osteomalacia*, softening of the bones, and *osteoporosis*, decreased bone mass. Bone cysts may develop. Manifestations of osteodystrophy include bone tenderness, pain and muscle weakness, which all increase the risk of spontaneous fractures (Amerman, 2018).

Endocrine and metabolic effects

Accumulated waste products of protein metabolism are a primary factor involved in the effects and manifestations of uraemia. Serum creatinine and urea levels are significantly elevated. Uric acid levels are increased, contributing to an increased risk of gout.

Tissues become resistant to the effects of insulin in uraemia, leading to glucose intolerance. High blood triglyceride levels and lower than normal high-density lipoprotein (HDL) levels contribute to the accelerated atherosclerotic process.

Reproductive function is affected. Pregnancies are rarely carried to term and menstrual irregularities are common. Reduced testosterone levels, low sperm counts and impotence affect men with ESKD.

Dermatological effects

Anaemia and retained pigmented metabolites cause pallor and a yellowish hue to the skin in uraemia. Dry skin with poor turgor, a result of dehydration and sweat gland atrophy, is common. Bruising and excoriations are frequently seen. Metabolic wastes not eliminated by the kidneys may be deposited in the skin, contributing to itching or pruritus. In advanced uraemia, high levels of urea in the sweat may result in *uraemic frost*, crystallised deposits of urea on the skin.

INTERPROFESSIONAL CARE

Management of CKD (kidney failure) regardless of its aetiology focuses on identifying and slowing the progression of the underlying disease process, preserving renal function, preventing and managing complications, and providing psychological support. This aim is achieved through the collaboration of all members of the healthcare team.

Diagnostics

Laboratory and diagnostic testing are valuable to identify the cause of CKD, monitor kidney function and evaluate the efficacy of treatment. A number of tests and procedures may be performed to determine the underlying renal disease. (See Table 27.7 for normal laboratory values for commonly requested blood and urine tests.) Once the diagnosis is established, renal function is monitored primarily through blood levels of metabolic wastes and electrolytes. Imaging investigations provide information about the size and shape of the kidneys, possible tumours or cysts, the nature of the renal parenchyma and the presence of any obstruction. See the chapter 'A person-centred approach to assessing the renal system' for the nursing implications of selected tests.

The following studies may be ordered to help identify the underlying cause or aetiology:

- *eGFR* provides an estimation of the GFR. eGFR is used to evaluate renal function and may be reduced despite serum creatinine levels being in the normal range.

TABLE 27.7 Changes in laboratory values associated with kidney disease

TEST	NORMAL VALUE	ASSOCIATED WITH KIDNEY DISEASE
Urea, serum	3.5–7.2 mmol/L Slightly higher in older adults	Elevated in hypovolaemia, AKI, later stages of CKD Decreased in hypervolaemia and malnutrition
Creatinine, serum	Female: 50–110 µmol/L Male: 60–120 µmol/L Slightly lower in older adults	Elevated in hypovolaemia, AKI, later stages of CKD
eGFR	> 90 mL/min (young adults) eGFR declines naturally with age	See Figure 27.3 eGFR is not validated for use in children, Indigenous populations or AKI
Serum albumin	33–41 g/L	Decreased in nephrotic syndrome
Serum electrolytes	Potassium 3.7–5.2 mmol/L Sodium 136–144 mmol/L Calcium 2.18–2.49 mmol/L Ionised calcium 1.16–1.30 mmol/L Phosphorus 0.88–1.46 mmol/L	Increased in renal insufficiency Decreased in nephrotic syndrome Decreased in later stages of CKD and malabsorption Elevated in hypocalcaemia and later stages of CKD
Haemoglobin	115–165 g/L	Decreased in later stages of CKD. Target concentration of 110 g/L for stage 4 and 5 CKD/ESKD
Red blood cell count	Female: 3.8–5.8 × 10^{12}/L Male: 4.5–6.5 × 10^{12}/L	Decreased in later stages of CKD
Urinary ACR	Female: 3.5–35 mg/mmol Male: 2.6–25 mg/mmol Female: > 35 mg/mmol Male: > 25 mg/mmol	Microalbuminuria Macroalbuminuria
Urinary PCR	> 30 mg/mmol	Proteinuria
Urine red blood cells	< 2–3/HPF; no RBC casts	Present in glomerular disorders

- *Urea* is the end product of protein metabolism. It is created by the breakdown and metabolism of both dietary and body proteins. Urea is eliminated from the body by filtration in the glomerulus; minimal amounts are reabsorbed in the renal tubules. Glomerular diseases interfere with filtration and elimination of urea nitrogen, causing blood levels to rise. Increased protein catabolism (destruction), which may occur with GI bleeding or tissue breakdown, can also raise the urea level.
- *Serum creatinine* measures the amount of creatinine in the blood. Creatinine is the metabolic by-product of muscle metabolism and is produced in relatively constant amounts by skeletal muscles. It is excreted entirely by the kidneys, making serum creatinine a good indicator of kidney function. Normal values are lower in the older adult because of decreased muscle mass.
- *Serum electrolytes* are monitored throughout the course of CKD because impaired kidney function alters their excretion. The serum sodium may be within normal limits or low because of water retention. Potassium levels are elevated but usually remain below 6.5 mmol/L. Serum phosphate is elevated and the calcium level is decreased. Metabolic acidosis is identified by a low pH, low CO_2 and low bicarbonate levels.
- *Full blood count (FBC)* provides information about the degree of anaemia, with most people with stage 4 and 5 CKD showing decreased haematocrit, haemoglobin, RBCs and platelets.
- *Erythrocyte sedimentation rate (ESR)* is a general indicator of inflammatory response. It is generally elevated in conditions such as vasculitis, acute post-streptococcal glomerulonephritis and lupus nephritis.
- *C-reactive protein (CRP)* is a non-specific inflammatory marker and is used to indicate the presence of inflammatory states. It may be elevated in infective processes and in lupus nephritis.
- *Urinalysis* often reveals red blood cells (RBCs) and proteins in the urine of people with CKD. These substances, which normally are too large to enter glomerular filtrate, escape due to the increased permeability of the glomerular basement membrane.

PATIENT SAFETY COMPETENCY FRAMEWORK

6 Evidence-based practice

The Patient Safety Competency Framework indicates that nursing students should demonstrate evidence-based practice by their ability to plan and provide care that takes into account best available evidence and to assess, appraise and critique multiple sources of evidence (Levett-Jones et al., 2017).

In CKD, urinary specific gravity may be fixed at approximately 1.010, equivalent to that of plasma. This fixed specific gravity is due to impaired tubular secretion, reabsorption and urine concentrating ability. Abnormal proteins (e.g. Bence-Jones proteins), blood cells and cellular casts may also be noted in the urine.

- *Albumin:creatinine (ACR)* and *protein:creatinine ratio (PCR)* evaluates the urinary excretion of either albumin or protein and is considered best practice in the primary screening of CKD.
- *24-hour timed urine* enables the measurement of urinary protein and/or creatinine excretion over a 24-hour time period. Urine creatinine levels decrease when renal function is impaired because it is not effectively eliminated from the body.
- *Urine microbial culture and sensitivity* may be ordered to identify any urinary tract infection that may hasten the progress of CKD.
- *Throat or skin cultures* detect infection by group A beta-haemolytic *Streptococcus*. Although post-streptococcal glomerulonephritis typically follows the acute infection by 1 to 2 weeks, treatment to eradicate any remaining organisms is initiated to minimise antibody production.
- *Antistreptolysin O (ASO) titre* and other tests detect streptococcal exoenzymes (bacterial enzymes that stimulate the immune response in acute post-streptococcal glomerulonephritis). Other titres such as antistreptokinase (ASK) or antideoxyribonuclease B (ADNAase B) may be obtained as well.
- *Kidney biopsy*, microscopic examination of kidney tissue, assists in determining the cause of CKD, its prognosis and appropriate treatment. It is usually done percutaneously, by inserting a biopsy needle through the skin into the kidney to obtain a tissue sample. Open biopsy, which requires surgery, may also be done. Biopsy is not justified when clinical evidence makes diagnosis almost certain—for example, polycystic kidney disease. Other contraindications include small kidneys, single kidney, uncontrolled blood pressure and/or uraemia.
- *Kidney, ureter, bladder (KUB) ultrasound* is considered a first-line imaging technique and is used to evaluate kidney size and identify potential obstructions. It is a useful non-invasive technique to differentiate acute kidney injury from chronic kidney disease. In AKI, the kidneys may be enlarged, whereas they typically appear small and shrunken with decreased cortical width in CKD. Ultrasound can also detect renal masses and differentiate polycystic kidney disease from renal carcinoma.
- *Kidney scan*, a nuclear medicine procedure, allows visualisation and functional assessment of the kidneys after intravenous administration of a radioisotope.
- *Intravenous pyelogram (IVP), retrograde pyelography* or *antegrade pyelography* may also be used to evaluate kidney structure and function. Radiological contrast media are used with extreme caution because of their potential nephrotoxicity. Retrograde pyelography, in which contrast dye is injected into the ureters, and antegrade pyelography, in which the contrast medium is injected percutaneously into the renal pelvis, are preferred because they have fewer nephrotoxic effects than IVP.
- *Renal angiography* is used to investigate and evaluate renal blood flow and the major vasculature of the kidney and affords the opportunity for simultaneous interventional procedures such as stenting or angioplasty.
- *Computed tomography (CT) scan* is used to detect and differentiate kidney masses such as cystic disease or tumours. CT can determine tumour density, local extension of the tumour and any regional lymph node or vascular involvement.
- *Bone density scan* is used to assess bone mineral density, see the chapter 'A person-centred approach to assessing the musculoskeletal system' for more information.

See the chapter 'A person-centred approach to assessing the renal system' for nursing implications of tests used in renal medicine.

CONSIDERATION FOR PRACTICE

People with pre-existing kidney disease, volume depletion or advanced age are at high risk of contrast nephropathy if exposed to radiocontrast. Alert the treating team prior to any imaging procedure that requires radiocontrast if person is in high-risk category. It should also be noted if the patient is prescribed metformin, an oral antidiabetic agent. There is a risk of lactic acidosis if the drug is continued and the patient has renal issues related to the contrast. The drug should be withheld for 48 hours post administration of the contrast medium. Preventive methods surround adequate hydration. If not contraindicated, ensure the person remains well hydrated pre- and post procedure.

Medications

CKD affects both the pharmacokinetic and pharmacodynamic effects of drug therapy. Many medications are excreted primarily by the kidney. The half-life and plasma levels of many drugs increase in CKD. Drug absorption may be decreased when phosphate-binding agents are administered concurrently. Proteinuria can significantly reduce plasma protein levels, leading to toxicity when highly protein-bound drugs are given. In addition, any potentially nephrotoxic agent is avoided or used with extreme caution in people with CKD. Dose reductions may be required and/or dosing intervals are lengthened in CKD according to individual GFR.

As renal function declines, medications become an integral component of replacing diminished kidney function. Medications are used to treat underlying disorders, reduce inflammatory processes, manage symptoms and attempt to slow the progression of CKD.

Diuretics such as frusemide may be prescribed to reduce extracellular fluid volume and oedema. Diuretic therapy can also reduce hypertension and lower potassium levels. Thiazides such as hydrochlorothiazide, which are commonly used in combination with some antihypertensive classes, are less effective as diuretics when the eGFR falls below 25–30 mL/min but still remain effective in reducing hypertension as they reduce blood pressure through a vasodilatory effect.

ANTIHYPERTENSIVE AGENTS Antihypertensive agents are used to maintain the blood pressure within normal levels, slow the progression of CKD and prevent complications of coronary heart disease and cerebral vascular disease. Angiotensin-converting-enzyme (ACE) inhibitors and angiotensin receptor blockers (ARB) are the recommended classes of antihypertensive agents for the management of CKD, although any class of antihypertensive agent may be prescribed (see the chapter 'Nursing care of people with vascular and lymphatic disorders'). ACE inhibitors and ARBs have been demonstrated to reduce decline in renal function, particularly in people with moderate albuminuria (KDIGO, 2021b). In individuals with diabetes, this protection extends to individuals with a normal GFR who are potentially not yet showing signs of kidney disfunction, as well as providing further cardiovascular protection (KDIGO, 2021b).

DRUGS FOR ACID–BASE IMBALANCE AND ELECTROLYTE DISTURBANCES Other drugs may be used to manage electrolyte imbalances and acid–base imbalances. Sodium bicarbonate may be used to correct mild acidosis.

If the serum potassium rises to dangerously high levels, a combination of bicarbonate, insulin and glucose may be given intravenously to promote potassium movement into the cells. Sodium polystyrene sulfonate (Resonium), a potassium-ion exchange resin, can be given either orally or rectally (as an enema).

PHOSPHATE BINDERS AND AGENTS FOR RENAL OSTEODYSTROPHY Oral phosphate binding agents such as calcium carbonate are taken with food to lower serum phosphate levels and before or after food to normalise serum calcium levels. Aluminium hydroxide has a stronger phosphate binding potency, but its use is limited by complications such as encephalopathy and osteodystrophy associated with long-term administration (Coulson, 2022). Vitamin D analogues such as calcitriol may be given to improve gastrointestinal calcium absorption and normalise calcium levels. Bisphosphonates such as alendronate are contraindicated when the eGFR falls below 35 mL/min and are also contraindicated in hypocalcaemia. Cinacalcet belongs to a drug class termed 'calcimimetic' as it imitates calcium at the parathyroid gland to decrease output of parathyroid hormone due to secondary hyperparathyroidism. This slows down excessive bone turn-over and remodelling and lowers the chance of harmful metastatic calcification.

ERYTHROPOIETIN STIMULATING AGENTS AND MEDICATIONS USED IN ANAEMIA Folic acid and iron supplements are given to combat anaemia associated with CKD due to impaired erythropoiesis and shortened red blood cell survival. A multivitamin preparation is also often prescribed due to anorexia, nausea and dietary restrictions limiting nutrient intake. Recombinant human erythropoietin stimulates the proliferation and differentiation of erythroid progenitors, which in turn increase haemoglobin synthesis and accelerate the release of reticulocytes (young RBCs) from the bone marrow. There are five erythropoietin stimulating agents (ESAs) currently on the Australian market. These are epoetin alfa (Eprex), epoetin beta (NeoRecormon), epoetin lambda (Novicrit), methoxy polyethylene glycol-epoetin beta (Mircera) and darbepoetin (Aranesp). There is little difference between the agents in terms of efficacy and the choice is governed by factors such as frequency and route of administration.

ANTIBIOTICS Antibiotics, usually from the penicillin family, are prescribed for the person with post-streptococcal glomerulonephritis to eradicate any remaining bacteria, removing the stimulus for antibody production. Nephrotoxic antibiotics such as aminoglycosides are avoided but will be administered in cases where the benefit outweighs the risk. Both vancomycin and gentamicin are cleared by the kidneys, so re-dosing is titrated according to serum levels.

ANALGESIA Non-steroidal anti-inflammatory medications such as ibuprofen may be avoided due to their nephrotoxic nature. Pethidine is avoided altogether as its metabolite is cleared by the kidneys and accumulation will cause seizures. Morphine may be avoided due its metabolite, M6G, accumulating in kidney disease but may be administered sparingly and with caution for acute pain episodes such as chest pain. Fentanyl and oxycodone are generally preferred due to the liver metabolising them into inactive metabolites.

IMMUNOSUPPRESSANTS Aggressive immunosuppressive therapy is used to treat acute inflammatory processes such as rapidly progressive glomerulonephritis, Goodpasture's syndrome and exacerbations of SLE. When commenced early, immunosuppressive therapy significantly reduces the risk of ESKD (kidney failure (CKD stage 5)). Corticosteroids such as prednisolone are often used in large doses for several months, sometimes in combination with other immunosuppressants such as azathioprine and cyclophosphamide. Corticosteroids may also be used to induce remission of nephritic syndrome. However, in post-streptococcal glomerulonephritis, they may actually worsen the condition, so are usually avoided. See the transplant section of this chapter and the chapter 'Nursing care of people with altered immunity' for more information about corticosteroids and other immunosuppressive drugs.

Nutrition and fluid management

As renal function declines, the elimination of water, solutes and metabolic wastes is impaired. Accumulation of these wastes in the body leads to uraemic symptoms. Instituted early in the course of CKD, dietary modifications can reduce uraemic symptoms and help prevent complications.

Unlike carbohydrates and fats, the body is unable to store excess proteins. Unused dietary proteins are degraded into urea and other nitrogenous wastes, which are then eliminated by the kidneys. Protein-rich foods also contain inorganic ions such as hydrogen ion, phosphate and sulfites that are eliminated by the kidneys. Consequently, dietary protein intake should be assessed by a renal dietitian with a bias towards optimising nutritional status.

A daily protein intake of 0.6–0.8 g/kg/day of ideal body weight provides the amino acids necessary for tissue repair in order to maintain body composition for people with CKD, provided the protein is of high biological value (Ko et al., 2017).

TABLE 27.8 Foods high in potassium or phosphate and some low-value alternatives

HIGH POTASSIUM	LOW POTASSIUM
Fruit and vegetable juices (except cranberry, lemon), bananas, apricots, plums, dried fruit, nuts and seeds, legumes, potatoes, avocados, tomatoes and tomato paste	Cranberry juice, apples, pears, blueberries, lychees, green beans, zucchinis, onions, strawberries, raspberries, lettuce, lemons
HIGH PHOSPHATE	**LOW PHOSPHATE**
Milk, eggs, cheese, meats, offal, poultry, fish, cola drinks and soy	Pasta, rice, corn cereals, popcorn, green beans, non-cola-based drinks and cordial

Carbohydrate and fat intake may need to be increased to maintain ideal body weight and energy requirements and is dependent on the rate of physical activity.

Water and sodium intake are regulated to maintain the extracellular fluid volume at normal levels. Water intake of 1,000 to 2,000 mL per day is generally recommended to maintain water balance. Sodium is restricted to 100 mmol or 2,300 mg per day initially and equates to the equivalent of a 'no added salt' diet. More stringent fluid and sodium restrictions may be necessary as CKD progresses. An individual's fluid retention may be monitored by observing and identifying rapid changes in body weight, as well as other signs of fluid retention such as oedema and increased respiratory effort.

When the GFR falls to less than 10 to 20 mL/min, potassium and phosphorus intake may also be restricted. Potassium intake is generally limited to 1 mmol/kg of ideal body weight per day. The person is cautioned to avoid using salt substitutes, which typically contain high levels of potassium chloride. See Table 27.8 for foods high in potassium and phosphorus and some low-potassium and low-phosphorus alternatives.

It is vital that any recommended dietary changes are made in consultation with a specialty dietitian.

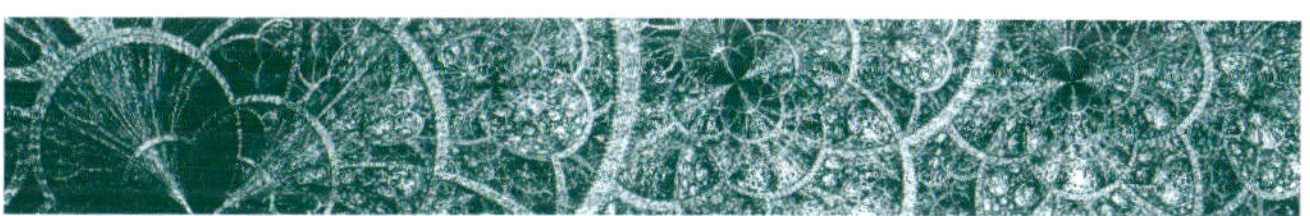

Nursing care

The clinical setting, whether it is in the community or a secondary or tertiary referral hospital, determines the nursing care.

Upon diagnosis of CKD, regardless of the clinical setting, the teaching of self-management principles begins. The principal nursing diagnosis at this time may be *Deficient knowledge* in relation to understanding of disease process and measures to help preserve kidney function. The nurse, in partnership with the person, should establish priorities for management and collaborate with other members of the interprofessional team as required. Ensure that the person and family understand and are able to discuss the following topics.

- information about the disease and the prognosis
- prescribed treatment, including activity and diet restrictions; the use and potential effects, both beneficial and adverse, of all medications
- risks, manifestations, prevention and management of complications such as fluid retention and infection
- signs, symptoms and implications of declining kidney function
- measures to prevent further kidney damage, including eliminating modifiable risk factors and avoiding nephrotoxic drugs
- community resources, such as home care providers and support groups.

Assist people with CKD to learn about the underlying pathology of their specific disease process, its treatment and usual course. Discuss measures to maintain optimal kidney function and the importance of avoiding additional insults to their kidneys. Include extra information about preventing UTI (such as hygiene measures) and early manifestations of UTI. Stress the importance of seeking treatment to prevent further kidney damage. Advise to avoid drugs that are potentially toxic to the kidneys and to check with the primary care provider before taking any new drug, including over-the-counter and complementary medicines.

For those with polycystic kidney disease, discuss the potential benefits of genetic counselling and screening of family members for evidence of the disease. This is particularly important if kidney transplantation is contemplated and family members are potential donors.

Health promotion

Measures to reduce the risk of CKD focus on preventing kidney disease, particularly in those with diabetes and hypertension. The rates of obesity in Australia demonstrate an independent risk factor linking increased BMI to type 2 diabetes, hypertension and cardiovascular disease. Deal with modifiable risk factors promptly, including the maintenance of a healthy diet, regular exercise and smoking cessation. Promote early and effective treatment of all infections, including skin and pharyngeal infections caused by streptococcal bacteria. Discuss measures to reduce the risk of urinary tract infections and stress the importance of prompt treatment to eradicate the infecting organism. Discuss the relationship between diabetes, hypertension and kidney disease. Emphasise that maintaining blood glucose levels and blood pressure within the recommended ranges reduces the risk of adverse effects on the kidneys. Reiterate the importance of avoiding drugs and substances that are potentially toxic to the kidneys. Ensure that all people with reduced kidney function are well hydrated, particularly when a potentially nephrotoxic drug is prescribed or anticipated. Finally, encourage people approaching ESKD (kidney failure (CKD stage 5)) to discuss their options for transplantation, dialysis modalities and supportive care with their nephrologist, Nurse Practitioner and/or CKD educator.

Assessment

Review the chapter 'A person-centred approach to assessing the renal system' for complete assessment of the kidney and urinary systems. Focused assessment data related to CKD include the following:

- *Health history*: complaints of facial or peripheral oedema or weight gain, fatigue, nausea and vomiting, headache, general malaise, abdominal or flank pain; cough or shortness of breath; changes in amount, colour or character of urine (e.g. frothy urine); history of skin or pharyngeal streptococcal infection, diabetes, SLE or kidney disease; current medications.
- *Physical examination*: general appearance; vital signs; weight; fluid balance; presence of periorbital, facial or peripheral oedema; skin for lesions, infection; inspect throat, obtain culture as indicated; urine specimen for colour, character, odour.

Nursing diagnoses and interventions

Nursing care is supportive and educational. Monitoring kidney function and fluid volume status is a key component of care, as is protecting the person from infection. Both manifestations of CKD and its treatment can interfere with a person's ability to maintain usual roles and responsibilities.

Excess fluid volume

Excess fluid volume and resulting oedema are common manifestations of glomerular disorders. When proteins are lost in the urine, the oncotic pressure of plasma falls and fluid shifts into the interstitial spaces. The body responds to this fluid shift by retaining sodium and water to maintain intravascular volume, leading to excess fluid volume.

- Monitor vital signs, including blood pressure, apical pulse, respirations and breath sounds 4-hourly or as indicated by acuity of presentation. Report significant changes. *Excess fluid increases the cardiac workload and the blood pressure. Tachycardia may result. Associated electrolyte imbalances can cause arrhythmias. Increased pulmonary vascular pressure can lead to pulmonary oedema, tachypnoea, dyspnoea and crackles (rales) in the lungs.*
- Record fluid intake and output as indicated. *Accurate fluid balance records help determine fluid volume status.*

> **CONSIDERATION FOR PRACTICE**
> **Weigh daily, using consistent technique (time of day, scale and clothing). Accurate daily weights are the best indicator of approximate fluid balance.**

- Monitor serum electrolytes, haemoglobin and haematocrit, urea, creatinine and eGFR. *Glomerular disorders affect fluid balance and may alter electrolyte balance as well, potentially leading to complications such as cardiac arrhythmias (see the chapter 'Nursing care of people with altered fluid, electrolyte and acid–base balance'). Increased intravascular volume can result in low haemoglobin and haematocrit values. Low haemoglobin may also be due to impaired erythropoietin production. Urea, creatinine and eGFR provide information about renal function.*
- Maintain fluid restriction as ordered. Offer ice chips (in limited and measured amounts) and frequent mouth care to relieve thirst. With the person, develop a fluid intake schedule. *Fluids may be restricted to reduce fluid overload, oedema and hypertension. Ice chips and frequent mouth care moisten mucous membranes and help relieve thirst while maintaining oral tissue integrity. Including the person in planning fluid intake promotes a sense of autonomy and understanding of the treatment regimen.*

> **CONSIDERATION FOR PRACTICE**
> **Carefully monitor and regulate intravenous infusions; include fluid used to dilute IV medications as intake. Significant 'hidden' fluid intake can occur with intravenous medication administration.**

- Arrange dietary consultation regarding sodium-, potassium- or protein-restricted diets. Include the person and dietitian in planning to allow individualisation of the diet to person preferences. *The glomerular disorder may reduce appetite; considering food preferences can help maintain adequate nutrition.*
- Monitor for desired and adverse effects of prescribed medications. *Diuretic therapy helps reduce excess fluid volume; however, glomerular disorders can affect the person's response to treatment. In addition, diuretics can exacerbate the electrolyte imbalances and muscle weakness often associated with glomerular disorders.*
- Provide frequent position changes and good skin care. *Perfusion may be altered by tissue oedema, increasing the risk of breakdown.*

Fatigue

Fatigue is a common manifestation of CKD. Anaemia, loss of plasma proteins, headache, anorexia and nausea compound this fatigue. The ability to maintain usual physical and mental activities may be impaired.

- Schedule activities and procedures to provide adequate rest and energy conservation. Prevent unnecessary fatigue. *Adequate rest and energy conservation reduce fatigue and improve the person's ability to tolerate and cope with required treatments and activities.*
- Assist with ADLs as needed. The goal is to conserve limited energy reserves.
- Discuss the relationship between fatigue and the disease process with the person and family. *Understanding the nature of the disease and associated fatigue helps the person and family cope with reduced energy and comply with prescribed rest.*
- Reduce energy demands with frequent, small meals and short periods of activity. *Small, frequent meals reduce the energy needed for eating and digestion. In addition, nurses can assist the fatigued person who may be reluctant to ask visitors to leave by limiting visits and numbers of visitors as discussed with the person.*

Ineffective protection

People with CKD are at high risk of infection. The use of some drug classes in specific treatments can depress the immune system further. The anti-inflammatory effect of corticosteroids may also mask early symptoms of infection.

CONSIDERATION FOR PRACTICE

Monitor vital signs, temperature and mental status 4 hourly or as indicated. An elevated temperature may indicate infection; anti-inflammatory drugs may moderate this response. Tachycardia, increasing lethargy or confusion may be the initial signs of infection.

- Assess frequently for other signs of infection such as purulent wound drainage, productive cough, adventitious breath sounds and red or inflamed lesions. Monitor for manifestations of UTI, such as dysuria, frequency and urgency, and cloudy, foul-smelling urine. *Early identification and treatment of infection is important to prevent systemic complications in the susceptible person.*
- Monitor FBC, focusing on the WCC and differential. *An elevated WCC and increased numbers of immature white cells in the blood (left shift) may be early indicators of infection.*
- Use standard precautions and good hand hygiene. Protect from cross-infection by providing a single room, where possible, and restricting ill visitors. *People with decreased resistance to infection need increased protection.*
- Avoid or minimise invasive procedures. *Maintaining the protective skin barrier is especially important for the person with altered immune status.*
- If catheterisation is required, use sterile intermittent straight catheterisation or maintain a closed drainage system for an indwelling catheter. Prevent urine reflux from the drainage system to the bladder or the bladder to the kidneys by ensuring a patent, gravity flow system. *The urinary tract is a frequent entry point for infection, particularly in the hospitalised person. Maintaining strict asepsis during catheterisation is vital. Intermittent catheterisation is associated with a lower risk of UTI than an indwelling catheter.*
- Provide a nutritionally sound diet with complete proteins. *A well-balanced, nutritionally sound diet is important to maintain nutritional status and support immune function.*
- Teach measures to prevent infection. *Care is often provided in the home, requiring the person and family to use appropriate infection control measures.*

Ineffective role performance and anticipatory grieving

Strategies to support people with ineffective role performance and anticipatory grieving are similar and revolve around support processes. The manifestations and treatment of CKD can affect the ability to maintain usual roles and activities. In addition, the person may express feelings associated with the loss of function and lifestyle. Fatigue and muscle weakness may limit physical and social activities. If uraemia is present, malaise, nausea and mental status changes can interfere with role function. Facial and periorbital oedema affect the person's self-esteem and may lead to isolation.

- Establish a strong therapeutic relationship. *It is important to gain the person's trust and confidence to afford them the opportunity to share their feelings.*
- Encourage self-care and participation in decision making. *Increased autonomy helps to restore self-confidence and reduce powerlessness.*
- Provide time for verbalisation of thoughts and feelings; listen actively, acknowledging and accepting fears and concerns. *Adequate time and active listening encourage expression of concerns and the effect of the disease or treatments on daily life. This helps the person deal with the illness, its treatment and associated losses.*
- Support coping skills, helping the person identify personal strengths. *This support helps the person gain confidence.*
- When possible, enlist the support of family, other people and friends. *These people can provide physical, psychological, emotional and social support.*
- Discuss the effect of the disease and treatments on roles and relationships, helping identify potential changes in roles, relationships and lifestyle. Help the person and family develop a plan for alternative behaviours and relationships, encouraging the person to maintain usual roles to the extent possible. *Developing a plan helps reduce the strain of role changes and maintain a sense of dignity and control.*
- Provide accurate and optimistic information about the disorder and its short- and long-term effects. *The person and family need accurate information to plan for the future.*
- Evaluate the need for additional support and social services for the person and family. Provide referrals as indicated. *Depending on the person and family strengths, the severity of the disorder and its treatment and prognosis, ongoing social support services may be necessary to facilitate coping and adaptation.*

Community-based care

Whereas hospital-based care is focused on treating the complications of CKD symptomology, community care is focused on primary prevention, screening practices and the teaching of self-management principles. The cornerstone of any primary prevention program is the screening of people in 'at-risk' categories (see Box 27.2). Screening programs, whether they are opportunistic or systematic, assist in identifying people with CKD and afford the opportunity to initiate timely intervention to prevent the progression to ESKD (kidney failure (CKD stage 5)). Nurses are ideally placed to identify at-risk people and implement screening strategies to identify people with CKD. One of the wonders of screening strategies for CKD is that they are predominantly non-invasive and non-expensive (see Box 27.3). Urinalysis and blood pressure measurements are key screening techniques for detecting glomerular dysfunction (i.e. microalbuminuria or proteinuria) and hypertension. Kidney function can also be measured through eGFR from a simple blood test. CKD is progressive in nature; its course is generally lengthy but may also progress rapidly in some cases.

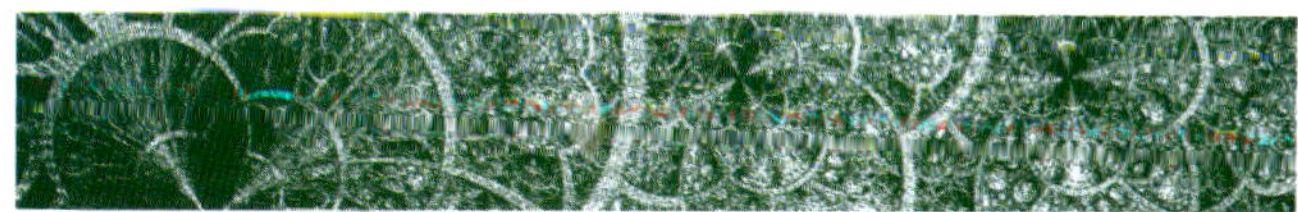

BOX 27.2 Major risk factors for chronic kidney disease (CKD)

- Diabetes
- High blood pressure
- Aged over 60 years
- Smoking
- Obesity
- Family history of kidney disease
- Aboriginal and/or Torres Strait Islander origin
- Established cardiovascular disease

BOX 27.3 The kidney health check

1. Blood test for eGFR to check kidney function
2. Urine test for albumin:creatinine ratio (ACR)
3. Check blood pressure for presence of hypertension

THE PERSON WITH END-STAGE KIDNEY DISEASE (KIDNEY FAILURE (CKD STAGE 5))

Kidney replacement therapy

Kidney replacement therapy (KRT) (previously referred to as renal replacement therapy (RRT)), used to treat ESKD (kidney failure (CKD stage 5)), is provided through haemodialysis, peritoneal dialysis or kidney transplantation. ESKD (kidney failure (CKD stage 5)) is reached when glomerular function decreases to a level of less than 15 mL/min (KDIGO, 2013). In Australia, dialysis and transplantation have been available since the early 1960s. The first dialysis was performed in Brisbane in 1954 (Dique, 1955). The first successful transplant was performed in Adelaide in 1965 (Lawrence, 1994).

KRT involves considerable individual and healthcare burdens. In 2020, Australia had 3,259 new KRT patients and an overall incidence rate of 127 per million population. The rate has remained stable for several years (ANZDATA Registry, 2021). In 2020, 885 kidney transplants were performed in Australia, a decrease on preceding years when over 1,000 kidney transplants had been performed each year (ANZDATA Registry, 2021). This was likely a result of the COVID-19 pandemic. The number of people receiving KRT will likely continue to increase, placing an enormous burden on future Australian healthcare resources.

Dialysis

Dialysis is the diffusion of solute molecules across a semipermeable membrane from an area of higher solute concentration to one of lower concentration. It is used to remove excess fluid and metabolic waste products in kidney failure. During dialysis, blood is separated from a dialysis solution by a semipermeable membrane. Both haemodialysis and peritoneal dialysis rely on the principle of diffusion to remove wastes from people during KRT. Dialysis is a life-sustaining treatment and an alternative when kidney transplant is not an option or not the chosen KRT of the person with kidney failure.

Of the 14,554 people receiving dialysis for treatment of kidney failure in 2020, approximately 83% were receiving haemodialysis and 17% were receiving peritoneal dialysis (ANZDATA Registry, 2021). Care involving dialysis is by far the most common reason for hospital admissions in Australia (AIHW, 2018). Unfortunately, there are significantly higher rates of admission for dialysis in Aboriginal and Torres Strait Islander populations and lower socioeconomic groups (AIHW, 2018).

Both peritoneal dialysis and haemodialysis can be undertaken safely at home. Benefits of home-based dialysis include greater flexibility for the person, improved mortality and decreased cost of overall for treatment of kidney failure (Choo et al., 2019; Marshall et al., 2021; Wong et al., 2019). Home dialysis can be performed more frequently and can suit the person's lifestyle (Sauve, Digel Vandyk & Fothergill Bourbonnais, 2016). Despite this, rates have not increased significantly in recent years (ANZDATA Registry, 2021). Employment and availability of a dialysis centre become the primary factors influencing the choice of haemodialysis or peritoneal dialysis (Bennett, Schatell & Shah, 2015).

People on long-term dialysis have a higher risk of complications and death than the general population. Mortality rates are higher with older age, diabetes, Indigenous status and coronary artery disease (ANZDATA Registry, 2021). Although dialysis and transplantation can provide lifesaving treatment, another option for people approaching kidney failure is supportive care.

Supportive care

The decision to initiate dialysis is not easy as dialysis only manages the symptoms of ESKD and is not a cure. Although many people on dialysis still maintain jobs, dialysis requires considerable support from healthcare professionals and significant others as people can be challenged with the day-to-day stress that accompanies dialysis treatment. Many people live with constant lethargy, never feeling truly well and may feel powerless because of their dependence on others for treatment. In the end, the person may choose supportive care rather than undergoing dialysis or transplantation.

Supportive care in the context of ESKD describes the active therapy that is delivered without dialysis or transplantation. Due to the high symptom burden in ESKD, renal supportive care includes appropriate symptom management, care coordination and ongoing education for patients, families and health professional staff. Although supportive care is increasingly being offered in Australia and globally, patients commonly report a greater emphasis on dialysis and transplant over supportive care (Hole et al., 2020; Moustakas, Bennett & Tranter, 2015). Given that quality of life is often compromised by dialysis and the mortality rates over 65 years are comparable to supportive care (Hole et al., 2020), supportive care is a legitimate therapy option for any person with ESKD (kidney failure (CKD stage 5)).

Haemodialysis

Haemodialysis uses the principles of diffusion and ultrafiltration to remove electrolytes, waste products and excess water from the body. Blood is pumped from the person via a vascular access to the dialyser (see Figure 27.7). The porous semi-permeable membranes of the dialyser allow small molecules such as water, glucose and electrolytes to pass through, but block larger molecules such as serum proteins and blood cells. The **dialysate**, a solution of approximately the same composition and temperature as normal extracellular fluid, passes along the other side of the membrane allowing small solute molecules to move freely across the membrane by diffusion.

The direction of movement for any substance is determined by the concentrations of that substance in the blood and the dialysate. Electrolytes and waste products such as urea and creatinine diffuse from the blood into the dialysate. Essential electrolytes such as calcium or potassium may be added to the dialysate to reduce excessive removal. Excess water is removed by creating a negative pressure onto the blood moving through the dialyser. This process is known as **ultrafiltration**.

Haemodialysis is predominantly performed three times a week, varying from 3 to 8 hours per treatment with the majority of people receiving 4 to 5 hours per treatment or 12 to 15 hours per week (ANZDATA Registry, 2021). Haemodialysis is performed most frequently in satellite, or community, settings that are nurse run and require little nephrologist management input (Damasiewicz & Polkinghorne, 2020). The most frequent complications during dialysis (intradialytic) are hypotension and muscle cramps (Karimi, Dideban & Heidari, 2022). Infection, malnutrition and vascular access problems are common long-term complications of haemodialysis.

Following are complications associated with haemodialysis:

- Hypotension, the most common complication of haemodialysis, is related to changes in serum osmolality, rapid removal of fluid from the vascular compartment, vasodilation and other factors.
- Bleeding is related to altered platelet function associated with uraemia, use of anticoagulation during dialysis and complications of vascular access.
- Infection (local or systemic) is related to WBC damage and immune system suppression. *Staphylococcus aureus* septicaemia is commonly associated with contamination of the vascular access site.

See the accompanying box for nursing care of the person undergoing intermittent haemodialysis.

Haemodiafiltration combines the processes of haemodialysis and greater ultrafiltration in an attempt to better mimic the function of the healthy kidney (Ward, 2022). Large amounts of fluid are removed from the blood and then replaced before and/or after the haemofilter. Both diffusion and convection occurs during this process. The advantage of haemodiafiltration is that a greater range of solutes can be removed through increased convection. Continuous haemodiafiltration, known as CVVHDF, is used in acutely ill people through continuous therapy.

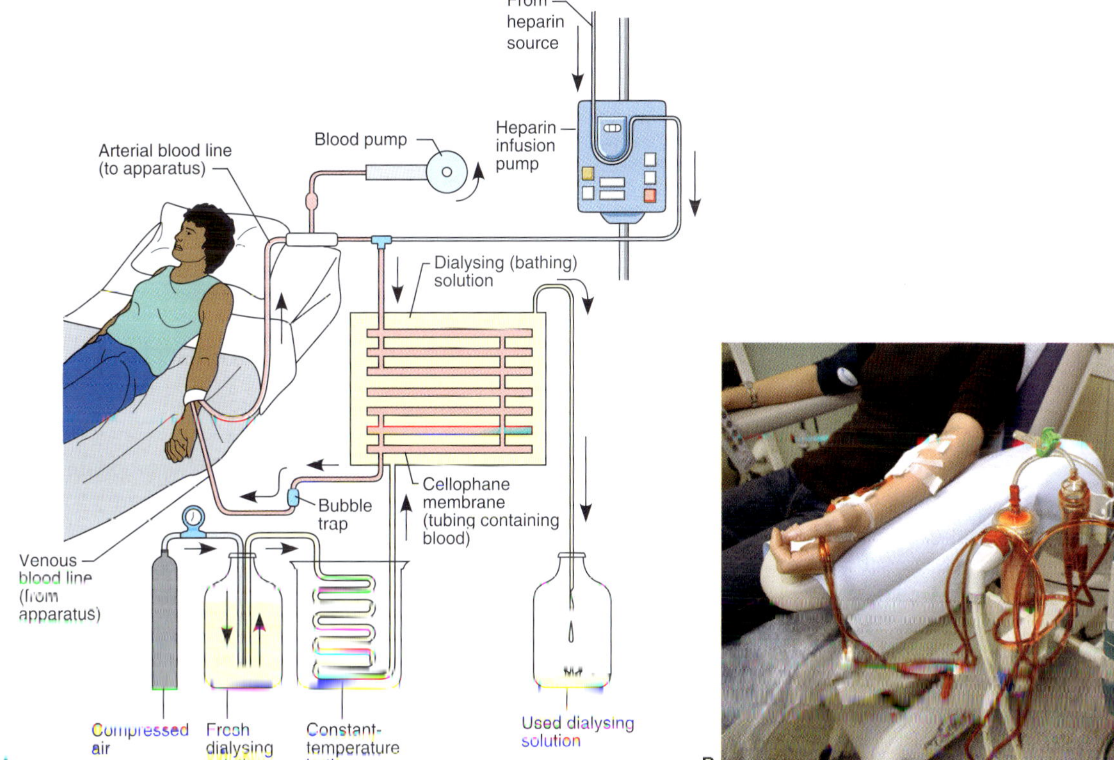

FIGURE 27.7 *A, The components of a haemodialysis system. B, A person receiving haemodialysis*

Source: B, © AJ Photo/Science Photo Library.

NURSING CARE OF THE PERSON undergoing intermittent haemodialysis

PRE-DIALYSIS CARE

- Assess vital signs, including blood pressures as required (lying, sitting and standing), pulse, respirations and lung sounds. *These data provide baseline information to help evaluate the effects of haemodialysis. Hypertension or hypotension may indicate excess fluid volume. The person who is hypotensive may not tolerate rapid fluid volume changes during dialysis. Abnormal heart sounds (e.g. a gallop or murmur) and changes in heart rate or rhythm may indicate excess fluid volume or electrolyte imbalance. Fluid overload may also cause dyspnoea, tachypnoea and rales or crackles in the lungs.*
- Record weight. *Weight changes are an indicator of fluid volume and nutritional status and assist in determining amount of ultrafiltration required.*
- Assess vascular access site for a palpable thrill and bruit, and for inflammation. *Infection and thrombus formation are the most common problems affecting the access site in haemodialysis people.*
- Alert all staff to avoid using the extremity with the AVF or AVG (or the non-dominant arm, if long-term access has not been established) for blood pressures or venepuncture. *These procedures may damage vessels and lead to failure of the arteriovenous fistula.*

INTRADIALYTIC CARE

- Assess and document vital signs during dialysis treatment. *Fluid removal may lead to hypotension.*
- Assess and treat other signs of volume depletion such as cramp, headaches, dizziness and nausea. Reset ultrafiltration as required. *Hypotension may lead to cramp and/or nausea and vomiting, among other symptoms. Severe episodes may lead to loss of consciousness.*
- Respond to dialysis machine blood circuit alarms. *Arterial pressure and/or venous pressure may indicate access or volume status complications.*
- Assess access sites for signs of bleeding. *Dialysis anticoagulation and/or complications of access may contribute to bleeding around access sites.*
- Use aseptic technique during cannulation technique and when accessing the blood circuit. *Poor aseptic technique may lead to infection.*

POST-DIALYSIS CARE

- Assess and document vital signs, weight and vascular access site condition. *Weight and vital signs are used to assess fluid removal goals. Fluid removal during dialysis can lead to hypotension.*
- Review urea, serum creatinine, serum electrolyte and haemoglobin levels between dialysis treatments. *These values determine the prescription of dialysis therapy, medications and dietary restrictions, including fluid.*
- Assess for other adverse effects of dialysis, such as hypovolaemia, nausea and vomiting, muscle cramps, neurological symptoms or altered levels of consciousness. *Excess fluid removal and rapid changes in electrolyte balance can lead to complications including fluid deficit, electrolyte imbalances or dialysis disequilibrium syndrome.*
- Assess for bleeding at the access site or elsewhere. Use standard precautions at all times. *Kidney failure and anticoagulation during dialysis increase the risk of bleeding.*
- Provide psychological support and listen actively. Address concerns and accept responses such as anger and depression. Reinforce person and family strengths in coping with kidney failure and haemodialysis. *Grieving is a normal response to loss of organ function. The person may feel hopeless or helpless and resent dependence on a machine. The nurse can help the person and family work through these responses and focus on positive aspects of living.*
- Refer to social services and counselling as indicated. *People with kidney failure may need additional support services to help them adapt to and live with their disease.*

Links to National Patient Safety Standards

NSQHS: Recognising and Responding to Acute Deterioration Standard

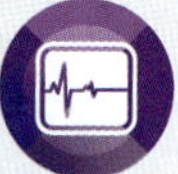

The intention of this standard is 'to ensure a person's acute deterioration is recognised promptly and appropriate action is taken' (ACSQHC, 2021, p. 67).

Implementing this standard is achieved by the establishment of systems to assist with recognition, initiating appropriate responses and ensuring meaningful and appropriate communication between all individuals involved in a person's care (including patients, families and carers).

Comprehensive and ongoing assessment of a person's kidney function should be undertaken and documented as frequently as clinically necessary to facilitate rapid, responsive action in the event of a person's deterioration. Treatment may be pharmacological but may also include acute kidney replacement therapy. Advanced planning should be undertaken prior to the potential rapid deterioration of kidney function to ensure treatment decisions are patient centred.

Source: ACSQHC (2021). *National Safety and Quality Health Service Standards* (2nd ed.). Sydney: ACSQHC. © Australian Commission on Safety and Quality in Health Care.

Vascular access

Access to the blood is required for haemodialysis and is commonly termed 'vascular access'. Vascular access can be in the form of arteriovenous fistula (AVF), arteriovenous graft (AVG) or central venous access device (CVAD). AVF is the preferred vascular access with decreased complications compared with grafts and catheters. In Australia, prevalent haemodialysis access comprises AVFs and AVGs at 83% and CVADs at 17% (ANZDATA Registry, 2021).

An AVF is formed by creating a surgical connection between an artery and a vein. In preparation for fistula formation, the access limb should not be used for venipuncture or blood pressure monitoring. The preferred vessels used to create an AVF are the radial artery and cephalic vein; however, other veins and arteries can be used. It takes approximately 4 to 6 weeks for the pressure in the artery to engorge and enlarge the veins. Once the veins are large enough and providing an adequate blood flow, the fistula can be used for circulation of blood during haemodialysis. A functional AVF has a palpable thrill and a bruit on auscultation. Ultrasound may be used as a further tool for assessment and to guide accurate cannulation (Schoch et al., 2019).

AVFs are cannulated with a specialty large-gauge dialysis needle to prevent the destruction of red blood cells during the long hours and high blood flows required for dialysis (Kumbar, Ramani & Brouwer-Maier, 2020). The needle is most often metal; however, plastic cannulae for dialysis have become available in recent years (Kumbar et al., 2020). A method of cannulation called 'rope ladder', where cannulation sites are rotated across the full length of the AVF, is recommended to decrease risks of infection, prolonged bleeding and aneurysm (Kumbar et al., 2020).

An arteriovenous graft may be created if AVF construction is not possible, often as a result of poor blood vessel condition. AVGs are most commonly made of polytetrafluoroethelene (PTFE) material. The graft is surgically implanted, connecting blood flow from the artery to the vein, thus providing sites for cannulation and adequate blood flow for haemodialysis. AVGs can be constructed in the arm or leg. Unlike AVFs, grafts can often be used soon after surgery. However, they are associated with higher infection and thrombosis rates (Thwaites, Holt & Yii, 2020). Haemodialysis Reliable Outflow (HeRO) grafts are a further option, comprising a of PTFE graft connecting an artery to a silicone lumen that returns blood directly to the right atrium (Hunter et al., 2019).

Central venous access devices (CVADs) are double-lumen catheters inserted into the internal jugular or femoral vein (see Figure 27.8). CVADs for dialysis can be temporary, inserted percutaneously and sutured in situ for use over a few weeks, or long-term tunnelled and cuffed catheters for indefinite long-term use (Lok et al., 2020). All CVADs draw blood into the catheter through small openings in the proximal portion of one lumen and return to the circulation through a second lumen to minimise recirculation of the blood that has just been dialysed.

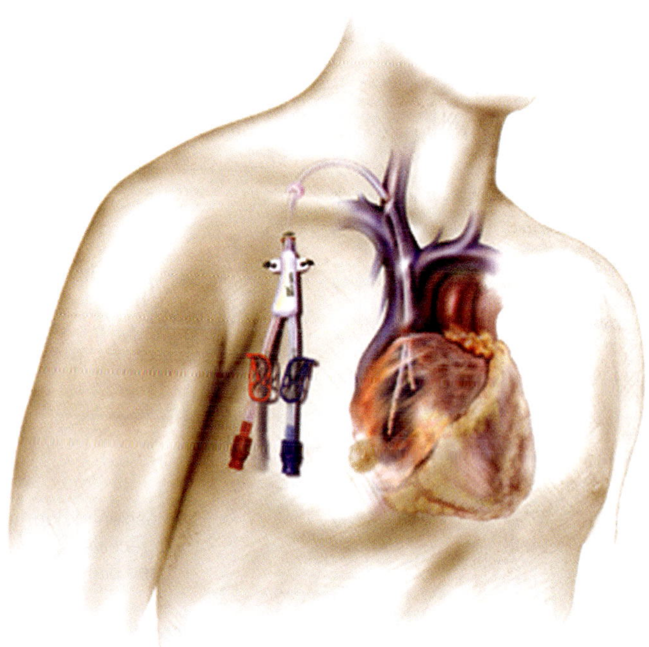

FIGURE 27.8 ***Central venous dialysis catheter***

The two most frequent complications of CVADs are infection and clotting. To reduce risk of infection, strict aseptic technique and regular exit site dressings are vital in caring for the CVAD (Lok et al., 2020). To reduce intraluminal clotting, insertion of anticoagulant lock (heparin, sodium citrate) is required between dialysis sessions. The anticoagulant lock is removed prior to the next treatment to avoid unnecessary anticoagulation.

Peritoneal dialysis

Peritoneal dialysis is a kidney replacement therapy that is mostly performed by the person with kidney failure, or a caregiver, in the home environment. It is often chosen by the individual due to increased independence and flexibility (Chan et al., 2019). Peritoneal dialysis uses the highly vascular peritoneal membrane, which surrounds the surfaces of the peritoneal cavity, as the dialysing surface (see Figure 27.9). Warmed sterile dialysate is instilled into the peritoneal cavity through a peritoneal dialysis cathcter (PDC) inserted into the peritoneal cavity. Metabolic waste products and excess electrolytes diffuse into the dialysate while it remains in the abdomen. Water movement is controlled using dextrose-based fluids as osmotic agents to draw it into the dialysate, a process known as ultrafiltration. The two most common forms of peritoneal dialysis are continuous ambulatory peritoneal dialysis and automated peritoneal dialysis

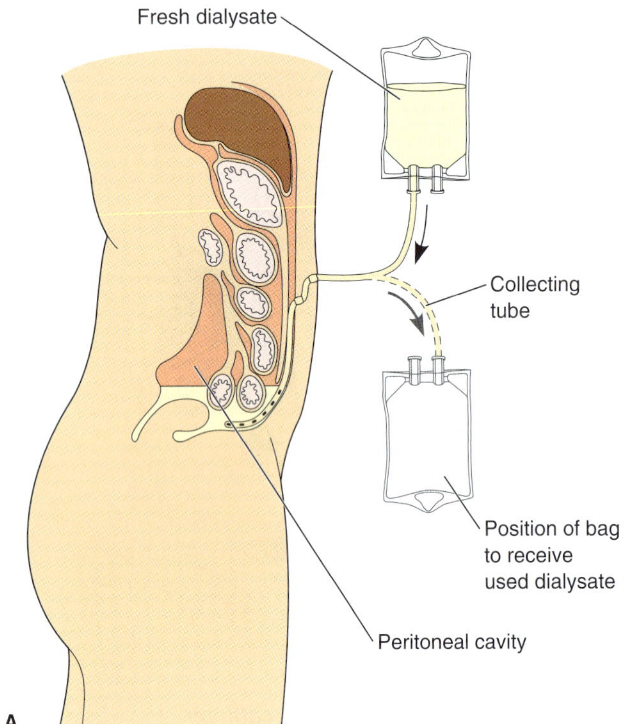

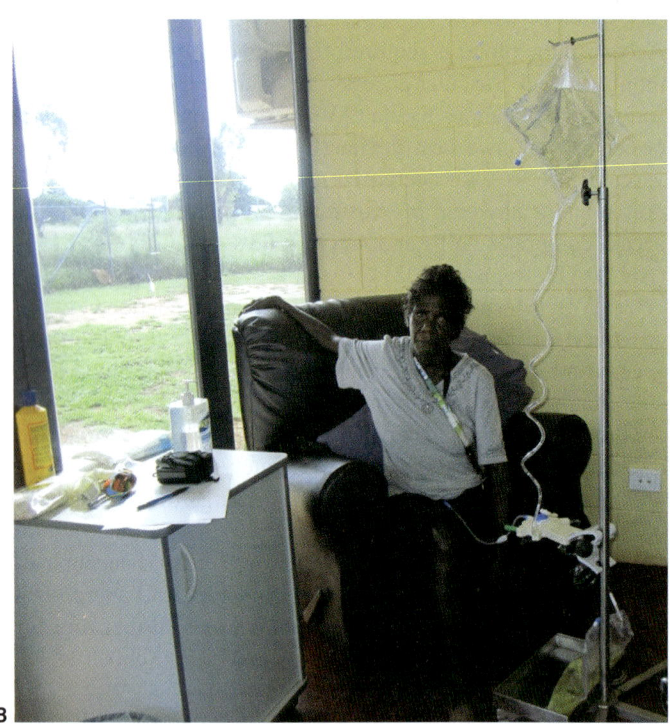

FIGURE 27.9 ***A, Peritoneal dialysis. B, A person receiving peritoneal dialysis***

Through peritoneal dialysis, the vascular complications and requirements for anticoagulation associated with haemodialysis are avoided. The clearance of metabolic waste is slower and more continuous, avoiding rapid fluctuations in extracellular fluid composition and associated symptoms. Less limited intake of fluids and nutrients may be possible for the person undergoing peritoneal dialysis. Glucose from the dialysate can be absorbed and can increase blood glucose levels. This requires monitoring and there is the potential for an increased need for hypoglycaemic medications, including insulin, particularly for those people suffering from diabetes.

A major complication of peritoneal dialysis is peritonitis, infection of the peritoneum. This can severely limit the effect of peritoneal dialysis, decrease the life of the peritoneal membrane and cause life-threatening infection if not treated early (Li et al., 2022). Other complications include exit site infection, mechanical flow restrictions, abdominal pain and peritoneal membrane dysfunction. (See the accompanying box for nursing care for the person undergoing peritoneal dialysis.) The presence of an indwelling peritoneal catheter may cause a body image disturbance; however, the presence of an AVF or CVAD in haemodialysis may also cause body image issues.

Continuous ambulatory peritoneal dialysis (CAPD) is performed manually. Due to portability, it can be performed at home, work or other locations. For CAPD, 1.5–3 L of dialysate fluid is infused into the abdomen and left to dwell for prescribed intervals. The fluid is then drained by gravity out of the peritoneal cavity into a sterile bag. This process of dialysate infusion, dwell time of the solution in the abdomen and drainage is repeated four to five times per day and is referred to as 'exchanges'. Excess fluid and solutes are removed more gradually in CAPD, minimising large blood pressure and solute variations. Depending on comfort, clearance and ultrafiltration measures, people receiving CAPD may leave a bag of dialysate fluid in their peritoneum overnight.

Automated peritoneal dialysis (APD) uses a machine (see Figure 27.10) to cycle dialysate fluid in and out of the peritoneum over a continuous period of 8 to 12 hours. This is most commonly undertaken overnight and at home.

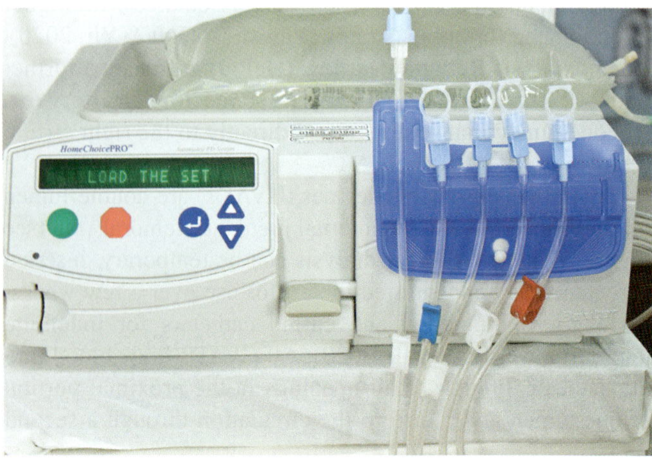

FIGURE 27.10 ***Automated peritoneal dialysis machine***

Source: Life in View/Science Photo Library.

NURSING CARE OF THE PERSON undergoing peritoneal dialysis

CONTINUOUS CARE

- Document vital signs including temperature, orthostatic blood pressures (lying, sitting and standing), pulse, respirations and lung sounds. *Data helps assess fluid volume status and tolerance of the dialysis procedure. Hypertension, abnormal heart or lung sounds, or dyspnoea may indicate excess fluid volume. Poor respiratory function may affect the ability to tolerate peritoneal dialysis. Temperature measurement is vital as infection is a common complication of peritoneal dialysis.*
- Assess weight daily and effluent drain volume between exchanges. *Weight is an accurate indicator of fluid volume status. Effluent volume enables assessment of ultrafiltration achieved by each exchange.*
- Monitor urea, serum electrolyte and creatinine levels. *These values are used to assess the effectiveness of dialysis.*
- Encourage healthy eating while assisting the person to maintain fluid and dietary restrictions as required. *Healthy eating while maintaining fluid and diet restrictions helps nutritional status and reduces hypervolaemia.*
- Warm the prescribed dialysate solution to the prescribed temperature using a designated heating pad. *Dialysate is warmed to prevent hypothermia and promote solute movement.*
- Explain all procedures and potential sensations. *Knowledge helps reduce anxiety and enhance understanding.*
- Use strict aseptic technique during the exchange procedure and when caring for the peritoneal dialysis catheter. *Peritonitis is a common complication of peritoneal dialysis; aseptic technique reduces the risk.*
- Add prescribed medications to the dialysate as required; prime the tubing with solution and connect it to the peritoneal dialysis catheter, avoiding kinks. *This allows dialysate to flow freely into the abdominal cavity and prevents leaking or contamination.*
- Instil dialysate into the abdominal cavity over a period of approximately 10 minutes. Clamp tubing and allow the dialysate to remain in the abdomen for the prescribed dwell time. Keep drainage tubing clamped at all times during instillation and dwell time. *Dialysate should flow freely into the abdomen if the peritoneal catheter is patent.*
- During instillation and dwell time, observe closely for signs of respiratory distress, such as dyspnoea, tachypnoea or crackles. Cease instillation and consider draining dialysis fluid to relieve respiratory distress if it develops. In this instance, seek further medical advice. *Respiratory compromise may result from overly rapid filling or overfilling of the abdomen or from a diaphragmatic defect that allows fluid to enter the thoracic cavity.*
- After prescribed dwell time, open drainage tubing clamps and allow dialysate to drain. Note the clarity, colour and odour of returned dialysate. *Cloudy dialysate may indicate an infection.*
- Accurately record amount and type of dialysate instilled (including any added medications), dwell time and amount and character of the drainage. *When more dialysate drains than has been instilled, excess fluid has been lost (output), the positive net difference between dialysate infused and effluent returned is termed the 'ultrafiltration volume'. If less dialysate is returned than has been instilled, a fluid gain has occurred (intake) and is referred to as 'fluid retained'.*
- Troubleshoot for possible problems during dialysis:
  a. Slow dialysate instillation. Increase the height of the dialysate bag and reposition the person. Check tubing and catheter for kinks. Check exit site dressing for wetness, indicating leakage around the catheter. Check the person has regular bowel motions. *Slow dialysate flow may be related to a partially obstructed tube or catheter. Constipation can cause obstruction of the catheter.*
  b. Excess dwell time. *Prolonged dwell time may lead to dialysate absorption and hyperglycaemia.*
  c. Poor dialysate drainage. Lower the drainage container, reposition, check for tubing kinks. Check abdominal dressing. Check the person is not constipated. *Tubing or catheter obstruction can also interfere with dialysate drainage.*

FAST FACTS

- Infective complications of peritoneal dialysis are the second most common cause of technique failure after withdrawal and/or death.
- A diagnosis of peritonitis is established if the person presents with two or more of the following: cloudy effluent with a WCC > 100 μL (with a neutrophil count > 50%), abdominal pain, fever or positive Gram stain.
- Fungal peritonitis generally requires the removal of the peritoneal dialysis catheter and temporary haemodialysis.

Continuous renal replacement therapy

Continuous renal replacement therapy (CRRT) is used for people with acute kidney injury (AKI) and is most commonly undertaken in a critical care or high-dependency setting. Initially, people with AKI typically undergo continuous haemodialysis, then intermittently as indicated. Intermittent haemodialysis is not used if the person is haemodynamically unstable (e.g. with hypotension or low cardiac output). Access to a blood flow of at least 200 mL/min is required for CRRT (see Figure 27.11), predominantly using a double-lumen venous catheter.

During CRRT, blood is continuously circulated through a highly porous haemofilter from artery to vein, or vein to vein, for a period of 12 or more hours. People are treated with CRRT for acute kidney dysfunction when unable to tolerate haemodialysis and rapid fluid removal with an unstable cardiovascular status (e.g. due to trauma, major surgery, heart failure, septicaemia). CRRT allows more gradual fluid and solute removal. Excess water and solutes such as electrolytes, urea, creatinine, uric acid and glucose are removed,

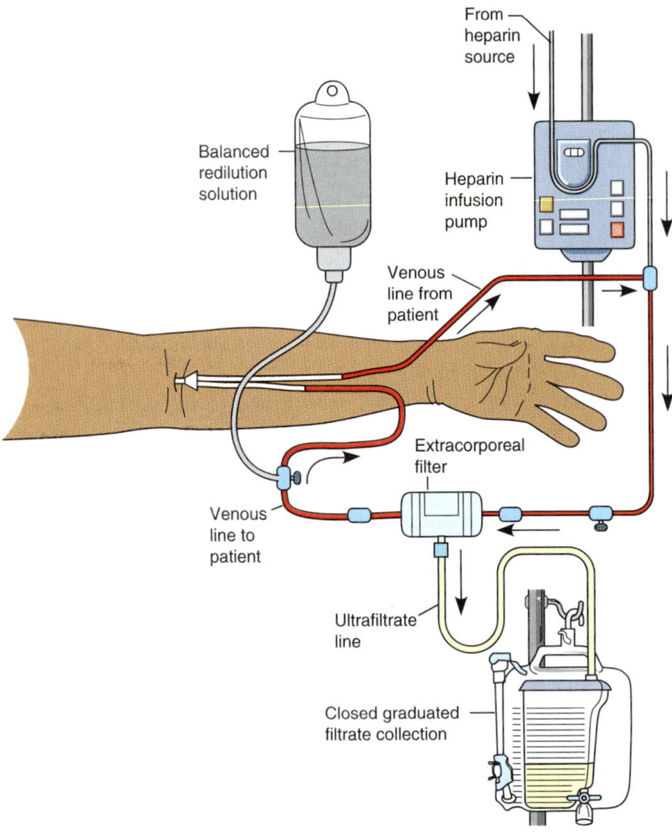

FIGURE 27.11 ***Continuous renal replacement therapy***

Source: Gambro.

and fluid may be replaced with a balanced electrolyte solution as needed.

CRRT is a slower process than maintenance haemodialysis and helps maintain haemodynamic stability and avoid complications associated with rapid changes in extracellular fluid composition. Continuous therapies include continuous venovenous haemofiltration (CVVH), continuous venovenous haemodialysis (CVVHD), continuous venovenous haemodiafiltration (CVVHDF) and slow continuous ultrafiltration (SCUF). Intermittent therapies include sustained low-efficiency dialysis (SLED) and intermittent haemodiafiltration (IHD). See Table 27.9.

KIDNEY TRANSPLANTATION

The first kidney transplant was performed in 1954 in Seattle, in the US; the donor and recipient were identical twins. Not long after, the first kidney transplants in Australia were performed in Melbourne and Adelaide. Kidney transplantation is limited primarily by the availability of organs. In Australia at the end of 2020, a total of 1,158 people were on the transplant waiting list (ANZDATA Registry, 2021).

Kidney transplantation can improve survival and quality of life for people with ESKD (kidney failure (CKD stage 5)). In Australia, a person who has received a transplant has a significantly increased survival rate over a person on dialysis (ANZDATA Registry, 2021). While medication and lifestyle regimens are required to maintain function and health with a kidney transplant, the person does not have the burden of frequent dialysis treatment, dietary and fluid restrictions and maintaining dialysis access (Tucker et al., 2019).

Kidneys are donated by living and deceased donors. In Australia in 2020, 20% of transplanted kidneys were donated by living donors, of whom most were genetically related to the recipient (ANZDATA Registry, 2021). For both deceased and living donor transplants, a close match between blood and tissue type is desired. Human leucocyte antigens (HLAs) are compared between the donor and recipient, with six antigens in common being considered to be a 'perfect' match. Close tissue typing may account for the better outcomes with living donors. Pre-emptive transplants (prior to commencement of dialysis) accounted for 40% of transplants in Australia in 2020 (ANZDATA Registry, 2021).

People with healthy kidneys who are in very good physical health may be candidates for donating a kidney. Pre-donation education is vital. A nephrectomy (removal of the kidney) is a substantial surgery and living with a single kidney involves some risk to the donor. If the transplant fails, the psychological impact on the donor can also be significant.

Deceased donor kidneys are accepted for donation after brain death (DBD) or donation after circulatory death (DCD) (ANZOD Registry, 2022). Donation of the person's two kidneys can be made to two separate recipients. A kidney is preserved by hypothermia and is transplanted within 24 hours. The system used to allocate cadaver kidneys for transplantation is outlined in Box 27.4.

TABLE 27.9 Continuous renal replacement therapies

TYPE	INDICATIONS	DESCRIPTION
Slow continuous ultrafiltration (SCUF)	Primarily removes fluid	Blood circulates through dialyser and fluid is removed through negative pressure.
Continuous venovenous haemofiltration (CVVH)	Remove fluid and some solutes	Blood circulates through a haemofilter, then returns to person; ultrafiltrate collects in a drainage bag through convection.
Continuous arteriovenous haemodialysis (CVVHD)	Remove fluid and waste products	Venous blood circulates through a haemofilter surrounded by dialysate, then returns to the person through a double-lumen venous catheter; ultrafiltrate collects in a drainage bag following diffusion and osmosis.
Continuous venovenous haemodiafiltration (CVVHDF)	Remove fluid and waste products	Venous blood circulates through a haemofilter surrounded by dialysate, then returns to the person through a double-lumen venous catheter; ultrafiltrate collects in a drainage bag. Sterile dialysate is infused and removed through convection and diffusion.

BOX 27.4 Donor kidney allocation in Australia: OrganMatch

The scarcity of organs for transplant raises questions about how deceased donor kidneys are allocated. Past inequities in the allocation process (e.g. more men than women, more Caucasians than people of colour, more rich than poor and more young than old) led to the development of the United Network for Organ Sharing (UNOS) in 1986. UNOS developed policies for organ distribution, including kidneys, hearts, livers and other transplanted organs. The Transplantation Society of Australia and New Zealand (TSANZ) has developed Australian processes based on UNOS principles.

In Australia, the allocation of kidneys from donors to people on the waiting list is determined by the national program OrganMatch, which identifies compatibility between donor kidneys and potential recipients, and is administered by the Australian Red Cross. The criteria that are used by OrganMatch to decide who will receive the kidneys include:

- blood group (most kidneys are donated to a person who is ABO compatible)
- tissue typing or 'matching' with the donor
- immunological sensitisation (antibodies the donor has developed against other people's tissue types)
- how long the person has been on dialysis
- whether the person is a child—children have priority (Transplantation Society of Australia and New Zealand (TSANZ), 2021).

People who are highly sensitised are can be more difficult to match (TSANZ, 2021). Immunological sensitisation is caused by exposure to cells and tissues of other people through pregnancy, blood transfusion and previous organ transplants (TSANZ, 2021). OrganMatch aims to match younger recipients who may require more than one kidney transplant in their lifetime with an organ that is least likely to create high levels of sensitisation to subsequent donor kidneys in the future. Via OrganMatch, kidneys are matched and sent between states and territories. However, a balance is maintained in the number of kidneys shared between jurisdictions (TSANZ, 2021).

The Australia and New Zealand Paired Kidney Exchange Program (ANZKX) is also coordinated through OrganMatch. This program matches incompatible donor-recipient pairs across Australia and New Zealand (Donate Life, n.d.). For example, Person A requires a kidney transplant and may have a willing donor (genetically or emotionally related) (Donor A). However, they are immunologically incompatible. Their transplanting unit can enrol them into ANZKX and OrganMatch will attempt to match them with a donor who is compatible with Person A and a recipient who is compatible with Donor A (Donate Life, n.d.). The exchange may not be directly between two pairs, but instead involve exchanges of kidneys between multiple pairs. ANZKX enables an increase in live donation and therefore an increase in kidneys available for transplantation.

During the transplant surgery the donor kidney is placed in the lower abdominal cavity of the recipient and the renal artery, vein and ureter are anastomosed (see Figure 27.12). The renal artery of the donor kidney is connected to the external iliac artery and the renal vein to the external iliac vein (Alexopoulos, Matsuoka & Karp, 2019). The ureter is connected to one of the recipient's ureters or directly to the bladder, using a tunnel technique to prevent reflux.

Nursing care for the person receiving a kidney transplant is outlined in the accompanying box.

The grafted kidney may stimulate an immune response to reject the transplanted kidney. Immunosuppressive drugs are used to minimise the immune response. These drugs suppress a portion of the immune system and the inflammatory response, increasing the risk of infections and cancers with long-term therapy. The nursing implications of immunosuppressive therapy are outlined in the chapter 'Nursing care of people with altered immunity'.

Maintenance immunotherapy for kidney transplant involves the person taking a combination of medications. Initial recommendations for immunosuppressive medications include the use of a calcineurin inhibitor (e.g. tacrolimus or cyclosporine) and an antiproliferative agent (e.g. mycophenolate mofetil or azathioprine), with or without a corticosteroid (Chadban et al., 2012; Lasmar et al., 2019). Once immunosuppression is established, calcineurin inhibitors or antiproliferative agents may be replaced with an mTOR inhibitor, such as sirolimus or everolimus (Chadban et al., 2012; Lasmar et al., 2019). While effective at preventing organ rejection, immunosuppressive

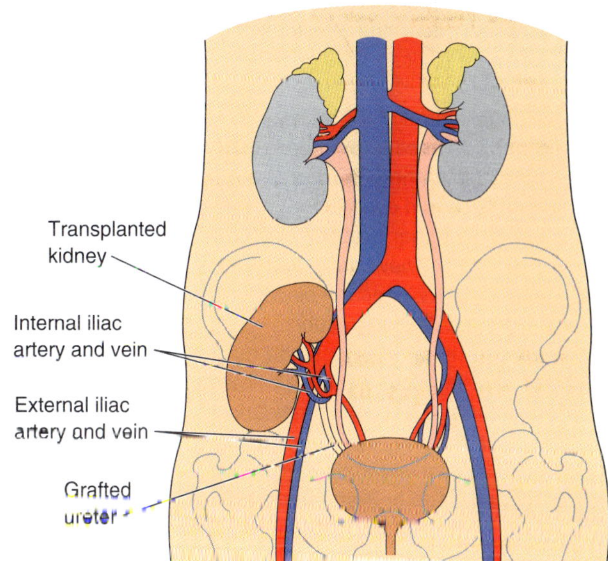

FIGURE 27.12 Placement of a transplanted kidney in the iliac fossa with anastomosis to the iliac artery, iliac vein and bladder

NURSING CARE OF THE PERSON receiving a kidney transplant

PREOPERATIVE CARE

- Provide routine preoperative care as outlined in the chapter 'Nursing care of people having surgery'.
- Assess knowledge and feelings about the procedure, answering questions and clarifying information as needed. Listen and address concerns about surgery, the source of the donor organ and possible complications. *Addressing concerns and reducing preoperative anxiety improve post-operative recovery.*
- Continue dialysis as prescribed. *Intermittent or continuous renal replacement therapy may be necessary to manage fluid and electrolyte balance and prevent uraemia prior to surgery.*
- Administer immunosuppressive medications as ordered before surgery. *Immunosuppression is initiated before transplantation to prevent immediate graft rejection.*

POSTOPERATIVE CARE

- Provide routine postoperative care as outlined in the chapter 'Nursing care of people having surgery'.
- Maintain urinary catheter patency and a closed system. *Catheter patency is vital to keep the bladder decompressed and prevent pressure on suture lines. A closed drainage system minimises the risk of urinary tract infection.*
- Measure urine output every 30 to 60 minutes initially. Careful assessment of urine output helps determine fluid balance and transplant function. *Acute tubular necrosis is a common early complication, usually due to tissue ischaemia during the period between removal of the kidney from the donor and transplantation. Oliguria is an early sign.*
- Monitor vital signs and haemodynamic pressures closely. *Diuresis may occur immediately, resulting in hypovolaemia, low cardiac output and impaired perfusion of the transplanted kidney.*
- Maintain fluid replacement, generally calculated to replace urine output over the previous 30 or 60 minutes. *Fluid replacement is vital to maintain vascular volume and tissue perfusion.*
- Administer diuretics as ordered. *Loop and/or osmotic diuretics may be used to promote postoperative diuresis.*
- Remove the catheter within 2 to 3 days or as ordered. Encourage to void every 1 to 2 hours and assess frequently for signs of urinary retention following catheter removal. *The bladder may have atrophied prior to surgery, reducing its capacity. Urinary retention places stress on suture lines and increases the risk of infection.*
- Monitor serum electrolytes and renal function tests. *These tests are used to monitor graft function and fluid and electrolyte status. Electrolyte imbalances may develop as the transplanted kidney begins to function and diuresis occurs. Elevated serum creatinine and urea levels may be early signs of rejection or graft failure.*
- Monitor for possible complications:
  a. *Haemorrhage* from an arterial or venous anastomosis can be either acute or insidious. Indicators include swelling at the operative site, increased abdominal girth and signs of shock, including changes in vital signs and level of consciousness. *Haemorrhage is a surgical emergency, requiring prompt recognition and treatment to preserve the graft.*
  b. *Ureteral anastomosis failure* causes urine leakage into the peritoneal cavity. It may be marked by decreased urine output with abdominal swelling and tenderness. *Failure of the ureteral anastomosis requires surgical intervention.*
  c. *Renal artery thrombosis* is characterised by an abrupt onset of hypertension and reduced GFR. *Renal artery thrombosis can result in transplant failure.*
  d. *Infection* due to immunosuppression is an immediate and continuing risk. The inflammatory response is diminished and infection may not significantly elevate the temperature. Monitor for signs such as change in level of consciousness, cloudy or malodorous urine, or purulent drainage from the incision. *Prevention and prompt treatment of infections is particularly important in the immunosuppressed person.*
- Include the following in pre-discharge teaching for the person and family:
  a. The use and effects of prescribed medications, including antihypertensive medications, immunosuppressive agents, prophylactic antibiotics and others as ordered.
  b. Monitoring vital signs (including temperature) and weight.
  c. Manifestations of organ rejection, such as swelling and tenderness over the graft site, fever, joint aching, weight gain and decreased urinary output. Stress the importance of promptly reporting signs and symptoms to the person's nephrologist.
  d. Ordered or recommended dietary restrictions such as restricted carbohydrate and sodium intake and increased protein intake. Encourage good nutritional habits.
  e. Measures to prevent infection, such as avoiding crowds and obviously ill individuals.

  The person and family will manage care after discharge and therefore need a good understanding of what to expect, how to monitor graft status and measures to reduce the adverse effects of medications.
- Provide psychological support, address concerns and provide information as needed. The person has often been managing a chronic disease independently and is used to having a degree of control. *Providing information and allowing the person to retain control relieves anxiety and improves recovery.*

medications have substantial potential side effects including gingival hyperplasia, hirsutism, gastrointestinal symptoms, dyslipidaemia, hypertension, increased risk of diabetes and malignancy, neurotoxicity and nephrotoxicity (Aiyegbusi et al., 2022). Being immunosuppressed leaves the individual at higher risk of infections. Glucocorticoids such as prednisone and methylprednisolone are used for both maintenance immunosuppression and to treat acute rejection episodes.

Side effects of long-term corticosteroid use include impaired wound healing, emotional disturbances, osteoporosis and Cushingoid effects on glucose, protein and fat metabolism.

Even with immunosuppressive therapy, the transplanted kidney can be rejected at any time. Either acute or chronic rejection may develop. *Acute rejection* develops within days to the first few months of the transplant and can be cell mediated, antibody mediated or a combination of both (Dunsmore, 2019). Few manifestations may be apparent other than a rise in serum creatinine and possible oliguria. *Chronic rejection*, which may develop months to years following the transplant, is a major cause of graft loss. Both humoral and cellular immune responses are involved in chronic rejection. It may not respond to increased immunosuppression. The presenting manifestations of chronic rejection—progressive uraemia, proteinuria and hypertension—are those of progressive CKD.

Hypertension is a common complication after kidney transplantation, contributing to high rates of morbidity and mortality from cardiovascular disease. Causes of hypertension are complex and can be multifactorial including immunosuppressive medications, fluid retention, renal artery stenosis and/or chronic graft rejection, as well as existing comorbidities (Tantisattamo et al., 2020). Management includes regular monitoring of blood pressure, antihypertensive medication, diuretics, diet and exercise (Tantisattamo et al., 2020).

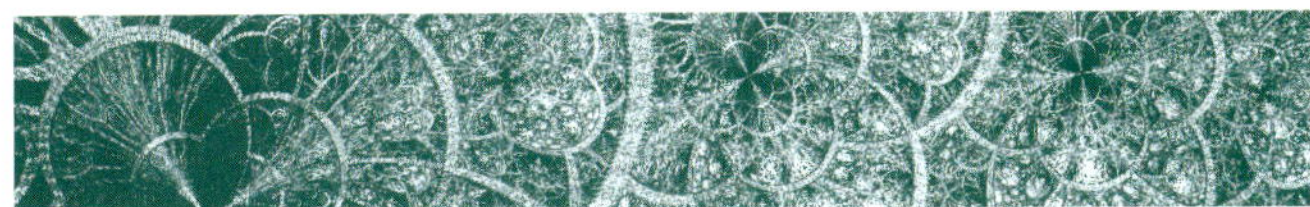

Nursing care

Assessment

Both subjective and objective data are used to assess the person with CKD approaching ESKD (kidney failure (Stage 5 CKD)):

- *Health history*: complaints of anorexia, nausea, weight gain or oedema; current treatment (if any), including type and frequency of dialysis or previous kidney transplant; chronic diseases such as diabetes, heart failure or kidney disease.
- *Physical examination*: mental status; vital signs, including temperature, heart and lung sounds, and peripheral pulses; urine output (if any); weight; skin colour, moisture, condition; presence of oedema (periorbital or dependent); bowel sounds; presence and location of an arteriovenous fistula or graft or CVAD or peritoneal dialysis catheter.

Nursing diagnosis and interventions

Whether the person with ESKD (kidney failure) is requiring long-term dialysis, kidney transplantation or supportive care, a number of nursing care needs can be identified. This section focuses on nursing care related to impaired kidney function nutritional deficits due to dietary restrictions and nausea, increased risk of infection and changes in body image. Also see the accompanying nursing care plan for nursing care of the person with ESKD.

Ineffective kidney perfusion

Capillaries are an integral part of the nephron. As nephrons are destroyed, kidney perfusion progressively declines. As kidney perfusion and nephron function fall, the kidney is less able to maintain fluid and electrolyte balance and eliminate waste products from the body.

- Monitor intake and output, vital signs including orthostatic blood pressures and weight. *These provide important data to identify changes in fluid volume.*
- Restrict fluids as ordered. *As kidney function declines, the ability to eliminate excess fluid is impaired.*

> **CONSIDERATION FOR PRACTICE**
> **Weight changes are a more accurate indicator of fluid volume status in the oliguric or anuric person than intake and output measurements.**

- Monitor respiratory status, including lung sounds as indicated. *Fluid volume overload may lead to heart failure and possible pulmonary oedema.*
- Monitor urea, serum creatinine, pH, electrolytes and FBC. Report significant changes. As kidney function declines, urea and serum creatinine increase. *Metabolic acidosis develops as the kidney is unable to eliminate hydrogen ions and conserve bicarbonate. Hyponatraemia, hyperkalaemia, hyperphosphataemia and hypocalcaemia are associated with kidney failure. The RBC count and haemoglobin decline due to deficient erythropoietin to stimulate cell production in the bone marrow. An acute fall in haemoglobin may also indicate GI bleeding, a risk in people with kidney failure.*
- Report manifestations of electrolyte imbalances, such as cardiac arrhythmias and other ECG changes, muscle tremors and possible tetany and Kussmaul's respirations. *Manifestations of electrolyte imbalance may indicate the need for intervention.*

> **CONSIDERATION FOR PRACTICE**
> **Monitor clarity of dialysate return. Dialysate should return clear in the person undergoing peritoneal dialysis. Cloudy dialysate may indicate peritonitis, the most common complication of peritoneal dialysis, and should be reported and cultured.**

- Administer medications to treat electrolyte imbalances as ordered. *Medications may be prescribed to help maintain electrolyte and acid–base balance and prevent adverse effects of imbalances.*
- Administer antihypertensive medications as ordered. *Hypertension management is an important factor in slowing the progression of CKD.*
- Time activities and procedures to allow rest periods. *Anaemia associated with CKD may cause significant fatigue and activity intolerance.*

Imbalanced nutrition: less than body requirements

Anorexia, nausea and vomiting are common manifestations of ESKD (kidney failure) and uraemia. The person often has a metallic taste and bad breath, which also diminish appetite. A diet restricted in protein and sodium will compound these problems. Food intake may be insufficient to meet metabolic needs. Catabolism, the breakdown of body proteins to meet energy needs, exacerbates uraemia.

- Monitor food and nutrient intake as well as episodes of vomiting. *Careful monitoring helps determine the adequacy of intake.*
- Weigh daily before breakfast. This provides the most accurate measurement. *Remember that a gain of 1 kg or more over a 24-hour period is more likely to reflect fluid retention than a gain in body mass.*
- Administer anti-emetic agents 30 to 60 minutes before eating. *Anti-emetics reduce nausea and the risk of vomiting with food intake.*
- Assist with mouth care prior to meals and at bedtime. *Mouth care improves taste, stimulates the appetite and maintains the integrity of oral mucous membranes.*
- Serve small meals and provide between-meal snacks. *Small meals are less likely to prompt nausea and can help improve food intake.*
- Arrange for a dietary consultation. Provide preferred foods to the extent possible and involve the person in planning daily menus. Encourage family members to bring food as dietary restrictions allow. *Providing preferred foods within restrictions promotes intake.*
- Monitor nutritional status by tracking weight, laboratory values such as serum albumin, and urea and anthropometric measurements (see the chapters 'A person-centred approach to assessing the gastrointestinal system' and 'Nursing care of people with nutritional disorders'). *Indicators of impaired nutrition develop gradually and may be subtle. Careful assessment is important.*

Risk of infection

People with kidney failure have altered immune systems and leucocyte function and have increasing susceptibility to infection. Invasive devices required for haemodialysis or peritoneal dialysis add to this risk. The person who has had a kidney transplant remains on immunosuppressive therapy for life, further depressing the immune system and increasing the risk of infection.

- Use standard precautions and good handwashing technique at all times. Handwashing is a primary means of preventing the transfer of organisms. *People who are on haemodialysis have an increased risk of vancomycin-resistant* Enterococcus *(VRE), methicillin-resistant* Staphylococcus aureus *(MRSA), hepatitis B, hepatitis C and HIV infection.*
- Monitor temperature and vital signs at least every 4 hours. *A low-grade fever or increased pulse rate may indicate an infection in the immunosuppressed person.*
- Monitor WBC count and differential. *Increased WBCs may indicate a bacterial infection; decreased WBCs may indicate a viral infection. A shift in the differential showing more immature WBCs (bands) in circulation is another indicator of infection.*
- Culture peritoneal dialysis fluid and other drainage as indicated. *Culture is done to verify the presence of pathogens and actively treat early signs of peritonitis.*
- Provide good respiratory hygiene, including position changes, coughing and deep breathing. *These measures improve clearance of respiratory secretions, reducing the risk of infection.*

> **CONSIDERATION FOR PRACTICE**
>
> **Monitor carefully for desired and adverse effects of all medications. Impaired kidney function affects drug elimination and increases the risk of toxic effects.**

- Restrict visits from people who may be infective or unwell. Teach the person and family about the risk of infection and measures to reduce the spread of infection. *The person's resistance to infection is impaired, necessitating extra caution in preventing unnecessary exposures.*

Disturbed body image

Chronic disease and impaired kidney function can affect the person's body image. Haemodialysis requires an arteriovenous fistula or shunt; a permanent peritoneal catheter is required for peritoneal dialysis. While kidney transplant can restore an image of wholeness, a visible scar remains and the organ may be perceived as 'foreign'.

- Involve the person in care, including meal planning, dialysis, and catheter, port or incision care, to the extent possible. *Involvement improves acceptance and stimulates discussion about the effect of the disease and treatment measures on the person's life.*
- Encourage expression of feelings and concerns, accepting perceptions and feelings without criticism. *Self-expression enhances the person's self-worth and acceptance.*
- Include the person in decision making and encourage self-care. *Increased autonomy enhances the person's sense of control, independence and self-worth.*
- Support positive gains, but do not support denial. *The person may have difficulty accepting the kidney failure, but adaptation to the loss is important.*
- Help the person develop and achieve realistic goals. *Realistic goals allow the person to see progress.*
- Provide positive reinforcement and feedback. *These measures support growth and adaptation.*
- Reinforce effective coping strategies. *Reinforcement helps the person develop positive versus negative strategies for coping.*
- Facilitate contact with a support group, such as Kidney Health Australia or other community members. *The person benefits by providing and receiving support in a group of people going through similar circumstances.*

NURSING CARE PLAN **A person with end-stage kidney disease**

Walter Cohen, 45 years old, is the librarian at a local university. He has had type 1 diabetes since the age of 20 and was diagnosed with diabetic nephropathy 10 years ago. Despite blood pressure control, ACE inhibitor medications and frequent blood glucose monitoring with insulin coverage, he developed overt proteinuria 5 years ago and has now progressed to ESKD (kidney failure (CKD stage 5)). He is admitted to the nephrology ward and will undertake haemodialysis while waiting for a peritoneal dialysis catheter to be inserted to perform CAPD. Mr Cohen's desire to continue working is the primary factor in his choice of CAPD over haemodialysis.

ASSESSMENT

Richard Gray, Mr Cohen's nurse, obtains a nursing assessment. Mr Cohen states that his diabetes has always been difficult to control. He has had numerous hypoglycaemic episodes and has been hospitalised 'four or five times' for ketoacidosis. Recently he has developed symptoms of peripheral neuropathy and increasing retinopathy. He attributed his lack of appetite, nausea, vomiting and fatigue over the past month to 'a touch of the flu'. His weight remained stable, so he did not worry about not eating much.

Physical assessment findings include T 36.5°C, P 96, R 20 and BP 178/100. His skin is cool and dry, with minor excoriations on forearms and lower legs. His breath has a strong offensive odour. Scattered fine rales noted in bilateral lung bases. He has bilateral pitting oedema of lower extremities to just below the knees; fingers and hands also oedematous. Abdominal assessment essentially normal, with hypoactive bowel sounds. Urinalysis shows a specific gravity of 1.011, gross proteinuria and multiple cell casts. FBC results: RBC 2.9 million/mm^3; haemoglobin 9.4 g/dL. Blood chemistry abnormalities include urea 32 mmol/L; creatinine 621 µmol/L; eGFR 9 mL/min; sodium 125 mmol/L; potassium 6.2 mmol/L; albumin 31 g/L; calcium 2.3 mmol/L; phosphate 3.5 mmol/L. A temporary jugular central venous access device will be inserted for haemodialysis the next day, followed by a peritoneal dialysis catheter insertion later in the week.

DIAGNOSES

- *Excess fluid volume* related to failure of kidneys to eliminate excess body fluid.
- *Imbalanced nutrition: less than body requirements* related to effects of uraemia.
- *Impaired skin integrity* of lower extremities related to dry skin and itching.
- *Risk of infection* related to invasive catheters and impaired immune function.

PLANNING

- Plan fluid balance to a restriction of 750 mL per day.
- Plan a nutrition and fluid education program.
- Plan skin care program.
- Plan peritoneal exit site and catheter care education.

Expected outcomes

- Adhere to the prescribed fluid restriction of 750 mL per day.
- Demonstrate reduced extracellular fluid volume by reduced body weight, decreased peripheral oedema, clear lung sounds and normal heart sounds.
- Consume and retain 100% of prescribed diet, including snacks.
- Demonstrate healing of lower extremity skin lesions.
- Support skin integrity and moisture.
- Remain free of infection.
- Demonstrate appropriate peritoneal exit site and catheter care.

IMPLEMENTATION

- Space person's fluid intake. For example, 400 mL from 0700 to 1500, 200 mL from 1500 to 2300, and 100 mL from 2300 to 0700.
- Encourage and provide mouth care at least every 4 hours and before every meal.
- Weigh daily before breakfast; monitor vital signs every 4 hours.
- Document intake and output accurately.
- Arrange dietary consultation for menu planning.
- If required, administer prescribed anti-emetic 1 hour before meals.
- Monitor food intake, noting percentage and types of food consumed.
- Clean lesions on lower extremities and visualise every 8 hours to monitor healing.
- Encourage moisturiser as appropriate to assist reduction in itch and dryness of skin.
- If possible, begin to teach CAPD procedure and peritoneal exit site care.
- Assist to identify strengths and needs in health regimen management.

EVALUATION

Mr Cohen was hospitalised for 2 weeks, undergoing four haemodialysis sessions to reduce uraemic symptoms. An arteriovenous fistula was created in his left arm in case he should need haemodialysis in the future. He begins peritoneal dialysis at the end of the second week and by discharge he is able to manage the catheter care and dialysis runs with the help of his wife and community nursing support. His heart and lung sounds are normal and he has minimal peripheral oedema on discharge. The excoriations on his legs have healed. His temperature is normal and no evidence of infection is noted. Mr Cohen remains anorexic and slightly nauseated but is eating most of his prescribed diet and snacks. He has lost 5 kg with excess fluid removal by dialysis, but his weight remains stable during the second week. Mr Cohen and his wife have been introduced to another person who has been on CAPD for several years to offer social support.

CRITICAL THINKING IN THE NURSING PROCESS

1. How does diabetes mellitus damage the kidneys and lead to ESKD (kidney failure)? Why is this more significant for a person with type 1 diabetes than for someone with type 2 diabetes (see the chapter 'Nursing care of people with diabetes mellitus')?
2. Why do high levels of urea in the blood often cause changes in cognition and mental status? What manifestations of encephalopathy would you expect to see?
3. How might Mr Cohen's insulin dosage and diet need to be changed with the institution of peritoneal dialysis? Why?
4. Develop a care plan for the nursing diagnosis *Disturbed body image*.

REFLECTION ON THE NURSING PROCESS

1. What impact does Mr Cohen's cognitive status have on his ability to contribute to a planned education program?
2. How has the nursing process influenced Mr Cohen's nutrition status?

TRANSLATION TO PRACTICE Evidence-based practice: minimising hypotension during dialysis

The effects of pre-emptively pausing fluid removal to minimise dialysis hypotension have been explored. As it is understood that a sudden drop in blood pressure occurs in between 15% and 55% of all treatments, this is the most common serious side effect seen in haemodialysis (Murdeshwar & Anjum, 2021). In an interventional pre- and post-test study involving 864 individual dialysis treatments, fluid removal was paused for a minimum of 10 minutes if the following criteria were met: (1) mean arterial pressure was less than or equal to 70 mmHg, or (2) the mean arterial pressure dropped by 30 mmHg or more. The results demonstrated that a pre-emptive nursing intervention decreased the odds of an intradialytic episode.

IMPLICATIONS FOR NURSING

Pre-emptively pausing fluid removal according to specific mean arterial pressure parameters is a method to decrease intradialytic hypotensive episodes. This may be particularly useful for dialysis units without biofeedback or profiling machine technology.

CRITICAL THINKING IN PERSON-CENTRED CARE

1. Identify blood pressure assessment that is required throughout the dialysis treatment tools.
2. Identify a contextually appropriate intervention based on evidence to minimise hypotension.
3. Develop a teaching plan for people receiving dialysis, families and significant others to help them develop strategies to identify the early signs of hypotension.

- Refer for mental health counselling as indicated or desired. *Counselling can help the person develop effective coping and adaptation strategies.*

Emerging nursing roles

Nurses have undertaken various roles in caring for people with kidney disease. Traditionally, these have involved renal ward care, haemodialysis care, peritoneal dialysis care and transplant care. Various specialty nursing roles have emerged for the many areas that the person with ESKD (kidney failure) has to address, including vascular access/renal access, anaemia and transplant liaison. These roles can be undertaken at an advanced practice nurse or Nurse Practitioner level.

The vascular access nurse can also coordinate renal access surgical lists, access surveillance and vascular access education. Primarily, the nurse provides a fluent communication channel between the renal services department, vascular surgery, allied health and other relevant units within the healthcare system and is an important member of the multidisciplinary team (MDT).

The renal anaemia nurse, also known as the renal anaemia coordinator, provides specialised anaemia-related support for people living with CKD and ESKD (kidney failure). This support includes education for people with kidney disease, monitoring and management of renal anaemia, administration of IV iron and blood transfusions, liaison with physicians, GPs and community nursing support, and education for nurses and other health professionals.

The transplant liaison nurse coordinates the evaluation and preparation of the person who has identified the request for a kidney transplant. Evaluation for kidney transplantation involves complete physical assessment to determine that the person is suitable to undergo a surgical procedure and to identify potential issues that will need to be managed post transplant. Cardiovascular evaluation is especially important, as cardiovascular disease is the leading cause of death post transplant of people with functioning renal grafts (ANZDATA Registry, 2021). It is also during the workup that contraindications to transplantation, such as malignancy, are identified. Preparation involves focused education, as the person's understanding, willingness and ability to manage their own care throughout the entire transplant process will have a major impact on the success and outcome of their transplant. Preparation also involves blood group typing and tissue typing. The transplant liaison nurse plays a pivotal role in encouraging the person to engage in healthy behaviours. Encouraging the person to be infection-free, adherent to medication and maintain a healthy body mass index is important to prevent post-transplant complications.

PATIENT SAFETY COMPETENCY FRAMEWORK

7 Preventing, minimising and responding to adverse events

The Patient Safety Competency Framework indicates that nursing students must demonstrate the ability to prevent, minimise and respond to adverse events by conducting regular and appropriate risk assessments (Levett-Jones et al., 2017).

Community-based care

CKD and ESKD (kidney failure) are long-term conditions that require self-management. No matter what treatment option is chosen (haemodialysis, peritoneal dialysis, kidney transplantation, supportive care), day-to-day management falls to the person and family. Teaching for home care includes the following topics:

- Nature of the kidney disease and kidney failure, including expected progression and effects.
- Monitoring weight, vital signs and temperature.
- Prescribed dietary and fluid restrictions. (Involve the person, a dietitian and the family member usually responsible for cooking. Include strategies to manage nausea and relieve thirst within allowed fluid limits.)

- How to assess and protect a fistula or graft for haemodialysis (or the extremity to be used if one is anticipated).
- Peritoneal dialysis (PD) catheter care and the procedure for peritoneal dialysis as indicated. (Include a family member or significant other, in case the person is unable to perform the procedure independently at some time.)
- Following kidney transplant, prescribed medications, adverse effects and their management, infection prevention, graft protection and manifestations of organ rejection.
- Refer to a dietitian for diet planning and counselling. If home haemodialysis is planned, refer the designated dialysis helper for formal training. Kidney Health Australia can provide support and educational materials for the person with ESKD (kidney failure) (visit https://kidney.org.au). Local and state trained representatives of these organisations can provide additional support.

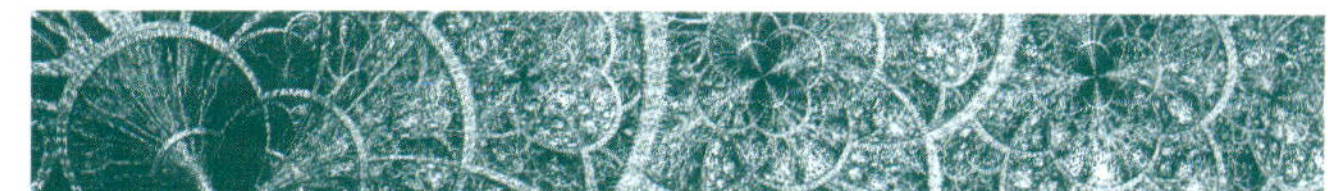

CHAPTER HIGHLIGHTS

- Glomerulonephritis, inflammation of the glomerulus of the kidney, leads to loss of proteins and blood cells in the urine, a decrease in the glomerular filtration rate and severe oedema.
- The renal and cardiovascular systems are closely interrelated. Vascular disorders, such as hypertension, renal artery stenosis or obstruction of the renal artery or vein, can have serious consequences in terms of kidney function.
- Acute kidney injury is a frequent complication of critical illnesses, typically occurring in people with no prior history of kidney disorders. Ischaemic and nephrotoxic damage to the kidney are the most common precipitating factors for AKI.
- Chronic kidney disease is the end-stage of numerous systemic and kidney disorders, such as diabetes mellitus, systemic lupus erythematosus and chronic glomerulonephritis.
- When the kidneys are no longer able to maintain homeostasis, kidney replacement therapies are necessary to eliminate metabolic waste products and sustain life. Dialysis and kidney transplant are the primary kidney replacement therapies used.
- Home dialysis therapy is the preferred treatment for people with ESKD (kidney failure).

CONCEPT CHECK

1 The physician orders digoxin 0.125 mg 3 times per week for an 82-year-old person with heart failure. The nurse should:

1 question the order because older people frequently require larger doses of the drug due to impaired ability of the kidneys to concentrate urine
2 administer the drug as ordered, monitoring the person for manifestations of toxicity
3 assess the person's urine specific gravity and pH before administering the drug at this dose
4 use 0.25 mg digoxin tablets, cutting the tablet in half to save money for the person

2 A person newly diagnosed with polycystic kidney disease asks if there is anything his children need to know about their risk of getting the disorder. The appropriate response by the nurse is:

1 Because the condition was just diagnosed, it is due to a new genetic mutation and there is no risk of passing the condition on to his children.
2 When his children prepare to marry, they and their potential partners should undergo genetic testing to determine if their children will be at risk.
3 The adult form of this disorder is transmitted as a dominant gene; each child has a 50% risk of having inherited the defective gene.
4 His children would have developed symptoms of the disorder in utero or shortly after birth if they had inherited the defective gene.

3 In obtaining a nursing history from a 22-year-old person admitted with a diagnosis of acute glomerulonephritis, the nurse specifically asks the person about a recent history of which of the following?

1 urinary tract infection
2 strep throat
3 x-ray using contrast media
4 illicit drug use

4 The nurse evaluates his teaching for a person with acute glomerulonephritis as effective when the person:

1 chooses soy or animal proteins for allowed grams of protein in the diet
2 states the need to remain on bed rest until his urine returns to clear yellow
3 demonstrates care for the vascular shunt or peritoneal catheter
4 limits fluid intake to less than 1,500 mL per day

5 Appropriate postoperative nursing interventions for the person who has had a partial or total nephrectomy include:

1 connecting all catheters and drains to a single collection device
2 routine irrigation of all catheters with sterile normal saline
3 administering cough suppressant medication as needed
4 labelling and securing all catheters, tubes and drains

6 Important nursing interventions to prevent acute kidney dysfunction in the critically ill person include:

1 maintaining fluid volume and cardiac output
2 avoiding all potentially nephrotoxic drugs
3 administering antihypertensive drugs
4 assessing for a history of diabetes or systemic lupus erythematosus

7 The nurse evaluates their teaching as effective when the person recovering from acute kidney dysfunction states that he will:

1 limit his fluid intake to 1,500 mL or less per day
2 consume only vegetable proteins
3 avoid taking drugs that may be nephrotoxic
4 self-catheterise for residual urine at least once a week

8 The nurse caring for a person preparing to undergo haemodialysis includes which of the following in the plan of care? (Select all that apply.)
1 Obtain weight and orthostatic vital signs.
2 Assess blood pressure of extremity where fistula has been created.
3 Monitor serum creatinine, urea and haemoglobin levels.
4 Determine urine specific gravity and pH.
5 Restrict fluid and protein intake.

9 An appropriate goal of nursing care for a person with end-stage kidney disease is the person will be able to:
1 identify a live-in caregiver
2 state the advantages and disadvantages of haemodialysis, peritoneal dialysis and kidney transplant as kidney replacement therapies
3 demonstrate the ability to independently perform haemodialysis in the home
4 relate the hospice philosophy and identify indicators of the need for hospice care

10 Following a kidney transplant, the nurse notes that the person's urine is cloudy. The most appropriate response by the nurse is to:
1 record the finding
2 increase the intravenous flow rate
3 irrigate the urinary catheter
4 notify the physician

BIBLIOGRAPHY

Alexopoulos, S., Matsuoka, L. & Karp, S. J. (2019). Surgical management of the renal transplant recipient. In J. Himmelfarb & T. Alp Ikizler (eds), *Chronic kidney disease, dialysis, and transplantation* (4th ed., pp. 582–590). Philadelphia: Elsevier.

Alscher, M. D., Erley, C. & Kuhlmann, M. K. (2019). Acute renal failure of nosocomial origin. *Deutsches Ärzteblatt International*, *116*(9), 149–158. doi: 10.3238/arztebl.2019.0149

Aiyegbusi, O., McGregor. E., McManus, S. K. & Stevens, K. I. (2022). Immunosuppression therapy in kidney transplantation. *Urologic Clinics of North America*, *49*(2), 345–360.

Amerman, E. C. (2018). *Human anatomy and physiology*. London: Pearson Education Limited.

ANZDATA Registry (2021). *44th annual report*. Adelaide: ANZDATA. Retrieved from https://www.anzdata.org.au

ANZOD Registry (2022). *Section 5: Deceased donor kidney donation. 2022 annual report*. Retrieved from www.anzdata.org.au;

Australian Commission on Safety and Quality in Health Care (ACSQHC) (2021). *National Safety and Quality Health Service Standards* (2nd ed.). Sydney: ACSQHC.

Australian Institute of Health and Welfare (AIHW) (2018). *Australia's health, 2018*. Retrieved from https://www.aihw.gov.au/

Australian Institute of Health and Welfare (AIHW) (2020). *Chronic kidney disease*. Retrieved from https://www.aihw.gov.au/

Australian Institute of Health and Welfare (AIHW) (2021). *Profile of Indigenous Australians*. Retrieved from https://www.aihw.gov.au/

Australian Institute of Health and Welfare (AIHW) (2022). *Cancer data in Australia*. Retrieved from https://www.aihw.gov.au/

Bagga, A. & Menon, S. (2016). Rapidly progressive glomerulonephritis. In D. F. Geary & F. Schaefer (eds), *Pediatric kidney disease* (pp. 567–580). Berlin: Springer.

Balasubramanian, R. & Marks, S. D. (2017). Post-infectious glomerulonephritis. *Paediatrics and International Child Health*, *37*(4), 240–247.

Bennett, P. N., Schatell, D. & Shah, K. D. (2015). Psychosocial aspects in home hemodialysis: A review. *Hemodialysis International*, *19*(S1), S128–S134.

Cass, A., Chadban, S. & Gallagher, M. (2020). *The economic impact of end-stage kidney disease in Australia: Projections to 2020*. Melbourne: Kidney Health Australia.

Chadban, S. J., Barraclough, K. A., Campbell, S. B. et al. (2012). KHA-CARI guideline: KHA-CARI adaptation of the KDIGO clinical practice guideline for the care of kidney transplant recipients. *Nephrology*, *17*(3), 204–214.

Chakraborty, R. K. & Burns, B. (2022). Systemic inflammatory response syndrome. *StatPearls* [Internet]. Treasure Island (FL): StatPearls Publishing.

Chan, C. T., Blankestijn, P. J., Dember, L. M. et al. (2019). Dialysis initiation, modality choice, access, and prescription: Conclusions from a Kidney Disease: Improving Global Outcomes (KDIGO) controversies conference. *Kidney International*, *96*(1), 37–47.

Choo, S. Z., See, E. J., Simmonds, R. E., Somerville, C. A. & Agar, J. W. M. (2019). Nocturnal home haemodialysis: The 17 year experience of a single Australian dialysis service. *Nephrology*, *24*, 1050–1055.

Conway, J., Lawn, S., Crail, S. & McDonald, S. (2018). Indigenous patient experiences of returning to country: A qualitative evaluation on the Country Health SA Dialysis bus. *BMC Health Services Research*, *18*(1), 1010.

Coulson, J. M. (2022). Dose-response relationships in aluminium toxicity in humans. *Clinical Toxicology*, *60*(4), 415–428. doi: 10.1080/15563650.2022.2029879

Damasiewicz, M. J. & Polkinghorne, K. R. (2020). Global dialysis perspective: Australia. *Kidney 360*, *1*, 48–51.

Dart, A. (2022). Sociodemographic determinants of chronic kidney disease in Indigenous children. *Pediatric Nephrology*, *37*, 547–553.

Dique, J. C. (1955). The artificial kidney in the treatment of severe puerperal infection due to *Clostridium welchii*, with report of a case. *Medical Journal of Australia*, *I*, 781–789.

Donate Life (n.d.). *Information for transplant units—ANZKX program*. Donate Life. Retrieved from https://www.donatelife.gov.au/

Dunsmore, V. (2019). Renal transplantation. In N. Thomas (ed.), *Renal nursing* (5th ed., pp. 277–334). New York: John Wiley & Sons.

Haas, M. (2017). Glomerular disease pathology in the era of proteomics: From pattern to pathogenesis. *Journal of the American Society of Nephrology*, *29*(1), 2–4.

Hole, B., Hemmelgarn, B., Brown, E. et al. (2020). Supportive care for end-stage kidney disease: An integral part of kidney services across a range of income settings around the world. *Kidney International Supplements*, *10*(1), e86–e94. doi: 10.1016/j.kisu.2019.11.008

Hoy, W. E., Mott, S. A. & McDonald, S. P. (2016). An expanded nationwide view of chronic kidney disease in Aboriginal Australians. *Nephrology*, *21*(11), 916–922.

Hunter, J. P., Knight, S. R., Inston, N. et al. (2019). The United Kingdom and Ireland experience of the Haemodialysis Reliable Outflow graft for vascular access. *The Journal of Vascular Access*, *20*(1), 12–18.

Jankowski, J., Floege, J., Fliser, D., Böhm, M. & Marx, N. (2021). Cardiovascular disease in chronic kidney disease: Pathophysiological insights and therapeutic options. *Circulation*, *143*, 1157–1172.

Karimi, M., Dideban, D. & Heidari, H. (2022). Using the intelligent system to improve the delivered adequacy of dialysis by preventing intradialytic complications. *Journal of Healthcare Engineering*, *2022*, 1–10. https://doi.org/10.1155/2022/8160269

Kashani, K., Rosner, M. H., Haase, M. et al. (2019). Quality improvement goals for acute kidney injury. *Clinical Journal of the American Society of Nephrology*, *14*(6), 941–953. doi: 10.2215/CJN.01250119

Khan, Y., Deepak, P. & Kumar, A. (2017). Study of etiology, clinical profile and outcome of acute kidney injury (AKI) in medical intensive care unit. *International Journal of Contemporary Medical Research*, *4*(11), 2225–2228.

Kidney Disease: Improving Global Outcomes (KDIGO) (2013). KDIGO 2012 Clinical practice guideline for the evaluation and management of chronic kidney disease. *Kidney International Supplements*, *3*(1), 1–150.

Kidney Disease: Improving Global Outcomes (KDIGO) (2021a). KDIGO 2021 Clinical practice guideline for the management of glomerular diseases. *Kidney International*, *100*(4S), S1 – S276.

Kidney Disease: Improving Global Outcome (KDIGO) (2021b). KDIGO 2021 Clinical practice guideline for the management of blood pressure in chronic kidney disease. *Kidney International*, *99*(3S), S1–S87.

Kidney Disease: Improving Global Outcomes (KDIGO) Acute Kidney Injury Workgroup (2012). KDIGO clinical practice guideline for acute kidney injury. *Kidney International Supplements*, *2*, 1–138.

Kidney Health Australia (2018). *Kidney fast facts*. Retrieved from https://kidney.org.au/

Kirkpatrick, J. J. & Leslie, S. W. (2022). Horseshoe kidney. *StatPearls* [Internet]. Treasure Island (FL): StatPearls Publishing.

Ko, G. J., Obi, Y., Tortorici, A. R. & Kalantar-Zadeh, K. (2017). Dietary protein intake and chronic kidney disease. *Current Opinion in Clinical Nutrition & Metabolic Care*, *20*(1), 77–85. doi: 10.1097/MCO.0000000000000342

Kumbar, L., Ramani, K. & Brouwer-Maier, D. (2020). Considerations in access cannulation: Traditional and evolving approaches. *Advances in Chronic Kidney Disease*, *27*(3), 199–207.

Lasmar, M. F., Dutra, R. S., Nogueira-Machado, J. A., Fabreti-Oliveira, R. A., Gomes Siqueira, R. & Nascimento, E. (2019). Effects of immunotherapy induction on outcome and graft survival of kidney-transplanted patients with different immunological risk of rejection. *BMC Nephrology*, *20*, 314. https://doi.org/10.1186/s12882-019-1497-5

Lauschke, A., Teichgräber, U. K. M., Frei, U. et al. (2006). 'Low-dose' dopamine worsens renal perfusion in patients with acute renal failure. *Kidney International*, *69*(9), 1669–1674.

Lawrence, J. R. (1994). The evolution of the end-stage renal disease program in Australia. *Renal Failure*, *16*, 133–146.

Levett-Jones, T., Dwyer, T., Reid-Searl, K., Heaton, L., Flenady, T., Applegarth, J., Guinea, S. & Andersen, P. (2017). *Patient Safety Competency Framework (PSCF) for Nursing Students*. Sydney. Retrieved from http://psframework.wpengine.com/

Levey, A. S., Eckardt, K.-U., Dorman, N. M. et al. (2020). Nomenclature for kidney function and disease: Report of a Kidney Disease: Improving Global Outcomes (KDIGO) Consensus Conference. *Kidneys International*, *97*, 1117–1129. https://doi.org/10.1016/j.kint.2020.02.010

Li, P. K.-T., Chow, K. M., Cho, Y. et al. (2022). ISPD peritonitis guideline recommendations: 2022 update on prevention and treatment. *Peritoneal Dialysis International*, *42*(2), 110–153.

Lok, C. E., Huber, T. S., Lee, T. et al. (2020). KDOQI clinical practice guideline for vascular access: 2019 update. *American Journal of Kidney Diseases*, *75*(4), S1–S164.

Loscalzo, J., Fauci, A. S., Kasper, D. L., Hauser, S. L. & Longo, D. (2022). *Harrison's principles of internal medicine* (21st ed.). New York: McGraw Hill Medical.

Marshall, M. R., Polkinghorne, K. R., Boudville, N. & McDonald, S. P. (2021). Home versus facility dialysis and mortality in Australia and New Zealand. *American Journal of Kidney Disease*, *78*(6), 826–837.

McCance, K. L. & Huether, S. E. (2019). *Pathophysiology: The biologic basis for disease in adults and children*. St Louis, MO: Elsevier Health Sciences.

Moustakas, J., Bennett, P. N. & Tranter, S. (2015). The information needs of older people who choose supportive care over dialysis: A case study approach. *Renal Society of Australasia Journal*, *11*(1), 6–11.

Murdeshwar, H. N. & Anjum, F. (2021) Hemodialysis. *StatPearls* [Internet]. Treasure Island (FL): StatPearls Publishing.

Ostermann, M., Macedo, E. & Oudemans-van Straaten, H. (2019). How to feed a patient with acute kidney injury. *Intensive Care Medicine*, *45*, 1006–1008. https://doi.org/10.1007/s00134-019-05615-z

O'Sullivan, E. D., Hughes, J. & Ferenbach, D. A. (2017). Renal aging: Causes and consequences. *Journal of the American Society of Nephrology*, *28*(2), 407–420. doi: 10.1681/ASN.2015121308

Rosenberg, A. Z. & Kopp, J. B. (2017). Focal segmental glomerulosclerosis. *Clinical Journal of the American Society of Nephrology*, *12*(3), 502–517.

Sauve, C., Digel Vandyk, A. & Fothergill Bourbonnais, F. (2016). Exploring the facilitators and barriers to home dialysis: A scoping review. *Nephrology Nursing Journal*, *42*(4), 295–308.

Schnuelle, P., Benck, U. & Yard, B. A. (2018). Dopamine in transplantation: Written off or comeback with novel indication? *Clinical Transplantation*, *32*(7), e13292. https://doi.org/10.1111/ctr.13292

Schoch, M., Currey, J., Bennett, P., Orellana, L., Smith, V. & Hutchinson, A. (2019). Asking the hard questions: Are dialysis nurses ready for point-of-care ultrasound guided cannulation? *Renal Society of Australasia Journal*, *15*, 3.

Singh, S. & Sookraj, K. (2022). Kidney trauma. *StatPearls* [Internet]. Treasure Island (FL): StatPearls Publishing.

Tantisattamo, E., Molnar, M. Z., Ho, B. T. et al. (2020). Approach and management of hypertension after kidney transplantation. *Frontiers in Medicine*, *7*, 229–229.

Thwaites, S. E., Holt, S. G. & Yii, M. K. (2020). Inferiority of arteriovenous grafts, in comparison to autogenous fistulas, is underestimated by standard survival measures alone. *ANZ Journal of Surgery*, *91*(1–2), 162–167.

Tran, J. & Ornstein, M. C. (2021). Clinical review on the management of metastatic renal cell carcinoma. *Journal of Oncology Practice*, *18*(3), 187–196. https://ascopubs.org/doi/pdf/10.1200/OP.21.00419

Transplantation Society of Australia and New Zealand (TSANZ) (2021). *Changes to Australian deceased donor kidney allocation*. Transplantation Society of Australia and New Zealand. Retrieved from https://transplant.org.au

Tucker, E. L., Smith, A. R., Daskin, M. S. et al. (2019). Life and expectations post-kidney transplant: A qualitative analysis of patient responses. *BMC Nephrology*, *20*(1), 175.

Ward, R. A. (2022). Basic prerequisites for on-line, high-volume hemodiafiltration. *Seminars in Dialysis*, online. https://doi.org/10.1111/sdi.13073

Wiesen, P. & Preiser, J. (2014). *Nutritional support of critically ill patients with renal failure*. Cambridge: Cambridge University Press.

Wong, C. K. H., Chen, J., Fung, S. K. S. et al. (2019). Direct and indirect costs of end-stage renal disease patients in the first and second years after initiation of nocturnal home haemodialysis, hospital haemodialysis and peritoneal dialysis. *Nephrology Dialysis Transplantation*, *34*(9), 1565–1576.

Wu, Q. & Zhang, H. (2018). Carbon dioxide pneumothorax following retroperitoneal laparoscopic partial nephrectomy: A case report and literature review. *BMC Anesthesiology*, *18*, 202. doi: 10.1186/s12871-018-0662-x

Yang, X., We, H. & Li, H. (2020). Dehydration-associated chronic kidney disease: A novel case of kidney failure in China. *BMC Nephrology*, *21*(159), 1–5. https://doi.org/10.1186/s12882-020-01804-x

UNIT 7 BUILDING CLINICAL COMPETENCE

Responses to altered urinary elimination

Clinical scenario

You have been assigned to work with the following four people for the 0700 shift on a renal medical–surgical unit. Significant data obtained during report are as follows:

- Phillip Connor is a 45-year-old who was admitted 2 days ago after a fall from a ute. He experienced a bruised right kidney and numerous ecchymotic areas on his right side from the fall. His vital signs are T 37.2°C, P 98, R 28, BP 110/68. He is complaining of abdominal pain and difficulty urinating.
- Agnes Gibson is an 84-year-old who was admitted 2 hours ago with manifestations of urinary incontinence, anorexia, confusion and lethargy. Her vital signs on admission were T 36.1°C, P 88, R 20, BP 148/90. The physician ordered trimethoprim-sulfamethoxazole (Bactrim) to be started as soon as possible.
- Joseph Rouse is a 45-year-old who is to undergo surgery for removal of uric acid stones after having a failed lithotripsy. His vital signs are T 37.5°C, P 94, R 24, BP 112/68. His skin is pale, cool and clammy. He is complaining of nausea, severe left-sided flank pain with spasms and light-headedness.
- Angela Baldwin is a 34-year-old who has a medical history of systemic lupus erythematosus (SLE). She was admitted with complaints of left flank pain and generalised oedema. Urinalysis results indicate haematuria and proteinuria. Vital signs are T 37.8°C, P 88, R 26, BP 144/90. She is admitted for aggressive immunosuppressive therapy.

Critical-thinking questions

1 In what order would you visit these people after report?

1.
2.
3.
4.

2 What top two priority nursing diagnoses would you choose for each of the people presented above? Can you explain, if asked, the rationale for your choices?

	Priority Nursing Diagnosis #1	Priority Nursing Diagnosis #2
Phillip Connor		
Agnes Gibson		
Joseph Rouse		
Angela Baldwin		

3 The physician ordered trimethoprim-sulfamethoxazole (Bactrim) for Agnes Gibson's uncomplicated cystitis. Mrs Gibson understands the length of antibiotic therapy when she verbalises which statement?

1. 'I will need to complete the full course of Bactrim.'
2. 'I can be discharged after 5 days of antibiotics.'
3. 'I need to stay in the hospital for 1 week to finish the antibiotics.'
4. 'I can stay in the hospital for 5 days of antibiotics and take 5 days of antibiotics at home.'

4 The physician orders phenazopyridine (Pyridium) for relief of pain and burning with cystitis. Which does the nurse teach the person about the use of this medication?

1. Take the medication with antacids to prevent stomach upset.
2. Drink less fluid to allow the drug to concentrate in the bladder.
3. Wear a sanitary pad to protect your clothing from stains while taking this drug.
4. Stop taking the drug if nausea and diarrhoea occur.

5 The person diagnosed with uric acid stones is ordered to follow a diet low in purines. Which is the meal plan lowest in purines?

1. liver with onions and potatoes
2. chicken burger with chips
3. spaghetti with Bolognese sauce
4. macaroni and cheese with stewed tomatoes

6 When assessing a person with glomerulonephritis, which manifestations are indicative of an early disease process?

1. pyuria, leucocytosis and hyperthermia
2. haematuria, proteinuria and hypertension
3. dysuria, hyperglycaemia and hypertension
4. oliguria, flank pain and hypotension

7 Which are risk factors of urinary tract infections? (Select all that apply.)

1. circumcision in males
2. decreased cervicovaginal antibodies
3. sexual intercourse in women
4. short urethra in men
5. ageing in men
6. urinary catheterisation

8 Which is the most accurate indicator of fluid volume status in the oliguric or anuric person?

1. intake and output
2. weight changes
3. restricted fluids
4. urea and creatinine levels

9 The most reliable diagnostic procedure to determine glomerular disorders is which diagnostic test?

1. kidney scan
2. antistreptolysin O titre
3. kidney biopsy
4. blood urea nitrogen

10 A female postoperative person is complaining of inability to void. A bladder ultrasound indicates that there is a significant amount of urine in the bladder. Which interventions does the nurse perform?

1. Insert a urinary catheter and completely drain the bladder at once.
2. Insert a urinary catheter and drain urine in 500 mL increments.
3. Ambulate person to the bathroom to try to void and run water in the sink.
4. Give the person a glass of water to drink to encourage voiding.

11 Which nursing actions are instituted for the person with kidney trauma?

1. Monitor level of consciousness and urine output.
2. Monitor vital signs for hypotension and bradycardia.
3. Observe for hypertension and check urine for haematuria.
4. Observe urine for oliguria and proteinuria.

12 After a person has returned from surgery, the nurse needs to report which urinary output?

1. 20 mL per hour
2. 40 mL per hour
3. 300 mL per 8 hours
4. 400 mL per 8 hours

Case study

Steven McEvoy is a 45-year-old Indigenous male who has been a truck driver for the past 20 years. Increasing shortness of breath has prompted him to attend the ED. He is admitted to the hospital with a further history of nausea for several weeks, weakness, fatigue and loss of appetite. He has been feeling very depressed. He has a past medical history of type 1 diabetes mellitus, hypertension and diabetic nephropathy. On admission, his vital signs are T 37.1°C, P 96, R 20, BP 170/110. He has bilateral pitting oedema of the lower extremities. His fingers and hands are also oedematous. He complains of dry and itching skin. His urine is dark, frothy and scanty. A specimen is collected for a urinalysis and blood is taken and sent to the laboratory. Results returned with the urinalysis show a specific gravity of 1.011, gross haematuria and 3+ protein. His blood work reveals a urea of 32.6 mmol/L, creatinine of 832 µmol/L and eGFR of 6.2 mL/min. Based on his past medical history of diabetes, hypertension and diabetic nephropathy and the current findings, a medical diagnosis of end-stage kidney disease (kidney failure (CKD (stage 5)) is established.

Based on Mr McEvoy's assessment and past medical history, the nursing diagnosis of *Impaired urinary elimination* is identified as one of the high priorities for planning nursing care.

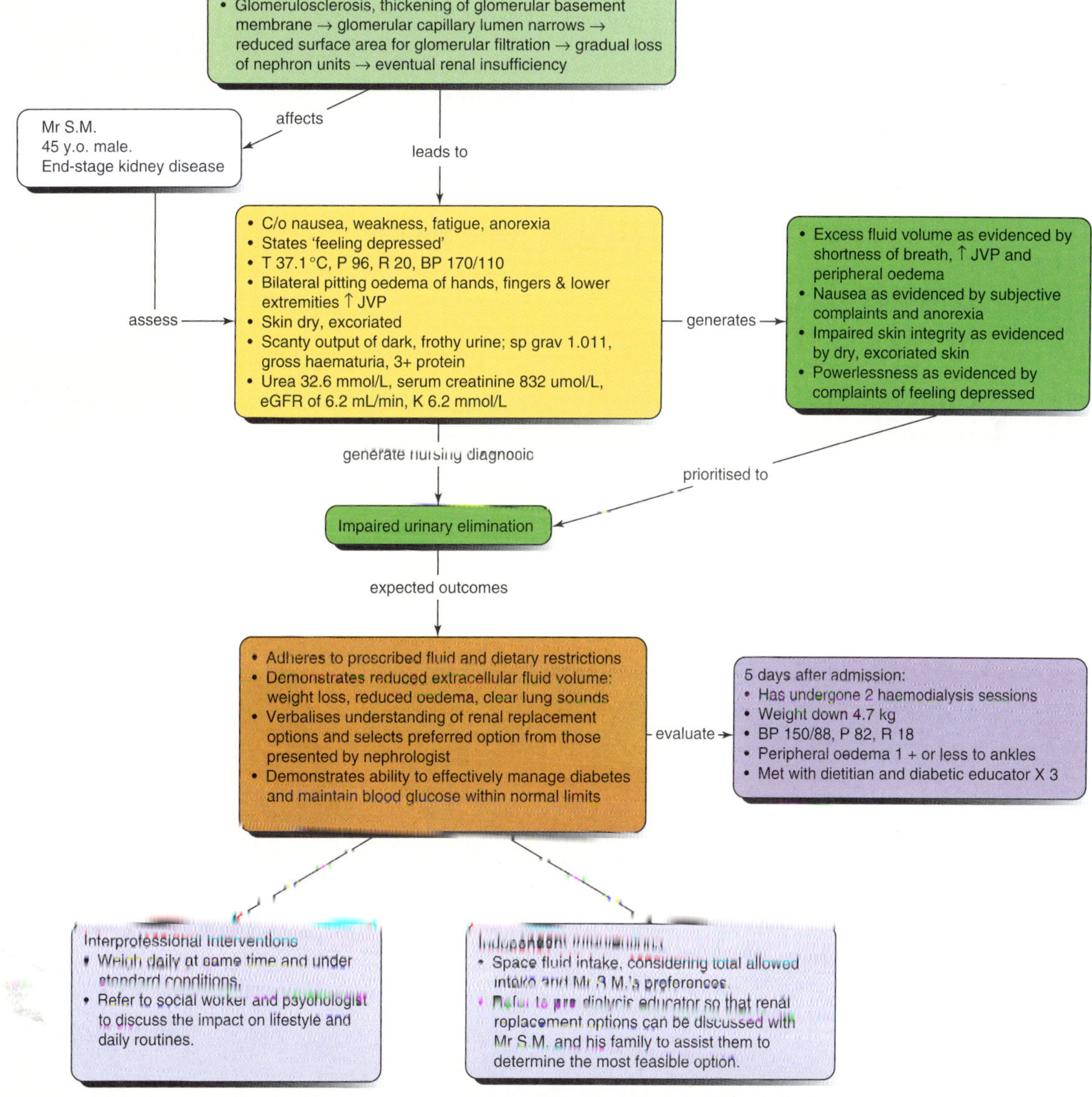

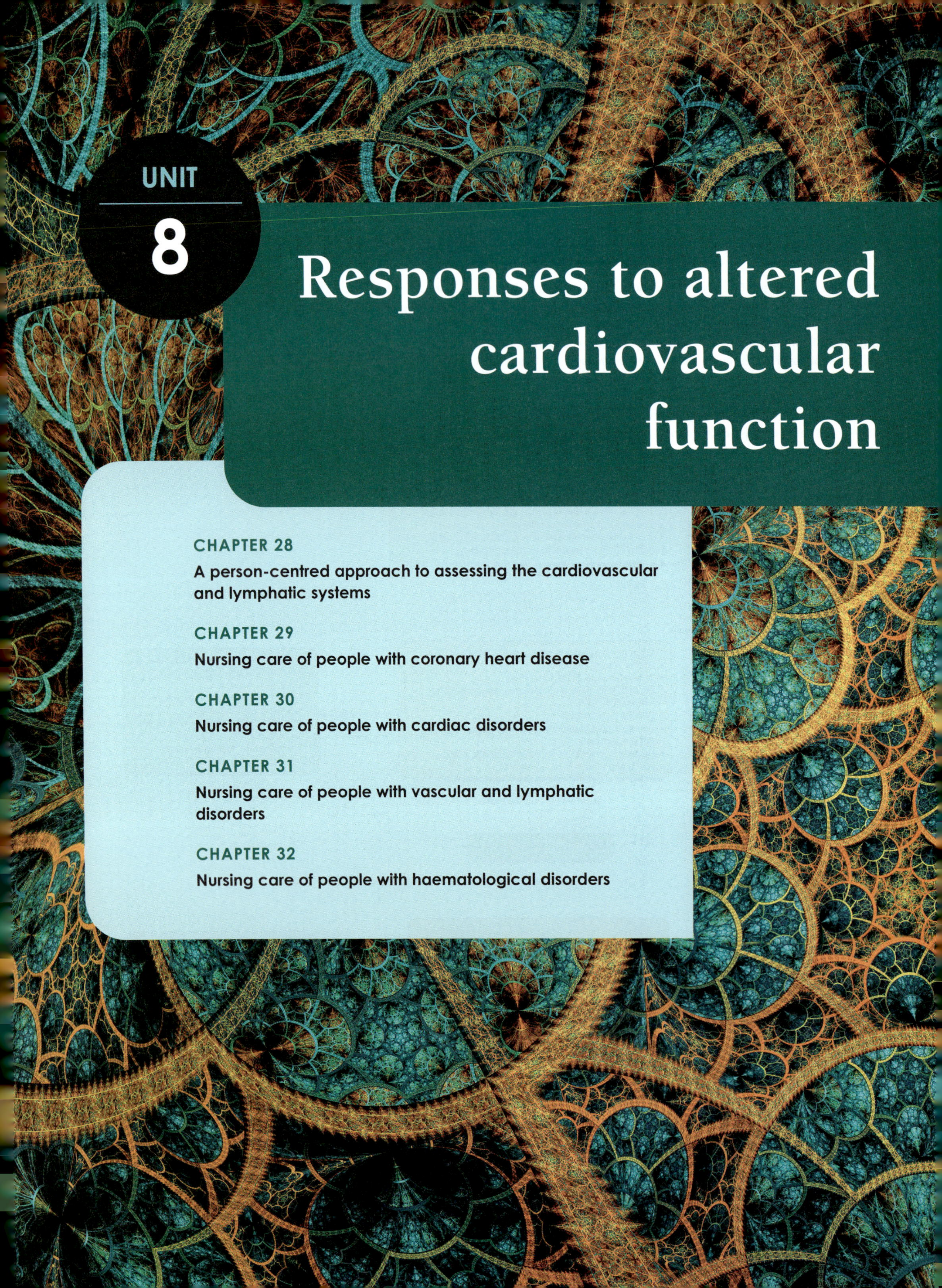

UNIT

8

Responses to altered cardiovascular function

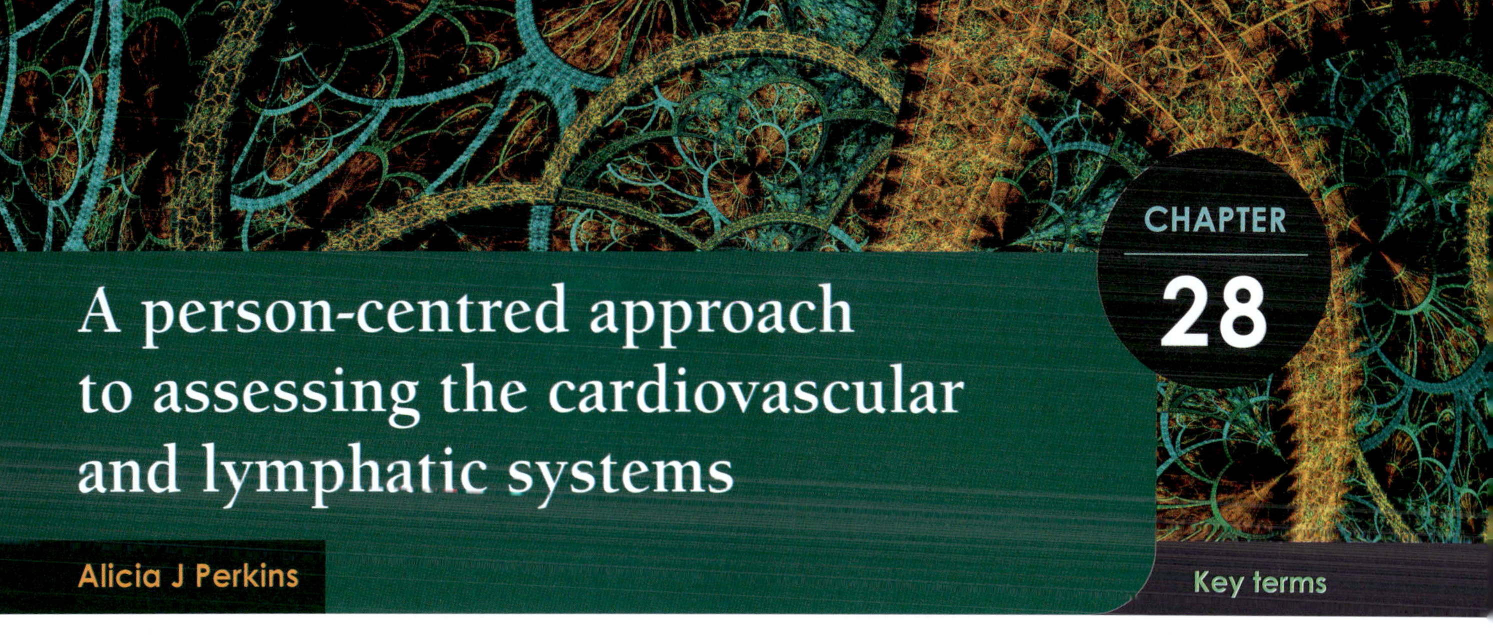

CHAPTER 28

A person-centred approach to assessing the cardiovascular and lymphatic systems

Alicia J Perkins

Learning outcomes

- Describe the anatomy and physiology of the cardiovascular and lymphatic systems.
- Examine investigations and observations important for assessing a person's cardiovascular and lymphatic system function.
- Accurately interpret normal and aberrant data gained from assessment of a person's cardiovascular and lymphatic system.
- Discuss manifestations of impaired cardiovascular and lymphatic systems.

Clinical competencies

- Assess an ECG strip and identify normal cardiac function and abnormal rhythm.
- Conduct and document a health history for people having or at risk of alterations in the structure and function of the cardiovascular, haematological or lymphatic systems.
- Conduct and document a physical assessment of cardiovascular, haematological and lymphatic status.
- Monitor the results of diagnostic tests and report abnormal findings.

Equipment needed

- Stethoscope with diaphragm and bell
- Blood pressure cuff
- Tape measure
- Metric ruler
- Doppler ultrasound device (if needed) and transducer gel

Key terms

afterload 933
apical impulse 960
arrhythmia 962
blood flow 937
blood pressure 937
cardiac index (CI) 933
cardiac output (CO) 931
cardiac reserve 931
contractility 932
ejection fraction 931
erythropoiesis 938
haemolysis 938
ischaemic 931
Korotkoff's sounds 964
leucocytosis 941
leucopenia 941
lymphadenopathy 970
lymphoedema 964
mean arterial pressure (MAP) 937
murmur 945
orthostatic hypotension 964
preload 933
pulse 934
pulse pressure 937
stem cell 938
stroke volume (SV) 931
thrill 961
total peripheral vascular resistance (TPVR) 937

The cardiovascular system comprises the heart (the system's pump), the peripheral vascular system (a network of arteries, veins and capillaries) and the haematological system (blood and blood components). The lymphatic system (lymph, lymph nodes and spleen) is a special vascular system that helps maintain sufficient blood volume in the cardiovascular system by collecting extracellular fluid from the tissues and returning it to the bloodstream. The heart beats an average of 70 times per minute. This continuous pumping moves blood through the body, nourishing tissue cells and removing wastes. Deficits in the structure or function of the heart affect all body tissues. Changes in cardiac rate, rhythm or output may limit almost all human functions, including self-care, mobility and the ability to maintain tissue perfusion, fluid volume status, respirations and comfort. Cardiac changes may also affect self-concept, sexuality and role performance.

STRUCTURE AND FUNCTION OF THE CARDIOVASCULAR SYSTEM

The heart is a hollow, cone-shaped organ approximately the size of an adult's fist, weighing less than 500 grams. It is located in the mediastinum of the thoracic cavity, between the vertebral column and the sternum, and is flanked laterally by the lungs. Two-thirds of the heart mass lies to the left of the sternum; the upper base lies beneath the second rib and the pointed apex is approximate with the fifth intercostal space, midpoint to the clavicle (see Figure 28.1).

The heart is covered by the pericardium, a double layer of fibroserous membrane (see Figure 28.2). The pericardium encases the heart and anchors it to the mediastinum, forming the pericardial sac. The snug fit of the pericardium prevents the heart from overfilling with blood. The fibrous outer layer is the parietal pericardium; the serous inner layer is the visceral pericardium (or epicardium) and adheres to the heart surface. The small space between the visceral and parietal layers of the pericardium is the pericardial cavity. A serous lubricating fluid secreted by the serous layer of the pericardium prevents friction as the heart contracts.

The heart wall consists of three layers of tissue: the epicardium, the myocardium and the endocardium (see Figure 28.2). The epicardium covers the entire heart and great vessels and then folds over to form the parietal layer that lines the pericardium and adheres to the heart surface. The myocardium, which is the middle layer of the heart wall, consists of specialised cardiac muscle cells (myofibrils) that provide the bulk of contractile heart muscle. The endocardium, which is the innermost layer, is a thin membrane composed of three layers; the inner layer consists of smooth endothelial cells that line the inside of the heart's chambers, the great vessels and the valves.

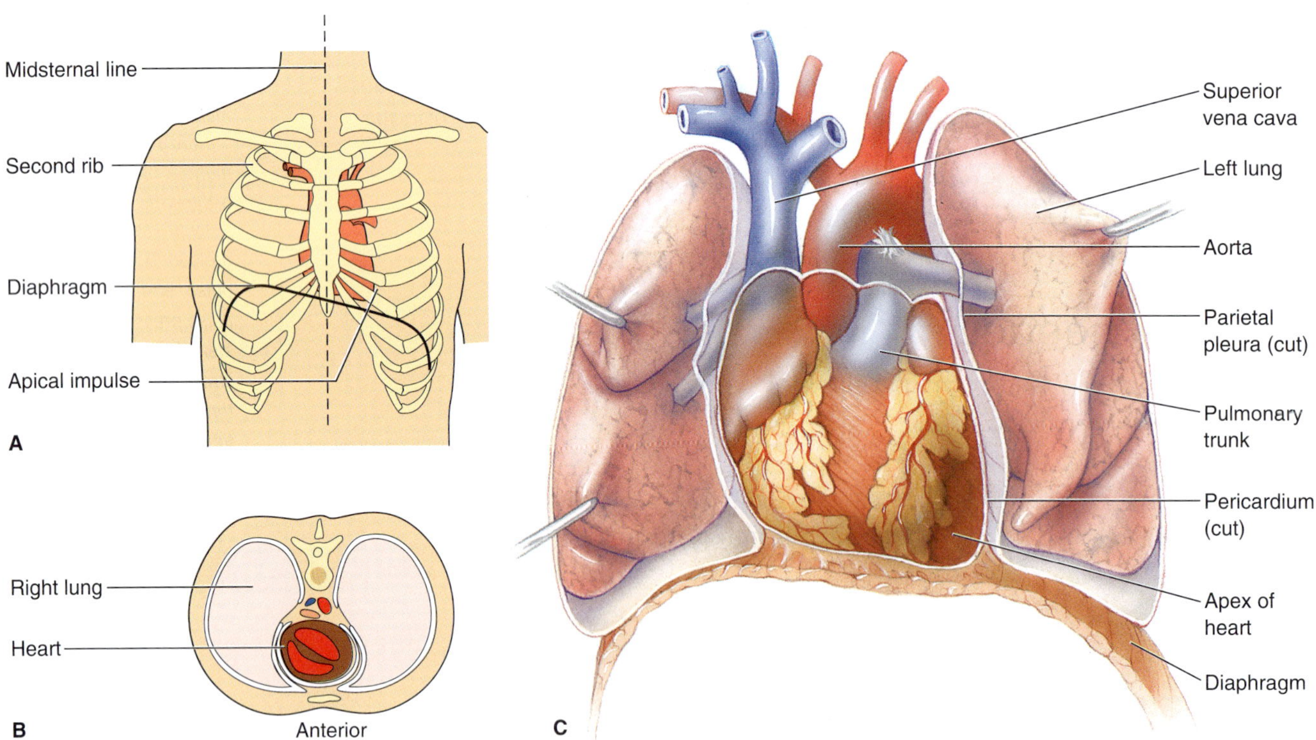

FIGURE 28.1 *Location of the heart in the mediastinum of the thorax. A, Relationship of the heart to the sternum, ribs and diaphragm. B, Cross-sectional view showing relative position of the heart in the thorax. C, Relationship of the heart and great vessels to the lungs*

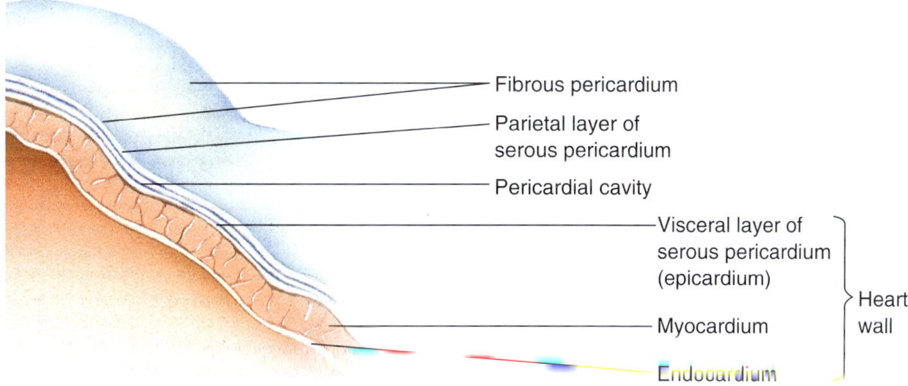

FIGURE 28.2 *Coverings and layers of the heart*

Chambers and valves of the heart

The heart has four hollow chambers, two upper atria and two lower ventricles. They are separated longitudinally by the interatrial septum and the interventricular septum (see Figure 28.3).

The right atrium receives oxygen-poor blood via three main veins:

1. The superior vena cava returns blood from the upper extremities, head, neck and thorax.
2. The inferior vena cava returns blood from the abdomen and lower extremities.
3. The coronary sinus drains blood from the coronary circulation.

(Note that the terms 'deoxygenated' and 'oxygen-poor' are often used interchangeably; however, 'oxygen-poor' is more technically correct. Haemoglobin will never become fully devoid of all oxygen—i.e. 'deoxygenated'—even at the tissues.)

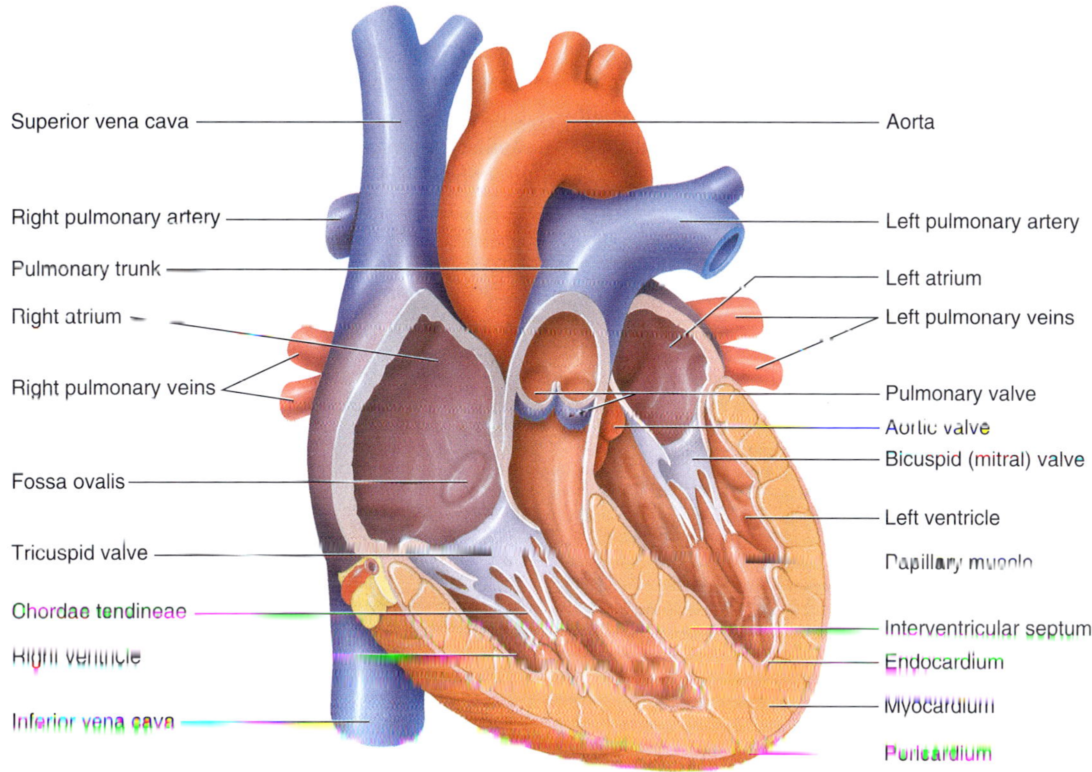

FIGURE 28.3 *The internal anatomy of the heart, frontal section*

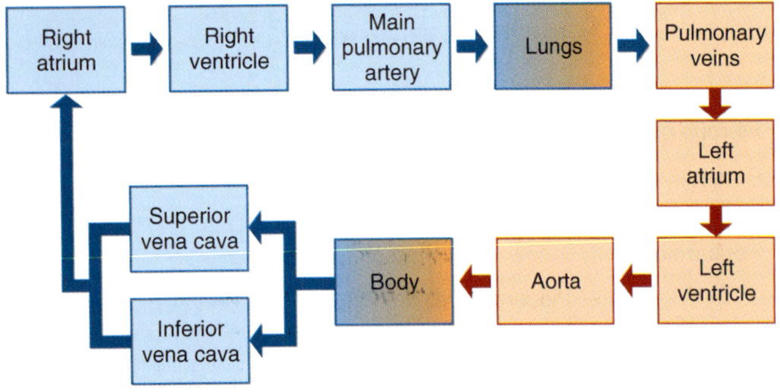

FIGURE 28.4 *Blood flow around the systemic circuit*

The left atrium receives oxygenated blood from the lungs via the pulmonary veins.

Oxygen-poor blood flows from the right atrium, through the tricuspid valve, into the right ventricle where it is pumped through the pulmonary artery to the pulmonary capillary bed for oxygenation. The newly oxygenated blood then travels through the pulmonary veins to the left atrium. It then flows through the mitral (bicuspid) valve into the left ventricle. Blood is then pumped out of the aorta to the arterial circulation (see Figure 28.4).

The chambers of the heart are separated by valves that allow unidirectional blood flow to the next chamber or great vessel. The atria are separated from the ventricles by the two atrioventricular (AV) valves; the tricuspid valve is on the right side and the bicuspid (or mitral) valve is on the left. The flaps of each of these valves are anchored to the papillary muscles of the ventricles by the chordae tendineae. These structures control the movement of the AV valves to prevent backflow of blood. The ventricles are connected to their great vessels by the semilunar valves. The pulmonary (pulmonic) valve joins the right ventricle with the pulmonary artery. The aortic valve joins the left ventricle to the aorta (see Figure 28.5).

Closure of the AV valves at the onset of contraction (systole) produces the first heart sound, or S_1 (characterised by the syllable 'lub'); closure of the semilunar valves at the onset of relaxation (diastole) produces the second heart sound, or S_2 (characterised by the syllable 'dub').

Systemic, pulmonary and coronary circulation

Because each side of the heart both receives and ejects blood, the heart is often described as a double pump, with the right and left sides pumping synchronously. The circulatory system has two parts: the pulmonary circulation (moving blood through the capillary bed surrounding the lungs to form the alveolar–capillary bed, where gas exchange occurs) and the systemic circulation, which supplies blood to all other body tissues. In addition, the heart muscle itself is supplied with blood via the coronary circulation.

Systemic circulation

The systemic circulation consists of the left side of the heart, the aorta and its branches, the capillaries that supply the brain and peripheral tissues, the systemic venous system and the vena cavae. The systemic system moves blood to peripheral areas of the body, via thick, muscular vessels. It is a high-pressure system.

Pulmonary circulation

The pulmonary circulation consists of the right side of the heart, the pulmonary artery, the pulmonary capillaries and the pulmonary veins. Because the pulmonary vessels are thinner and less muscular, the pulmonary circulation is a low-pressure system. Pulmonary circulation begins with the right side of the heart. Oxygen-poor blood from the venous system enters the right atrium through three large veins, the superior and inferior venae cavae and the coronary sinus, and is transported to the lungs via the pulmonary artery and its branches (see Figure 28.6). After oxygen and carbon dioxide are exchanged at the alveolar–capillary membrane, oxygen-rich blood returns to the left atrium through several pulmonary veins.

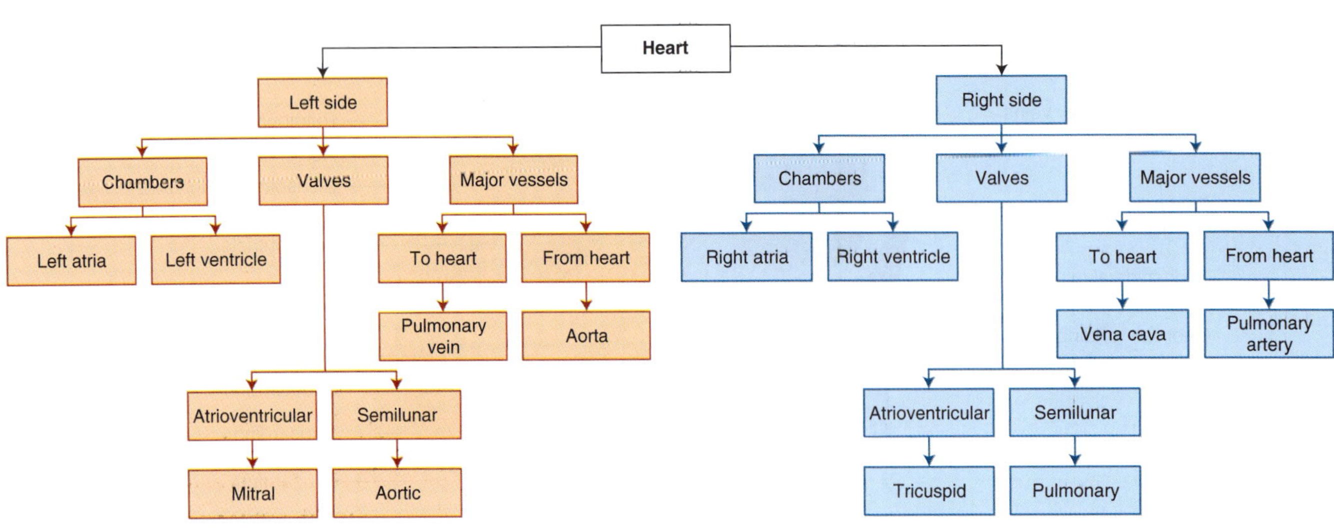

FIGURE 28.5 *Summary of key components of the heart*

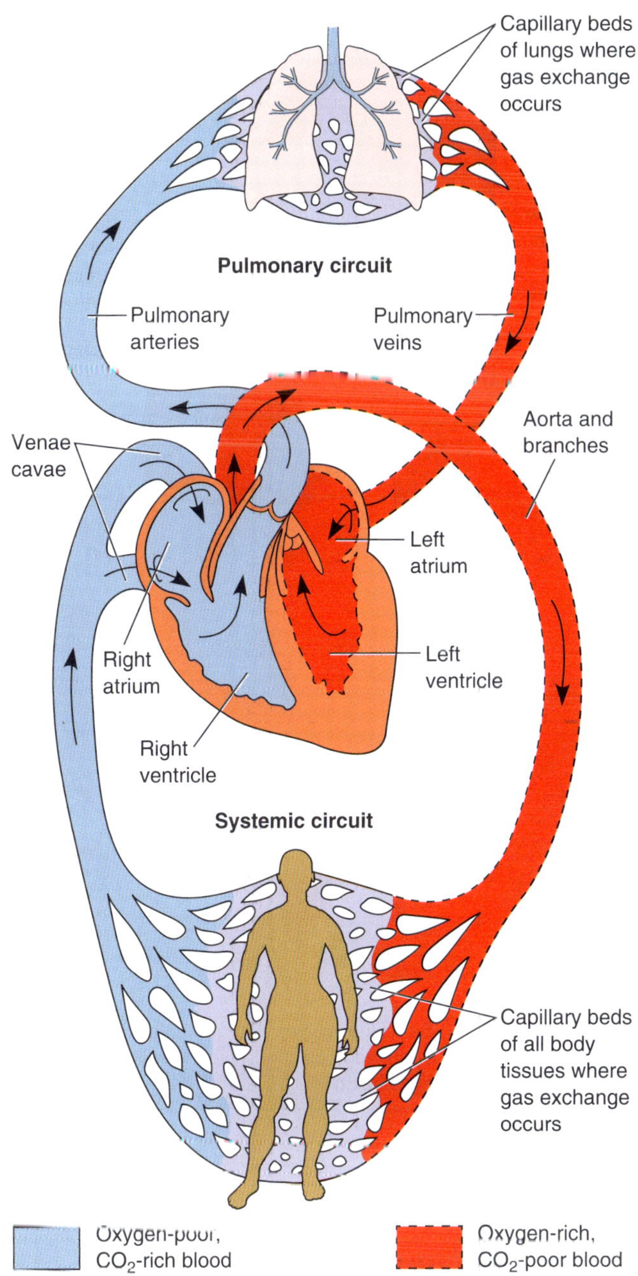

FIGURE 28.6 ***Pulmonary and systemic circulation***

Coronary circulation

The heart muscle itself is supplied by its own network of vessels through the coronary circulation. The left and right coronary arteries originate at the base of the aorta in the sinuses of Valsalva and branch out to encircle the myocardium (see Figure 28.7A), supplying blood, oxygen and nutrients to the myocardium. The left main coronary artery divides to form the anterior descending and circumflex arteries. The anterior descending artery supplies the interventricular septum and the anterior wall of the left ventricle. The circumflex branch supplies the lateral wall of the left ventricle and the left atrium. The right coronary artery, which branches into the posterior descending artery, supplies the inferior and posterior wall of the left ventricle, the right ventricle and right atrium (Marieb & Hoehn, 2019). While ventricular contraction delivers blood through the pulmonary circulation and the systemic circulation, it is during ventricular relaxation that the coronary arteries fill with oxygen-rich blood. After the blood perfuses the heart muscle, the cardiac veins drain the blood into the coronary sinus, which empties into the right atrium of the heart (see Figure 28.7B).

Blood flow through the coronary arteries is regulated by several factors. Aortic pressure is the primary factor. Other factors include the heart rate (most flow occurs during diastole, when the muscle is relaxed), metabolic activity of the heart and blood vessel tone (constriction).

The cardiac cycle and cardiac output

The contraction and relaxation of the heart constitutes one heartbeat and is called the cardiac cycle (see Figure 28.8). Ventricular filling is followed by ventricular systole, a phase during which the ventricles contract and eject blood into the pulmonary and systemic circuits. Systole is followed by diastole, the relaxation phase, during which the ventricles refill, the atria contract and the myocardium is perfused. Normally, the complete cardiac cycle occurs about 70 to 80 times per minute, measured as the heart rate (HR).

During diastole, the volume in the ventricles is increased to approximately 120 mL (end-diastolic volume); at the end of systole, approximately 40 mL of blood remains in the ventricles (end-systolic volume). The difference between the end-diastolic volume and the end-systolic volume is called the **stroke volume (SV)** (see Figure 28.9). Normal SV is 60 to 100 mL/beat and averages about 80 mL/beat in an adult. The **cardiac output (CO)** is the amount of blood pumped by the ventricles into the pulmonary and systemic circulations in 1 minute. Therefore:

$$CO = HR \times SV.$$

Ejection fraction (EF) is the SV divided by the end-diastolic volume and represents the fraction or percentage of the diastolic volume that is ejected from the heart during systole (Marieb & Hoehn, 2019). For example, an end-diastolic volume of 120 mL divided by a stroke volume of 80 mL equals an ejection fraction of 66% (see Figure 28.9). Normal EF ranges from 50% to 70%.

The average person's CO varies significantly, from 4 to 8 L/min, and is largely determined by body surface area (BSA). Therefore, to accurately evaluate CO, it must be corrected to BSA. This correction is called the cardiac index (CI). CO is an indicator of how well the heart is functioning as a pump. If the heart cannot pump effectively, cardiac output and tissue perfusion are decreased. Body tissues that do not receive enough blood and oxygen (carried in the blood on haemoglobin) become **ischaemic** (deprived of oxygen). If the tissues do not receive enough blood flow to maintain the functions of the cells, the cells die. (Cellular death results in necrosis or infarction.)

In addition to BSA, activity level, metabolic rate, physiological and psychological stress responses and age all influence CO. CO is then determined by the interaction of four main factors: heart rate, preload, afterload and contractility. Changes in each of these variables influence CO intrinsically and each can also be manipulated to affect CO. The heart's ability to respond to the body's changing need for CO is called **cardiac reserve**.

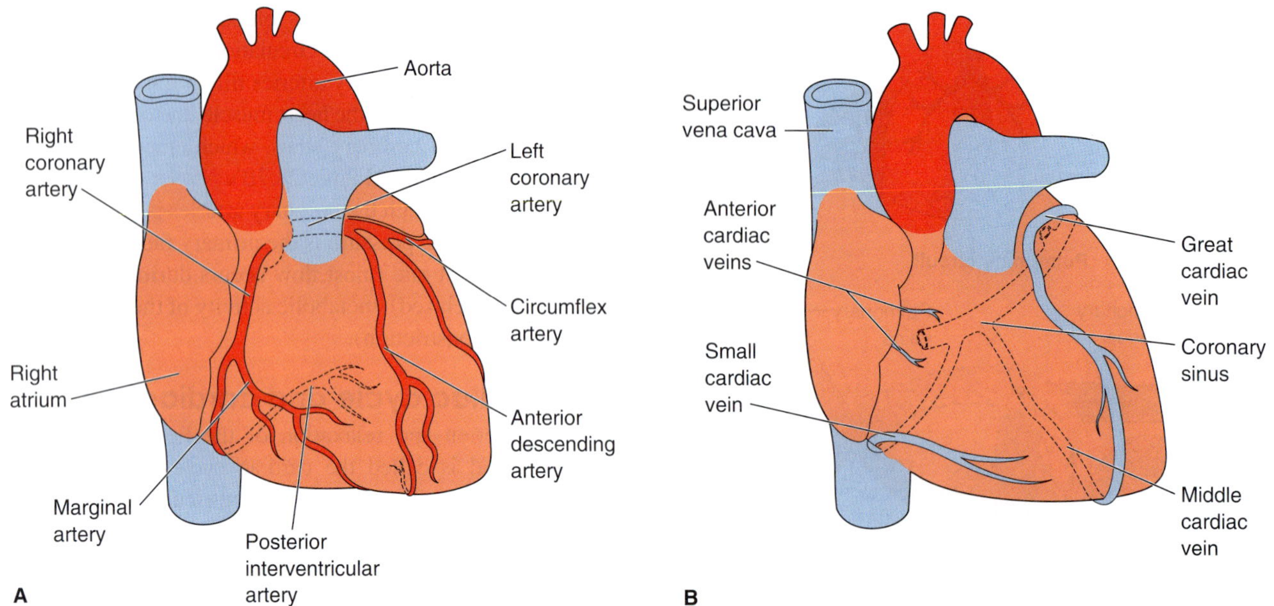

FIGURE 28.7 ***Coronary circulation. A, Coronary arteries; B, coronary veins***

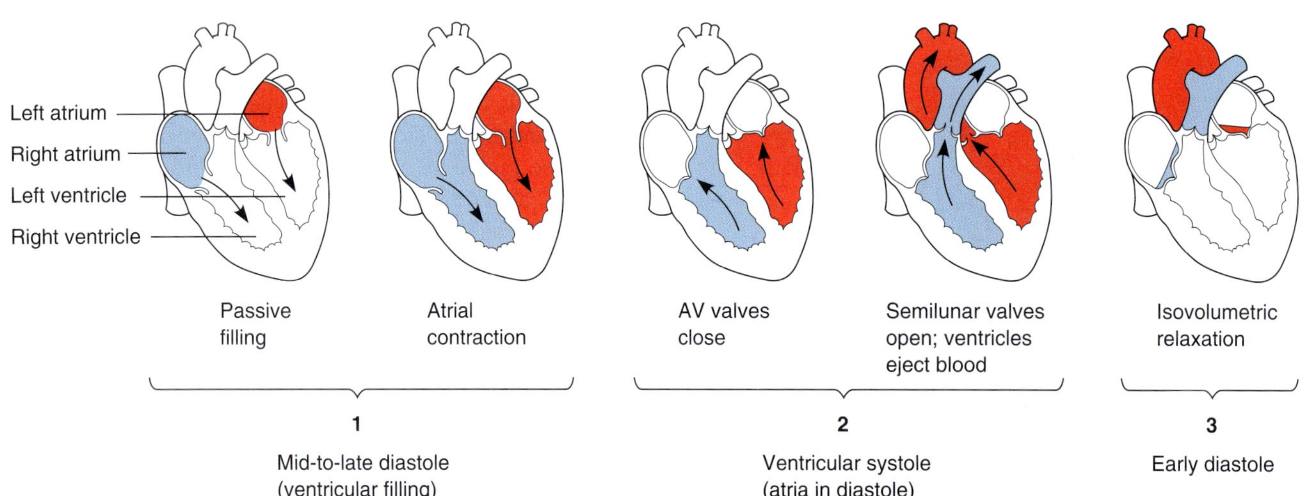

FIGURE 28.8 ***The cardiac cycle has three events: (1) ventricular filling in mid-to-late diastole, (2) ventricular systole, and (3) isovolumetric relaxation in early diastole***

Heart rate

Heart rate is affected by both direct and indirect autonomic nervous system stimulation. Direct stimulation is accomplished through the innervation of the heart muscle by sympathetic and parasympathetic nerves. The sympathetic nervous system increases the heart rate, whereas the parasympathetic vagal tone slows the heart rate. Reflex regulation of the heart rate in response to systemic blood pressure also occurs through activation of sensory receptors known as baroreceptors or pressure receptors located in the carotid sinus, aortic arch, venae cavae and pulmonary veins (Marieb & Hoehn, 2019).

If heart rate increases, cardiac output also increases when there is no change in stroke volume. However, rapid heart rate leads to a shorter diastolic time; that is, a decrease in ventricular filling time. This in turn decreases stroke volume, with a subsequent fall in cardiac output. Because coronary artery filling occurs primarily during diastole, this decrease in diastolic time may significantly impair coronary perfusion.

If heart rate decreases, cardiac output decreases (if stroke volume remains unchanged) because the number of cardiac cycles is decreased.

Contractility

Contractility is the inherent capability of the cardiac muscle fibres to shorten. Poor contractility of the heart muscle reduces the forward flow of blood from the heart, increases the ventricular pressures from accumulation of blood volume and reduces cardiac output. Increased contractility due to positive inotropic factors may cause fatigue and myocardial stress.

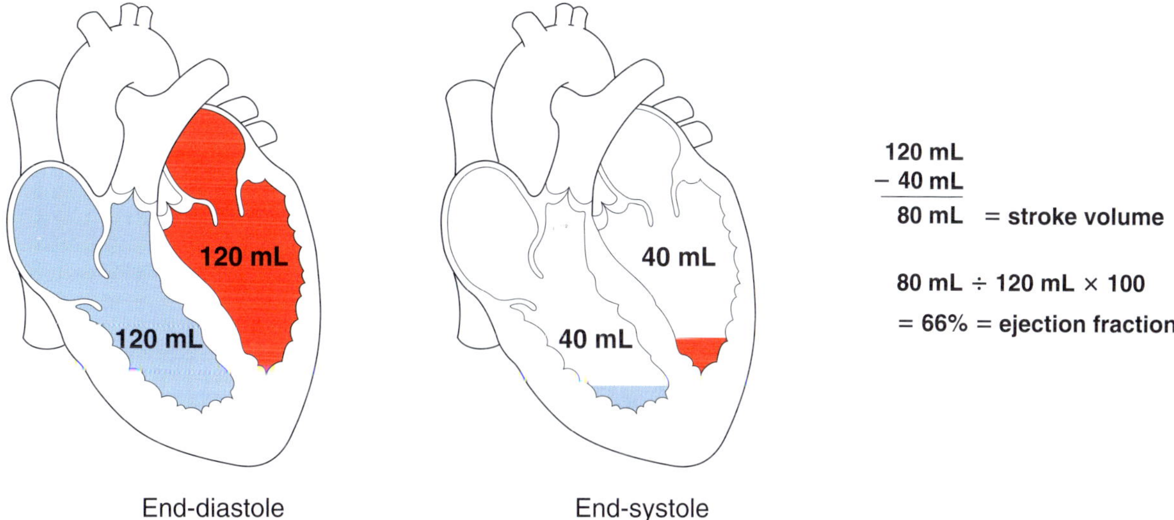

FIGURE 28.9 *Stroke volume is end-diastole volume minus end-systole volume; ejection fraction is stroke volume divided by end-diastole volume, expressed as a percentage*

Preload

Preload is the amount of cardiac muscle fibre tension or stretch that exists at the end of diastole, just before contraction of the ventricles. Preload is influenced by venous return and the compliance of the ventricles. It is related to the total volume of blood in the ventricles: the greater the volume, the greater the stretch of the cardiac muscle fibres and the greater the force with which the fibres contract to accomplish emptying. This principle is called the Frank–Starling law (Muir & Hamlin, 2020).

This mechanism has a physiological limit. Just as continuous overstretching of a rubber band causes the band to relax and lose its ability to recoil, overstretching of the cardiac muscle fibres eventually results in ineffective contraction. Disorders such as kidney disease and congestive heart failure result in sodium and water retention and increased preload. Vasoconstriction also increases venous return and preload.

Reduced circulating blood volume results in decreased venous return and therefore decreased preload. A decrease in preload reduces stroke volume and thus cardiac output. Decreased preload may result from haemorrhage or maldistribution of blood volume, as occurs in 'third spacing' (see the chapter 'Nursing care of people with altered fluid, electrolyte and acid–base balance').

Afterload

Afterload is the resistance the ventricles must overcome to eject the blood volume. The higher the afterload, the harder the ventricle must work. The right ventricle must generate enough tension to open the pulmonary valve and eject its volume into the low-pressure pulmonary arteries. Right ventricle afterload is measured as pulmonary vascular resistance (PVR). Similarly, the left ventricle needs to generate enough energy to open the aortic valve and pump blood into the aorta. Afterload of the left ventricle is measured as systemic vascular resistance (SVR) or by the older term total peripheral resistance (TPR). Aortic pressure is much higher than pulmonary artery pressure; thus, the workload of the left ventricle is much harder than that of the right ventricle (Muir & Hamlin, 2020).

Alterations in vascular tone affect afterload and ventricular work. As the pulmonary or arterial blood pressure increases (e.g. through vasoconstriction), PVR and/or SVR increases and the work of the ventricles increases. As workload increases, consumption of myocardial oxygen also increases. A compromised heart cannot effectively meet this increased oxygen demand and a vicious cycle ensues. By contrast, a very low afterload decreases the forward flow of blood into the systemic circulation and the coronary arteries. Afterload is also increased due to stenosis of the semilunar valves (i.e. pulmonary valve stenosis and aortic valve stenosis).

Clinical indicators of cardiac output

For many people who are critically ill, invasive haemodynamic monitoring catheters or echocardiography are used to measure cardiac output in quantifiable numbers. However, advanced technology is not the only way to identify and assess compromised blood flow. Tissue perfusion is the direct outcome of adequate cardiac output; therefore, clinical indicators of low cardiac output may be manifested by changes in organ function that result from compromised blood flow. For example, a decrease in blood flow to the brain presents as a change in level of consciousness. Other manifestations of decreased cardiac output are discussed in the chapters 'Nursing care of people with altered fluid, electrolyte and acid–base balance' and 'Nursing care of people with coronary heart disease'.

Cardiac index (CI) is the cardiac output adjusted for the person's body size, also called the person's body surface area (BSA). Because it takes into account the person's BSA, the cardiac index provides more meaningful data about the heart's ability to perfuse the tissues and therefore is a more accurate indicator of the effectiveness of the circulation.

BSA is stated in square metres (m^2) and cardiac index is calculated as CO divided by BSA. Results are considered adequate when they fall within the range of 2.5 to 4.0 L/min/m^2. Cardiac index has value in understanding a person's cardiac function, normalising for the person's body size.

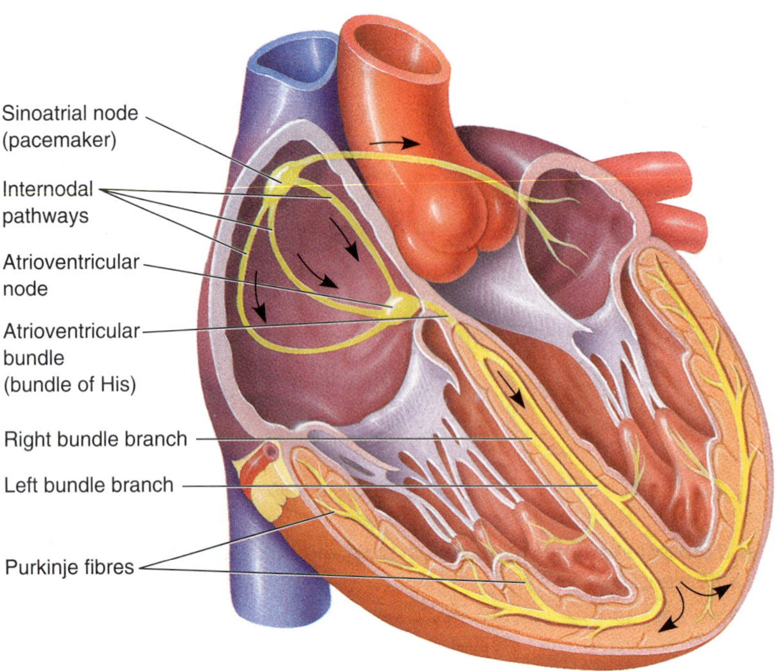

FIGURE 28.10 ***The intrinsic conduction system of the heart***

The conduction system of the heart

The cardiac cycle is perpetuated by a complex electrical circuit commonly known as the intrinsic conduction system of the heart. Cardiac muscle cells possess an inherent characteristic of self-excitation, which enables them to initiate and transmit impulses independent of a stimulus. However, specialised areas of myocardial cells typically exert a controlling influence in this electrical pathway.

One of these specialised areas is the sinoatrial (SA) node, located at the junction of the superior vena cava and right atrium (see Figure 28.10). The SA node acts as the normal 'pacemaker' of the heart, usually generating an impulse 60 to 100 times per minute. This impulse travels across the atria via internodal pathways to the atrioventricular (AV) node, in the floor of the interatrial septum. The AV node is the electrical connection between the atria and the ventricles. It consists of two pathways: a fast pathway and a slow pathway with refractory periods that effectively prevent rapid conduction in the ventricles in the presence of atrial arrhythmias. From the AV node, the impulse then passes through the bundle of His at the atrioventricular junction and continues down the interventricular septum through the right and left bundle branches and out to the Purkinje fibres in the ventricular muscle walls (Marieb & Hoehn, 2019).

THE PERIPHERAL VASCULAR SYSTEM

The two main components of the peripheral vascular system are the arterial and venous networks. The arterial network begins with the major arteries that branch from the aorta. The major arteries of the systemic circulation are illustrated in Figure 28.11. These major arteries branch into successively smaller arteries, which in turn subdivide into the smallest of the arterial vessels, called *arterioles*. The smallest arterioles feed into beds of hair-like capillaries in the body's organs and tissues.

In the *capillary* beds, oxygen and nutrients are exchanged for metabolic wastes, and deoxygenated blood is transported back towards the heart through venules, the smallest vessels of the venous network. Venules join the smallest of veins, which in turn flow into larger veins. Large veins empty into the superior and inferior venae cavae entering the right side of the heart. The major veins of the systemic circulation are shown in Figure 28.12.

Structure of blood vessels

The structure of blood vessels reflects their different functions within the circulatory system (see Figure 28.13). Except for the micro vessels, blood vessel walls have three layers: the tunica intima, the tunica media and the tunica adventitia. The tunica intima, the innermost layer, is made of simple squamous epithelium (the endothelium); this provides a slick surface to facilitate the flow of blood. In arteries the middle layer, or tunica media, is made of smooth muscle and is thicker than the tunica media of veins. This makes arteries more elastic than veins and allows the arteries to alternately expand and recoil as the heart contracts and relaxes, producing an arterial pressure waveform, which can be felt as a **pulse** over an artery. The smaller arterioles are less elastic than arteries but contain more smooth muscle, which promotes constriction and dilation, and subsequently are the major controllers of arterial blood pressure. The tunica adventitia, or outermost layer, is made of connective tissue and serves to protect and anchor the vessel. Veins have a thicker tunica adventitia than arteries to prevent the veins from collapsing and to provide protection to superficial veins.

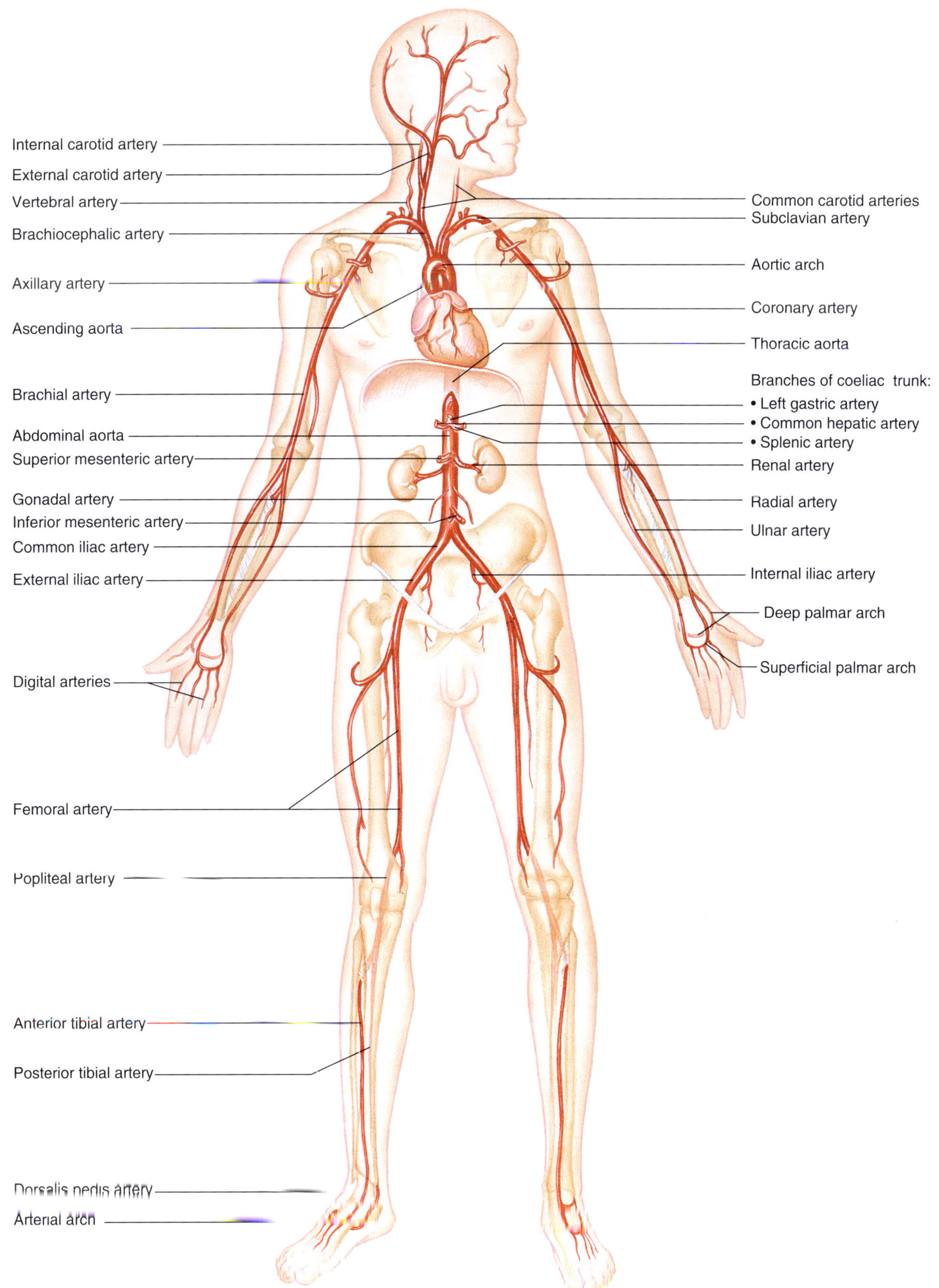

FIGURE 28.11 ***Major arteries of the systemic circulation***

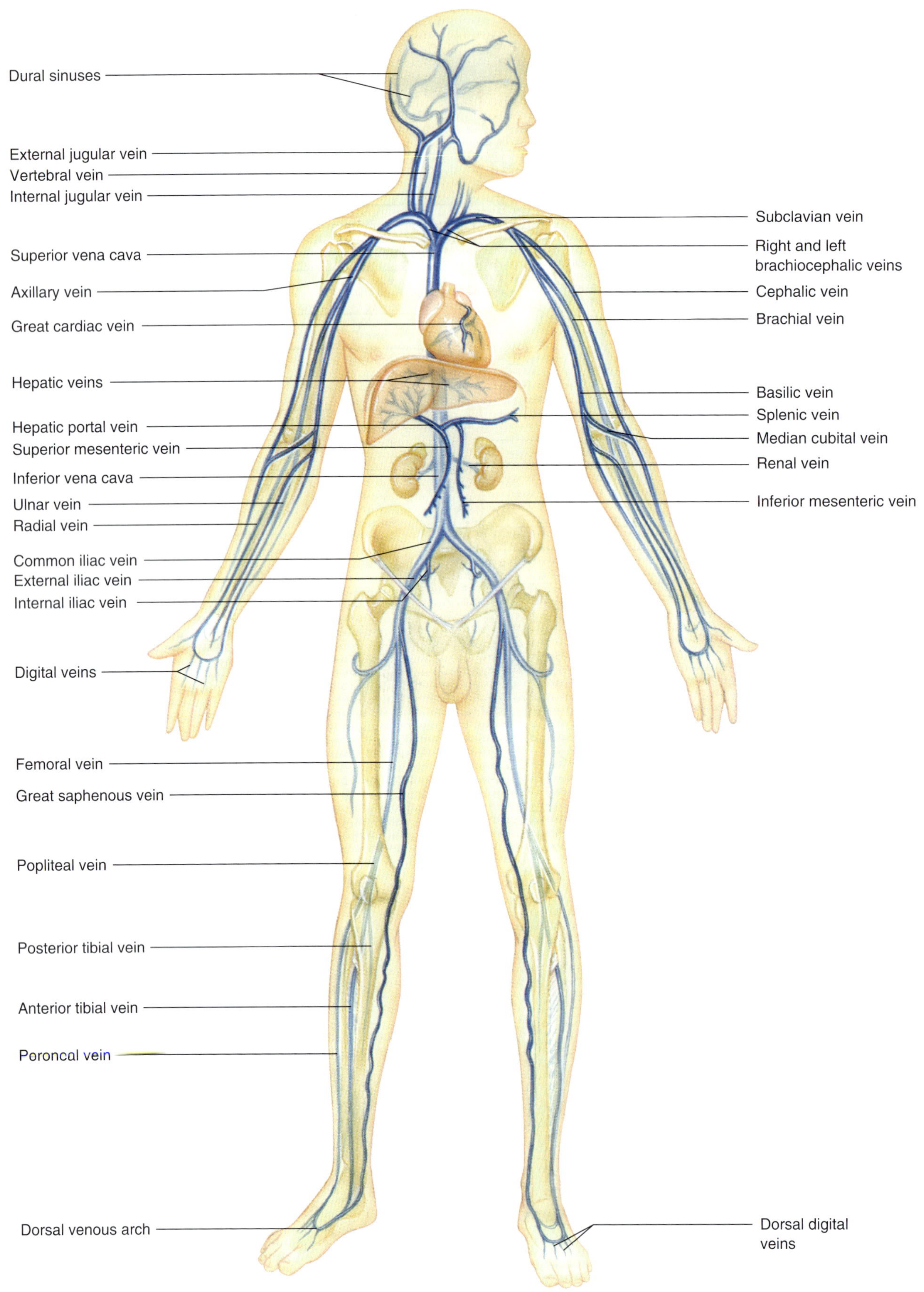

FIGURE 28.12 *Major veins of the systemic circulation*

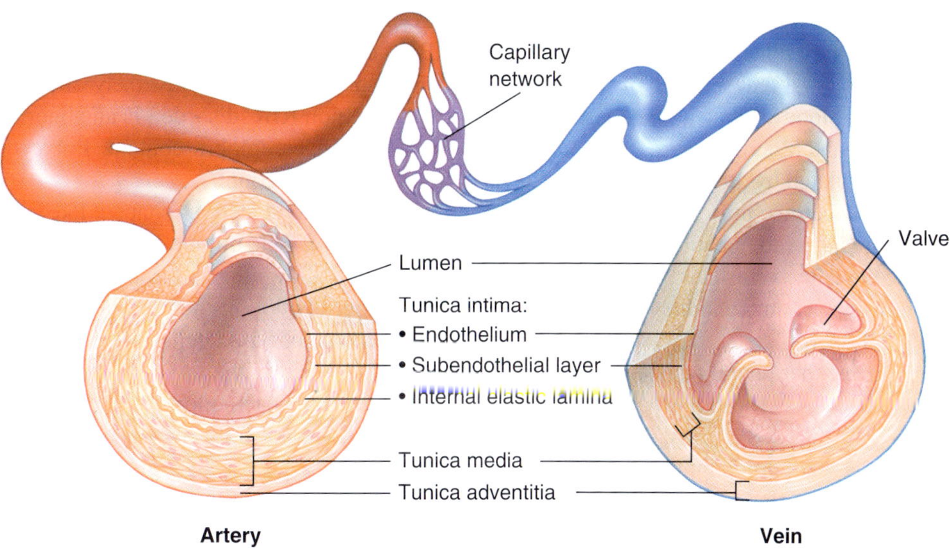

FIGURE 28.13 ***Structure of arteries, veins and capillaries. Capillaries are composed of only a fine tunica intima. Notice that the tunica media is thicker in arteries than in veins***

Blood in the veins travels at a much lower pressure than blood in the arteries. Veins have thinner walls, a larger lumen and greater capacity, and many have valves that help blood flow against gravity back to the heart. The 'milking' action of skeletal muscle contraction (called the muscular pump) also supports venous return. When skeletal muscles contract against veins, the valves proximal to the contraction open and blood is pushed towards the heart. The abdominal and thoracic pressure changes that occur with breathing (called the respiratory pump) also facilitate venous return to the heart.

The tiny capillaries that connect the arterioles and venules contain only one thin layer of tunica intima, which is permeable to the gases and molecules exchanged between blood and tissue cells. Capillaries typically are found in interwoven networks. They filter and shunt blood from pre capillary arterioles to post-capillary venules.

Physiology of arterial circulation

The factors that affect arterial circulation are blood flow, peripheral vascular resistance and blood pressure. **Blood flow** refers to the volume of blood transported in a vessel, in an organ or throughout the entire circulation over a given period of time. It is commonly expressed as litres or millilitres per minute or cubic centimetres per second.

Total peripheral vascular resistance (TPVR) refers to the opposing forces or impedance to blood flow as the arterial channels become more and more distant from the heart. Peripheral vascular resistance is determined by three factors:

1. *Blood viscosity*: the greater the viscosity, or thickness of the blood, the greater its resistance to moving and flowing.
2. *Length of the vessel*: the longer the vessel, the greater the resistance to blood flow.
3. *Diameter of the vessel*: the smaller the diameter of a vessel, the greater the friction against the walls of the vessel and, thus, the greater the impedance to blood flow.

Blood pressure is the force exerted against the walls of the arteries by the blood as it is pumped from the heart. It is most accurately referred to as **mean arterial pressure (MAP)**. The highest pressure exerted against the arterial walls at the peak of ventricular contraction (systole) is called the systolic blood pressure. The lowest pressure exerted during ventricular relaxation (diastole) is the diastolic blood pressure.

Mean arterial blood pressure is regulated mainly by cardiac output (CO) and peripheral vascular resistance (PVR), as represented in this formula: $MAP = CO \times PVR$. For clinical use, the MAP may be estimated by calculating the diastolic blood pressure plus one-third of the **pulse pressure** (the difference between the systolic and diastolic blood pressure).

Factors influencing arterial blood pressure

Blood flow, peripheral vascular resistance and blood pressure, which influence arterial circulation, are in turn influenced by various factors, as follows:

- The sympathetic and parasympathetic nervous systems are the primary mechanisms that regulate blood pressure. Stimulation of the sympathetic nervous system exerts a major effect on peripheral resistance by causing vasoconstriction of the arterioles, thereby increasing blood pressure. Parasympathetic stimulation causes vasodilation of the arterioles, lowering blood pressure.
- Baroreceptors and chemoreceptors in the aortic arch, carotid sinus and other large vessels are sensitive to pressure and chemical changes and cause reflex sympathetic stimulation, resulting in vasoconstriction, increased heart rate and increased blood pressure.
- The kidneys help maintain blood pressure by excreting or conserving sodium and water. When blood pressure decreases, the kidneys initiate the renin–angiotensin mechanism. This stimulates vasoconstriction, resulting in the release of the hormone aldosterone from the adrenal

cortex, increasing sodium ion reabsorption and water retention. In addition, pituitary release of antidiuretic hormone (ADH) promotes renal reabsorption of water. The net result is an increase in blood volume and a consequent increase in cardiac output and blood pressure.

- Blood pressure is also regulated by atrial natriuretic peptide (ANP) secreted by cardiac muscle cells in the atrial appendages and by brain natriuretic peptide (BNP) secreted from cardiac muscle cells in the ventricles. ANP and BNP in response to hypertension act on the kidneys to increase sodium and water excretion.
- Temperature may also affect peripheral resistance: cold causes vasoconstriction, whereas warmth produces vasodilation.
- Many chemicals, hormones and drugs influence blood pressure by affecting CO and/or PVR. For example, adrenaline causes vasoconstriction and increased heart rate; prostaglandins dilate blood vessel diameter (by relaxing vascular smooth muscle); endothelin, a chemical released by the inner lining of vessels, is a potent vasoconstrictor; nicotine causes vasoconstriction; and alcohol and histamine cause vasodilation.
- Dietary factors, such as intake of salt, saturated fats and cholesterol, elevate blood pressure by affecting blood volume and vessel diameter.
- Race, gender, age, weight, time of day, position, exercise and emotional state may also affect blood pressure.

These factors influence the arterial pressure. Systemic venous pressure, though it is much lower, is also influenced by such factors as blood volume, venous tone and right atrial pressure.

STRUCTURE AND FUNCTION OF BLOOD

Blood is an exchange medium between the external environment and the body's cells. Blood consists of plasma, solutes (e.g. proteins, electrolytes and organic constituents), red blood cells, white blood cells and platelets (which are fragments of cells). The haematopoietic (blood-forming) system includes the bone marrow (myeloid) tissues, where blood cells form, and the lymphoid tissues of the lymph nodes, where white blood cells mature and circulate. All blood cells originate from cells in the bone marrow called **stem cells** or *haemocytoblasts*. The origin of the cellular components of blood is illustrated in Figure 28.14.

Regulatory mechanisms cause stem cells to differentiate into families of parent cells, each of which gives rise to one of the formed elements of the blood (red blood cells, platelets and white blood cells). The functions of blood include transporting oxygen, nutrients, hormones and metabolic wastes; protecting against invasion of pathogens; maintaining blood coagulation; and regulating fluids, electrolytes, acids, bases and body temperature (Marieb & Hoehn, 2019).

Red blood cells

Red blood cells (RBCs, erythrocytes) and the haemoglobin molecules they contain are required to transport oxygen to body tissues. Haemoglobin also binds with some carbon dioxide, carrying it to the lungs for excretion. Abnormal numbers of RBCs, changes in their size and shape, or altered haemoglobin content or structure can adversely affect health. Anaemia, the most common RBC disorder, is an abnormally low RBC count or reduced haemoglobin content. Polycythaemia is an abnormally high RBC count.

The red blood cell is shaped like a biconcave disk (see Figure 28.15). This unique shape increases the surface area of the cell and allows the cell to pass through very small capillaries without disrupting the cell membrane. RBCs are the most common type of blood cell.

Haemoglobin is the oxygen-carrying protein within RBCs. It consists of the haem molecule and globin, a protein molecule. Globin is made of four polypeptide chains—two alpha chains and two beta chains (see Figure 28.16). Each of the four polypeptide chains contains a haem unit containing an iron atom. Thus, each haemoglobin molecule, when 100% saturated with oxygen, will be carrying four oxygen molecules. The iron atom binds reversibly with oxygen, allowing it to transport oxygen as *oxyhaemoglobin* to the cells. Haemoglobin is synthesised within the RBCs. The rate of synthesis depends on the availability of iron (Bullock & Hales, 2019).

Normal adult laboratory values for RBCs are defined and identified in Table 28.1. The size, colour and shape of stained RBCs also may be analysed. RBCs may be normocytic (normal size), smaller than normal (microcytic) or larger than normal (macrocytic). Their colour may be normal (normochromic) or diminished (hypochromic).

Red blood cell production and regulation

In adults, RBC production (**erythropoiesis**) (see Figure 28.17) begins in red bone marrow of the vertebrae, sternum, ribs and pelvis and is completed in the blood or spleen. Erythroblasts begin forming haemoglobin while they are in the bone marrow, a process that continues throughout the RBC lifespan. Erythroblasts differentiate into *normoblasts*. As these slightly smaller cells mature, their nucleus and most organelles are ejected, eventually causing normoblasts to collapse inward and assume the characteristic biconcave shape of RBCs. The cells enter the circulation as *reticulocytes*, which fully mature in about 48 hours. The complete sequence from stem cell to RBC takes 3 to 5 days.

The stimulus for RBC production is tissue hypoxia. The hormone erythropoietin is released by the kidneys in response to hypoxia. Erythropoietin stimulates the bone marrow to produce RBCs. However, the process of RBC production takes about 5 days to maximise. During periods of increased RBC production, the percentage of reticulocytes (immature RBCs) in the blood exceeds that of mature cells.

Red blood cell destruction

RBCs have a life span of about 120 days. Old or damaged RBCs are lysed (destroyed) by phagocytes in the spleen, liver, bone marrow and lymph nodes. The process of RBC destruction is called **haemolysis**. Phagocytes save and reuse amino acids and iron from haem units in the lysed RBCs. Most of the haem unit is converted to bilirubin, an orange-yellow pigment that is

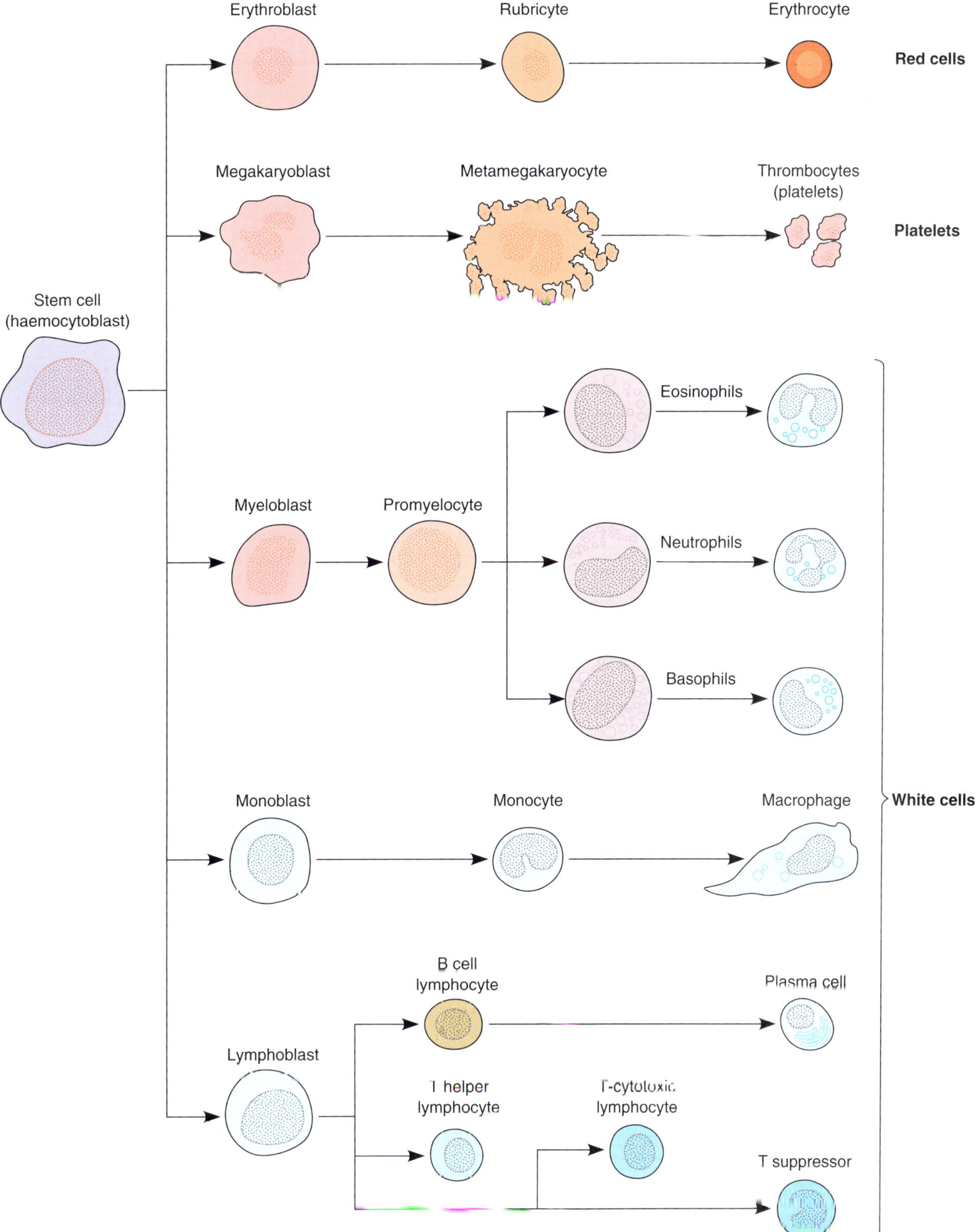

FIGURE 28.14 *Blood cell formation from stem cells. Regulatory factors control the differentiation of stem cells into blasts. Each of the five kinds of blasts is committed to producing one type of mature blood cell. Erythroblasts, for example, can differentiate only into RBCs, megakaryoblasts can differentiate only into platelets*

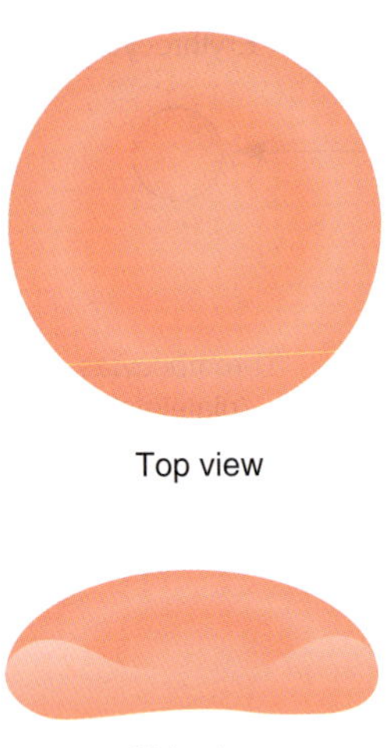

FIGURE 28.15 *Top and side view of a red blood cell (erythrocyte). Note the distinctive biconcave shape*

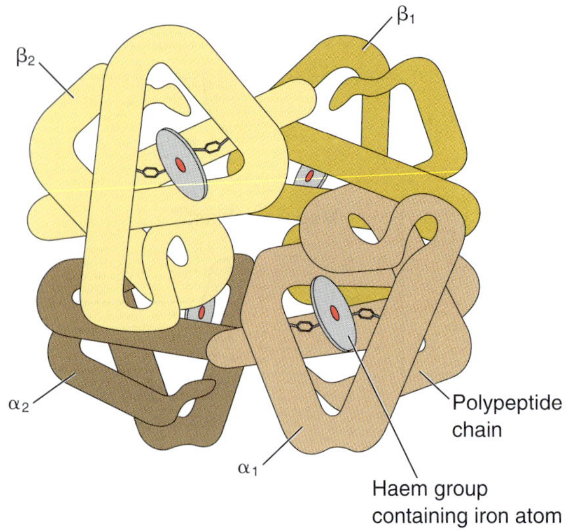

FIGURE 28.16 *The haemoglobin molecule includes globin (a protein) and haem, which contains iron. Globin is made of four subunits, two alpha and two beta polypeptide chains. A haem disk containing an iron atom (red dot) nests within the folds of each protein subunit. The iron atoms combine reversibly with oxygen, transporting it to the cells*

TABLE 28.1 Full blood count (FBC)

COMPONENT	PURPOSE	NORMAL VALUES
Haemoglobin (Hb)	Measures the capacity of the haemoglobin to carry gases	Women: 115–155 g/L Men: 130–170 g/L
Haematocrit (HCT)	The haematocrit represents the percentage of whole blood volume composed of erythrocytes	Women: 0.33–0.45 L/L Men: 0.36–0.50 L/L
Total RBC count	Counts number of circulating RBCs	Women: $3.8–5.8 \times 10^{12}$/L Men: $4.5–6.5 \times 10^{12}$/L
Red cell indices: Mean cell volume (MCV) Mean cell haemoglobin (MCH) Mean cell haemoglobin concentration (MCHC)	Determines relative size of cell Average haemoglobin inside an RBC Evaluates content of Hb in the RBC	80–100 fL 27–32 pg 300–350 g/L
WBC count (leucocytes aka white blood cells)	Measures total number of leucocytes (total count) and whether each kind of WBC is present in proper proportion (differential)	Total WBC count: $4.3–11 \times 10^{9}$/L WBC differential: Neutrophils: $2.0–7.5 \times 10^{9}$/L Eosinophils: $0.04–0.4 \times 10^{9}$/L Basophils: $0.0–0.2 \times 10^{9}$/L Lymphocytes: $1.5–4 \times 10^{9}$/L Monocytes: $0.2–0.8 \times 10^{9}$/L
Platelets	Measures number of platelets available to maintain clotting functions	$150–400 \times 10^{9}$/L

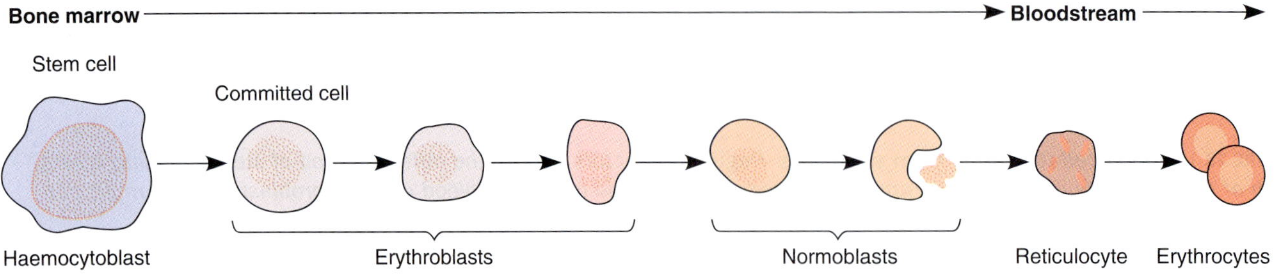

FIGURE 28.17 *Erythropoiesis. RBCs begin as erythroblasts within the bone marrow, maturing into normoblasts, which eventually eject their nucleus and organelles to become reticulocytes. Reticulocytes mature within the blood or spleen to become erythrocytes*

removed from the blood by the liver and excreted in the bile. During disease processes causing increased haemolysis or impaired liver function, bilirubin accumulates in the serum, causing a yellowish appearance of the skin and sclera (jaundice).

White blood cells

White blood cells (WBCs, leucocytes) are a part of the body's defence against microorganisms and constitute approximate 1% of total blood volume. **Leucocytosis** is a higher than normal WBC count; **leucopenia** is a WBC count that is lower than normal.

WBCs originate from haemopoietic stem cells in the bone marrow. These stem cells differentiate into the various types of WBCs (see Figure 28.14).

The two basic types of WBCs are granular leucocytes (or granulocytes) and non-granular leucocytes. Granulocytes have horseshoe-shaped nuclei and contain large granules in the cytoplasm. Stimulated by granulocyte-macrophage colony-stimulating factor (GM-CSF) and granulocyte colony-stimulating factor (G-CSF), granulocytes mature fully in the bone marrow before being released into the bloodstream. The three types of granulocytes are as follows:

- Neutrophils (also called *polymorphonuclear (PMN)* or segmented (*segs*) leucocytes) comprise 60–70% of the total circulating WBCs. Their nuclei are divided into three to five lobes. Neutrophils are active phagocytes, the first cells to arrive at a site of injury. Their numbers increase during inflammation. Immature forms of neutrophils (bands) are released during inflammation or infections and are referred to as having a shift to the left (so named because immature cell frequencies appear on the left side of the graph) on a differential blood count. Neutrophils have a lifespan of only about 10 hours and are constantly being replaced.
- Eosinophils comprise 1–3% of circulating WBCs but are found in large numbers in the mucosa of the intestines and lungs. Their numbers increase during allergic reactions, eosinophilic asthma and parasitic infestations.
- Basophils, which comprise less than 1% of the WBC count, contain histamine, heparin and other inflammatory mediators. Basophils increase in number during allergic and inflammatory reactions.

Non-granular WBCs (agranulocytes) include the monocytes and lymphocytes. They enter the bloodstream before final maturation.

- Monocytes are the largest of the WBCs and constitute approximately 3–8% of the total WBC count. Monocytes contain powerful bactericidal substances and proteolytic enzymes. They are phagocytic cells that mature into macrophages. Macrophages dispose of foreign and waste material, especially in inflammation. They are an active part of the immune response.
- Lymphocytes constitute 20–30% of the WBC count and mature in lymphoid tissue into B cells and T cells. B cells are involved in the humoral immune response and antibody formation, whereas T cells take part in the cell-mediated immunity process (see the chapter 'Nursing care of people with altered immunity'). Plasma cells (which arise from B cells) are lymphoid cells found in bone marrow and connective tissue; they also are involved in immune reactions.

Platelets

Platelets (thrombocytes) are cell fragments that have no nucleus and cannot replicate but are metabolically active. Platelets produce ATP and release mediators required for clotting. They are formed in the bone marrow as pinched-off portions of large megakaryocytes (see Figure 28.14). Platelet production is controlled by *thrombopoietin*, a protein produced by the liver, kidney, smooth muscle and bone marrow. Thrombopoietin release is determined by the number of circulating platelets. Once released from the bone marrow, platelets remain in the spleen for approximately 8 hours before entering the circulation. Platelets live up to 10 days in circulation. An excess of platelets is *thrombocytosis*. A deficit of platelets is *thrombocytopenia*.

Haemostasis

Platelet and coagulation disorders affect haemostasis (control of bleeding). Haemostasis is a series of complex interactions between platelets and clotting mechanisms that maintains a relatively steady state of blood volume, blood pressure and blood flow through injured vessels. The five stages of haemostasis are: (1) vessel spasm, (2) formation of the platelet plug, (3) development of an insoluble fibrin clot, (4) clot retraction, and (5) clot dissolution.

Vessel spasm

When a blood vessel is damaged, thromboxane A_2 (TXA_2) is released from platelets and cells, causing *vessel spasm*. This spasm constricts the damaged vessel for about 1 minute, reducing blood flow.

Formation of the platelet plug

Platelets attracted to the damaged vessel wall change from smooth disks to spiny spheres. Receptors on the activated platelets bind with *von Willebrand's factor*, a protein molecule, and exposed collagen fibres at the site of injury to form the platelet plug (see Figure 28.18). The platelets release adenosine diphosphate (ADP) and TXA_2 to activate nearby platelets, adhering them to the developing plug. Activation of the clotting pathway on the platelet surface converts fibrinogen to fibrin. Fibrin, in turn, forms a meshwork that binds the platelets and other blood cells to form a stable plug (see Figure 28.19).

Development of the fibrin clot

The process of coagulation creates a meshwork of fibrin strands that cements the blood components to form an insoluble clot. Coagulation requires many interactive reactions and two clotting pathways (see Figure 28.20). The slower intrinsic pathway is activated when blood contacts collagen in the injured vessel wall; the faster extrinsic pathway is activated when blood is exposed to tissues. The final outcome of both pathways is fibrin clot formation. Each procoagulation substance is activated in sequence, the activation of one coagulation factor activates another in turn. Table 28.2 lists known factors, their origin and their function or pathway. A deficiency of one or more factors or inappropriate inactivation of any factor alters normal coagulation (Marieb & Hoehn, 2019).

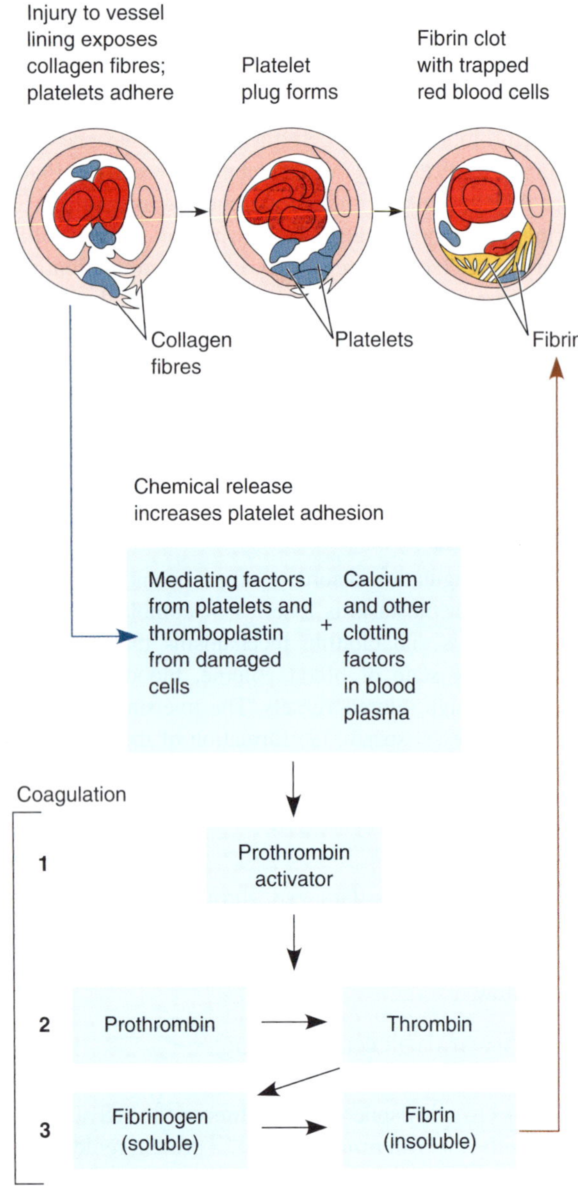

FIGURE 28.18 ***Platelet plug formation and blood clotting. The flow diagram summarises the events leading to fibrin clot formation***

Clot retraction

After the clot is stabilised (within about 30 minutes), trapped platelets contract, much like muscle cells. Platelet contraction squeezes the fibrin strands, pulling the broken portions of the ruptured blood vessel closer together. Growth factors released by the platelets stimulate cell division and tissue repair of the damaged vessel.

Clot dissolution

Fibrinolysis, the process of clot dissolution, begins shortly after the clot has formed, restoring blood flow and promoting tissue repair. Like coagulation, fibrinolysis requires a sequence of interactions between activator and inhibitor substances. Plasminogen, an enzyme that promotes fibrinolysis, is converted into plasmin, its active form, by chemical mediators released from vessel walls and the liver. Plasmin dissolves the clot's fibrin strands and certain coagulation factors. Stimuli such as exercise, fever and vasoactive drugs promote plasminogen activator release. The liver and endothelium also produce fibrinolytic inhibitors.

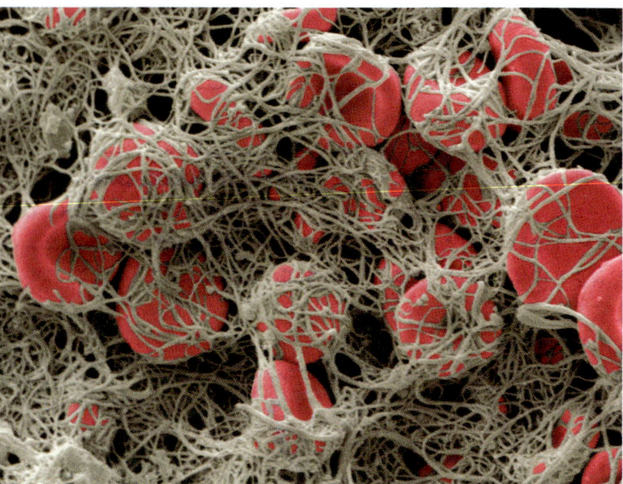

FIGURE 28.19 ***Scanning electron micrograph of an RBC trapped in a fibrin mesh***

Source: Steve Gschmeissner/Science Photo Library/Alamy Stock Photo.

STRUCTURE AND FUNCTION OF THE LYMPHATIC SYSTEM

The structures of the lymphatic system include the lymphatic vessels and several lymphoid organs (see Figure 28.21). The organs of the lymphatic system are the lymph nodes, the spleen, the thymus, the tonsils and the Peyer's patches of the small intestine. Lymph nodes are small aggregates of specialised cells that assist the immune system by removing foreign material, infectious organisms and tumour cells from lymph. Lymph nodes are distributed along the lymphatic vessels, forming clusters in certain body regions, such as the neck, axilla and groin (see Figure 28.21). The spleen, the largest lymphoid organ, is in the upper left quadrant of the abdomen under the thorax. The main function of the spleen is to filter the blood by breaking down old RBCs and storing or releasing to the liver their by products (such as iron). The spleen also synthesises lymphocytes, stores platelets for blood clotting and serves as a reservoir of blood. The thymus gland is located in the mediastinum, in the upper anterior chest, directly behind the sternum, and is most active in childhood, producing hormones (such as thymosin) that facilitate the immune action of lymphocytes. The tonsils of the pharynx and Peyer's patches of the small intestine are lymphoid organs that protect the upper respiratory and digestive tracts from foreign pathogens.

The lymphatic vessels, or lymphatics, form a network around the arterial and venous channels and interweave at the capillary beds. They collect and drain excess tissue fluid, called *lymph*, that 'leaks' from the cardiovascular system and accumulates at the venous end of the capillary bed. The lymphatic network

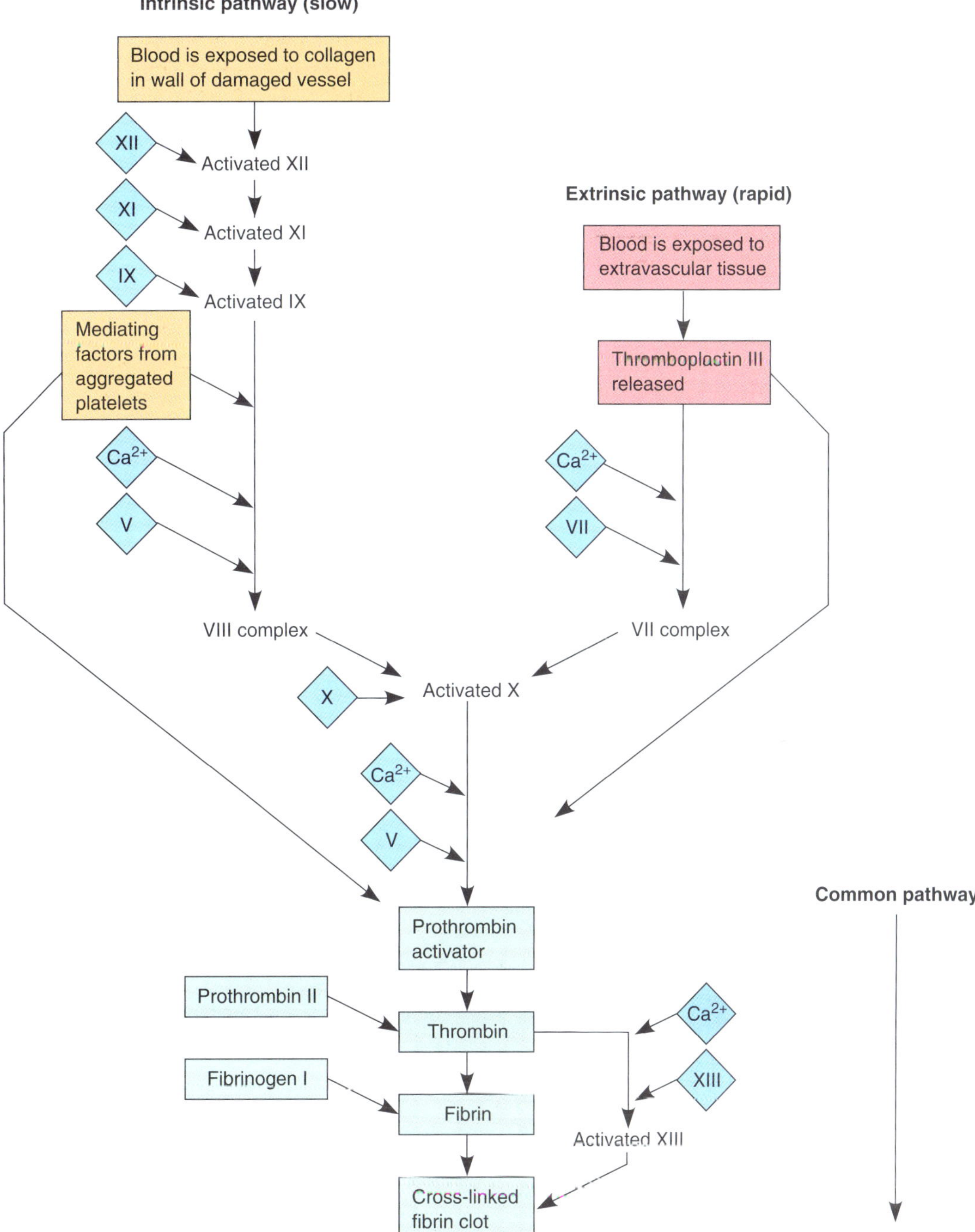

FIGURE 28.20 *Clot formation. Both the slower intrinsic pathway and the more rapid extrinsic pathway activate factor X. Factor X then combines with other factors to form prothrombin activator. Prothrombin activator transforms prothrombin into thrombin, which then transforms fibrinogen into long fibrin strands. Thrombin also activates factor XIII, which draws the fibrin strands together into a dense meshwork. The complete process of clot formation occurs within 3 to 6 minutes after blood vessel damage*

returns this fluid to the heart through a one-way system of lymphatic venules and veins that eventually drain into the right lymphatic duct and left thoracic duct, both of which empty into their respective subclavian veins (Standring & Gray, 2021). The lymphatic system is a low pressure system without a pump; their fluid transport depends on the rhythmic contraction of their smooth muscle and the muscular and respiratory pumps that assist venous circulation.

Lymphatic system and the human brain

Despite the presence of cerebral blood vessels, until recently it was believed that there was no lymphatic system in the brain. Recent advances in brain scanning, however, have demonstrated the existence of three lymphatic drainage systems in the outer layer of the brain (Wang et al., 2023). This discovery may lead to a better understanding of neurological diseases, such as multiple sclerosis and Alzheimer's disease, and future treatments.

TABLE 28.2 Blood coagulation factors

FACTOR	NAME	FUNCTION OR PATHWAY
I	Fibrinogen	Converted to fibrin strands
II	Prothrombin	Converted to thrombin
III	Thromboplastin	Catalyses conversion of thrombin
IV	Calcium ions	Needed for all steps of coagulation
V	Proaccelerin	Extrinsic/intrinsic pathways
VI	Derived from proaccelerin	A hypothetical agent said to be derived from proaccelerin
VII	Serum prothrombin conversion accelerator	Extrinsic pathway
VIII	Antihaemophilic factor	Intrinsic pathway
IX	Plasma prothrombin component	Intrinsic pathway
X	Stuart factor	Extrinsic/intrinsic pathways
XI	Plasma prothrombin antecedent	Intrinsic pathway
XII	Hageman factor	Intrinsic pathway
XIII	Fibrin stabilising factor	Cross-links fibrin strands to form insoluble clot

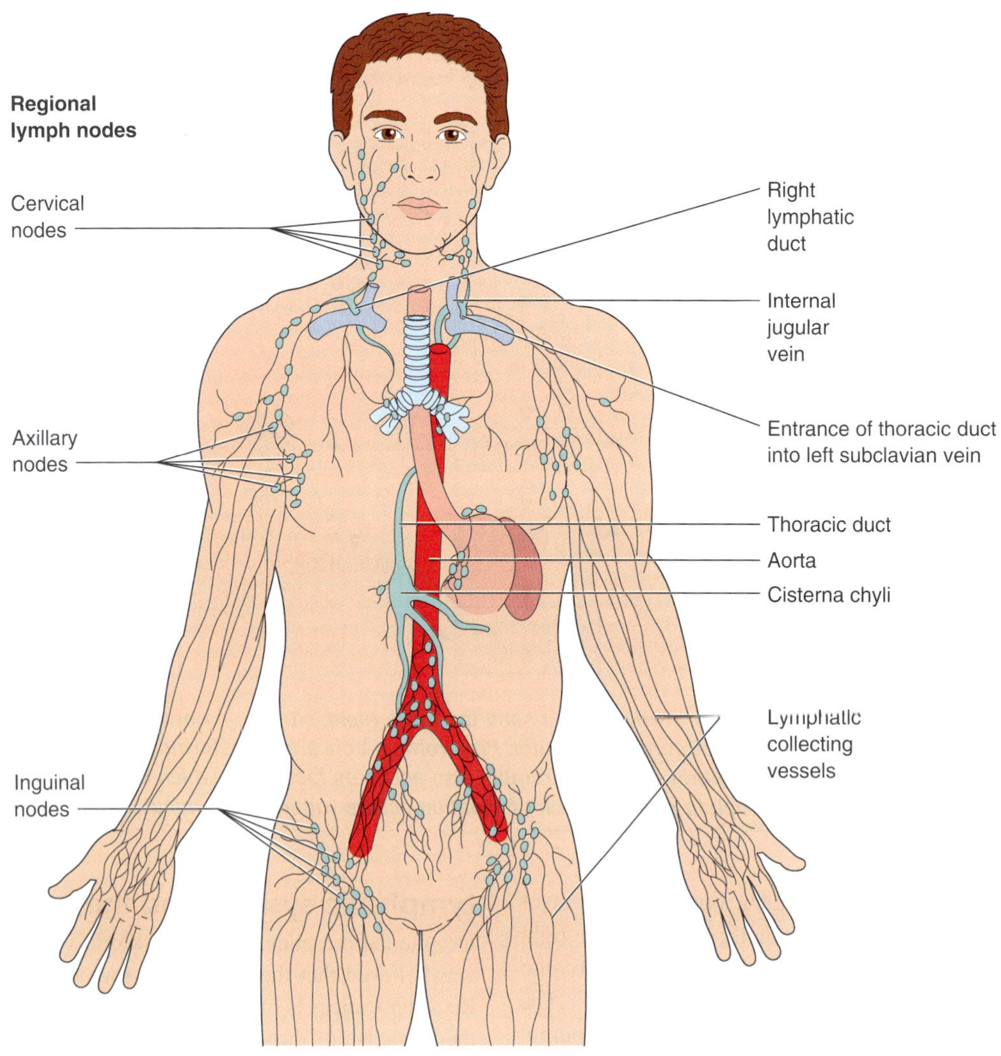

FIGURE 28.21 *The lymphatic system*

HEALTH ASSESSMENT AND DOCUMENTATION

Cardiovascular, haematological and lymphatic function is assessed by findings from a health assessment interview during which subjective data is collected. A physical assessment and various diagnostic tests elucidate objective data. Consideration of all the data that contributes to understanding a person's absolute cardiovascular disease (CVD) risk should be considered. The National Vascular Disease Prevention Alliance (2012) has produced comprehensive guidelines to assist clinicians with assessment of CVD risk.

Health assessment interview

A health assessment interview to determine problems with the structure and functions of the cardiovascular and/or lymphatic systems may be conducted during a health screening, may focus on a chief complaint (such as chest pain, fatigue and bleeding) or may be part of a total health assessment.

During the assessment of a person with suspected cardiovascular or lymphatic dysfunction, the use of the mnemonic SOCRATES is beneficial to ensure comprehensive data collection (Harcharran, 2022). The letters stand for **S**ite, **O**nset, **C**haracteristics, **R**adiation, **A**ssociated symptoms, **T**iming, **E**xacerbating factors and **S**everity. For example, ask the person:

- Site: 'Where is your pain?'
- Onset: 'When did the pain begin?'
- Characteristics: 'Is it burning, crushing stabbing or …?'
- Radiation: 'Does the pain go anywhere? Into your arm? Your back? Your neck?'
- Associated symptoms: 'Do you get nauseous, sweaty, light-headed or …? Have you developed swelling anywhere?'
- Time: 'Is your pain there all the time or does it come and go? Does it stay the same or is it getting worse over time?'
- Exacerbating factors: 'Is it worse (or better) when you take a breath or move or …?'
- Severity: 'Out of 10, if 0 is no pain and 10 is the worst pain you've ever had in your whole life, how would you score the pain now?'

Explore the person's history for heart disorders such as angina, myocardial infarction (MI), congestive heart failure (CHF), hypertension (HTN), arrhythmia or valvular disease. Ask the person about previous heart surgery or illnesses, such as COVID-19, rheumatic fever or recurrent streptococcal throat infections. Also ask about the presence and treatment of other chronic illnesses such as diabetes mellitus, bleeding disorders or endocrine disorders. Review the person's family history for coronary artery disease (CAD), HTN, cerebrovascular accident (CVA—stroke), hyperlipidaemia, diabetes mellitus, congenital heart disease or sudden death.

Ask the person about past or present occurrence of various cardiac symptoms, such as chest pain, shortness of breath, difficulty breathing, cough, palpitations, fatigue, light headedness or dizziness, fainting, heart murmur, blood clots or swelling. Because cardiac function affects all other body systems, a full history may need to explore other related systems, such as respiratory function and/or peripheral vascular function.

Review the person's personal habits and nutritional history, including body weight; eating patterns; dietary intake of fats, salt and fluids; dietary restrictions; hypersensitivities or intolerances to food or medication; and the use of caffeine and alcohol. If the person uses tobacco/nicotine products, ask about type (cigarettes, patches, pipe, cigars, snuff), duration, amount and efforts to quit. If the person uses illicit drugs, ask about type, method of administration (e.g. inhaled or injected), duration of use and efforts to quit. Include questions about the person's activity level and tolerance, recreational activities and relaxation habits. Assess the person's sleep patterns for interruptions in sleep due to dyspnoea, cough, discomfort, urination or stress. Ask how many pillows the person uses when sleeping.

Also consider psychosocial factors that may affect the person's stress level:

- What is the person's marital status, family composition and role within the family?
- Have there been any changes?
- What is the person's occupation, level of education and socioeconomic level?
- Are resources for support available?
- What is the person's emotional disposition and personality type?
- How does the person perceive their state of health or illness, and how able is the person to comply with treatment?

See the 'Functional health pattern interview' box for a list of interview questions categorised by functional health patterns.

Diagnostic tests of the cardiovascular and lymphatic systems

The results of diagnostic tests of cardiovascular and lymphatic function are used to support the diagnosis of a specific disease, to provide information to identify or modify the appropriate medications or therapy used to treat the disease and to help nurses monitor the person's responses to treatment and nursing care interventions. Diagnostic tests to assess the structures and functions of the heart are described below and summarised in the following bulleted list. More information is included in the discussion of specific disorders in the chapters 'Nursing care of people with coronary heart disease' and 'Nursing care of people with cardiac disorders'.

- The primary test used to identify the risk of coronary artery disease or to monitor treatment for alterations in lipid levels is a measurement of lipid components of cholesterol, triglycerides and lipoproteins in the blood.
- Non-invasive tests of cardiac structure and function include a chest x-ray and stress/exercise tests. The treadmill test is the most basic exercise test, with diagnostic ability to measure cardiac perfusion enhanced by administering IV radioisotopes during the test. A treadmill exercise test is often combined with other tests to evaluate cardiac function under stress. The exercise thallium or technetium test is a useful non-invasive test to monitor and diagnose CAD.

Links to National Patient Safety Standards

NSQHS: Recognising and Responding to Acute Deterioration Standard

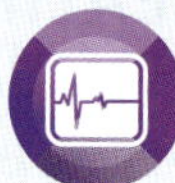

The intention of this standard is to 'ensure that a person's acute deterioration is recognised promptly and appropriate action is taken. Acute deterioration includes physiological changes, as well as acute changes in cognition and mental state' (Australian Commission on Safety and Quality in Health Care (ACSQHC), 2021, p. 67).

Implementing this standard is achieved by the establishment of systems to assist with recognition, initiating appropriate responses and ensuring meaningful and appropriate communication between all individuals involved in a person's care (including patients, families and carers).

Comprehensive and ongoing assessment of a person's cardiovascular system function should be undertaken and documented as frequently as clinically necessary to facilitate rapid, responsive action in the event of a person's deterioration.

Source: ACSQHC (2021). *National Safety and Quality Health Service Standards* (2nd ed.). Sydney: ACSQHC.

FUNCTIONAL HEALTH PATTERN INTERVIEW **Cardiovascular, haematological and lymphatic systems**

FUNCTIONAL HEALTH PATTERN	INTERVIEW QUESTIONS AND LEADING STATEMENTS
Health perception–Health management	■ Have you ever had any problems with your heart, such as angina (pain), 'heart attack' (MI) or valve disease? If so, describe. What was used to treat these problems?
	■ Describe any problems you have had with bleeding, bruising, swollen glands and circulation (e.g. heart disease, high cholesterol, high blood pressure or stroke, clots).
	■ Have you been diagnosed with high blood pressure? If so, how is it treated?
	■ Have you had your cholesterol checked recently? What is it? If you have high cholesterol, how is it treated?
	■ Have you ever been diagnosed with a health problem involving the blood, heart, blood vessels or lymph glands? If so, what were they and how were they treated?
	■ Is there a family history of bleeding, cancer or anaemia? Explain.
	■ What medications, vitamins, dietary supplements, complementary theories or over-the-counter drugs do you take now?
	■ Do you, or have you ever, smoked? If so, what, for how long and how many a day?
Nutritional–Metabolic	■ Describe your usual intake of food and fluids in a 24-hour period.
	■ Do you drink coffee, tea, cola or other caffeinated drinks? If so, how much?
	■ Do you drink alcohol? If so, what type, how much and how often?
	■ Describe how much salt you use on your food.
	■ Describe what type of fatty foods you eat. How often?
	■ Have you had a recent weight gain or loss? Explain.
	■ Have you noticed any change in the colour, temperature or appearance of the skin on your arms, hands, legs or feet? If so, what were they?
	■ Have you noticed any glands that are sore and swollen? What do you think causes this?
	■ Have you noticed an increase in the time it takes your blood to clot if you cut yourself or how easily you bruise?
	■ Have you noticed loss of hair, bulging veins, sores that will not heal on your legs or thicker toenails? Have you ever worn support stockings?
	■ Do your feet ever swell or your shoes feel tight? If so, when does this happen and what do you do to decrease the swelling?

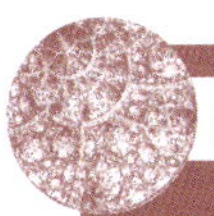

FUNCTIONAL HEALTH PATTERN INTERVIEW Cardiovascular, haematological and lymphatic systems (continued)

FUNCTIONAL HEALTH PATTERN	INTERVIEW QUESTIONS AND LEADING STATEMENTS
Elimination	■ Has a health problem interfered with your usual bowel and bladder movements? Explain.
	■ Have your bowel movements been a dark black colour?
Activity–Exercise	■ Has there been any change in your ability, energy or strength to perform your usual activities (such as bathing, housework, gardening, shopping)? If so, explain.
	■ Describe your activities in a typical day.
	■ Do you exercise regularly? Describe what you do when you exercise.
	■ Have your activities or exercise abilities changed? If so, explain.
	■ Do you notice shortness of breath with certain activities? If so, what are they? How long does this last? What do you do to breathe better?
	■ Do you have leg pain when you walk? If so, where is it located? How far do you walk before you have pain? Describe the pain. What do you do to relieve it?
	■ Do you ever have to stop and rest while doing daily activities? Explain.
	■ Do you feel tired even after sleep and rest? Describe the feeling.
Sleep–Rest	■ How much rest and sleep do you get each day?
	■ Does your health problem interfere with your ability to sleep and rest? Explain.
	■ Do leg cramps ever wake you at night? If so, describe the pain and what you do to relieve it.
	■ Have you experienced any numbness or tingling, dizziness or light-headedness, or palpitations? Describe if so.
	■ Do you ever feel short of breath while you are resting or sleeping? Does this wake you up if so? Explain.
Cognitive–Perceptual	■ Describe any chest pain you have experienced. When did it occur? Where was it located? On a scale of 0 to 10, with 10 being the worst pain you have ever had, rate the pain and describe it (e.g. burning, crushing, stabbing, squeezing, heavy, tight).
	■ Did you have any other symptoms with the pain, such as nausea or vomiting, sweating, racing heart, pale skin, palpitations?
	■ What made the pain worse? What did you do to try to relieve the pain? Did that work?
	■ Do you have any of these sensations in your legs or feet: pain, cramps, burning, numbness, tingling?
	■ If you have these sensations, when do they occur, how long do they last and what do you do to relieve them?
Self-perception– Self-concept	■ How does having this health problem make you feel about yourself?
Role–Relationships	■ How has having this health problem affected your relationships with others?
	■ Has having this health problem interfered with your ability to work? Explain.
	■ Does your work environment bring you into contact with any chemicals? Describe them.
Sexuality–Reproductive	■ Has this condition interfered with your usual sexual activity?
	■ Have you ever had chest pain during sexual activity? What do you do for it?
	■ *For women:* Have you noticed any changes in your menstrual cycle? (*For older women:* Have you gone through menopause?) If so, describe them.
Coping–Stress–Tolerance	■ Has having this condition created stress for you?
	■ Have you experienced any kind of stress that makes the condition worse? Explain.
	■ Describe what you do when you feel stressed.
Value–Belief	■ Describe how specific relationships or activities help you cope with this problem.
	■ Describe specific cultural beliefs or practices that affect how you care for and feel about this problem.
	■ Are there any specific treatments (such as blood transfusions) that you would not use to treat this problem?

- Coronary artery calcium (CAC) scores using computed tomography (CT) scans have quickly developed as an outstanding tool to not only diagnose symptomatic individuals with cardiovascular disease, but also predict potential outcomes of asymptomatic individuals (Gupta et al., 2022).
- Abnormal areas of the heart may be identified and evaluated by an MRI to locate areas of myocardial infarction or a positron emission tomography (PET) test to evaluate myocardial perfusion and myocardial metabolic function.
- Echocardiograms (ECGs) are conducted in conjunction with Dopplers and colour flow imaging to produce audio and graphical data about the motion, wall thickness and chamber size of the heart and of the blood flow and velocity.
- A dobutamine stress echocardiogram is performed in instances where exercising on a treadmill is not appropriate. Dobutamine infusion is administered intravenously to replicate exercise stress on the heart and transthoracic echocardiogram is performed to measure myocardial function.
- A transoesophageal echocardiogram (TOE) allows visualisation of structures adjacent to the oesophagus to visualise cardiac and extracardiac structures, including cardiac valve pathology, intracardiac thrombus, aortic dissection, endocarditis and ventricular function.
- A cardiac catheterisation with coronary angiography may be performed to identify CAD or cardiac valvular disease, to determine pulmonary artery or intracardiac pressures, to obtain a myocardial biopsy, to evaluate artificial valves or to perform percutaneous coronary intervention.
- Pericardiocentesis is a procedure undertaken to remove fluid from the pericardial sac for diagnostic or therapeutic purposes. It may also be an emergency procedure to treat cardiac tamponade.
- A physical assessment of the lymphatic system includes specific problems such as lymph node enlargement or swollen glands, as well as other more general complaints about infection or impaired immunity.

Regardless of the type of diagnostic test, the nurse is responsible for explaining the procedure and any special preparation needed, for assessing for medication use that may affect the outcome of the tests, for supporting the person during the examination as necessary, for documenting the procedures as appropriate and for monitoring the results of the tests.

See Box 28.1 for insights into the effect of COVID-19 on cardiac rhythm.

BOX 28.1 Arrhythmia and COVID-19

Infection with severe acute respiratory syndrome coronavirus 2 (SARS-CoV-2) has been associated with a number of cardiac arrhythmias including atrial fibrillation (AF), atrial flutter, ventricular ectopy and ventricular tachycardia, cardiac arrest and, most commonly, sinus tachycardia. An increased risk of developing long QTc has also been observed.

The arrhythmogenicity effect of a SARS-CoV-2 infection increases the risk of AF, especially in severe cases, where individuals experience a 19% increased risk of AF compared to non-severe episodes (3%).

It should also be noted that some countries with significant infection rates early in the outbreak experienced an increase between 52% and 60% in out-of-hospital arrest rates during peak infection periods. An increase in in-hospital cardiac arrests was also observed, with the primary cause being respiratory, and most commonly resulting in asystole.

Some arrhythmias may be attributed to the increased presence of hypoxia, electrolyte disturbance and fever. Therefore, active prevention and management of these states should ultimately mitigate the increased risk.

Source: Prutkin (2022). COVID-19: Arrhythmias and conduction system disease. *UpToDate*. Retrieved from https://www.uptodate.com/.

DIAGNOSTIC TESTS Cardiac disorders

NAME OF TEST Lipids

PURPOSE AND DESCRIPTION Blood lipids are cholesterol, triglycerides and phospholipids. They circulate bound to proteins and so are known as lipoproteins. Lipids are measured to evaluate risk of CAD and to monitor effectiveness of anti-cholesterol medications.

Normal values:

Cholesterol: < 4.0 mmol/L
Triglycerides: < 2.0 mmol/L (fasting)
HDL: Men = 0.9-2.0 mmol/L
Women = 1.0-2.2 mmol/L
LDL: < 2.0-3.4 mmol/L

(*Note:* Normal values may vary by laboratory.)

RELATED NURSING CARE Cholesterol levels alone may be measured at any time of the day, regardless of food or fluid intake. When measuring triglycerides and lipoproteins (HDL and LDL), fasting for 12 hours (except for water) with no alcohol intake for 24 hours prior to the test is recommended.

DIAGNOSTIC TESTS Cardiac disorders (continued)

NAME OF TEST Electrocardiogram (ECG) **PURPOSE AND DESCRIPTION** See Boxes 28.2 and 28.3.	**RELATED NURSING CARE** No special preparation is needed.
NAME OF TEST Chest x-ray **PURPOSE AND DESCRIPTION** An x-ray of the thorax can illustrate the contours, placement and chambers of the heart. It may be done to identify heart displacement or hypertrophy, or fluid in the pericardial sac.	**RELATED NURSING CARE** No special preparation is needed.
NAME OF TEST Stress/exercise tests ■ Treadmill test **PURPOSE AND DESCRIPTION** Stress testing is based on the theory that CAD results in depression of the ST segment with exercise. Depression of the ST segment and depression or inversion of the T wave indicates myocardial ischaemia. When the person is walking on a treadmill machine, the work rate of the heart is changed every 3 minutes for 15 minutes by increasing the speed and degree of incline by 3% each time. People exercise until they are fatigued, develop symptoms or reach their maximum predicted heart rate.	**RELATED NURSING CARE** *For all stress/exercise tests:* ask the person to wear comfortable shoes and to avoid food, fluids and smoking for 2 to 3 hours before the test. Assess for events that contraindicate the tests: recent myocardial infarction; severe, unstable angina; controlled arrhythmias; congestive heart failure or recent pulmonary embolism.
NAME OF TEST Thallium/technetium stress test (Myocardial perfusion scan, Cardiac blood pool imaging) **PURPOSE AND DESCRIPTION** *Thallium stress test:* thallium-201, a radioisotope that accumulates in myocardial cells, is used during the stress test to evaluate myocardial perfusion. Second scans are done 2 to 3 hours later when the heart is at rest; this is to differentiate between an ischaemic area and an infarcted or scarred area of myocardium. *Exercise technetium perfusion test:* technetium-99m-laced compounds are administered and a scan is done to evaluate cardiac perfusion, wall motion and ejection fraction. This is probably the most useful non-invasive test to diagnose and monitor CAD.	**RELATED NURSING CARE** Assess medications; those that affect the blood pressure or heart rate should be discontinued for 24 to 36 hours prior to the test (unless the test is being done to monitor the effectiveness of the medications).
NAME OF TEST Nuclear persantin (dipyridamole) stress test (Myocardial perfusion scan) **PURPOSE AND DESCRIPTION** This test is used when the person is not physically able to walk on the treadmill. Persantin, given IV, dilates the coronary arteries and increases myocardial blood flow. Coronary arteries that are narrowed from CAD cannot dilate to increase myocardial perfusion.	**RELATED NURSING CARE** Person is nil by mouth (NBM) after midnight except for water. Food, fluids and drugs that contain caffeine should be avoided for 24 hours prior to the test, as should decaffeinated fluids. Some drugs, such as theophylline preparations, are discontinued for 36 hours prior to the test.

(continued)

DIAGNOSTIC TESTS **Cardiac disorders (continued)**

NAME OF TEST Nuclear dobutamine stress test

PURPOSE AND DESCRIPTION Dobutamine is an adrenergic drug that increases myocardial contractility, heart rate and systolic blood pressure, which increases coronary oxygen consumption and thus increases coronary blood flow.

RELATED NURSING CARE Person is NBM after midnight except for water. Discontinue beta-blockers, calcium channel blockers and ACE inhibitors for 36 hours prior to the test. Do not administer nitrates for 6 hours prior to the test.

NAME OF TEST Magnetic resonance imaging (MRI)

PURPOSE AND DESCRIPTION An MRI may be used to identify and locate areas of myocardial infarction.

RELATED NURSING CARE Assess for any metallic implants (such as pacemaker, body piercing or artificial joint), which would contraindicate the test.

NAME OF TEST Computed tomography (CT) scan for coronary artery calcium (CAC) scoring

PURPOSE AND DESCRIPTION A CT scan may be conducted to quantify calcium deposits in coronary arteries. CAC scoring is a non-invasive procedure and a tool for primary prevention of coronary artery disease, whereby coronary artery calcification is quantified with the use of CT. The scan is very quick (acquisition in less than 10 seconds), there is very low radiation exposure and no intravenous contrast or special preparation is required. Calcium deposits appear bright on CT imaging. Not only does CAC provide an indication of atherosclerotic plaque burden, its main use is to reliably predict the risk of future myocardial infarction and mortality. The Cardiac Society of Australia and New Zealand (CSANZ) (2017) recommends CAC for intermediate-risk people who are asymptomatic, do not have known coronary artery disease and are aged 45 to 75 years, as CAC has the ability to reclassify these people into lower- or higher-risk groups. The CSANZ also recommends CAC for lower-risk people where traditional risk scores may underestimate cardiac risk, particularly those people who have a family history of premature CVD and/or people with diabetes aged 40 to 60 years. CAC is not recommended for people who are very high or very low risk, currently symptomatic or with diagnosed CVD.

CAC scores are interpreted as follows:

1. CAC = 0. A zero score confers a very low risk of death, < 1% at 10 years.
2. CAC = 1–100. Low risk, < 10% at 10 years.
3. CAC = 101–400. Intermediate risk, 10–20% at 10 years.
4. CAC = 101–400 and > 75th percentile. Moderately high risk, 15–20% at 10 years.
5. CAC > 400. High risk, > 20% at 10 years.

RELATED NURSING CARE No special preparation is required. Explain the procedure to the person including the physical aspect of going into the CT scanner. Reassure the person, particularly those who have claustrophobia, that it is very quick.

NAME OF TEST Cardiolite—technetium-99m sestamibi (Myocardial perfusion scan)

PURPOSE AND DESCRIPTION Used to evaluate blood flow in different parts of the heart. Cardiolite (technetium-99m sestamibi) is injected IV. In a dipyridamole cardiolite scan, dipyridamole (Persantin) is injected to increase blood flow to coronary arteries. These scans may be done in conjunction with a treadmill test.

RELATED NURSING CARE As for stress/exercise tests, above. Instruct the person to avoid intake of caffeine for 12 hours before having a test with dipyridamole cardiolite.

NAME OF TEST positron emission tomography (PET)

PURPOSE AND DESCRIPTION Two scans are performed following injection of radionuclides and the resulting images compared for myocardial perfusion and myocardial metabolic function. A stress test (treadmill) may be a part of the test. If the myocardium is ischaemic or damaged, the images will be different. Normally, the images will be the same.

RELATED NURSING CARE Assess person's blood glucose: for accurate metabolic activity images, the blood glucose level must be between 60 and 140 mg/dL. If exercise is included in the test, the person will need to be NBM and avoid smoking and caffeine for 24 hours prior to the test.

DIAGNOSTIC TESTS Cardiac disorders (continued)

NAME OF TEST Blood pool imaging

PURPOSE AND DESCRIPTION Following intravenous injection of technetium-99m pertechnetate, sequential evaluation of the heart can be performed for several hours. Useful for evaluation of cardiac status following myocardial infarction and congestive heart failure and assessing effectiveness of cardiac medications. Can be done at the person's bedside.

RELATED NURSING CARE No special preparation is needed. Following the procedure, explain that the dose is very low and the biological elimination of the technetium-99m is virtually complete by 6 hours. It is best to refrain from breastfeeding during this time.

NAME OF TEST Echocardiogram

- M-mode
- Two-dimensional (2-D)
- Cardiac Doppler
- Colour Doppler
- Stress echocardiogram

PURPOSE AND DESCRIPTION Echocardiograms use a transducer to record waves that bounce or 'echo' off the heart and to record the direction and flow of blood through the heart in audio and graphical data. An *M-mode (motion-mode) echocardiogram* records the motion, wall thickness and chamber size of the heart.

A *2-D echocardiogram* provides a cross-sectional view of the heart. *Colour flow imaging* combines 2-D echocardiography and Doppler technology to evaluate the speed and direction of blood flow through the heart, which can identify pathology such as leaky valves. *Stress echocardiography* combines a treadmill test with ultrasound images to evaluate segmental function and wall motion. If the person is not physically able to exercise, IV dobutamine may be administered and ultrasound images taken.

RELATED NURSING CARE No special preparation is needed; see related nursing care for the person having a treadmill test for a stress echocardiogram.

NAME OF TEST Transoesophageal echocardiography (TOE)

PURPOSE AND DESCRIPTION Allows visualisation of adjacent cardiac and extracardiac structures to identify or monitor cardiac valve pathology, intracardiac thrombus, aortic dissection, endocarditis, perioperative left ventricular function and intracardiac repairs during surgery. A transducer (probe) attached to an endoscope is inserted into the oesophagus and images are taken. Concurrent Doppler ultrasound and colour flow imaging may be used.

RELATED NURSING CARE Twilight anaesthesia administered by an anaesthetist is the safest option to ensure airway patency and decrease the risk of oesophageal perforation. Continuous cardiac monitoring must be available with cycling non-invasive blood pressure monitoring. Local anaesthetic is applied to the oropharynx.

Following the procedure, protect airway and assess conscious state. Explain that it may be difficult to swallow for a few hours. Nil orally for 2 hours after application of local anaesthetic.

NAME OF TEST Cardiac catheterisation

PURPOSE AND DESCRIPTION A cardiac catheterisation may be performed to identify CAD or cardiac valvular disease, to determine pulmonary artery or intracardiac pressures (right heart catheterisation), to obtain a myocardial biopsy, to evaluate artificial valves or to perform percutaneous coronary intervention (PCI). The test is performed by inserting a long catheter into a large vein (for pulmonary artery pressures/right heart studies) or the radial, femoral or brachial artery (for coronary angiography and PCI).

Coronary angiography and left heart catheterisation: using fluoroscopy, the catheter is advanced into the coronary arteries and radiopaque contrast media is injected. Blood is not visible on x-ray but blood flow is replicated with contrast media; coronary artery disease is evident as partial or complete obstruction to coronary blood flow. The findings on coronary angiography guide therapy—medical therapy, PCI +/− coronary stenting or coronary artery bypass grafting. Other left heart cardiac catheterisation procedures demonstrate aortic valve disease, intracardiac shunts and ventricular failure to guide appropriate therapy.

Right cardiac catheterisation: the catheter is inserted into the femoral vein or antecubital vein and then advanced, under fluoroscopic guidance, through the vena cava into

(continued)

DIAGNOSTIC TESTS Cardiac disorders (continued)

the right atrium, then floated through the right ventricle, right ventricular outflow tract and into the pulmonary artery. Pressures are measured in right heart chambers, pulmonary artery and pulmonary capillary wedge (as an estimation of left atrial pressure). Blood samples can be obtained to measure oxygen saturation for the purposes of evaluating intracardiac shunts and for measurement of cardiac output using the Fick equation. Right heart catheterisation also allows evaluation of pulmonary valve, tricuspid and mitral valve stenosis.

RELATED NURSING CARE See the 'Nursing care' box.

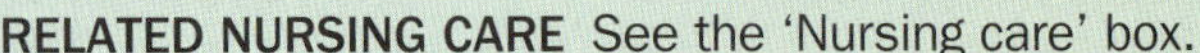

NAME OF TEST Pericardiocentesis

PURPOSE AND DESCRIPTION This procedure is performed to remove fluid from the pericardial sac for diagnostic or therapeutic purposes for people with pericardial effusions or it may be performed as an emergency procedure for the person with pericardial tamponade. *Note*: pericardiocentesis is the only treatment for pericardial tamponade. A large-gauge 10 cm needle is inserted in the sub-xiphoid process and a pigtail catheter is advanced using Seldinger technique into the pericardial sac. Excess fluid is withdrawn (see Figure 28.22). An ECG lead is clipped onto the needle to indicate if the needle contacts the epicardial surface (ST elevation will be evident), thus preventing perforation of the myocardium or coronary arteries.

RELATED NURSING CARE See the 'Nursing care' box.

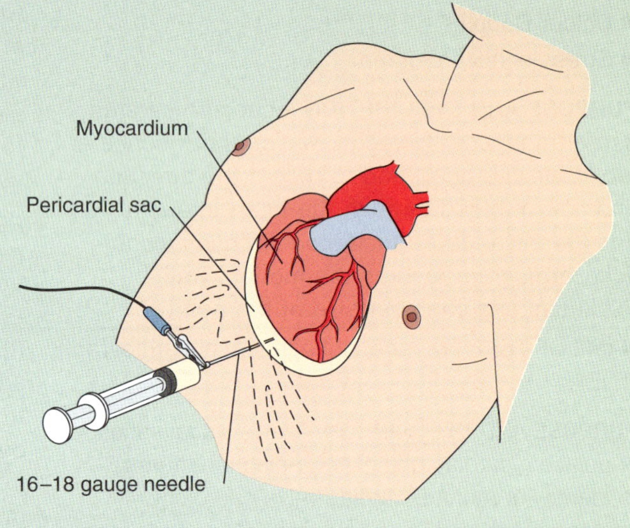

FIGURE 28.22 *Pericardiocentesis*

BOX 28.2 Electrocardiogram

The *electrocardiogram (ECG)* is a graphical record of the heart's electrical activity. Electrodes applied to the body surface are used to obtain a graphical representation of cardiac electrical activity. These electrodes detect the magnitude and direction of electrical currents produced in the heart. They attach to the electrocardiograph by an insulated wire called a *lead*. The electrocardiograph converts the electrical impulses it receives into a series of waveforms that represent cardiac depolarisation and repolarisation. Placement of electrodes on different parts of the body allows different views of this electrical activity, much like turning the head while holding a camera provides different views of the scenery. ECG waveforms and patterns are examined to detect arrhythmias as well as myocardial damage, the effects of drugs and electrolyte imbalances.

ECG waveforms reflect the direction of electrical flow in relation to a positive electrode. Current flowing towards the positive electrode produces an upward (positive) waveform; current flowing away from the positive electrode produces a downward (negative) waveform. Current flowing perpendicular to the positive pole produces a biphasic (both positive and negative) waveform. Absence of electrical activity is represented by a straight line called the *isoelectric line*.

ECG waveforms are recorded by a heated stylus on heat-sensitive paper. The paper is marked at standard intervals that represent time and voltage or amplitude (see Figure 1). Each small box is 1 mm^2. The recording speed of the standard ECG is 25 mm/second, so each small box represents 0.04 second. Five small boxes horizontally and vertically make one large box, equivalent to 0.20 second. Five large boxes represent 1 full second. Measured vertically, each small box represents 0.1 mV.

Both bipolar and unipolar leads are used in recording the ECG. A bipolar lead uses two electrodes of opposite polarity (negative and positive). In a *unipolar* lead, one positive electrode and

BOX 28.2 Electrocardiogram (continued)

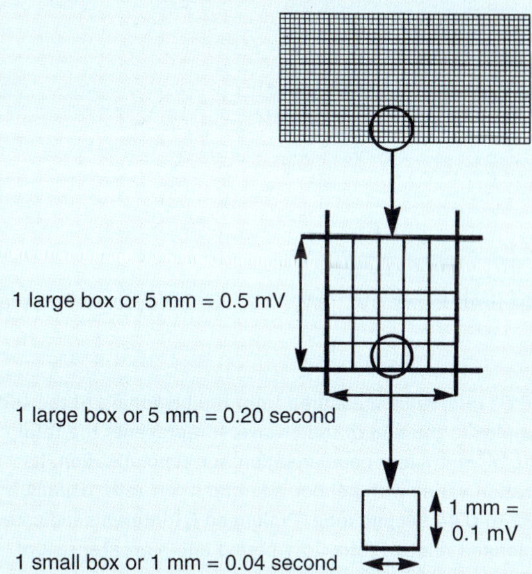

(1) Time and voltage measurements on ECG paper at a recording speed of 25 mm/second

a negative reference point at the centre of the heart are used. The electrical potential between the two monitoring points is graphically recorded as the ECG waveform.

The heart can be viewed from both the frontal plane and the horizontal plane (see Figure 2). Each plane provides a unique perspective of the heart muscle. The frontal plane is an imaginary cut through the body that views the heart from top to bottom (superior–inferior) and side to side (right–left). This perspective of the heart is analogous to a paper doll cut-out. It provides information about the inferior and lateral walls of the heart. The horizontal plane is a cross-sectional view of the heart from front to back (anterior–posterior) and side to side (right–left). Information regarding the anterior, septal and lateral walls of the heart, as well as the posterior wall, is obtained from this view.

A standard 12-lead ECG provides a simultaneous recording of six limb leads and six precordial leads (see Figure 3). The limb leads provide information about the heart in the frontal plane and include three bipolar leads (I, II, III) and three unipolar leads (aV_R, aV_L and aV_F). The bipolar limb leads measure electrical activity between a negative lead on one extremity and a positive lead on another. The unipolar limb leads (called augmented leads) measure the electrical activity between a single positive electrode on a limb (right arm (R), left arm (L) or left leg (F for foot)) and the centre of the heart.

The *precordial leads*, also known as chest leads or V leads, view the heart in the horizontal plane. They include six unipolar leads (V_1, V_2, V_3, V_4, V_5 and V_6), which measure electrical

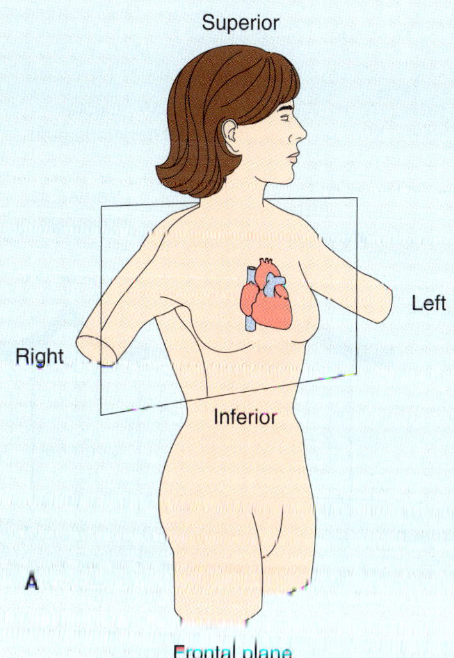

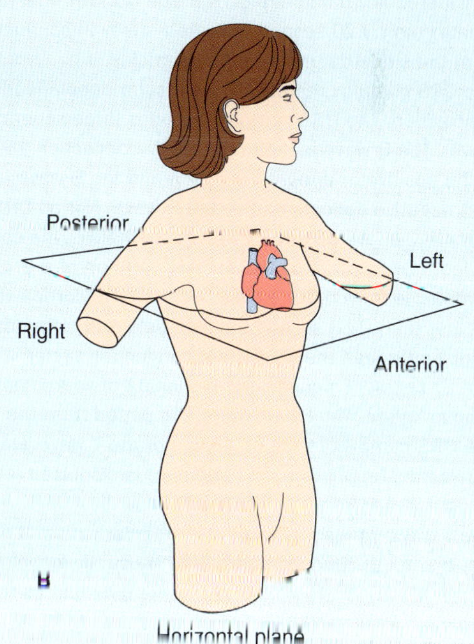

(2) Planes of the heart. A, Frontal plane. B, Horizontal plane

(continued)

BOX 28.2 Electrocardiogram (continued)

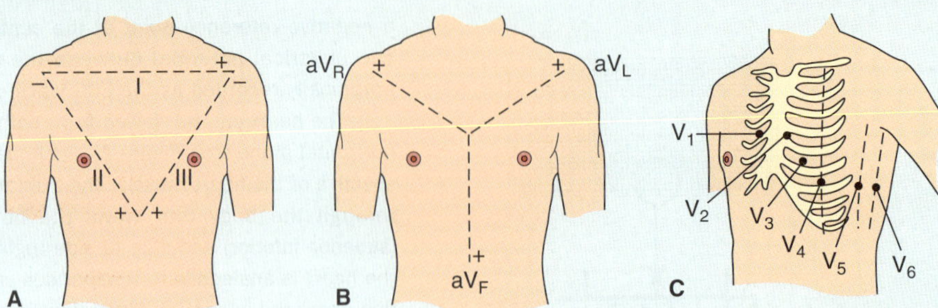

(3) Leads of the 12-lead ECG. A, Bipolar limb leads I, II, III; B, Unipolar limb leads aV_R, aV_L, aV_F; C, Unipolar precordial leads V_1 to V_6

activity between the centre of the heart and a positive electrode on the chest wall.

The cardiac cycle is depicted as a series of waveforms, the P, Q, R, S and T waves (see Figure 4).

- The *P wave* represents atrial depolarisation and contraction. The impulse is from the sinoatrial (or sinus) node. The P wave precedes the QRS complex and is normally smooth, round and upright. P waves may be absent when the sinoatrial node is not acting as the pacemaker. Atrial repolarisation occurs during ventricular depolarisation and usually is not seen on the ECG.
- The *PR interval* represents the time required for the sinus impulse to travel to the atrioventricular node and into the Purkinje fibres. This interval is measured from beginning of P wave to beginning of QRS complex. If no Q wave is seen, the beginning of the R wave is used. The PR interval is normally 0.12 to 0.20 second. (Up to 0.24 second is considered normal in adults over age 65.) PR intervals greater than 0.20 second indicate a delay in conduction from the sinoatrial node to the ventricles.
- The *QRS complex* represents ventricular depolarisation and contraction. The QRS complex includes three separate waves: the Q wave is the first negative deflection, the R wave is the positive or upright deflection and the S wave is the first negative deflection after the R wave. Not all QRS complexes have all three waves; nonetheless, the complex is called a QRS complex. The normal duration of a QRS complex is from 0.06 to 0.10 second. QRS complexes greater than 0.10 second indicate delays in transmitting the impulse through the ventricular conduction system.
- The *ST segment* signifies the beginning of ventricular repolarisation. The ST segment, the period from the end of the QRS complex to the beginning of the T wave, should be isoelectric. An abnormal ST segment is displaced (elevated or depressed) from the isoelectric line.
- The *T wave* represents ventricular repolarisation. It normally has a smooth, rounded shape that is usually less than 10 mm tall. It usually points in the same direction as the QRS complex. Abnormalities of the T wave may indicate myocardial ischaemia or injury or electrolyte imbalances.
- The *QT interval* is measured from the beginning of the QRS complex to the end of the T wave. It represents the total time of ventricular depolarisation and repolarisation. Its duration varies with gender, age and heart rate; usually, it is 0.32 to 0.44 second long. Prolonged QT intervals indicate a prolonged relative refractory period and a greater risk of arrhythmias. Shortened QT intervals may result from medications or electrolyte imbalances.
- The *U wave* is not normally seen. It is thought to signify repolarisation of the terminal Purkinje fibres. If present, the U wave follows the same direction as the T wave. It is most commonly seen in hypokalaemia.

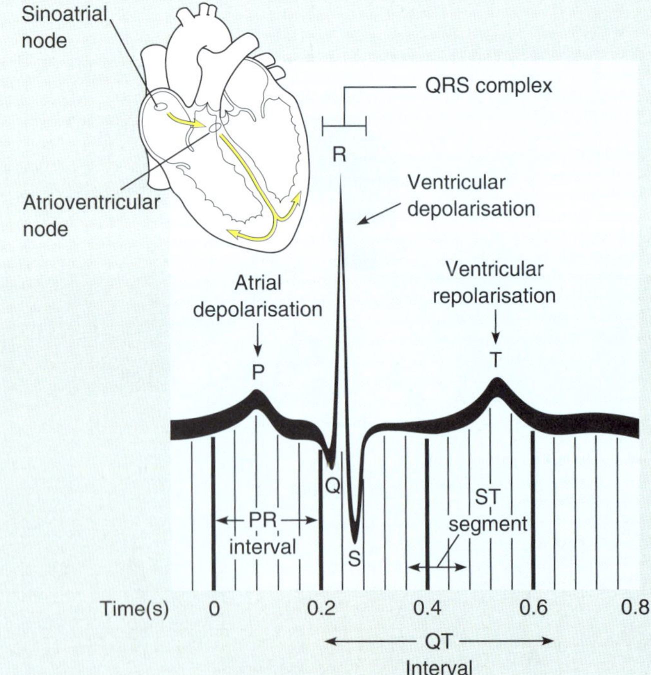

(4) Normal ECG waveform and intervals

BOX 28.3 Interpreting an ECG

Interpreting an ECG strip to determine the cardiac rhythm is a skill that takes practice to learn and master. Many methods are used to analyse ECGs. It is important to use a consistent method for ECG analysis. Identifying and interpreting complex arrhythmias requires advanced skills and knowledge obtained through further training. One method follows.

- **Step 1: Determine rate**. Assess heart rate. Use P waves to determine the atrial rate and R waves for the ventricular rate. Several approaches can be used to determine the heart rate.
  - Count the number of complexes in a 6-second rhythm strip (the top margin of ECG paper is marked at 3-second intervals) and multiply by 10. This provides an estimate of the rate and is particularly valuable if rhythms are irregular.
  - Count the number of large boxes between two consecutive complexes and divide 300 (the number of large boxes in 1 minute) by this number. For example, there are 6 large boxes between two R waves; 300 divided by 6 equals a ventricular rate of 50 bpm. Memorise the following sequence for rapid rate determination: 300, 150, 100, 75, 60, 50, 43. One large box between complexes equals a rate of 300; two, a rate of 150; three, a rate of 100; and so on.
  - Count the number of small boxes between two consecutive complexes and divide 1,500 (the number of small boxes in 1 minute) by this number. For example, there are 19 small boxes between two R waves; 1,500 divided by 19 equals a ventricular rate of 79 bpm. This is the most precise measurement of heart rate.
  - Use a commercially available rate ruler, following strictly the instructions on the device (see Figure 1).
- **Step 2: Determine regularity**. Regularity is the consistency with which the P waves or QRS complexes occur. In a regular rhythm, all waves occur at a consistent rate. Rhythm regularity is determined by measuring the interval between consecutive waves. Place one point of an ECG calliper (a measuring device) on the peak of the P wave (for atrial rhythm) or the R wave (for ventricular rhythm). Adjust the other point to the peak of the next wave, P to P or R to R (see Figure 2). Keeping the callipers set at this distance, evaluate intervals between consecutive waves. The rhythm is *regular* if all calliper points fall on succeeding wave peaks. Alternately, use a strip of blank paper on top of the ECG strip, marking the peaks of two or three consecutive waves. Then move the paper along the strip to consecutive waves. Wave peaks that vary by more than one to three small boxes (depending on the rate) are *irregular*. Irregular rhythms may be *irregularly irregular* (if the intervals have no pattern) or *regularly irregular* (if a consistent pattern to the irregularity can be identified).
- **Step 3: Assess P wave**. The presence or absence of P waves helps determine the origin of the rhythm. All the P waves should be alike in size and shape (*morphology*). If P waves are not seen or they differ in shape, the rhythm may not originate in the sinoatrial node.
- **Step 4: Assess P to QRS relationship**. Determine the relationship between P waves and QRS complexes. There should be one and only one P wave for every QRS complex, because the normal stimulus for ventricular contraction originates in the sinoatrial node.
- **Step 5: Determine interval durations**. To evaluate impulse transmission through the cardiac conduction system, measure the PR interval, QRS duration and QT interval. To measure, count the number of small boxes from the beginning of the interval to the end and multiply by 0.04 second. Then determine whether the interval duration is within its normal limits. For example, the PR interval is 3.5 small boxes wide, or 0.14 second. This is within the normal limits of 0.12 to 0.20 second. This interval should be consistent, not varying from beat to beat. A PR interval greater than 0.20 second or one that varies from beat to beat is abnormal.

  The QRS complex duration is normally between 0.06 and 0.10 second. A QRS complex greater than 0.12 second indicates delayed ventricular conduction.

  The QT interval is normally 0.32 to 0.44 second. It varies inversely with the heart rate: the faster the heart rate, the shorter the QT interval. As a general rule, the QT interval should be no more than half the previous R–R interval. A prolonged QT interval indicates a prolonged relative refractory period of the heart.
- **Step 6: Identify abnormalities**. Note the presence and frequency of ectopic (extra) beats, deviation of the ST segment above or below the baseline and abnormalities in waveform shape and duration.

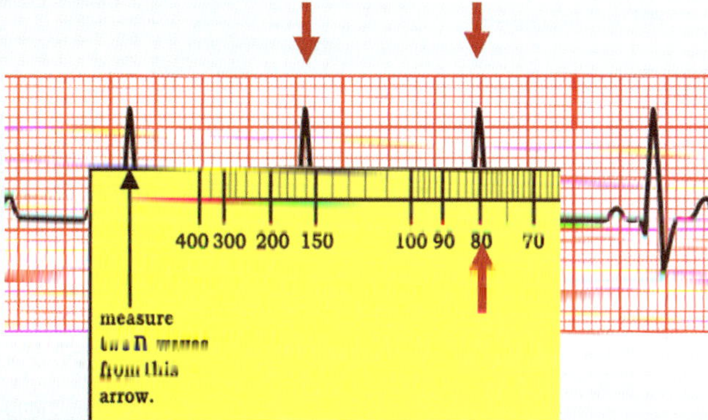

(1) Example of commercially available rate ruler

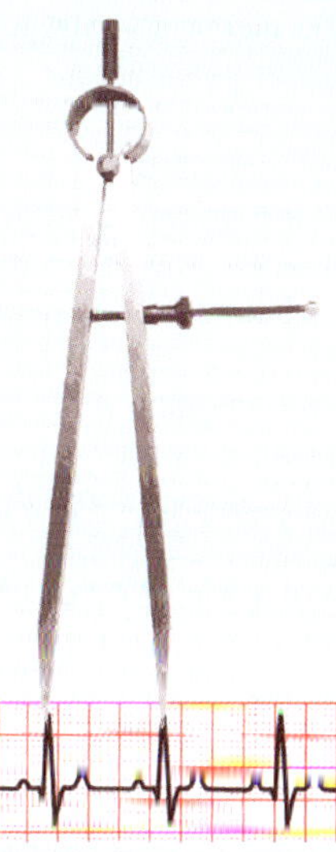

(2) Use of callipers to determine rate

NURSING CARE OF THE PERSON having cardiac catheterisation

BEFORE THE PROCEDURE

- Explain the procedure to the person.
- No food or fluids are allowed for 4 to 6 hours before the test.
- Assess for allergies to seafood, iodine or iodine contrast dyes (if previous tests have been done). If a previous known allergic response to the contrast is recorded, oral and intravenous steroid therapy may be administered the evening before and the morning of the test. There is no evidence that antihistamines provide any therapeutic or prophylactic benefit (Australasian Society of Clinical Immunology and Allergy, 2022).
- Assess for use of NSAIDs (risk of bleeding).
- Assess kidney function—glomerular filtration rate and creatinine levels. Contrast media is nephrotoxic and pre-hydration with IV fluids should be initiated for people with renal impairment.
- Discontinue oral anticoagulant medications as ordered by cardiologist. Withhold subcutaneous low-molecular-weight heparin on the morning of the procedure.
- Continue aspirin as usual.
- Establish intravenous access.
- Establish baseline of peripheral pulses.
- Measure and record baseline vital signs.
- Clip hair from access site.

PROCEDURE

- The person is positioned on the catheter laboratory procedure table. IV sedation is administered as ordered.
- ECG leads are applied and continuous haemodynamic monitoring is performed during the procedure, which takes 30 minutes to 3 hours.
- Local anaesthetic is administered to the site of sheath insertion.
- Continuous reassurance is provided to the person throughout the procedure.

AFTER THE PROCEDURE

- Monitor vital signs every 15 minutes for the first hour and then every 30 minutes until stable. Assess cardiac rhythm and rate for alterations. Assess peripheral pulses distal to the insertion site.
- Assess the person for chest heaviness, shortness of breath and abdominal or groin pain.
- Monitor catheter insertion site for bleeding or haematoma. In case of bleeding/haematoma, apply enough pressure to the insertion site to compress the artery or vein. Call for assistance and follow local protocol for management of vascular access site complications.
- Administer pain medications as prescribed.
- Instruct the person to remain on bed rest for 2 to 3 hours post sheath removal dependent upon site of insertion.
- Encourage oral fluids unless contraindicated (i.e. if the person has congestive heart failure).

NURSING CARE OF THE PERSON having pericardiocentesis

BEFORE THE PROCEDURE

- Gather all supplies:
  a. Pericardiocentesis tray
  b. ECG machine and electrode patches
  c. Emergency cart with defibrillator
  d. Dressing
  e. Culture bottles (if indicated).
- Reinforce teaching and answer questions about the procedure or associated care. Provide emotional support.
- Ensure that informed consent has been obtained.
- Provide for privacy.
- Obtain and document baseline vital signs.
- Connect the person to a cardiac monitor; obtain a baseline rhythm strip for comparison during and after the procedure.
- Connect the precordial ECG lead of the hub of the aspiration needle using an alligator clamp.

DURING THE PROCEDURE

- Follow standard precautions.
- Position seated at a 45- to 60-degree angle. Place a dry towel under the rib cage to catch blood or fluid leakage.
- Observe the ST segment for elevation and the ECG monitor for signs of myocardial irritability (PVCs) during the procedure. These indicate that the needle is touching the myocardium.
- Notify the physician of changes in cardiac rhythm, blood pressure, heart rate, level of consciousness and urine output. These may indicate cardiac complications.
- Monitor central venous pressure (CVP) and blood pressure closely. As the effusion is relieved, CVP will decrease and BP will increase.

AFTER THE PROCEDURE

- Document the procedure and the person's response to and tolerance of the procedure.
- Continue to monitor vital signs and cardiac rhythm every 15 minutes during the first hour, every 30 minutes during the next hour and every hour for the next 24 hours.
- Record the amount of fluid removed as output on the intake and output record.
- If indicated, send a sample of aspirated fluid for microbiology, cytology or histology.
- Assess heart and breath sounds.

DIAGNOSTIC TESTS Haematological, peripheral vascular and lymphatic disorders

NAME OF TEST Full blood count (FBC)

PURPOSE AND DESCRIPTION This is a blood test involving several measurements of blood components. See Table 28.1.

RELATED NURSING CARE No special preparation is needed.

NAME OF TEST Erythrocyte sedimentation rate (ESR)

PURPOSE AND DESCRIPTION This blood test is done as a measure of inflammation; the ESR is increased in many illnesses, including cancer, heart disease and kidney disease. This test is performed to detect and monitor inflammation in both acute and chronic medical conditions. The findings are used to assist in identifying the cause of inflammation, infections, cancers and autoimmune diseases. It is a non-specific test; therefore, it is typically used in conjunction with other tests, such as FBC, to determine a specific cause of ill health.

Normal values:
Women: 1–12 mm in 1 hour; men: 1–14 mm in 1 hour; pregnant women: > 30 mm in the first hour (due to elevated levels of plasma globulins and fibrinogen)—therefore, ESR cannot be used as an inflammatory marker in pregnancy.

RELATED NURSING CARE No special preparation is needed.

NAME OF TEST Bone marrow biopsy

PURPOSE AND DESCRIPTION Conducted to evaluate blood-forming tissue; to diagnose multiple myeloma, leukaemia and some lymphomas; and to assess effectiveness of therapy for leukaemia. Bone marrow is removed from a site such as the posterior iliac crest with needle aspiration.

RELATED NURSING CARE See the following 'Nursing care' box.

NAME OF TEST Magnetic resonance angiography (MRA)

PURPOSE AND DESCRIPTION Used to visualise vascular occlusive disease and aneurysms of the abdominal aorta. The procedure is done by using a gadolinium contrast medium injected IV.

RELATED NURSING CARE Assess for any metallic implants, such as a pacemaker or body piercings. Pacemakers and implantable defibrillators implanted after the year 2000 are now generally considered safe for MRA and MRI. If in doubt, the device manufacturer should be contacted for advice.

NAME OF TEST Magnetic resonance imaging (MRI)

PURPOSE AND DESCRIPTION A radiological study used to visualise liver, spleen and lymph nodes. Does not require injection of contrast medium.

RELATED NURSING CARE As above.

NAME OF TEST Computed tomography (CT) scan

PURPOSE AND DESCRIPTION A radiological study used to evaluate the lymph nodes. Contrast medium may be used when assessing the nodes of the abdomen.

RELATED NURSING CARE Assess for allergy to iodine if contrast medium is to be administered.

NAME OF TEST Liver and/or spleen scan

PURPOSE AND DESCRIPTION A radiological study used to assess the liver and/or spleen. A radioisotope is injected IV prior to the scan.

RELATED NURSING CARE Assess for allergy to iodine.

(continued)

DIAGNOSTIC TESTS Haematological, peripheral vascular and lymphatic disorders (continued)

NAME OF TEST Lymphangiography (lymphangiogram)

PURPOSE AND DESCRIPTION This is an x-ray examination of the lymphatic vessels and lymph nodes, used to assess metastasis of the lymph nodes, to identify malignant lymphoma and to identify the cause of lymphoedema. An iodine contrast, Evans blue dye or contrast is injected at various sites and fluoroscopy is used to visualise lymphatic filling.

RELATED NURSING CARE Ask the person about allergies to iodine or contrast medium used in a previous x-ray test. Tell the person that the blue contrast dye discolours the urine and possibly the skin for a few days.

NAME OF TEST Lymph node biopsy

PURPOSE AND DESCRIPTION Done to obtain tissue for histological examination for diagnosis and treatment. May be open (performed in the operating room) or closed (needle) by needle aspiration of tissue from a lymph node.

RELATED NURSING CARE Use sterile technique when changing dressings.

Disorders of the arteries and veins are diagnosed by various non-invasive examinations, including echocardiography, ultrasound and Doppler studies. A magnetic resonance angiography (MRA) may be done to visualise vascular occlusive disease and abdominal aorta aneurysms.

Tests of the lymphatic system, including a lymphangiogram and a lymph node biopsy, may be done to identify malignancies, assess metastasis of cancer to lymph nodes, identify the causes of lymphoedema and obtain tissue for diagnosis and treatment.

NURSING CARE OF THE PERSON having bone marrow studies

Bone marrow specimens are obtained by either aspiration or biopsy. The preferred site for bone marrow aspiration is the posterior iliac crest; the anterior iliac crest or the sternum may also be used. The procedure is performed by inserting a needle into the bone and drawing out a sample of the blood in the marrow. A bone marrow biopsy is performed by making a small incision over the bone and screwing a core biopsy instrument into the bone to obtain a specimen. Bone marrow studies are used to diagnose leukaemias, metastatic cancer, lymphoma, aplastic anaemia and Hodgkin's disease.

PREPARATION OF THE PERSON

- Explain the purpose and procedure of the test.
- Ensure presence of a signed consent for the procedure.
- Offer sedation (neuroleptic or tranquillising) and/or pain relief before the procedure to alleviate discomfort.
- Record vital signs.
- Ask the person to void.
- Support person into the supine position if the specimen will be obtained from the sternum or anterior iliac crest; prone position if the posterior iliac crest will be used.
- Assist the person to remain still during the procedure.

AFTER THE PROCEDURE

- Apply pressure to the puncture site for 5 to 10 minutes.
- Assess vital signs and compare results with pre-procedure readings.
- Apply a dressing to the puncture site and monitor for bleeding and infection for 24 hours.

HEALTH EDUCATION FOR THE PERSON AND FAMILY

- The procedure (either aspiration or biopsy) takes about 20 minutes.
- A sedative may be given prior to the procedure.
- It is important the person remains very still during the procedure to prevent accidental injury.
- Although the area will be anaesthetised with a local anaesthetic, insertion of the needle will be painful for a short time. Taking deep breaths may make this part of the procedure less painful for the person. (In certain circumstances, such as with confused or paediatric patients, sedation or a short-acting general anaesthetic may be used to prevent excessive movement during the procedure.)
- The aspiration site may ache for 1 or 2 days.
- Ask the person to report any unusual bleeding immediately.

Physical assessment

Physical assessment of cardiovascular and lymphatic function may be performed either as part of a total assessment or alone for people with suspected or known problems with cardiovascular or lymphatic function. Assess the heart through inspection, palpation and auscultation over the precordium (the area of the chest wall overlying the heart). Normal age-related findings for the older person are summarised in Table 28.3.

The techniques used to assess these systems include inspection of the skin for such changes as oedema, ulcerations or alterations in colour and temperature; auscultation of blood pressure; and palpation of the major pulse points of the body (see Figure 28.23) and lymph nodes. The person may be assessed in the supine, sitting and standing positions. Normal age-related findings for the older adult are summarised in Table 28.4.

Before beginning the assessment, collect all required equipment and explain the techniques to the person to decrease anxiety. A quiet environment is essential to hear and assess heart sounds accurately.

The person may sit or lie in the supine position. Movements over the precordium may be more easily seen with tangential lighting (in which the light is directed at a right angle to the area being observed, producing shadows). Assess the following types of movements:

- The **apical impulse** is a normal, visible pulsation in the area of the midclavicular line in the left fifth intercostal space. It can be seen on inspection in about half of the adult population. (The apical impulse was previously called the point of maximal impulse (PMI), but this term is no longer used because a maximal impulse may occur in other areas of the precordium as a result of abnormal conditions.)

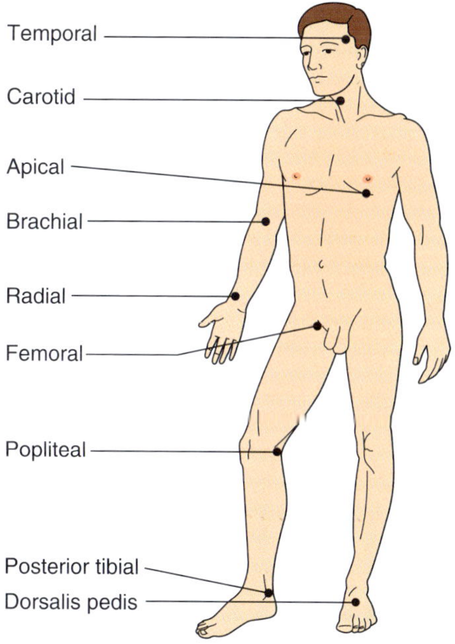

FIGURE 28.23 *Body sites at which peripheral pulses are most easily palpated*

TABLE 28.3 Age-related changes in the heart

AGE-RELATED CHANGE	SIGNIFICANCE
Myocardium: ↓ efficiency and contractibility. Sinoatrial node: ↑ in thickness of shell surrounding the node and a ↓ in the number of pacemaker cells.	• Decreased cardiac output when under physiological stress with resulting tachycardia that lasts longer. The person may require rest time between physical activities.
Left ventricle: slight hypertrophy, prolonged isometric contraction phase and relaxation time; ↑ time for diastolic filling and systolic emptying cycle.	• Stroke volume may increase to compensate for tachycardia, leading to increased blood pressure.
Valves and blood vessels: aorta is elongated and dilated, valves are thicker and more rigid and resistance to peripheral blood flow increases by 1% per year.	• Blood pressure increases to compensate for increased peripheral resistance and decreased cardiac output.

TABLE 28.4 Age-related changes in the haematological, peripheral vascular and lymphatic systems

AGE-RELATED CHANGE	SIGNIFICANCE
Bone marrow: ↓ ability of bone marrow to respond to need for increased RBCs, WBCs and platelets.	• Anaemia may result.
Blood vessels: • *Tunica intima*: fibrosis, calcium and lipid accumulation, cellular proliferation.	• As a result of age-related changes, the systolic blood pressure rises. Decreased arterial elasticity results in vascular changes in the heart, kidneys and pituitary gland. Decreased baroreceptor function results in postural hypotension. Vessels in the head, neck and extremities are more prominent.
• *Tunica media*: thins, elastin fibres calcify; increase in calcium results in stiffening. Baroreceptor function is impaired and peripheral resistance increases.	• Inefficient vasoconstriction, decreased cardiac output and reduced muscle mass and subcutaneous tissue lead to a reduced ability to respond to cold temperatures. • With a decrease in blood pressure and changes in blood vessel walls, tissue perfusion may be inadequate, leading to oedema, inflammation, pressure ulcers and changes in effects of medications.
• [illegible]	
Immune system: • Impaired function of B and T lymphocytes. • Decreased production of antibodies. • Unable to distinguish 'self' from 'non-self'. • Phagocytic immune response delayed.	• Increased risk of infection, with decreased manifestations of an actual infection. • Increased incidence of cancers. • Altered response to antigens (such as Mantoux tuberculin test). • May have reactivation of tuberculosis.

- Retraction is a pulling in of the tissue of the precordium; a slight retraction just medial to the midclavicular line at the area of the apical impulse is normal and is more likely to be visible in people who are thin.
- Pulsations (other than the normal apical pulsations), which may be called heaves or lifts, are considered abnormal. They may occur as the result of cardiomyopathy.

Genetic considerations

When conducting a health assessment interview and a physical assessment, it is important for the nurse to consider genetic influences on the health of the person. During the health assessment interview, ask about family members with health problems affecting cardiovascular and lymphatic function, or about a family history of high cholesterol levels or early-onset coronary artery disease. Ensure that the person considers both alive and deceased relatives in their family history. In addition, ask about a family history of high blood pressure, haemophilia, chronic myeloid leukaemia, porphyria and/or atherosclerosis. Depending on the racial and ethnic background of the person, ask about any family members with sickle cell anaemia or thalassaemia. During the physical assessment, assess for any manifestations that might indicate a genetic disorder (see the 'Genetic considerations' box). If data are found to indicate genetic risk factors or alterations, ask about genetic testing and refer for appropriate genetic counselling and evaluation. The chapter 'Genetic implications of adult health nursing' provides further information about genetics in medical–surgical nursing.

GENETIC CONSIDERATIONS Cardiovascular, haematological and lymphatic system disorders

Cardiovascular disorders

- Familial hypercholesterolaemia is a single gene disorder that results in atherosclerosis and CAD, which may occur at an earlier age than in the general population (i.e. before age 55 in men and age 65 in women). However, increased cholesterol levels may also be inherited and are a risk factor for CAD in both men and women.
- Marfan's syndrome is an autosomal dominant inherited disorder that affects the connective tissue with specific characteristics affecting the heart, blood vessels, bones, joints (hypermobility) and eyes (retinal detachment). Aortic dilatation can be life threatening as it leads to aortic dissection or rupture. The lungs, skin and nervous system may also be affected.
- Supraventricular aortic stenosis (SVAS) is a genetic vascular disorder resulting in an hourglass-shaped stenosis of the ascending aorta. It may also affect other major arteries, including the pulmonary, carotid, cerebral, renal and coronary arteries.
- Hypertrophic obstructive cardiomyopathy, a disease of sarcomere proteins, has a genetic transmission. The interventricular septum becomes enlarged and obstructs the left ventricular outflow tract.
- Williams syndrome is a rare genetic disorder characterised by characteristic 'elfin-like' features and heart and blood vessel problems (as well as other physical problems).
- Long QT syndrome (LQTS) is an inherited genetic disorder that results from structural abnormalities of the potassium channels in the heart, leading to arrhythmias. This can result in loss of consciousness and may cause sudden cardiac death in teenagers and young adults when exposed to stressors ranging from exercise to loud sounds.

Haematological, peripheral vascular and lymphatic disorders

- There is a genetic link in 30–40% of people with primary hypertension.
- Sickle cell anaemia is an inherited genetic disorder seen in people of Mediterranean, Caribbean, Central and South American, Arab or East Indian ancestry. As Australia is an increasingly multicultural society, healthcare professionals need to be aware of its existence among people with these racial backgrounds.
- Gaucher disease, more common in descendants of Eastern European Jewish people, is an inherited illness caused by a gene mutation. The gene is responsible for an enzyme that breaks down a specific fat. When the fat is not broken down, it accumulates in the liver, spleen and bone marrow, causing pain, fatigue, jaundice, bone damage, anaemia and even death.
- Haemophilia A is a hereditary blood disorder, primarily affecting males, characterised by a deficiency of the blood clotting factor named factor VIII. Abnormal bleeding results.
- Chronic myeloid leukaemia (CML), a cancer of blood cells, is characterised by replacement of bone marrow with malignant, leukaemic cells. Leukaemic cells also circulate in the blood, causing enlargement of the spleen, liver and other organs. This leukaemia is the result of a chromosomal abnormality called the Philadelphia chromosome.
- Porphyria is a group of genetic blood diseases in which haem production is disrupted. When haem production is disrupted, porphyrins (a part of haem) are overproduced and cause illnesses; they also give urine a reddish-purple colour.
- Thalassaemia, an inherited disease of abnormal haemoglobin synthesis, is prevalent in descendants of people living near the Mediterranean Sea, Africa, the Middle East and Asia. It comprises a group of disorders that range from very mild blood abnormalities to severe or fatal anaemia.
- Atherosclerosis is characterised by narrowing of arteries by cholesterol-rich plaques of immune system cells. Risk factors may be genetic and/or environmental.

INTERPRETATION OF NORMAL AND ABERRANT DATA OBTAINED FROM CARDIOVASCULAR AND LYMPHATIC SYSTEM ASSESSMENT

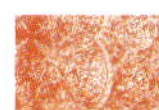

CARDIAC ASSESSMENTS

Technique/normal findings	Abnormal findings
Apical impulse assessment **First using the palmar surface and then repeating with finger pads, palpate the precordium for symmetry of movement and the apical impulse for location, size, amplitude and duration. The sequence for palpation is shown in Figure 28.24. To locate the apical impulse, ask the person to assume a left lateral recumbent position. Simultaneous palpation of the carotid pulse may also be helpful.** *The apical impulse is not palpable in all people. The apical impulse may be palpated in the mitral area and has only a brief small amplitude.*	■ An enlarged or displaced heart is associated with an apical impulse lateral to the midclavicular line (MCL) or below the fifth left intercostal space (ICS). ■ Increased size, amplitude and duration of the apical impulse are associated with left ventricular volume overload (increased afterload) in conditions such as hypertension (HTN) and aortic stenosis, and with pressure overload (increased preload) in conditions such as aortic or mitral regurgitation. ■ Increased amplitude alone may occur with hyperkinetic states, such as anxiety, hyperthyroidism and anaemia. ■ Decreased amplitude is associated with dilated heart cardiomyopathy. ■ Displacement alone may also occur with dextrocardia, diaphragmatic hernia, gastric distension or chronic lung disease. ■ A **thrill** (a palpable vibration over the precordium or an artery) may accompany severe valve stenosis. ■ A marked increase in amplitude of the apical impulse at the right ventricular area occurs with right ventricular volume overload in atrial septal defect. ■ An increase in amplitude and duration occurs with right ventricular pressure overload in pulmonary valve stenosis and pulmonary hypertension. A lift or heave may also be seen in these conditions (and in chronic lung disease). ■ A palpable thrill in this area occurs with ventricular septal defect.
Palpate the subxiphoid area with the index and middle finger. *No pulsations or vibrations should be palpated.*	■ Right ventricular enlargement may produce a downward pulsation against the fingertips. ■ An accentuated pulsation at the pulmonary area may be present in hyperkinetic states. ■ A prominent pulsation reflects increased flow or dilation of the pulmonary artery. ■ A thrill may be associated with aortic or pulmonary stenosis, aortic stenosis, pulmonary HTN or atrial septal defect. ■ Increased pulsation at the aortic area may suggest aortic aneurysm. ■ A palpable second heart sound (S_2) may be noted with systemic HTN.

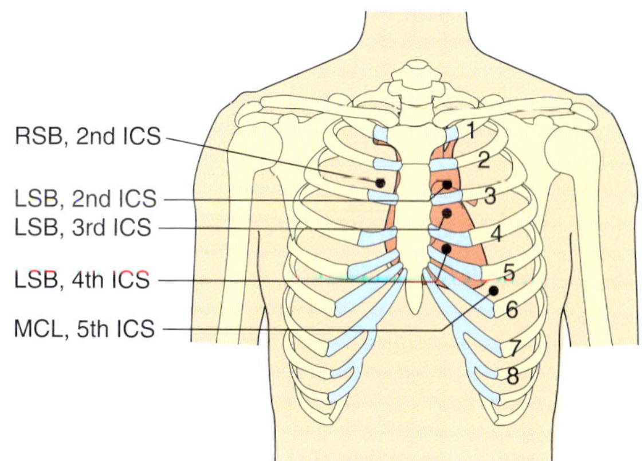

FIGURE 28.24 ***Areas for inspection and palpation of the precordium, indicating the sequence for palpation (ICS = intercostal space; LSB = left sternal border; MCL = midclavicular line RSB = right sternal border)***

(continued)

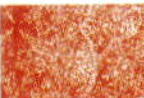

CARDIAC ASSESSMENTS (continued)

Technique/normal findings	Abnormal findings
Cardiac rate and rhythm assessment	
Auscultate heart rate. The heart rate should be 60 to 100 beats per minute with regular rhythm (in an adult).	■ A heart rate exceeding 100 beats per minute (beats/min) is tachycardia. A heart rate less than 60 beats/min is bradycardia.
Simultaneously palpate the radial pulse while listening to the apical pulse. *The radial and apical pulses should be equal.*	■ If the radial pulse falls behind the apical rate, the person has a pulse deficit, indicating weak, ineffective contractions of the left ventricle.
Auscultate heart rhythm. *The heart rhythm should be regular.*	■ **Arrhythmias** (abnormal heart rate or rhythm) may be regular or irregular in rhythm; their rates may be slow or fast. Irregular rhythms may occur in a pattern (e.g. an early beat every second beat, called bigeminy), sporadically or with frequency and disorganisation (e.g. atrial fibrillation). A pattern of gradual increase and decrease in heart rate that is within the normal heart rate and that correlates with inspiration and expiration is called sinus arrhythmia.
Heart sounds assessment	
See guidelines for cardiac auscultation in Box 28.4.	
Identify S_1 (first heart sound) and note its intensity. At each auscultatory area, listen for several cardiac cycles. See Figure 28.25 for auscultation areas. *S_1 is loudest at the apex of the heart.*	■ An accentuated S_1 occurs with tachycardia, states in which cardiac output is high (fever, anxiety, exercise, anaemia, hyperthyroidism), complete heart block and mitral stenosis. ■ A diminished S_1 occurs with first-degree heart block, mitral regurgitation, CHF, CAD and pulmonary or systemic HTN. The intensity is also decreased with obesity, emphysema and pericardial effusion. Varying intensity of S_1 occurs with complete heart block and grossly irregular rhythms.
Listen for splitting of S_1. *Splitting of S_1 may occur during inspiration.*	■ Abnormal splitting of S_1 may be heard with right bundle branch block and premature ventricular contractions.

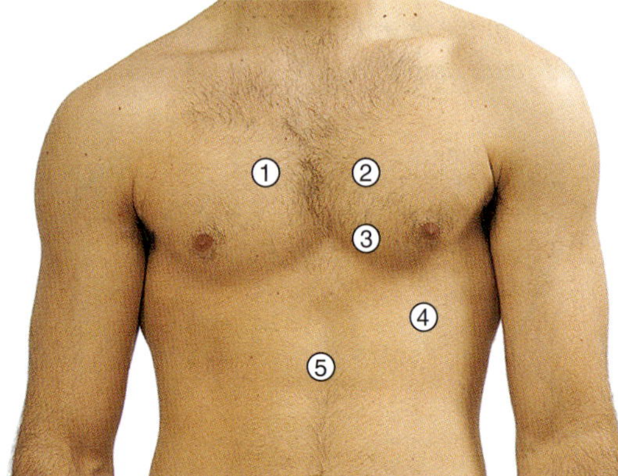

FIGURE 28.25 *Areas for auscultation of the heart*

BOX 28.4 Guidelines for cardiac auscultation

1. Locate the major auscultatory areas on the precordium.
2. Choose a sequence of listening. Either begin from the apex and move upward along the sternal border to the base or begin at the base and move downward to the apex.
3. Listen first with the person in the sitting or supine position. Then ask the person to lie on the left side and focus on the apex. Lastly, ask the person to sit up and lean forward. These position changes bring the heart closer to the chest wall and enhance auscultation. Carry out the following steps when the person assumes each of these positions:
   a. First, auscultate each area with the diaphragm of the stethoscope to listen for high-pitched sounds: S_1, S_2, murmurs, pericardial friction rubs.
   b. Next, auscultate each area with the bell of the stethoscope to listen for lower-pitched sounds: S_3, S_4, murmurs.
   c. Listen for the effect of respirations on each sound; while the person is sitting up and leaning forward, ask the person to exhale and hold the breath while you listen to heart sounds.

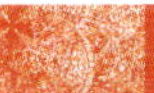

CARDIAC ASSESSMENTS (continued)

Technique/normal findings	Abnormal findings
Identify S_2 (second heart sound) and note its intensity. *S_2 immediately follows S_1 and is loudest at the base of the heart.*	▪ An accentuated S_2 may be heard with HTN, exercise, excitement and conditions of pulmonary HTN such as CHF and cor pulmonale. ▪ A diminished S_2 occurs with aortic stenosis, a fall in systolic blood pressure (shock) and increased anteroposterior chest diameter.
Listen for splitting of S_2. *No splitting of S_2 should be heard.*	▪ Wide splitting of S_2 is associated with delayed emptying of the right ventricle, resulting in delayed pulmonary valve closure (e.g. mitral regurgitation, pulmonary stenosis and right bundle branch block). ▪ Fixed splitting occurs when right ventricular output is greater than left ventricular output and pulmonary valve closure is delayed (e.g. with atrial septal defect and right ventricular failure). ▪ Paradoxical splitting occurs when closure of the aortic valve is delayed (e.g. left bundle branch block).
Identify extra heart sounds in systole. *Extra heart sounds are not present in systole.*	▪ Ejection sounds (or clicks) result from the opening of deformed semilunar valves (e.g. aortic and pulmonary stenosis). ▪ A midsystolic click is heard with mitral valve prolapse (MVP).
Identify the presence of extra heart sounds in diastole. *Extra heart sounds are not present in diastole.*	▪ An opening snap results from the opening sound of a stenotic mitral valve. ▪ A pathological S_3 (a third heart sound that immediately follows S_2, called a ventricular gallop) results from myocardial failure and ventricular volume overload (e.g. CHF, mitral or tricuspid regurgitation). ▪ An S_4 (a fourth heart sound that immediately precedes S_1, called an atrial gallop) results from increased resistance to ventricular filling after atrial contraction (e.g. HTN, CAD, aortic stenosis and cardiomyopathy). ▪ A combined S_3 and S_4 is called a summation gallop and occurs with severe CHF.
Identify extra heart sounds in both systole and diastole. *No extra heart sounds should be heard during systole and diastole.*	▪ A pericardial friction rub results from inflammation of the pericardial sac, as with pericarditis.
Murmur assessment	
Identify any murmurs. Note location, timing, presence during systole or diastole, and intensity. Use the following scale to grade murmurs: **I = Barely heard** **II = Quietly heard** **III = Clearly heard** **IV = Loud** **V = Very loud** **VI = Loudest; may be heard with stethoscope off the chest.** **A thrill may accompany murmurs of grade IV to grade VI.** **Note pitch (low, medium, high) and quality (harsh, blowing or musical). Note pattern/shape, crescendo, decrescendo and radiation/transmission (to axilla, neck).** *No murmurs should be heard.*	▪ Midsystolic murmurs are heard with semilunar valve disease (e.g. aortic and pulmonary stenosis) and with hypertrophic cardiomyopathy. ▪ Pansystolic (holosystolic) murmurs are heard with AV valve disease (e.g. mitral and tricuspid regurgitation, ventricular septal defect). ▪ A late systolic murmur is heard with MVP. ▪ Early diastolic murmurs occur with regurgitant flow across incompetent semilunar valves (e.g. aortic regurgitation). ▪ Mid-diastolic and presystolic murmurs, such as with mitral stenosis, occur with turbulent flow across the AV valves. ▪ Continuous murmurs throughout systole and all or part of diastole occur with patent ductus arteriosus.

(continued)

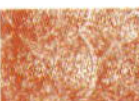

CARDIAC ASSESSMENTS (continued)

Technique/normal findings | **Abnormal findings**

Blood pressure and pulse pressure assessment

See Box 28.5 for blood pressure measurement guidelines.

Auscultate blood pressure in each arm with the person seated. *The normal blood pressure is considered to be <120/>80, with readings of 120–139/80–89 diagnosed as prehypertension.*

- Consistent BP readings over 140/90 in adults under age 40 are considered hypertension.
- BP under 90/60 is considered hypotension.
- An auscultatory gap—a temporary disappearance of sound between the systolic and diastolic BP—may be a normal variation or it may be associated with systolic HTN or a drop in diastolic BP due to aortic stenosis.
- **Korotkoff's sounds** (see Box 28.5) may be heard down to zero with cardiac valve replacements, hyperkinetic states, thyrotoxicosis and severe anaemia, as well as after vigorous exercise.
- The sounds of aortic regurgitation may obscure the diastolic BP.
- A difference of over 10 mmHg between arms suggests arterial compression on the side of the lower reading, aortic dissection or coarctation of the aorta.

Auscultate blood pressure in each arm with the person standing. If orthostatic changes occur, measure the BP with the person supine, legs dangling, and again with the person standing, 1 to 3 minutes apart. *A decrease in systolic BP is expected but should be < 10 mmHg; diastolic BP should not drop on standing.*

- A decrease in systolic BP of over 10 to 15 mmHg and a drop in diastolic BP on standing is called **orthostatic hypotension**. Causes include antihypertensive medications, volume depletion, peripheral vascular disease, prolonged bed rest and ageing.

> **CONSIDERATION FOR PRACTICE**
>
> If unable to auscultate blood pressure or palpate pulses, a Doppler ultrasound device may be used to evaluate blood flow. Apply a five-cent-piece amount of gel over the blood vessel to be assessed and lightly place the probe over the gel. Listen for a whooshing (artery) or rushing (vein) sound.

Observe the pulse pressure. The pulse pressure is the difference between the systolic and diastolic BP. For example, if the BP is 140/80, the pulse pressure is 60. *A normal pulse pressure is one-third the systolic measurement.*

- A widened pulse pressure with an elevated systolic BP occurs with exercise, arteriosclerosis, severe anaemia, thyrotoxicosis, increased intracranial pressure and increased age.
- A narrowed pulse pressure with a decreased systolic BP occurs with shock, pericardial tamponade, cardiac failure and pulmonary embolus.

Skin assessment

Inspect the colour of the skin. *The skin colour should be appropriate to the person's age and race.*

- Pallor reflects constriction of peripheral blood flow (e.g. due to syncope or shock) or decreased circulating oxyhaemoglobin (e.g. due to haemorrhage or anaemia).
- Central cyanosis of the lips, earlobes, oral mucosa and tongue suggests chronic cardiopulmonary disease. (See Box 28.6 for abnormal findings associated with peripheral vascular and lymphatic assessment.)

Inspect the skin of the extremities and over the regional lymph nodes, noting any oedema, erythema, red streaks or skin lesions. *There should be no oedema, redness or lesions over the regional lymph nodes.*

- Lymphangitis (inflammation of a lymphatic vessel) may produce a red streak with induration (hardness) following the course of the lymphatic collecting duct; infected skin lesions may be present, particularly between the digits.
- **Lymphoedema** (swelling due to lymphatic obstruction) occurs with congenital lymphatic anomaly (Milroy's disease) or with trauma to the regional lymphatic ducts from surgery or metastasis (e.g. arm lymphoedema after radical mastectomy with axillary node removal).

BOX 28.5 Guidelines for blood pressure assessment

Review of Korotkoff's sounds

The first sound heard is the systolic pressure; at least two consecutive sounds should be clear. If the sound disappears and then is heard again 10 to 15 mmHg later, an auscultatory gap is present; this may be a normal variant, or it may be associated with hypertension. The first diastolic sound is heard as a muffling of the Korotkoff's sound and is considered the best approximation of the true diastolic pressure. The second diastolic sound is the level at which sounds are no longer heard.

Key issues relating to blood pressure assessment are listed below.

Technique reminders

- Choose a cuff of an appropriate size: the cuff should snugly cover two-thirds of the upper arm and the bladder should completely encircle the arm. The bladder should be centred over the brachial artery, with the lower edge 2 to 3 cm above the antecubital space.
- The person's arm should be slightly flexed and supported (on a table or by the examiner) at heart level.
- To determine how high to inflate the cuff, palpate the brachial pulse and inflate the cuff to the point on the manometer at which the pulse is no longer felt; then, add 30 mmHg to this reading and use the sum as the target for inflation. Wait 15 seconds before reinflating the cuff to auscultate the BP.
- To recheck a BP, wait at least 30 seconds before attempting another inflation.
- Always inflate the cuff completely, then deflate it. Once deflation begins, allow it to continue; do not try to reinflate the cuff if the first systolic sound is not heard or if the cuff inadvertently deflates.
- The bell of the stethoscope more effectively transmits the low-pitched sounds of BP.

Sources of error

- Falsely high readings can occur if the cuff is too small or too loose, or if the person supports their own arm.
- Falsely low readings can occur if a standard cuff is used on a person with thin arms.
- Inadequate inflation may result in underestimation of the systolic pressure or overestimation of the diastolic pressure if an auscultatory gap is present.
- Rapid deflation and repeated or slow inflations (causing venous congestion) can lead to underestimation of the systolic BP and overestimation of the diastolic BP.

Factors altering blood pressure

- A change from the horizontal to upright position causes a slight decrease (5 to 10 mmHg) in systolic BP; the diastolic BP remains unchanged or rises slightly.
- BP taken in the arm is lower when the person is standing.
- If the BP is taken with the person in the lateral recumbent position, a lower BP reading may be obtained in both arms; this is especially apparent in the right arm with the person in the left lateral position.
- Factors that increase BP include exercise, caffeine, cold environment, eating a large meal, painful stimuli and emotions.
- Factors that lower BP include sleep (by 20 mmHg) and very fast, slow or irregular heart rates.
- BP tends to be higher in people who are taller or heavier.

Alternative methods of blood pressure measurement

- The palpatory method may be necessary if severe hypotension is present and the BP is inaudible. Palpate the brachial pulse and inflate the cuff 30 mmHg above the point where the pulse disappears; deflate the cuff and note the point on the manometer where the pulse becomes palpable again. Record this as the palpatory systolic BP.
- Leg BP measurement may be needed when there is injury of the arms or to rule out coarctation of the aorta or aortic insufficiency when arm diastolic BP is over 90 mmHg. Place the person in the prone or supine position with the leg slightly flexed. Place a large leg cuff on the thigh with the bladder centred over the popliteal artery. Place the bell of the stethoscope over the popliteal space. Normal leg systolic BP is higher than arm BP; diastolic BP should be equal to or lower than arm BP. Abnormally low leg BP occurs with aortic insufficiency and coarctation of the aorta.

BOX 28.6 Abnormal findings associated with peripheral vascular and lymphatic assessment

- *Pallor* is an absence of colour of the skin. The degree of pallor depends on the person's normal skin colour and health status. Dark skin may appear ashen or have a yellowish tinge.
- *Cyanosis* is a bluish discolouration of the skin and mucous membranes in people with light skin. In people with dark skin, cyanosis may be difficult to observe. Inspect the nail beds and conjunctiva.
- *Oedema* is an abnormal accumulation of fluid in the interstitial spaces of tissues. It is often most apparent in the lower extremities.
- *Varicose veins* are tortuous and dilated veins that have incompetent valves. The superficial leg veins are most commonly affected.
- *Enlarged lymph nodes* result from infection or malignancy.
- *Atrophic changes* are changes in size or activity of body tissues as the result of pathology or injury. Decreased blood flow and oxygenation of the lower extremities often cause atrophic changes of loss of hair, thickened toenails, changes in pigmentation and ulcerations.
- *Gangrene* is the necrosis (or death) of tissue, most often the result of loss of blood supply and infection. Gangrene often begins in the most distal of the tissues of the extremities.
- *Pressure ulcers*, also called decubitus ulcers or bed sores, are the result of ischaemia and hypoxia of tissue following prolonged pressure. These ulcers often are located over bony prominences. If untreated, the tissue changes proceed from red skin to deep, crater-like ulcers.

CARDIAC ASSESSMENTS (continued)

Technique/normal findings	Abnormal findings
	■ Oedema of lymphatic origin is usually not pitting and the skin may be thickened; one example is the taut swelling of the face and body that occurs with myxoedema, associated with hypothyroidism.
Artery and vein assessment **Palpate the temporal arteries.** *There should be no redness, swelling, nodules or variations in pulse amplitude.*	■ Redness, swelling, nodularity and variations in pulse amplitude may occur with temporal arteritis.
Inspect and palpate the carotid arteries. Note symmetry, the pulse rate, rhythm, volume and amplitude. Note any variation with respiration. Describe all pulses as increased, normal, diminished or absent. Scales ranging from 0 to 4+ are sometimes used as follows: 0 = Absent 1+ = Diminished 2+ = Normal 3+ = Increased 4+ = Bounding **Pulse waveforms are shown in Box 28.7.**	**BOX 28.7 Types of pulse patterns** 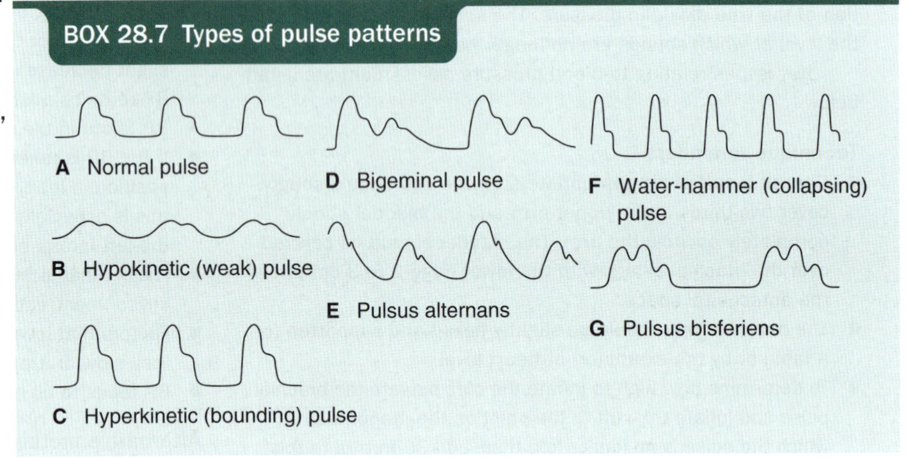
Remember that carotid pulses should never be assessed simultaneously as this can cause vagal stimulation and potentially result in decreased cerebral perfusion. *The carotid pulses should be bilaterally equal in rate, rhythm, volume and amplitude.*	■ A unilateral pulsating bulge is seen with a tortuous or kinked carotid artery. ■ Alterations in pulse rate or rhythm are due to cardiac arrhythmias. ■ An absent pulse indicates arterial occlusion. ■ A hypokinetic (weak) pulse is associated with decreased stroke volume (see Box 28.7B). This may be due to congestive heart failure (CHF), aortic stenosis or hypovolaemia; to increased peripheral resistance, which may result from cold temperatures; or to arterial narrowing, commonly found with atherosclerosis. ■ A hyperkinetic (bounding) pulse occurs with increased stroke volume and/or decreased peripheral resistance (see Box 28.7C). This may result from states in which cardiac output is high or from aortic regurgitation. It also may occur with anaemia, hyperthyroidism, bradycardia or reduced compliance, as with atherosclerosis. ■ A bigeminal pulse is marked by decreased amplitude of every second beat (see Box 28.7D). This may be due to premature contractions (usually ventricular). ■ Pulsus alternans is a regular pulse with alternating strong and weak beats (see Box 28.7E). This may be due to left ventricular failure and severe HTN. ■ Pulsus paradoxus is a > 10 mmHg drop in systolic pressure during inspiration. It is an indicator of pericardial tamponade.
Auscultate the carotid arteries, using the bell of the stethoscope. *No bruits should be heard.*	■ A murmuring or blowing sound heard over stenosed peripheral vessels is known as a *bruit*. A bruit heard over the middle to upper carotid artery suggests atherosclerosis.
Inspect and palpate the internal and external jugular veins for venous pressure. *See Box 28.8 for guidelines for assessing jugular venous pressure (JVP).*	■ An increase in jugular venous pressure (JVP) over 3 cm and located above the sternal angle reflects increased right atrial pressure. This occurs with right ventricular failure or, less commonly, with constrictive pericarditis, tricuspid stenosis and superior venae cavae obstruction.
If venous pressure is elevated, assess the hepatojugular reflex. (Compress the liver in the right upper abdominal quadrant with the palm of the hand for 30 to 60 seconds while observing the jugular veins.)	■ A decrease in venous pressure reflects reduced left ventricular output or blood volume. ■ Unilateral neck vein distension suggests local compression or anatomic anomaly. ■ A rise in the column of neck vein distension over 1 cm with liver compression indicates right heart failure.

BOX 28.8 Assessing jugular venous pressure

When a person with normal venous pressure lies in the supine position, full neck veins are normally visible, but as the head of the bed is elevated, the pulsations disappear. In the person with greatly elevated venous pressure, visible pulsations of the jugular vein are present even in the upright position. To conduct the inspection:

1. Remove clothing from the person's neck and chest. Elevate the head of the bed 30 to 45 degrees (semi-Fowler's position) and turn the person's head to the opposite side. As jugular venous pressure is the measurement of pressure in the right atrium, it is best to examine the right jugular vein. This is because it has a more direct anatomical path to the right atrium.
2. Make sure the neck and the upper thorax are exposed. Avoid neck flexion or hyperextension which may cause the jugular vein to become kinked or stretched, causing compression pulsations.
3. Assess venous pressure by measuring the vertical distance between the angle of St Louis and the highest visible level of pulsation in the internal jugular vein. Using two rulers, line up the bottom edge with the top of the area of pulsation in the jugular vein. Then align another ruler perpendicular to the first at the level of the sternal angle. In centimetres, measure the distance between the second ruler and the sternal angle.
4. Repeat this technique on the other side. Bilateral pressures higher than 2.5 cm are considered elevated and are a sign of right-sided heart failure. One-sided pressure elevation can be a sign of obstruction.
5. If jugular distension is present, assess the JVP by measuring from the highest point of visible distension to the sternal angle (the point at which the clavicles meet) on both sides of the neck (see the accompanying figure). Bilateral measurements above 3 cm are considered elevated and indicate increased venous pressure; distension on only one side may indicate obstruction.

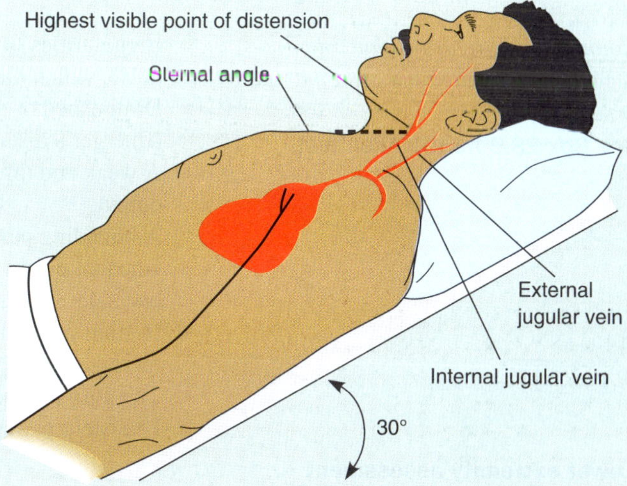

Assessment of the highest point of jugular vein distension

CARDIAC ASSESSMENTS (continued)

Technique/normal findings	Abnormal findings
Upper extremity assessment	
Inspect and palpate the arms and hands, noting size and symmetry, skin colour and temperature. *Arms and hands should be symmetrical in size and shape, warm and of appropriate skin colour.*	■ Unilateral swelling with venous prominence occurs with venous obstruction. ■ Extreme localised pallor of the fingers is seen with Raynaud's disease. ■ Cyanosis of the nail beds reflects chronic cardiopulmonary disease. ■ Cold temperature of the hands and fingers occurs with vasoconstriction.
Palpate the nail beds for capillary refill. (Apply pressure to the person's fingertips. Watch for blanching of the nail beds. Release the pressure. Note the time it takes for capillary refill, indicated by the return of pink colour on release of the pressure.) *Capillary refill should be less than 2 seconds (i.e. immediate).*	■ Capillary refill that takes more than 2 seconds reflects circulatory compromise, such as hypovolaemia or anaemia.
Assess venous pattern and pressure. (Elevate one of the person's arms over the head for a few seconds. Slowly lower the arm. Observe the filling of the person's hand veins.) *Hand veins should fill equally and immediately.*	■ Distension of hand veins at elevations over 9 cm above heart level reflects an increase in systemic venous pressure.

(continued)

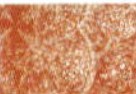

CARDIAC ASSESSMENTS (continued)

Technique/normal findings	Abnormal findings
Palpate the radial and brachial pulses. Note rate, rhythm, volume amplitude, symmetry, variations with respiration. (See Box 28.7 for pulse patterns.) *Radial and brachial pulses should have equal and normal rate, be strong and not vary with respirations.*	■ Alterations in pulse rate or rhythm are due to cardiac arrhythmias (such as atrial fibrillation, atrial flutter and premature ventricular contractions). A pulse rate over 100 bpm is tachycardia; a pulse rate below 60 bpm is bradycardia. ■ A pulse deficit (slower radial rate than apical rate) occurs with arrhythmias and CHF.
Colour should return within 3 to 5 seconds in both the ulnar and the radial arteries. **See Box 28.9 for the Allen test.**	■ Irregularities of rhythm produce early beats and pauses (skipped beats) in the pulse, which may be regular in pattern, sporadic or grossly irregular. ■ Diminished or absent radial pulses may be due to thromboangiitis obliterans (Buerger's disease) or acute arterial occlusion. ■ A weak and thready pulse, often with tachycardia, reflects decreased cardiac output. ■ A bounding pulse occurs with hyperkinetic states and atherosclerosis. ■ Unequal pulses between extremities suggest arterial narrowing or obstruction on one side. ■ In sinus arrhythmia (a normal variant, especially in young adults), the pulse rate increases with inspiration and decreases with expiration. ■ The normal ulnar artery may or may not have a palpable pulse. ■ Persistent pallor with the Allen test suggests ulnar artery occlusion.
Lower extremity assessment	
Inspect and palpate each leg, noting size, shape and symmetry; arterial pattern; skin colour, temperature and texture; hair pattern; pigmentation; rashes; ulcers, sensation; and capillary refill. *Legs should be symmetrical in size and shape, arterial pattern, appropriate colour, warm, without lesions. Capillary refill on toenails should be immediate.*	■ Chronic arterial insufficiency may be due to arteriosclerosis or autonomic dysfunction, or to acute occlusion resulting from thrombosis, embolus or aneurysm. ■ Signs of arterial disruption include pallor, dependent rubor (dusky redness); cool to cold temperature; and atrophic changes, such as hair loss with shiny and smooth texture, thickened nails, sensory loss, slow capillary refill and muscle atrophy. ■ Ulcers with symmetric margins, a deep base, black or necrotic tissue and absence of bleeding may occur at pressure points on or between the toes, on the heel, on the lateral malleolar or tibial area, over the metatarsal heads or along the side or sole of the foot. ■ Gangrene due to complete arterial occlusion presents as black, dry, hard skin; pre-gangrenous colour changes include deep cyanosis and purple-black discolouration.
With the person supine, assess the venous pattern of the legs. Repeat with the person standing. *Venous pattern on both legs should be symmetrical and there should be no oedema, cyanosis or lesions.*	■ Signs of venous insufficiency include swelling, thickened skin, cyanosis, stasis dermatitis (brown pigmentation, erythema and scaling) and superficial ankle ulcers located predominantly at the medial malleolus with uneven margins, ruddy granulation tissue and bleeding. ■ Varicose veins appear as dilated, tortuous and thickened veins, which are more prominent in a dependent position.

BOX 28.9 Allen test

If arterial insufficiency is suspected, palpate the ulnar pulse and perform the Allen test:

- Have the person make a tight fist.
- Compress both the radial and ulnar arteries.
- Have the person open the hand to a slightly flexed position.
- Observe for pallor and manifestations of pain.
- Release the ulnar artery and observe for the return of pink colour within 3 to 5 seconds.
- Repeat the procedure on the radial artery.

CARDIAC ASSESSMENTS (continued)

Technique/normal findings	Abnormal findings
Palpate the femoral, popliteal, posterior tibial and dorsalis pedis pulses for volume, amplitude and symmetry (see Figure 28.23). *All lower extremity pulses should be strong and equal in amplitude.*	▪ Diminished or absent leg pulses suggest partial or complete arterial occlusion of the proximal vessel and are often due to arteriosclerosis obliterans. ▪ Increased and widened femoral and popliteal pulsations suggest aneurysm. ▪ Watson's water hammer pulse, also known as collapsing pulse (or Corrigan's pulse when observed in the carotid artery), is a bounding, high-amplitude pulse with rapid upstroke and descent that manifests with aortic valve regurgitation. It can be seen (or felt) in the radial, ulnar or brachial arteries when slightly lifting the person's arm. ▪ Absence of a posterior tibial pulse with signs and symptoms of arterial insufficiency is usually due to acute occlusion by thrombosis or embolus. ▪ Diminished or absent pedal pulses are often due to popliteal occlusion associated with diabetes mellitus.
If pulses are diminished, observe for postural colour changes. Elevate both legs 60 degrees and observe the colour of the soles of the feet. Have the person sit and dangle the legs; note the return of colour to the feet.	▪ Extensive pallor on elevation is suggestive of arterial insufficiency. ▪ Rubor (dusky redness) of the toes and feet along with delayed venous return (over 45 seconds) suggests arterial insufficiency.
If arterial insufficiency is suspected, auscultate the femoral arteries. *No bruits should be heard.*	▪ Femoral bruits suggest arterial narrowing due to arteriosclerosis.
Inspect and gently palpate the calves. *There should be no redness or swelling, heat or pain in the calves of the legs.*	▪ Redness, warmth, swelling, tenderness and cords along a superficial vein suggest thrombophlebitis or deep venous thrombosis.

Inspect and palpate for oedema. Use your thumb to compress the dorsum of the person's foot, around the ankles and along the tibia (see Figure 28.26A). *A depression in the skin that does not immediately refill is called pitting oedema. Normally, there is no oedema.*	▪ Oedema can be graded on a scale from 1+ to 4+ (Figure 28.26B):
	  ▪ 1+ (−2 mm depression)—No visible change in the leg; slight pitting
	  ▪ 2+ (−4 mm depression)—No marked change in the shape of the leg; pitting slightly deeper
	  ▪ 3+ (−6 mm depression)—Leg visibly swollen; pitting deep
	  ▪ 4+ (−8 mm depression)—Leg very swollen; pitting very deep
	▪ Oedema may be caused by disease of the cardiovascular system such as CHF; by renal, hepatic or lymphatic problems; or by infection.
	▪ Venous distension suggests venous insufficiency or incompetence.

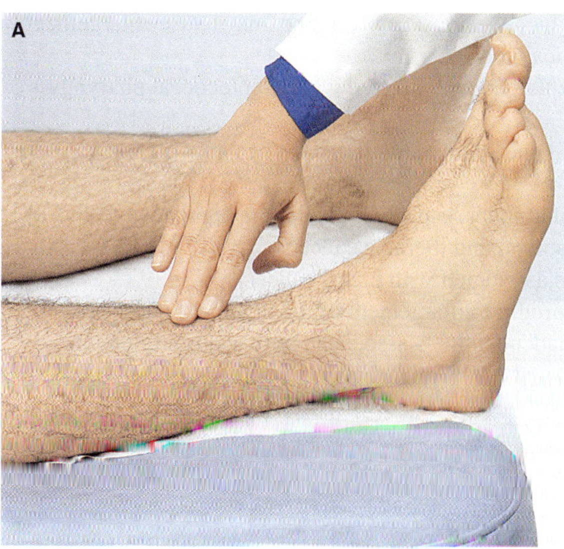

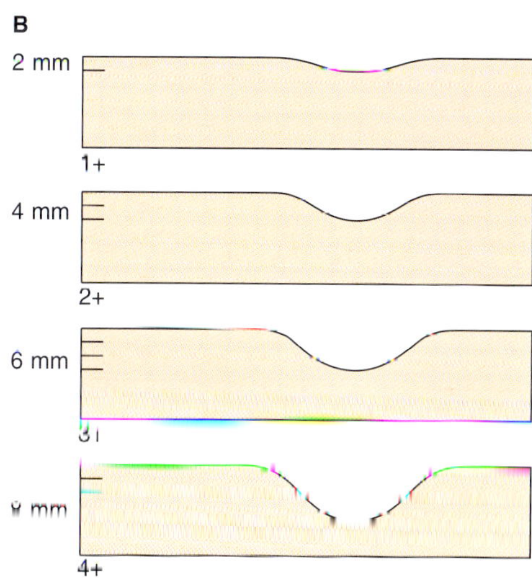

FIGURE 28.26 *Evaluation of oedema. A, Palpating for oedema over the tibia. B, Four-point scale for grading oedema*

(continued)

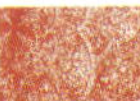

CARDIAC ASSESSMENTS (continued)

Technique/normal findings	Abnormal findings
Abdominal assessment	
Inspect and palpate the abdominal aorta. Note size, width and any visible pulsations or bulging. *Abdominal aorta should be of appropriate size without visible pulsations or bulging.*	■ A pulsating mass in the upper abdomen suggests an aortic aneurysm, particularly in the older adult. ■ An aorta greater than 2.5 to 3 cm in width reflects pathological dilation, secondary to chronic hypertension and/or arteriosclerosis.
Auscultate the epigastrium and each abdominal quadrant, using the bell of the stethoscope (see Figure 28.27). *No bruits should be heard over the abdominal aorta.*	■ Abdominal bruits reflect turbulent blood flow associated with partial arterial occlusion. ■ A bruit heard over the aorta suggests an aneurysm. ■ A bruit heard over the epigastrium and radiating laterally, especially with HTN, suggests renal artery stenosis. ■ Bruits heard in the lower abdominal quadrants suggest partial occlusion of the iliac arteries.
Lymph node assessment	
Palpate the regional lymph nodes of the head and neck, axillae, arms and groin. Use firm, circular movements of the finger pads and note size, shape, symmetry, consistency, delineation, mobility, tenderness, sensation and condition of overlying skin. *Nodes should not be enlarged or painful.*	■ **Lymphadenopathy** refers to the enlargement of lymph nodes (over 1 cm) with or without tenderness. It may be caused by inflammation, infection or malignancy of the nodes or the regions drained by the nodes. ■ Lymph node enlargement with tenderness suggests inflammation (*lymphadenitis*). With bacterial infection, the nodes may be warm and matted with localised swelling. ■ Malignant or metastatic nodes may be hard, indicating lymphoma; rubbery, indicating Hodgkin's disease; or fixed to adjacent structures. Usually they are not tender. ■ Ear infections and scalp and facial lesions, such as acne, may cause enlargement of the pre-auricular and cervical nodes. ■ Anterior cervical nodes are enlarged and infected with streptococcal pharyngitis and mononucleosis. ■ Lymphadenitis of the cervical and submandibular nodes occurs with herpes simplex lesions. ■ Enlargement of supraclavicular nodes, especially the left, is highly suggestive of metastatic disease from abdominal and thoracic cancer. ■ Axillary lymphadenopathy is associated with breast cancer. ■ Lesions of the genitals may produce enlargement of the inguinal nodes. ■ Persistent generalised lymphadenopathy is associated with acquired immune deficiency syndrome (AIDS) and AIDS-related complex.

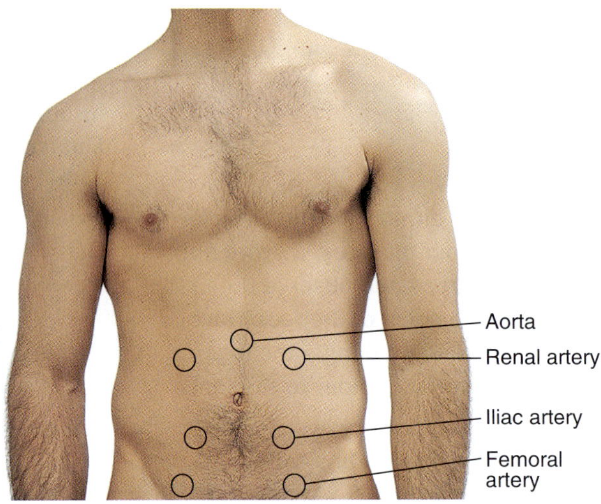

FIGURE 28.27 ***Auscultation sites of the abdominal aorta and its branches***

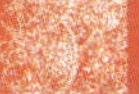

CARDIAC ASSESSMENTS (continued)

Technique/normal findings	Abnormal findings
Spleen assessment	
Palpate for the spleen, in the upper left quadrant of the abdomen. *The spleen is normally not palpable.*	■ A palpable spleen in the left upper abdominal quadrant of an adult may indicate abnormal enlargement (splenomegaly) and may be associated with cancer, blood dyscrasias and viral infection, such as mononucleosis.
Percuss for splenic dullness in the lowest left intercostal space (ICS) at the anterior axillary line or in the ninth to tenth ICS at the midaxillary line (see Figure 28.28). *Normally, tympany is heard.*	■ A dull percussion note in the lowest left ICS at the anterior axillary line or below the tenth rib at the midaxillary line suggests splenic enlargement.

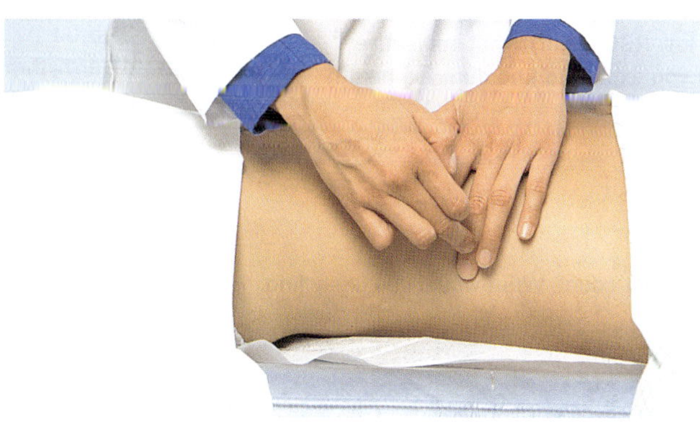

FIGURE 28.28 *Percussing the spleen*

TRANSLATION TO PRACTICE: A systematic review of assessment and management of preventive cardiovascular care in primary health for Aboriginal and Torres Strait Islander women and men

A gender gap in cardiovascular health exists between Aboriginal and Torres Strait Islander woman and men. Sixteen studies reporting gender-specific data were reviewed. Although these studies identified the existence of a health gap, the review was unable to find evidence of how to incorporate social and emotional wellbeing into cardiovascular care. There was also little identification of factors that may contribute to improved cardiovascular health (McBride et al., 2022).

IMPLICATIONS FOR NURSING

This article highlights a significant need for further research into the factors that contribute to the gender disparity in cardiovascular health within Aboriginal and Torres Strait Islander Australians.

CRITICAL THINKING IN PERSON-CENTRED CARE

1 What factors contribute to worse cardiovascular health outcomes for Aboriginal and Torres Strait Islander woman? How do these factors differ from those of Aboriginal and Torres Strait Islander men?
2 What research methods would elucidate the parameters contributing to this disparity? How does social and emotional wellbeing contribute to cardiovascular health?
3 What can nurses do to help identify and reduce the disparities for people requiring assistance to develop, maintain or improve cardiovascular health?

CONCEPT CHECK

1 The amount of blood pumped by the ventricles in 1 minute is known as:

1 heart rate
2 ventricular contraction
3 stroke volume
4 cardiac output

2 During what part of the cardiac cycle is the myocardium perfused?

1 prior to atrial filling
2 prior to ventricular relaxation
3 during diastole
4 during pulmonary perfusion

3 What physiological process is responsible for the electrical impulse that stimulates myocardial contraction?

1 action potential
2 cardiac reserve
3 cardiac potential
4 ventricular contraction

4 The intensity of chest pain may be assessed by asking which question?

1 'Did the pain move into your left arm?'
2 'Was your pain relieved by [illegible] busy?'
3 'On a scale of 0 (no pain) to 10 (worst pain), what number was your pain?'
4 'Was the pain a pressure, a burning or a tightness?'

5 At what anatomical location would you assess the apical impulse?
1 left midclavicular, fifth intercostal space
2 left substernal, sixth intercostal space
3 right midaxillary, second intercostal space
4 right nipple line, any intercostal space

6 A person's heart rate is 50. You would document this as:
1 tachycardia
2 bradycardia
3 hypertension
4 hypotension

7 A person has a very low RBC count. What subjective manifestation would you expect to find during a health history?
1 sore throat
2 chest pain
3 fatigue
4 nausea

8 A person has a low platelet count. What would you likely find on physical assessment?
1 enlarged lymph nodes
2 excessive bruising
3 varicose veins
4 changes in pulse pressure

9 An older person is severely dehydrated and, as a result, has increased blood viscosity. How will this affect the peripheral vascular resistance (PVR)?
1 increased PVR
2 decreased PVR
3 no change
4 depends on gender

10 When auscultating the abdominal aorta, you hear a murmuring or blowing sound. You would document this sound as a:
1 hypokinetic pulse
2 bigeminal pulse
3 bruit
4 arrhythmia

11 Swelling of a body part as a result of lymphatic obstruction is labelled:
1 lymphoedema
2 lymphadenopathy
3 atrophic change
4 central cyanosis

12 You are assessing a man who has severe leg pain. The leg is cool and cyanotic. You are unable to palpate a femoral pulse. What would be your priority intervention based on these assessments?
1 Document your findings.
2 Ask the family about this problem.
3 Teach the man relaxation techniques.
4 Notify the medical officer immediately.

BIBLIOGRAPHY

Australasian Society of Clinical Immunology and Allergy (2022). *Radiocontrast media hypersensitivity*. Retrieved from https://www.allergy.org.au/

Australian Commission on Safety and Quality in Health Care (ACSQHC) (2021). *National Safety and Quality Health Service Standards* (2nd ed.). Sydney: ACSQHC.

Bullock, S. & Hales, M. (2019). *Principles of pathophysiology* (2nd ed.). Sydney: Pearson.

Cardiac Society of Australia and New Zealand (CSANZ) (2017). *Coronary artery calcium scoring*. Position statement. Retrieved from http://www.csanz.edu.au/

Gupta, A., Bera, K., Kikano, E. et al. (2022). Coronary artery calcium scoring: Current status and future directions. *RadioGraphics*, *42*, 4. https://pubs.rsna.org/doi/epdf/10.1148/rg.210122

Harcharran, M. (2022). Assessment and examination of the cardiovascular system. *Practice Nursing*, *33*(3), 98–104. https://doi.org/10.12968/pnur.2022.33.3.98

Marieb, E. M. & Hoehn, K. (2019). *Human anatomy and physiology* (11th ed.). San Francisco: Pearson Benjamin Cummings.

McBride, K., Nguyen, J., Dowling, A. et al. (2022). A systematic review on assessment and management of preventive cardiovascular care in primary health for Aboriginal and Torres Strait Islander women and men. *Australian Journal of Primary Health*, *28*(3), 179–199. https://doi.org/10.1071/PY21219

Muir, W. W. & Hamlin, R. L. (2020). Myocardial contractility: Historical and contemporary considerations. *Frontiers in Physiology*, *11*, 222. https://doi.org/10.3389/fphys.2020.00222

National Vascular Disease Prevention Alliance (2012). *Guidelines for the management of absolute cardiovascular disease risk*. Retrieved from http://strokefoundation.com.au/

Prutkin, J. (2022). COVID-19: Arrhythmias and conduction system disease. *UpToDate*. Retrieved from https://www.uptodate.com/

Standring, S. & Gray, H. (2021). *Gray's anatomy: The anatomical basis of clinical practice* (42nd ed.). Philadelphia: Elsevier.

Wang, Y.-J., Sun, Y.-R., Pei, Y.-H., Ma, H.-W., Mu, Y.-K., Qin, L.-H. & Yan, J.-H. (2023). The lymphatic drainage systems in the brain: A novel target for ischemic stroke? *Neural Regeneration Research*, *18* (In press).

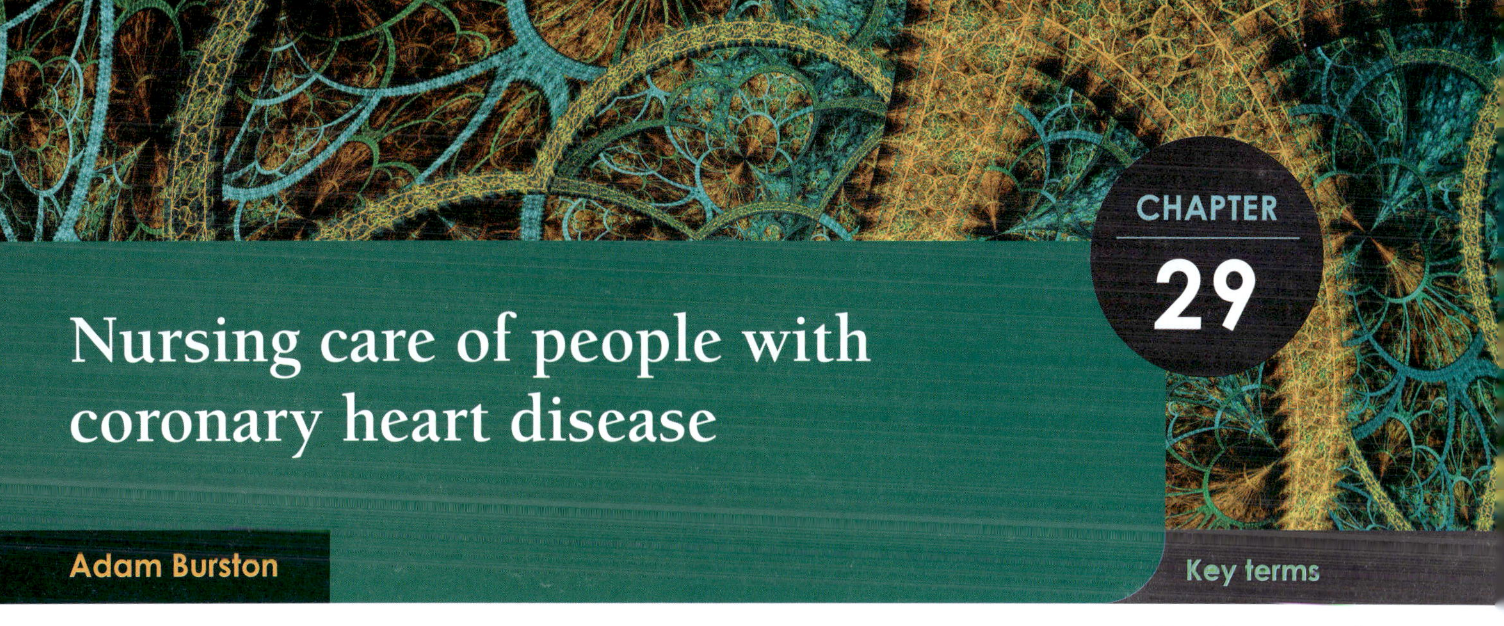

CHAPTER 29

Nursing care of people with coronary heart disease

Adam Burston

Key terms

acute coronary syndrome (ACS) 990
acute myocardial infarction (AMI) 998
angina pectoris 983
arrhythmia 1000
atherosclerosis 974
atrioventricular block 1012
cardiac arrest 1018
cardiac rehabilitation 1006
cardiovascular disease (CVD) 974
collateral vessels 974
coronary heart disease (CHD) 974
ectopic beats 1012
ischaemia 983
normal sinus rhythm (NSR) 1012
pacemaker 1023
sudden cardiac death (SCD) 1031

Learning outcomes

- Discuss how alterations to myocardial perfusion contribute to the development of a person's heart disease.
- Relate interprofessional care principles for a person with stable and unstable angina to the course and manifestations of the condition.
- Summarise the assessment and evaluation and then the course, management and outcomes when caring for a person with acute coronary syndrome.
- Compare and contrast the potential complications for a person experiencing an acute myocardial infarction.
- Differentiate between various cardiac arrhythmia in the context of influence on lifestyle and management principles.
- Discuss the interprofessional care and implications for a person following sudden cardiac death.

Clinical competencies

- Assess functional health status of the person with coronary heart disease and/or an arrhythmia, including the impact of the disorder on the person's ability to perform the activities of daily living.
- Apply knowledge of the normal anatomy and physiology of the heart to improve care of the person with coronary heart disease.
- Interpret assessment data, determine priorities of care and develop and implement individualised nursing interventions for the person with coronary heart disease and arrhythmias.
- Monitor the person with coronary heart disease or arrhythmias for expected and unexpected manifestations, reporting and recording findings as indicated.
- Administer medications and treatments to the person with coronary heart disease and arrhythmias safely and knowledgeably.
- Integrate interprofessional care into nursing care planning and implementation for the person with coronary heart disease and arrhythmias.
- Collaborate with the patient to discuss prevention, health promotion and self-care related to coronary heart disease and arrhythmias.
- Evaluate the effectiveness of nursing interventions, revising or modifying the plan of care as needed to promote, maintain or restore functional health for the person with coronary heart disease or arrhythmias.

Irrespective of the underlying cause, impaired cardiac function affects the person's ability to participate in exercise and activities of daily living. When the functioning of other systems becomes affected by problems such as impaired blood flow to the myocardium, changes in the conduction of electrical impulses through the heart or structural changes in the heart itself, it becomes unable to pump enough blood to meet the body's demand for oxygen and nutrients, and death may result.

Cardiovascular disease (CVD) is a generic term for disorders of the heart and blood vessels. CVD is the leading cause of death and disability in many developed countries and affects over 1.9 million Australians. In Australia, CVD kills one person every 12 minutes and represented 10% of all deaths in 2020. Nationally, approximately $5 billion is spent on CVD annually, representing 19.6% of the total allocated health expenditure (Australian Institute of Health and Welfare (AIHW), 2018). It is the leading cause of death for Indigenous Australians (AIHW, 2022a).

Coronary heart disease (CHD) refers more specifically to an ischaemic pathology related to disease of the blood vessels, causing myocardial oxygenation issues. Angina and myocardial infarction are the two main clinical forms of this disease. Cardiovascular disease carries one of the highest burdens of disease at 13%, but through increased funding, research and public education campaigns, deaths from CHD have reduced by 63% since 2003 (AIHW, 2018). Although obesity is still a major concern, education involving the reduction of fat intake, increasing exercise and lowering cholesterol levels has made Australians more aware of risk factors associated with CHD.

This chapter focuses on disorders of myocardial blood flow (coronary heart disease) and cardiac rhythm. Disorders of cardiac structure and function are discussed in the chapter 'Nursing care of people with cardiac disorders'. Review the normal anatomy and physiology and nursing assessment of the heart in the chapter 'A person-centred approach to assessing the cardiovascular and lymphatic systems' before proceeding with this chapter.

FAST FACTS

- Coronary heart disease accounted for approximately 16,600 deaths in Australia in 2022.
- One in 9 adult Australians aged 75 and over has CHD.
- Aboriginal and Torres Strait Islander people are twice as likely as non-Indigenous Australians to experience CHD (AIHW, 2022a).

Disorders of myocardial perfusion

THE PERSON WITH CORONARY HEART DISEASE

Coronary heart disease or *coronary artery disease (CAD)* is caused by impaired blood flow to the myocardium. Accumulation of atherosclerotic plaque in the coronary arteries is the usual cause. Coronary heart disease may be asymptomatic or may lead to angina pectoris, acute coronary syndrome, myocardial infarction (MI), arrhythmias, heart failure and even sudden death.

Incidence and prevalence

Many risk factors for CHD can be controlled through lifestyle modification. In fact, with increased public awareness of risk factors related to CHD, mortality rates have declined by over 80% since the 1980. Nevertheless, CHD remains a major public health problem. Nurses are in a prime position to encourage and support positive lifestyle changes by teaching and promoting healthy living practices.

Both men and women are affected by CHD; however, in women the onset is about 10 years later because of the heart-protective effects of oestrogen. After menopause, women's risk is equal to that of men.

Physiology review

The two main coronary arteries, the left and the right, supply blood, oxygen and nutrients to the myocardium. They originate in the root of the aorta, just outside the aortic valve. The *left main coronary artery* divides to form the anterior descending and circumflex arteries. The *anterior descending* artery supplies the anterior interventricular septum and the left ventricle, including the apex of the heart. The *circumflex* branch supplies the lateral wall of the left ventricle. The *right coronary artery* supplies the right ventricle and forms the *posterior descending artery*. The posterior descending artery supplies the posterior portion of the heart (see Figure 28.7).

Blood flow through the coronary arteries is regulated by several factors, the primary one being aortic pressure. Other factors include the heart rate (most flow occurs during diastole, when the muscle is relaxed), metabolic activity of the heart, blood vessel tone (constriction) and collateral circulation. Although there are no connections between the large coronary arteries, small arteries are joined by **collateral vessels**. If large vessels are gradually occluded, the collateral vessels enlarge, providing alternative routes for blood flow.

Pathophysiology

Coronary atherosclerosis is the most common cause of reduced coronary blood flow.

Atherosclerosis

Atherosclerosis is a progressive disease characterised by *atheroma* (plaque) formation, which affects the intimal and medial layers of large and midsize arteries. See 'Pathophysiology illustrated: coronary heart disease'.

Atherosclerosis is initiated by unknown precipitating factors that cause lipoproteins and fibrous tissue to accumulate in the arterial wall. Although the precise mechanisms are unknown, endothelial dysfunction, abnormal lipid metabolism and injury to or inflammation of endothelial cells lining the artery appear to be key to its development.

Endothelial dysfunction is mediated by various factors including endothelial tone and vascular remodelling. An imbalance of endothelial-derived relaxing factors (EDRFs) and endothelial-derived constricting factors (EDCFs) results in augmented constriction intake (Peyter et al., 2021). This continued workload results in arterial hypertrophy within the media and perpetuates local hypertension, increasing shear stress and contributing to further endothelial damage and remodelling.

In the bloodstream, lipids are transported attached to proteins called apoproteins. High levels of certain *lipoproteins*, a type of apoprotein, increase the risk of atherosclerosis. *Low-density lipoproteins*, which are high in cholesterol, carry cholesterol to peripheral tissues where some of it is released to be taken up and incorporated into cells for use in producing energy. *Very-low-density lipoproteins*, large molecules primarily composed of triglycerides and cholesterol, carry triglycerides to muscle and fat cells. When the triglycerides are released into these tissues, the remainder of the molecule is a low-density lipoprotein. *High-density lipoproteins*, in contrast, attract cholesterol, returning it from peripheral tissues to the liver (Bullock & Hales, 2019).

Hyperlipidaemia itself may damage arterial endothelium. Endothelial damage promotes platelet adhesion and aggregation and attracts leucocytes to the area. At the site of injury, *atherogenic* (atherosclerosis-promoting) lipoproteins collect in the intimal lining of the artery. These lipoproteins appear to actually bind with the extracellular portion of the vessel endothelium. Macrophages migrate to the injured site as part of the inflammatory process. Contact with platelets, cholesterol and other blood components stimulates smooth muscle cells and connective tissue within the vessel wall to proliferate abnormally. Although blood flow is not affected at this stage, this early lesion appears as a yellowish fatty streak on the inner lining of the artery. Fibrous plaque develops as smooth muscle cells enlarge, collagen fibres proliferate and blood lipids accumulate. The lesion protrudes into the arterial lumen and is fixed to the inner wall of the intima. It may invade the muscular media layer of the vessel as well. The developing plaque not only gradually occludes the vessel lumen but also impairs the vessel's ability to dilate in response to increased oxygen demands. Fibrous plaque lesions often develop at arterial bifurcations or curves or in areas of narrowing. As the plaque expands, it can produce severe stenosis or total occlusion of the artery.

The final stage of the process is the development of *atheromas*, complex lesions consisting of lipids, fibrous tissue, collagen, calcium, cellular debris and capillaries. These calcified lesions can ulcerate or rupture, stimulating thrombosis. The vessel lumen may be rapidly occluded by the thrombus or it may embolise to occlude a distal vessel.

Plaque formation may be *eccentric*, located in a specific, asymmetric region of the vessel wall, or *concentric*, involving the entire vessel circumference. Manifestations of the process usually do not appear until about 75% of the arterial lumen has been occluded.

Atherosclerosis tends to develop where arteries bifurcate or branch, which encourages atheroma-prone conditions such as high shear forces, less ordered endothelial cell alignment and inferior shear-resistant endothelial cell morphology, ultimately promoting a pro-inflammatory microenvironment (Perrotta, 2022). Certain vessels have a higher likelihood of being affected, including the coronary arteries (the left anterior descending artery, in particular), the renal arteries, the bifurcation of the carotid arteries and branching sections of peripheral arteries. In addition to obstructing or occluding blood flow, atherosclerosis weakens arterial walls and is a major cause of aneurysm in vessels such as the aorta and iliac arteries.

Myocardial ischaemia

Myocardial cells become ischaemic when the oxygen *supply* is inadequate to meet metabolic *demands*. The critical factors in meeting the metabolic demand of cardiac cells are coronary perfusion and myocardial workload. Coronary perfusion can be affected by several different mechanisms:

- One or more vessels may be partially occluded by large, stable areas of plaque.
- Platelets can aggregate in narrowed vessels, forming a thrombus.
- Normal or already narrowed vessels may spasm.
- A drop in blood pressure may lead to inadequate flow through coronary vessels.
- Normal autoregulatory mechanisms that increase flow to working muscles may fail.

Workload is affected by the heart rate, myocardial contractility, preload (the amount of blood in the ventricles just prior to systole) and afterload (the peripheral pressure that must be overcome to move blood out of the heart into the circulation). The oxygen content of the blood and haematocrit are contributing factors to myocardial ischaemia. Table 29.1 lists factors that may lead to myocardial ischaemia.

TABLE 29.1 Factors contributing to myocardial ischaemia

CORONARY PERFUSION	MYOCARDIAL WORKLOAD	BLOOD OXYGEN CONTENT
• Atherosclerosis • Thrombosis • Vasospasm • Inadequate perfusion pressure	• Rapid heart rate • Increased preload, afterload or contractility • Increased metabolic demands (e.g. hyperthyroidism)	• Reduced atmospheric oxygen pressure • Impaired gas exchange • Low red blood cells and haemoglobin content

Coronary heart disease

Coronary heart disease usually is due to *athero-sclerosis*, occlusion of the coronary arteries by fibrous, fatty plaque. Coronary heart disease is manifested by *angina pectoris, acute coronary syndrome* and/or *myocardial infarction*. Risk factors for coronary heart disease include age (over 50 years), heredity, smoking, obesity, high serum cholesterol levels, hypertension and diabetes mellitus. Other factors, such as diet and lack of exercise, also contribute to the risk of CHD.

Atherosclerosis

In atherosclerosis, lipids accumulate in the intimal layer of arteries. Fibroblasts in the area respond by producing collagen, and smooth muscle cells proliferate, together forming a complex lesion called plaque. Plaque consists mostly of cholesterol, triglycerides, phospholipids, collagen and smooth muscle cells.

Plaque reduces the size of the lumen of the affected artery, impairing blood flow. In addition, plaque may ulcerate, causing a thrombus to form that may completely occlude the vessel.

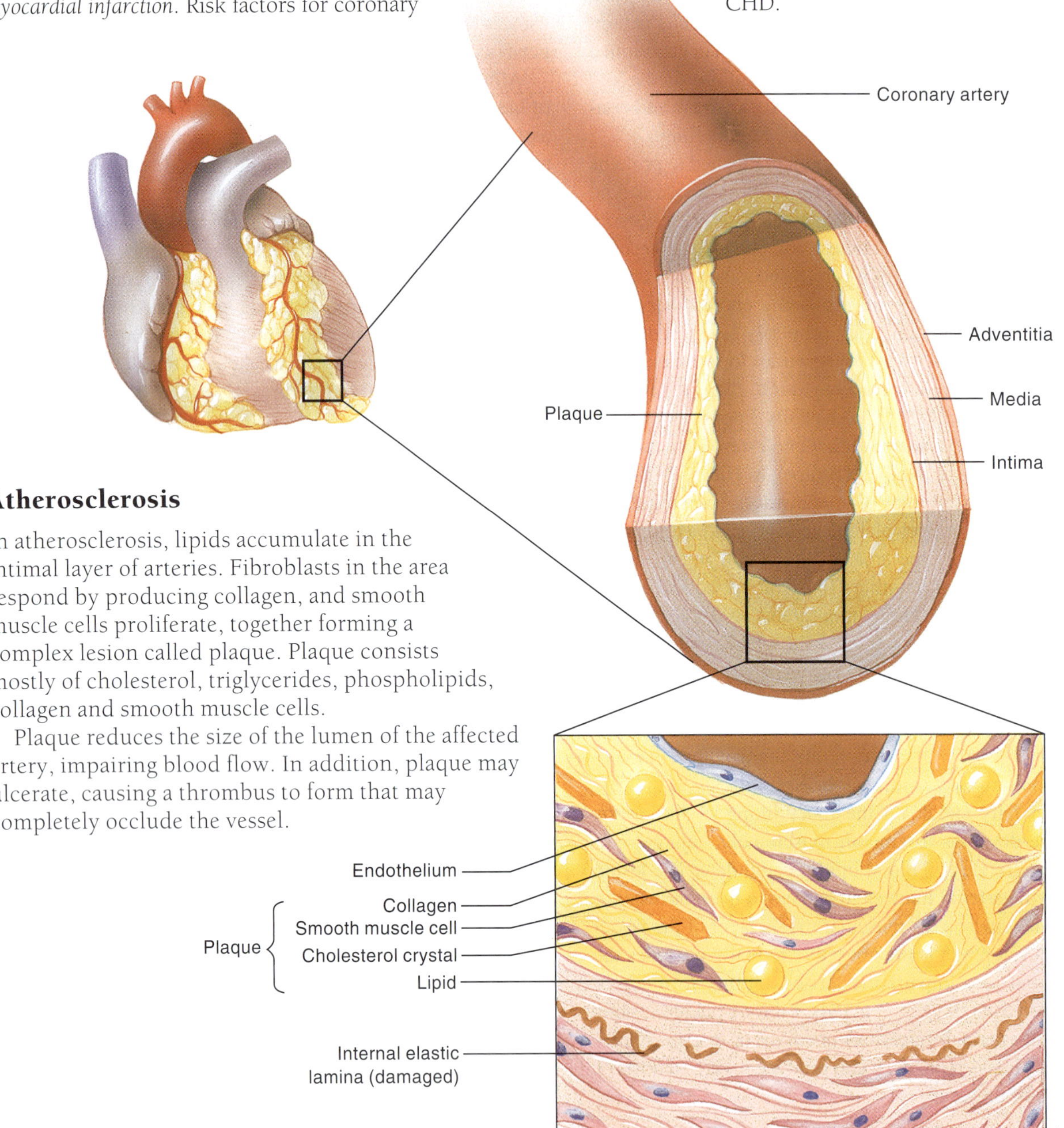

Angina pectoris

Angina is characterised by episodes of chest pain, usually precipitated by exercise and relieved by rest. When myocardial oxygen needs are greater than partially occluded vessels can supply, myocardial cells become ischaemic and shift to anaerobic metabolism. Anaerobic metabolism produces lactic acid that stimulates nerve endings in the muscle, causing pain. The pain subsides when the oxygen supply again meets myocardial demand.

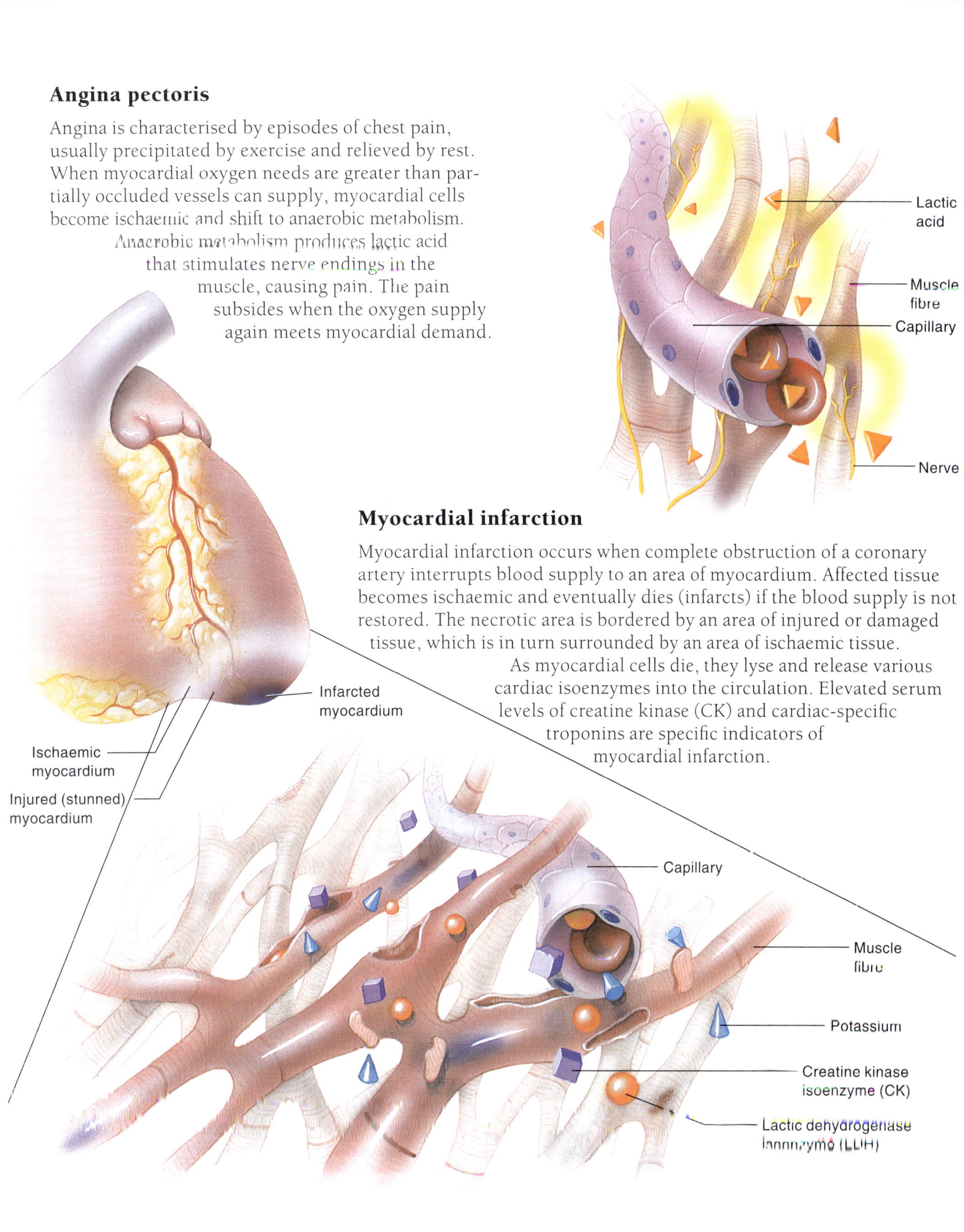

Myocardial infarction

Myocardial infarction occurs when complete obstruction of a coronary artery interrupts blood supply to an area of myocardium. Affected tissue becomes ischaemic and eventually dies (infarcts) if the blood supply is not restored. The necrotic area is bordered by an area of injured or damaged tissue, which is in turn surrounded by an area of ischaemic tissue.

As myocardial cells die, they lyse and release various cardiac isoenzymes into the circulation. Elevated serum levels of creatine kinase (CK) and cardiac-specific troponins are specific indicators of myocardial infarction.

Myocardial cells have limited supplies of adenosine triphosphate (ATP) for energy storage. When myocardial workload increases or the supply of blood and oxygen falls, cellular ATP stores are quickly depleted, affecting their contractility. Cellular metabolism switches from an efficient aerobic process to anaerobic metabolism. Lactic acid accumulates and cells are damaged. If blood flow is restored within 20 minutes, aerobic metabolism and contractility are restored and cellular repair begins (Bullock & Hales, 2019). Continued ischaemia results in cell necrosis and death (infarction).

Coronary heart disease is generally divided into two categories: chronic ischaemic heart disease and acute coronary syndromes. *Chronic ischaemic heart disease* includes stable and unstable angina pectoris and silent myocardial ischaemia. In women, angina is the most common presenting symptom of CHD. *Acute coronary syndromes* range from unstable angina to myocardial infarction (Coven, 2020). Acute coronary syndromes and myocardial infarction are the most common manifestations of CHD in men. These disorders are discussed in the following sections of this chapter.

Risk factors

The causes of atherosclerosis are not known, but certain risk factors have been linked with the development of atherosclerotic plaques. The seminal Framingham Heart Study (FHS) provided vital research into the relationship between risk factors and the development of heart disease (see the 'Translation to practice' box). Research into CHD is ongoing, looking at causative factors, manifestations and protective measures for many populations. Risk factors for CHD are frequently classified as *non-modifiable*, factors that cannot be changed, and *modifiable*, those factors that can be changed (see Table 29.2).

Non-modifiable risk factors

Age is a non-modifiable risk factor. In Australia, approximately 6.7% of all male deaths and 2.7% of all female deaths attributable to CHD occur in individuals under 55. Although showing signs of decreasing from preceding years, just over 1 in 4 Australians over the age of 75 had heart disease in 2017–2018, with men evidencing higher rates (31.5%) than women (20.4%) (Australian Bureau of Statistics (ABS), 2018). *Genetic factors* and *gender* also are non-modifiable risk factors for CHD. A family history of CHD is considered a significant risk factor of the development of coronary artery disease. Men are affected by CHD at an earlier age than women, yet women are still at risk of CHD, despite the perception otherwise. Discordance in CHD risk perception continues to exist (Beussink-Nelson et al., 2022). It is clear that there is still a need to improve CHD information campaigns, encompassing factors such as risk, prevention and identification.

Modifiable risk factors

Modifiable risk factors include lifestyle factors and pathological conditions that predispose the person to developing CHD. Disease conditions that contribute to CHD include hypertension, diabetes mellitus and hyperlipidaemia. Although these conditions are not a matter of choice, they are modifiable risk factors that can often be controlled through medication, weight control, diet and exercise.

Behavioural or lifestyle factors can be controlled or completely eliminated if appropriate supports are available. Lifestyle changes require significant commitment by the person; ongoing support from the healthcare team is vital for success.

TRANSLATION TO PRACTICE Evidence-based practice: Framingham Heart Study

The Framingham Heart Study (FHS) is an ongoing, significant clinical research study that has provided data about cardiovascular disease for over 60 years. The study was initiated in 1948 with an original study group of 5,209 participants in the town of Framingham, Massachusetts, in the United States (Framingham Heart Study (FHS), 2022). Every 2 years, this original group is evaluated for cardiovascular 'events' via their medical history, physical findings and diagnostic testing. Children and grandchildren of the original group have also been studied as part of the Framingham Offspring Study. It was in reports of the Framingham study that the term 'risk factor' first appeared.

IMPLICATIONS FOR NURSING

Data collected from the Framingham Heart Study and the Framingham Offspring Study provide a rich database from which to develop evidence-based approaches for people with heart disease. A major application of these research findings to practice is in primary preventive education—for example, through community cardiovascular health programs. Although research shows that increased public awareness of cardiovascular risk factors has lowered morbidity and mortality from heart disease, it remains a leading cause of premature death in Australia. For cardiovascular disease to be reduced on a large scale, education about the effects of lifestyle on the cardiovascular system must begin in the early school years and be reinforced throughout the formative years where healthy choices can become habit.

A second application of these findings is in interprofessional management. Nurses should keep up to date on the latest strategies for medical treatment so that they can provide accurate rationales to individuals and formulate effective nursing care plans that complement medical management strategies. The result is better communication, a sense of collegiality and teamwork, and positive health outcomes.

CRITICAL THINKING IN PERSON-CENTRED CARE

1 What kinds of strategies can be used in primary school settings to teach cardiovascular health in a fun, informative manner?
2 Which healthcare providers should be included in a multidisciplinary effort to encourage individuals to modify their lifestyles?
3 What are some of the structural barriers to effective and sustained lifestyle changes?

TABLE 29.2 Risk factors for coronary heart disease

NON-MODIFIABLE	MODIFIABLE	PATHOPHYSIOLOGICAL
Age	Cigarette smoking	Hyperlipidaemia
Men ≥ 45 years	Obesity	Elevated LDL cholesterol
Women ≥ 55 years	Sedentary behaviour	Elevated triglycerides
Gender	Insufficient fruit and vegetable intake	Low HDL cholesterol
Heredity	Excessive alcohol intake	Hypertension
	Women only: use of oral contraceptives, hormone replacement therapy	Diabetes mellitus
		Kidney disease
		Women only: premature menopause
		Emerging risk factors:
		Elevated homocysteine levels
		Thrombogenic factors
		Inflammatory factors
		Impaired fasting glucose

HYPERTENSION *Hypertension* is a condition associated with consistent blood pressure readings greater than 140 mmHg systolic or 90 mmHg diastolic. Hypertension affects approximately 31% of Australians, with Indigenous Australians experiencing higher rates of hypertension than non-Indigenous Australians. Aboriginal and Torres Strait Islander people develop hypertension earlier (AIHW, 2022b). Hypertension damages arterial endothelium, and inflammatory responses stimulate the development of atherosclerotic plaque. Individuals can reduce hypertension through lifestyle changes and appropriate support.

TABLE 29.3 Serum cholesterol and triglyceride targets

Total cholesterol	< 4 mmol/L
High-density lipoprotein cholesterol (HDL-C)	≥ 1 mmol/L
Low-density lipoprotein cholesterol (LDL-C)	< 2 mmol/L
Non-high-density lipoprotein cholesterol (non-HDL-C)	< 2.5 mmol/L
Triglycerides (TG)	< 2 mmol/L

Source: Royal Australian College of General Practitioners (RACGP) (2022a). *Prevention of vascular and metabolic disease: Cholesterol and other lipids*. Retrieved from https://www.racgp.org.au/.

DIABETES *Diabetes mellitus* contributes to CHD in several ways. Diabetes is associated with several risk factors, including hyperlipidaemia, a higher incidence of hypertension and obesity. In addition, diabetes affects vascular endothelium, which contributes to the development of atherosclerosis. Hyperglycaemia and hyperinsulinaemia, altered platelet function, elevated fibrinogen levels and inflammation also are thought to play a role in the development of atherosclerosis in people with diabetes.

ABNORMAL BLOOD LIPIDS *Hyperlipidaemia* is an abnormally high level of blood lipids and lipoproteins. Lipoproteins carry cholesterol in the blood. Low-density lipoproteins (LDLs) are the primary carriers of cholesterol. High levels of LDL promote atherosclerosis because LDLs deposit cholesterol on artery walls. By contrast, high density lipoproteins (HDLs) help clear cholesterol from the arteries by transporting it to the liver for excretion. HDL levels above 0.4 mmol/L have a protective effect, reducing the risk of CHD; by contrast, HDL levels lower than 0.4 mmol/L are associated with an increased risk of CHD. Triglycerides are compounds of fatty acids bound to glycerol. They are used for fat storage by the body and are carried on very low density lipoprotein (VLDL) molecules. Elevated triglycerides also contribute to the risk of CHD. Table 29.3 lists the aims for lipid lowering therapy as recommended by National Vascular Disease Prevention Alliance.

TOBACCO USE *Tobacco use*, in particular smoking, is an independent risk factor for CHD. The effects of nicotine and other toxins from cigarette smoke negatively affect the cardiovascular system. Individuals who smoke are significantly more at risk of developing CHD than non-smokers (Khan et al., 2021). Research suggests that stopping smoking by the age of 45 removes almost all mortality risks associated with smoking (Greenhalgh, Stillman & Ford, 2020). Cigarette smoking promotes CHD in several ways. The carbon monoxide damages vascular endothelium, promoting cholesterol deposition, and nicotine stimulates catecholamine release and increases blood pressure, heart rate and myocardial oxygen demand. Nicotine also causes arterial vasoconstriction, which reduces tissue perfusion. In addition, nicotine reduces HDL levels, increases platelet aggregation and increases the risk of thrombus formation.

FAST FACT

Cigarette smoking is the leading independent risk factor for coronary heart disease and is a primary target of risk factor management.

OBESITY *Obesity* (excess adipose tissue) is generally defined as a body mass index (BMI) of 30 kg/m^2 or greater. Obese people have higher rates of hypertension, diabetes and hyperlipidaemia. In the Framingham Study (FHS, 2022), obese men over age 50 had twice the incidence of CHD and acute myocardial infarction (MI) of those who were within 10% of their ideal weight. Central obesity, or intra-abdominal fat, is associated with an increased risk of CHD. The best indicator of central obesity is the waist circumference. A waist-to-hip ratio of greater than 0.8 (women) or 0.9 (men) increases the risk of CHD.

PHYSICAL INACTIVITY *Physical inactivity* is associated with a higher risk of CHD. Research data indicate that people who maintain a regular program of physical activity are less prone to developing CHD than sedentary people. Cardiovascular benefits of exercise include increased availability of oxygen to the heart muscle, decreased oxygen demand and cardiac workload, and increased myocardial function and electrical stability. Other positive effects of regular physical activity include decreased blood pressure and blood lipids, and a decrease in insulin resistance, platelet aggregation and weight (van Trier et al., 2022).

DIET Diet is a risk factor for CHD, independent of fat and cholesterol intake. Diets high in fruits, vegetables, whole grains and unsaturated fatty acids appear to have a protective effect. The underlying factors are not clear, but probably relate to nutrients such as antioxidants, folic acid, other B vitamins, omega-3 fatty acids and other unidentified micronutrients (Zhu et al., 2022).

Emerging risk factors

The link between *elevated serum homocysteine levels*, *deficiencies in folic acid* and *deficiencies in vitamins such as* B_6 and B_{12} and CHD is long established (Bajac et al., 2022). Up until menopause, women have lower homocysteine levels than men, which may partially explain their lower risk of CHD. Increased homocysteine levels negatively correlate with serum folate and dietary folate intake. Increasing folate intake can reduce homocysteine levels. However, currently, studies do not show benefits of folic acid supplementation. As an alternative, a balanced diet including two serves of fruit and five serves of vegetables a day is recommended to provide adequate vitamin and nutrient supply.

Based on evidence that aspirin and antiplatelet therapies reduce the risk of MI, *clot-promoting factors* are identified as CHD risk factors. *Inflammation* has also recently been identified as a risk factor. Inflammatory processes may increase the development of atherosclerotic plaque (Bullock & Hales, 2019). Inflammation also promotes clot formation at the site of ruptured plaque.

Metabolic syndrome

Metabolic syndrome, a group of metabolic risk factors occurring in an individual, is a strong risk factor for CHD (see Box 29.1). Metabolic syndrome has emerged as a risk factor for premature CHD that is equal to cigarette smoking. Three underlying causes of metabolic syndrome have been identified: overweight/obesity, physical inactivity and genetic factors. It is closely associated with *insulin resistance*, where tissue responds poorly to insulin signalling. Both genetic and acquired factors play a role in insulin resistance, including the presence of abdominal obesity, physical inactivity, and dietary and lifestyle choices.

BOX 29.1 Characteristics of the metabolic syndrome

- Abdominal obesity
- Abnormal blood lipids (low HDL, high triglycerides)
- Hypertension
- Elevated fasting blood glucose
- Clotting tendency
- Inflammatory factors

Risk factors unique to women

Risk factors unique to women include *premature menopause*, *oral contraceptive use* and *hormone replacement therapy (HRT)*. At menopause, serum HDL levels drop and LDL levels rise, increasing the risk of CHD (see the 'Translation to practice' box). Early menopause (natural or surgically induced) increases the risk of CHD and MI. Women who have undergone bilateral oophorectomy before age 35 without hormone replacement are eight times more likely than women experiencing natural menopause to have an MI. Oestrogen replacement therapy reduces the risk of CHD and MI in these women. Oral contraceptives with unopposed oestrogen (oestrogen without progestogen), by contrast, increase the risk of MI, particularly in women who also smoke. This increased risk is due to the tendency of oral contraceptives to promote clotting and their effects on blood pressure, serum lipids and glucose tolerance (Momeni et al., 2020).

FAST FACTS

- Risk factors for coronary heart disease are those factors that promote atherosclerosis and plaque development.
- Angina pectoris, acute coronary syndromes and myocardial infarction are the manifestations of myocardial ischaemia and coronary heart disease due to atherosclerosis.
- Atherosclerosis also is the primary underlying cause of stroke and peripheral vascular disease; therefore, the risk factors for atherosclerosis are also the risk factors for coronary heart disease, including angina, acute coronary syndromes and myocardial infarction.

Risk factors unique to Indigenous Australians

Some significant cardiovascular risk factors include obesity, diabetes, smoking, inactivity and chronic kidney disease. Indigenous Australians experience CVD-related risk factors more than non-Indigenous Australians. Prevalence of type 2 diabetes is three times greater and chronic kidney disease is two times greater in Indigenous Australians than in non-Indigenous Australian populations (AIHW, 2022b). There are stark demographic differences between Indigenous and non-Indigenous Australians (see Table 29.4 and the 'Focus on cultural diversity' box).

TRANSLATION TO PRACTICE Evidence-based practice: underrepresentation of women in cardiovascular trials

It has long been thought that women are poorly represented in cardiovascular research. A review by Tobb, Kocher & Bullock-Palmer (2022) considered the magnitude of disparity, the possible causes and potential solutions to address the situation.

IMPLICATIONS FOR NURSING

Nurses are informed by research. If current research practices regarding cardiovascular issues are not equally inclusive of women, incorrect assumptions can be made about results when extrapolation of data collected is erroneously applied. This action may result in nurses misinterpreting clinical observations, developing flawed care plans or undertaking inappropriate clinical interventions. Nurses should understand limitations of knowledge stemming from cardiovascular research biasing male participation.

CRITICAL THINKING IN PERSON-CENTRED CARE

1 Why might women be less inclined or willing to participate in cardiovascular research?
2 How do presentation, imaging and pathophysiology of cardiovascular disease differ in women?
3 What role can a nurse play in influencing change in promoting a more equitable representation of women in cardiovascular research?

TABLE 29.4 Comparison of demographic characteristics between Indigenous and non-Indigenous Australians

	INDIGENOUS AUSTRALIANS	NON-INDIGENOUS AUSTRALIANS
Percentage of population	3.3%	74.9%
Current smokers–% of population (15 years and above)	43%	14%
Median age	24 years old	38 years old
Life expectancy (years)	Male–71.6, Female–80.2	Male–75.6, Female–83.4
Obesity	1.6 times higher	
Hypertension	1.6 times higher	
Diabetes	2.7 times higher	
CVD-related deaths	23%	11%

Sources: Adapted from data from ABS (2022a). *Aboriginal and Torres Strait Islander people: Census*. Retrieved from https://www.abs.gov.au/; ABS (2022b). *Regional population by age and sex*. Retrieved from https://www.abs.gov.au/; AIHW (2017). *Aboriginal and Torres Strait Islander Health Performance Framework*. Retrieved from https://www.aihw.gov.au/.

FOCUS ON CULTURAL DIVERSITY Cardiovascular disease risk factors

Cardiovascular mortality in Aboriginal and Torres Strait Islander people has reduced to 1.5 times that of non-Indigenous Australians and constitutes a significant health burden on Indigenous Australians. Myocardial infarctions account for almost 56% of cardiovascular-related deaths in males and almost 50% of cardiovascular-related deaths in females. All cardiovascular-disease-associated risk factors are higher for Aboriginal and Torres Strait Islander Australians than they are for non-Indigenous Australians (AIHW, 2022b).

Ethnicity has a strong role in the development of cardiovascular disease. People from some countries experience fewer risk factors by virtue of their diet and genetics.

Implications for nursing

Australia is a multicultural country and an understanding of how ethnicity and structural discrimination may increase or decrease an individual's risk factors for coronary artery disease is important in not only the assessment of an individual presenting with symptoms of cardiovascular dysfunction, providing holistic care and administering medications, but also in individualised planning of education sessions.

Critical thinking in person-centred care

1 It is well established that an individual's diet will influence cardiovascular risk factors. Choose four different ethnicities commonly found in Australia. Research a typical diet of these four different groups.
2 Of the four ethnic groups that you have chosen, predict how the diets might influence cardiovascular risk factors. Pay particular attention to fat, cholesterol and triglycerides.
3 Genetics can have an influence on the pharmacology of antihyperlipidaemic agents. Research the influence of genetics/ethnicity on lipid lowering medications. Relate this to the answers you have given for question 2.

PATIENT SAFETY COMPETENCY FRAMEWORK

6 Evidence-based practice

The Patient Safety Competency Framework indicates that nursing students must appropriately utilise evidence-based practice by including patient values and preferences as valid evidence sources and explaining how evidence-based practice influences the choice of interventions in the provision of effective cardiac care (Levett-Jones et al., 2017).

INTERPROFESSIONAL CARE

Care of people with coronary heart disease focuses on aggressive risk factor management to slow the atherosclerotic process and maintain myocardial perfusion. Until manifestations of chronic or acute ischaemia are experienced, the diagnosis often is presumptive, based on history and the presence of risk factors.

Diagnosis

Laboratory testing is used to assess for risk factors such as an abnormal blood lipid profile (elevated triglyceride and LDL levels and decreased HDL levels).

- *Total serum cholesterol* is elevated in hyperlipidaemia. A *lipid profile* includes triglyceride (TG), HDL and LDL levels. Calculations are made of the ratio of HDL to total cholesterol. The ratio should be at least 1:5, with 1:3 being the ideal ratio. Elevated lipid levels are associated with an increased risk of atherosclerosis. In people with a strong family history of premature CHD or familial hypercholesterolaemia, *lipoprotein (a)* (Lp(a)) may also be measured. Elevated levels of Lp(a) may independently increase the risk of CHD. Other subsets of blood lipids may also be measured in selected individuals. See the 'Diagnostic tests' boxes in the chapter 'A person-centred approach to assessing the cardiovascular and lymphatic systems' for nursing care related to lipid profile studies.

Diagnostic tests to identify subclinical (asymptomatic) CHD may be indicated when multiple risk factors are present.

- *C-reactive protein* is a serum protein associated with inflammatory processes. Recent evidence suggests that elevated blood levels of this protein may be predictive of CHD.
- *The ankle–brachial blood pressure index (ABI)* is an inexpensive, non-invasive test for peripheral vascular disease that may be predictive of CHD. The systolic blood pressure in the brachial, posterior tibial and dorsalis pedis arteries is measured by Doppler. An ABI of < 0.9 in either leg indicates the presence of peripheral arterial disease and a significant risk of CHD.
- *Exercise ECG testing* may be performed. ECGs are used to assess the response to increased cardiac workload induced by exercise. The test is considered 'positive' for CHD if myocardial ischaemia is detected on the ECG (depression of the ST segment by greater than 3 mm) (see Figure 29.1), the person develops chest pain or the test is stopped due to excess fatigue, arrhythmias or other symptoms before the predicted maximal heart rate is achieved.
- *Electron beam computed tomography (EBCT)* creates a three-dimensional image of the heart and coronary arteries that can reveal plaque and other abnormalities. This non-invasive test requires no special preparation and can identify individuals at risk of developing myocardial ischaemia.
- *Myocardial perfusion imaging* (scintigraphy), see the section on angina that follows, may be used to evaluate myocardial blood flow and perfusion, both at rest and during stress testing (exercise or mental stress). These diagnostic tests are further explained the chapter 'A person-centred approach to assessing the cardiovascular and lymphatic systems' and the section on angina. Perfusion imaging studies are costly and therefore are not recommended for routine CHD risk assessment.

Risk factor management

Conservative management of CHD focuses on risk factor modification, including smoking, diet, exercise and management of contributing conditions.

SMOKING Individuals who smoke are 6.6 times more likely to develop atherosclerosis, 5.9 times more likely to develop an aortic aneurysm and dissection and are up to five times more at risk of dying from coronary artery disease than non-smokers (Briffa et al., 2021). Smoking cessation reduces the risk of CHD within months after quitting and improves cardiovascular status (RACGP, 2022b). In addition, stopping smoking improves HDL levels, lowers LDL levels and reduces blood viscosity. All smokers are advised to quit. Health promotion activities focus on preventing children, teenagers and adults

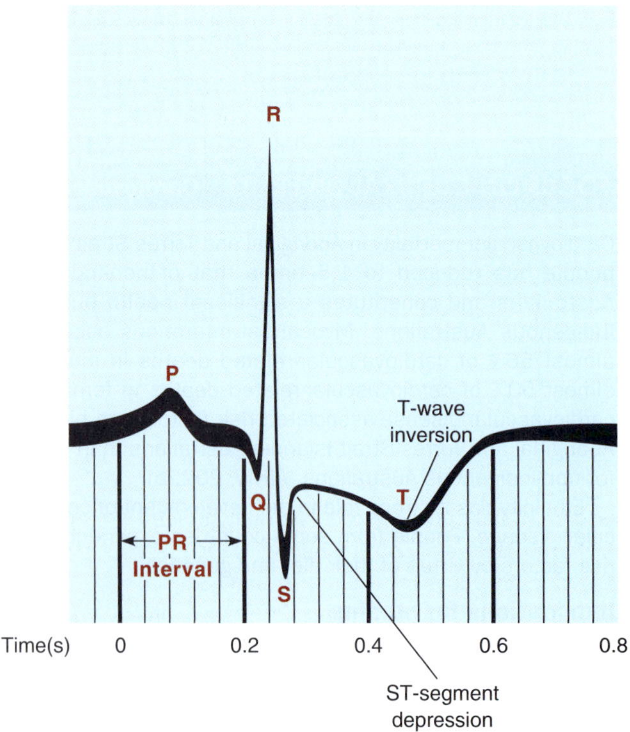

FIGURE 29.1 ***ECG changes during an episode of angina. Note characteristic T-wave inversion and ST-segment depression of myocardial ischaemia***

from starting to smoke. Specific attention should also be paid to pregnant women in order to assist them to quit smoking.

DIET Dietary recommendations for cardiovascular health should include strategies to lower LDL levels and the need to reduce saturated fat and cholesterol intake. Most fats are a mixture of saturated and unsaturated fatty acids. The highest proportions of saturated fat are found in whole-milk products, red meats and coconut oil. Non-fat dairy products, fish and poultry as primary protein sources are recommended. Solidified vegetable fats (e.g. margarine, shortening) contain *trans* fatty acids, which behave more like saturated fats. Soft margarines and vegetable oil spreads contain low levels of trans fatty acids and should be used instead of butter, margarine and shortening. Monounsaturated fats, found in olive, canola and peanut oils, actually lower LDL and cholesterol levels. Certain cold-water fish, such as tuna, salmon and mackerel, contain high levels of omega-3 fatty acids, which help raise HDL levels and decrease serum triglycerides, total serum cholesterol and blood pressure (Singer et al., 2021).

In addition, increased intake of soluble fibre (found in oats, psyllium, pectin-rich fruit and beans) and insoluble fibre (found in whole grains, vegetables and fruit) is recommended. Folic acid and vitamins B_6 and B_{12} affect homocysteine metabolism, reducing serum levels. Leafy green vegetables (e.g. spinach and broccoli) and legumes (e.g. black-eyed peas, dried beans and lentils) are rich sources of folate. Meat, fish and poultry are rich in vitamins B_6 and B_{12}. Vitamin B_6 also is found in soy products; B_{12} is in fortified cereals. Increased intake of antioxidant nutrients (vitamin E, in particular) and foods rich in antioxidants (fruits and vegetables) appear to increase HDL levels and have a protective effect on CHD (National Heart Foundation of Australia, 2019).

In middle-aged and older adults, low levels of alcohol consumption (½ standard drink a day) may reduce the risk of CHD. Consumption of no more than two drinks per day for men or one drink per day for women is recommended. People who do not drink alcohol, however, should not be encouraged to start consuming it as a heart-protective measure as any benefit from alcohol consumption can be gained more readily from healthy diet and exercise (RACGP, 2022b).

People who are overweight or obese are encouraged to lose weight through a combination of reduced kilojoule intake (maintaining a nutritionally sound diet) and increased exercise. High-protein, high-fat weight-loss programs are not recommended for weight reduction.

EXERCISE Regular physical exercise reduces the risk of CHD in several ways. It lowers VLDL, LDL and triglyceride levels and raises HDL levels. Regular exercise reduces blood pressure and insulin resistance. National guidelines for physical activity for adults between 18 and 64 years of age have recently changed to accumulate between 150 and 300 minutes of moderate intensity or 75–150 minutes of intense physical intensity (or a combination) each week. Several themes are fostered in the new guidelines, including doing any physical activity is better than none, trying to be active most days and gradually building to the recommended amount (RACGP, 2022b).

HYPERTENSION Although hypertension often cannot be prevented or cured, it can be controlled. Hypertension control (maintaining a blood pressure lower than 140/90 mmHg) is vital to reduce its atherosclerosis-promoting effects and to reduce the workload of the heart. Management strategies include reducing sodium intake, increasing calcium intake, regular exercise, stress management and medications. Hypertension management is discussed in the chapter 'Nursing care of people with vascular and lymphatic disorders'.

DIABETES Diabetes increases the risk of CHD by accelerating the atherosclerotic process. Weight loss (if appropriate), reduced fat intake and exercise are particularly important for the person with diabetes. Because hyperglycaemia also contributes to atherosclerosis, consistent blood glucose management is vital. See the chapter 'Nursing care of people with diabetes mellitus' for a detailed discussion of diabetes and blood glucose management.

Medications

Drug therapy to lower total serum cholesterol and LDL levels and to raise HDL levels is now an integral part of CHD management. It is used in conjunction with diet and other lifestyle changes and is based on the individual's overall risk of CHD.

Drugs used to treat hyperlipidaemia act specifically by lowering LDL levels and increasing HDLs. The goal of treatment is to achieve an LDL level of < 2 mmol/L (RACGP, 2022a). Medications to treat hyperlipidaemia are not inexpensive, and high-risk patients are able to access statins through the Pharmaceutical Benefits Scheme, but the cost–benefit ratio needs to be considered because long-term treatment may be required. The four main classes of cholesterol-lowering drugs are statins, bile acid sequestrants, nicotinic acid and fibrates (see 'Medication administration' box).

People at high risk of MI are often started on prophylactic low-dose aspirin therapy. The usual dose is 100 mg/day. In women, the benefit of low-dose aspirin in reducing the risk of CHD is not clear prior to age 65. Aspirin is contraindicated for individuals who have a history of aspirin sensitivity, bleeding disorders or active peptic ulcer disease. Angiotensin-converting-enzyme (ACE) inhibitors or angiotensin receptor blockers also may be prescribed for high-risk individuals, including diabetics with other CHD risk factors (Bullock & Manias, 2022).

THE PERSON WITH ANGINA PECTORIS

Angina pectoris, or *angina*, is chest pain resulting from reduced coronary blood flow, which causes a temporary imbalance between myocardial blood supply and demand. The imbalance may be due to coronary heart disease, atherosclerosis or vessel constriction that impairs myocardial blood supply. Hypermetabolic conditions such as exercise, thyrotoxicosis, stimulant use (e.g. cocaine), hyperthyroidism and emotional stress can increase myocardial oxygen demand, precipitating angina. Anaemia, heart failure, ventricular hypertrophy or pulmonary diseases may also affect blood and oxygen supplies as well, causing angina. Angina is considered one of the acute coronary syndromes.

Pathophysiology

The imbalance between myocardial blood supply and demand causes temporary and reversible myocardial ischaemia. **Ischaemia**, deficient blood flow to tissue, may be caused by

MEDICATION ADMINISTRATION Cholesterol-lowering drugs

STATINS

Statins inhibit the enzyme HMG-CoA reductase in the liver, lowering LDL synthesis and serum levels. The statins are first-line treatment for elevated LDL, used in conjunction with diet and lifestyle changes. Although their side effects are minimal, they may cause increased serum liver enzyme levels and myopathy.

Nursing responsibilities

- Monitor serum cholesterol and liver enzyme levels before and during therapy. Report elevated liver enzyme levels.
- Assess for muscle pain and tenderness. Monitor creatine phosphokinase (CPK) level if present.
- Monitor for and report digoxin toxicity in any person receiving concurrent digoxin therapy.

Health education for the person and family

- Promptly report muscle pain, tenderness or weakness; skin rash or hives or changes in skin colour; abdominal pain, nausea or vomiting.
- Drugs should not be used when pregnant or if pregnancy is planned.
- Inform the medical officer if taking any other medications concurrently.

BILE ACID SEQUESTRANTS

Bile acid sequestrants lower LDL levels by binding bile acids in the intestine, reducing LDL reabsorption and cholesterol production in the liver. They are used in combination therapy regimens and for women who are considering pregnancy. Their primary disadvantages are inconvenience of administration due to bulk and gastrointestinal side effects such as constipation.

Nursing responsibilities

- Store in a tightly sealed container.

Health education for the person and family

- Promptly report constipation, severe gastric distress with nausea and vomiting, unexplained weight loss, black or bloody stools, or sudden back pain.
- Drinking ample amounts of fluid while taking these drugs reduces problems of constipation and bloating.
- Do not omit doses as this may affect the absorption of other drugs the person is taking.

NICOTINIC ACID

Nicotinic acid in both prescription and non-prescription forms lowers total and LDL cholesterol and triglyceride levels. The crystalline form and the extended-release tablet also raise HDL levels. Because the doses required to achieve significant cholesterol-lowering effects are associated with multiple side effects, nicotinic acid generally is used in combination therapy, particularly with statins.

Nursing responsibilities

- Give oral preparations with meals and accompanied by a cold beverage to minimise GI effects.
- Administer with caution to individuals with active liver disease, peptic ulcer disease, gout or type 2 diabetes.
- Monitor blood glucose, uric acid levels and liver function tests during treatment.

Health education for the person and family

- Flushing of face, neck and ears may occur within 2 hours following dose; these effects generally subside as treatment continues. Alcohol use during nicotinic acid therapy may worsen this effect.
- Report weakness or dizziness with changes in posture (lying to sitting; sitting to standing). Change positions slowly to reduce the risk of injury.

FIBRIC ACID DERIVATIVES

The fibrates are used to lower serum triglyceride levels; they have only a slight to modest effect on LDL. They affect lipid regulation by blocking triglyceride synthesis. They are used to treat very high triglyceride levels and may be used in combination with statins.

Nursing responsibilities

- Monitor serum LDL and VLDL levels, electrolytes, glucose, liver enzymes, renal function tests and full blood count (FBC) during therapy. Report abnormal values.
- Up to 2 months of treatment may be required to achieve a therapeutic effect; rebound, with decreasing benefit, may occur in the second or third month of treatment.

Health education for the person and family

- Take with meals if the drug causes gastric distress.
- Promptly report flu-like symptoms (fatigue, muscle aching, soreness or weakness).
- Drug should not be used in pregnancy. Use reliable birth control measures while taking this drug.
- Consultation with a medical officer is required before stopping this drug and before taking any over-the-counter preparations.

partial obstruction of a coronary artery, coronary artery spasm or a thrombus. Obstruction of a coronary artery deprives cells in the region of the heart normally supplied by that vessel of oxygen and nutrients needed for metabolic processes. Cellular processes are compromised as ATP stores are depleted. Reduced oxygen causes cells to switch from aerobic metabolism to anaerobic metabolism. Anaerobic metabolism causes lactic acid to accumulate in the cells. It also affects cell membrane permeability, releasing substances such as histamine, kinins and specific enzymes that stimulate terminal nerve fibres in the cardiac muscle and send pain impulses to the central nervous system. The pain radiates to the upper body because the heart shares the same dermatome as this region. Return of adequate circulation provides the nutrients needed by cells and clears the waste products. More than 30 minutes of ischaemia irreversibly damages myocardial cells (necrosis).

Three types of angina have been identified:

1. *Stable angina* is the most common and predictable form of angina. It occurs with a predictable amount of activity or stress and is a common manifestation of CHD. Stable

angina usually occurs when the work of the heart is increased by physical exertion, exposure to cold or by stress. Stable angina is relieved by rest and nitrates.

2. *Prinzmetal's (variant) angina* is atypical angina that occurs unpredictably (unrelated to activity) and often at night. It is caused by coronary artery spasm with or without an atherosclerotic lesion. The exact mechanism of coronary artery spasm is unknown. It may result from hyperactive sympathetic nervous system responses, altered calcium flow in smooth muscle or reduced prostaglandins that promote vasodilation.
3. *Unstable angina* occurs with increasing frequency, severity and duration. Pain is unpredictable and occurs with decreasing levels of activity or stress and may occur at rest. People with unstable angina are at risk of myocardial infarction. Unstable angina is discussed further in the section on acute coronary syndromes that follows.

Silent myocardial ischaemia, or asymptomatic ischaemia, is thought to be common in people with CHD, especially with the comorbidity diabetes mellitus. Silent ischaemia may occur with either activity or mental stress. Mental stress increases the heart rate and blood pressure, increasing myocardial oxygen demand (Bullock & Hales, 2019). Like symptomatic angina, silent myocardial ischaemia is associated with an increased chance of myocardial infarction and death.

FAST FACTS

- Stable angina occurs with a predictable amount of activity or stress.
- Unstable angina occurs with increasing frequency and severity; it may occur at times unrelated to activity or stress.
- Prinzmetal's angina is the only type of angina not necessarily related to coronary heart disease and atherosclerosis; it develops due to coronary artery spasm.

Course and manifestations

The cardinal manifestation of angina is chest pain. The pain typically is precipitated by an identifiable event, such as physical activity, emotional distress, stress, eating a heavy meal or exposure to cold. The classic sequence of angina is activity = pain, rest = relief. The person may describe the pain as tight, squeezing, heavy pressure or a constricting sensation. It characteristically begins beneath the sternum and may radiate leftwards to the jaw, neck, shoulder or arm. Less characteristically, the pain may be felt in the jaw, epigastric region or back. Anginal pain usually occurs in a crescendo–decrescendo pattern (increasing to a peak, then gradually decreasing) and typically lasts 2 to 5 minutes. It generally is relieved by rest. Additional manifestations of angina include dyspnoea, pallor, tachycardia, and significant anxiety and fear.

Females frequently present with atypical symptoms of angina, including indigestion or nausea, vomiting and upper back pain. The manifestations of angina are summarised in the 'Manifestations' box.

MANIFESTATIONS Angina

- *Chest pain*: substernal or precordial (across the chest wall); may radiate to neck, arms, shoulders or jaw.
- *Quality*: tight, squeezing, constricting or heavy sensation; may also be described as burning, aching, choking, dull or constant.
- *Associated manifestations*: dyspnoea, pallor, tachycardia, anxiety and fear.
- *Atypical manifestations*: indigestion, nausea, vomiting, upper back pain.
- *Precipitating factors*: exercise or activity, strong emotion, stress, cold, heavy meal
- *Relieving factors*: rest, position change; glyceryl trinitrate.

The severity of angina can be graded by the degree to which it limits the individual's activities. Class I angina does not occur with ordinary physical activities. It is prompted by strenuous, rapid or prolonged physical exertion. Class II angina may develop with rapid or prolonged walking or stair climbing, whereas class III angina significantly limits ordinary physical activities. The person with class IV angina may have angina at rest, as well as with any physical activity (Haber, 2021).

INTERPROFESSIONAL CARE

The management of a person experiencing stable angina focuses on maintaining coronary blood flow and cardiac function. Stable angina often can be managed by medical therapy. Measures to restore coronary blood flow are discussed in the section on acute coronary syndrome. As for CHD, risk factor management is a vital component of care for the person with angina.

Diagnosis

The diagnosis of angina is based on the person's past medical history and family history, a comprehensive description of the chest pain and physical assessment findings. Laboratory tests may confirm the presence of risk factors, such as an abnormal blood lipid profile and elevated blood glucose. Diagnostic tests provide information about overall cardiac function.

Common diagnostic tests to assess for coronary heart disease and angina include electrocardiography, stress testing, nuclear medicine studies, echocardiography (ultrasound) and coronary angiography

ELECTROCARDIOGRAPHY A resting ECG may be normal, may show non-specific changes in the ST segment and T wave, or may show evidence of previous myocardial infarction. Characteristic ECG changes are seen during anginal episodes. During periods of ischaemia, the ST segment is depressed or down-sloping and the T wave may flatten or invert (see Figure 29.1). These changes reverse when ischaemia is relieved. For more details about the ECG, its waveforms and its uses, see the chapter 'A person-centred approach to assessing the cardiovascular and lymphatic systems'.

STRESS ELECTROCARDIOGRAPHY Stress electrocardiography (exercise stress test) uses ECGs to monitor the cardiac response to an increased workload during progressive exercise. See the 'Diagnostic tests' box in the chapter 'A person-centred approach to assessing the cardiovascular and lymphatic systems' for more information about exercise stress tests.

RADIONUCLIDE TESTING Radionuclide testing is a safe, non-invasive technique to evaluate myocardial perfusion and left ventricular function. The amount of radioisotope injected is very small; no special radiation precautions are required during or after the scan. Thallium-201 or a technetium-based radio compound is injected intravenously and the heart is scanned with a radiation detector. Ischaemic or infarcted cells of the myocardium do not take up the substance normally, appearing as a 'cold spot' on the scan. If the ischaemia is transient, these spots gradually fill in, indicating the reversibility of the process. With severe ischaemia or a myocardial infarction, these areas may remain devoid of radioactivity.

Left ventricular function can also be evaluated. Whereas the ejection fraction or portion of blood ejected from the left ventricle during systole normally increases during exercise, it may actually decrease in coronary heart disease and stress-induced ischaemia.

Radionuclide testing may be combined with pharmacological stress testing for individuals who are physically unable to exercise or to detect subclinical myocardial ischaemia. A vasodilator is injected to induce the same ischaemic changes that occur with exercise in the diseased heart. Coronary arteries unaffected by atherosclerosis dilate in response to the drugs, increasing blood flow to already well-perfused tissue. This reduces flow to ischaemic muscle, called *myocardial steal syndrome*.

ECHOCARDIOGRAPHY *Echocardiography* is a non-invasive test that uses ultrasound to evaluate cardiac structure and function. It may be done at rest, during supine exercise or immediately following upright exercise to evaluate movement of the myocardial wall and assess for possible ischaemia or infarction.

Transoesophageal echocardiography (TOE) uses ultrasound to identify abnormal blood flow patterns as well as cardiac structures. In TOE, the probe is on the tip of an endoscope inserted into the oesophagus, positioning it close to the posterior heart (especially the left atrium and the aorta). It avoids interference by breasts, ribs or lungs. This diagnostic intervention generally requires light sedation.

See the 'Diagnostic tests' box in the chapter 'A person-centred approach to assessing the cardiovascular and lymphatic systems' for more information about nursing care of the person undergoing these tests.

CORONARY ANGIOGRAPHY *Coronary angiography* is the gold standard for evaluating the coronary arteries (Chew et al., 2016). Guided by fluoroscopy, a catheter introduced into the femoral or brachial artery is threaded into the coronary artery. Dye is injected into each coronary opening, allowing visualisation of the main coronary branches and any abnormalities, such as stenosis or obstruction. Narrowing of the vessel lumen by more than 50% is considered significant; most lesions that cause symptoms involve more than 70% narrowing. Vessel obstructions are noted on a coronary artery 'map' that provides a guide for tracking disease progression and for elective treatment with angioplasty or cardiac surgery. See the 'Diagnostic tests' box in the chapter 'A person-centred approach to assessing the cardiovascular and lymphatic systems' for the nursing care of the person undergoing coronary angiography. See the 'Translation to practice' box regarding research related to extracardiac findings from angiography.

Medications

Drugs may be used for both acute and long-term relief of angina. The goal of drug treatment is to reduce oxygen demand and increase oxygen supply to the myocardium. Three main classes of drugs are used to treat angina: nitrates, beta-blockers and calcium channel blockers.

NITRATES Nitrates, including glyceryl trinitrate (GTN) and longer-acting nitrate preparations, are used to treat acute anginal attacks and prevent angina.

Sublingual glyceryl trinitrate (Anginine) is the drug of choice to treat acute angina. It acts within 1 to 2 minutes, decreasing myocardial work and oxygen demand through venous and arterial dilation, which in turn reduces preload and

TRANSLATION TO PRACTICE Possible non-invasive alternative to angiography to determine the presence of coronary artery disease

Recent research sought to explore the benefits of coronary computed tomography angiography compared to invasive coronary angiography in identifying extracardiac findings (ECF). The aim was to analyse potential clinical benefits to the patient from identification of ECFs, particularly in patients with atypical chest pain, and to further clarify different beliefs in existing research (Laskowski et al., 2021).

IMPLICATIONS FOR NURSING

Nurses are often required to coordinate and advocate for care for individuals with chest pain requiring angiography. Knowledge of the attendant benefits of all treatment options available is necessary. This research indicates that computed tomographic angiography may be more useful than invasive coronary angiography in many instances.

CRITICAL THINKING IN PERSON-CENTRED CARE

1 What are the potential benefits from the identification of extracardiac findings through angiography?
2 What role does the nurse play in coordinating and advocating care for individuals with chest pain?

afterload. It may also improve myocardial oxygen supply by dilating collateral blood vessels and reducing stenosis. Rapid-acting glyceryl trinitrate is also available as a buccal/sublingual spray in a metered system. For some individuals, this may be easier to handle than small glyceryl trinitrate tablets. The spray has a longer storage life, reducing the need to discard and repurchase fresh medication every 3 months.

Longer-acting glyceryl trinitrate preparations (oral tablets, ointment or transdermal patches) are used to prevent attacks of angina, rather than treat an acute attack. The primary problem with long-term nitrate use is the development of *tolerance*, a decreasing effect from the same dose of medication. Tolerance can be limited by a dosing schedule that allows a nitrate-free period of at least 8 to 10 hours daily. This is usually scheduled at night, when angina is less likely to occur.

Headache is a common side effect of nitrates and may limit their usefulness. Nausea, dizziness and hypotension are also common effects of therapy.

> **CONSIDERATION FOR PRACTICE**
> **Sublingual glyceryl trinitrate tablets and glyceryl trinitrate spray are the only medications appropriate to treat an acute anginal attack.**

BETA-BLOCKERS Beta-blockers, including propranolol, metoprolol and atenolol, are considered first-line drugs to treat stable angina. They block the cardiac-stimulating effects of noradrenaline and adrenaline, preventing anginal attacks by reducing heart rate, myocardial contractility and blood pressure, thus reducing myocardial oxygen demand. Beta-blockers may be used alone or with other medications to prevent angina.

Beta-blockers are contraindicated for people with asthma or severe COPD (see the chapter 'Nursing care of people with gas exchange disorders') because they may cause severe bronchospasm. They are not used in people with significant bradycardia or atrioventricular (AV) conduction blocks and are used cautiously in heart failure. Beta-blockers are not used to treat Prinzmetal's angina because they may worsen the condition.

CALCIUM CHANNEL BLOCKERS Calcium channel blockers reduce myocardial oxygen demand and increase myocardial blood and oxygen supply. These drugs, which include verapamil, diltiazem and nifedipine, lower blood pressure, reduce myocardial contractility and, in some cases, lower the heart rate, decreasing myocardial oxygen demand. They are also potent coronary vasodilators, effectively increasing oxygen supply. Like beta-blockers, calcium channel blockers act too slowly to effectively treat an acute attack of angina; they are used for long-term prophylaxis. Because they may actually increase ischaemia and mortality in people with heart failure or left ventricular dysfunction, these drugs are not usually prescribed in the initial treatment of angina. They are used cautiously in individuals with arrhythmias, heart failure or hypotension.

The nursing implications of anti-anginal medications are summarised in the 'Medication administration' box.

ASPIRIN The person with angina, particularly unstable angina, is at risk of myocardial infarction because of significant narrowing of the coronary arteries. Low-dose aspirin (100 mg/day) is often prescribed to reduce the risk of platelet aggregation and thrombus formation.

MEDICATION ADMINISTRATION Anti-anginal medications

ORGANIC NITRATES

Nitrates dilate both arterial and venous vessels, depending on the dose. Coronary artery vasodilation increases myocardial oxygen supply. Venous dilation allows peripheral blood pooling, reducing venous return, preload and cardiac work. Arterial dilation reduces vascular resistance and afterload, also reducing cardiac work. Sublingual glyceryl trinitrate (GTN) is used to treat and prevent acute anginal attacks (when taken prophylactically before activity). Nitrates are administered sublingually by buccal spray, or intravenously for immediate effect. For a sustained effect, oral or topical administration is recommended.

Nursing responsibilities

- Dilute intravenous glyceryl trinitrate before infusing; use glass bottles only for the mixture. Glyceryl trinitrate will adsorb onto many infusion lines and PVC bags, affecting the amount of drug that is delivered. Special GTN infusion tubing must be used.
- Wear gloves when opening ampoules and drawing up glyceryl trinitrate infusions to prevent inadvertent administration to self through direct skin absorption.
- Remove glyceryl trinitrate patches daily (or when required) reducing tolerance by providing GTN-free time.

Health education for the person and family

- Use only the sublingual, buccal and spray forms of nitrates to treat acute angina.
- If the first nitrate dose does not relieve angina within 5 minutes, take a second dose. After 5 more minutes, the person may take a third dose if needed. If the pain is unrelieved, seek medical assistance immediately.
- Advise the person to carry a supply of glyceryl trinitrate tablets with them. Dissolve sublingual glyceryl trinitrate tablets under the tongue or between the upper lip and gum. The patient should not eat, drink or smoke until the tablet is completely dissolved.
- Keep sublingual tablets in their original amber glass bottle to protect them from heat, light and moisture. Replacement should occur every 3 months after opening the supply (tablets). Spray can be kept for a year.
- Burning or tingling sensation may be felt under the tongue and the person may develop a transient headache on taking the drug. These effects are expected; the headache will diminish over time.
- Use caution when standing from a sitting position; glyceryl trinitrate may cause light-headedness.

(*continued*)

MEDICATION ADMINISTRATION **Anti-anginal medications (continued)**

- Rotate the application sites of the transdermal patches. Apply to a hairless area so that the drug can reach the skin. Remove the patch at bedtime daily (or as ordered). Apply a fresh dose in the morning (or as ordered).
- If using a long-acting nitrate, a supply of immediate-acting nitrates should be kept to treat acute angina.

BETA-BLOCKERS

Beta-blockers decrease cardiac workload by blocking beta receptors on the heart muscle, thus decreasing heart rate, contractility, myocardial oxygen consumption and blood pressure. Beta-blockers also reduce *reflex tachycardia* (an increased heart rate in response to stimuli such as increased sympathetic nervous system activity or vasodilation), which may develop with other anti-anginal drugs. Beta-blockers are frequently prescribed as anti-anginal and antihypertensive agents. Some examples include metoprolol and carvedilol.

Nursing responsibilities

- Document heart rate and blood pressure before administering the beta-blockers. Withhold the drug if the heart rate is below 50 bpm or the blood pressure is below prescribed limits. Notify the medical team.
- Assess for and report possible contraindications to therapy, including heart failure, bradycardia, AV block, asthma or chronic obstructive pulmonary disease (COPD).
- Concurrent use of beta-blockers and calcium channel blockers increases the risk of heart failure; notify the medical team if these drugs are prescribed together.
- Do not abruptly discontinue these drugs after long-term therapy, as this can increase heart rate, contractility and blood pressure, and cause fatal arrhythmia, myocardial infarction or stroke.

Health education for the person and family

- Beta-blockers help prevent angina but will not relieve an acute attack. The person should keep a supply of fast-acting nitrates on hand for acute anginal attacks.
- The person should not suddenly stop taking this medication, but instead should discuss discontinuing medication with medical officers.
- Teach the person to check their pulse before administration. The person should not take the drug and should contact the doctor if the heart rate is below 50 bpm. Check blood pressure frequently.
- Report a slow or irregular pulse, swelling or weight gain, or difficulty breathing.

CALCIUM CHANNEL BLOCKERS

Calcium channel blockers are used to control angina, hypertension and arrhythmias. By blocking the entry of calcium into cells, these drugs reduce contractility, slow the heart rate and conduction, and cause vasodilation. Calcium channel blockers increase myocardial oxygen supply by dilating the coronary arteries; they decrease the workload of the heart by lowering vascular resistance and oxygen demand. Calcium channel blockers are often prescribed for people with coronary artery spasm (Prinzmetal's angina). Some examples include verapamil and nifedipine.

Nursing responsibilities

- Do not mix verapamil in any solution containing sodium bicarbonate. Administer verapamil as an intravenous bolus over 2 to 3 minutes.
- Document blood pressure and heart rate before administering the drug. Withhold the drug if the heart rate is below 50 bpm. Notify the medical team.
- The nifedipine capsule may be punctured and administered by extracting the liquid with a syringe and squirting the dose under the person's tongue. (Discard the needle first!)
- Use caution when giving a calcium channel blocker with other cardiac depressants, such as beta-blockers. Concomitant administration with nitrates may cause excessive vasodilation.
- Manifestations of toxicity include nausea, generalised weakness, signs of decreased cardiac output, hypotension, bradycardia and AV block. Report these findings immediately. Maintain intravenous access and slowly administer intravenous calcium chloride. Do not infuse large volumes of fluid to treat hypotension as heart failure may result.

Health education for the person and family

- Take pulse before taking the drug. Do not take the drug and notify doctor if the heart rate drops below 50 bpm.
- Keep a fresh supply of immediate-acting nitrate available to treat acute anginal attacks. Calcium channel blockers are not sufficiently rapid acting to relieve an acute attack.

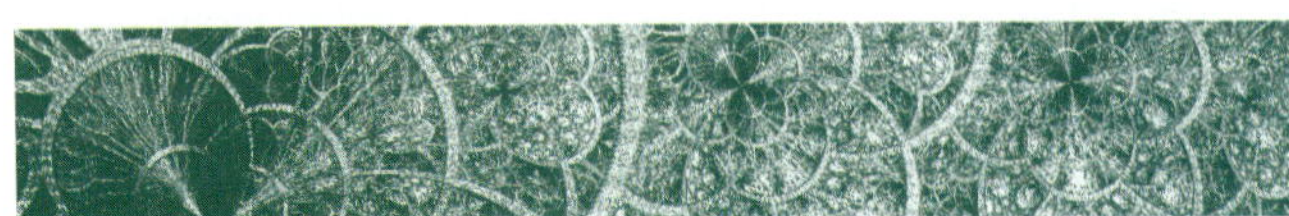

Nursing care

The focus of nursing care for the person with angina is similar to the interprofessional care focus: to reduce myocardial oxygen demand and improve the oxygen supply. Angina usually is treated in community settings; the primary nursing focus is education.

Health promotion

In addition to health promotion measures identified for CHD, emphasise the importance of active CHD risk factor management to slow progression of the disease. Encourage the person to stop smoking. Discuss the use of cholesterol-lowering drug therapy with people who have hypercholesterolaemia.

Encourage regular aerobic exercise and a diet based on the National Heart Foundation guidelines.

Assessment

Focused assessment data for the person with angina include the following:

- *Health history*: chest pain—Onset, Location, Duration, Characteristics, Aggravating symptoms, methods to Relieve the pain, current Treatment (OLDCART); history of other cardiovascular disorders, peripheral vascular disease or stroke; current medications and treatment; usual diet, exercise and alcohol intake patterns; smoking history; use of other recreational drugs.
- *Physical assessment*: vital signs and heart sounds; strength and equality of peripheral pulses; skin colour and temperature (central and peripheral); physical appearance during pain episode (e.g. shortness of breath, apparent anxiety, colour, diaphoresis).

Nursing diagnoses and interventions

High-priority nursing problems for individuals with angina include ineffective cardiac tissue perfusion and management of the prescribed therapeutic regimen.

Ineffective tissue perfusion: cardiac

The pain of angina results from impaired blood flow and oxygen supply to the myocardium. Nursing interventions can both prevent ischaemia and shorten the duration of pain.

- Keep prescribed glyceryl trinitrate tablets (or spray) at the person's side so that this can be taken at the onset of pain. Anginal pain indicates *myocardial ischaemia. Glyceryl trinitrate causes vasodilation improving myocardial oxygen supply, relieving ischaemia and pain.*
- Start oxygen at 2 to 4 L/min per nasal prongs if the person is showing signs of hypoxia. *Supplemental oxygen reduces myocardial hypoxia by increasing oxygen supply.*
- Plan activities to allow rest between them. *Activity increases myocardial oxygen demand and may precipitate angina. Spacing activities reduces the risk of exceeding myocardial oxygen supply.*
- Teach about prescribed medications to maintain myocardial perfusion and reduce cardiac work. Emphasise that beta-blockers, calcium channel blockers and long-acting nitrates are used to *prevent* anginal attacks, not to *treat* an acute attack. *It is important for the person to understand the purpose and use of prescribed drugs to maintain optimal myocardial perfusion.*
- Instruct to take sublingual glyceryl trinitrate before engaging in activities that precipitate angina (e.g. climbing stairs, sexual intercourse). *This prophylactic dose of glyceryl trinitrate helps maintain cardiac perfusion (by improving myocardial oxygen supply) when increased work (myocardial oxygen demand) is anticipated; this reduces ischaemia and chest pain.*
- Encourage the person to implement and maintain a progressive exercise program under the supervision of the primary care provider or a cardiac rehabilitation professional. *Exercise slows the atherosclerotic process and helps develop collateral circulation to the heart muscle.*
- Refer individual to a smoking cessation program as indicated. *Nicotine causes vasoconstriction, increases the heart rate, decreases myocardial perfusion and increases cardiac workload.*

Risk of ineffective therapeutic regimen management

Denial may be strong in the person with angina pectoris. Because many people think of the heart as the locus of life itself, problems such as angina remind people of their mortality, an uncomfortable fact. Denial may lead to 'forgetting' to take prescribed medications or to attempting activities that will precipitate angina. Some people, by contrast, may become afraid to engage in activities because of anticipated chest pain. Their inactivity may actually hasten the atherosclerotic process and inhibit collateral circulation development, worsening angina.

- Assess knowledge and understanding of angina. *Assessment allows tailoring of teaching and interventions to the needs of the person.*
- Teach the individual about angina and atherosclerosis, building on current knowledge base. *This can help the person understand that angina is a manageable disease and that pain can usually be controlled and the disease progress slowed.*
- Provide written and verbal instructions about prescribed medications and their use. *Written instructions reinforce teaching and are available to the person for future reference.*
- Stress the importance of taking chest pains seriously while maintaining a positive attitude. *Although it is vital to recognise the significance of chest pain and deal with it appropriately, it is also important to maintain a positive outlook.*
- Refer to a cardiac rehabilitation program or other organised activities and support groups for individuals with coronary heart disease. *Programs such as these help the person develop risk factor management strategies, maintain a program of supervised activity and gain coping skills.*

Community-based care

Many people with stable angina manage their pain effectively, continuing to live active and productive lives. To promote effective management of this disorder, include the following topics in teaching for home care:

- coronary heart disease and the processes that cause chest pain, including the relationship between the pain and reduced blood flow to the heart muscle
- use and effects (desired and adverse) of prescribed medications; importance of not discontinuing medications abruptly
- glyceryl trinitrate use for acute angina: always carry tablets, use prophylactically before activities that often cause chest pain, take tablet at first indication of pain rather than waiting to see if the pain develops; seek immediate medical

assistance if three glyceryl trinitrate tablets over 15 minutes do not relieve the pain

- the importance of calling 000 or going to the emergency department immediately for unrelieved chest pain
- appropriate storage of glyceryl trinitrate: this unstable compound needs to be stored in a cool, dry, dark place; no more than a 3-month supply should be kept on hand.

For the person who has undergone cardiac surgery, also include the following:

- respiratory care, activity and pain management
- the importance of actively participating in rehabilitation
- manifestations of infection or other potential complications and their management.

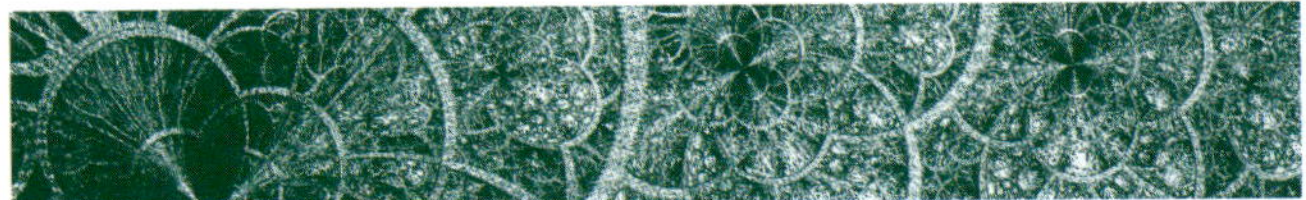

THE PERSON WITH ACUTE CORONARY SYNDROME

Acute coronary syndrome (ACS) is a cluster of conditions, including unstable angina and myocardial infarction, that lead to or result from cardiac ischaemia. ACS includes unstable angina and acute myocardial ischaemia with or without significant injury of myocardial tissue. Although the term ACS may, in some cases, be applied to acute myocardial infarction (AMI) (myocardial tissue death), myocardial infarction is discussed separately in the next section of this chapter.

> **FAST FACTS**
>
> - Acute coronary syndrome (severe cardiac ischaemia), a common cause of hospital admission, includes unstable angina and acute myocardial infarction.
> - Unstable angina is characterised by injury to myocardial cells. With prompt restoration of blood flow, muscle tissue recovers.
> - Myocardial infarction is characterised by necrosis and death of myocardial cells; scar tissue forms and functional muscle is lost.

Pathophysiology

ACS is a dynamic state in which coronary blood flow is acutely reduced, but not fully occluded. Myocardial cells are injured by the acute ischaemia that results. Most people affected by ACS have significant stenosis of one or more coronary arteries.

ACS is precipitated by any number of pathophysiological causes, including partial occlusion and clot formation of myocardial blood vessels, an oxygen demand versus supply issue or acute changes in the patency of critical myocardial vessels (Coven, 2020). Changes in haemodynamic factors such as increased heart rate, blood flow and blood pressure occur in response to a surge of sympathetic nervous system (SNS) activity. Increased SNS activity also is thought to contribute to the higher incidence of plaque rupture (Mohanta et al., 2022).

When atherosclerotic plaque ruptures or erodes, the exposed lipid core of the plaque stimulates platelet aggregation and the extrinsic clotting pathway. Thrombin is generated and fibrin is deposited, forming a clot that severely impairs or obstructs blood flow to tissue distal to the area of plaque rupture. As a result, these cells become ischaemic.

Injured myocardial cells contract less effectively, potentially reducing cardiac output if a large area of myocardium is affected. Lactic acid released from ischaemic cells stimulates pain receptors, causing chest pain. Ischaemia and injury affect electrical impulse conduction, producing inversion of the T wave and possibly elevation of the ST segment on the ECG.

Manifestations

The cardinal manifestation of ACS is chest pain, usually substernal or epigastric. The pain often radiates to the neck, left shoulder and/or left arm. The pain may occur at rest and typically lasts longer than 10 to 20 minutes. In ACS, the chest pain is more severe and prolonged than that previously experienced by the individual. It may be a new onset of pain or may represent a pattern of increasing frequency and severity of anginal pain. Dyspnoea, diaphoresis, pallor and cool skin may be present. Tachycardia and hypotension may occur. The person may be nauseated or feel light-headed.

INTERPROFESSIONAL CARE

The person with ACS generally presents at the emergency department or general practice with complaints of severe chest pain. The pain may be unrelieved by glyceryl trinitrate or may be more severe and of longer duration than previous anginal episodes. An ECG is used in conjunction with blood levels of cardiac markers (troponin) to differentiate between unstable angina and acute myocardial infarction. People with unstable angina generally are admitted to an acute care unit on bed rest with cardiac monitoring for 12 to 24 hours. Coronary revascularisation procedures may be performed within 48 hours if significant CHD is identified, but best evidence suggests that within 60 to 90 minutes of chest pain onset provides the best outcomes (Chew et al., 2016).

Diagnosis

The ECG and serum cardiac markers are the primary tests used to establish the diagnosis of ACS. Serum cardiac markers, proteins released from injured and necrotic heart muscle, can be measured. (See the following section on acute myocardial infarction and Table 29.5 for more information about serum cardiac markers.)

- Cardiac muscle troponins, *cardiac-specific troponin* T (cT_nT) and *cardiac-specific troponin* I (cT_nI), are sensitive indicators of myocardial damage. Troponins may be elevated in ACS or may be within normal limits if chest pain is due to unstable angina. Troponin assay can now be checked at the bedside in acute situations.

TABLE 29.5 Serum cardiac markers

MARKER	NORMAL LEVEL	PRIMARY TISSUE LOCATION	SIGNIFICANCE OF ELEVATION	CHANGES OCCURRING WITH MI		
				APPEARS	PEAKS	DURATION
CK (CPK)	< 270 U/L	Cardiac muscle, skeletal muscle, brain	Injury to muscle cells	3 to 6 hours	12 to 24 hours	24 to 48 hours
CK-MB	< 10 U/L	Cardiac muscle	MI, cardiac ischaemia, myocarditis, cardiac contusion, defibrillation	4 to 8 hours	18 to 24 hours	72 hours
cT_nT	< 0.1 μg/L	Cardiac and skeletal muscle	Acute MI, unstable angina	2 to 4 hours	24 to 36 hours	10 to 14 days
cT_nI	0.4 μg/L (ACS) > 01.5 μg/L (AMI)	Cardiac muscle	Acute MI, unstable angina	2 to 4 hours	24 to 36 hours	7 to 10 days

- Creatine kinase (CK) and CK-MB (specific to myocardial muscle) levels are likely to be within normal limits or demonstrate transient elevation, returning to normal levels within 12 to 24 hours.

The ECG, particularly when recorded during an acute episode of chest pain, is a valuable diagnostic tool for ACS. ST-segment changes (elevation or depression) during chest pain that resolve when the pain abates usually indicate acute myocardial ischaemia and severe underlying CHD.

Medications

Medications include drugs to reduce myocardial ischaemia and to reduce the risk of blood clotting. Thrombolytic drugs (i.e. drugs that break down the fibrin in blood clots) may be given prior to or on admission to the emergency department. These drugs restore blood flow to ischaemic cardiac muscle and can prevent permanent damage. See the section on myocardial infarction for more information about thrombolytic drugs and their nursing implications.

Nitrates and beta-blockers are used to restore blood flow to the ischaemic myocardium and reduce the workload of the heart. Glyceryl trinitrate is given by sublingual tablet or buccal spray. If chest pain is unrelieved after three doses 5 minutes apart, an intravenous glyceryl trinitrate infusion is initiated. The infusion may be continued until the chest pain is relieved or for 12 to 24 hours. Topical or oral nitrates are then initiated. Beta-adrenergic blockers are initially given intravenously, followed by oral beta-blockers. See the 'Medication administration: anti-anginal medications' box for the nursing implications of these drugs.

Aspirin, other antiplatelet drugs and heparin are given to inhibit blood clotting and reduce the risk of thrombus formation. Aspirin and clopidogrel are given to people with ACS who do not have an excessive bleeding risk. Aspirin and clopidogrel suppress platelet aggregation, interrupting the process of forming a stable blood clot. Both increase the risk of serious haemorrhage; for most people, however, the benefit outweighs the risk. Intravenous antiplatelet drugs such as abciximab, eptifibatide or tirofiban may be used when an invasive coronary revascularisation procedure is anticipated in the immediate or near future. Nursing implications for the antiplatelet drugs are outlined in the 'Medication administration: antiplatelet drugs' box.

MEDICATION ADMINISTRATION Antiplatelet drugs

ORAL ANTIPLATELET DRUGS

Antiplatelet drugs suppress platelet aggregation in arteries, preventing the development of an arterial thrombus. Aspirin and clopidogrel block different platelet activation pathways to inhibit platelet aggregation and clot formation. The dose of aspirin given to achieve antiplatelet effects is low, 100 mg/day.

Nursing responsibilities

- Inquire about a history of intracranial haemorrhage, upper gastrointestinal bleeding, peptic ulcer disease or known bleeding tendency.
- Observe for and report increased bruising, petechiae, purpura, apparent or occult bleeding (e.g. melaena, haematemesis).
- Do not administer concurrently with warfarin.

Health education for the person and family

- Take as directed. Take aspirin with food or milk; clopidogrel may be taken at any time of day.
- Do not use non-steroidal anti-inflammatory drugs (NSAIDs) or other over-the-counter drugs that may contain aspirin or an NSAID unless prescribed by the doctor.
- Advise the person to check with their pharmacist before taking any herbal remedies such as evening primrose oil, feverfew, garlic, ginkgo biloba or grapeseed extract.
- Report unusual bruising or excessive bleeding.
- Inform all healthcare providers (including dental professionals) of use of these drugs.

INTRAVENOUS ANTIPLATELET DRUGS

The intravenously administered antiplatelet drugs, abciximab, epifibatide and tirofiban, block the final common pathway of

(continued)

MEDICATION ADMINISTRATION **Antiplatelet drugs (continued)**

platelet activation and thus are more effective. However, the risk of bleeding is greater than with the orally administered antiplatelet drugs.

Nursing responsibilities

- Assess risk of and determine history of bleeding disorders, intracranial haemorrhage, recent trauma or surgery.
- Inquire about recent use of oral antiplatelet or anticoagulant drugs.
- Monitor FBC, including haemoglobin, haematocrit and platelet count; clotting studies, including prothrombin time (PT), International Normalized Ratio (INR), activated partial thromboplastin time (aPTT); vital signs; and ECG during therapy.
- Maintain a separate intravenous line for venesection and administration of other drugs during infusion.
- Closely observe for and immediately report anaphylaxis or bleeding uncontrolled by pressure. Keep resuscitation equipment readily available.
- Maintain bed rest during infusion.

Health education for the person and family

- This drug is given to reduce the risk of clotting and myocardial infarction. It helps maintain blood flow through the affected vessel following angioplasty and stent placement.
- Immediately report any chest tightness, difficulty breathing, shortness of breath or itching that develops during the infusion.
- The risk of bleeding should return to normal within about 2 days following the infusion.
- Immediately report any unusual bruising or bleeding.

Revascularisation procedures

Several procedures may be used to restore blood flow and oxygen to ischaemic tissue. Non-surgical techniques include transluminal coronary angioplasty, laser angioplasty, coronary atherectomy and intracoronary stents. Coronary artery bypass grafting (CABG) is a surgical procedure that may be used.

PERCUTANEOUS TRANSLUMINAL CORONARY REVASCULARISATION *Percutaneous transluminal coronary revascularisation (PTCA)* procedures are used to restore blood flow to the ischaemic myocardium in the person with CHD. There are over 48,000 percutaneous coronary interventions a year performed in Australia (AIHW, 2022c). PTCA is used to treat the person with:

- moderately severe, chronic stable angina unrelieved by medical therapy
- unstable angina
- acute myocardial infarction
- significant stenosis of the left anterior descending coronary artery
- stenosis of a coronary artery bypass graft.

PTCA procedures are similar to the procedure used for coronary angiography. A catheter introduced into the arterial circulation is guided into the opening of the narrowed coronary artery. A flexible guide wire is inserted through the catheter lumen into the affected vessel. The guide wire is then used to thread an angioplasty balloon, arterial stent or other therapeutic device into the narrowed segment of the artery (see Figure 29.2). The procedure is performed in the cardiac catheterisation laboratory using local anaesthesia. The hospital stay is short (1 to 2 days), minimising costs.

Intracoronary stents are metallic scaffolds used to maintain an open arterial lumen. Stents are now used in the majority of all PTCA procedures. Some stents are drug-eluting and release chemicals known to reduce restenosis (Shurmur, 2022). The stent is placed over a balloon catheter, guided into position and expanded as the balloon is inflated. It then remains in the artery as a prop after the balloon is removed. Endothelial cells will completely line the inner wall of the stent to produce a smooth inner lining. Antiplatelet medications (aspirin and ticlopidine) are given following stent insertion to reduce the risk of thrombus formation at the site.

In contrast to stent procedures, which enlarge the artery by displacing plaque, atherectomy procedures remove plaque from the identified lesion. The directional atherectomy catheter shaves the plaque off vessel walls using a rotary cutting head, retaining the fragments in its housing and removing them from the vessel. Rotational atherectomy catheters pulverise plaque into particles small enough to pass through the coronary microcirculation. Laser atherectomy devices use laser energy to remove plaque.

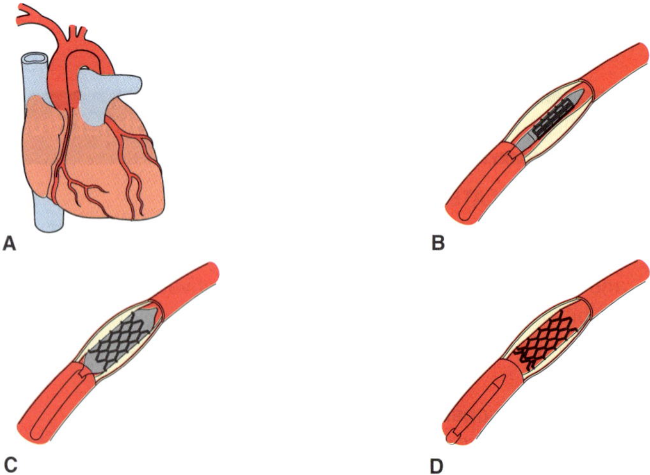

FIGURE 29.2 ***Percutaneous coronary revascularisation. A, The balloon catheter with the stent is threaded into the affected coronary artery. B, C, The stent is positioned across the blockage and expanded. D, The balloon is deflated and removed, leaving the stent in place***

Complications following PTCA procedures include haematoma at the catheter insertion site, pseudoaneurysm, embolism, hypersensitivity to contrast dye, arrhythmias, bleeding and vessel perforation. Other complications include restenosis or reocclusion of the treated vessel.

Nursing care of the person undergoing PTCA is outlined in the accompanying box.

CORONARY ARTERY BYPASS GRAFTING Surgery for coronary heart disease involves using a section of a vein or an artery to create a connection (or bypass) between the aorta and the coronary artery beyond the obstruction (see Figure 29.3). This then allows blood to perfuse the ischaemic portion of the heart. The internal mammary artery in the chest and the saphenous vein from the leg are the vessels most commonly used for CABG.

Bypass grafts are safe and effective. Angina is totally relieved or significantly reduced in 90% of people who undergo complete revascularisation. While anginal pain may recur within 3 years, it rarely is as severe as before surgery. Coronary artery bypass graft has a positive effect on mortality in many cases. It is recommended for people who have multiple vessel disease and impaired left ventricular function or diabetes, and for people who have significant obstruction of the left main coronary artery (Kalyanasundaram, 2020).

A median sternotomy commonly is used to access the heart. The heart is usually stopped during surgery by administration of a transient paralysing agent called cardioplegia. The *cardiopulmonary bypass (CPB) pump* is used to maintain perfusion to the rest of the organs during open-heart surgery. Venous blood is removed from the body through a cannula placed in the right

NURSING CARE OF THE PERSON **undergoing PTCA**

BEFORE THE PROCEDURE

- Assess the person's knowledge of the procedure and expectations of treatment. *This allows information to be tailored to the person's needs and provides an opportunity to clarify misconceptions.*
- Describe the cardiac catheterisation laboratory and the planned PTCA procedure, including:
  - preoperative preparation (see the chapter 'Nursing care of people having surgery')
  - planned anaesthesia or sedation to be used
  - drugs that may be given during the procedure, such as anticoagulants to reduce the risk of thrombus formation; intravenous glyceryl trinitrate; and a calcium channel blocker to dilate coronary arteries and prevent anginal pain.
- Discuss possible sensations during the procedure, including flushing or warmth and a metallic taste in the mouth as the contrast dye is injected, and a feeling of pressure or chest pain during balloon inflation. *Advanced preparation for expected sensations reduces anxiety and improves outcomes.*
- Perform a comprehensive assessment, including hydration status (skin and mucous membrane moisture, turgor) and peripheral circulation (colour, warmth, sensation, pulses and capillary refill).

AFTER THE PROCEDURE

- Complete a head-to-toe assessment. Note any complaints of chest pain or evidence of decreased cardiac output or myocardial infarction. *Assessment provides a baseline for subsequent assessments and allows early identification of possible complications.*
- Monitor vital signs and cardiac rhythm continuously. Treat arrhythmias as ordered. Obtain a 12-lead ECG if signs of ischaemia develop and notify the treating team. *Vital signs reflect cardiac output. Arrhythmias may develop with reperfusion of the ischaemic myocardium. ECG changes may indicate infarction or restenosis of the affected vessel.*
- Maintain intravenous glyceryl trinitrate infusion. Administer anticoagulant and antiplatelet medications, nitrates and calcium channel blockers as ordered. *These drugs decrease oxygen demand and increase oxygen supply by dilating the coronary arteries and systemic vasculature. They also reduce the risk of thrombus formation.*
- Monitor for and treat or report chest pain as indicated. *Chest pain may indicate ischaemia and possible myocardial infarction.*
- Maintain bed rest as ordered with the head of the bed at 30 degrees or less. Prevent flexion of the leg on the affected side. Following sheath removal, follow protocol for pressure dressing or device or sandbag placement. *A large puncture wound occurs at the insertion site. Immobilisation allows the wound to seal; a pressure dressing helps prevent bleeding.*
- Monitor distal pulses, colour, movement, sensation and temperature of the affected leg and insertion site every 15 minutes for the first hour, every 30 minutes for the next hour, every hour for the next 8 hours, then every 4 hours. A clot may form at the site, reducing perfusion of the affected leg. The site and dressing are monitored for excessive bleeding, haematoma formation or pseudoaneurysm. *Pseudoaneurysm occurs as a result of inadequate haemostasis after catheter removal.*
- Monitor intake and output, serum electrolytes, urea, creatinine, full blood count (FBC), activated partial thromboplastin time (aPTT) and cardiac enzymes. Report abnormal results to the medical officer. *Contrast dye causes osmotic diuresis and may cause kidney damage or a hypersensitivity reaction. Electrolyte imbalances increase the risk of arrhythmias. Cardiac enzymes are monitored for indications of possible myocardial damage during the procedure. The aPTT monitors the effectiveness of heparin therapy.*
- Monitor for bradycardia, light-headedness, hypotension, diaphoresis and loss of consciousness during sheath removal. Keep atropine at bedside during sheath removal. Bradycardia and signs of decreased cardiac output may occur during sheath removal because of a vasovagal reaction. *Atropine decreases vagal tone and increases heart rate.*

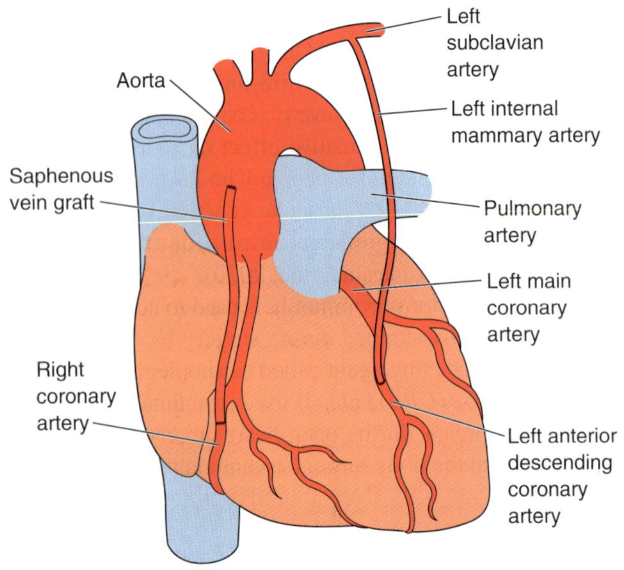

FIGURE 29.3 ***Coronary artery bypass grafting using the internal mammary artery and a saphenous vein graft***

atrium or the superior and inferior venae cavae. Blood then circulates through the CPB pump, where it is oxygenated, its temperature is regulated and it is filtered. Oxygenated blood is returned to the body through a cannula in the ascending aorta (see Figure 29.4). Cardiopulmonary bypass enables surgeons to operate on a still heart and a relatively bloodless field. Hypothermia can be maintained to reduce the metabolic rate and decrease oxygen demand during surgery.

Newer techniques have been developed that allow surgeons to perform CABG without cardioplegia (stopping the heart) and CPB. Off-pump coronary artery bypass (OPCAB) allows use of a smaller incision for access. Although cardiopulmonary bypass is employed for the majority of coronary artery bypass procedures, OPCAB is a promising alternative. OPCABs reduce mortality and morbidity rates and result in faster recovery for the person undergoing OPCAB as compared to CABG with cardiopulmonary bypass (Kalyanasundaram, 2020).

Even more recently, a technique known as robotic CABG has emerged. The surgeon uses a computer to manipulate robotic arms to undertake surgery on anterior vessels in a more endoscopic approach (Kalyanasundaram, 2020). Early evidence is suggesting that this intervention may become a valuable and less traumatic option for selected individuals.

When the saphenous vein is used, it is excised from its normal attachments in the leg and flushed with a cold heparinised saline solution. It is then reversed so that its valves do not interfere with blood flow. When appropriate, a laparoscopic approach may be used to remove the vein. The vein is *anastomosed* (grafted) to the aorta and the coronary artery, distal to

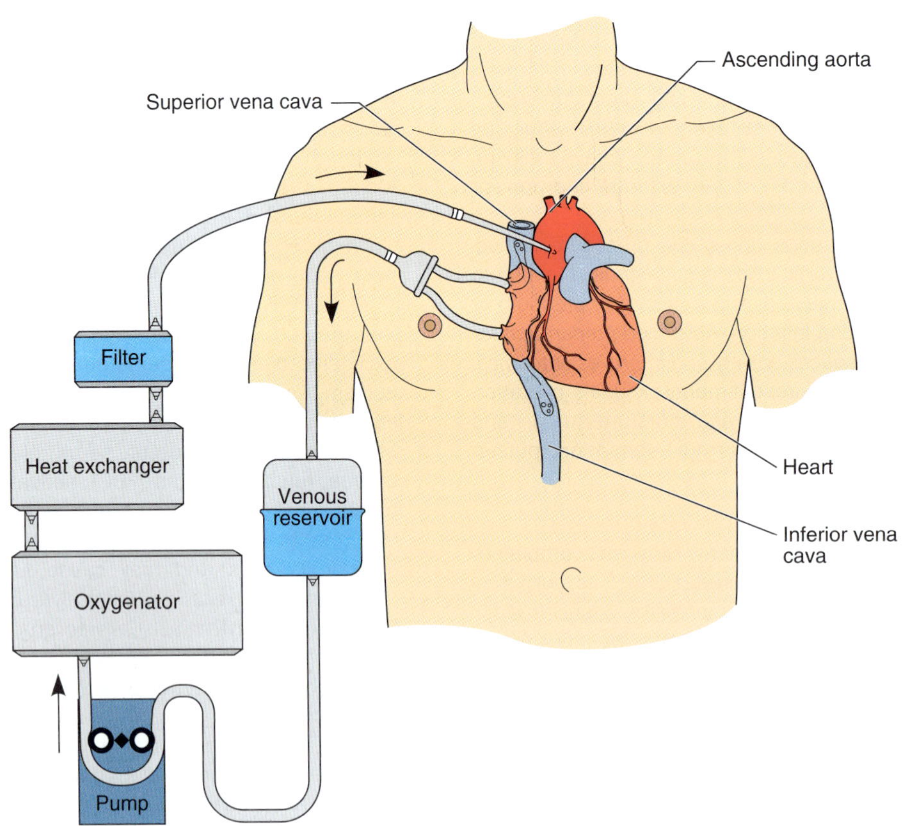

FIGURE 29.4 ***A diagrammatic representation of cardiopulmonary bypass. A cannula in the superior and inferior venae cavae removes venous blood, which is then pumped through an oxygenator and heat exchanger. After filtering, oxygenated blood is returned to the ascending aorta***

the occlusion (see Figure 29.3). This provides a bridge or conduit for blood flow past the obstruction. If the internal mammary artery (IMA) is used, its distal end is excised and anastomosed to the coronary artery distal to the obstruction. The IMA often is used to revascularise the left coronary artery because of the greater oxygen demand of the left ventricle.

Once grafting is completed, cardiopulmonary bypass is discontinued and the person is rewarmed. Rewarming stimulates the heart to resume beating. Temporary pacing wires are sutured in place and passed through the chest wall in case temporary pacing is necessary. Chest tubes are placed in the pleural space and mediastinum to drain blood and re-establish negative pressure in the thoracic cavity, and to drain bleeding as a result of the operation. The sternum is closed using heavy wires and bone wax, the skin is closed with sutures or staples, and sterile dressings are applied over sternal and leg incisions.

Pre- and postoperative nursing care and teaching for the person having a coronary artery bypass graft or other open-heart surgery are outlined in the 'Nursing care of the person' box.

NURSING CARE OF THE PERSON **having coronary artery bypass grafts**

PREOPERATIVE CARE

- Provide routine preoperative care and teaching as outlined in the chapter 'Nursing care of people having surgery'.
- Verify presence of laboratory and diagnostic test results in the chart, including full blood count (FBC), serum electrolytes, coagulation profile, urinalysis, chest x-ray and coronary angiogram. *These baseline data are important for comparison of postoperative results and values.*
- Type and crossmatch four or more units of blood as ordered or establish arrangements for existing autologous transfusion. *Blood is made available for use during and after surgery as needed.*
- Collaborate with the person and their family with specific teaching related to procedure and postoperative care. Include the following topics:
  - cardiac recovery unit; sensory stimuli, personnel; noise and alarms; visiting policies
  - tubes, drains and general appearance
  - monitoring equipment, including cardiac and haemodynamic monitoring systems
  - respiratory support: ventilator, endotracheal tube, suctioning; communication while intubated
  - incisions and dressings
  - pain management.

  Preoperative teaching reduces anxiety and prepares the person and family for the postoperative environment and expected sensations.

POSTOPERATIVE CARE

Provide routine postoperative care as outlined in the chapter 'Nursing care of people having surgery'. In addition to the care needs of all individuals having major surgery, the person having cardiac surgery has specific care needs related to open-heart and thoracic surgery. These are outlined under the nursing diagnoses identified below.

Decreased cardiac output

Cardiac output may be compromised postoperatively due to bleeding and fluid loss; depression of myocardial function by drugs, hypothermia and surgical manipulation; arrhythmias; increased vascular resistance; and a potential complication, *cardiac tamponade*, compression of the heart due to collected blood or fluid in the pericardium.

- Cardiac rhythm, intra-arterial blood pressure, ventilation, oxygen saturation and haemodynamic parameters are monitored continuously. Note trends and report significant changes to the treating team. *Initial hypothermia and bradycardia are expected; the heart rate should return to the normal range with rewarming. The blood pressure may fall during rewarming as peripheral vasodilation occurs. Hypotension and tachycardia, however, may indicate low cardiac output. Pulmonary artery pressure (PAP), pulmonary artery wedge pressure (PAWP), cardiac output and oxygen saturation are often monitored to evaluate fluid volume, cardiac function and gas exchange.* Haemodynamic monitoring is further discussed in the chapter 'Nursing care of people with cardiac disorders'.
- Auscultate heart and breath sounds on admission and at least every 4 hours. *A ventricular gallop, or S_3, is an early sign of heart failure; an S_4 may indicate decreased ventricular compliance. Muffled heart sounds may be an early indication of cardiac tamponade. Adventitious breath sounds (wheezes or rales—crackles) may be a manifestation of heart failure or respiratory compromise.*
- Assess skin colour and temperature, peripheral pulses and level of consciousness with vital signs. *Pale, mottled or cyanotic colouring, cool and clammy skin, and diminished pulse amplitude are indicators of decreased cardiac output.*
- Continuously monitor and document cardiac rhythm. *Arrhythmias are common and may interfere with cardiac filling and contractility, decreasing the cardiac output.*
- Measure intake and output hourly. Report urine output less than 0.5 mL/kg per hour for 2 consecutive hours. *Intake and output measurements help evaluate fluid volume status. A fall in urine output may be an early indicator of decreased cardiac output.*
- Record chest tube output hourly. *Chest tube drainage greater than 70 mL/h or that is warm, bright red and free flowing indicates haemorrhage and may necessitate a return to surgery. A sudden drop in chest tube output may indicate impending cardiac tamponade.* Monitoring for the presence of pulsus paradoxis and pulsus alternans should occur.
- Monitor haemoglobin, haematocrit and serum electrolytes. *A drop in haemoglobin and haematocrit may indicate haemorrhage that is not otherwise obvious. Electrolyte imbalances—potassium, calcium and magnesium, in particular—affect cardiac rhythm and contractility.*
- Administer intravenous fluids, fluid boluses and blood transfusions as ordered. *Fluid and blood replacement helps ensure adequate blood volume and oxygen-carrying capacity.*

(continued)

NURSING CARE OF THE PERSON having coronary artery bypass grafts (continued)

- Administer medications as ordered. *Medications ordered in the early postoperative period to maintain the cardiac output include inotropic drugs (e.g. dopamine, dobutamine) to increase the force of myocardial contractions; vasodilators (e.g. nitroprusside or glyceryl trinitrate) to decrease vascular resistance and afterload; and anti-arrhythmic agents to correct arrhythmias that affect cardiac output.*
- Keep a temporary pacemaker at the bedside; initiate pacing as indicated. *Temporary pacing may be needed to maintain the cardiac output with bradyarrhythmias, such as high-level AV blocks.*

CONSIDERATION FOR PRACTICE

Assess for signs of cardiac tamponade: increased heart rate, decreased BP, decreased urine output, increased central venous pressure, a sudden decrease in chest tube output, muffled/distant heart sounds and diminished peripheral pulses. Institute an emergency response call immediately. Cardiac tamponade is a life-threatening complication that may develop postoperatively. Cardiac tamponade interferes with ventricular filling and contraction, decreasing cardiac output. Untreated, cardiac tamponade leads to cardiogenic shock and possible cardiac arrest.

Hypothermia

Hypothermia is maintained during cardiac surgery to reduce the metabolic rate and protect vital organs from ischaemic damage. Although rewarming is instituted on completion of the surgery, the person often remains hypothermic on admission to cardiac recovery. Gradual rewarming is necessary to prevent profound and rapid peripheral vasodilation and hypotension.

- Monitor core body temperature for the first 8 hours following surgery. Often an oesophageal temperature probe will be put in beside the nasogastric tubes. *Oral temperature measurements are not reliable indicators of core body temperature during this period. Tympanic temperature monitoring is indicated.*
- Institute rewarming measures (e.g. warmed intravenous solutions or blood transfusion, warm blankets, warm inspired gases, radiant heat lamps) as needed to maintain a temperature above 36°C. Administer medication (clonidine or fentanyl) to relieve shivering (as ordered). *Low body temperature may cause shivering, increasing oxygen demand. Hypothermia also increases the risk of hypoxia, metabolic acidosis, vasoconstriction and increased cardiac work, altered clotting and arrhythmias. If shivering cannot be controlled with opioid agents, paralysing agents may be needed if the individual's haemodynamic stability is compromised. This intervention is not desirable, but is occasionally necessary. Shivering and hypothermia increase oxygen demand by up to 400%.*

Acute pain

Following a CABG, pain is experienced due to both the thoracic incision and removal of the saphenous vein from the leg. Dissection of the internal mammary artery (usually the left IMA) from the chest wall also causes chest pain on the affected side. Chest tube sites are also uncomfortable. The leg from which the saphenous vein graft was obtained may be more painful than the chest incision.

- Frequently assess for pain, including its location and character. Document its intensity using a standard pain scale. Assess for verbal and non-verbal indicators of pain. Validate pain cues with the individual. *Pain is subjective and differs among individuals. Incisional pain is expected; however, anginal pain also may develop. It is important to differentiate the type of pain.*
- Administer analgesics on a scheduled basis, by patient-controlled analgesia (PCA), or by continuous infusion for the first 24 to 48 hours. *Research demonstrates that adequate pain management in the immediate postoperative period reduces complications from sympathetic stimulation and allows faster recovery. Pain causes muscle tension and vasoconstriction, impairing circulation and tissue perfusion, slowing wound healing and increasing cardiac work.*
- Pre-medicate 30 minutes before activities or planned procedures. *Pre-medication and the subsequent reduction of pain improve the person's participation and their cooperation with care.*

CONSIDERATION FOR PRACTICE

Promptly report chest pain. Cardiac pain may indicate a perioperative or postoperative myocardial infarction.

Ineffective airway clearance/Impaired gas exchange

Atelectasis due to impaired ventilation and airway clearance is a common pulmonary complication of cardiac surgery. Gas exchange may also be affected by blood loss and decreased oxygen-carrying capacity following surgery. Phrenic nerve paralysis is a potential complication of cardiac surgery which may also contribute to impaired ventilation and gas exchange.

- Evaluate respiratory rate, depth, effort, symmetry of chest expansion and breath sounds frequently. *Pain, anxiety, excess fluid volume, surgical injury, narcotics and anaesthesia, and altered homeostasis can affect respiratory rate, depth and effort postoperatively. Decreased chest expansion or asymmetrical movement may indicate impaired ventilation of one lung and needs further evaluation.*
- Note endotracheal tube (ETT) placement on chest x-ray. Mark tube position and secure in place. *The chest x-ray documents correct ETT placement above the carina (bifurcation to the right and left mainstem bronchus). Marking its appropriate placement allows evaluation of potential tube movement. Secure the tube firmly in place to prevent slippage or inadvertent removal.*
- Maintain ventilator settings to optimise respiratory function and oxygenation. Monitor arterial blood gases (ABGs). *Mechanical ventilation promotes optimal lung expansion and oxygenation postoperatively. ABGs are used to evaluate oxygenation and acid–base balance.*
- Suction as needed. *Suctioning is performed only as indicated to clear airway secretions.*
- Prepare for ventilator weaning and extubation, as appropriate. *The individual is removed from the ventilator and*

NURSING CARE OF THE PERSON having coronary artery bypass grafts (continued)

extubated as soon as possible to reduce complications associated with mechanical ventilation and intubation.

- After extubation, and when appropriately alert, teach use of the incentive spirometer and encourage use every 2 hours. Encourage deep breathing; advise against vigorous coughing. Teach use of a 'cough pillow' to splint chest incision and decrease pain. Assist in frequent pressure area care and encourage movement. *Deep breathing, controlled coughing and position changes improve ventilation and airway clearance and help prevent complications. Vigorous coughing may excessively increase intrathoracic pressure and cause sternal instability.*

Risk of infection

Following an open chest procedure, a sternal infection may develop that can progress to involve the mediastinum. Incisions for removal of the saphenous vein also may become infected. People with IMA grafts who are diabetic, older or malnourished are at high risk: harvesting of IMA disrupts blood supply to the sternum, and these individuals have impaired immune responses and healing.

- Assess sternal incision and leg wounds frequently each shift. Document redness, warmth, swelling and/or drainage from the site. Note wound approximation. *These assessments provide indicators of inflammation and healing.*
- Depending on the type of dressing applied in the operating suite, it might be necessary to maintain a sterile dressing for the first 48 hours and then leave the incision exposed. Use wound approximation strips as needed to maintain approximation of the wound edges. Alternatively, an occlusive dressing may be left in situ longer. *Care to reduce the risk of wound infection is paramount.*
- Report signs of wound infection: a swollen, erythematous area that is hot and painful to the touch; drainage from the wound; impaired healing or healed areas that reopen. *Evidence of infection or impaired healing requires further evaluation and treatment. Individuals with a subclinical infection will often report greater pain from the surgical wound.*
- Sample wound drainage for microscopy, culture and sensitivity if indicated. *Identifying the infective organism facilitates appropriate antibiotic therapy.*
- Collaborate with the dietitian to promote nutrition and fluid intake. *Good nutritional status is vital to healing and immune function.*

Psychological alterations

Many factors affect neuropsychological function after CABG, including the length of cardiopulmonary bypass, age, pre-surgery organic brain dysfunction, severity of illness and decreased cardiac output. Sensory overload and deprivation, sleep disruption and numerous drugs also affect thinking and mental clarity.

- Frequently reorient during initial recovery period. Remind the person that surgery is over and that the person is in the recovery area. *Frequent reorientation provides emotional support.*
- Explain all procedures before performing them. Speak in a clear, calm voice. Encourage questions and give honest answers. *These measures provide information, decrease anxiety and establish trust.*
- Secure all intravenous lines and invasive catheters/tubes (e.g. ETT, urinary catheter, nasogastric tube). *Disoriented individuals may tug or pull at invasive equipment, disrupting them and increasing the risk of injury.*
- Note verbal responses to questions. Correct misconceptions immediately. *False beliefs or confused impressions regarding care may result in further confusion or refusal to accept necessary care.*
- Orientate the individual to person, place and time (PPT). *This reduces confusion and assists the person to participate more in recovery.*
- Involve family members in providing reorientation. Place familiar objects and photographs within view. Encourage family presence. *The family provides reassurance and contact with the familiar, assisting with orientation.*
- Promote participation in their own care and decision making as appropriate. *This allows the person to maintain a degree of power and control and enables the individual to take an active role in recovery.*
- Report signs of hallucinations, delusions, depression or agitation. *These may indicate progressive deterioration of mental status.*
- Administer sedatives cautiously. *Mild sedation may help prevent injury. Some sedatives may, however, have adverse effects, such as respiratory depression, increasing confusion and disorientation.*
- Re-evaluate neurological status every shift or whenever change is noted. *These data allow evaluation of the effect of interventions.*

MINIMALLY INVASIVE CORONARY ARTERY SURGERY

Minimally invasive coronary artery surgery is a potential future alternative to CABG. Two approaches may be used. *Port-access coronary artery bypass* uses several small holes, or 'ports', in the chest wall to access vessels for connection to the CPB pump and the surgical site. Alternatively, the femoral artery and femoral vein may be used for CPB. CPB is avoided altogether using the *minimally invasive direct coronary artery bypass* (MIDCAB) approach. With MIDCAB, a small surgical incision and several chest wall ports are used to graft a chest wall artery to the affected coronary vessel while the heart continues to beat. Beta-blockers are often used to reduce the heart rate to reduce movement in the surgical site.

TRANSMYOCARDIAL LASER REVASCULARISATION A new development in myocardial revascularisation techniques is called *transmyocardial laser revascularisation (TMLR)*. In this procedure, a laser is used to drill tiny holes into the myocardial muscle itself to provide collateral blood flow to ischaemic muscle. Individuals whose coronary artery obstructions are too diffuse to bypass are candidates for this new surgical treatment.

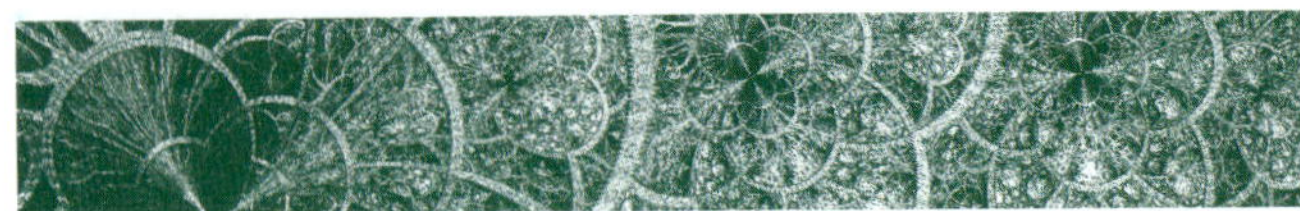

Nursing care

Health promotion, assessment, nursing diagnoses and interventions for the person with ACS are similar to those identified for people with angina and with acute myocardial infarction. See the preceding and subsequent sections of this chapter for specific nursing care activities, as well as the nursing care plan.

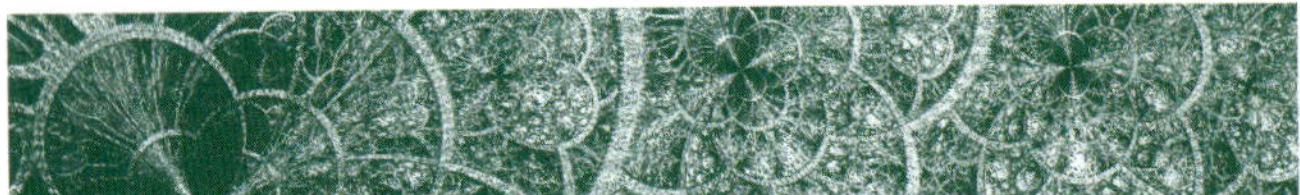

THE PERSON WITH ACUTE MYOCARDIAL INFARCTION

An **acute myocardial infarction (AMI)**—necrosis (death) of myocardial cells—is a life-threatening event. If circulation to the affected myocardium is not promptly restored, loss of functional myocardium affects the heart's ability to maintain an effective cardiac output. This may ultimately lead to cardiogenic shock and death.

Many deaths from MI occur during the first few hours after symptoms begin. Heightening public awareness of the manifestations of MI, the importance of seeking immediate medical assistance and training in cardiopulmonary resuscitation (CPR) techniques are vital to decrease deaths due to MI.

Myocardial infarction rarely occurs in people without pre-existing coronary heart disease. While no specific cause

NURSING CARE PLAN A person having coronary artery bypass surgery

Six weeks ago, John Clements, aged 50, was discharged from the hospital after emergency triple bypass surgery. Despite having emergency surgery, his postoperative recovery was uneventful and he was discharged 6 days after admission. He returns to the clinic for a postoperative stress test and to discuss his cardiac rehabilitation program.

ASSESSMENT

Mr Clements' medical history reveals significant CHD and an anterior wall myocardial infarction that led to his emergency triple bypass, and hyperlipidaemia. Current medications include diltiazem, isosorbide mononitrate, aspirin and a glyceryl nitrate patch. The ECG reveals sinus rhythm with some ST segment and T wave flattening, resting heart rate 68 and blood pressure 136/84.

Mr Clements has a family history of CHD. He does not smoke and uses alcohol occasionally in social situations. He enjoys takeaway fried chicken and watching television. Mr Clements states his only regular exercise used to be an evening of indoor volleyball about once a month, 'But I get short of breath walking around the block now, so I guess I can't play anymore!'

Mr Clements owns his own contracting business and states that he typically works about 50 to 60 hours per week. He doesn't know what the cardiac rehabilitation program is supposed to do for him. 'I have got to get back to work! You just can't sit around in my business—you have to make sure that the work is getting done on time and you have to check on supplies and equipment and the like. But I feel like a weakling—I need to get my energy back!'

DIAGNOSIS

- *Activity intolerance* related to general weakness and fatigue and manifested by inability to perform activities.
- *Ineffective role performance* related to health crisis manifested by inability to return to work.

PLANNING

- Define the purpose and components of a cardiac rehabilitation program.
- Enrol in 'cardiac rehabilitation' classes, including cardiac anatomy, physiology and coronary heart disease; exercise and activity prescriptions; lifestyle modifications, including diet counselling and stress management; emotional reactions to CAD; sexual activity; use of cardiac medications; and self-responsibility for health.
- Plan an exercise program based on stress test results, physical examination and interview.
- Encourage to schedule rest periods before and after activity/exercise.
- Review signs and symptoms of overexertion.
- Provide information about community resources for emotional and educational support.
- Assist to identify strategies for dealing with concerns about his business role.

Expected outcomes

- Verbalise an understanding of the definition and components of his structured cardiac rehabilitation program.
- Verbalise a desire to make lifestyle changes.
- Identify resources available in the community to assist with lifestyle changes.

IMPLEMENTATION

- Participate in his activity program without suffering any complications.
- Report an increase in energy after 6 weeks on the program.
- Manage the temporary change in his usual work responsibilities in a way that is appropriate for him.

EVALUATION

Mr Clements decides to 'give the rehab program a try'. Together, the cardiac rehabilitation team work with him to plan an individualised exercise/activity program. A dietitian provides dietary counselling. Stress management strategies are emphasised. Mr Clements is able to list manifestations of overexertion and states that he realises the need for gradual activity progression.

After 6 weeks, Mr Clements has reported a significant increase in energy and strength. 'I am feeling much stronger and have been sleeping better. Mary and I are taking evening walks around the neighbourhood. My chest soreness is also gone.' He has completed the 12-week cardiac rehabilitation program and another stress test indicates that his cardiac function is adequate. Mr Clements has joined the local National Heart Foundation 'Just Walk

NURSING CARE PLAN **A person having coronary artery bypass surgery (continued)**

It' group and states that he is now incorporating 'heart-healthy' considerations into his daily routines.

CRITICAL THINKING IN THE NURSING PROCESS

1 Develop a personalised risk factor reduction plan for Mr Clements.
2 How might denial affect Mr Clements' ability to: (a) accept the need for cardiac rehabilitation, (b) comply with the proposed lifestyle changes, and (c) make permanent adjustments to his daily life?
3 How does partner support influence an individual's engagement with and adherence to a structured cardiac rehabilitation program?
4 Mr Clements tells you that since the surgery, his wife has been afraid that sexual activity will induce another heart attack. How would you respond to these concerns?

CRITICAL THINKING IN PERSON-CENTRED CARE

1 Given the significance of cardiovascular function on exercise tolerance, is there a risk that Mr Clements may further damage his myocardium if demand outweighs supply? If so, what are the risks and how can they be avoided?
2 Outline what you have learned from this case study that you will apply to your clinical practice.

has been identified, the risk factors for MI are those for coronary heart disease: age, gender, heredity, race, smoking, obesity, hyperlipidaemia, hypertension, diabetes, sedentary lifestyle, diet and others. See the previous section of this chapter on coronary heart disease for further discussion of these risk factors.

Pathophysiology

Atherosclerotic plaque may form stable or unstable lesions. *Stable* lesions progress by gradually occluding the vessel lumen, whereas *unstable* (or *complicated*) lesions are prone to rupture and thrombus formation (Bullock & Hales, 2019). Stable lesions often cause angina (discussed previously); unstable lesions often lead to acute coronary syndromes or acute ischaemic heart diseases. Acute coronary syndromes include unstable angina, myocardial infarction and sudden cardiac death.

Myocardial infarction occurs when blood flow to a portion of cardiac muscle is completely blocked, resulting in prolonged tissue ischaemia and irreversible cell damage. Coronary occlusion is usually caused by ulceration or rupture of a complicated atherosclerotic lesion. When an atherosclerotic lesion ruptures or ulcerates, substances are released that stimulate platelet aggregation, thrombin generation and local vasomotor tone. As a result, the vessel constricts and a thrombus (clot) forms, occluding the vessel and interrupting blood flow to the myocardium distal to the obstruction.

Cellular injury occurs when the cells are denied adequate oxygen and nutrients. When ischaemia is prolonged, lasting more than 20 to 45 minutes, irreversible hypoxaemic damage causes cellular death and tissue necrosis. Oxygen, glycogen and ATP stores of ischaemic cells are rapidly depleted. Cellular metabolism shifts to an anaerobic process, producing hydrogen ions and lactic acid. Cellular acidosis increases cells' vulnerability to further damage. Intracellular enzymes are released through damaged cell membranes into interstitial spaces.

Cellular acidosis, electrolyte imbalances and hormones released in response to cellular ischaemia affect impulse conduction and myocardial contractility. The risk of arrhythmias increases and myocardial contractility decreases, reducing stroke volume, cardiac output, blood pressure and tissue perfusion.

The subendocardium suffers the initial damage, within 20 minutes of injury, because this area is the most susceptible to changes in coronary blood flow. If blood flow is restored at this point, the infarction is limited to subendocardial tissue (a *subendocardial* or *non-Q-wave infarction*). The damage progresses to the epicardium within 1 to 6 hours. When all layers of the myocardium are affected, it is known as a *transmural infarction*. A significant Q wave develops with a transmural infarction, so this may also be called a *Q-wave MI*. Complications such as heart failure are more frequently associated with Q-wave MIs; however, individuals with non-Q-wave MIs frequently experience recurrent ischaemia or subsequent MI within weeks or months of the event (Burke, 2021).

The necrotic, infarcted tissue is surrounded by regions of injured and ischaemic tissues. Tissue in this ischaemic area is potentially viable; restoration of blood flow minimises the amount of tissue lost. This surrounding tissue also undergoes metabolic changes. It may be *stunned*, its contractility impaired for hours to days following reperfusion, or *hibernating*, a process that protects myocytes until perfusion is restored. *Myocardial remodelling* also may occur, with cellular hypertrophy and loss of contractility in regions distant from the infarction. Rapid restoration of blood flow limits these changes (Bullock & Hales, 2019).

When a larger artery is compromised, *collateral vessels* connecting smaller arteries in the coronary system dilate to maintain blood flow to the cardiac muscle. The degree of collateral circulation helps determine the extent of myocardial damage from ischaemia. Acute occlusion of a coronary artery without any collateral flow results in massive tissue damage and possible death. Progressive narrowing of the larger coronary arteries allows collateral channels to develop and enlarge, meeting the demand for blood flow. Good collateral circulation can limit the size of an MI.

Myocardial infarctions are described by the damaged area of the heart. The coronary artery that is occluded determines the area of damage. Myocardial infarction usually affects the left ventricle because it is the major 'workhorse' of the heart; its muscle mass is greater, as are its oxygen demands. Occlusion of the left anterior descending (LAD) artery affects blood flow to the anterior wall of the left ventricle (an *anterior MI*) and part of the interventricular septum. Occlusion of the left circumflex artery (LCA) causes a lateral MI. *Right ventricular, inferior* and *posterior infarcts* involve occlusions of the right coronary artery (RCA) and posterior descending artery (PDA). Occlusion of the left main coronary artery is the most devastating, causing ischaemia of the entire left ventricle and a grave prognosis. Identifying the infarct site helps predict possible complications and determine appropriate therapy.

Cocaine-induced MI

Acute myocardial infarction may develop due to cocaine intoxication. Cocaine increases sympathetic nervous system activity by both increasing the release of catecholamines from central and peripheral stores and interfering with the reuptake of catecholamines. This increased catecholamine concentration stimulates the heart rate and increases its contractility, increases the automaticity of cardiac tissues and the risk of arrhythmias, and causes vasoconstriction and hypertension. The person with cocaine-induced MI may present with an altered level of consciousness, confusion and restlessness, seizure activity, tachycardia, hypotension, increased respiratory rate and respiratory crackles.

Manifestations

Pain is a classic manifestation of myocardial infarction. Chest pain secondary to MI may be more severe than anginal pain. However, it is not the intensity of the chest pain that distinguishes MI from angina or acute coronary syndrome, but its duration and its continuous nature. The onset of pain is sudden and usually is not associated with activity. In fact, most MIs occur in the early morning. People with a history of angina may have more frequent anginal attacks in the days or weeks prior to an MI (unstable angina or ACS). Chest pain may be described as crushing and severe; as a pressure, heavy or squeezing sensation; or as chest tightness or burning. The pain often begins in the centre of the chest (*substernal*) and may radiate to the shoulders, neck, jaw or arms. It lasts more than 15 to 20 minutes and is not relieved by rest or glyceryl trinitrate.

Women and older adults often experience atypical chest pain, presenting with complaints of indigestion, heartburn, nausea and vomiting. The greater diversity of clinical manifestations experienced by women having a cardiovascular event decreases the likelihood of healthcare professionals recognising an event, and also reduces the likelihood of the woman seeking assistance (Cardeillac et al., 2022).

Compensatory mechanisms cause many of the other symptoms of MI. Sympathetic nervous system stimulation causes anxiety, tachycardia and vasoconstriction. This results in cool, clammy, mottled skin. Pain and blood chemistry changes stimulate the respiratory centre, causing tachypnoea. The person often has a sense of impending doom and death. Tissue necrosis causes an inflammatory reaction that increases the white blood cell count and elevates the temperature. Serum cardiac enzyme levels rise as enzymes are released from necrotic myocytes.

Other manifestations may vary, depending on the location and amount of infarcted tissue. Hypertension, hypotension or signs of heart failure may develop. Vagal stimulation may cause nausea and vomiting, bradycardia and hypotension. Hiccupping may develop due to diaphragmatic irritation. Inferior infarction often causes vomiting due to vagus nerve proximity. If a large vessel is occluded, the first sign of MI may be sudden death. Typical manifestations of MI are listed in the 'Manifestations' box.

Complications

The risk of complications associated with myocardial infarction is related to the size and location of the MI.

Arrhythmias

Arrhythmias, disturbances or irregularities of heart rhythm, are the most frequent complication of MI. Arrhythmias are discussed in detail in the next section of this chapter.

Infarcted tissue is *arrhythmogenic*; that is, it affects the generation and conduction of electrical impulses in the heart, increasing the risk of arrhythmias. Premature ventricular contractions (PVCs) are common following an MI and may be predictive of more dangerous arrhythmias such as ventricular tachycardia or ventricular fibrillation (Burke, 2021). The risk of ventricular fibrillation is greatest the first hour after MI; it is a frequent cause of sudden cardiac death associated with acute MI. Its incidence declines with time. If the infarct affects a conduction pathway, electrical conduction may be affected. Any degree of AV block may occur following MI, especially when the anterior wall is infarcted. First-degree and Mobitz I (Wenckebach) blocks are most common, although complete

MANIFESTATIONS Acute myocardial infarction

- Chest pain: substernal or precordial (across the entire chest wall); may radiate to neck, jaw, shoulder(s) or left arm
- Tachycardia, tachypnoea
- Dyspnoea, shortness of breath
- Nausea and vomiting
- Anxiety, sense of impending doom
- Diaphoresis
- Cool, mottled skin; diminished peripheral pulses
- Hypotension or hypertension
- Palpitations, arrhythmias
- Signs of left heart failure
- Decreased level of consciousness

MEETING INDIVIDUALISED NEEDS **Recognising acute myocardial infarction in women and older adults**

Women and older adults often present with atypical manifestations of MI. However, heart disease is the number one cause of death in both groups, making early recognition and aggressive treatment vital.

Women are more likely than men to have a 'silent' or unrecognised heart attack or to present in cardiac arrest or with cardiogenic shock. Women often experience epigastric pain and nausea, causing them to blame their discomfort on heartburn. Shortness of breath is common, as is fatigue and weakness of the shoulders and upper arms.

Older people often seek treatment for vague complaints of difficulty breathing, confusion, fainting, dizziness, abdominal pain or cough. They often attribute their symptoms to a stroke. The prevalence of silent ischaemia is greater in older adults.

Stress the importance of seeking medical help promptly for atypical manifestations of MI. Prompt diagnosis and intervention reduces the mortality and morbidity of MI in women and older adults, just as it does in men. Despite this fact, both women and older adults are more likely to delay seeking treatment and are less likely to be accurately diagnosed and aggressively treated for CHD. Women are almost three times more likely to die from heart disease than from breast cancer (National Heart Foundation, 2021).

heart block may develop. Bradyarrhythmias (abnormal slow rhythms) also may develop, particularly when the inferior wall of the ventricle is affected.

Pump failure

Myocardial infarction reduces myocardial contractility, ventricular wall motion and compliance. Impaired contractility and filling may produce heart failure. The risk of heart failure is greatest when large portions of the left ventricle are infarcted. Heart failure may be more severe with an anterior infarction. Loss of 20–30% of the left ventricular muscle mass may cause manifestations of left-sided heart failure, including dyspnoea, fatigue, weakness and respiratory crackles on auscultation. Inferior or right ventricular MI may lead to right-sided heart failure with manifestations such as neck vein distension and peripheral oedema. Haemodynamic monitoring including cardiac output is often initiated for people with evidence of heart failure. Heart failure and its manifestations are discussed in greater depth in the chapter 'Nursing care of people with cardiac disorders'.

CARDIOGENIC SHOCK *Cardiogenic shock*, impaired tissue perfusion due to pump failure, results when functioning myocardial muscle mass decreases by more than 40%. The heart is unable to pump enough blood to meet the needs of the body and maintain organ function. Low cardiac output due to cardiogenic shock also impairs perfusion of the coronary arteries and myocardium, further increasing tissue damage. Mortality from cardiogenic shock is greater than 70%, although this can be reduced by prompt intervention with revascularisation procedures (Ren, 2019). See the chapter 'Nursing care of people experiencing trauma and shock' for a more extensive discussion of cardiogenic shock.

Infarct extension

Approximately 10% of people experience extension or reinfarction in the area of the original infarction during the first 10 to 14 days after an MI. *Extension* of the MI is characterised by increased myocardial necrosis from continued blood flow impairment and ongoing injury. *Expansion* of the MI is described as a permanent expansion of the infarcted area from thinning and dilation of the muscle. Infarct extension and expansion may cause manifestations such as continuing chest pain, haemodynamic compromise and worsening heart failure.

Structural defects

Necrotic muscle is replaced by scar tissue that is thinner than the ventricular muscle mass. This can lead to such complications as ventricular aneurysm, rupture of the interventricular septum or papillary muscle, and myocardial rupture. A *ventricular aneurysm* is a weakening and bulging of the ventricular wall. It may develop when a large section of the ventricle is replaced by scar tissue. Because it does not contract during systole, stroke volume decreases. Blood may pool within the aneurysm, causing clots to form. Ischaemia of the papillary muscle or chordae tendineae may cause structural damage leading to papillary muscle dysfunction or rupture. This affects AV valve function (usually the mitral valve), causing *regurgitation*, backflow of blood into the atria during systole. The interventricular septum may perforate or rupture due to ischaemia and infarction. Myocardial rupture is a risk between days 4 and 7 after MI, when the injured tissue is soft and weak. This potential complication of MI is often fatal.

Pericarditis

Tissue necrosis prompts an inflammatory response. *Pericarditis*, inflammation of the pericardial tissue surrounding the heart, may complicate AMI, usually within 2 to 3 days. Pericarditis causes chest pain that may be aching or sharp and stabbing, aggravated by movement or deep breathing. A *pericardial friction rub* may be heard on auscultation of heart sounds.

Dressler's syndrome, thought to be a hypersensitivity response to necrotic tissue or an autoimmune disorder, may develop days to weeks after AMI. It is a symptom complex characterised by fever, chest pain and dyspnoea. Dressler's syndrome may spontaneously resolve or recur over several months, causing significant discomfort and distress.

FAST FACTS

- Arrhythmias are the most common complication of AMI.
- Heart failure also is a common complication or consequence of myocardial infarction, developing due to loss of functional muscle tissue.

INTERPROFESSIONAL CARE

Immediate treatment goals for the person with an MI are to:

- relieve chest pain
- reduce the extent of myocardial damage
- maintain cardiovascular stability
- decrease cardiac workload
- prevent complications.

Slowing the process of coronary heart disease and reducing the risk of future MI is a major long-term management goal for the person.

Rapid assessment and early diagnosis are important in treating AMI. 'Time is muscle' is a clinical truism for the person with AMI. The evolution of an AMI is dynamic: the quicker the artery is reopened (medically, surgically or spontaneously), the more myocardium can be salvaged. Survival and long-term outcomes following AMI are improved by rapidly restoring blood flow to the 'stunned' myocardium surrounding the infarcted tissue, reducing myocardial oxygen demand and limiting the accumulation of toxic by-products of necrosis and reperfusion (Del Buono et al., 2021).

The major problem interfering with timely reperfusion is delay in seeking medical care following the onset of symptoms. Up to 44% of people with symptoms of chest discomfort or pain wait more than 4 hours before seeking treatment. Many factors are cited as reasons for treatment delay, including advanced age, the perception of the seriousness of symptoms, denial, access to medical care, the availability of an emergency response system and in-hospital delays. Immediate evaluation of the person presenting with manifestations of myocardial infarction is essential to early diagnosis and treatment.

Diagnosis

Diagnostic testing is used to establish the diagnosis of AMI.

- *Serum cardiac markers* are proteins released from necrotic heart muscle. The proteins most specific for diagnosis of MI are the cardiac-specific troponins and creatine kinase (CK or creatine phosphokinase, CPK) (see Table 29.5).
- *Creatine kinase* is an important enzyme for cellular function, found principally in cardiac and skeletal muscle and the brain. CK levels rise rapidly with damage to these tissues, appearing in the serum 4 to 6 hours after AMI, peaking within 12 to 24 hours, and then declining over the next 48 to 72 hours. The CK level correlates with the size of the infarction; the greater the amount of infarcted tissue, the higher the serum CK level.
- *CK-MB* (also called MB-bands) is a subset of CK specific to cardiac muscle. This isoenzyme of CK is considered the most sensitive indicator of MI. Elevated CK alone is not specific for MI; elevated CK-MB greater than 5% is considered a positive indicator of MI. CK-MB levels do not normally rise with chest pain from angina or causes other than MI.
- Cardiac muscle troponins, *cardiac-specific troponin T* (cT_nT) and *cardiac-specific troponin I* (cT_nI), are proteins released during myocardial infarction that are sensitive indicators of myocardial damage. These proteins are part of the actin–myosin unit in cardiac muscle and normally are not detectable in the blood. With necrosis of cardiac muscle, troponins are released and blood levels rise. The specificity of cT_nT and cT_nI to cardiac muscle necrosis makes these markers particularly useful when skeletal muscle trauma contributes to elevated CK levels (e.g. when CPR has been performed or traumatic injury occurred at the time of the MI). They are sensitive enough to detect very small infarctions that do not cause significant CK elevation. Both cT_nT and cT_nI remain in the blood for 10 to 14 days after an MI, making them useful to diagnose MI when medical treatment is delayed.

Serum levels of cardiac markers are ordered on admission and for 3 succeeding days. Serial blood levels help establish the diagnosis and determine the extent of myocardial damage.

Other laboratory tests may include the following:

- *Myoglobin* is one of the first cardiac markers to be detectable in the blood after an MI. It is released within 2 to 4 hours of symptom onset. However, its lack of specificity to cardiac muscle and rapid excretion (blood levels return to normal within 24 to 36 hours) limit its use (Gursahani, 2021).
- *Full blood count (FBC)* shows an elevated white blood cell (WBC) count due to inflammation of the injured myocardium. The erythrocyte sedimentation rate (ESR) also rises because of inflammation, although ESR is a non-specific marker of inflammation.
- *Arterial blood gases (ABGs)* may be ordered to assess blood oxygen levels and acid–base balance, and electrolytes such as potassium levels are also helpful.

Electrocardiography, echocardiography and myocardial nuclear scans are the most common diagnostic tests performed when AMI is suspected. With the exception of the ECG, the timing of these tests depends on the individual's immediate condition. Haemodynamic monitoring may be initiated in the unstable person following MI.

- The *electrocardiogram* reflects changes in conduction due to myocardial ischaemia and necrosis. Classic ECG changes seen in AMI include T-wave inversion, ST-segment elevation and formation of a Q wave. Ischaemic changes in the heart are seen as depression of the ST segment or inversion of the T wave (see Figure 29.1). With myocardial injury, elevation of the ST segment occurs (see Figure 29.5A). Significant Q-wave development (see Figure 29.5B) indicates a transmural or full-thickness infarction. Myocardial damage can be localised using the 12-lead ECG. Current Australian Resuscitation Council (ARC) guidelines (2016) recommend ECG measurement as soon as possible after patient contact. See the chapter 'A person-centred approach to assessing the cardiovascular and lymphatic systems' for more information about ECGs.

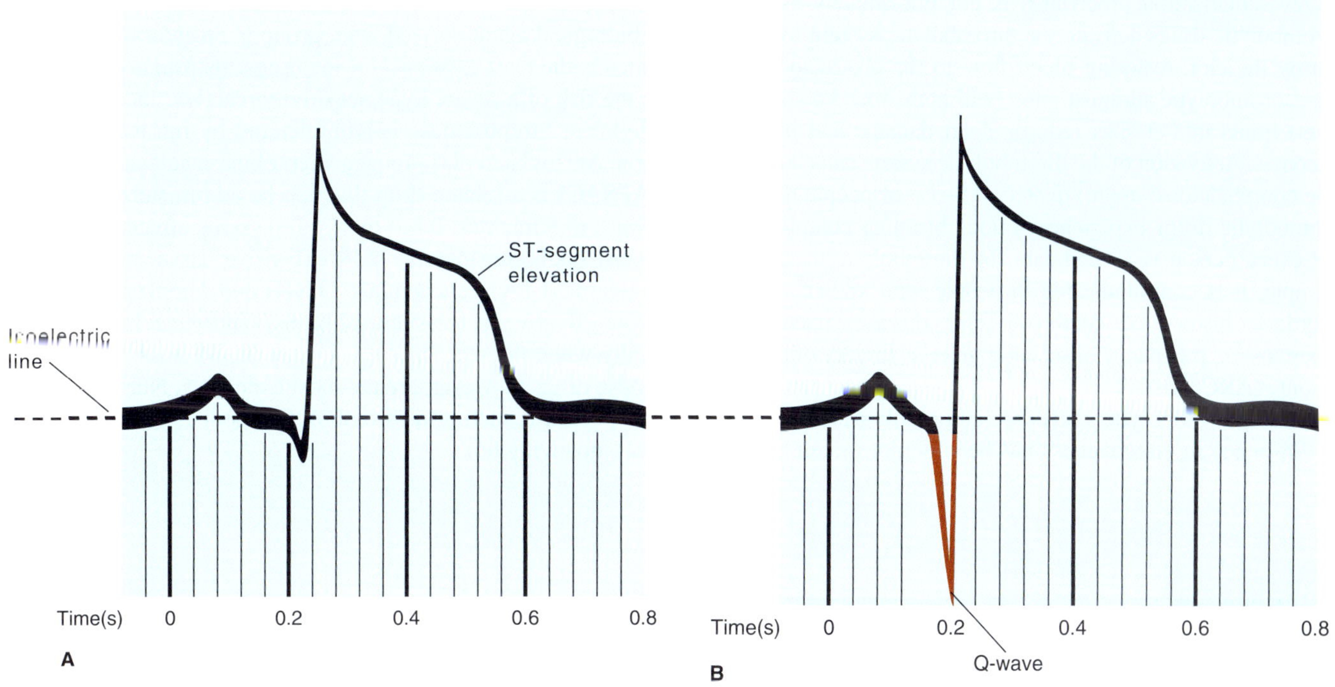

FIGURE 29.5 ***ECG changes characteristic of MI. A, ST-segment elevation characteristic of myocardial injury. B, Clinically significant Q-wave characteristic of a transmural infarction***

- *Echocardiography* is used to evaluate cardiac wall motion and left ventricular function. Stunned and infarcted tissue does not contract as effectively (if at all) as healthy myocardium.
- *Radionuclide imaging* may be used to evaluate myocardial perfusion. These studies cannot differentiate between an acute MI and old scar tissue but do help identify the specific area of myocardial ischaemia and damage.
- *Haemodynamic monitoring* may be initiated when AMI significantly affects cardiac output and haemodynamic status. These invasive procedures are described in the chapter 'Nursing care of people with cardiac disorders'.

Medications

Aspirin, a platelet inhibitor, is now considered an essential part of treating AMI. A 300 mg aspirin tablet is given by emergency personnel, with the instruction that it is to be chewed (for buccal absorption). This initial dose is followed by a daily oral dose of 100 mg of aspirin.

Thrombolytic agents, analgesics and anti-arrhythmic agents are among the principal classes of drugs used in treating AMI.

ANALGESIA Pain relief is vital in managing the care of a person with AMI. Pain stimulates the sympathetic nervous system, increasing the heart rate and blood pressure and, in turn, myocardial workload. Sublingual glyceryl trinitrate may be given (up to three 0.4 mg doses at 5-minute intervals). Intravenous glyceryl trinitrate may be continued for the first 24 to 48 hours to reduce myocardial work. In addition to pain relief, glyceryl trinitrate decreases myocardial oxygen demand and may increase the supply of oxygen to the myocardium. Glyceryl trinitrate is a peripheral and arterial vasodilator that reduces afterload. It dilates coronary arteries and collateral channels in the heart, increasing coronary blood flow to save myocardial tissue at risk. Nitrates may, however, cause reflex tachycardia or excessive hypotension, so close monitoring is necessary during administration. It also is important to ask the person about use of sildenafil (Viagra) within the previous 24 hours before administering glyceryl trinitrate, as the combination can precipitate a significant drop in blood pressure. See the 'Medication administration: anti-anginal medications' box for the nursing implications of glyceryl trinitrate and other drugs given to reduce myocardial work following AMI.

Opioids are the drug of choice for pain unrelieved by glyceryl trinitrate for sedation and the reduction of sympathetic stress and catecholamine release. Fentanyl has gained popularity as morphine is thought to decrease absorption of oral antiplatelet medications. Intravenous doses of 25 to 50 micrograms should be administered every 5 to 10 minutes, titrated to effect. It is important to assess frequently for pain relief and possible adverse effects of analgesia, such as excessive sedation. Pain unrelieved by expected or usual doses should be reported to the doctor as it may indicate a complication such as extension of the infarct. See the chapter 'Nursing care of people in pain' for more details about morphine administration. Anxiolytic agents such as diazepam may also be administered to promote rest.

THROMBOLYTIC THERAPY Thrombolytic agents, drugs that dissolve or break up blood clots, are first-line drugs used to treat acute MI when access to a cardiac catheterisation lab for revascularisation procedures is not immediately available. Thrombolytic drugs activate the thrombolytic system to *lyse* or destroy the clot, restoring blood flow to the obstructed artery. Early thrombolytic administration (within the first 3 hours of MI onset) limits infarct size, reduces heart damage and improves outcomes. Activation of the thrombolytic system can cause multiple complications; approximately 0.5–5% of people receiving thrombolytic drugs experience serious bleeding complications. Not every person is a candidate for thrombolytic therapy; for example, it is contraindicated in people with known bleeding disorders, history of cerebrovascular disease, uncontrolled hypertension, pregnancy or recent trauma or surgery of the head or spine (ARC, 2016).

Several thrombolytic agents are commonly used today. Little difference in effectiveness has been demonstrated between these; there are, however, big differences in cost. Streptokinase, a biological agent derived from group C *Streptococcus* organisms, is the least expensive of the drugs. Its primary drawback is the risk of a severe hypersensitivity reaction, including anaphylaxis. Streptokinase is administered by intravenous infusion. Anisoylated plasminogen streptokinase activator complex (APSAC) is a related drug that can be administered by bolus over 2 to 5 minutes. It has many of the same effects as streptokinase but is considerably more expensive. Tissue plasminogen activator (t-PA), tenecteplase (TNK) and reteplase (rPA) are more effective in re-establishing myocardial perfusion, especially when the pain developed more than 3 hours previously. These drugs, however, are the most expensive. Nursing care of the person receiving a thrombolytic agent is outlined in the accompanying box.

NURSING CARE OF THE PERSON receiving thrombolytic therapy

PRE-INFUSION CARE

- Obtain nursing history and perform a physical assessment. Information obtained from the history and physical exam helps determine whether thrombolytic therapy is appropriate. *The goal is to initiate thrombolytic therapy within 30 minutes of arrival.*
- Evaluate for contraindications to thrombolytic therapy: recent surgery or trauma (including prolonged CPR), bleeding disorders or active bleeding, cerebral vascular accident, neurosurgery within the last 2 months, gastrointestinal ulcers, diabetic haemorrhagic retinopathy and uncontrolled hypertension. *Thrombolytic agents dissolve clots and therefore may precipitate intracranial, internal or peripheral bleeding.*
- Inform the person of the purpose of the therapy. Discuss the risk of bleeding and the need to keep the extremity immobile during and after the infusion. *Minimal movement of the extremity is necessary to prevent bleeding from the infusion site.*

DURING THE INFUSION

- Assess and record vital signs and the infusion site for haematoma or bleeding every 15 minutes for the first hour, every 30 minutes for the next 2 hours and then hourly until the intravenous catheter is discontinued. Assess pulses, colour, sensation and temperature of both extremities with each vital sign check. *Vital signs and the site are frequently assessed to detect possible complications.*
- Remind the person to keep the extremity still and straight. Do not elevate head of bed above 15 degrees. *Extremity immobilisation helps prevent infusion site trauma and bleeding. Hypotension may develop; keeping the bed flat helps maintain cerebral perfusion.*
- Maintain continuous cardiac monitoring during the infusion. Keep anti-arrhythmic drugs and the emergency trolley readily available for treatment of significant arrhythmias. *Ventricular arrhythmias commonly occur with reperfusion of the ischaemic myocardium.*

POST-INFUSION CARE

- Assess vital signs, distal pulses and infusion site frequently as needed. *The person remains at high risk of bleeding following thrombolytic therapy.*
- Evaluate response to therapy: normalisation of ST segment, relief of chest pain, reperfusion arrhythmias, early peaking of the CK and CK-MB. *These are signs that the clot has been dissolved and the myocardium is being reperfused.*
- Maintain bed rest for 6 hours. Keep the head of the bed at or below 15 degrees. Reinforce the need to keep the extremity straight and immobile. Avoid any injections for 24 hours after catheter removal. *Precautions such as these are important to prevent bleeding.*
- Assess puncture sites for bleeding. On catheter removal hold direct pressure over the site for at least 30 minutes. Apply a pressure dressing to any venous or arterial sites as needed. Perform routine care in a gentle manner to avoid bruising or injury. *Thrombolytic therapy disrupts normal coagulation. Peripheral bleeding may occur at puncture sites and there may not be sufficient fibrin to form a clot. Direct or indirect pressure may be needed to control the bleeding.*
- Assess body fluids, including urine, vomit and faeces, for evidence of bleeding; frequently assess for changes in level of consciousness and manifestations of increased intracranial pressure, which may indicate intracranial bleeding. Assess surgical sites for bleeding. Monitor haemoglobin and haematocrit levels, prothrombin time (PT) and activated partial thromboplastin time (aPTT). *These provide additional means of assessing for bleeding.*
- Administer platelet-modifying drugs (e.g. aspirin, dipyridamole) as ordered. *Platelet inhibitors decrease platelet aggregation and adhesion and are used to prevent reocclusion of the artery.*
- Report manifestations of reocclusion, including changes in the ST segment, chest pain or arrhythmias. *Early recognition of reocclusion is vital to save myocardial tissue.*

ANTI-ARRHYTHMICS Arrhythmias are a common complication of AMI, particularly in the first 12 to 24 hours. While dysrhythmia is the correct term (arrhythmia means *absence* of rhythm), arrhythmia is in widespread use. Anti-arrhythmic medications are used as needed to treat arrhythmias. They also may be given prophylactically to prevent arrhythmias. Ventricular arrhythmias are treated with a class I or class III anti-arrhythmic drug (see the 'Medication administration: anti-arrhythmic drugs' box). Symptomatic bradycardia (bradycardia with associated hypotension and other signs of low cardiac output) is treated with intravenous atropine, 0.5 to 1 mg. Intravenous verapamil or the short-acting beta-blocker esmolol may be ordered to treat atrial fibrillation or other supraventricular tachyarrhythmias.

OTHER MEDICATIONS Beta-blockers such as propranolol, atenolol and metoprolol limit infarct size and decrease the incidence of serious ventricular arrhythmias in AMI. However, *routine* use in emergency settings is not supported by evidence (ARC, 2016). They may also reduce the risk of papillary muscle rupture. These drugs decrease the heart rate, reducing cardiac work and myocardial oxygen demand. Initial doses are given intravenously. Oral beta-blocker therapy is continued to reduce the risk of reinfarction and death related to cardiovascular causes (Bullock & Manias, 2022; Coven, 2020).

ACE inhibitors also reduce mortality associated with AMI. These drugs reduce ventricular remodelling following an MI, reducing the risk of subsequent heart failure. They also may reduce the risk of re-infarction (Bullock & Manias, 2022; Coven, 2020).

Anticoagulants and antiplatelet medications often are prescribed to maintain coronary artery patency following thrombolysis or a revascularisation procedure. Abciximab reduces platelet aggregation and the risk of re-occlusion following angioplasty. It also improves vessel opening with thrombolytic therapy, permitting lower doses of thrombolytic drugs. Standard or low-molecular-weight heparin preparations often are given to a person with AMI. Heparin helps establish and maintain patency of the affected coronary artery. It also is used, along with long-term warfarin, to prevent systemic or pulmonary embolism in people with significant left ventricular impairment or atrial fibrillation following AMI. See the 'Medication administration: antiplatelet drugs' box for the nursing implications of antiplatelet drugs and the chapter 'Nursing care of people with haematological disorders' for more information about anticoagulant therapy.

Individuals with pump failure and hypotension may receive intravenous dopamine, a vasopressor. At low doses (less than 5 mg/kg/min), it improves blood flow to the kidneys, preventing renal ischaemia and possibly acute kidney injury (see the chapter 'Nursing care of people with kidney disorders'). With increasing doses, dopamine increases myocardial contractility and causes vasoconstriction, improving blood pressure and cardiac output.

Antihyperlipidaemic agents are used for the person with hyperlipidaemia. A stool softener such as docusate sodium is prescribed to maintain normal bowel function and reduce straining.

Treatments

The individual with a suspected or confirmed MI is monitored continuously. Care is provided in the intensive coronary care unit for the first 24 to 48 hours, after which time less intensive monitoring (e.g. telemetry) may be required. At least one intravenous line is established to allow rapid administration of emergency medications.

Bed rest is prescribed for the first 12 hours to reduce the cardiac workload. The bedside commode generally is allowed; studies have shown this to be less stressful than using a bedpan. If the person's condition is stable, sitting in a chair at the bedside is permitted after 12 hours. Activities are gradually increased as tolerated. A quiet, calm environment with limited outside stimuli is preferred. Visitors are limited to promote rest. Oxygen is administered by nasal prongs at 2 to 4 L/min to improve oxygenation of the myocardium and other tissues.

A liquid diet may be prescribed for the first 4 to 12 hours to reduce gastric distension and myocardial work. Following that, a low-fat, low-cholesterol, reduced-sodium diet is allowed. Sodium restrictions may be lifted after 2 to 3 days if no evidence of heart failure is present. Small, frequent feedings are often recommended. Drinks containing caffeine, and very hot and cold foods, may also be limited.

Revascularisation procedures

Many people with AMI are treated with immediate or early coronary revascularisation such as angioplasty and stent placement. Percutaneous transluminal coronary revascularisation (PCTA) may follow thrombolytic therapy or be used in place of thrombolytic therapy to restore blood flow to ischaemic myocardium. For successful revascularisation, PCTA should be performed ('door to balloon') within 60 minutes if the person presents within an hour of onset of chest pain, or 90 minutes if they present later (Sweis & Jivan, 2022). Where PTCA is not immediately available, alternative therapies such as fibrinolysis may prove to be equally beneficial. When compared with thrombolytic therapy, prompt PTCA reduces hospital mortality (Kalyanasundaram, 2020). In some cases, coronary artery bypass grafting (CABG) surgery may be performed. The choice of procedure depends on the person's age and immediate condition, the time elapsed from the onset of manifestations and the extent of myocardial disease and damage. These procedures and related nursing care are covered in more depth in the preceding section on acute coronary syndrome.

Other invasive procedures

For individuals with large MIs and evidence of pump failure, invasive devices may be used to temporarily take over the function of the heart, allowing the injured myocardium to heal. The intra-aortic balloon pump is widely used to augment cardiac output. Ventricular assist devices are indicated for people requiring more or longer-term artificial support than the intra-aortic balloon pump provides.

INTRA-AORTIC BALLOON PUMP The *intra-aortic balloon pump (IABP)*, also called intra-aortic balloon counter-pulsation, is a mechanical circulatory support device that may be used after cardiac surgery or to treat cardiogenic shock following AMI. The IABP temporarily supports cardiac function, allowing the heart gradually to recover by decreasing myocardial workload and oxygen demand and increasing perfusion of the coronary arteries. The IABP supports left ventricular function by decreasing afterload.

A catheter with a 30 to 40 mL balloon is introduced into the aorta, usually via the femoral artery. The balloon catheter is connected to a console that regulates the inflation and deflation of the balloon. The IABP catheter inflates with helium gas during diastole, increasing perfusion of the coronary and renal arteries, and deflates just prior to systole, decreasing afterload and cardiac workload (see Figure 29.6). The inflation–deflation sequence is triggered by the ECG pattern. During the most acute period, the balloon inflates and deflates with each heartbeat (1:1 ratio), providing maximal assistance to the heart. As the person's condition improves, the IABP is weaned to inflate–deflate at varying intervals (e.g. 1:2, 1:4, 1:8). This provides a continually decreasing amount of support as the heart muscle recovers. When mechanical assistance is no longer required, the IABP catheter is removed.

VENTRICULAR ASSIST DEVICES Use of *ventricular assist devices (VADs)* to aid the failing heart is becoming more common with advances in technology. Whereas the IABP can supplement cardiac output by approximately 10–15%, the VAD temporarily takes partial or complete control of cardiac function, depending on the type of device used. VADs may be used as temporary or complete assist in AMI and cardiogenic shock when there is a chance for recovery of normal heart function after a period of cardiac rest. The device also may be used as a bridge in heart transplant. Nursing care for the person with a VAD is supportive and includes assessing haemodynamic status and for complications associated with the device. People with VADs *in situ* are at considerable risk of infection; strict aseptic technique is used with all invasive catheters and dressing changes. Pneumonia also is a risk due to immobility and ventilatory support. Mechanical failure of the VAD is a life-threatening event that requires immediate intervention (Varshney et al., 2022).

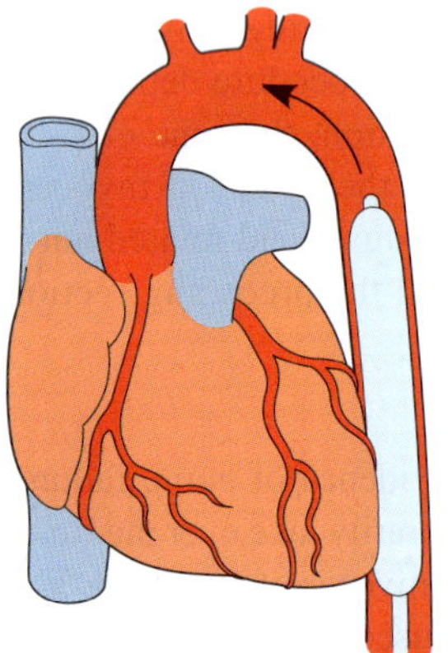

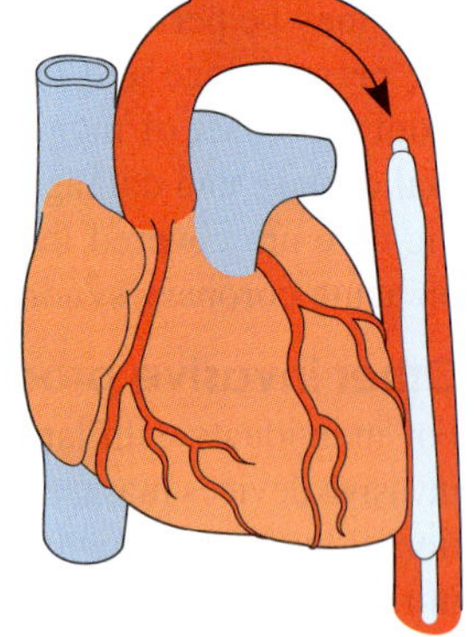

FIGURE 29.6 ***The intra-aortic balloon pump. A, When inflated during diastole, the balloon supports cerebral, renal and coronary artery perfusion. B, The balloon deflates during systole, so cardiac output is unimpeded***

Cardiac rehabilitation

Cardiac rehabilitation is a long-term program of medical evaluation, exercise, risk factor modification, education and counselling designed to limit the physical and psychological effects of cardiac illness and improve the person's quality of life. Cardiac rehabilitation begins with admission for a cardiac event such as AMI or a revascularisation procedure. Phase 1 of the program is the inpatient phase. A thorough assessment of the person's history, current status, risk factors and motivation is obtained. During this phase, activity progresses from bed rest to independent performance of activities of daily living (ADLs) and ambulation within the facility. Both subjective and objective responses to increasing activity levels are evaluated. Excess fatigue, shortness of breath, chest pain, tachypnoea, tachycardia or cool, clammy skin indicates activity intolerance. Phase 2, immediate outpatient cardiac rehabilitation, begins within 3 weeks of the cardiac event. The goals for the outpatient program are to increase activity level, participation and capacity; improve psychosocial status and treat anxiety or depression; and provide education and support for risk factor reduction. Continuation programs, phase 3 of cardiac rehabilitation, are directed at providing a transition to independent exercise and exercise maintenance. During this final phase, the person may 'check in' every 3 months to evaluate risk factors, quality of life and exercise habits.

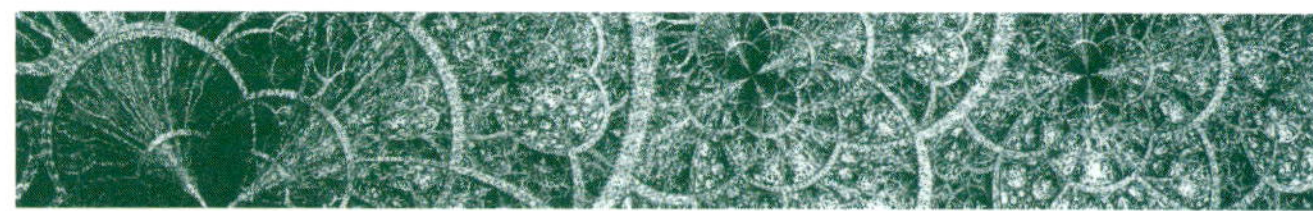

Nursing care

Nursing care of the person with an acute myocardial infarction focuses on reducing cardiac work, identifying and treating complications in a timely manner, and preparing the person for rehabilitation. See the accompanying nursing care plan for a person with an AMI.

Health promotion

Health promotion activities to prevent AMI are those outlined for coronary heart disease and angina in previous sections of this chapter. In addition, discuss risk factor management, use of prescribed medications and cardiac rehabilitation to reduce the risk of complications or future infarctions.

Assessment

Nursing assessment for the person with AMI must be both timely and ongoing. Assessment data related to AMI include the following:

- *Health history*: complaints of chest pain, including its location, intensity, character, radiation and timing;

NURSING CARE PLAN **A person with acute myocardial infarction**

Lyn Williams, a 62-year-old office worker, is admitted to the emergency department with complaints of severe substernal chest pain. Mrs Williams states that the pain began after lunch, about 4 hours ago. She initially attributed the pain to indigestion. She described the pain, which now radiates to her jaw and left arm, as 'really severe heartburn'. It is accompanied by a 'choking feeling', severe shortness of breath and diaphoresis. The pain is unrelieved by rest, antacids or three sublingual glyceryl trinitrate tablets (0.4 mg).

Oxygen is started per nasal prongs at 5 L/min because SpO_2 is noted to be 92%. Central and peripheral intravenous lines are inserted. A 12-lead ECG and the following pathology are obtained: cardiac troponins, CK and CK isoenzymes, ABGs, FBC and both a chemistry panel and coagulation profile. Intravenous morphine relieves Mrs Williams' pain.

Mrs Williams' medical history includes type 2 diabetes, stable angina and hypertension. She has a 45-year history of cigarette smoking, averaging 1.5 to 2 packets per day. Family history reveals that Mrs Williams' father died at age 42 of AMI and her paternal grandfather died at age 65 of AMI. Mrs Williams is taking the following medications: tolbutamide, hydrochlorothiazide and isosorbide mononitrate.

Based on ECG changes and cardiac markers, an acute anterior MI is diagnosed. Mrs Williams has no contraindications to thrombolytic therapy and is deemed an appropriate candidate. Intravenous alteplase (t-PA) is given by bolus followed by intravenous infusions of alteplase and heparin. She is transferred to the coronary care unit (CCU).

ASSESSMENT

Mrs Williams is alert and oriented to person, place and time. Vital signs are T 37.5°C, P 118, R 24 with adequate depth and BP 172/92. Auscultation reveals an S_4 and fine crackles in the bases of both lungs. The ECG shows sinus tachycardia with occasional premature ventricular contractions (PVCs). Her skin is cool and slightly diaphoretic. Capillary refill is less than 3 seconds and peripheral pulses are strong and equal. Her nail beds are pink.

A triple-lumen central line is in place. Glyceryl trinitrate is infusing at 200 µg/min in the distal lumen; the alteplase infusion is in the middle lumen; and a heparin infusion is in the proximal lumen. The peripheral intravenous line has a saline lock. Mrs Williams states, 'The pain is better since the nurse in the ED gave me a needle. But it has been coming and going. I would rate it a 4 right now, but it was terrible before. The doctor told me that this drug I'm getting will quickly open up the artery that is blocked. I hope it works! Do many people get this drug?'

DIAGNOSIS

- *Acute pain* related to ischaemic myocardial tissue.
- *Anxiety* and *Fear* related to change in health status.
- *Ineffective protection* related to the risk of bleeding secondary to thrombolytic therapy.
- *Risk of decreased cardiac output* related to altered cardiac rate and rhythm.

PLANNING

The following interventions are planned during the immediate phase of Mrs Williams' hospitalisation.

- Instruct her to report all chest pain. Monitor and evaluate pain using a scale of 0 to 10. Titrate intravenous glyceryl trinitrate infusion for chest pain; stop infusion if systolic BP is below 100 mmHg. Administer 2 to 4 mg of morphine intravenously for chest pain unrelieved by glyceryl trinitrate infusion.
- Encourage verbalisation of fears and concerns. Respond honestly and establish understanding about the disease, therapeutic interventions or prognosis.
- Assess knowledge of CHD. Explain the purpose of thrombolytic therapy to dissolve the fresh clot and reperfuse the heart muscle, limiting heart damage.
- Explain the need for frequent monitoring of vital signs and potential bleeding.
- Assess for manifestations of internal or intracranial bleeding, such as complaints of back or abdominal pain, headache, decreased level of consciousness, dizziness, bloody secretions or excretions, or pallor. Test all stools, urine and vomit for occult blood. Notify the medical team immediately of any abnormal findings.

Expected outcomes

- Rate chest pain as 0 on a pain scale of 0 to 10.
- Report reduced anxiety and fear.
- Demonstrate no signs of internal or external bleeding.
- Maintain an adequate cardiac output during and following reperfusion therapy.

IMPLEMENTATION

- Monitor for signs of reperfusion: decreased chest pain, return of ST segment to baseline, reperfusion arrhythmias (e.g. PVCs, bradycardia and heart block).
- Continuously monitor ECG for changes in cardiac rate, rhythm and conduction. Assess vital signs.
- Treat dangerous arrhythmias or other cardiac events per protocol. Notify the medical officer.
- Discuss continuing cardiac care and rehabilitation.

EVALUATION

The initial morphine dose reduces Mrs Williams' chest pain from a rating of 8 to 4. The glyceryl trinitrate infusion and thrombolytic therapy further reduce her pain to 2. The glyceryl trinitrate infusion is gradually discontinued after 24 hours. As her pain subsides, Mrs Williams states that she feels 'much better now that the pain is gone. I was afraid it would just get worse'. She verbalises an understanding of thrombolytic therapy to limit myocardial damage. No indication of bleeding problems is noted. Reperfusion is indicated by relief of chest pain, return of the ST segment to baseline on the ECG, early peaking of CK levels and increased frequency of PVCs but no significant arrhythmias. Mrs Williams remains in the CCU for 36 hours until she is transferred to the cardiac medical ward.

CRITICAL THINKING IN THE NURSING PROCESS

1 How would the initial plan of care have changed if Mrs Williams was not a candidate for thrombolytic therapy?

2 Two days after her initial therapy, Mrs Williams complains of palpitations. You identify frequent PVCs on the ECG monitor. What do you do?

3 What health promotion topics would you discuss with Mrs Williams before discharge?

4 Mrs Williams states, 'I've been smoking for 45 years and I'm not going to stop now! Besides, it calms me down when I'm anxious.' How would you respond to this statement?

(continued)

NURSING CARE PLAN **A person with acute myocardial infarction (continued)**

REFLECTION ON THE NURSING PROCESS

1 Outline what you have learned from this case study that you will apply to your future practice.
2 Cardiovascular disease in women presents many challenges for assessment and diagnosis, resulting in higher mortality and morbidity statistics. Explore the factors that complicate the identification of cardiovascular disease in women. How will this information modify your practice when next assessing a woman presenting with chest pain?

associated symptoms such as nausea, heartburn, shortness of breath and anxiety; treatment measures taken since onset of pain; past medical history, especially cardiac related; chronic diseases; current medications and any known allergies to medications; smoking history and use of recreational drugs and alcohol.

- *Physical examination*: general appearance, including obvious signs of distress; vital signs; peripheral pulses; skin colour, temperature, moisture; level of consciousness; heart and breath sounds; cardiac rhythm (on bedside monitor); bowel sounds, abdominal tenderness.

Nursing diagnoses and interventions

Priorities of nursing care include relieving chest pain, reducing cardiac work and promoting oxygenation. Psychosocial support is especially important because an acute myocardial infarction can be devastating, bringing the person face to face with their own mortality for the first time.

Acute pain

Chest pain occurs when the oxygen supply to the myocardium does not meet the demand. Myocardial ischaemia and infarction causes pain, as does reperfusion of an ischaemic area following thrombolytic therapy or emergent PTCA. Pain stimulates the sympathetic nervous system, increasing cardiac work. Pain relief is a priority of care for the person with AMI.

- Assess for verbal and non-verbal signs of pain. Document characteristics and the intensity of the pain, using a standard pain scale. Verify non-verbal indicators of pain with the person. Frequent, careful pain assessment allows early intervention to reduce the risk of further damage. *Pain is a subjective experience; its expression may vary with location and intensity, previous experiences and cultural and social background. Pain scales provide an objective tool for measuring pain and a way to assess pain relief or reduction.*
- Administer oxygen at 2 to 5 L/min per nasal prongs if clinical hypoxia is present ($SpO_2 < 95\%$). *Supplemental oxygen increases oxygen supply to the myocardium, decreasing ischaemia and pain.*
- Promote physical and psychological rest. Provide information and emotional support. *Rest decreases cardiac workload and sympathetic nervous system stimulation, promoting comfort. Information and emotional support help decrease anxiety and provide psychological rest.*
- Titrate intravenous glyceryl trinitrate as ordered to relieve chest pain, maintaining a systolic blood pressure greater than 100 mmHg. *Glyceryl trinitrate decreases chest pain by dilating peripheral vessels, reducing cardiac work and dilating coronary vessels, including collateral circulation, improving blood flow to ischaemic tissue.*

CONSIDERATION FOR PRACTICE

Intravenous glyceryl trinitrate (GTN) causes peripheral vasodilation, which may lead to hypotension, reduced coronary blood flow and tachycardia. Reduce the GTN flow rate and notify the medical officer if this occurs.

- Administer 2 to 4 mg morphine by intravenous push for chest pain as needed. *Morphine is an effective narcotic analgesic for chest pain. It acts as a venodilator and decreases the respiratory rate, anxiety and the perception of pain. The resulting reduction in preload and sympathetic nervous system stimulation reduces cardiac work and oxygen consumption.*

CONSIDERATION FOR PRACTICE

Reassess for relief of chest pain. The goal of care is to achieve absolute pain relief, not simply a reduction in pain to a 'manageable' level. Any chest pain of cardiac origin indicates myocardial ischaemia.

Ineffective tissue perfusion

Cardiac muscle damage affects compliance, contractility and cardiac output. The extent of the effect on tissue perfusion depends on the location and amount of damage. Anterior wall infarcts have a greater effect on cardiac output than do right ventricular infarcts. Infarcted muscle also increases the risk of cardiac arrhythmias, which can also affect the delivery of blood and oxygen to the tissues.

- Assess and document vital signs. Report increases in heart rate and changes in rhythm, blood pressure and respiratory rate. *Decreased cardiac output activates compensatory mechanisms that may cause tachycardia and vasoconstriction, increasing cardiac work.*
- Assess for changes in level of consciousness (LOC); decreased urine output; moist, cool, pale, mottled or cyanotic skin; dusky or cyanotic mucous membranes and nail beds; diminished to absent peripheral pulses; delayed capillary refill. *These are manifestations of impaired tissue*

perfusion. A change in LOC is often the first manifestation of altered perfusion because brain tissue and cerebral function depend on a continuous supply of oxygen.

- Auscultate heart and breath sounds. Note abnormal heart sounds (e.g. an S_3 or S_4 gallop or a murmur) or adventitious lung sounds. *Abnormal heart sounds or adventitious lung sounds may indicate impaired cardiac filling or output, increasing the risk of decreased tissue perfusion.*
- Monitor ECG rhythm continuously. *Arrhythmias can further impair cardiac output and tissue perfusion.*

CONSIDERATION FOR PRACTICE

Obtain a 12-lead ECG to assess complaints of chest pain. Report marked changes to the doctor. Continued or unrelieved chest pain may indicate further myocardial ischaemia and extension of the infarct; an ECG during episodes of chest pain provides a valuable diagnostic tool to assess myocardial perfusion. A repeat ECG on subsidence of pain is also very valuable.

- Monitor oxygen saturation levels. Administer oxygen as ordered. Obtain and assess ABGs as indicated. *Oxygen saturation is an indicator of gas exchange, tissue perfusion and the effectiveness of oxygen administration. ABGs provide a more precise measurement of blood oxygen levels and allow assessment of acid–base balance.*
- Administer anti-arrhythmic medications as needed. *Arrhythmias affect tissue perfusion by altering cardiac output.*
- Obtain serial CK, isoenzyme and troponin levels as ordered. *Levels of cardiac markers—CK isoenzymes, in particular—correlate with the extent of myocardial damage.*
- Plan for invasive haemodynamic monitoring. *Haemodynamic monitoring facilitates AMI management and treatment evaluation by providing a means of assessing pressures in the systemic and pulmonary arteries, the relationship between oxygen supply and demand, cardiac output and cardiac index.*

CONSIDERATION FOR PRACTICE

Continuously evaluate the response to interventions such as thrombolytic therapy, drugs to improve cardiac output and tissue perfusion, and drugs to reduce cardiac work. Adverse effects of therapy may reduce the effectiveness of treatment. Bleeding due to thrombolytic therapy may affect vascular volume and cardiac output; reperfusion arrhythmias also may affect cardiac output. Drugs used to improve cardiac output may also increase cardiac work, whereas those given to reduce cardiac work may significantly affect contractility and cardiac output.

Ineffective coping

Coping mechanisms help a person deal with a life-threatening event or with acute changes in health. However, certain coping mechanisms may be detrimental to restoring health, particularly if the person relies on them for a prolonged period. Denial, for example, is a common coping mechanism among people following an MI. In the initial stages, denial can reduce anxiety. Continued denial, however, can interfere with learning and treatment adherence.

- Establish an environment of caring and trust. Encourage the person to express feelings. *Establishing a trusting relationship provides a safe environment for the person to discuss feelings of helplessness, powerlessness, anxiety and hopelessness. The nurse may then be able to provide additional resources to meet the person's needs.*
- Accept denial as a coping mechanism, but do not reinforce it. *Denial may initially help by diminishing the psychological threat to health, decreasing anxiety. However, its prolonged use can interfere with acceptance of reality and cooperation, possibly delaying treatment and hindering recovery.*
- Note aggressive behaviours, hostility or anger. *Document any reluctance to engage with treatments. These signs can indicate anxiety and denial.*
- Support the person in identifying positive coping skills used in the past (e.g. problem-solving skills, verbalisation of feelings, asking for help, prayer). *Reinforce use of positive coping behaviours. Coping behaviours that have been successful in the past can help the person deal with the current situation. These familiar methods can decrease feelings of powerlessness.*
- Provide opportunities for the person to make decisions about the plan of care, as far as possible. *This promotes self-confidence and independence. Participating in care planning gives the person a sense of control and the opportunity to use positive coping skills.*
- Provide privacy for the person and significant other to share their questions and concerns. *Privacy provides an opportunity for the person and their partner to share their feelings and fears, offer support and encouragement to one another, relieve anxiety and establish effective coping methods.*

Fear

The fear of death and disability can be a paralysing emotion that adversely affects the person's recovery from acute myocardial infarction.

- Assess the person's level of fear, noting verbal and non-verbal signs. This information enables the nurse to plan appropriate interventions. *Individuals may not voice concerns; attention to non-verbal indicators is important. Controlling fear helps decrease sympathetic nervous system responses and catecholamine release that may increase feelings of fear and anxiety.*
- Acknowledge the person's perception of the situation. Allow individuals to verbalise concerns. *A sudden change in health status causes anxiety and fear of the unknown. Verbalising these fears may help the person cope with change and allow the healthcare team to provide information and correct misconceptions.*
- Encourage questions and provide consistent, factual answers. Repeat information as needed. *Accurate and consistent information can reduce fear. Honest explanations help strengthen the patient–nurse relationship and help the person develop realistic expectations. Anxiety and fear*

decrease the ability to concentrate and retain information; therefore, information may need to be repeated.

- Encourage self-care. Allow the individual to make decisions regarding the plan of care. *This promotes personal responsibility for health and allows some control over the situation. The person's confidence increases as their dependence decreases.*
- Administer anxiolytic medications as ordered. *These medications promote rest and relaxation and decrease feelings of anxiety, which may act as barriers to health restoration.*
- Teach non-pharmacological methods of stress reduction (e.g. relaxation techniques, mental imagery, music therapy, breathing exercises, meditation, massage). *Stress management techniques can help reduce tension and anxiety, provide a sense of control and enhance coping skills.*

Community-based care

Cardiac rehabilitation begins with admission to the healthcare facility and continues through the inpatient stay and after discharge into the rehabilitative period. The emphasis is on realistic application of information to maintain lifestyle changes.

Assessing readiness to learn is an important first step in preparing for home care. The person in strong denial may not identify any relevance to the information being taught. Evaluate ability to learn, assessing physiological and psychological health, beliefs regarding personal responsibility for health and expectations of the healthcare system. Also assess developmental level, ability to perform psychomotor skills, cognitive function, learning disabilities, existing knowledge base and the influence of previous learning experiences. Provide written material to supplement teaching and encourage questions.

Include the following topics in teaching for home care:

- the normal anatomy and physiology of the heart and the specific area of heart damage
- the process of CHD and implications of MI
- purposes and side effects of prescribed medications
- the importance of complying with the medical regimen and cardiac rehabilitation program and of keeping follow-up appointments
- information about community resources such as the National Heart Foundation.

After discharge, follow up by telephone within 1 week and periodically thereafter during the recovery period. Provide telephone numbers of resource personnel who are available to respond to questions and concerns after discharge. Research demonstrates the value of motivational and social support in adopting healthier behaviours after AMI (see the 'Translation to practice' box).

Because the person who has had an MI is at high risk of sudden cardiac death, encourage family members to learn CPR and provide information about community resources for CPR training.

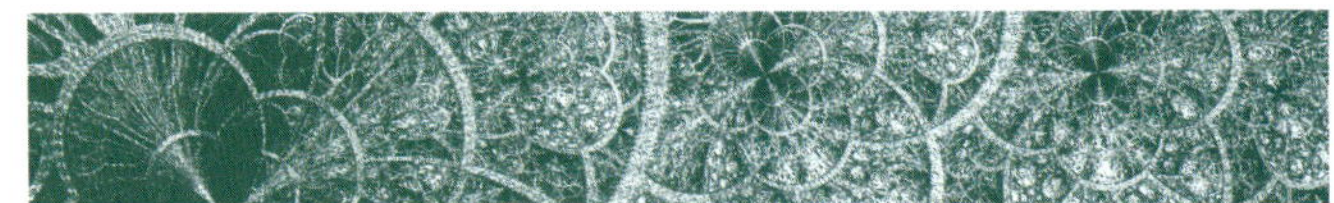

TRANSLATION TO PRACTICE Evidence-based practice: the prevalence and pathophysiology of MINOCA

Most people who experience a myocardial infarction have angiographically recordable atherosclerotic disease. However, there are a small number of individuals who are diagnosed with an MI yet, strangely, demonstrate no evidence of obstructive atherosclerotic lesion. Consequently, a new diagnosis is emerging from the literature: myocardial infarction with non-obstructive coronary arteries (MINOCA).

In a systematic review by Merlo et al. (2022), a meta-analysis of 14 publications revealed that the prevalence of MINOCA is approximately 6–9%. The pathogenesis is still under investigation. However, there are currently two mechanisms postulated: epicardial causes involving coronary artery plaque, spasm or dissection; and microvascular causes involving microvascular spasm or thromboembolism. Individuals diagnosed with MINOCA tend to be younger, have lower LDLs and less often smoke and have diabetes. Mortality rates differ depending on the mechanism.

IMPLICATIONS FOR NURSING

When working with younger females or individuals with no distinct hyperlipidaemia, the risk for developing non-obstructive coronary artery disease resulting in myocardial ischaemia or infarction should not be ignored. Education promoting healthy lifestyle choices, including nutrition and activity levels, remains paramount in the prevention of CHD.

CRITICAL THINKING IN PERSON-CENTRED CARE

1. Which clinical manifestations might a person experiencing a myocardial infarction experience?
2. How might a woman's description of clinical manifestations differ from a man's when experiencing a myocardial infarction?
3. Which assessments would you undertake and what data might you collect from a person you suspect is experiencing an MI?
4. How will the findings of this meta-analysis influence your clinical practice?

Source: Based on Merlo et al. (2022). Myocardial infarction with non-obstructive coronary arteries: Risk factors and associated comorbidities. *Frontiers in Cardiovascular Medicine*, 9, 895053. https://doi.org/10.3389/fcvm.2022.895053.

Cardiac rhythm disorders

Heart muscle contracts in response to electrical stimulation. In the normal heart, electrical stimulation produces a synchronised, rhythmic heart muscle contraction that propels blood into the vascular system. Changes in cardiac rhythm affect this synchronised activity and the heart's ability to effectively pump blood to body tissues.

THE PERSON WITH A CARDIAC ARRHYTHMIA

A cardiac arrhythmia is a disturbance or irregularity in the electrical system of the heart. Cardiac arrhythmias may be benign or have lethal consequences. Prompt recognition of a lethal arrhythmia and quick action can be lifesaving.

Arrhythmias develop for many reasons. Not all are pathological; some alterations in cardiac rhythm occur in response to events such as exercise or fear. For example, a rapid heart rate due to exercise, fever or excitement is a normal response to the body's demand for oxygen or to stimulation of the sympathetic nervous system. Slow heart rates also may be normal. Athletic heart syndrome, which results from long-term training on the heart muscle, allows the heart to beat more slowly and forcefully while maintaining cardiac output and tissue perfusion. Many athletes have a heart rate of less than 60 beats per minute (beats/min or bpm). Ageing affects cardiac rhythm as well (see the 'Nursing care of the older adult' box).

Regardless of cause, an arrhythmia can significantly affect cardiac performance, depending on myocardial health. The person's response to the arrhythmia is key to determining the urgency and type of treatment needed.

Physiology review

The unique properties of cardiac cells allow effective heart function. Four properties are electrical; the fifth is cardiac muscle's mechanical response to electrical stimulation.

1. *Automaticity* is the ability of pacemaker cells to spontaneously initiate an electrical impulse (action potential). The sinoatrial (SA) node is the dominant pacemaker, generating impulses at 60 to 100 times a minute. Myocardial muscle cells do not possess this ability.
2. *Excitability* is the ability of myocardial cells to respond to stimuli generated by pacemaker cells.
3. *Conductivity* is the ability to transmit an impulse from cell to cell. When one cell is stimulated, the impulse rapidly spreads throughout the heart muscle.
4. *Refractoriness* is the inability of cardiac cells to respond to additional stimuli immediately following

NURSING CARE OF THE OLDER ADULT Cardiac arrhythmias

Ageing affects the heart and the cardiac conduction system, increasing the incidence of arrhythmias and conduction defects. Older adults may experience arrhythmias even when no evidence of heart disease is found.

Older adults have a higher incidence of both ventricular and supraventricular arrhythmias without detrimental effects than younger people. Ectopic beats, including short runs of ventricular tachycardia, occur more commonly during exercise in older adults. These arrhythmias do not affect cardiac morbidity or mortality. Fibrosis of the bundle branches can lead to atrioventricular blocks, and a prolonged PR interval is common in people over the age of 65. Older adults also have a higher incidence of diseases that may affect heart rhythm. An older adult person with hyperthyroidism, for example, may present with atrial fibrillation, syncope and confusion instead of the usual manifestations of goitre, tremor and exophthalmos.

ASSESSING FOR HOME CARE

Assessing older adults for problems related to cardiac arrhythmias focuses on the effect of the arrhythmia on functional health status

- Ask about a history of cardiovascular disease and current medications.
- Inquire about symptoms such as episodes of presyncope, syncope, palpitations, chest pain or dyspnoea.
- Ask about relationship of symptoms such as palpitations to intake of certain foods and caffeine-containing beverages.
- Evaluate for other contributing factors such as smoking or alcohol intake.
- Inquire about a history of falls, particularly those occurring without apparent reason.

HEALTH EDUCATION FOR THE PERSON AND FAMILY

Teach measures to reduce the risk of cardiac arrhythmias and potential adverse consequences of arrhythmias.

- Emphasise the importance of taking medications as prescribed. Discuss possible effects of over-the-counter medications on the heart.
- Encourage reducing or eliminating caffeine intake. Caffeine increases the risk of ectopic beats and rapid heart rates.
- Encourage participation in a smoking cessation program and reduction or elimination of alcohol intake if appropriate.
- Encourage engaging in regular exercise. Discuss the beneficial effects of exercise in maintaining muscle mass, including cardiac muscle and cardiovascular health.
- Instruct the individual to contact the primary healthcare provider for evaluation of symptoms such as dizziness, fainting, frequent palpitations, dyspnoea, unexplained falls or chest pain.

depolarisation. In the absolute refractory period, depolarisation will not occur in response to any stimulus. A stronger than normal stimulus is required to initiate depolarisation during the relative refractory period. This is followed by the supernormal period, during which a mild stimulus will cause depolarisation.

5. *Contractility* is the ability of myocardial fibres to shorten in response to a stimulus. Heart muscle responds in an all-or-nothing manner: stimulation of one muscle fibre causes the entire muscle mass to contract to its fullest extent as one unit.

Electrical activity of the heart is normally controlled by the cardiac conduction. The SA node, the primary pacemaker of the heart, usually generates impulses at a regular rate of 60 to 100 bpm. The impulse spreads through the atria, is briefly delayed at the AV node, then spreads through conduction pathways of the ventricles and to ventricular muscle. The AV nodal delay allows the atria to contract, delivering an extra bolus of blood to the ventricles before they contract (the atrial kick). The AV node also controls the number of impulses that reach the ventricles, preventing extremely rapid heart rates.

Pathophysiology

Arrhythmias arise through disruption of the very properties that stimulate and control the heartbeat: automaticity, excitability, conductivity and refractoriness.

Arrhythmias due to altered impulse formation include changes in rate and rhythm and the development of ectopic beats. This category includes *tachyarrhythmias* (rapid heart rates), *bradyarrhythmias* (slow heart rates) and ectopic rhythms. These arrhythmias result from a change in the automaticity of cardiac cells. The rate of impulse formation may abnormally increase or decrease. Aberrant (abnormal) impulses may originate outside normal conduction pathways, causing **ectopic beats**. Ectopic beats interrupt the normal conduction sequence and may not initiate a normal muscle contraction. Depending on the site and timing of abnormal impulses, they may have little effect on the person or pose a significant threat.

Ischaemia, injury and infarction of myocardial tissue affect its excitability and ability to conduct and respond to an electrical stimulus. Conduction abnormalities cause varying degrees of **atrioventricular block**, a block in the normal conduction pathways. Myocardial injury or infarction can obstruct or delay impulse conduction. Bundle branch blocks are common in acute myocardial infarction.

The *re-entry phenomenon*, a phenomenon of normal and slow conduction, is a major cause of tachyarrhythmias. A stimulus such as an ectopic beat triggers the re-entry phenomenon. The impulse is delayed in one area of the heart (e.g. an area of ischaemia or injury) but conducted normally through the rest. Muscle that has been depolarised by the normally conducted impulse is repolarised by the time the impulse travelling through the area of slow conduction reaches it, thus initiating another cycle of depolarisation (Norris, 2018). The result is an arrhythmia that propagates itself.

Several forms of re-entry may occur. The impulse may travel through a set pathway to re-enter repolarised tissue. Many atrial arrhythmias follow this pattern, including atrial flutter. In functional re-entry, local differences in the conduction of an impulse interrupt the normal wave of depolarisation, sending it back upon itself in a spiral pattern and setting up a permanent rotation. This type of pattern suppresses normal pacemaker activity and can lead to atrial fibrillation (Olshansky, 2022).

Cardiac rhythms are classified according to the site of impulse formation or the site and degree of conduction block. Supraventricular rhythms arise above the ventricles. These rhythms usually produce a QRS complex within the normal range. Sinus rhythms, atrial rhythms and junctional (arising from the AV junction) rhythms are all supraventricular rhythms. Ventricular rhythms originate in the ventricles and may prove fatal if left untreated. AV conduction blocks result from a defect in impulse transmission from the atria to the ventricles. The major normal and abnormal cardiac rhythms are summarised in Table 29.6.

FAST FACTS

- The normal sinus rhythm is 60 to 100 bpm. Each complex includes a P wave, QRS and T wave.
- Supraventricular arrhythmias arise in the sinus node or the atria. A P wave may be present; the QRS appears normal and a T wave may be seen.
- Junctional arrhythmias arise in tissue just above or just below the AV node. The P wave may be inverted and may precede, follow or be buried in the QRS complex. The QRS usually appears normal and is followed by a T wave.
- Ventricular arrhythmias arise in ventricular myocardium. They do not reset the SA node or activate the atria. QRS complexes are wide and bizarre.

Supraventricular rhythms

NORMAL SINUS RHYTHM **Normal sinus rhythm (NSR)** is the normal heart rhythm, in which impulses originate in the SA (sinus) node and travel through all normal conduction pathways without delay. All waveforms are of normal configuration, look alike and have consistent (fixed) durations. The rate is between 60 and 100 bpm.

SINUS NODE ARRHYTHMIAS *Sinus node arrhythmias* may occur as a normal compensatory response (e.g. to exercise) or because of altered automaticity. In these rhythms, as in NSR, the initiating impulse is from the sinus node. They differ from NSR in the rate or regularity of the rhythm. Sinus arrhythmias include sinus arrhythmia, sinus tachycardia and sinus bradycardia.

Sinus arrhythmia *Sinus arrhythmia* is a sinus rhythm in which the rate varies with respirations, causing an irregular rhythm. The rate increases during inspiration and decreases with expiration. Sinus arrhythmia is common in the very young and the very old. It can also be caused by an increase in vagal tone, by digoxin toxicity or by morphine administration.

TABLE 29.6 Characteristics of selected cardiac rhythms and arrhythmias

RHYTHM/ECG APPEARANCE	ECG CHARACTERISTICS	MANAGEMENT
Supraventricular rhythms		
Normal sinus rhythm (NSR)	Rate: 60 to 100 beats/min Rhythm: regular P:QRS: 1:1 PR interval: 0.12 to 0.20 sec QRS complex: 0.6 to 0.10 sec	None; normal heart rhythm.
Sinus arrhythmia	Rate: 60 to 100 beats/min Rhythm: irregular, varying with respirations P:QRS: 1:1 PR interval: 0.12 to 0.20 sec QRS complex: 0.6 to 0.10 sec	Generally none; considered a normal rhythm in the very young and very old.
Sinus tachycardia	Rate: 101 to 150 beats/min Rhythm: regular P:QRS: 1:1 (With very fast rates, P wave may be hidden in preceding T wave) PR interval: 0.12 to 0.20 sec QRS complex: 0.6 to 0.10 sec	Treated only if symptomatic or person is at risk for myocardial damage. Treat underlying cause (e.g. hypovolaemia, fever, pain). Beta-blockers or verapamil may be used.
Sinus bradycardia	Rate: < 60 beats/min Rhythm: regular P:QRS: 1:1 PR interval: 0.12 to 0.20 sec QRS complex: 0.6 to 0.10 sec	Treated only if symptomatic. Intravenous atropine or isoprenaline, and/or pacemaker therapy may be used.
Premature atrial contractions (PACs)	Rate: variable Rhythm: irregular, with normal rhythm interrupted by early beats arising in the atria P:QRS: 1:1 PR interval: 0.12 to 0.20 sec, but may be prolonged QRS complex: 0.6 to 0.10 sec	Usually require no treatment. Advise to reduce alcohol and caffeine intake, to reduce stress and to stop smoking. Beta-blocker may be prescribed.
Paroxysmal supraventricular tachycardia (PSVT)	Rate: 100 to 280 beats/min (usually 150 to 200 beats/min) Rhythm: regular P:QRS: P waves often not identifiable PR interval: not measured QRS complex: 0.6 to 0.10 sec	Treat if symptomatic. Treatment may include vagal manoeuvres (Valsalva, carotid sinus massage); oxygen therapy; adenosine or a beta-blocker; temporary pacing or synchronised cardioversion.

(continued)

TABLE 29.6 Characteristics of selected cardiac rhythms and arrhythmias (continued)

RHYTHM/ECG APPEARANCE	ECG CHARACTERISTICS	MANAGEMENT
Atrial flutter 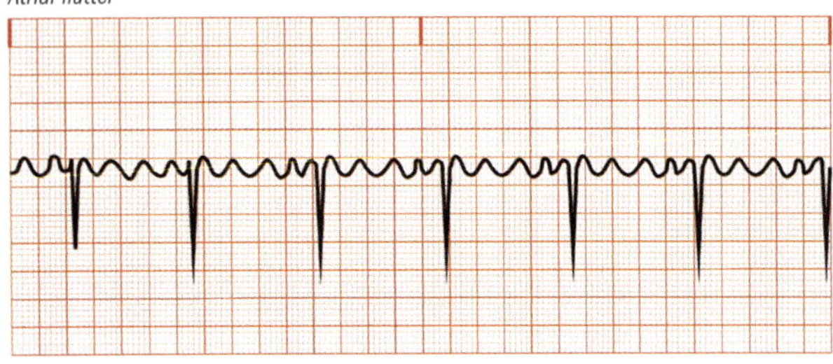	Rate: atrial 240 to 360 beats/min, ventricular rate depends on degree of AV block and usually is < 150 beats/min Rhythm: atrial regular; ventricular usually regular P:QRS: 2:1, 4:1, 6:1; may vary PR interval: not measured QRS complex: 0.6 to 0.10 sec	Synchronised cardioversion; medications to slow ventricular response such as a beta-blocker or calcium channel blocker, followed by a class I anti-arrhythmic agent or amiodarone.
Atrial fibrillation 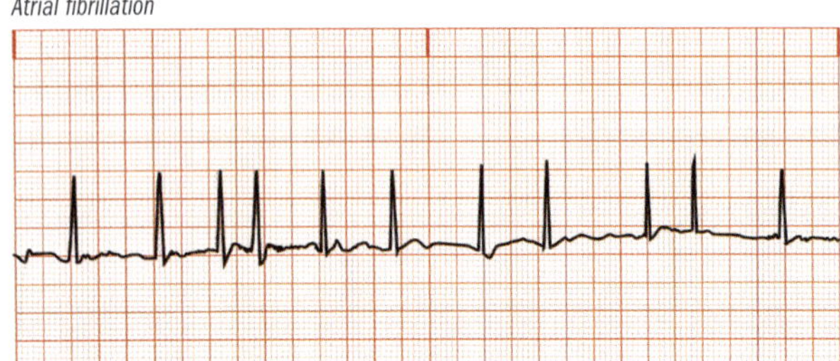	Rate: atrial 300 to 600 beats/min (too rapid to count); ventricular 100 to 180 beats/min in untreated people Rhythm: irregularly irregular P:QRS: variable PR interval: not measured QRS complex: 0.06 to 0.10 sec	Synchronised cardioversion; medications to reduce ventricular response rate: metaprolol, diltiazem or digoxin; anticoagulant therapy to reduce risk of clot formation and stroke.
Junctional escape rhythm 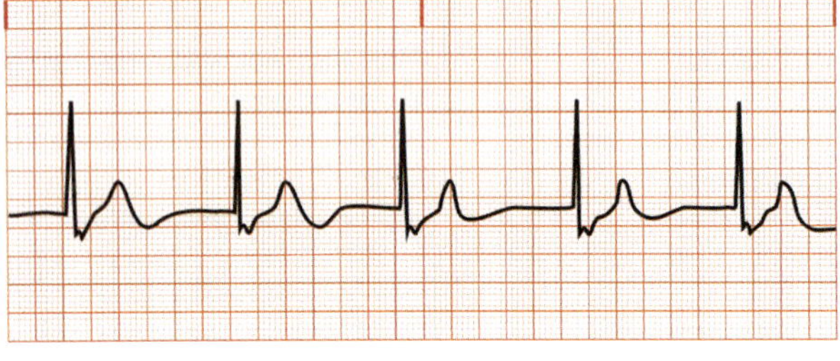	Rate: 40 to 60 beats/min; junctional tachycardia 60 to 140 beats/min Rhythm: regular P:QRS: P waves may be absent, inverted and immediately preceding or succeeding QRS complex or hidden in QRS complex PR interval: < 0.10 sec QRS complex: 0.06 to 0.10 sec	Treat cause if symptomatic.
Ventricular rhythms		
Premature ventricular contractions (PVCs) 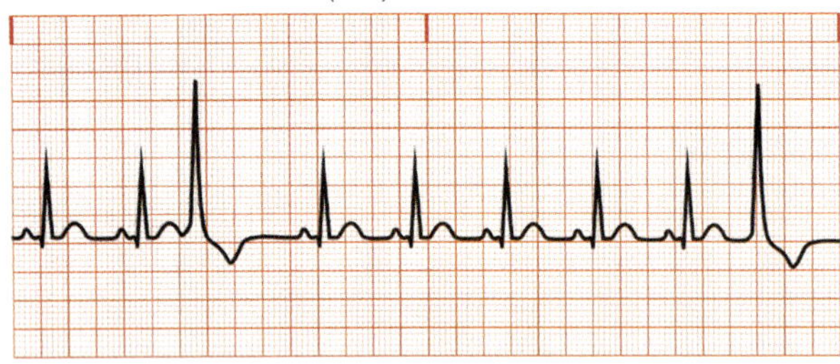	Rate: variable Rhythm: irregular, with PVC interrupting underlying rhythm and followed by a compensatory pause P:QRS: No P wave noted before PVC PR interval: absent with PVC QRS complex: wide (> 0.12 sec) and bizarre in appearance; differs from normal QRS complex	Treat if symptomatic or in presence of severe heart disease. Advise against stimulant use (caffeine, nicotine). Beta-blockers or class I or III anti-arrhythmic agents (see the 'Medication administration: anti-arrhythmic drugs' box) may be used in people with severe heart disease who are symptomatic.
Ventricular tachycardia (VT, V tach) 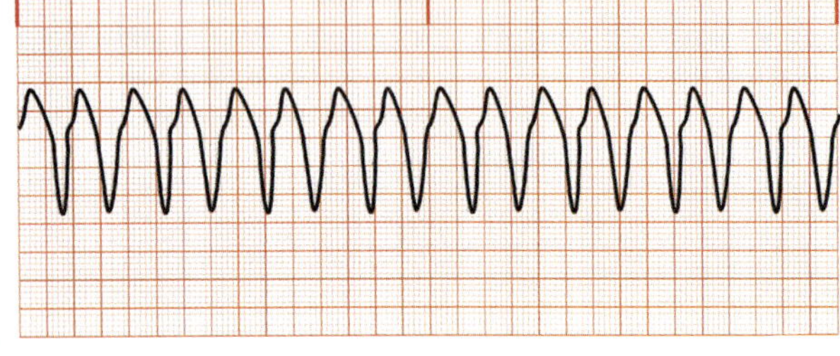	Rate: 100 to 250 beats/min Rhythm: regular P:QRS: P waves usually not identifiable PR interval: not measured QRS complex: 0.12 sec or greater; bizarre shape	Treat if VT is sustained, symptomatic or associated with organic heart disease. Treatment includes DC cardioversion or intravenous procainamide, lignocaine or a class III anti-arrhythmic agent if haemodynamic instability accompanies. Surgical ablation or pacing with an implanted cardioverter-defibrillator (ICD) for repeated episodes.
Ventricular fibrillation (VF, V fib) 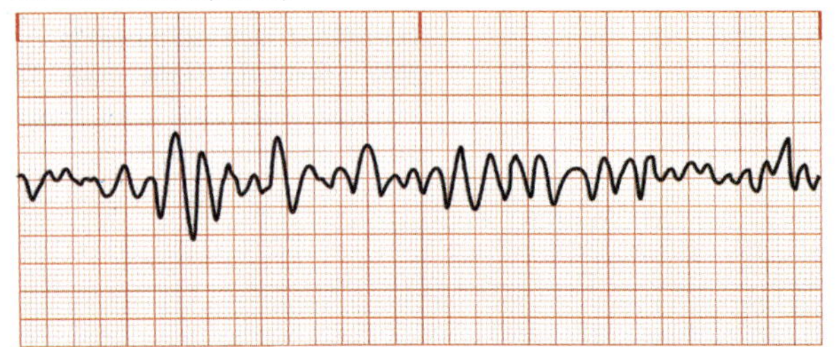	Rate: no real rate to count Rhythm: grossly irregular P:QRS: no identifiable P waves PR interval: none QRS: bizarre, varying in shape and direction	Immediate cardioversion/defibrillation.

TABLE 29.6 Characteristics of selected cardiac rhythms and arrhythmias (continued)

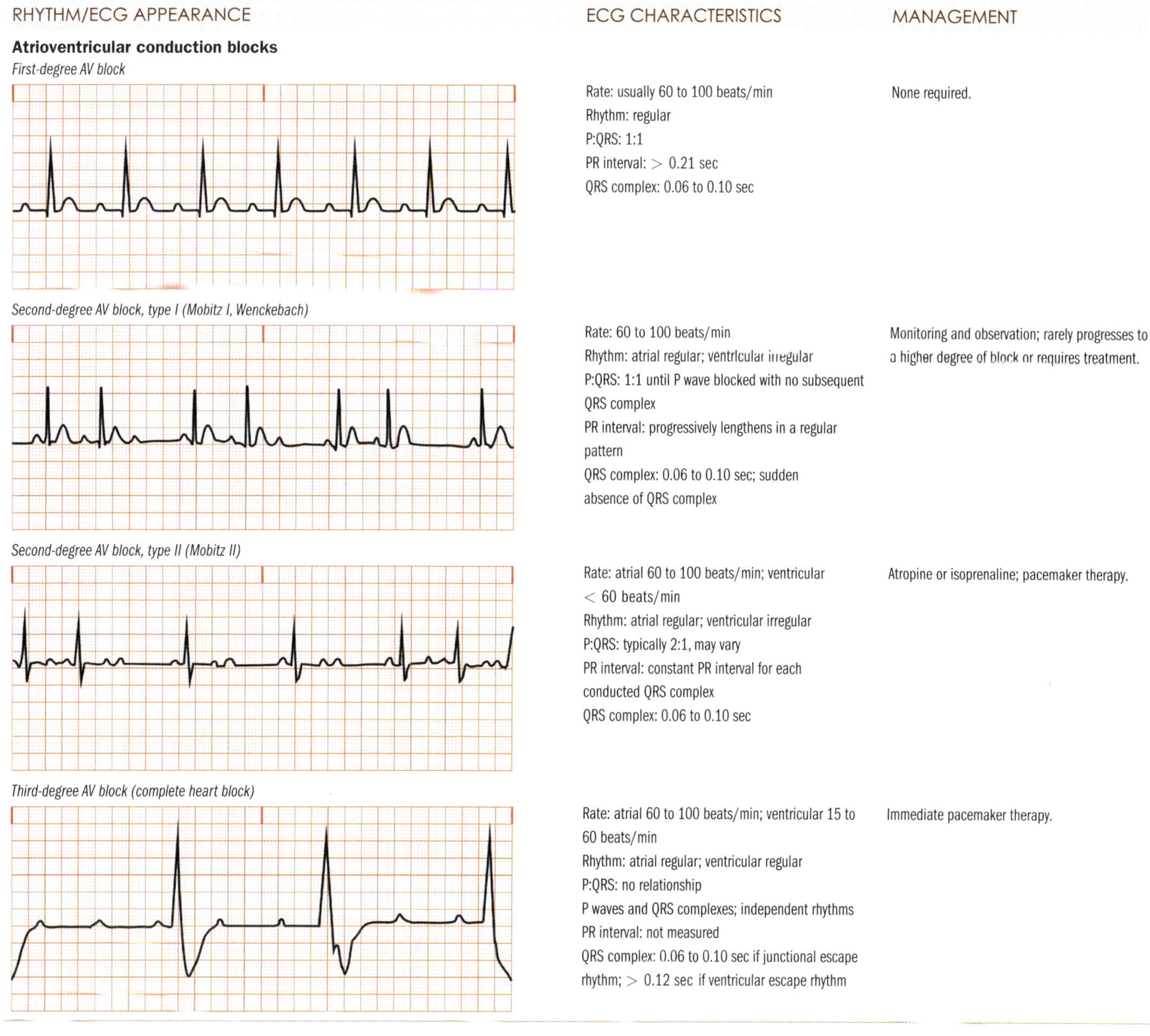

RHYTHM/ECG APPEARANCE	ECG CHARACTERISTICS	MANAGEMENT
Atrioventricular conduction blocks		
First-degree AV block	Rate: usually 60 to 100 beats/min Rhythm: regular P:QRS: 1:1 PR interval: > 0.21 sec QRS complex: 0.06 to 0.10 sec	None required.
Second-degree AV block, type I (Mobitz I, Wenckebach)	Rate: 60 to 100 beats/min Rhythm: atrial regular; ventricular irregular P:QRS: 1:1 until P wave blocked with no subsequent QRS complex PR interval: progressively lengthens in a regular pattern QRS complex: 0.06 to 0.10 sec; sudden absence of QRS complex	Monitoring and observation; rarely progresses to a higher degree of block or requires treatment.
Second-degree AV block, type II (Mobitz II)	Rate: atrial 60 to 100 beats/min; ventricular < 60 beats/min Rhythm: atrial regular; ventricular irregular P:QRS: typically 2:1, may vary PR interval: constant PR interval for each conducted QRS complex QRS complex: 0.06 to 0.10 sec	Atropine or isoprenaline; pacemaker therapy.
Third-degree AV block (complete heart block)	Rate: atrial 60 to 100 beats/min; ventricular 15 to 60 beats/min Rhythm: atrial regular; ventricular regular P:QRS: no relationship P waves and QRS complexes; independent rhythms PR interval: not measured QRS complex: 0.06 to 0.10 sec if junctional escape rhythm; > 0.12 sec if ventricular escape rhythm	Immediate pacemaker therapy.

Sinus tachycardia *Sinus tachycardia* has all of the characteristics of NSR, except that the rate is greater than 100 bpm. Tachycardia arises from enhanced automaticity in response to changes in the internal environment. Sympathetic nervous system stimulation or blocked vagal (parasympathetic) activity increases the heart rate. Tachycardia is a normal response to any condition or event that increases the body's demand for oxygen and nutrients, such as exercise or hypoxia. If the person on bed rest or someone who has done little to increase oxygen demand has tachycardia, this is an ominous sign. Sinus tachycardia may be an early sign of cardiac dysfunction, such as heart failure. Tachycardia is detrimental in the person with cardiac disease because it increases oxygen demand and decreases oxygen supply (due to decreased diastole reducing coronary artery filling time).

Common causes of sinus tachycardia include exercise, excitement, anxiety, pain, fever, hypoxia, hypovolaemia, anaemia, hyperthyroidism, myocardial infarction, heart failure, cardiogenic shock, pulmonary embolism, caffeine intake and certain drugs, such as atropine, adrenaline or isoprenaline.

Manifestations of sinus tachycardia include a rapid pulse rate. The person may complain of feeling that the heart is 'racing', shortness of breath and dizziness. In the presence of heart disease, sinus tachycardia may precipitate chest pain.

Sinus bradycardia *Sinus bradycardia* has all of the characteristics of NSR, but the rate is less than 60 bpm. Sinus bradycardia may result from increased vagal (parasympathetic) activity or from depressed automaticity due to injury or ischaemia to the sinus node. Sinus bradycardia may be normal (e.g. in the person with athletic heart syndrome). The heart rate also normally slows during sleep because the parasympathetic nervous system is dominant at this time. Other causes of sinus bradycardia include pain, increased intracranial pressure, sinus node disease, AMI (especially with inferior wall damage), hypothermia, acidosis and certain drugs.

Sinus bradycardia may be asymptomatic; it is important to assess the person before treating the rhythm. Manifestations of decreased cardiac output, such as decreased level of consciousness, syncope (faintness) or hypotension, indicate a need for intervention.

Sick sinus syndrome *Sick sinus syndrome (SSS)* results from sinus node disease or dysfunction that causes problems with impulse formation, transmission and conduction. Sick sinus syndrome is often found in older adults. It may be caused by direct injury to sinus tissue, fibrosis of conduction fibres associated with ageing and such drugs as digoxin, beta-blockers and calcium channel blockers.

ECG characteristics of SSS include sinus bradycardia, sinus arrhythmia, sinus pauses or arrest, and atrial tachyarrhythmias such as atrial fibrillation, atrial flutter or atrial tachycardia. Bradycardia–tachycardia syndrome, characterised either by paroxysmal (abrupt onset and termination) atrial tachycardia followed by prolonged sinus pauses or alternating periods of bradycardia and tachycardia, also may indicate sinus node dysfunction.

Manifestations of sinus node dysfunction often are intermittent, related to a drop in cardiac output caused by the irregular rhythm. Fatigue, dizziness, light-headedness and syncope are common. The heart rate may not increase in response to stressors such as exercise or fever.

SUPRAVENTRICULAR ARRHYTHMIAS When an action potential originates in atrial tissue outside the sinus node, the resulting rhythm is classified as a *supraventricular rhythm*. In these arrhythmias, an ectopic pacemaker takes over or overrides the SA node. They may also occur when the SA node fails; an *escape rhythm* develops as a fail-safe mechanism to maintain the heart rate. The most common supraventricular arrhythmias are premature atrial contractions, paroxysmal supraventricular tachycardia, atrial flutter and atrial fibrillation. These rhythms may be paroxysmal; that is, occur in bursts with an abrupt beginning and end.

Premature atrial contractions *A premature atrial contraction (PAC)* is an ectopic atrial beat that occurs earlier than the next expected sinus beat. PACs can arise anywhere in the atria. They are usually asymptomatic and benign, but they may initiate paroxysmal supraventricular tachycardia in susceptible individuals. PACs are common in older adults, often occurring without an obvious cause. Strong emotions, excessive alcohol intake, tobacco and stimulants such as caffeine can precipitate PACs. They also may be associated with myocardial infarction, heart failure and other cardiac disorders, hypoxaemia, pulmonary embolism, digoxin toxicity and electrolyte or acid–base imbalances. In people with underlying heart disease, PACs may precede a more serious arrhythmia.

The ECG tracing shows interruption of the underlying rhythm by a premature complex that looks similar to the underlying beats. The ectopic impulse of the PAC is usually conducted normally, leading to depolarisation of cardiac muscle and a normal QRS complex. Because the impulse arises above the ventricles, it follows normal conduction pathways through the ventricles. The QRS complex is narrow or matches those of the underlying rhythm. The shape of the P wave of a PAC differs from normal P waves because its impulse arises outside the sinus node. A *non-compensatory pause* usually follows, as the PAC resets the SA node rhythm. Occasionally, the ectopic impulse may not be conducted through the heart, resulting in a lone P wave without a QRS or a non-conducted PAC.

PACs cause few manifestations. If frequent, they may cause palpitations or a fluttering sensation in the chest. Early beats may be noted on auscultating or palpating the pulse.

Paroxysmal supraventricular tachycardia *Paroxysmal supraventricular tachycardia (PSVT)* is tachycardia of sudden onset and termination. PSVT is usually initiated by a re-entry loop in or around the AV node; that is, an impulse re-enters the same section of tissue over and over, causing repeated depolarisations.

PSVT occurs more frequently in women. Sympathetic nervous system stimulation and stressors such as fever, sepsis and hyperthyroidism may precipitate PSVT. It also may be associated with heart diseases such as CHD, myocardial infarction, rheumatic heart disease, myocarditis or acute pericarditis. Abnormal conduction pathways associated with Wolff–Parkinson–White (WPW) syndrome may account for PSVT.

PSVT affects ventricular filling and cardiac output and decreases coronary artery perfusion. Its manifestations include complaints of palpitations and a 'racing' heart, anxiety, dizziness, dyspnoea, anginal pain, diaphoresis, extreme fatigue and polyuria. (Urine output may reach up to 3 L in the first few hours after PSVT onset.)

Atrial flutter *Atrial flutter* is a rapid and regular atrial rhythm thought to result from an intra-atrial re-entry mechanism. Causes include sympathetic nervous system stimulation due to anxiety or caffeine and alcohol intake; thyrotoxicosis; coronary heart disease or myocardial infarction; pulmonary embolism; and abnormal conduction syndromes, such as WPW syndrome. Older people with rheumatic heart disease and/or valvular disease are especially vulnerable.

Two types of atrial flutter have been identified. Type I atrial flutter has an atrial rate of 240 to 340 bpm. It develops due to a re-entry mechanism in the right atrium. The mechanism leading to type II atrial flutter has not been identified. In this type of flutter, the atrial rate is faster, to 350 bpm.

People with atrial flutter may complain of palpitations or a fluttering sensation in the chest or throat. If the ventricular rate is rapid, manifestations of decreased cardiac output, such as decreased level of consciousness, hypotension, decreased urinary output and cool, clammy skin, may be noted. The atrial kick (additional ventricular filling with atrial contraction) is lost because of inadequate atrial filling.

ECG characteristics include a 'sawtooth' or 'picket fence' appearance of P waves, which are labelled flutter (F) waves. The atrial rate is rapid, often around 300 bpm. As a protective mechanism, many impulses are blocked at the AV node and the ventricular rate is rarely greater than 150 to 170 bpm. Usually, atrial impulses are evenly conducted through the AV node; for example, two impulses to one QRS complex (2:1), four impulses to one QRS complex (4:1) or six impulses to one QRS complex (6:1). A constant conduction ratio results in a regular ventricular rhythm; the ventricular rhythm is irregular if the conduction ratio varies. The ventricular rate usually ranges from 150 to 170 bpm in 2:1 conduction and from 60 to 75 bpm for lower conduction ratios. The T wave is usually hidden by overriding F waves; some F waves may be hidden in the QRS complex.

Atrial fibrillation *Atrial fibrillation* is a common arrhythmia characterised by disorganised atrial activity without discrete atrial contractions. Multiple small re-entry circuits develop in the atria. Atrial cells cannot repolarise in time to respond to the next stimulus (Norris, 2018). Extremely rapid atrial impulses bombard the AV node, resulting in an irregularly irregular ventricular response which may be rapid > 100 bpm or slow < 60 bpm. Atrial fibrillation may occur suddenly and recur or it may persist as a chronic arrhythmia. Atrial fibrillation is commonly associated with heart failure, rheumatic heart disease, coronary heart disease, hypertension and hyperthyroidism.

Manifestations of atrial fibrillation are dependent on the ventricular rate. With rapid ventricular response rates, manifestations of decreased cardiac output such as hypotension, dyspnoea, fatigue and angina may develop. People with extensive heart disease may develop syncope or heart failure. Peripheral pulses are irregular and of variable amplitude (strength).

The specific ECG characteristics of atrial fibrillation include an irregularly irregular rhythm and the absence of identifiable P waves. The atrial rate is so rapid that it is not measurable. The ventricular rate varies.

Atrial fibrillation increases the risk of formation of thromboemboli. Organ infarction may occur as a result; the incidence of stroke is high.

Junctional arrhythmias

Rhythms that originate in AV nodal tissue are termed *junctional*. The AV junction includes the AV node and the bundle of His, which branches into the right and left bundle branches. An impulse arising from the AV junction may occur in response to failure of higher pacemakers, as in a *junctional escape rhythm*, or may result from an abnormal mechanism, such as altered automaticity. An impulse arising from the AV junction may or may not be conducted back up to the atria. This conduction against the normal flow or pattern is called *retrograde conduction*. The resulting atrial wave, called a P wave, may be found before, during or after the QRS complex, depending on the speed of conduction. The P wave is inverted in some ECG leads because the impulse moves from the AV node up to the atria, instead of from the SA node down towards the AV node. In addition, the PR interval is shorter than normal (less than 0.12 sec). The QRS complex is typically narrow.

A junctional rhythm may be due to drug toxicity (e.g. digoxin, beta-blockers or calcium channel blockers) or other causes such as hypoxaemia, hyperkalaemia, increased vagal tone or damage to the AV node, myocardial infarction and heart failure. Loss of synchronised atrial contraction and the atrial kick may affect cardiac output, leading to manifestations of decreased cardiac output and impaired myocardial tissue perfusion. Heart failure may develop.

Premature junctional contractions (PJCs) occur before the next expected beat of the underlying rhythm. Isolated PJCs may occur in healthy people and are insignificant. *Junctional tachycardia* is a junctional rhythm with a rate greater than 60 bpm. It is caused by increased automaticity of AV nodal tissue. The ventricular rate is usually less than 140 bpm. Both rhythms are most commonly associated with digoxin toxicity, hypoxia, ischaemia or electrolyte imbalances.

Ventricular arrhythmias

Ventricular arrhythmias originate in the ventricles. Because the ventricles pump blood into the pulmonary and systemic vasculature, any disruption of their rhythm can affect cardiac output and tissue perfusion. A wide and bizarre QRS complex (greater than 0.12 sec) is a characteristic feature of ventricular arrhythmias. This occurs because ventricular ectopic impulses begin and travel outside normal conduction pathways. Other characteristics include no relationship of the QRS complex to a P wave, increased amplitude of the QRS complex, an abnormal ST segment and a T wave deflected in the opposite direction from the QRS complex.

PREMATURE VENTRICULAR CONTRACTIONS

Premature ventricular contractions (PVCs) are ectopic ventricular beats that occur before the next expected beat of the underlying rhythm. They usually do not reset the atrial rhythm and are followed by a full compensatory pause. PVCs often have no significance in people without heart disease. Frequent, recurrent or multifocal PVCs may be associated with an increased risk of lethal arrhythmias. PVCs result from either enhanced automaticity or a re-entry phenomenon. They may be triggered by anxiety or stress; tobacco, alcohol or caffeine use; hypoxia, acidosis and electrolyte imbalances; sympathomimetic drugs; coronary heart disease; heart failure; mechanical stimulation of the heart (e.g. the insertion of a cardiac catheter); or reperfusion after thrombolytic therapy. The incidence and significance of PVCs is greatest after myocardial infarction.

PVCs may be isolated or occur in a specific pattern. Two PVCs in a row are called a *couplet* or *paired* PVCs. Three consecutive PVCs (a *triplet* or *salvo*) is a short run of ventricular tachycardia. *Ventricular bigeminy* is characterised by a PVC following each normal beat; a PVC noted every third beat is called *ventricular trigeminy*. When the ventricular impulse arises from one ectopic site, all PVCs look the same (*monomorphic*) and are called *unifocal* PVCs. *Multifocal* PVCs arise from different ectopic sites and appear different from one another on the ECG (*polymorphic*).

The frequency and patterns of PVCs can be indicative of myocardial irritability and the risk of a lethal arrhythmia. The following are considered warning signs in the person with acute heart disease (e.g. an acute MI):

- PVCs that develop within the first 4 hours of an MI
- frequent PVCs (six or more per minute)
- couplets or triplets
- multifocal PVCs
- R-on-T phenomenon (PVCs or ventricular pacing falling on the T wave).

In people without heart disease, isolated PVCs usually are insignificant and do not require treatment. Individuals may complain of feeling that their hearts 'skip a beat' or of palpitations. In a person with pre-existing heart disease, PVCs may indicate a drug toxicity or an increased risk of lethal arrhythmias and cardiac arrest. The risk is greatest following acute MI.

VENTRICULAR TACHYCARDIA *Ventricular tachycardia (VT, V tach)* is a rapid ventricular rhythm defined as three or more consecutive PVCs. Ventricular tachycardia may occur in short bursts, or 'runs', or may persist for more than 30 seconds (sustained ventricular tachycardia). The rate is greater than 100 bpm and the rhythm is usually regular. Re-entry is the usual electrophysiological mechanism responsible for VT. Myocardial ischaemia and infarction are the most common predisposing factors for VT. It also is associated with cardiac structural disorders such as valvular disease, rheumatic heart disease or cardiomyopathy. It may occur in the absence of heart disease and with anorexia nervosa, metabolic disorders and drug toxicity.

Non-sustained VT may occur paroxysmally and convert back to an effective rhythm spontaneously. The person may experience a fluttering sensation in the chest or complain of palpitations and brief shortness of breath. People in sustained VT generally develop signs and symptoms of decreased cardiac output and haemodynamic instability, including severe hypotension, a weak or non-palpable pulse, and loss of consciousness. Allowed to continue, VT can deteriorate into ventricular fibrillation. Sustained ventricular tachycardia is a medical emergency that requires immediate intervention, particularly in people with cardiac disease.

Torsades de pointes is a type of ventricular tachycardia associated with *long QT syndrome*, a prolongation of the QT interval. Long QT syndrome may be genetic or acquired, occurring secondarily to electrolyte disruptions, myocardial infarction, cocaine use, liquid protein diets, medications or other conditions. In torsades de pointes, the QRS complexes vary in size, shape and amplitude (see Figure 29.7). Individuals with torsades de pointes may have multiple bursts or episodes of ventricular tachycardia or may develop ventricular fibrillation and sudden cardiac death (Dave, 2022).

VENTRICULAR FIBRILLATION *Ventricular fibrillation (VF, V fib)* is extremely rapid, chaotic ventricular depolarisation causing the ventricles to quiver and cease contracting; the heart does not pump. This is known as **cardiac arrest**; it is a medical emergency requiring immediate intervention with cardiopulmonary resuscitation (CPR). VF is the most common initial rhythm and is found in 60–80% of all cardiac arrests.

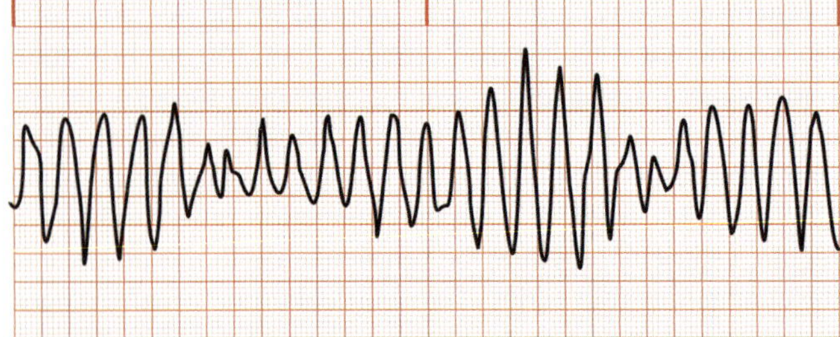

FIGURE 29.7 ***Torsades de pointes. Note the wide and bizarre QRS complexes of varying size, shape (morphology) and amplitude***

Survival rates are poor. However, the presence of a shockable rhythm, reduced CPR duration and quick return of spontaneous circulation (ROSC) increase the likelihood of survival (Bertic et al., 2022).

Ventricular fibrillation is usually triggered by severe myocardial ischaemia or infarction. It is the terminal event in many disease processes or traumatic conditions. Ventricular fibrillation may be precipitated by a single PVC or may follow VT. Other causes of VF include digoxin toxicity, reperfusion therapy, anti-arrhythmic drugs, hypokalaemia and hyperkalaemia, hypothermia, metabolic acidosis, mechanical stimulation (as with the insertion of cardiac catheters or pacing wires) and electrocution.

Clinically, loss of ventricular contractions results in absence of a palpable or audible pulse. The person loses consciousness and stops breathing as perfusion ceases. The ECG shows grossly irregular, bizarre complexes with no discernible rate or rhythm.

Atrioventricular conduction blocks

Conduction defects that delay or block transmission of the sinus impulse through the AV node are called *atrioventricular conduction blocks*. Impaired conduction may result from tissue injury or disease, increased vagal (parasympathetic) tone, drug effects or a congenital defect. AV conduction blocks vary in severity from benign to severe.

FAST FACTS

- First-degree AV block = delayed conduction through the AV node and a long PR interval.
- Second-degree AV block = complete blockage of *some* impulses through the AV node; some P waves are not followed by a QRS complex.
- Third-degree AV block = complete blockage of *all* impulses through the AV node; no relationship between P waves and QRS complexes.

FIRST-DEGREE AV BLOCK *First-degree AV block* is a benign conduction delay that generally poses no threat, has no symptoms and requires no treatment. Impulse conduction through the AV node is slowed, but all atrial impulses are conducted to the ventricles. It may result from injury or infarct of the AV node, other cardiac diseases or drug effects. The ECG shows all characteristics of NSR, except the PR interval is greater than 0.20 second.

SECOND-DEGREE AV BLOCK *Second-degree AV block* is characterised by failure to conduct one or more impulses from the atria to the ventricles. Two patterns of second-degree AV block are seen, identified as type I and type II.

Second-degree AV block—type I *Type I second-degree AV block (Mobitz type I* or *Wenckebach phenomenon)* is characterised by a repeating pattern of increasing AV conduction delays until an impulse fails to conduct to the ventricles. On the ECG, PR intervals progressively lengthen until one QRS complex is not conducted or dropped. The ventricular rate remains adequate to maintain cardiac output and the person usually is asymptomatic. Mobitz type I AV block usually is transient, associated with acute MI or drug intoxication (e.g. digoxin, beta-blockers or calcium channel blockers). It rarely progresses to complete heart block.

Second-degree AV block—type II *Type II second-degree AV block (Mobitz type II)* involves intermittent failure of the AV node to conduct an impulse to the ventricles without preceding delays in conduction. The PR interval remains constant, but not all P waves are followed by QRS complexes (e.g. there may be two P waves for every QRS). Conduction through the His–Purkinje system usually is delayed as well, causing a widened QRS complex. Mobitz type II block is frequently associated with acute anterior wall MI and a high rate of mortality (Norris, 2018). Manifestations of Mobitz type II block depend on the ventricular rate. Pacemaker therapy may be required to maintain the cardiac output.

THIRD-DEGREE AV BLOCK *Third-degree AV block (complete heart block)* occurs when atrial impulses are completely blocked at the AV node and fail to reach the ventricles. As a result, the atria and ventricles are controlled by different and independent pacemakers, with separate rates and rhythms. The ventricular impulse arises from either junctional fibres (with a rate of 40 to 60 bpm) or a ventricular pacemaker at a rate of less than 40 bpm. The width of the QRS complex depends on the location of the escape pacemaker. The QRS is wide and the rate is slow when the rhythm arises distal to the bundle of His.

Third-degree block is frequently associated with an inferior or anteroseptal myocardial infarction. Other causes include congenital conditions, acute or degenerative cardiac disease or damage, drug effects and electrolyte imbalances. The slow escape rhythm significantly affects cardiac output, causing manifestations such as syncope (known as a *Stokes–Adams attack*), dizziness, fatigue, exercise intolerance and heart failure. Third-degree AV block is life threatening and requires immediate intervention to maintain adequate cardiac output.

AV DISSOCIATION Complete dissociation of atrial and ventricular rhythms can occur in conditions other than third-degree AV block. The two primary factors leading to AV dissociation are severe sinus bradycardia and a lower pacemaker (junctional or ventricular) that competes with or exceeds the normal sinus rhythm. AV dissociation may result from acute myocardial ischaemia or infarction, cardiac surgery or drug effects. The ECG shows separate and competing atrial (P waves) and ventricular (QRS complexes) rhythms.

Intraventricular conduction blocks

Once the impulse enters the ventricles, its conduction through the right and left bundle branches may be impaired (*bundle branch block*). As a result, the impulse is conducted more slowly than normal through the ventricles. On the ECG, the QRS complex is prolonged. Its appearance varies, depending on the affected bundle (right or left). Typically, no clinical manifestations are associated with bundle branch block unless it occurs in conjunction with an AV block.

INTERPROFESSIONAL CARE

Cardiac arrhythmias may be either benign or critical: recognising lethal arrhythmias is a matter of life and death. Major goals of care include identifying the arrhythmia, evaluating its effect on physical and psychosocial wellbeing and treating underlying causes. This may involve correcting fluid and electrolyte or acid–base imbalances; treating hypoxia, pain or anxiety; administering anti-arrhythmic medications; or mechanical and surgical interventions.

Diagnosis

Diagnostic tests for arrhythmias include the electrocardiogram, cardiac monitoring and electrophysiology studies. Laboratory tests such as serum electrolytes, drug levels and ABGs may be done to help identify the cause of the arrhythmia.

ELECTROCARDIOGRAM The 12-lead ECG may be required to accurately diagnose an arrhythmia. It also provides information about underlying disease processes, such as myocardial infarction or other cardiac disease. The ECG may also be used to monitor the effects of treatment. See the chapter 'A person-centred approach to assessing the cardiovascular and lymphatic systems' for more information about the 12-lead ECG.

CARDIAC MONITORING Cardiac monitoring allows continuous observation of the cardiac rhythm. It is used in many different circumstances (see Box 29.2). Different types of ECG monitoring are employed for different situations.

Continuous cardiac monitoring Continuous monitoring of the cardiac rhythm is provided by bedside and central monitoring stations. Electrodes placed on the person's chest attach to cables connected to a monitor. The heart rate and rhythm is displayed on a bedside monitor connected to a central monitoring station. The central station allows simultaneous monitoring of many individuals within a nursing unit. Alarms on both bedside and central monitors warn of potential problems such as very rapid or very slow heart rates. Alarm limits are

BOX 29.2 Indications for cardiac monitoring

- Perioperative monitoring of heart rate and rhythm
- Detecting and identifying arrhythmias
- Monitoring the effects of cardiac and non-cardiac diseases on the heart
- Monitoring people with potentially life-threatening conditions:
  a. Major trauma (especially cardiac trauma)
  b. Dissecting aneurysm
  c. Acute myocardial infarction
  d. Heart failure
  e. Shock
  f. Other emergency conditions
- Evaluating responses to procedures and interventions:
  a. Drug therapies
  b. Diagnostic procedures
  c. Ablative techniques
  d. Angioplasty or cardiac catheterisation
  e. Cardiac surgery
  f. Pacemaker function
  g. Automatic implantable cardioverter-defibrillator function

preset by the nurse for the individual. Procedure 29.1 describes how to place a person on cardiac monitoring.

Telemetry may be used in acute care settings when the person is ambulatory. Chest electrodes are connected to a portable transmitter worn around the neck or waist; the ECG is transmitted electronically to a central monitoring station for continuous monitoring.

Holter monitoring Individuals often complain of palpitations or other heart symptoms but are asymptomatic during evaluation in a hospital or community-based setting. Ambulatory or Holter monitoring may be used to identify intermittent arrhythmias, to detect silent ischaemia, to monitor the effects of treatment and to assess pacemaker or automatic cardioverter-defibrillator function. Electrodes are applied and the leads attached to a portable telemetry monitor that records and stores all electrical activity. Individuals are instructed to leave the electrode pads in place during monitoring, record any cardiac symptoms or events in a journal (such as chest pain, palpitations, syncope) and are told when to return to the clinic. After the prescribed period, usually 48 to 72 hours, the person returns and the monitor is removed. Diary entries are compared to the recorded heart rhythms to identify the effects of arrhythmias.

PROCEDURE 29.1 Initiating cardiac monitoring

GATHER SUPPLIES

- Bedside monitor and cable or telemetry unit with fresh battery
- Electrodes—self-adherent, pre-gelled, disposable
- Lead wires
- Washcloth, soap and towel
- Alcohol prep pads
- Dry gauze pads or ECG prep pads

BEFORE THE PROCEDURE

Explain the reason for ECG monitoring. Reassure person that changes in heart rhythm can be noted and immediately treated if necessary. Explain that loose or disconnected lead wires, poor electrode contact, excessive movement, electrical interference or equipment malfunction may trigger alarms and alert the staff, allowing correction of the problem. Reassure that movement is allowed, within activity restrictions, while on the monitor. Explain skin preparation procedure. Provide for privacy and drape appropriately.

PROCEDURE

1 Follow standard precautions.
2 Check equipment for damage (i.e. fraying, bent or broken wires). Connect lead wires to cable and secure connections.
3 Select electrode sites on the chest wall, avoiding areas of excessive movement, joints, skin creases, scar tissue or other lesions.
4 Clean sites with soap and water and dry thoroughly. Alcohol may be used to remove skin oils; allow the skin to dry for 60 seconds after use.
5 Gently rub the site with a dry gauze pad or ECG prep pad to remove dead skin cells, debris and residue.
6 Open the electrode package; peel the backing from the electrode and check to ensure that the centre of the pad is moist with conductive gel.
7 Apply electrode pads, pressing firmly to ensure contact.
8 Attach leads and position cable with sufficient slack for comfort. Place the telemetry unit (if used) in gown pouch or pocket.
9 Assess ECG tracing on the monitor, adjusting settings as needed.
10 Set monitor alarm limits typically at 20 bpm higher and lower than the person's baseline rate. Turn alarms on and leave on at all times. Assess immediately if an alarm is triggered.
11 Time and date pads with every change.

AFTER THE PROCEDURE

Monitor periodically for comfort. Assess electrode and lead wire connections as needed. Remove and apply new pads every 24 to 48 hours or whenever the pad becomes dislodged or non-adherent. Clean gel residue from previous site and document skin condition under the pads. Choose an alternative site if the skin appears irritated or blistered. Document ECG strips according to unit policy and/or doctor's order, as well as when the cardiac rhythm or the person's condition changes (especially with complaints of chest pain, decreased level of consciousness or changes in vital signs). Note the date, time, personal identification, monitor lead, duration of PR and QT intervals, and rhythm interpretation on each ECG strip.

ELECTROPHYSIOLOGY STUDIES *Diagnostic cardiac electrophysiology (EP) procedures* are used to identify arrhythmias and their causes. EP studies are used to analyse components of the conduction system, identify sites of ectopic stimulation and evaluate the effectiveness of treatment. EP procedures can be used both for diagnosis and as a therapeutic intervention.

In the electrophysiology laboratory, electrode catheters are guided by fluoroscopy into the heart through the femoral or brachial vein. The timing and sequence of electrical activation during normal and abnormal (aberrant) rhythms is observed and measured. Electrical stimulation may be used to induce arrhythmias similar to the person's clinical arrhythmia (Greenberg, 2022). Following diagnosis, an EP procedure may be used to treat the arrhythmia—for example, by overdrive pacing (stimulating the person's heart rate to a rate faster than that of the tachyarrhythmia) to break the arrhythmia's cycle or to perform ablative therapy to destroy the ectopic site. See the section on cardiac mapping and catheter ablation for further information.

Nursing care for the individual undergoing an EP procedure is similar to that for a percutaneous coronary revascularisation (see 'Nursing care of the person undergoing PTCA' box). The procedure and expected sensations are explained. The person remains awake during the procedure; anxiolytic medications or sedatives are given to reduce apprehension. Intravenous heparin may be given during the procedure to reduce the risk of thromboembolism.

Complications of EP procedures are infrequent, but include fatal ventricular fibrillation, cardiac perforation and major venous thrombosis (Greenberg, 2022). Careful post-procedure monitoring is vital.

Medications

The goal of drug therapy is to suppress arrhythmia formation. No drug has been found to be completely safe and effective. Anti-arrhythmic drugs are primarily used for acute treatment of arrhythmias, although they may also be used to manage chronic conditions. The overall goal of therapy is to maintain an effective cardiac output by stabilising cardiac rhythm.

It is important to remember that virtually all anti-arrhythmic drugs also have proarrhythmic effects; that is, they can worsen existing arrhythmias and precipitate new ones. Because of this tendency, the higher mortality rates demonstrated in people receiving anti-arrhythmic medications, and the increasing safety and availability of interventional techniques, anti-arrhythmic medications are used sparingly.

Most anti-arrhythmic drugs are classified by their effects on the cardiac action potential. Most are class I drugs or fast sodium channel blockers. By blocking sodium channels, these drugs slow impulse conduction in the atria and ventricles. This class is further divided into subclasses A, B and C. Class II drugs are beta-blockers, which decrease SA node automaticity, AV conduction velocity and myocardial contractility. Class III agents block potassium channels, delaying repolarisation and prolonging the relative refractory period. Class IV drugs are calcium channel blockers. Their effect is similar to that of beta-blockers. Adenosine and digoxin do not fit within the major classes. Both drugs reduce SA node automaticity and slow AV conduction. Magnesium also falls outside the major classes but is used to treat arrhythmias. The 'Medication administration' box identifies common anti-arrhythmic drugs within each class and the nursing implications in caring for people receiving these drugs.

Drugs that affect the autonomic nervous system may also be used to treat arrhythmias. Sympathomimetics, such as adrenaline, stimulate the heart, increasing both heart rate and contractility. Anticholinergic agents such as atropine are used to decrease vagal tone and increase the heart rate. Magnesium sulfate is an unclassified drug that has been shown to be safe and effective in the treatment of ventricular tachycardias.

MEDICATION ADMINISTRATION Anti-arrhythmic drugs

CLASS I DRUGS: SODIUM CHANNEL BLOCKERS

Class IA

Class IA drugs decrease the flow of sodium into the cell and prolong the action potential. This decreases automaticity, slows the rate of impulse conduction and prolongs refractoriness. They are used to treat both supraventricular and ventricular tachycardias.

Class IB

Class IB, or lignocaine-like, drugs decrease the refractory period but have little effect on automaticity. Drugs in this class are used primarily to treat ventricular arrhythmias, including PVCs and ventricular tachycardia.

Class IC

Class IC drugs slow impulse conduction velocity but have little effect on refractoriness. They are used to reduce or eliminate tachyarrhythmias associated with re-entry. Their significant proarrhythmic effects limit their usefulness, but they may be used to treat supraventricular tachycardia.

CLASS II DRUGS: BETA-BLOCKERS

Class II drugs are beta-blockers that decrease automaticity and conduction through the AV node. They also reduce the heart rate and myocardial contractility. They are used to treat supraventricular tachycardia and to slow the ventricular response rate to atrial fibrillation. These drugs may cause bronchospasm and are contraindicated for people with asthma, chronic obstructive pulmonary disease (COPD) or other restrictive or obstructive lung diseases.

CLASS III DRUGS: POTASSIUM CHANNEL BLOCKERS

Class III drugs block potassium channels, prolonging repolarisation and the refractory period. Drugs in this class are used primarily to treat ventricular tachycardia and ventricular fibrillation. Amiodarone may also be used for supraventricular tachycardias.

(continued)

MEDICATION ADMINISTRATION Anti-arrhythmic drugs (continued)

CLASS IV DRUGS: CALCIUM CHANNEL BLOCKERS

Calcium channel blockers decrease automaticity and AV nodal conduction. They are used to manage supraventricular tachycardias. Like the beta-blockers, calcium channel blockers reduce myocardial contractility.

OTHER DRUGS

Adenosine and digoxin decrease conduction through the AV node and are used to treat supraventricular tachycardias.

Nursing responsibilities

- Obtain baseline data, including vital signs, cardiac rhythm (including rate, PR and QT intervals, and QRS duration) and physical assessment (especially cardiac, neurological and respiratory status).
- Assess medication regimen to identify drugs that may interfere with anti-arrhythmic therapy.
- Monitor ECG to evaluate the effectiveness of therapy and to assess for possible arrhythmias precipitated by treatment.
- Immediately report manifestations of drug toxicity:
  - Procainamide—signs of heart failure; conduction delays or ventricular arrhythmias; skin rash, myalgias or arthralgias, flu-like symptoms.
  - Lignocaine—changes in neurological status, such as agitation, confusion, dizziness, nervousness.
  - Amiodarone—pulmonary fibrosis (increasing dyspnoea, cough, hepatic dysfunction—changes in liver function tests, jaundice); vision changes, photosensitivity.
  - Digoxin—anorexia, nausea, vomiting; blurred or double vision; yellow–green halos; new-onset arrhythmias.
- Use an infusion pump to administer intravenous infusions. Monitor the dose and assess its appropriateness (in mg/min or μg/kg/min).

Health education for the person and family

- Take the drug exactly as prescribed. Do not skip or double doses. Check with the medical officer regarding instructions for a missed dose.
- Pulse rates should be taken and recorded daily before rising. The record should be brought to all appointments with healthcare professionals.
- Report irregular pulse rates or rhythms, dizziness, eye pain, changes in vision, skin rashes or colour changes, wheezing or other respiratory problems, or changes in behaviour to the medical officer.

Countershock

Countershock is used to interrupt cardiac rhythms that compromise cardiac output and the person's welfare. Delivery of a direct current charge depolarises all cardiac cells at the same time. This simultaneous depolarisation may stop a tachyarrhythmia and allow the sinus node to recover control of impulse formation. There are two types of countershock: synchronised cardioversion and defibrillation.

SYNCHRONISED CARDIOVERSION *Synchronised cardioversion* delivers direct electrical current synchronised with the person's heart rhythm. Synchronisation of the shock with the QRS complex prevents ventricular fibrillation by avoiding current delivery during the vulnerable period of repolarisation. Cardioversion is usually done as an elective procedure to treat supraventricular tachycardia, atrial fibrillation, atrial flutter or haemodynamically stable ventricular tachycardia.

The nurse assists with cardioversion by preparing the individual before the procedure; obtaining any laboratory tests ordered; obtaining and documenting rhythm strips prior to, during and after treatment; setting up the equipment; and monitoring the person's response. Procedure 29.2 describes synchronised cardioversion.

People in atrial fibrillation are at high risk of thromboembolism following cardioversion. Loss of atrial contractions with atrial fibrillation leads to blood pooling in the atria, increasing the risk of clot formation. When the atria begin to contract following successful cardioversion, clots may be dislodged, embolising to the pulmonary or systemic circulation. If possible, anticoagulants are given for several weeks before cardioversion is attempted.

DEFIBRILLATION Unlike carefully synchronised cardioversion, *defibrillation* is an emergency procedure that delivers direct current without regard to the cardiac cycle. Ventricular fibrillation is immediately treated as soon as the arrhythmia is recognised. Early defibrillation does improve survival in people experiencing VF; however, VF can still re-occur post defibrillation (Sassen et al., 2019).

Defibrillation can be delivered by external or internal paddles or pads. Conductive gel pads or paste is applied and external paddles or pads are placed on the chest wall at the apex and base of the heart (see Figure 29.8). Internal paddles are applied directly on the heart and may be used in surgery, the emergency

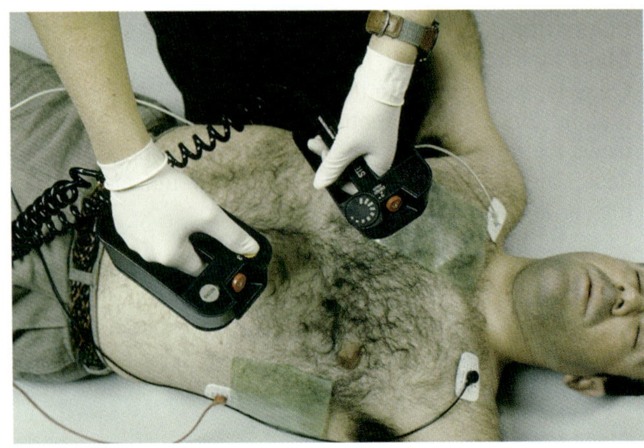

FIGURE 29.8 ***Placement of pads for defibrillation***

Source: Floyd Jackson/Pearson Education.

PROCEDURE 29.2 Elective synchronised cardioversion

GATHER SUPPLIES

- Cardioverter-defibrillator with ECG cable and monitor
- Conductive gel pads or paste
- Dry gauze pads
- Emergency drug kit and resuscitation equipment
- IV supplies (catheter, solution, administration set)

BEFORE THE PROCEDURE

Explain the purpose of the procedure (to restore an effective cardiac rhythm). Describe the procedure in simple non-threatening terms. Advise that some discomfort may be felt with each countershock, but a light anaesthetic will be given to minimise discomfort. Witness the signature on the procedure consent form. Document pre-procedure rhythm on an ECG strip. Ensure a patent intravenous access site for emergency drug administration. Keep nil by mouth (NBM) as specified prior to the procedure. Assess acid–base and electrolyte levels (especially potassium, magnesium and calcium) and drug levels if appropriate. Report abnormalities to the medical team prior to the procedure. Document vital signs, level of consciousness and peripheral pulses. Remove any medication patches from the chest and all metallic objects. Assist where necessary with the airway and medications for level of consciousness. Ensure privacy and position the person supine.

PROCEDURE

1. Use standard precautions.
2. Turn on the defibrillator and ECG monitor.
3. Connect the person's ECG cable to the defibrillator. Select a lead with prominent R waves for monitoring (generally lead II).
4. Set defibrillator to 'synchronise' mode. Observe the ECG waveform on the monitor for indications of synchronisation, such as a flashing bold line or a blip. Many units also display the message 'synchronised mode' on the monitor.
5. Place all-in-one conductive pads/leads on the chest below the right clavicle to the right of the sternum and in the midaxillary line on the left.
6. Turn on the ECG recording strip for a continuous printout during the procedure.
7. Turn oxygen off and remove it.
8. Charge the defibrillator to the prescribed energy dose (joules). The machine will beep to indicate that the selected energy level has been reached and that the paddles are ready for discharge.
9. Ensure that no one is touching the person or the bed prior to discharge of the electrical shock. There may be a slight delay in shock delivery as the machine synchronises with the R wave.
10. Assess person's status and ECG rhythm. Assure a patent airway and the presence of a pulse.
11. The procedure may be repeated if unsuccessful. The energy level may be increased with each attempt.
12. Remove conductive pads. Ensure that the skin is clean and dry.

AFTER THE PROCEDURE

Assess the individual for return of consciousness from sedative or cardioversion. Evaluate neurological, cardiovascular and respiratory status. Assess for possible complications, including emboli (especially cerebral), respiratory depression and arrhythmias. Document postcardioversion rhythm strip. Assess skin for burns. Document the procedure and the person's response in the medical record.

department or critical care. Internal defibrillation is done only by a doctor; external defibrillation may be performed by any healthcare provider who has been trained in the procedure. Automatic external defibrillators (AEDs) are available on most hospital units to allow early defibrillation for cardiac arrest (see Procedure 29.3).

Pacemaker therapy

A **pacemaker** is a pulse generator used to provide an electrical stimulus to the heart when the heart fails to generate or conduct on its own at a rate that maintains the cardiac output. The pulse generator is connected to *leads* (insulated wires) passed intravenously into the heart or sutured directly to the epicardium. The leads sense intrinsic electrical activity of the heart and provide an electrical stimulus to the heart when necessary (pacing).

Pacemakers are used to treat both acute and chronic conduction defects such as third-degree AV block. They also may be used to treat bradyarrhythmias and tachyarrhythmias.

Temporary pacemakers use an external pulse generator (see Figure 29.9) attached to a lead threaded intravenously into the right ventricle, to temporary pacing wires implanted during cardiac surgery or to external conductive pads placed on the chest wall for emergency pacing.

Permanent pacemakers use an internal pulse generator placed in a subcutaneous pocket in the subclavian space or abdominal wall. The generator connects to leads sewn directly onto the heart (*epicardial*) or passed transvenously into the heart (*endocardial*). Epicardial pacemakers (see Figure 29.10) require surgical exposure of the heart. Leads may be placed during cardiac surgery or using a small subxiphoid incision to expose the heart. Transvenous pacemaker leads are positioned in the right heart via the cephalic, subclavian or jugular vein (see Figure 29.11). Local anaesthesia can be used for permanent pacemaker insertion.

Pacemakers are programmed to stimulate the atria or the ventricles (*single-chamber pacing*) or both (*dual-chamber pacing*). Table 29.7 defines terms used to describe pacemaker

PROCEDURE 29.3 Emergency external defibrillation

GATHER SUPPLIES

- Automatic external defibrillator or defibrillator with ECG cable and monitor
- Conductive gel pads or paste
- Dry gauze pads
- Emergency medications and emergency trolley with pacemaker, airway management equipment and oxygen supplies

BEFORE THE PROCEDURE

Verify the lethal arrhythmia, such as pulseless VT, VF or asystole. Initiate the cardiac arrest (code) procedure and obtain the defibrillator. If one is not immediately available, begin CPR until the emergency cart and defibrillator are brought to the bedside. Place person in supine position on a firm surface.

PROCEDURE

1. Chest compressions should continue during preparation and time off the chest should be minimised.
2. Turn on the defibrillator. Set it in *defibrillation* mode.
3. Turn ECG recording on for a continuous printout of events during the procedure.
4. Set the energy level and charge the paddles. Monophasic—360 J for all shocks. Biphasic—200 J for all shocks.
5. Place conductive adhesive pads on the chest.
6. Perform a visual check that no one is touching the person or the bed. State: 'All clear.'
7. Depress the shock/discharge button on the defibrillator to discharge the energy.
8. Immediately resume CPR.
9. If there are signs of life, evaluate cardiac rhythm and for a pulse after approximately 2 minutes but do not delay CPR.
10. Implement ACLS protocols.

AFTER THE PROCEDURE

If the arrhythmia is successfully converted, evaluate and support neurological, cardiovascular and respiratory status. Monitor and titrate any intravenous infusions as ordered. Maintain ventilatory support as needed. Evaluate skin for burns. Obtain blood for laboratory analysis as ordered. Monitor vital signs and ECG continuously. Transfer to the critical care unit as indicated. Provide support and information to the individual and their family.

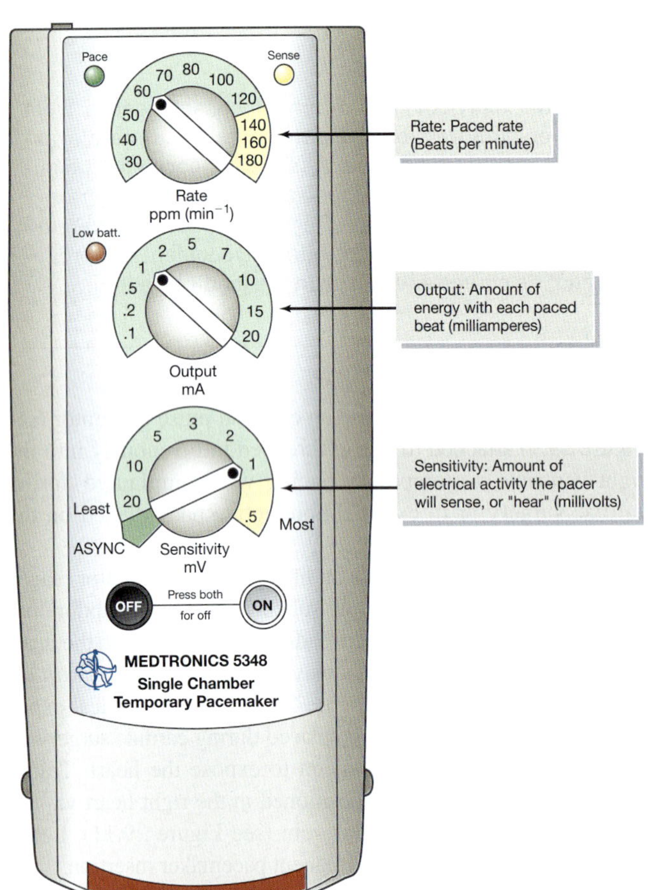

FIGURE 29.9 ***Programmable settings on a temporary pacemaker***

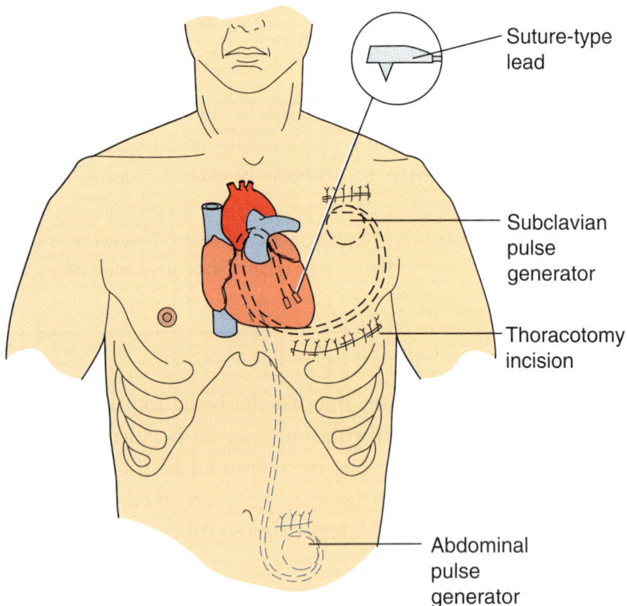

FIGURE 29.10 ***A permanent epicardial pacemaker. The pulse generator may be placed in subcutaneous pockets in the subclavian or abdominal regions***

modes and functions. The most commonly used pacemakers either: (1) sense activity in and pace the ventricles only, or (2) sense activity in and pace both the atria and the ventricles. Dual-chamber or *atrioventricular sequential pacing* stimulates both chambers of the heart in sequence. AV pacing imitates the normal sequence of atrial contraction followed by ventricular contraction, improving cardiac output.

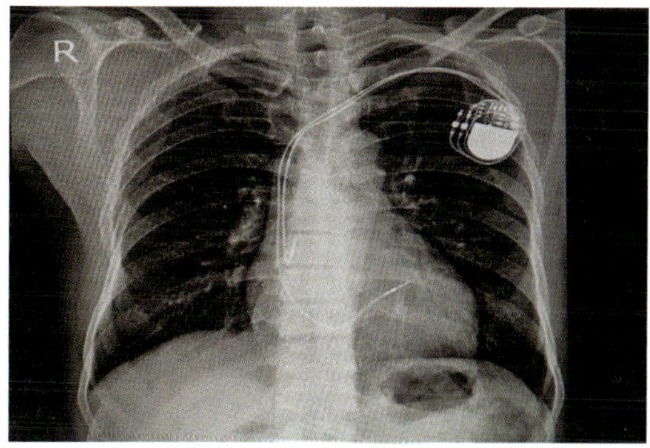

FIGURE 29.11 ***A permanent transvenous (endocardial) pacemaker with the lead placed in the right ventricle via the subclavian vein***

Source: Richman Photo/Shutterstock.

Pacing is detected on the ECG strip by the presence of pacing artefacts (see Figure 29.12). A sharp spike is noted before the P wave with atrial pacing and before the QRS complex with ventricular pacing. Pacing spikes are seen before both the P wave and QRS complex in AV sequential pacing. Capture is noted if there is a contraction of the chamber immediately following the pacer spike. Problems in sensing, pacing and capture are noted in Table 29.8.

Care of the person with a temporary or permanent pacemaker focuses on monitoring for pacemaker malfunctioning, maintaining safety (see Box 29.3) and preventing infection and postoperative complications.

Implantable cardioverter-defibrillator

The true incidence of sudden cardiac death in Australia and New Zealand is unknown. The implantable cardioverter-defibrillator (ICD) detects life-threatening changes in the cardiac rhythm and

BOX 29.3 Safety for the person with a temporary pacemaker

- Wear gloves when handling the pacemaker electrodes or wires (to prevent microshock).
- Ensure that all electrical equipment in use has a grounded plug; do not use adapters or extension cords.
- Encourage the use of battery-powered equipment (e.g. electric razor).
- Remove any damaged electrical equipment from the unit, including equipment that:
  a. has been abused (e.g. has been dropped or in which liquid has been spilled)
  b. has given anyone a shock
  c. has damaged electrical cords or plugs
  d. has other evidence of impaired function, such as a hot smell during use, or control knobs that are loose or do not consistently produce the expected response.
- Insulate pacemaker terminals and pacing wires with non-conductive, moisture proof material (e.g. a rubber glove).
- Test the pacemaker battery prior to use.
- Keep a spare pacemaker, cable, batteries and battery tester available at all times.
- Immediately report any apparent deviation from expected pacemaker function.

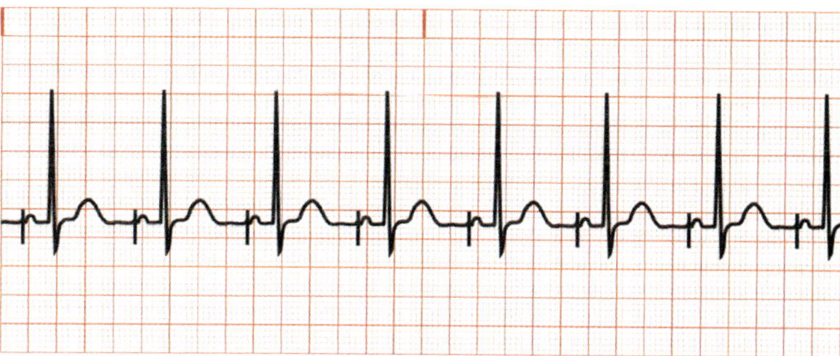

A

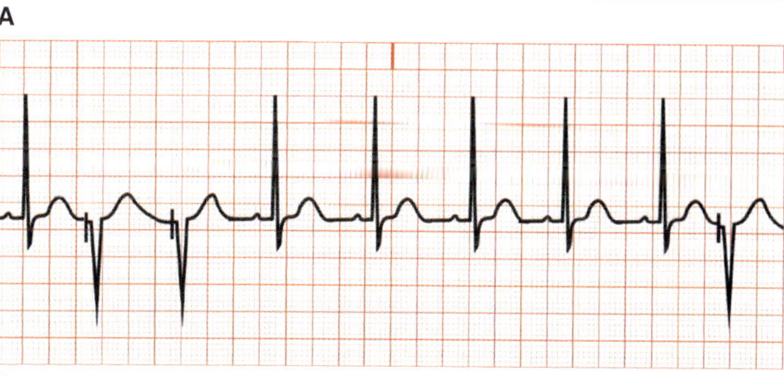

B

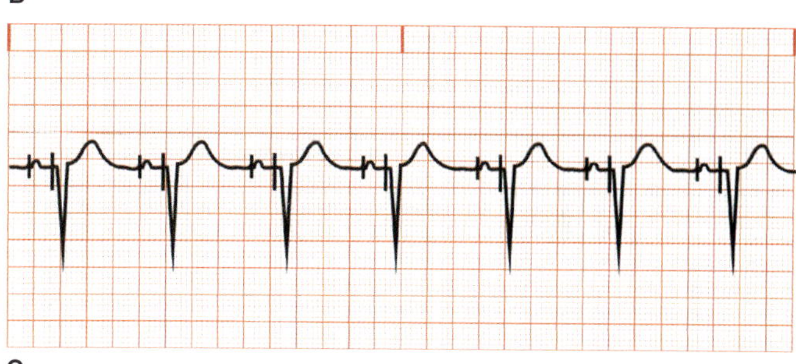

C

FIGURE 29.12 ***Pacing artefacts. A, Atrial pacing and ventricular sensing. Note the pacer spike preceding the P wave. B, Ventricular demand pacing. Note the absence of pacer spikes when the person's natural rhythm predominates. C, Atrioventricular pacing. Note the pacer spikes preceding both P waves and QRS complexes***

TABLE 29.7 Terms used to describe pacemaker functions

TERM	DEFINITION
Asynchronous pacing	A setting that results in delivery of a pacing stimulus at a set rate regardless of intrinsic cardiac activity.
Base rate	The rate at which the unit paces when no intrinsic cardiac activity is detected.
Capture	The ability of the stimulus to generate depolarisation through the myocardium.
Demand pacing	A setting that results in delivery of a pacing stimulus only when the intrinsic rate falls below the unit's base rate.
Dual-chamber pacing	The pacing of both atria and ventricles; mode most often used in permanent implanted pacing devices.
Lead	An insulated wire that is capable of sensing intrinsic cardiac activity and delivering a pacing stimulus.
Output	The electrical stimulus delivered by the unit.
Pacing spike	A vertical line occurring on the ECG with every pacemaker stimulus.
Sensing	The unit's ability to sense and respond to intrinsic cardiac activity.
Single-chamber pacing	The pacing of only atria or ventricles; mode most often used in the context of temporary pacing activities.

Source: Adapted from Link (2022). Modes of cardiac pacing: Nomenclature and selection. *UpToDate*. Retrieved from https://www.uptodate.com/.

automatically delivers an electric shock to convert the arrhythmia back into a normal rhythm. ICDs are used for sudden death survivors, people with recurrent ventricular tachycardia and individuals with demonstrated risk factors for sudden death. ICDs can deliver a shock as needed, provide pacing on demand and can store ECG records of tachycardic episodes (Beyerbach, 2019).

A pulse generator connected to lead electrodes for rhythm detection and current delivery is implanted in the left pectoral region. The lead is threaded transvenously to the apex of the right ventricle. The ICD is programmed to sense a change in heart rate or rhythm. When it detects a potentially lethal rhythm, it shocks the heart to convert the rhythm. The device can be programmed or reprogrammed at the bedside as necessary. The ICD may be tested prior to discharge.

Local or general anaesthesia is used and the individual may be discharged within 24 hours. The lithium-powered battery must be surgically replaced every 5 years. Complications and

TABLE 29.8 Selected pacing problems

PROBLEM	POSSIBLE CAUSE	RESOLUTION
Failure to capture **Pacer 'fires' but fails to initiate myocardial depolarisation** **Native rhythm** Occurs when there is no atrial (or ventricular complex–whichever is appropriate) following the pacing spike. The pacing unit has delivered an impulse but the target myocardium did not achieve depolarisation.	The output mA* is set too low on the pacing unit.	Support HR & BP†. Increase the mA* on the unit until capture is obtained.
	The tip may have migrated or is not well enough in contact with the target myocardium.	Support HR & BP†. Reposition the individual lying on the other side (sometimes this will facilitate capture again). Observe for other signs that the tip may have migrated (i.e. hiccupping–the tip may have migrated to the diaphragm).
	The lead may have fractured.	Support HR & BP†. Change pacing leads.
	The threshold in the target myocardium may have increased due to chemical or metabolic changes making the cells less responsive to the mA* set.	Support HR & BP†. Increase the mA* on the unit until capture is obtained. Change the polarity of the pacing wires in the pacing box (place the negative where the positive had been and the positive where the negative wire had been).
	The pacemaker unit's battery may be low.	Change pacing box to programmed replacement unit and then replace batteries in old unit ready for use.
Failure to sense (undersensing) 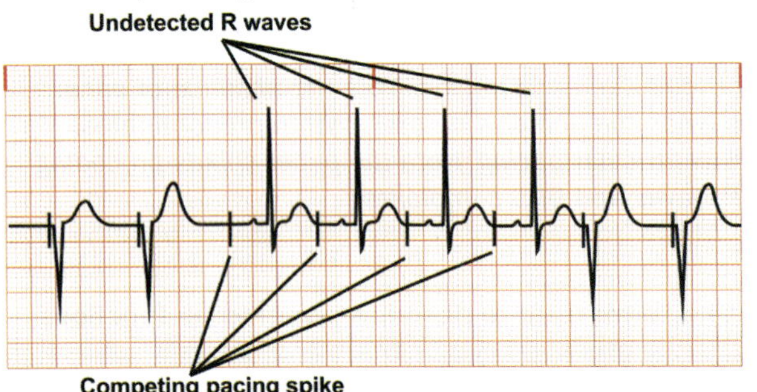 Occurs when the pacing unit does not detect the intrinsic/native event (P wave or QRS complex) and delivers an impulse. If the pacing unit delivers an impulse onto the myocardium during repolarisation it can cause fibrillation in the target tissue (i.e. if it occurs during atrial repolarisation it can cause atrial fibrillation and if it occurs during ventricular repolarisation it can cause ventricular fibrillation).	The person's intrinsic/native myocardial voltage is low. The sensitivity is set too low (mV‡ is set too high) on the pacing unit.	Increase the sensitivity of the pacing unit (decrease mV‡) until sensing is identified.
	A wire or lead may be dislodged, loose or fractured, or the pacemaker may be malfunctioning.	Check all connections and change pacing leads. Try another pacing unit.
	The pacemaker unit's battery may be low.	Change pacing box to programmed replacement unit and then replace batteries in old unit ready for use.
	The person may be experiencing an electrolyte imbalance.	Check the person's electrolytes.
Failure to pace (oversensing) 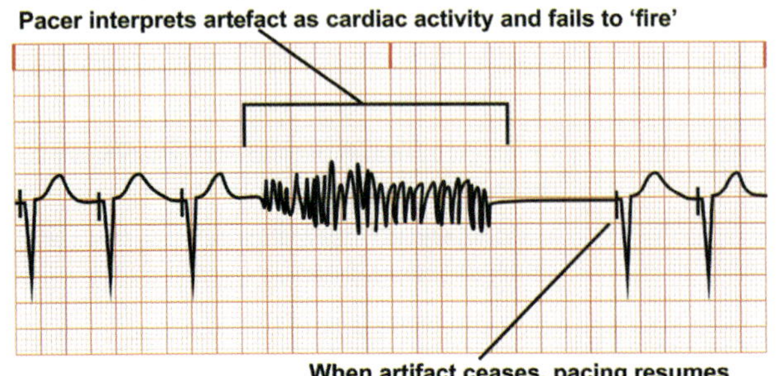 Occurs when the pacing unit does not deliver an impulse even though the person's intrinsic/native rhythm is inadequate.	The sensitivity is set too high (mV‡ is set too low) on the pacing unit.	Support HR & BP†. Decrease the sensitivity of the pacing unit (increase mV‡) until appropriate sensing is identified.
	A wire or lead may be dislodged, loose or fractured, or the pacemaker may be malfunctioning.	Support HR & BP†. Check all connections and change pacing leads. Try another pacing unit.
	The pacemaker unit's battery may be low.	Support HR & BP†. Change pacing box to programmed replacement unit and then replace batteries in old unit ready for use.
	The person may be experiencing some cellular or electrolyte issues.	Support HR & BP†. Change the polarity of the pacing wires in the pacing box. Check the person's electrolytes.

*mA = milliamperes. †Support HR & BP (i.e. support the person's heart rate and blood pressure by other means where possible). ‡mV = millivolts.

nursing care are similar to that for an individual having a permanent pacemaker implant.

The person may briefly lose consciousness before the device discharges, typically regaining consciousness quickly after the episode. Some people report significant discomfort with ICD discharge (like a 'blow to the chest'). A person in direct contact with the individual when the device discharges may experience a tingling sensation.

Cardiac mapping and catheter ablation

Cardiac mapping and catheter ablation are used to locate and destroy an ectopic focus. These diagnostic and therapeutic measures use electrophysiology techniques and can be performed in the cardiac catheterisation laboratory. *Cardiac mapping* is used to identify the site of earliest impulse formation in the atria or the ventricles. Intracardiac and extracardiac catheter electrodes and computer technology are used to pinpoint the ectopic site on a map of the heart. These same catheters can be used to deliver the ablative intervention.

Ablation destroys, removes or isolates an ectopic focus. In most instances, radiofrequency energy produced by high-frequency alternating current is used to create heat as it passes through tissue. Catheter ablation is used to treat supraventricular tachycardias, atrial fibrillation and flutter, and, in some cases, paroxysmal ventricular tachycardia.

Anticoagulant therapy may be started after catheter ablation to reduce the risk of clot formation at the ablation site.

Other therapies

In addition to medications and interventional techniques, other measures may be used to treat selected arrhythmias. Vagal manoeuvres that stimulate the parasympathetic nervous system may be used to slow the heart rate in supraventricular tachycardias. These manoeuvres include *carotid sinus massage* and the *Valsalva manoeuvre*. Carotid sinus massage is performed only by a medical officer during continuous cardiac monitoring. Excessive slowing of the heart rate may result. The Valsalva manoeuvre—forced exhalation against a closed glottis (e.g. bearing down)—increases intrathoracic pressure and vagal tone, slowing the pulse rate.

NURSING CARE OF THE PERSON **having a permanent pacemaker implant**

PREOPERATIVE CARE

- Provide routine preoperative care and teaching as outlined in the chapter 'Nursing care of people having surgery'.
- Assess knowledge and understanding of the procedure, clarifying and expanding on existing knowledge as needed. *Clarifying knowledge, providing information and conveying emotional support reduces anxiety and fear and allows the individual to develop a realistic outlook regarding pacer therapy.*
- Place ECG monitor electrodes away from potential incision sites. *This helps preserve skin integrity.*
- Teach range-of-motion (ROM) exercises for the affected side. *ROM exercises of the affected arm and shoulder prevent stiffness and impaired function following pacemaker insertion.*

POSTOPERATIVE CARE

- Provide postoperative monitoring, analgesia and care as outlined in the chapter 'Nursing care of people having surgery'.
- Obtain a chest x-ray as ordered. *A postoperative chest x-ray is used to identify lead location and detect possible complications, such as pneumothorax or pleural effusion.*
- Position for comfort. Minimise movement of the affected arm and shoulder during the initial postoperative period. *Restricting movement minimises discomfort on the operative side and allows the leads to become anchored, reducing the risk of dislodging.*
- Assist with gentle ROM exercises at least three times daily, beginning 24 hours after pacemaker implantation. *ROM exercises help restore normal shoulder movement and prevent contractures on the affected side.*
- Monitor pacemaker function with cardiac monitoring or intermittent ECGs. Report pacemaker problems to the doctor:
  - Failure to pace. *This may indicate battery depletion, damage or dislodgement of pacer wires or inappropriate sensing.*
  - Failure to capture (the pacemaker stimulus is not followed by ventricular depolarisation). *The electrical output of the pacemaker may not be adequate or the lead may be dislodged.*
  - Improper sensing (the pacemaker is firing or not firing, regardless of the intrinsic rate). *This increases the risk of decreased cardiac output and arrhythmias.*
  - Runaway pacemaker (a pacemaker firing at a rapid rate). *This may be due to generator malfunction or problems with sensing.*
  - Hiccups. A lead positioned near the phrenic nerve or diaphragm can stimulate it, causing hiccups. *Hiccups may occur in extremely thin individuals or may indicate a medical emergency with perforation of the right ventricle by the pacing electrode tip.*
- Assess for arrhythmias and treat as indicated. *Until the catheter is 'seated' or adheres to the myocardium, its movement may cause myocardial irritability and arrhythmias. Fibrotic tissue develops within 2 to 3 days.*
- Document the date of pacemaker insertion, the model and type, and settings. *This information is important for future reference.*
- Immediately report signs of potential complications, including myocardial perforation, cardiac tamponade, pneumothorax or haemothorax, emboli, skin breakdown, bleeding, infection, endocarditis or poor wound healing. (See the chapter 'Nursing

(continued)

NURSING CARE OF THE PERSON **having a permanent pacemaker implant (continued)**

care of people with cardiac disorders' for more information about cardiac tamponade and endocarditis, and the chapter 'Nursing care of people with ventilation disorders' for pneumothorax and haemothorax.) *Early identification of complications allows for aggressive intervention.*

- Provide a pacemaker identification card, including the manufacturer's name, model number, mode of operation, rate parameters and expected battery life. *This card provides a reference for the individual and future healthcare providers.*

HEALTH EDUCATION FOR THE PERSON AND FAMILY

Provide appropriate teaching for the person and their family about:

- Placement of the pacemaker generator and leads in relation to the heart.
- How the pacemaker works and the rate at which it is set.
- Battery replacement. Most pacemaker batteries last 6 to 12 years. Replacement requires an outpatient surgery to open the subcutaneous pocket and replace the battery.
- How to take and record the pulse rate. Instruct to assess pulse daily before arising and notify the doctor if 5 or more bpm slower than the preset pacemaker rate.
- Incision care and signs of infection. Bruising may be present following surgery.
- Signs of pacemaker malfunction to report, including dizziness, fainting, fatigue, weakness, chest pain or palpitations.
- Activity restrictions as ordered. This usually is limited to contact sports (which may damage the generator) and avoiding heavy lifting for 2 months after surgery.
- Resuming sexual activity as recommended by the medical officer. Avoid positions that cause pressure on the site.
- Avoiding tight-fitting clothing over the pacemaker site to reduce irritation and avoid skin breakdown.
- Carrying the pacemaker identification card at all times and wearing a MedicAlert® bracelet or tag.
- Notifying all care providers of the pacemaker.
- Not holding or using certain electrical devices over the pacemaker site, including household appliances or tools, garage door openers, antitheft devices or burglar alarms. Pacemaker will set off airport security detectors; notify security officials of its presence.
- Maintaining follow-up care with the doctor as recommended.

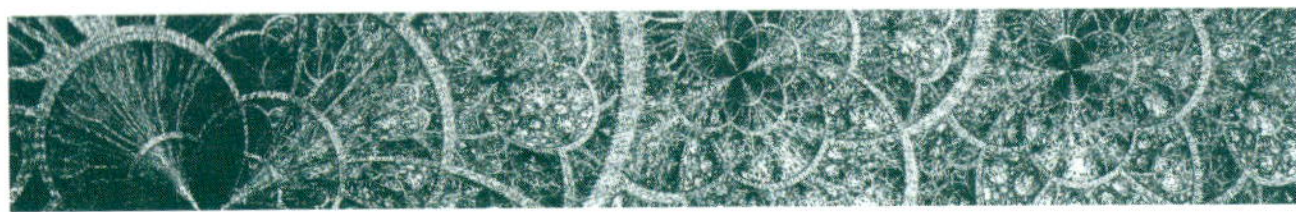

Nursing care

Caring for the person with cardiac arrhythmias requires the ability to recognise, identify and, in some cases, promptly treat the arrhythmia. The urgency of intervention is determined by the effects of the arrhythmia on the individual. Nursing care focuses on maintaining cardiac output, monitoring the response to therapy and teaching. See also the following nursing care plan for a person with superventricular tachycardia.

Health promotion

Health promotion measures to prevent coronary heart disease also reduce the risk of arrhythmias. In most cases, arrhythmias develop as a result of ischaemic or structural changes in the heart, rather than in isolation. Advise people who are at risk or who complain of occasional palpitations or 'flutters' in their chest to reduce their intake of caffeine and other sympathetic nervous system stimulants, such as excess chocolate.

Assessment

Assessment is vital before treating any suspected arrhythmia. What appears to be ventricular tachycardia on the monitor may be the individual scratching or brushing their teeth. Apparent asystole on the monitor may be due to a loose electrode patch. Similarly, a heart rate of 52 bpm may not affect the overall cardiac output in some individuals. Review the chapter 'A person-centred approach to assessing the cardiovascular and lymphatic systems' for complete assessment of the person with a cardiac problem.

- *Health history*: complaints of palpitations (ask for further definition of palpitations), 'fluttering' sensations or a sensation of the heart racing; episodes of dizziness, lightheadedness or syncope (fainting); timing (duration, time of day); correlation with food or beverage intake, activity; presence of chest pain, shortness of breath or other associated symptoms; history of heart or endocrine disease (such as hyperthyroidism); current medications.
- *Physical examination*: LOC; vital signs, including apical pulse for a full minute; regularity and amplitude of peripheral pulses; colour; presence of dyspnoea, adventitious lung sounds; ECG rhythm analysis; oxygen saturation levels.

Nursing diagnoses and interventions

The effect of the arrhythmia on cardiac output is the priority of nursing care. Other potential nursing diagnoses related to arrhythmias may include *Ineffective tissue perfusion*, *Activity intolerance*, and *Fear* or *Anxiety*.

Decreased cardiac output

Arrhythmias can affect cardiac output. Bradycardias decrease cardiac output if the stroke volume does not increase to compensate for the slow heart rate. Tachycardia reduces diastolic filling time, affecting stroke volume and coronary artery perfusion. Loss of the atrial kick in junctional rhythms, atrial fibrillation and AV blocks also decreases ventricular filling and cardiac output. In ventricular fibrillation, loss of ventricular contractions causes cardiac arrest and no cardiac output.

- Assess for decreased cardiac output: decreased LOC; tachycardia; tachypnoea; hypotension; low oxygen saturation; diaphoresis; low urine output; cool, clammy, mottled skin; pallor or cyanosis; diminished peripheral pulses. Initial signs of decreased cardiac output may be subtle, such as decreased LOC. *Early recognition of the arrhythmia's effect on cardiac output facilitates appropriate treatment and may prevent further adverse effects.*

> **CONSIDERATION FOR PRACTICE**
>
> **Before treating any arrhythmia, assess the individual, not just the monitor! Loose electrode pads, disconnected leads or cables, and muscle movement can simulate critical arrhythmias. The person's condition is the best indicator of the need for treatment.**

- Monitor ECG; obtain a rhythm strip and 'post-event' ECG strip every shift and when rhythm changes occur. Perform a daily (or as required) 12-lead ECG to track changes or detect ischaemia. *Documenting cardiac rhythm provides a record of disease progression and treatment effectiveness.*
- Assess for underlying causes of arrhythmias, such as hypovolaemia, hypoxia, anaemia, vagal stimulation or medications. *Sinus tachycardia often develops in response to tissue hypoxia. Vagal stimulation (such as the Valsalva manoeuvre) can precipitate bradycardia.*

NURSING CARE PLAN A person with supraventricular tachycardia

Sandra Banks, a 53-year-old woman from the Torres Strait Islands, is admitted to the cardiac unit with complaints of palpitations, light-headedness and dyspnoea. Her history reveals rheumatic fever at age 12 with subsequent rheumatic heart disease and mitral stenosis. An intravenous line is in place and she is receiving intranasal oxygen.

ASSESSMENT

Ms Banks is moderately anxious. Her ECG shows supraventricular tachycardia (SVT) with a rate of 154. Vital signs: T 37.1°C, R 26, BP 95/60. Peripheral pulses weak but equal, mucous membranes pale pink, skin cool and dry. Fine crackles noted in both lung bases. A loud S_3 gallop and a diastolic murmur are noted. Ms Banks is still complaining of palpitations and states that she 'feels so nervous and weak and dizzy'. Adenosine was trialled with no effect followed by an order for verapamil 2.5 mg IV. Preparations for synchronised cardioversion are planned if her ventricular rate does not respond to drug therapy.

DIAGNOSES

- *Decreased cardiac output* related to inadequate ventricular filling associated with rapid tachycardia.
- *Ineffective tissue perfusion: cerebral/cardiopulmonary/peripheral* related to decreased cardiac output.
- *Anxiety* related to unknown outcome of altered health state.

PLANNING

- Prepare propofol infusion (or intraprocedure medications as ordered).
- Document pretreatment vital signs, level of consciousness and peripheral pulses.
- Position the emergency trolley with drugs and airway management supplies near to the person's bed or trolley.

Expected outcomes

- Maintain adequate cardiac output and tissue perfusion.
- Demonstrate a ventricular rate within normal limits and stable vital signs.
- Verbalise reduced anxiety.
- Verbalise an understanding of the rationale for the treatment measures to control the heart rate.

IMPLEMENTATION

- Assist with cardioversion as indicated.
- Document procedure and postcardioversion rhythm and response to intervention.
- Provide oxygen per nasal prongs at 2 to 4 L/min.
- Explain the importance of rapidly reducing the heart rate. Explain the cardioversion procedure and encourage questions.
- Encourage verbalisation of fears and concerns. Answer questions honestly, correcting misconceptions about the disease process, treatment or prognosis.

EVALUATION

- Assess LOC, level of sedation, cardiovascular and respiratory status and skin condition following cardioversion.
- Continuously monitor ECG for rate, rhythm and conduction. Assess vital signs and associated symptoms with changes in ECG. Report findings to medical officer.

Intravenous verapamil lowers Ms Banks' heart rate to 138 for a short time, after which it increases to 164 with BP of 82/64. Her cardiologist performs carotid sinus massage. The ventricular rate slows to 126 for 2 minutes, revealing atrial flutter waves, and then returns to a rate of 150. Dr Mullins explains the treatment options, including synchronised cardioversion.

Ms Banks is lightly sedated and synchronised cardioversion is performed. One countershock converts Ms Banks to regular sinus rhythm at 96 bpm with BP 112/60.

Ms Banks is sleepy from the sedation but recovers without incident. She states that she feels 'much better', and her vital signs return to her normal levels. She remains in NSR with a rate of 86 to 92 for the remainder of her hospital stay. Ms Banks is commenced on frusemide to treat manifestations of mild heart failure.

CRITICAL THINKING IN THE NURSING PROCESS

1. What is the scientific basis for using carotid massage to treat supraventricular tachycardias? Was this an appropriate manoeuvre in the case of Ms Banks?
2. What other treatment options might the doctor have used to treat Ms Banks' supraventricular tachycardia if she had been asymptomatic with stable vital signs?
3. Why might the adenosine have failed? What critical interventions are required to increase the likelihood of success with this drug? (Hint: related to drug half life.)
4. Develop a teaching plan for Ms Banks related to her prescription for frusemide.

REFLECTION ON THE NURSING PROCESS

1. What is the likelihood of Ms Banks experiencing SVT again? What education is required for an individual who presents with SVT?
2. Outline what you have learned from this case study that you will apply to your future practice.

- Assess serum electrolytes (especially potassium, calcium and magnesium) and digoxin and anti-arrhythmic drug levels as indicated. Report abnormal values. *Electrolyte imbalances affect cardiac depolarisation and repolarisation and may cause arrhythmias. Toxic levels of digoxin and anti-arrhythmic drugs can precipitate further arrhythmias. Impaired renal or hepatic function increases the risk of toxicity, as does ageing.*

CONSIDERATION FOR PRACTICE

Assess vital signs, ECG and oxygen saturation every 5 to 15 minutes during acute arrhythmic episodes and during anti-arrhythmic drug infusions. These data provide a record of cardiac output during the arrhythmia. Anti-arrhythmic drugs can adversely affect heart rate, rhythm and blood pressure, further decreasing cardiac output.

- Be prepared to administer anti-arrhythmic medications as indicated. Implement *advanced* cardiac life support (ACLS) protocols as needed. *Emergency drugs should be readily available, especially on units with individuals at high risk of a life-threatening cardiac event.* See Table 29.6 and the 'Medication administration: anti-arrhythmic drugs' box for drugs used to treat common arrhythmias that may affect cardiac output.
- If appropriate, instruct to perform the Valsalva manoeuvre (bear down as if straining or coughing) for supraventricular tachycardia or ventricular tachycardia without angina. *Vagal manoeuvres stimulate the parasympathetic system and may terminate some arrhythmias. The Valsalva manoeuvre is contraindicated if chest pain occurs with the arrhythmia.*
- Prepare to assist with cardioversion. Prepare the individual per orders or hospital protocol (see Procedure 29.2). Explain the procedure to reduce anxiety. Have emergency equipment readily available. *Elective or emergency cardioversion is a treatment of choice for certain arrhythmias.*

CONSIDERATION FOR PRACTICE

On recognising ventricular fibrillation and cardiac arrest, begin emergency basic life support procedures. Call for help. Initiate advanced cardiac life support (ACLS) protocols if it is within your scope and training to do so. Assist with resuscitation measures as directed. Cardiac output ceases with ventricular fibrillation. Immediate or early defibrillation has been shown to have the greatest impact on survival following cardiac arrest.

- After cardiac arrest, transfer to critical care. Perform and document head-to-toe assessment; obtain laboratory tests, serial 12-lead ECGs and a chest x-ray as ordered; monitor and maintain oxygenation and intravenous infusions; and monitor vital signs and cardiac rhythm. *The period following resuscitation is critical, necessitating careful monitoring. Post-arrest assessment allows comparison of the individual's condition with pre-arrest status and may identify CPR-related injuries. Correcting electrolyte disturbances, hypoxia and acid–base imbalances is important to prevent further arrhythmias and potential adverse effects on cardiac output. Intravenous access is crucial to maintain drug infusions. Haemodynamic monitoring may be instituted. The 12-lead ECG documents myocardial status and the chest x-ray provides information about pulmonary status and possible thoracic injury due to CPR.*
- Notify the family of significant changes in the person's condition, providing up-to-date information. Prepare family members prior to visits by explaining interventions (such as invasive tubes, a ventilator or additional equipment) implemented since the last visit. *Concern for the family and significant others is part of holistic nursing. Researchers studying the needs of families have found that one of the most important needs was information about their loved one's condition. Individuals and their families need and appreciate honest communication and compassionate care. Preparing the family for critical changes in the person's condition and plan of care helps them to cope with a situational crisis.*

Community-based care

Arrhythmias have a significant physical and psychological impact on the person and all their family members. Many of these individuals and their families are under a great deal of stress from frequent hospitalisations, experimentation with therapies, frustration and the fear of sudden cardiac death. A major teaching effort focuses on coping strategies and lifestyle changes as well as specific management of prescribed therapies. Include the following topics as appropriate when teaching the person and their family for home care:

- function, maintenance, precautions and signs of malfunction or complications of any implanted device such as a pacemaker or ICD
- monitoring pulse rate and rhythm
- activity or dietary restrictions, and any potential effects of the arrhythmia or its treatment on lifestyle
- medication management to reduce the risk of arrhythmias, including the desired and potential adverse effects of anti-arrhythmic drugs
- specific instructions related to planned diagnostic tests or procedures
- the importance of follow-up visits with the cardiologist
- the importance of obtaining CPR training for the individual and their family members.

In addition, discuss fears related to treatment or implanted devices, such as that of shocking a significant other during close contact or sexual activity. Explain that if a shock occurs, the partner may feel a slight buzz or tingling but should not be harmed. Refer to and encourage the person and their family to attend a peer support group for the specific condition.

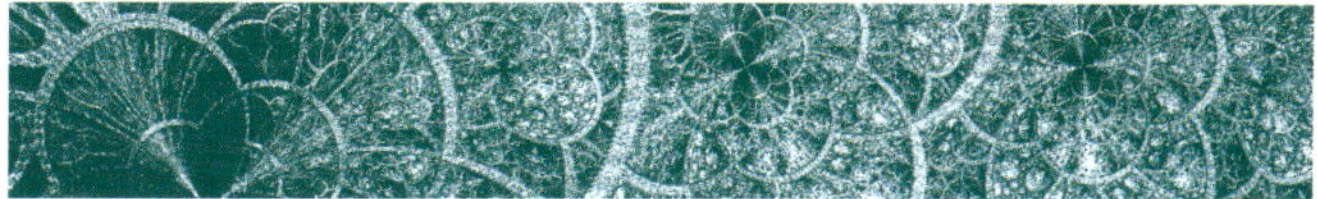

THE PERSON WITH SUDDEN CARDIAC DEATH

Sudden cardiac death (SCD) is defined as unexpected death occurring within 1 hour of the onset of cardiovascular symptoms. The presence of left ventricular dysfunction caused by any condition is the greatest predictor of SCD and usually results from ventricular fibrillation or pulseless ventricular tachycardia (Sovari, 2020). These rhythms are within the group of rhythms that cannot sustain life and can be called a cardiac arrest. *Cardiac arrest* is the sudden collapse, loss of consciousness and cessation of effective circulation that precedes biological death. Worldwide, fewer than 6% of out-of-hospital cardiac arrest victims survive.

Almost 50% of all deaths due to coronary heart disease are attributed to SCD. A significant per cent of sudden cardiac deaths can be attributed to CHD. Other cardiac pathologies such as cardiomyopathy and valvular disorders also may lead to SCD. Non-cardiac causes of sudden death include electrocution, pulmonary embolism and rapid blood loss from a ruptured aortic aneurysm.

Ventricular fibrillation is the most common arrhythmia associated with sudden cardiac death, accounting for the majority of cardiac arrests. Sustained severe bradyarrhythmias, *asystole* or cardiac standstill, and pulseless electrical activity (organised cardiac electrical activity without a mechanical response) are responsible for most of the remaining SCDs. Selected cardiac and non-cardiac causes of sudden cardiac death are listed in Box 29.4.

Risk factors for SCD are those associated with coronary heart disease (see the first section of this chapter). Advancing age and male gender are powerful risk factors. After age 65, the gap between male and female incidence of SCD narrows. Individuals with arrhythmias such as recurrent ventricular tachycardia (VT) may have a higher risk of SCD. Women with acute myocardial infarction, however, are more likely to present with cardiac arrest and cardiogenic shock than with ventricular tachycardia. Australian statistics demonstrate that in the first decade of the 21st century, even though deaths from cardiovascular diseases have decreased for both men and women, overall there are still more women dying of cardiac arrest and CVD than men (ABS, 2010).

Pathophysiology

Evidence of coronary heart disease with significant atherosclerosis and narrowing of two or more major coronary arteries is found in the majority of SCD victims. An acute change in cardiovascular status precedes cardiac arrest by up to 1 hour; however, often the onset is instantaneous or abrupt. An imbalance in electrolytes, or autonomic tone, irregular cellular activity, or functional blockages within the conduction system, may contribute to the development of ventricular tachycardiac or ventricular fibrillation (Sovari, 2020).

Various other factors can also contribute to the development of lethal arrhythmia, including abnormalities of myocardial structure or function. Structural abnormalities include infarction, hypertrophy and myopathy. Functional deviations are caused by such factors as ischaemia followed by reperfusion, altered homeostasis, pathological hormone interactions, and toxic effects. The interactions of the two cause myocardial instability and may precipitate fatal arrhythmias.

BOX 29.4 Selected causes of sudden cardiac death

Cardiac causes
- Coronary heart disease
- Reperfusion following ischaemia
- Myocardial hypertrophy
- Cardiomyopathy
- Inflammatory myocardial disorders
- Valve disorders
- Primary electrical disorders
- Dissecting or ruptured aortic or ventricular aneurysm
- Cardiac drug toxicity

Non-cardiac causes
- Pulmonary embolism
- Cerebral haemorrhage
- Autonomic dysfunction
- Choking
- Electrical shock
- Electrolyte and acid–base imbalances

Manifestations

Sudden cardiac death may be preceded by typical manifestations of acute coronary syndrome or myocardial infarction, including severe chest pain, dyspnoea or orthopnoea, and palpitations or light-headedness. The event itself is abrupt, with complete loss of consciousness and death within minutes. If ventricular tachycardia precedes cardiac arrest, consciousness and mentation may be impaired prior to collapse and loss of consciousness.

INTERPROFESSIONAL CARE

The goal of care is to restore cardiac output and tissue perfusion. Treatment measures are initiated as soon as clinical cardiac arrest is verified by the absence of respirations and carotid or femoral pulses. Basic life support and ACLS measures must be instituted within 2 to 4 minutes of cardiac arrest to prevent permanent neurological damage and ischaemic injury to other organs.

FIGURE 29.13 ***Schematic of an automated external defibrillator (AED) attached to an individual***

Where available, an *automated external defibrillator (AED)* should be used to immediately defibrillate the person in ventricular fibrillation. Self-adhesive conductive pads attached to connecting cables are positioned on the chest (see Figure 29.13). The Australian Resuscitation Council supports the use of public access defibrillation in association with emergency services and locally provided training.

Cardiopulmonary resuscitation is a mechanical attempt to maintain tissue perfusion and oxygenation using oral resuscitation and external cardiac compressions. All healthcare providers need to be proficient in CPR. The technique should be performed according to the Australian Resuscitation Council's most recent procedures. Healthcare personnel need to be familiar with these protocols and maintain up-to-date knowledge and skills, as the techniques and theory do change.

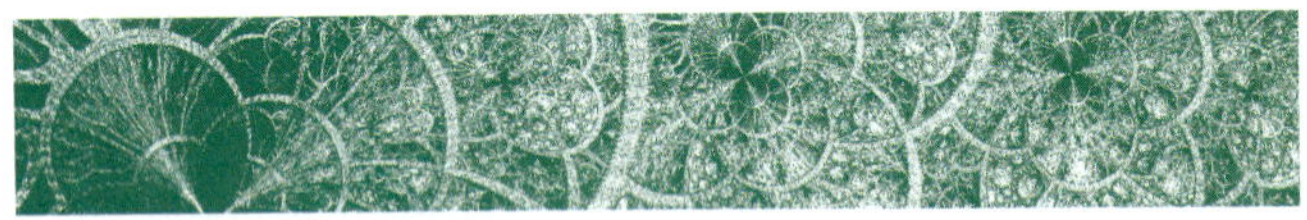

Nursing care

Nursing care of the person experiencing sudden cardiac death requires prompt recognition of the event and immediate initiation of basic lifesaving (BLS) and advanced lifesaving (ALS) protocols. As previously noted, fast and effective cardiac compressions and early defibrillation of unstable VT and VF are the most important keys to survival of cardiac arrest victims. Important concepts of emergency cardiac care are:

- Treat the person, not the monitor. If a bizarre rhythm is displayed on the monitor, it is important to determine if this is artefact, clinical deterioration or emergency. It is critical to look at the individual. If they are talking, well perfused and in no apparent discomfort, there may be other explanations for what is occurring on the monitor. Recognise signs and symptoms of cardiac compromise early.
- Activate the emergency medical services system (i.e. call a 'code', call 000 or 112 from a mobile phone—even if it has no credit).
- Begin and continue basic cardiac life support principles throughout the resuscitation effort.
- Continually assess the effectiveness of emergency interventions.
- Defibrillate ventricular fibrillation (VF) and pulseless ventricular tachycardia (VT) as soon as possible.
- Initiate advanced cardiac life support protocols early if within scope of practice.

The family should not be forgotten during resuscitation. If the family is present, a staff member needs to support significant others and offer a private room in which to await the outcome. If the family is not present, they should be notified that their family member is not doing well and asked to come to the hospital as soon as possible. The outcome should be presented in a careful manner to prevent the family from racing to the hospital, possibly precipitating an automobile crash. Pastoral care or the family's choice of spiritual support is offered to help during this difficult time. Attendance of family members during resuscitation efforts is controversial and depends on institutional protocols and family desires.

After successful resuscitation, the nurse provides care specific to the individual's underlying disease processes and needs. Intravenous infusions such as lignocaine, bretylium or dopamine may be ordered to prevent further arrhythmias and maintain haemodynamic stability.

If the person does not survive the arrest, the nurse provides postmortem care and emotional and spiritual support to the family.

Nursing diagnoses to consider for the person experiencing SCD include the following:

- *Ineffective tissue perfusion*: *cerebral* related to ineffective cardiac output.
- *Impaired spontaneous ventilation* related to cardiac arrest.

- *Spiritual distress* related to unexplained sudden cardiac death.
- *Disturbed thought processes* related to compromised cerebral circulation.
- *Fear* related to risk of future episodes of sudden cardiac death.

The risk of a future episode of sudden cardiac death requires careful and effective teaching for home care prior to discharge. Discuss the following topics with the person and family:

- risk factor reduction for coronary heart disease
- planned diagnostic studies to identify the cause of SCD and possible interventions
- the risks and benefits of an ICD if appropriate
- the importance of carrying a card at all times listing all current medications and the healthcare provider
- early manifestations or warning signs of cardiac arrest
- the importance of CPR training and maintaining proficiency in performing CPR. (Provide referral to local CPR training providers.)

Nurses can affect death rates from cardiac arrest through community teaching as well. Survival rates from sudden cardiac death improve in communities in which a significant portion of the population is trained in CPR and early response by emergency services is stressed. Work with community groups and individuals can help create a population of people able to perform effective CPR.

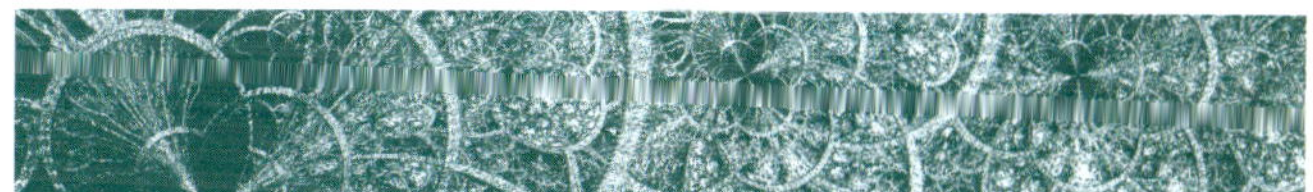

CHAPTER HIGHLIGHTS

- Atherosclerosis is the primary underlying process in coronary heart disease, and impaired perfusion of myocardial tissue.
- The risk factors for coronary heart disease are those for atherosclerosis: age, gender and genetic factors; hypertension, diabetes, abnormal blood lipids; cigarette smoking, obesity, physical inactivity and diet; and emerging risk factors such as the metabolic syndrome and homocysteine levels.
- Smoking cessation, exercise, diet modification, weight loss, medications to achieve desired blood lipid values and effective hypertension and diabetes management are the primary treatment measures for coronary heart disease.
- Atherosclerosis of coronary vessels impairs the supply of blood, oxygen and nutrients to the myocardium. Myocardial ischaemia results in the manifestations of coronary heart disease: angina pectoris, acute coronary syndrome and myocardial infarction.
- Stable angina develops with a predictable amount of activity or stress and typically follows an activity–pain, rest–relief pattern. Stable angina often can be managed effectively by medications and risk factor modification. The nursing focus is on education.
- Acute coronary syndrome or unstable angina is characterised by increasingly severe chest pain that occurs unpredictably. Acute coronary syndrome often requires aggressive interventions such as percutaneous coronary revascularisation or coronary artery bypass surgery.
- Myocardial infarction, necrosis of myocardial tissue, results from complete blockage of a coronary artery, usually due to atherosclerotic plaque rupture and thrombus formation. Prompt restoration of blood flow through a revascularisation procedure or administration of a thrombolytic drug to dissolve the blood clot is necessary to preserve functional muscle tissue.
- The nursing focus for individuals with acute coronary syndrome and myocardial infarction is on reducing myocardial work through measures such as pain relief and activity limitation, promoting blood flow and oxygenation through medication and oxygen administration and positioning, and early recognition and treatment of complications.
- Cardiac arrhythmias may arise anywhere in [illegible] tissue of the myocardium. Arrhythmias may be either benign or fatal, depending on their effect on cardiac output.
- Tachycardias increase the workload of the heart and may interfere with cardiac output if ventricular filling is impaired by the rapid rate.
- Bradycardias can affect cardiac output when the rate is too slow to meet the metabolic needs of the body.
- Atrial fibrillation is a common arrhythmia that can lead to formation of blood clots within the heart and subsequent stroke if these clots lodge in cerebral blood vessels.
- Frequent ventricular arrhythmias may indicate an increased risk of ventricular fibrillation and cardiac arrest.
- AV conduction blocks interfere with conduction of the sinus or atrial impulse through the AV node and to the ventricles.
- Although many anti-arrhythmic medications are available, all increase the risk of arrhythmia development, so they are used sparingly.
- The nurse's role in caring for a person with cardiac arrhythmias focuses on prompt identification of the rhythm disruption, assessment of its effect on the person, administration of medications and other treatment measures, and institution of life support procedures as indicated.

CONCEPT CHECK

1 The nurse evaluates her teaching as effective when an individual identifies which of the following modifiable risk factors for coronary heart disease (CHD) as contributing to the greatest extent?

1 obesity
2 diet
3 smoking
4 stress

2 When teaching an individual about simvastatin, the nurse instructs the person to:

1 promptly report muscle pain or tenderness to the doctor
2 consume a diet that includes no more than 20% of kilojoules from saturated fat
3 abstain from alcohol use while taking this drug
4 take the drug with meals to minimise gastric distress

3 When assessing a person with stable angina, the nurse would expect to find:

1 persistent ECG changes
2 correlation between activity level and pain
3 increasing nocturnal pain
4 evidence of impaired cardiac output such as weak peripheral pulses

4 The nurse caring for a person with acute coronary syndrome identifies which of the following nursing diagnoses to be of highest priority?
1 *Anxiety* related to unknown outcome of disorder.
2 *Ineffective health maintenance* related to lack of knowledge about coronary heart disease.
3 *Decreased cardiac output* related to myocardial ischaemia.
4 *Ineffective tissue perfusion: cardiopulmonary* related to underlying coronary heart disease.

5 The nurse caring for a person returning from a coronary angioplasty with stent placement plans which of the following interventions?
1 securing chest tubes to bedding
2 maintaining leg extension on the affected side
3 discontinuing intravenous lines when taking oral fluids
4 treating chest pain with intravenous morphine as needed

6 In planning care for the person with acute myocardial infarction (AMI), the nurse identifies the highest priority goal of care as:
1 stable ECG rhythm
2 ability to verbalise causes and effects of CHD
3 compliance with prescribed bed rest
4 relief of pain

7 Which of the following nursing diagnoses is of highest priority for the person undergoing thrombolytic therapy?
1 *Ineffective protection.*
2 *Ineffective health maintenance.*
3 *Risk of powerlessness.*
4 *Anxiety.*

8 In reviewing laboratory results for a person admitted with acute chest pain, the nurse is most concerned about which of the following?
1 haematocrit 35%
2 AST 65 U/L
3 CK 320 U/L
4 aPTT 35 seconds

9 The nurse recognises second-degree AV block, type II (Mobitz II) and intervenes appropriately when he:
1 records the finding in the chart
2 prepares for temporary pacemaker insertion
3 administers a class IB anti-arrhythmic drug
4 places the person in Fowler's position

10 On identifying sinus bradycardia at a rate of 45 bpm, the nurse should:
1 assess mental status and blood pressure
2 assess peripheral pulses on all four extremities
3 determine if an apical–radial pulse deficit is present
4 prepare to administer intravenous atropine

BIBLIOGRAPHY

Australian Bureau of Statistics (ABS) (2018). *Heart, stroke and vascular disease 2017–18*. Retrieved from https://www.abs.gov.au/

Australian Bureau of Statistics (ABS) (2022a). *Aboriginal and Torres Strait Islander people: Census*. Retrieved from https://www.abs.gov.au/

Australian Bureau of Statistics (ABS) (2022b). *Regional population by age and sex*. Retrieved from https://www.abs.gov.au/

Australian Institute of Health and Welfare (AIHW) (2017). *Aboriginal and Torres Strait Islander Health Performance Framework*. Retrieved from https://www.aihw.gov.au/

Australian Institute of Health and Welfare (AIHW) (2018). *Health expenditure Australia 2016–17*. Health and welfare expenditure series no. 64. (Cat. no. HWE 74.) Canberra: AIHW. Retrieved from https://www.aihw.gov.au/

Australian Institute of Health and Welfare (AIHW) (2022a). *Australia's health 2022: Topic health*. (Cat. no. AUS 241.) Canberra: AIHW. Retrieved from https://www.aihw.gov.au/

Australian Institute of Health and Welfare (AIHW) (2022b). *Aboriginal and Torres Strait Islander Health Performance Framework 2020 summary report*. (Cat. No. IHPF 2.) Canberra: AIHW. Retrieved from https://indigenoushpf.gov.au/

Australian Institute of Health and Welfare (AIHW) (2022c). *Admitted patient care 2020–21: Table S6.8: Differential access to hospital procedures*. Retrieved from https://www.aihw.gov.au/

Australian Resuscitation Council (ARC) (2016). *Section 14: Acute coronary syndromes*. Retrieved from https://www.resus.org.au/

Bajic, Z., Sobot, T., Skrbic, R., Stojiljkovic, M. P., Ponorac, N., Matavulj, A. & Djuric, D. M. (2022). Homocysteine, vitamins B6 and folic acid in experimental models of myocardial infarction and heart failure. How strong is that link? *Biomolecules, 12*(4), 536. https://doi.org/10.3390/biom12040536

Bertic, M., Worme, M., Foroutan, F., Rao, V., Ross, H., Billia, F. & Alba, A. (2022). Predictors of survival and favorable neurologic outcome in patients treated with eCPR: A systematic review and meta-analysis. *Journal of Cardiovascular Translational Research, 15*(2), 279–290. https://doi.org/10.1007/s12265-021-10195-9

Beussink-Nelson, L., Baldridge, A., Hibler, E. et al. (2022). Knowledge and perception of cardiovascular disease risk in women of reproductive age. *American Journal of Preventive Cardiology, 11*, 100364. https://doi.org/10.1016/j.ajpc.2022.100364

Beyerbach, D. (2019). Pacemakers and implantable cardioverter-defibrillators. *Emedicine*. Retrieved from http://emedicine.medscape.com/

Briffa, T., Winnall, W., Greenhalgh, E. & Winstanley, M. (2021). 3.1 Smoking and cardiovascular disease. In E. Greenhalgh, M. Scollo & M. Winstanley (eds), *Tobacco in Australia: Facts and issues*. Melbourne: Cancer Council Victoria. Retrieved from https://www.tobaccoinaustralia.org.au/

Bullock, S. & Hales, M. (2019). *Principles of pathophysiology* (2nd ed.). Frenchs Forest, NSW: Pearson.

Bullock, S. & Manias, E. (2022). *Fundamentals of pharmacology* (9th ed.). Frenchs Forest, NSW: Pearson.

Burke, A. (2021). Pathology of acute myocardial infarction. *Emedicine*. Retrieved from http://emedicine.medscape.com/

Cardeillac, M., Lefebvre, F., Baicry, F. et al. (2022). Symptoms of infarction in women: Is there a real difference compared to men? A systematic review of the literature with meta-analysis. *Journal of Clinical Medicine, 11*(5), 1319. https://doi.org/10.3390/jcm11051319

Chew, D., Scott, I., Cullen, L. et al. (2016). National Heart Foundation of Australia and Cardiac Society of Australia and New Zealand: Australian clinical guidelines for the management of acute coronary syndromes 2016. *Heart, Lung and Circulation, 25*(9), 895–951.

Coven, D. (2020). Acute coronary syndrome. *Emedicine*. Retrieved from http://emedicine.medscape.com/

Dave, J. (2022). Torsade de pointes. *Emedicine*. Retrieved from http://emedicine.medscape.com/

Del Buono, M. G., Montone, R. A., Camilli, M. et al. (2021). Coronary microvascular dysfunction across the spectrum of cardiovascular diseases: JACC state-of-the-art review. *Journal of the American College of Cardiology, 78*(13), 1352–1371. https://doi.org/10.1016/j.jacc.2021.07.042

Framingham Heart Study (FHS) (2022). *About the Framingham Heart Study*. Retrieved from https://www.framinghamheartstudy.org/

Greenberg, M. (2022). Catheter ablation. *Emedicine*. Retrieved from http://emedicine.medscape.com/

Greenhalgh, E., Stillman, S. & Ford, C. (2020). 7.1 Health and other benefits of quitting. In E. Greenhalgh, M. Scollo & M. Winstanley (eds), *Tobacco in Australia: Facts and issues*. Melbourne: Cancer Council Victoria. Retrieved from http://www.tobaccoinaustralia.org.au/

Gursahani, K. (2021). Cardiac markers. *Emedicine*. Retrieved from http://emedicine.medscape.com/

Haber, M. (2021). Angina pectoris in emergency medicine. *Emedicine*. Retrieved from http://emedicine.medscape.com/

Kalyanasundaram, A. (2020). Comparison of coronary artery grafting (CABG) and percutaneous coronary intervention (PCI). *Emedicine*. Retrieved from http://emedicine.medscape.com/

Khan, S., Ning, H., Sinha, A. et al. (2021). Cigarette smoking and competing risks for fatal and nonfatal cardiovascular disease subtypes across the life course. *Journal of the American Heart Association, 10*(23), e021751–e021751. https://doi.org/10.1161/JAHA.121.021751

Laskowski, D., Feger, S., Bosserdt, M. et al. (2021). Detection of relevant extracardiac findings on coronary computed tomography angiography vs.

invasive coronary angiography. *European Radiology*, *32*(1), 122–131. https://doi.org/10.1007/s00330-021-07967-x

Levett-Jones, T., Dwyer, T., Reid-Searl, K., Heaton, L., Flenady, T., Applegarth, J., Guinea, S. & Andersen, P. (2017). *Patient Safety Competency Framework (PSCF) for Nursing Students*. Sydney. Retrieved from http://psframework.wpengine.com/

Link, M. (2022). Modes of cardiac pacing: Nomenclature and selection. *UpToDate*. Retrieved from https://www.uptodate.com/

Merlo, A., Troccolo, A., Piredda, E., Porto, I. & Gil Ad, V. (2022). Myocardial infarction with non-obstructive coronary arteries: Risk factors and associated comorbidities. *Frontiers in Cardiovascular Medicine*, *9*, 895053. https://doi.org/10.3389/fcvm.2022.895053

Mohanta, S., Peng, L., Li, Y. et al. (2022). Neuroimmune cardiovascular interfaces control atherosclerosis. *Nature (London)*, *605*(7908), 152–159. https://doi.org/10.1038/s41586-022-04673-6

Momeni, Z., Dehghani, A., Fallahzadeh, H., Koohgardi, M., Dafei, M., Hekmatimoghaddam, S. H. & Mohammadi, M. (2020). The impacts of pill contraceptive low-dose on plasma levels of nitric oxide, homocysteine, and lipid profiles in the exposed vs. non exposed women: As the risk factor for cardiovascular diseases. *Contraception and Reproductive Medicine*, *5*(1), 7. https://doi.org/10.1186/s40834-020-00110-z

National Heart Foundation (2021). *Women and heart disease*. Retrieved from https://www.heartfoundation.org.au/

National Heart Foundation of Australia (2019). *Heart healthy eating patterns*. Retrieved from https://www.heartfoundation.org.au/

Norris, T. L. (2018). *Porth's pathophysiology: Concepts of altered health states* (10th ed.). Philadelphia: Lippincott Williams & Wilkins.

Olshansky, B. (2022). Atrioventricular nodal reentry tachycardia. *Emedicine*. Retrieved from http://emedicine.medscape.com/

Perrotta, I. (2022). Atherosclerosis: From molecular biology to therapeutic perspective. *International Journal of Molecular Sciences*, *23*(7), 3444. https://doi.org/10.3390/ijms23073444

Peyter, A.-C., Armengaud, J.-B., Guillot, E. & Yzydorczyk, C. (2021). Endothelial progenitor cells dysfunctions and cardiometabolic disorders: From mechanisms to therapeutic approaches. *International Journal of Molecular Sciences*, *22*(13), 6667. https://doi.org/10.3390/ijms22136667

[illegible] ([illegible]). Cardiogenic shock. *Emedicine*. Retrieved from http://emedicine.medscape.com/

Royal Australian College of General Practitioners (RACGP) (2022a). *Prevention of vascular and metabolic disease: Cholesterol and other lipids*. Retrieved from https://www.racgp.org.au/

Royal Australian College of General Practitioners (RACGP) (2022b). *Guidelines for preventive activities in general practice*. Retrieved from https://www.racgp.org.au/

Sassen, M. V., Spies, D. M., Kiekenap, J., Betz, S. & Kill, C. (2019). Defibrillation success in out-of-hospital cardiac arrest: Point in time of ventricular fibrillation recurrence after successful shock during early phase of cardiopulmonary resuscitation. *Resuscitation*, *142*, e32–e32. https://doi.org/10.1016/j.resuscitation.2019.06.079

Shurmur, S. (2022). Coronary drug-eluting stent. *Emedicine*. Retrieved from http://emedicine.medscape.com/

Singer, P., Richter, V., Singer, K. & Löhlein, I. (2021). Analyses and declarations of omega-3 fatty acids in canned seafood may help to quantify their dietary intake. *Nutrients*, *13*(9), 2970. https://doi.org/10.3390/nu13092970

Sovari, A. (2020). Sudden cardiac death. *Emedicine*. Retrieved from http://emedicine.medscape.com/

Sweis, R. & Jivan, A. (2022). Revascularization for acute coronary syndromes. *MSD Manual Professional Version*. Retrieved from https://www.msdmanuals.com/

Tobb, K., Kocher, M. & Bullock-Palmer, R. P. (2022). Underrepresentation of women in cardiovascular trials—It is time to shatter this glass ceiling. *American Heart Journal Plus*, *13*, 100109. https://doi.org/10.1016/j.ahjo.2022.100109

van Trier, T., Mohammadnia, N., Snaterse, M., Peters, R., Jørstad, H. & [illegible], W. ([illegible]). Lifestyle management to prevent atherosclerotic cardiovascular disease: Evidence and challenges. *Netherlands Heart Journal*, *30*(1), 3–14. https://doi.org/10.1007/s12471-021-01642-y

Varshney, A., DeFilippis, E., Cowger, J., Netuka, I., Pinney, S. & Givertz, M. (2022). Trends and outcomes of left ventricular assist device therapy: JACC focus seminar. *Journal of the American College of Cardiology*, *79*(11), 1092–1107. https://doi.org/10.1016/j.jacc.2022.01.017

Zhu, J., Xun, P.-C., Kolencik, M., Yang, K.-F., Fly, A. D. & Kahe, K. (2022). Do B vitamins enhance the effect of omega-3 polyunsaturated fatty acids on cardiovascular diseases? A systematic review of clinical trials. *Nutrients*, *14*(8), 1608. https://doi.org/10.3390/nu14081608

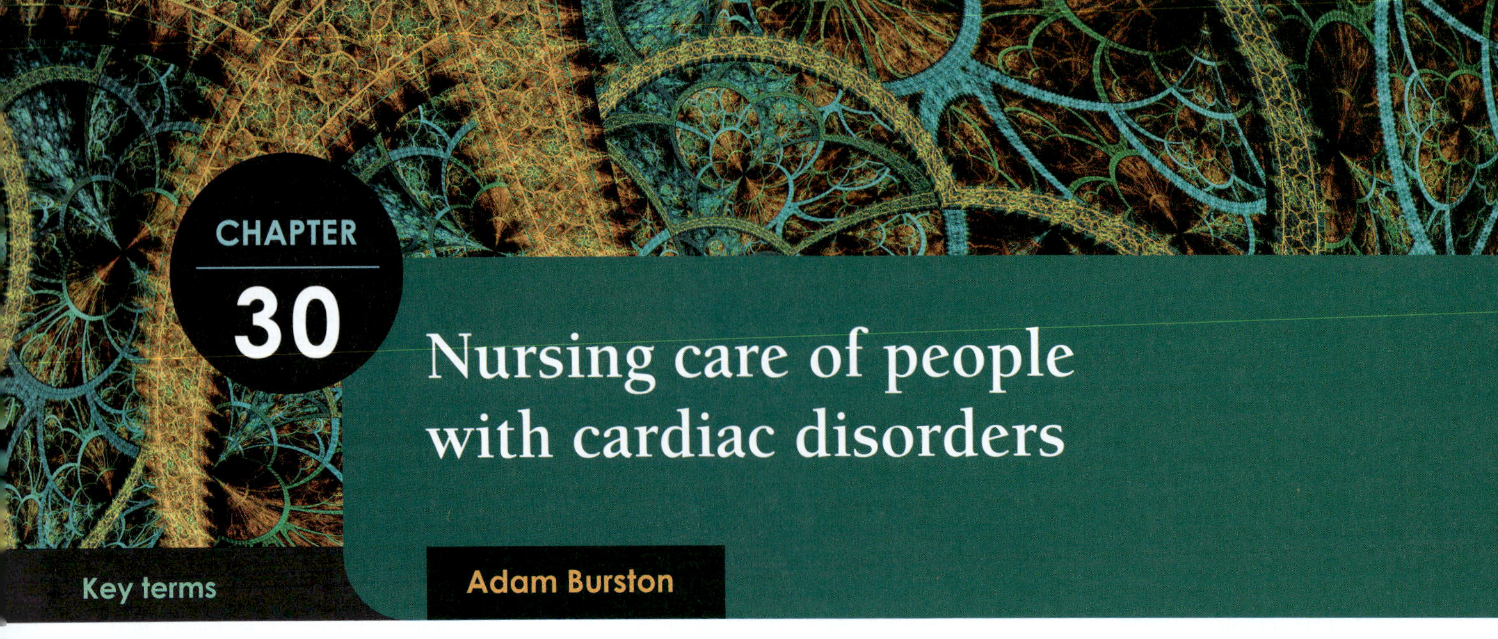

CHAPTER 30

Nursing care of people with cardiac disorders

Adam Burston

Key terms

Learning outcomes

- Relate the interprofessional care requirements for a person with heart failure to the pathophysiology of the condition.
- Explain the risk factors, course and interventions required to competently care for a person with pulmonary oedema.
- Differentiate between the various inflammatory and infective conditions resulting in a person's cardiac disorder.
- Compare and contrast the course and management principles for individuals experiencing various cardiomyopathies.

Clinical competencies

- Apply knowledge of normal cardiac anatomy and physiology and assessment techniques in caring for the person with cardiac disorders.
- Assess functional health status of individuals with cardiac disorders, documenting and reporting deviations to expected findings.
- Plan, prioritise and provide evidence-based, individualised care for the person with cardiac disorders.
- Administer prescribed medications and treatments to individuals with cardiac disorders.
- Actively participate in planning and coordinating interprofessional care for the person with cardiac disorders.
- Provide appropriate teaching and community-based care for people with cardiac disorders and their families.
- Evaluate the effectiveness of nursing care, revising the plan of care as needed to promote, maintain or restore functional health status of individuals with cardiac disorders.

Cardiac disorders affect the structure and/or function of the heart. These disorders interfere with the heart's primary purpose: to pump enough blood to meet the body's demand for oxygen and nutrients. Disruptions in cardiac function affect the performance of other organs and tissues, potentially leading to organ system failure and death.

Heart failure is the most common cardiac disorder. Pulmonary oedema is also discussed in this chapter. The inclusion and organisation of the inflammatory and infective cardiac disorders proves difficult as there is usually an intimate relationship between these conditions, either as a cause or effect. As such, although conditions such as rheumatic heart disease, the various carditises and cardiomyopathy are often related, they are treated as separate entities in this chapter in order to facilitate sufficient coverage of content.

Before continuing with this chapter, please review the heart's anatomy and physiology, nursing assessment and diagnostic tests in the chapter 'A person-centred approach to assessing the cardiovascular and lymphatic systems'.

Heart failure

Heart failure is a complex syndrome caused by conditions that impair the ejection of oxygen and nutrient-rich blood from the ventricles. The failure to pump sufficient blood into the systemic circulation results in an inability to meet the body's metabolic demands (Bullock & Hales, 2019). It is often a long-term effect of coronary heart disease (CHD) and myocardial infarction (MI) when left ventricular damage is extensive enough to impair cardiac output (see the chapter 'Nursing care of people with coronary heart disease'). Other diseases of the heart also may cause heart failure, including structural and inflammatory disorders. In normal hearts, failure can result from excessive demands placed on the heart. Heart failure may be acute or chronic.

THE PERSON WITH HEART FAILURE

When the heart cannot effectively fill or contract with adequate strength to meet the needs of the body, cardiac output falls and decreased tissue perfusion develops. Initially, compensatory mechanisms are activated to offset reduced cardiac output and restore tissue perfusion. The heart failure will often result in vascular congestion, resulting in oedema in either the lungs or the periphery, and is therefore commonly called *congestive heart failure (CHF)*. As the compensatory mechanisms are exhausted, morbidity and mortality risks increase.

Reduced cardiac function may occur due to *impaired myocardial contraction*, from CHD, myocardial ischaemia or infarction, or from a primary cardiac muscle disorder such as cardiomyopathy or myocarditis. Structural cardiac disorders, such as valve disorders or congenital heart defects, and hypertension also can lead to heart failure when the heart muscle is damaged by the long-standing *excessive workload* associated with these conditions. Individuals without a primary abnormality of myocardial function may present with manifestations of heart failure due to *acute excess demands* placed on the myocardium, such as volume overload, hyperthyroidism and massive pulmonary embolus (see Table 30.1). Hypertension and coronary heart disease are the leading causes of heart failure in Australia.

Incidence, prevalence and risk factors

In Australia in 2020, 1,472 male and 1,777 female deaths resulted from heart failure. It has dropped slightly to the 14th leading cause of death in males and the 11th leading cause of death in females (Australian Bureau of Statistics (ABS), 2021), an improvement over the past decade. Some explanation of the gender disparity in the statistics may be related to greater life expectancy in women, as a significant percentage of heart-failure-related deaths occur in older women (see the 'Nursing care of the older adult' box). The prognosis for an individual with heart failure depends on its underlying cause and how effectively precipitating factors can be treated.

Prevalence of heart failure in Aboriginal and Torres Strait Islander people is slowly decreasing but remains 1.4 times higher than in non-Indigenous Australians (ABS, 2021). Those admitted to hospital with heart failure are younger than non-Indigenous patients and have a higher number of comorbidities (McGee et al., 2021) (see the 'Focus on cultural diversity' box).

In Aboriginal and Torres Strait Islander people, rheumatic heart disease (RHD) plays a significant role in mortality. Rheumatic heart disease prevalence in Aboriginal and Torres Strait Islander people is significant, with over 81% of cases reported during 2015–2019 occurring in this population (Australian Institute of Health and Welfare (AIHW), 2021).

Physiology review

The mechanical pumping action of cardiac muscle propels the blood it receives to the pulmonary and systemic vascular systems for reoxygenation and delivery to the tissues. *Cardiac output (CO)* is the amount of blood pumped from the ventricles in 1 minute. Cardiac output is used to assess cardiac performance, especially left ventricular function. Effective cardiac

TABLE 30.1 Selected causes of heart failure

IMPAIRED MYOCARDIAL FUNCTION	INCREASED CARDIAC WORKLOAD	ACUTE NON-CARDIAC CONDITIONS
• Coronary heart disease	• Hypertension	• Volume overload
• Cardiomyopathies	• Valve disorders	• Hyperthyroidism
• Rheumatic fever	• Anaemias	• Fever, infection
• Infective endocarditis	• Congenital heart defects	• Massive pulmonary embolus

NURSING CARE OF THE OLDER ADULT with heart failure

Ageing affects cardiac function. Diastolic filling is impaired by decreased ventricular compliance. With ageing, the heart is less responsive to sympathetic nervous system stimulation. As a result, maximal heart rate, cardiac reserve and exercise tolerance are reduced. Concurrent health problems such as arthritis that affect stamina or mobility often contribute to a more sedentary lifestyle, further decreasing the heart's ability to respond to increased stress. Heart failure in this population is a significant predictor of frailty (Pandey et al., 2019).

ASSESSING FOR HOME CARE

The older adult with heart failure may not be dyspnoeic, instead presenting with weakness and fatigue, somnolence, confusion, disorientation or worsening dementia. Dependent oedema and respiratory crackles may or may not indicate heart failure in older adults.

Assess the diet of the older adult. Decreased taste may lead to increased use of salt to bring out food flavours. Limited mobility or visual acuity may cause the older adult to rely on prepared foods that are high in sodium, such as canned soups and frozen meals. Discuss normal daily activities and assess sleep and rest patterns. It is also important to assess the environment for:

- safe roads or neighbourhoods for walking
- access to pharmacy, medical care and assistive services
- a cardiac rehabilitation program or structured exercise programs designed for older adults.

HEALTH EDUCATION FOR THE PERSON AND FAMILY

Teaching for the older adult with heart failure focuses on maintaining function and promptly identifying and treating episodes of heart failure. Teach individuals how to adapt to changes in cardiovascular function associated with ageing, such as:

- allowing longer warm-up and cool-down periods during exercise
- engaging in regular exercise such as walking five or more times a week
- resting with feet elevated (e.g. in a recliner) when fatigued
- maintaining adequate fluid intake
- preventing infection through pneumococcal and influenza immunisations.

FOCUS ON CULTURAL DIVERSITY

Heart failure and rheumatic heart disease

- Aboriginal and Torres Strait Islander people are 1.7 times more likely than non-Indigenous Australians to experience CHF.
- Manifestations of heart failure develop at an earlier age.
- The disease progresses more rapidly.
- More hospital visits are attributed to heart failure.
- The mortality rate is higher than in non-Indigenous Australians.

Heart failure in overseas-born individuals living in Australia

- In proportion to percentage of population, hospital admission rates of Australian residents born in Italy, Poland and Greece are higher than for Australian-born individuals.
- Hospital admission rates of Australian residents born in most other countries are lower than those of Australian-born individuals in proportion to percentage of population.

Rheumatic heart disease (RHD) in the Aboriginal and Torres Strait Islander Australian population

- Aboriginal and Torres Strait Islander Australians are 25 times more likely than non-Indigenous Australians to develop RHD.
- Aboriginal and Torres Strait Islander women are almost twice as likely as Aboriginal and Torres Strait Islander men to develop RHD.

output depends on adequate functional muscle mass and the ability of the ventricles to work together. Cardiac output normally is regulated by the oxygen needs of the body: as oxygen use increases, cardiac output increases to maintain cellular function. *Cardiac reserve* is the ability of the heart to increase CO to meet metabolic demand (Marieb & Hoehn, 2019). Ventricular damage reduces the cardiac reserve.

Cardiac output is a product of heart rate and stroke volume. *Heart rate (HR)* affects cardiac output by controlling the number of ventricular contractions per minute. It is influenced by the autonomic nervous system, catecholamines and thyroid hormones. Activation of a stress response (e.g. hypovolaemia or fear) stimulates the sympathetic nervous system, increasing heart rate and contractility. Elevated heart rates increase cardiac output. However, very rapid heart rates shorten ventricular filling time (diastole), reducing stroke volume and cardiac output. On the other hand, a slow heart rate reduces cardiac output simply because of fewer cardiac cycles (Bullock & Hales, 2019).

Stroke volume, the volume of blood ejected with each heartbeat, is determined by preload, afterload and myocardial contractility. *Preload* is the volume of blood in the ventricles at end diastole (just prior to contraction). The blood in the ventricles exerts pressure on the ventricle walls, stretching muscle fibres. The greater the blood volume, the greater the force with which the ventricle contracts to expel the blood. End-diastolic volume depends on the amount of blood returning to the ventricles (*venous return*) and the distensibility or stiffness of the ventricles (*compliance*). See Box 30.1.

Afterload is the force needed to eject blood into the circulation. This force must be great enough to overcome arterial pressures within the pulmonary and systemic vascular systems. Increased systemic vascular resistance (e.g. hypertension) increases afterload, impairing stroke volume and increasing myocardial work.

Contractility is the natural ability of cardiac muscle fibres to shorten during systole. Contractility is necessary to overcome arterial pressures and eject blood during systole. Impaired contractility affects cardiac output by reducing stroke volume. The *ejection fraction (EF)* is the percentage of blood in the ventricle that is ejected during systole. A normal ejection fraction is approximately 60%.

BOX 30.1 Explaining physiological terms using practical examples

The concepts of preload, the Frank–Starling mechanism, compliance and afterload can be difficult to understand and to explain to people. Use common analogies to make these concepts easier to understand.

- ***Preload*: Think about a new rubber band. The further a rubber band is stretched, the greater the force with which it snaps back.**
- ***Frank–Starling mechanism*: When a rubber band is repeatedly stretched beyond its limit, it loses some elasticity and fails to return to its original shape and size.**
- ***Compliance*: A new balloon is not very compliant—it takes a lot of work (force) to inflate it. As the balloon is repeatedly inflated and stretched, it becomes more compliant, expanding easily with less force.**
- ***Afterload*: When a hose is crimped or plugged, more force is required to eject a stream of water out its end.**

Pathophysiology

When the heart begins to fail, mechanisms are activated to compensate for the impaired function and to maintain the cardiac output. The primary compensatory mechanisms are: (1) the Frank–Starling mechanism, (2) neuroendocrine responses including activation of the sympathetic nervous system and the renin–angiotensin system, and (3) myocardial hypertrophy. These mechanisms and their effects are summarised in Table 30.2.

Decreased cardiac output initially stimulates aortic baroreceptors, which in turn stimulate the sympathetic nervous system (SNS). SNS stimulation produces both cardiac and vascular responses through the release of noradrenaline. Noradrenaline increases heart rate and contractility by stimulating cardiac beta-receptors. Cardiac output improves as both heart rate and stroke volume increase. Noradrenaline also causes arterial and venous vasoconstriction, increasing venous return to the heart. Increased venous return increases ventricular filling and myocardial stretch, increasing the force of contraction (the Frank–Starling mechanism). An ineffective contraction results from overstretching the muscle fibres past their physiological limit (Marieb & Hoehn, 2019).

Blood flow is redistributed to the brain and the heart to maintain perfusion of these vital organs. Decreased renal perfusion causes renin to be released from the kidneys. Activation of the renin–angiotensin system produces additional vasoconstriction and stimulates the adrenal cortex to produce aldosterone and the posterior pituitary to release antidiuretic hormone (ADH). Aldosterone stimulates sodium reabsorption in renal tubules, promoting water retention. ADH acts on the distal tubule to inhibit water excretion and also causes

TABLE 30.2 Compensatory mechanisms activated in heart failure

MECHANISM	PHYSIOLOGY	EFFECT	COMPLICATIONS
Frank-Starling mechanism	The greater the stretch of cardiac muscle fibres, the greater the force of contraction.	• ↑ contractile force leading to ↑ CO	• ↑ myocardial oxygen demand • Limited by overstretching
Neuroendocrine response	↓ CO stimulates the sympathetic nervous system and catecholamine release.	• ↑ HR, BP and contractility • ↑ vascular resistance • ↑ venous return	• ↑ vascular resistance • Tachycardia with ↓ filling time and ↓ CO • ↑ myocardial workload and oxygen demand
	↓ CO and ↓ renal perfusion stimulate renin-angiotensin system. Angiotensin stimulates aldosterone release from adrenal cortex.	Vasoconstriction and ↑ BP	• Fluid retention • Pulmonary congestion • ↑ preload and afterload
	ADH is released from posterior pituitary. Atrial [illegible] peptide are released.	• ↓ sodium excretion • ↓ diuresis • ↓ [illegible]	• Fluid retention • Pulmonary congestion • ↑ myocardial workload
	Blood flow is redistributed to vital organs (heart and brain).	Vasodilation [illegible] locations Vasoconstriction other locations • ↓ perfusion of other organ systems • ↓ perfusion of skin and muscles	• Renal vasoconstriction and ↓ [illegible] • Renal failure • Anaerobic metabolism and lactic acidosis • ↑ preload and [illegible]
Ventricular hypertrophy	↑ cardiac workload causes myocardial muscle to hypertrophy and ventricles to dilate.	• ↑ contractile force to maintain CO	• ↑ myocardial oxygen demand • Myocyte enlargement

vasoconstriction. The effect of these hormones is significant vasoconstriction and salt and water retention, with a resulting increase in vascular volume. Increased ventricular filling increases the force of contraction, improving cardiac output. The effects of the renin–angiotensin–aldosterone system and ADH release are counterbalanced to a certain extent by two additional hormones. The increased vascular volume and venous return prompted by vasoconstriction and sodium and water retention increase the volume and pressures in the heart. Stimulation of stretch receptors in the atria and ventricles lead to the release of *atrial natriuretic peptide (ANP)* and *brain natriuretic peptide (BNP)* from stores in the atria (ANP and BNP) and ventricles (BNP). These hormones promote sodium and water excretion and inhibit the release of noradrenaline, renin and ADH, with resulting vasodilation. Although beneficial, the effects of these hormones are too weak to completely counteract the vasoconstriction and sodium and water retention that occurs in heart failure.

Ventricular remodelling occurs as the chambers and myocardium adapt to fluid volume and pressure increases. The chambers dilate to accommodate excess fluid resulting from increased vascular volume and incomplete emptying. Initially, this additional stretch causes more effective contractions. *Ventricular hypertrophy* occurs as existing cardiac muscle cells enlarge, increasing their contractile elements (actin and myosin) and force of contraction.

Although these responses may help in the short-term regulation of cardiac output, it is now recognised that they hasten the deterioration of cardiac function. The onset of heart failure is indicated by *decompensation*, the loss of effective compensation. Heart failure progresses due to the very mechanisms that initially maintained circulatory stability.

The rapid heart rate shortens diastolic filling time, compromises coronary artery perfusion and increases myocardial oxygen demand. Resulting ischaemia further impairs cardiac output. Beta-receptors in the heart become less sensitive to continued SNS stimulation, decreasing heart rate and contractility. As the beta-receptors become less sensitive, noradrenaline stores in the cardiac muscle become depleted. In contrast, alpha-receptors on peripheral blood vessels become increasingly sensitive to persistent stimulation, promoting vasoconstriction and increasing afterload and cardiac work.

Initially, ventricular hypertrophy and dilation increase cardiac output, but chronic distension causes the ventricular wall to eventually thin and degenerate. The purpose of hypertrophy is therefore defeated. In addition, chronic overloading of the dilated ventricle eventually stretches the fibres beyond the optimal point for effective contraction. The ventricles continue to dilate to accommodate the excess fluid, but the heart loses the ability to contract forcefully. The heart muscle may eventually become so large that the coronary blood supply is inadequate, causing ischaemia.

Chronic distension exhausts stores of ANP and BNP. The effects of noradrenaline, renin and ADH prevail and the renin–angiotensin pathway is continually stimulated. This mechanism ultimately raises the haemodynamic stress on the heart by increasing both preload and afterload. As heart function deteriorates, less blood is delivered to the tissues and to the heart itself. Ischaemia and necrosis of the myocardium further weaken the already failing heart and the cycle repeats.

In normal hearts, the cardiac reserve allows the heart to adjust its output to meet metabolic needs of the body, increasing the cardiac output by up to five times the basal level during exercise. People with heart failure have minimal to no cardiac reserve. At rest, they may be unaffected; however, any stressor (e.g. exercise, illness) tips the balance between oxygen demand and oxygen supply. Manifestations of activity intolerance when the person is at rest indicate a critical level of cardiac decompensation.

Classifications and manifestations of heart failure

Heart failure is commonly classified in several different ways, depending on the underlying pathology. Classifications include systolic versus diastolic failure, left-sided versus right-sided failure, high-output versus low-output failure, and acute versus chronic failure (Bullock & Hales, 2019).

FAST FACTS

Terms used to describe or classify heart failure:

- systolic or diastolic failure
- left ventricular (or sided) or right ventricular (or sided) failure
- low-output or high-output failure
- acute or chronic failure
- forward or backward effects.

Systolic versus diastolic failure

Systolic failure occurs when the ventricle fails to contract adequately to eject a sufficient blood volume into the arterial system. Systolic function is affected by loss of myocardial cells due to ischaemia and infarction, cardiomyopathy or inflammation. The manifestations of systolic failure are those of decreased cardiac output: weakness, fatigue and decreased exercise tolerance.

Diastolic failure results when the heart cannot completely relax in diastole, disrupting normal filling. Passive diastolic filling decreases, increasing the importance of atrial contraction to preload. Diastolic dysfunction results from decreased ventricular compliance due to hypertrophic and cellular changes and impaired relaxation of the heart muscle. Its manifestations result from increased pressure and congestion behind the ventricle: shortness of breath, tachypnoea and respiratory crackles if the left ventricle is affected; distended neck veins, liver enlargement, anorexia and nausea if the right ventricle is affected. Many individuals have components of both systolic and diastolic failure.

Left-sided versus right-sided failure

Depending on the pathophysiology involved, either the left or the right ventricle may be primarily affected. In chronic heart failure, however, both ventricles typically are impaired to some degree. Coronary heart disease and hypertension are common causes of *left-sided heart failure*, whereas *right-sided heart failure* often is caused by conditions that increase blood pressure in the pulmonary vasculature, such as acute or chronic pulmonary disease. Left-sided heart failure also can lead to right-sided failure as pressures in the pulmonary vascular system increase with congestion behind the failing left ventricle.

As left ventricular function fails, cardiac output falls. Pressures in the left ventricle and atrium increase as the amount of blood remaining in the ventricle after systole increases. These increased pressures impair filling, causing congestion and increased pressures in the pulmonary vascular system. Increased pressures in this normally low-pressure system increase fluid movement from the blood vessels into interstitial tissues and the alveoli (see Figure 30.1).

The manifestations of left-sided heart failure result from pulmonary congestion (*backward effects*) and decreased cardiac output (*forward effects*). Fatigue and activity intolerance are common early manifestations. Dizziness and syncope also may result from decreased cardiac output. Pulmonary congestion causes dyspnoea and cough. The person may develop orthopnoea (difficulty breathing while lying down), prompting use of two or three pillows or a recliner for sleeping. Cyanosis from impaired gas exchange may be noted. On auscultation of the lungs, inspiratory crackles (rales) and wheezes may be heard in lung bases. An S_3 gallop may be present, reflecting the heart's attempts to fill an already distended ventricle.

In right-sided heart failure, increased pressures in the pulmonary vasculature or right ventricular muscle damage impair the right ventricle's ability to pump blood into the pulmonary circulation. The right ventricle and atrium become distended and blood accumulates in the systemic venous system. Increased venous pressures cause abdominal organs to become congested and peripheral tissue oedema to develop (see Figure 30.2).

Dependent tissues tend to be affected because of the effects of gravity; oedema develops in the feet and legs or, if the person is bedridden, in the sacrum. Congestion of gastrointestinal tract vessels causes anorexia and nausea. Right upper quadrant pain may result from liver engorgement. Neck veins distend and become visible even when the person is upright, due to increased venous pressure.

Low-output versus high-output failure

People with heart failure due to coronary heart disease, hypertension, cardiomyopathy and other primary cardiac disorders develop *low-output failure* and manifestations such as those

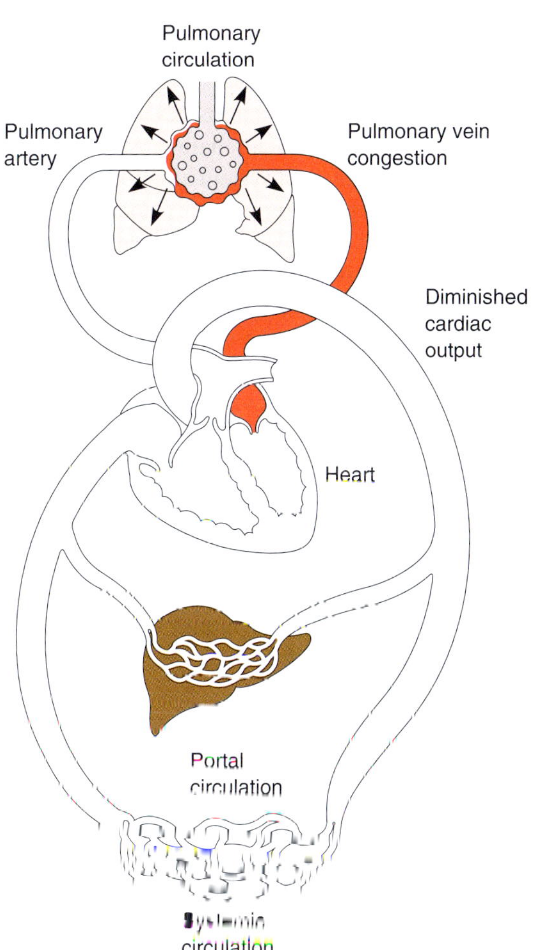

FIGURE 30.1 *The haemodynamic effects of left-sided heart failure*

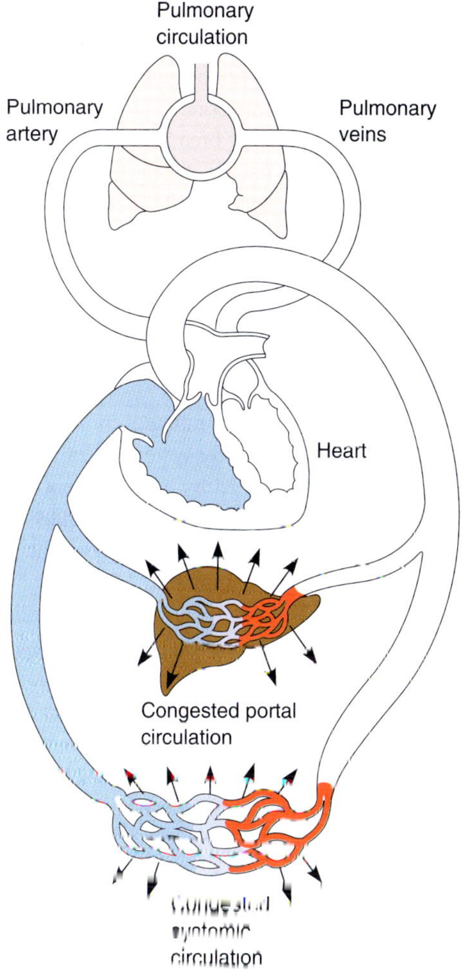

FIGURE 30.2 *The haemodynamic effects of right sided heart failure*

previously described. Individuals in hypermetabolic states (e.g. hyperthyroidism, infection, anaemia or pregnancy) require increased cardiac output to maintain blood flow and oxygen to the tissues. If the increased blood flow cannot meet the oxygen demands of the tissues, compensatory mechanisms are activated to further increase cardiac output, which in turn further increases oxygen demand. Thus, even though cardiac output is high, the heart is unable to meet increased oxygen demands. This condition is known as *high-output failure*.

Acute versus chronic failure

Acute failure is the abrupt onset of a myocardial injury (such as a massive MI) resulting in suddenly decreased cardiac function and signs of decreased cardiac output. *Chronic failure* is a progressive deterioration of the heart muscle due to cardiomyopathies, valvular disease or CHD (Bullock & Hales, 2019).

Other manifestations

In addition to the previous manifestations for the various classifications of heart failure, other signs and symptoms commonly are seen.

A fall in cardiac output activates mechanisms that cause increased salt and water retention. This causes weight gain and further increases pressures in the capillaries, resulting in oedema. *Nocturia*, voiding more than one time at night, develops as oedema fluid from dependent tissues is reabsorbed while the person is supine. **Paroxysmal nocturnal dyspnoea (PND)** may develop. PND is a frightening condition in which the person awakens at night acutely short of breath. PND occurs when fluid that has accumulated in the tissues during the day is reabsorbed into the circulation at night, causing fluid overload and pulmonary congestion. Severe heart failure with little or no cardiac reserve may cause dyspnoea at rest, as well as with activity. Both an S_3 and an S_4 gallop may be heard on auscultation.

See 'Multisystem effects of heart failure'.

Complications

The compensatory mechanisms initiated in heart failure can lead to complications in other body systems. Congestive hepatomegaly and splenomegaly caused by engorgement of the portal venous system result in increased abdominal pressure, ascites and gastrointestinal problems. With prolonged right-sided heart failure, liver function may be impaired. Myocardial distension can precipitate arrhythmias, further impairing cardiac output. Pleural effusions and other pulmonary problems may develop. Major complications of severe heart failure are cardiogenic shock (described in the chapter 'Nursing care of people experiencing trauma and shock') and acute pulmonary oedema, a medical emergency described in the next section of this chapter.

INTERPROFESSIONAL CARE

The main goals for care of heart failure are to slow its progression, reduce cardiac workload, improve cardiac function and control fluid retention. Treatment strategies are based on the evolution and progression of heart failure. The National Heart Foundation of Australia and the Cardiac Society of Australia and New Zealand (NHF & ACSANZ, 2018) produce guidelines for the prevention, detection and management of chronic heart failure. These guidelines are a comprehensive set of recommendations regarding the diagnosis and management of individuals with heart failure. A comprehensive online resource has also been developed for clinicians encompassing all aspects of heart failure assessment and management (National Heart Foundation of Australia, 2022).

In Australia, symptom classification is still achieved using the New York Heart Association (NYHA) grading of symptoms in chronic heart failure (see Table 30.3).

Diagnosis

Diagnosis of heart failure is based on the history, physical examination and diagnostic findings. The National Heart Foundation of Australia recommends an echocardiogram, electrocardiogram, chest x-ray, full blood count (FBC), plasma, urea, creatinine and electrolytes in all individuals suspected of heart failure (NHF & ACSANZ, 2018) (see Table 30.4).

The arterial blood pressure reflects the cardiac output and resistance to blood flow created by the elastic arterial walls (systemic vascular resistance, SVR). Cardiac output is determined by the blood volume and the ability of the ventricles to fill and effectively pump that blood. Systemic vascular resistance is primarily determined by vessel diameter and distensibility (compliance). Factors such as SNS input, circulating hormones (e.g. adrenaline, noradrenaline, ANP and vasopressin) and the renin–angiotensin system affect SVR.

The systolic blood pressure, normally about 120 mmHg in healthy adults, reflects the pressure generated during ventricular systole. During diastole, elastic arterial walls keep a minimum pressure within the vessel (diastolic blood pressure) to maintain blood flow through the capillary beds. The average diastolic pressure in a healthy adult is 80 mmHg. The mean arterial pressure (MAP) is the average pressure in the arterial circulation throughout the cardiac cycle. It reflects the driving pressure or perfusion pressure, an indicator of tissue perfusion. The formula $MAP = CO \times SVR$ is often used to show the relationships between factors determining the blood pressure. Mean arterial pressures of 70 to 90 mmHg are desirable. Perfusion to vital organs is severely jeopardised at MAPs of 50 or less; MAPs greater than 105 mmHg may indicate hypertension or vasoconstriction.

TABLE 30.3 NYHA grading of symptoms in chronic heart failure

CLASS	SEVERITY OF SYMPTOMS
I	No limitations in physical activity/asymptomatic
II	Symptoms with strenuous activity
III	Symptoms with mild activity
IV	Symptoms at rest

Source: American Heart Association (AHA). (2018). *Hypertrophic cardiomyopathy*. Retrieved from https://www.heart.org/idc/groups/heart-public/@wcm/@hcm/documents/downloadable/ucm_312225.pdf.

Multisystem effects of heart failure

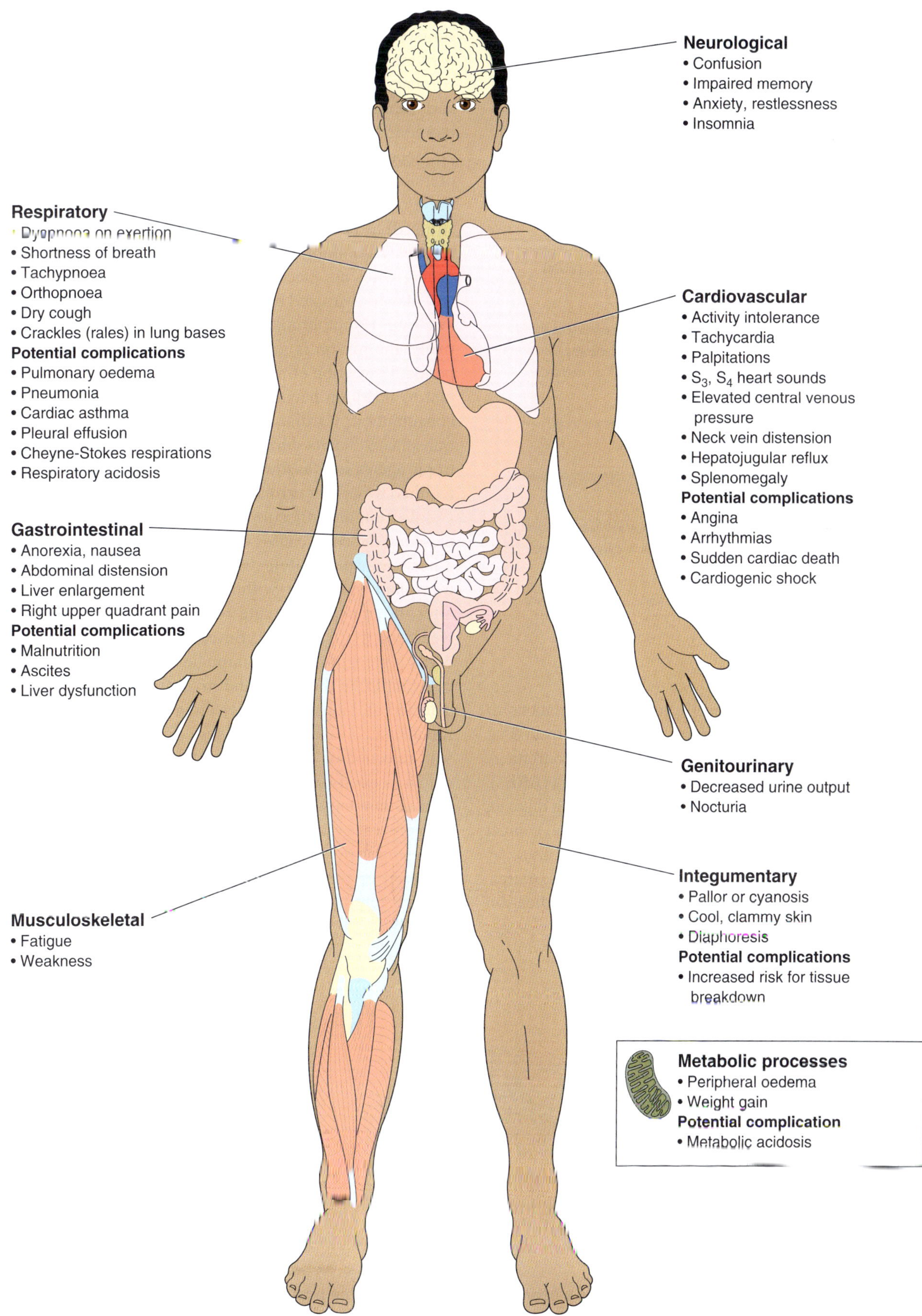

TABLE 30.4 Tests indicated for individuals suspected of heart failure

Blood glucose	Metabolic disorders not only increase the risk of cardiovascular disease but complicate its course and management.
BNP and NT-pro BNP	Natriuretic peptides released by the atria may detect deterioration in pump function as increases in these values correlate with worsening heart failure.
Chest x-ray (CXR)	Assesses structure; some inferences regarding function may be made.
Echocardiogram (ECHO)	Assesses structure and function of the myocardium.
Electrocardiogram (ECG)	May demonstrate possible contributing factor or resulting consequence (arrhythmia or chamber enlargement).
Full blood count (FBC)	May detect anaemia.
Urea and electrolytes (U&Es)	Urea and creatinine are markers of renal function and can suggest renal failure or cause of fluid retention. Electrolyte measures may detect fluid and electrolyte imbalances.
Liver function tests (LFTs)	May detect alterations in liver function which can demonstrate possible cause or effect.
Arterial blood gases (ABGs)	May detect hypoxia as a cause or consequence of heart failure.
Myocardial perfusion scans (MPS or sestamibi)	May detect changes in ventricular wall function, such as wall motion or perfusion anomalies, as causes or consequences of heart failure.
Coronary angiogram	May quantify vessel occlusion as a cause of heart failure.

Medications

People with heart failure often receive multiple medications to reduce cardiac work and improve cardiac function. The main drug classes used to treat heart failure are the angiotensin-converting-enzyme (ACE) inhibitors, angiotensin II receptor blockers (ARBs), beta-blockers, diuretics, inotropic medications (including digoxin, sympathomimetic agents and phosphodiesterase inhibitors), direct vasodilators and anti-arrhythmic drugs.

Nursing implications for ACE inhibitors and ARBs, diuretics and inotropic medications are found in the 'Medication administration' box.

Surgery

Nursing care of the person who has had a heart transplant (see Figure 30.3) is similar to care for a person who has had cardiac surgery (see box on the nursing care of person having a coronary artery bypass in the chapter 'Nursing care of people with coronary heart disease'). Bleeding is a major concern in the early postoperative period. Chest tube drainage is frequently monitored (initially every 15 minutes), as are the cardiac output, pulmonary artery pressures and CVP. Cardiac tamponade (compression of the heart) can develop, presenting as either a sudden event or a gradual process. Chest tubes are gently milked (not stripped) as needed to maintain patency. Atrial arrhythmias are relatively common following cardiac transplant. Temporary pacing wires are placed during surgery as the conduction system may be disrupted by surgical manipulation or postoperative swelling. Hypothermia is induced during surgery; postoperatively, the person is gradually rewarmed over a 1- to 2-hour period. Prevention of rapid rewarming and shivering are important to maintain haemodynamic stability and reduce oxygen consumption. Cardiac function is impaired in up to 50% of transplanted hearts during the early postoperative period. Inotropic agents such as low-dose dopamine or dobutamine may be required to support cardiac function and circulation.

Infection and rejection are major postoperative concerns; these are the chief causes of mortality in people who have had a heart transplant. Rejection may develop immediately after transplant (rarely) or within weeks to months or even years after the transplant. Acute rejection usually presents within weeks of the transplant, developing when the transplanted organ is recognised by the immune system as foreign. Lymphocytes infiltrate the organ and myocardial cell necrosis can be detected on biopsy. Acute rejection often can be treated using immunosuppressive drugs. These drugs also are given to prevent rejection of the transplanted organ, even when the tissue match is good (see the chapter 'Nursing care of people with altered immunity'). Although immunosuppressive medications help prevent organ rejection, they impair the person's defences against infection. Early postoperative infections commonly are bacterial or fungal (*Candida*). Multiple invasive lines, prolonged ventilator support and immunosuppressive therapy contribute to the transplant recipient's risk of infection.

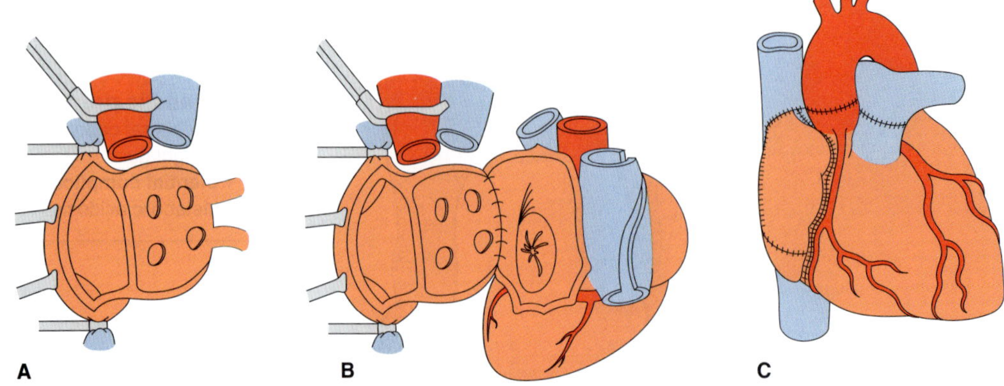

FIGURE 30.3 *Cardiac transplantation. A, The person's heart is removed, leaving the posterior walls of the atria intact. The donor heart is anastomosed to the atria, B, and the great vessels, C*

MEDICATION ADMINISTRATION Heart failure

ACE INHIBITORS AND ARBS

Angiotensin-converting-enzyme inhibitors (ACE inhibitors) and angiotensin II receptor blockers (ARBs) prevent acute coronary events and reduce mortality in heart failure. ACE inhibitors interfere with production of angiotensin II, resulting in vasodilation and reduced circulating blood volume, ultimately reducing blood pressure. In heart failure, ACE inhibitors reduce afterload, improve cardiac output and increase renal perfusion. They also reduce pulmonary congestion and peripheral oedema. ACE inhibitors suppress myocyte growth and reduce ventricular remodelling in heart failure. While the pharmacological effect of ARBs is similar, they block the action of angiotensin II at the receptor rather than interfering with its production. This mechanism of action results in fewer side effects as ACE is also required in the lungs to break down the substances responsible for increasing airway hyperreactivity, tachykinins and bradykinins.

Nursing responsibilities

- Do not administer these drugs to women in the second and third trimesters of pregnancy.
- Carefully monitor individuals who are volume depleted or who have impaired renal function.
- Use an infusion pump when administering ACE inhibitors intravenously.
- Monitor blood pressure closely for 2 hours following first dose and as indicated thereafter.
- Monitor serum potassium levels; ACE inhibitors can cause hyperkalaemia. (This is less of a concern with ARBs.)
- Monitor white blood cell (WBC) count for potential neutropenia. Report to the doctor.

Health education for the person and family

- Take the drug at the same time every day to ensure a stable blood level.
- Monitor blood pressure and weight weekly. Report significant changes to the doctor.
- Avoid making sudden position changes; for example, rise from bed slowly. Lie down if feeling dizzy or light-headed, particularly after the first dose.
- Report any signs of easy bruising and bleeding, sore throat or fever, oedema or skin rash. Immediately report swelling of the face, lips or eyelids, and itching or breathing problems.
- A persistent, dry cough may develop if taking an ACE inhibitor. Contact the doctor if this becomes a problem.

DIURETICS

Diuretics act on different portions of the kidney tubule to inhibit the reabsorption of sodium and water and promote their excretion. With the exception of the potassium-sparing diuretics—spironolactone and amiloride—diuretics also promote potassium excretion, increasing the risk of hypokalaemia. Spironolactone, an aldosterone receptor blocker, reduces symptoms and slows progression of heart failure. Aldosterone receptors in the heart and blood vessels promote myocardial remodelling and fibrosis, activate the sympathetic nervous system and promote vascular fibrosis (which decreases compliance) and baroreceptor dysfunction.

Nursing responsibilities

- Obtain baseline weight and vital signs.
- Monitor blood pressure, intake and output, weight, skin turgor and oedema as indicators of fluid volume status.
- Assess for volume depletion, particularly with loop diuretics (frusemide and ethacrynic acid—ethacrynic acid is primarily restricted to people who are either allergic to, or refractory to, frusemide or bumetanide): dizziness, orthostatic hypotension, tachycardia, muscle cramping.
- Report abnormal serum electrolyte levels to the doctor. Replace electrolytes as indicated.
- Do not administer potassium replacements to individuals receiving a potassium-sparing diuretic.
- Evaluate renal function by assessing urine output and serum urea and creatinine.
- Administer intravenous frusemide slowly, no faster than 20 mg/minute. Evaluate for signs of ototoxicity. Do not administer this drug or ethacrynic acid concurrently with aminoglycoside antibiotics (e.g. gentamicin), which are also ototoxic.

Health education for the person and family

- Drink at least 6 to 8 glasses of water per day.
- Take your diuretic at times that will be the least disruptive to your lifestyle, usually in the morning and early afternoon if a second dose is ordered. Take with meals to decrease gastric upset.
- Monitor your blood pressure, pulse and weight weekly. Report significant weight changes to your doctor.
- Report any of the following to your doctor: severe abdominal pain, jaundice, dark urine, abnormal bleeding or bruising, flu-like symptoms, signs of hypokalaemia, hyponatraemia and dehydration (thirst, salt craving, dizziness, weakness, rapid pulse). See the chapter 'Nursing care of people with altered fluid, electrolyte and acid–base balance' for manifestations of electrolyte imbalances.
- Avoid sudden position changes. They may cause dizziness, light-headedness or feelings of faintness.
- Unless taking a potassium-sparing diuretic, integrate foods rich in potassium into your diet (see the chapter 'Nursing care of people with altered fluid, electrolyte and acid–base balance'). Limit sodium use.

POSITIVE INOTROPIC AGENTS

Digoxin glycosides

Digoxin (Lanoxin)

Digoxin improves myocardial contractility by interfering with ATPase in the myocardial cell membrane and increasing the amount of calcium available for contraction. The increased force of contraction causes the heart to empty more completely, increasing stroke volume and cardiac output. Improved cardiac output improves renal perfusion, decreasing renin secretion. This decreases preload and afterload, reducing cardiac work. Digoxin also has electrophysiological effects, slowing conduction through the AV node and thus decreasing heart rate and reducing oxygen consumption.

(continued)

MEDICATION ADMINISTRATION **Heart failure (continued)**

Nursing responsibilities

- Assess apical pulse before administering. Withhold digoxin and notify the doctor if heart rate is below 60 bpm and/or manifestations of decreased cardiac output are noted. Record apical rate on medication record.
- Evaluate electrocardiogram (ECG) for scooped (spoon-shaped) ST segment, AV block, bradycardia and other arrhythmias (especially PVCs and atrial tachycardias).
- Report manifestations of digoxin toxicity: anorexia, nausea, vomiting, abdominal pain, weakness, vision changes (diplopia, blurred vision, yellow-green or white halos seen around objects) and new-onset arrhythmias.
- Assess potassium, magnesium, calcium and serum digoxin levels before giving digoxin. Hypokalaemia can precipitate toxicity even when the serum digoxin level is in the 'normal' range.
- Monitor individuals with renal insufficiency or renal failure and older adults carefully for digoxin toxicity.
- Prepare to administer digoxin immune Fab (Digibind) for digoxin toxicity.

Health education for the person and family

- Take pulse daily before taking the digoxin. Do not take the digoxin if the pulse is below 60 bpm or if weak, fatigued, light-headed, dizzy, short of breath or having chest pain. Notify the doctor immediately.
- Contact the doctor if any manifestations of digoxin toxicity occur: palpitations, weakness, loss of appetite, nausea, vomiting, abdominal pain, blurred or coloured vision, double vision.
- Avoid using antacids and laxatives; they decrease digoxin absorption.
- Notify the doctor immediately if any manifestations of potassium deficiency occur: weakness, lethargy, thirst, depression, muscle cramps or vomiting.
- Incorporate foods high in potassium into your diet: fresh orange or tomato juice, bananas, raisins, dates, figs, prunes, apricots, spinach, cauliflower and potatoes.

SYMPATHOMIMETIC AGENTS

Sympathomimetic agents stimulate the heart, improving the force of contraction. Dobutamine is preferred in managing heart failure because it does not increase the heart rate as much as dopamine and it has a mild vasodilatory effect. These drugs are given by intravenous infusion and may be titrated to obtain their optimal effects.

Nursing care directed at prevention of infection is vital and includes strict aseptic technique, early extubation to reduce the risk of ventilator-associated infections, limitation of individuals who may present an infection risk and early ambulation (Aitken, Marshall & Chaboyer, 2019).

The donor heart is denervated during the transplant procedure and therefore the person's heart rate is commonly between 90–100 bpm. This occurs because the slowing effects of the parasympathetic nervous system are lost. The endocrine system, position changes, exercise and certain drugs moderate heart rate following a heart transplant.

OTHER PROCEDURES A person with heart failure may benefit from coronary revascularisation, left ventricular aneurysmectomy or mitral valvuloplasty (NHF & ACSANZ, 2018). Other surgical procedures such as cardiomyoplasty and ventricular reduction surgery are not recommended because of unfavourable results.

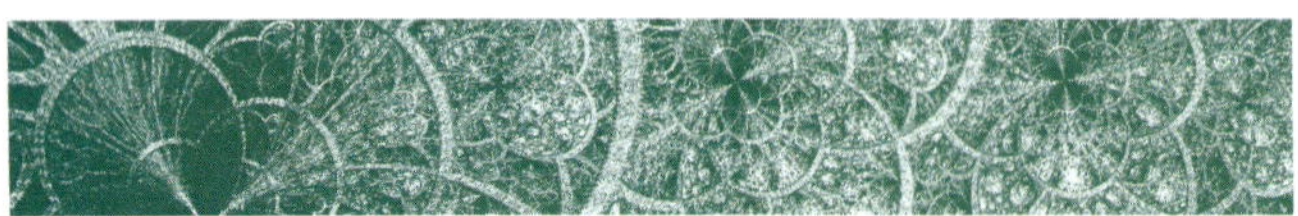

Nursing care

Health promotion

Health promotion activities to reduce the risk and incidence of heart failure should be directed at the risk factors. Teach individuals about coronary heart disease, the primary underlying cause of heart failure. Discuss CHD risk factors and ways to reduce those risk factors (see the chapter 'Nursing care of people with coronary heart disease').

Hypertension also is a major cause of heart failure. Routinely screen individuals for hypertension and refer them to a medical officer as required. Discuss the importance of effectively managing hypertension to reduce the future risk of heart failure. Likewise, stress the relationship between effective diabetes management and reduced risk of heart failure.

Assessment

Obtain both subjective and objective data when assessing the person with heart failure:

- *Health history*: complaints of increasing dyspnoea, decreasing activity tolerance or paroxysmal nocturnal dyspnoea; number of pillows used for sleeping; recent weight gain; presence of a cough; chest or abdominal pain; anorexia or nausea; history of cardiac disease, previous episodes of heart failure; other risk factors such as hypertension or diabetes; current medications; usual diet and activity and recent changes.
- *Physical examination*: general appearance; ease of breathing, conversing, changing positions; apparent anxiety; vital signs including apical pulse; colour of skin and mucous membranes; neck vein distension, peripheral pulses, capillary refill, presence and degree of oedema; heart and breath sounds; abdominal contour, bowel sounds, tenderness; right upper abdominal tenderness, liver enlargement.
- *Diagnostic tests*: serum electrolyte, urea, creatinine and digoxin levels; arterial blood gas (ABG) results; ECG, echocardiogram and chest x-ray reports.

Nursing diagnosis and interventions

Heart failure impacts on quality of life and interferes with activities of daily living (ADLs). Reducing myocardial oxygen demand is a major nursing care goal for the individual in acute heart failure. This includes providing rest and undertaking the prescribed interventions to reduce cardiac work, improve contractility and manage symptoms. See also the accompanying nursing care plan for additional nursing diagnoses and interventions for the individual with heart failure.

- Auscultate the person's heart and breath sounds regularly. *S_1 and S_2 may be diminished if cardiac function is poor. A ventricular gallop (S_3) is an early sign of heart failure; atrial gallop (S_4) may also be present. Crackles are often heard in the lung bases; increasing crackles and dyspnoea indicate worsening failure.*

Decreased cardiac output

Pump failure results in decreased upstroke volume and tissue perfusion.

- Monitor the person's vital signs and oxygen saturation as indicated. *Decreased cardiac output stimulates the SNS to increase the heart rate in an attempt to restore CO. Tachycardia at rest is common. Diastolic blood pressure may initially be elevated because of vasoconstriction; in late stages, compensatory mechanisms fail and the person's BP will fall. Oxygen saturation levels provide a measure of gas exchange and tissue perfusion.*
- Administer supplemental oxygen as needed. *This improves oxygenation of the blood, decreasing the effects of hypoxia and ischaemia.*

CONSIDERATION FOR PRACTICE

Report manifestations of decreased cardiac output and tissue perfusion including changes in mentation, decreased urine output, cool, clammy skin, diminished pulses, pallor or cyanosis, and arrhythmias.

- Administer prescribed medications as ordered. *Drugs are used to decrease the cardiac workload and increase contractility.*
- Encourage rest, explaining the rationale. Elevate the head of the bed to reduce the work of breathing. Provide a bedside commode and assist with ADLs. Instruct the person to avoid the Valsalva manoeuvre and encourage the use of stool softeners to reduce strain. *These measures reduce cardiac workload.*

CONSIDERATION FOR PRACTICE

Encourage the person to rest and teach methods to decrease anxiety. Maintain a quiet environment and encourage expression of fears and feelings. Explain care measures and their purpose. Reducing anxiety diminishes the sympathetic nervous system effects, resulting in an improved balance between oxygen demand and supply.

Excess fluid volume

As cardiac output falls, compensatory mechanisms cause salt and water retention, increasing blood volume. This increased fluid volume places additional stress on the already failing ventricles, making them work harder to move the fluid load.

- Assess respiratory status and auscultate lung sounds at least every 4 hours. Notify the doctor of significant changes in condition. *Declining respiratory status indicates worsening left heart failure.*

CONSIDERATION FOR PRACTICE

Immediately notify the doctor if the person develops dyspnoea, tachypnoea, severe orthopnoea, a cough productive of large amounts of pink, frothy sputum, or an overwhelming sense of impending doom or panic. Acute pulmonary oedema is a medical emergency and can develop rapidly. Immediate intervention is required to preserve life.

- Monitor the person's intake and output. Notify the doctor if urine output is less than 30 mL/h. Weigh daily. *Careful monitoring of fluid volume is important during treatment of heart failure. Diuretics may reduce circulating volume, producing hypovolaemia despite persistent peripheral oedema. A fall in urine output may indicate significantly reduced cardiac output and renal ischaemia. Weight is an objective measure of fluid status: 1 L of fluid is equal to 1 kg of weight.*
- Record abdominal girth every shift. Note complaints of a loss of appetite, abdominal discomfort or nausea. *Venous congestion can lead to ascites and may affect gastrointestinal function and nutritional status.*
- Monitor and record the person's haemodynamic measurements. Report significant changes and negative trends. *Haemodynamic measurements provide a means of monitoring condition and response to treatment.*
- Restrict fluids as ordered. Offer appropriate choices of fluid type and timing of intake, scheduling most fluid intake during morning and afternoon hours. Offer ice chips and frequent mouth care. *Providing choices increases the person's sense of control. Ice chips and frequent mouth care relieve dry mouth and thirst and promote comfort.*

Activity intolerance

People with heart failure have insufficient cardiac reserve to meet increased oxygen demands. As the disease progresses and cardiac function is further compromised, activity intolerance increases. The low cardiac output and inability to participate in activities may hinder self-care.

- Organise nursing care to allow rest periods. Grouping activities together allows adequate time to 'recharge'. However, care must be taken to avoid overtaxing the individual during the grouped activities. *Frequently gauge the person's capacity to continue and adjust the plans as required.*

NURSING CARE PLAN A person with heart failure

One year ago, Arthur Jackson, 67 years old, had a large anterior wall MI and underwent subsequent coronary artery bypass surgery. On discharge, he was started on a regimen of enalapril, digoxin, frusemide, warfarin and a potassium chloride supplement. He is now in the cardiac unit complaining of severe shortness of breath, haemoptysis and poor appetite for 1 week. He is diagnosed with acute heart failure.

ASSESSMENT

Mr Jackson refuses to settle in bed, preferring to sit in the bedside recliner in high-Fowler's position. He states, 'Lately, this is the only way I can breathe.' Mr Jackson states that he has not been able to work in his garden without getting short of breath. He complains of his shoes and belt being too tight.

Mr Jackson insists that he takes his medications regularly. He states that he normally works in his garden for light exercise. In his diet history, Mr Jackson admits fondness for bacon and takeaway food and sheepishly admits to snacking between meals 'even though I need to lose weight'.

Mr Jackson's vital signs are: BP 95/72 mmHg, HR 124 and irregular, R 28 and laboured, and T 36.5°C. The cardiac monitor shows atrial fibrillation. An S_3 is noted on auscultation; the cardiac impulse is left of the midclavicular line. He has crackles and diminished breath sounds in the bases of both lungs. Significant jugular venous distension, 3+ pitting oedema of feet and ankles and abdominal distension are noted. Liver size is within normal limits by percussion. His skin is cool and he is diaphoretic. Chest x-ray shows cardiomegaly and pulmonary infiltrates.

DIAGNOSES

- *Excess fluid volume* related to impaired cardiac pump and salt and water retention manifested by crackles and pitting oedema.
- *Risk of activity intolerance* related to impaired cardiac output manifested by inability to undertake activities of daily living.
- *Impaired health maintenance* related to lack of knowledge about diet restrictions manifested by frequent consumption of foods high in salt and fat.

PLANNING

- Hourly vital signs and haemodynamic pressure measurements.
- Monitor oxygen saturation continuously. Notify doctor if less than 94%.
- Administer and monitor effects of prescribed diuretics and vasodilators.
- Weigh daily; strict fluid balance monitoring.
- Enforce fluid restriction of 1,500 mL/24 hours.
- Auscultate heart and breath sounds every 4 hours and as indicated.

Expected outcomes

- Demonstrate loss of excess fluid by weight loss and decreases in oedema, jugular venous distension and abdominal distension.
- Demonstrate improved activity tolerance.
- Verbalise understanding of diet restrictions.

IMPLEMENTATION

- Administer oxygen per nasal prongs at 2 L/min.
- High-Fowler's or position of comfort.
- Notify doctor of significant changes in laboratory values.
- Teach about all medications and how to take and record pulse. Provide information about anticoagulant therapy and signs of bleeding.
- Design an activity plan with Mr Jackson that incorporates preferred activities and scheduled rest periods.
- Instruct about sodium-restricted diet. Allow meal choices within allowed limits.
- Consult dietitian for planning and teaching Mr and Mrs Jackson about a low-sodium diet.

EVALUATION

Mr Jackson is discharged after 3 days in the cardiac unit. He has lost 3.5 kilograms during his stay and states it is much easier to breathe and his shoes fit better. He is able to sleep in semi-Fowler's position with only one pillow. His peripheral oedema has resolved. Mr and Mrs Jackson met with the dietitian, who helped them develop a realistic eating plan to limit sodium, sugar and fats. The dietitian also provided a list of high-sodium foods to avoid. The physiotherapist designed a progressive activity plan with Mr Jackson that he will continue at home. He remains in atrial fibrillation, a chronic condition. His knowledge of digoxin and warfarin has been assessed and reinforced. The nurse confirms that he is able to accurately check his pulse and can identify signs of digoxin toxicity and excessive bleeding.

CRITICAL THINKING IN THE NURSING PROCESS

1. Mr Jackson's medication regimen remains the same after discharge. What specific teaching does he need related to potential interactions of these drugs?
2. Mr Jackson exclaims, 'Talk to my wife about my medications—she's Tarzan and I'm Jane, now.' How would you respond?
3. Mr Jackson tells you, 'Sometimes I forget whether I have taken my aspirin, so I'll take another just to be sure. After all, they are only baby aspirin. One or two extra a day shouldn't hurt, right?' What is your response?
4. Mr Jackson is admitted to the neurology unit 6 months later with a cerebral vascular accident (CVA). What are the possible contributing factors of his stroke?

REFLECTION ON THE NURSING PROCESS

1. Outline what you have learned from this case study that you will apply to your future practice.
2. Given that Mr Jackson has a cerebrovascular accident 6 months later, explore the influence of cardiovascular conditions on the development of other comorbidities and conditions. What other conditions/comorbidities are common in individuals who present with an ischaemic heart disease? Why? What specifically can a nurse do to influence a person with ischaemic heart disease to reduce the risk of developing these common comorbidities and conditions in the future?

CONSIDERATION FOR PRACTICE

Monitor vital signs and cardiac rhythm during and after activities. Tachycardia, arrhythmias, increasing dyspnoea, changes in blood pressure, diaphoresis, pallor, complaints of chest pain, excessive fatigue or palpitations indicate activity intolerance. Instruct to rest if manifestations are noted. The failing heart is unable to increase cardiac output to meet increased oxygen demands associated with activity. Assessing response to activities helps evaluate cardiac function. Decreasing activity tolerance may signal deterioration of cardiac function, not overexertion.

- Assist with ADLs as needed. Encourage independence within prescribed limits. *Assisting with ADLs helps ensure that care needs are met while reducing cardiac workload. Involving the individual promotes a sense of control and reduces helplessness.*
- Plan and implement progressive activities. Use passive and active range-of-motion (ROM) exercises as appropriate. Consult with physical therapist on activity plan. *Progressive activity slowly increases exercise capacity by strengthening and improving cardiac function without strain. Activity also helps prevent skeletal muscle atrophy. ROM exercises prevent complications of immobility in severely compromised individuals.*
- Provide written and verbal information about activity after discharge. *Written information provides a reference for important information. Verbal information allows clarification and validation of the material.*

Deficient knowledge: low-sodium diet

Diet is an important part of long-term management of heart failure to manage fluid retention.

- Discuss the rationale for sodium restrictions. *Understanding fosters compliance with the prescribed diet.*
- Consult with dietitian to plan and teach a low-sodium and, if necessary for weight control, low-kilojoule diet. Provide a list of high-sodium, high-fat, high-cholesterol foods to avoid. Provide National Heart Foundation of Australia materials. *Dietary planning and teaching increase the individual's sense of control and participation in disease management. Food lists are useful memory aids.*
- Assist the person to construct a 2 day meal plan, choosing foods low in sodium. *This allows learning assessment, clarification of misunderstandings and reinforcement of teaching.*
- Encourage small, frequent meals rather than three heavy meals per day. *Small, frequent meals provide continuing energy resources and decrease the work required to digest a large meal.*

CONSIDERATION FOR PRACTICE

Teach a person with cardiovascular pathology how to read food labels for nutritional information. Many processed foods contain 'hidden' sodium, which can be identified by careful label reading.

PATIENT SAFETY COMPETENCY FRAMEWORK

5 Clinical reasoning

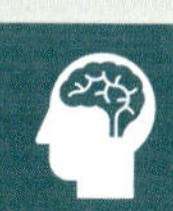

The Patient Safety Competency Framework supports the use of clinical reasoning in managing the person with heart failure. Heart failure management requires the nurse to conduct a cyclical process of data collection and processing of information, with a view to setting appropriate goals for the person. This process must include the person's values and preferences as valid sources of evidence and occurs within the context of an evolving evidence base requiring adaptation in the knowledge used to inform the reasoning process. Effective clinical reasoning leads to sound clinical decisions and enhances patient outcomes (Levett-Jones et al., 2017).

Community-based care

Heart failure is a chronic condition requiring active participation by the individual and family for effective management. In teaching for home care, include the following topics:

- the disease process and its effects on the individual's life
- warning signals of cardiac decompensation requiring treatment
- desired and adverse effects of prescribed drugs; monitoring for effects; importance of compliance with drug regimen to prevent acute and long-term complications of heart failure
- prescribed diet and sodium restriction; practical suggestions for reducing salt intake; recommend National Heart Foundation of Australia materials and recipes
- exercise recommendations to strengthen the heart muscle and improve aerobic capacity (see Box 30.2)
- the importance of keeping scheduled follow-up appointments to monitor disease progression and effects of therapy.

Provide referrals for home healthcare and household assistance (shopping, transportation, personal needs and housekeeping) as indicated. Referrals to community agencies, such as local cardiac rehabilitation programs, heart support groups or the National Heart Foundation of Australia, can provide the person and their family with additional materials and psychosocial support.

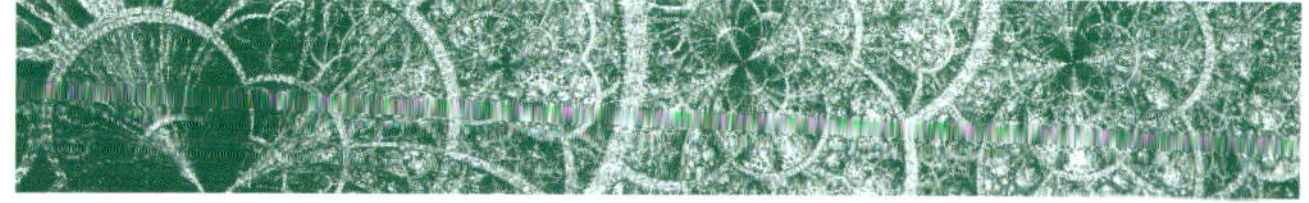

THE PERSON WITH PULMONARY OEDEMA

Pulmonary oedema is an abnormal accumulation of fluid in the interstitial tissue and alveoli of the lung. Both cardiac and non-cardiac disorders can cause pulmonary oedema. Cardiac

BOX 30.2 Home activity guidelines for the person with heart failure

- Perform as many activities as independently as possible.
- Space meals and activities.
  a. Eat six small meals a day.
  b. Allow time during the day for periods of rest and relaxation.
- Perform all activities at a comfortable pace.
  a. If tired during activity, stop and rest for 15 minutes.
  b. Resume activity only when capable.
- Stop any activity that causes chest pain, shortness of breath, dizziness, faintness, excessive weakness or sweating. Rest. Notify the doctor if activity tolerance changes and if symptoms continue after rest.
- Avoid straining. Do not lift heavy objects. Eat a high-fibre diet and drink plenty of water to prevent constipation. Use laxatives or stool softeners, as approved by the doctor, to avoid constipation and straining during bowel movements.
- Begin a graded exercise program. Walking is good exercise that does not require any special equipment (except a good pair of walking shoes). Exercise programs should be initiated by a medical officer and supervised by appropriately trained exercise prescription professionals taking into account the clinical status of the individual. Isometric activity is not recommended as it increases left ventricular afterload.

FAST FACTS

- Cardiogenic pulmonary oedema is a severe form of heart failure. Risk factors are those associated with heart failure and treatment focuses on maintaining oxygenation and improving cardiac function.
- Non-cardiogenic pulmonary oedema is a primary or secondary lung disorder. It usually occurs secondarily to a critical event such as major trauma, shock or disseminated intravascular coagulation (DIC). Treatment focuses on maintaining oxygenation and the primary, underlying disorder.

causes include acute myocardial infarction, acute heart failure and valvular disease. *Cardiogenic pulmonary oedema*, the focus of this section, is a sign of severe cardiac decompensation. Non-cardiac causes of pulmonary oedema include primary pulmonary disorders, such as acute respiratory distress syndrome (ARDS), trauma, sepsis, drug overdose or neurological sequelae. Pulmonary oedema due to ARDS is discussed in the chapter 'Nursing care of people with gas exchange disorders'.

Pulmonary oedema is a medical emergency: the person is literally drowning in the fluid in the alveolar and interstitial pulmonary spaces. Its onset may be acute or gradual, progressing to severe respiratory distress. Immediate treatment is necessary.

Pathophysiology

In cardiogenic pulmonary oedema, the contractility of the left ventricle is severely impaired. The ejection fraction falls because the ventricle is unable to eject the blood that enters it, causing a sharp rise in end-diastolic volume and pressure. Pulmonary hydrostatic pressures rise, ultimately exceeding the osmotic pressure of the blood. As a result, fluid leaking from the pulmonary capillaries congests interstitial tissues, decreasing lung compliance and interfering with gas exchange. As capillary and interstitial pressures increase further, the tight junctions of the alveolar walls are disrupted and the fluid enters the alveoli, along with large red blood cells (RBCs) and protein molecules. Ventilation and gas exchange are severely disrupted and hypoxia worsens.

Manifestations

The person with acute pulmonary oedema presents with classic manifestations (see the 'Manifestations' box). Dyspnoea and laboured respirations are acute and severe, accompanied by orthopnoea. Cyanosis is present and the skin is cool, clammy and diaphoretic. A productive cough with pink, frothy sputum develops due to fluid, RBCs and plasma proteins in the alveoli and airways. Crackles are heard throughout the lung fields on auscultation. As the condition worsens, lung sounds become harsher. The person often is restless and highly anxious, although severe hypoxia may cause confusion or lethargy.

As noted earlier, pulmonary oedema is a medical emergency. Without rapid and effective intervention, severe tissue hypoxia and acidosis will lead to organ system failure and death.

INTERPROFESSIONAL CARE

Immediate treatment for acute pulmonary oedema focuses on restoring effective gas exchange and reducing fluid and pressure in the pulmonary vascular system. The individual is placed in an upright sitting position with the legs dangling to reduce venous return by trapping some excess fluid in the lower extremities. This position also facilitates breathing.

MANIFESTATIONS Acute pulmonary oedema

RESPIRATORY
- Tachypnoea
- Laboured respirations
- Dyspnoea
- Orthopnoea
- Paroxysmal nocturnal dyspnoea
- Cough productive of frothy, pink sputum
- Crackles, wheezes

CARDIOVASCULAR
- Tachycardia
- Hypotension
- Cyanosis
- Cool, clammy skin
- Hypoxaemia
- Ventricular gallop (S_3)

NEUROLOGICAL
- Restlessness
- Anxiety
- Sense of impending doom

Diagnosis

Diagnostic testing is limited to assessment of the acute situation. *ABGs* are drawn to assess gas exchange and acid–base balance. Oxygen tension (PaO_2) is usually low. Initially, carbon dioxide levels ($PaCO_2$) may also be reduced because of rapid respirations. As the condition progresses, the $PaCO_2$ rises and respiratory acidosis develops (see the chapter 'Nursing care of people with altered fluid, electrolyte and acid–base balance'). *Oxygen saturation* levels also are continuously monitored. The *chest x-ray* shows pulmonary vascular congestion and alveolar oedema. Provided the person's condition allows, *haemodynamic monitoring* is instituted. In cardiogenic pulmonary oedema, the pulmonary artery wedge pressure is elevated, usually over 25 mmHg. Cardiac output may be decreased.

Medications

Morphine is administered intravenously to relieve anxiety and improve the efficacy of breathing. It also is a vasodilator that reduces venous return and lowers left atrial pressure. Although morphine is very effective for individuals with cardiogenic pulmonary oedema, naloxone, its antidote, should be kept readily available in case respiratory depression occurs.

Oxygen is administered using a positive-pressure system that can achieve a 100% oxygen concentration. A continuous positive airway pressure (CPAP) mask system may be used or the person may be intubated and mechanical ventilation employed (see the chapter 'Nursing care of people with gas exchange disorders'). Positive pressure increases alveolar pressures and gas exchange while decreasing fluid diffusion into the alveoli.

Potent loop diuretics such as frusemide are administered intravenously to promote rapid diuresis. Vasodilators such as intravenous glyceryl trinitrate may be given to improve cardiac output by reducing afterload. However, care must be taken to avoid profound hypotension. Positive inotropes may be administered to improve the myocardial contractility and cardiac output.

When the person's condition has stabilised, further diagnostic tests may be done to determine the underlying cause of pulmonary oedema and specific treatment measures directed at the cause instituted.

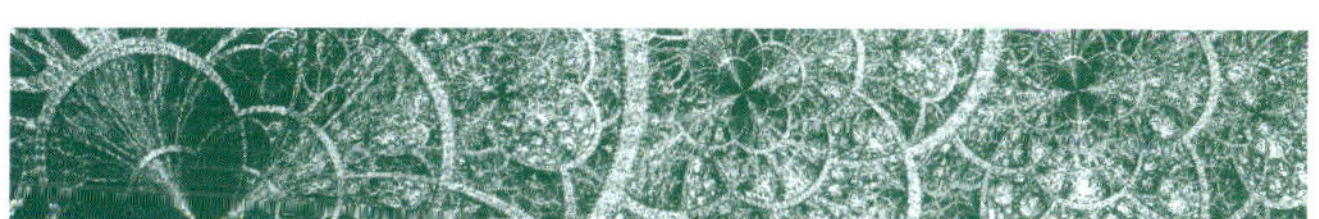

Nursing care

Nursing care of the person with acute pulmonary oedema focuses on relieving the pulmonary effects of the disorder. Interventions are directed towards improving oxygenation, reducing fluid volume and providing emotional support.

The nurse is often instrumental in recognising early manifestations of pulmonary oedema and initiating treatment. As with many critical conditions, emergent care is directed towards the ABCs: airway, breathing and circulation.

Nursing diagnoses and interventions

Promoting effective gas exchange and restoring an effective cardiac output are the priorities for nursing and interprofessional care of the person with cardiogenic pulmonary oedema. The experience of acute dyspnoea is terrifying for the individual; the nurse is instrumental in providing emotional support and reassurance.

Impaired gas exchange

Accumulated fluid in the alveoli and airways interferes with ventilation of the lungs. As a result, alveolar oxygen levels fall and carbon dioxide levels may rise. Reduced alveolar oxygen decreases diffusion of the gas into pulmonary capillaries. In addition, pulmonary oedema increases the distance over which gases must diffuse to cross the alveolar–capillary membrane, further reducing oxygen levels in the blood and oxygen delivery to the tissues.

- Ensure airway patency. *A patent airway is absolutely vital for pulmonary function, including ventilation and gas exchange.*

> **CONSIDERATION FOR PRACTICE**
>
> **Assess the effectiveness of respiratory efforts and airway clearance. Pulmonary oedema increases the work of breathing. This increased effort can lead to fatigue and decreased respiratory effort.**

- Assess respiratory status frequently, including rate, effort, use of accessory muscles, sputum characteristics, lung sounds and skin colour. *The status of a person in acute pulmonary oedema can change rapidly for the better or worse.*
- Place in high-Fowler's position with the legs dangling. *The upright position facilitates breathing and decreases venous return.*
- Administer oxygen as ordered by mask, CPAP mask or ventilator. *Supplemental oxygen promotes gas exchange; positive pressure increases the pressure within the alveoli, airways and thoracic cavity, decreasing venous return, pulmonary capillary pressure and fluid leak into the alveoli.*
- Encourage to cough up secretions; provide nasotracheal suctioning if necessary. *Coughing moves secretions from smaller airways into larger airways where they can be suctioned out or coughed up if necessary.*

> **CONSIDERATION FOR PRACTICE**
>
> **Have emergency equipment readily available in case of respiratory arrest. Be prepared to assist with intubation and initiation of mechanical ventilation. Fatigue, impaired gas exchange and respiratory acidosis can lead to respiratory and cardiac arrest.**

Decreased cardiac output

Cardiogenic pulmonary oedema usually is caused by either an acute decrease in myocardial contractility or increased workload that exceeds the ability of the left ventricle. The significant decrease in cardiac output increases pressure within the pulmonary vascular system and triggers compensatory mechanisms that increase the heart rate and blood volume. These compensatory mechanisms further increase the workload of the failing heart.

- Monitor vital signs, haemodynamic status and rhythm continuously. *Acute pulmonary oedema is a critical condition and cardiovascular status can change rapidly.*
- Assess heart sounds for possible S_3, S_4 or murmurs. *These abnormal heart sounds may be due to excess fluid.*
- Initiate an intravenous line for medication administration. Administer morphine, diuretics, vasodilators, bronchodilators and positive inotropic medications (e.g. digoxin, dopamine or dobutamine) as ordered. *These drugs reduce cardiac work and improve contractility.*
- Keep accurate intake and output records. Restrict fluids as ordered. *Fluids may be restricted to reduce vascular volume and cardiac work.*

Fear and anxiety

Acute pulmonary oedema is a very frightening experience for everyone (including the nurse).

- Provide emotional support for the person and their family members. *Fear and anxiety stimulate the sympathetic nervous system, which can lead to ineffective respiratory patterns and interfere with cooperation with care measures.*
- Explain all procedures and the reasons they are performed to the person and their family members. Keep information brief and to the point. Use short sentences and a reassuring tone. *Anxiety and fear interfere with the ability to assimilate information; brief, factual information and reassurance reduce anxiety and fear.*
- Maintain close contact and provide reassurance that recovery from acute pulmonary oedema is often as dramatic as its onset.

Answer questions and provide accurate information in a caring manner. *Knowledge reduces anxiety and psychological stress associated with this critical condition.*

CONSIDERATION FOR PRACTICE

Insert an indwelling catheter; record output hourly. Urine output of less than 30 mL/h indicates impaired renal perfusion due to severely impaired cardiac output and a risk of renal failure or other complications.

Community-based care

During the acute period, teaching is limited to immediate care measures. Once the acute episode of pulmonary oedema has resolved, teach the person and their family about its underlying cause and prevention of future episodes. If pulmonary oedema follows an acute MI, include information related to CHD and the acute AMI, as well as information related to heart failure. Review the teaching and home care needs for the person with these disorders.

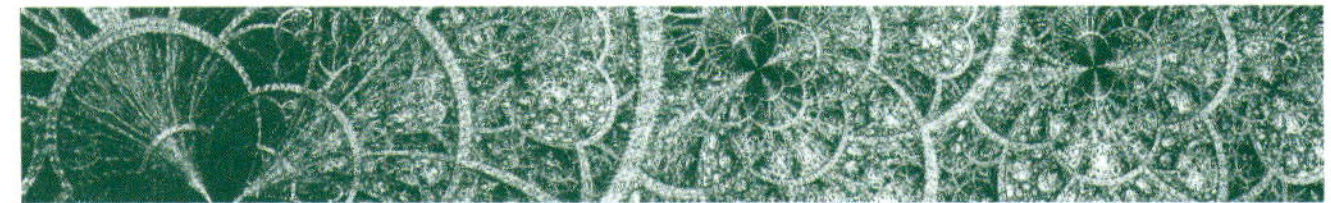

The person with an inflammatory or infective condition of the heart

Infective conditions include rheumatic heart disease and conditions that result in inflammation of any layer of the cardiac tissue. Manifestations of inflammatory heart disorders range from very mild to life threatening. This section discusses the causes and management of rheumatic heart disease, endocarditis, myocarditis and pericarditis.

THE PERSON WITH RHEUMATIC FEVER AND RHEUMATIC HEART DISEASE

Rheumatic fever is a systemic inflammatory disease caused by an abnormal immune response to pharyngeal infection by group A beta-haemolytic streptococci. Rheumatic fever usually is a self-limiting disorder, although it may become recurrent or chronic. The heart commonly is involved in the acute inflammatory process and approximately 60% of people with rheumatic fever develop rheumatic heart disease (Wallace, 2021). Rheumatic heart disease frequently damages the heart valves and is a major cause of mitral and aortic valve disorders discussed in the next section of this chapter.

Incidence, prevalence and risk factors

In Australia, rheumatic fever is more common than in most other developed countries. As described earlier, rheumatic heart disease (RHD) remains a significant problem for northern and central Indigenous Australians, although RHD is relatively uncommon in other Australian populations. Indigenous Australian females are 35 times and Indigenous males 30 times more likely to develop RHD than non-Indigenous Australians. The incidence of RHD is underreported as it is often difficult to diagnose (RHDAustralia, 2020).

Rheumatic fever and rheumatic heart disease remain significant public health problems in many developing countries. Globally it is estimated that there are over 15.6 million people with rheumatic heart disease.

Risk factors for streptococcal infections of the pharynx include environmental and economic factors such as crowded living conditions, malnutrition, immunodeficiency and poor access to healthcare (RHDAustralia, 2020).

Pathophysiology

The pathophysiology of rheumatic fever is not yet totally understood. It results from an abnormal immune response to M proteins on group A beta-haemolytic streptococcal bacteria. These antigens can bind to cells in the heart, muscles and brain. They also bind with receptors in synovial joints, provoking an autoimmune response (Wallace, 2021). The resulting immune response to the bacteria also leads to inflammation in tissues containing these M proteins. Inflammatory lesions develop in

FAST FACTS

- The Northern Territory has the highest prevalence of RHD, at just under 43%.
- Aboriginal and Torres Strait Islander people constitute 81% of the population diagnosed with RHD.
- The rate of diagnosis is almost two times higher in female than males.
- At time of diagnosis, 55% are under the age of 25 years.
- The median age at diagnosis for Aboriginal and Torres Strait Islander people is 22 years, compared to 50 years of age for non-Indigenous Australians (AIHW, 2021).

connective tissues on the heart, joints and skin. The antibodies may remain in the serum for up to 6 months following the initiating event. See the chapters 'Nursing care of people with infections' and 'Nursing care of people with altered immunity' for more information about the immune system and inflammatory response.

Carditis, inflammation of the heart, develops in 30–60% of people with rheumatic fever. The inflammatory process usually involves all three layers of the heart—the pericardium, myocardium and endocardium. *Aschoff bodies*, localised areas of tissue necrosis surrounded by immune cells, develop in cardiac tissues. Pericardial and myocardial inflammation tends to be mild and self-limiting. Endocardial inflammation, however, causes swelling and erythema of valve structures and small vegetative lesions on valve leaflets. As the inflammatory process resolves, fibrous scarring occurs, causing deformity.

Rheumatic heart disease (RHD) is a slowly progressive valvular deformity that may follow acute or repeated attacks of rheumatic fever. Valve leaflets become rigid and deformed; commissures (openings) fuse and the chordae tendineae fibrose and shorten. This results in stenosis or regurgitation of the valve. In **stenosis**, a narrowed fused valve obstructs forward blood flow. **Regurgitation** occurs when the valve fails to close properly (an *incompetent* valve), allowing blood to flow back through it. Valves on the left side of the heart are usually affected; the mitral valve is most frequently involved.

Manifestations

Manifestations of acute rheumatic fever (ARF) typically follow the initial streptococcal infection by about 2 to 3 weeks. Fever and migratory joint pain are often initial manifestations. The knees, ankles, hips and elbows are common sites of swelling and inflammation. *Erythema marginatum* is a temporary non-pruritic skin rash characterised by red lesions with clear borders and blanched centres usually found on the trunk and proximal extremities. Neurological symptoms of rheumatic fever, although rare in adults, may range from irritability and an inability to concentrate to clumsiness and involuntary muscle spasms. See the 'Manifestations' box.

Manifestations of carditis include chest pain, tachycardia, a pericardial friction rub or evidence of heart failure. On auscultation, an S_3, S_4 or heart murmur may be heard. Cardiomegaly or pericardial effusion may develop. See Table 30.6 for other manifestations.

MANIFESTATIONS Acute rheumatic fever

CARDIAC
- Chest pain
- Friction rub
- Heart murmur

MUSCULOSKELETAL
- *Migratory polyarthritis*: redness, heat, swelling, pain and tenderness of more than one joint
- Usually affects large joints of extremities

SKIN
- *Erythema marginatum*: transitory pink, non-pruritic, macular lesions on trunk or inner aspect of upper arms or thighs
- *Subcutaneous nodules* over extensors of wrist, elbow, ankle and knee joints

NEUROLOGICAL
- *Sydenham's chorea:* irritability, behaviour changes; sudden, jerky, involuntary movements

BLOOD TESTS
- Serum antistreptolysin O (ASO) antibodies titres are measured to confirm the diagnosis. Serum ASO rises within 1–2 weeks of infection and reaches a maximum at about 3–6 weeks after infection.
- Serum antideoxyribonuclease B (anti-DNase B) antibodies are also commonly measured to increase the sensitivity of the testing. It is produced by all group A beta-haemolytic streptococci. Serum anti-DNase B peaks 4 to 8 weeks after infection, remains elevated for several months and declines slowly.

INTERPROFESSIONAL CARE

Management of the person with rheumatic heart disease focuses on eradicating the streptococcal infection and managing the manifestations of the disease. Carditis and resulting heart failure are treated with measures to reduce the inflammatory process and manage the heart failure. Activities are limited, but bed rest is not generally ordered.

Diagnosis

As Australia has a significant incidence of rheumatic heart disease, RHDAustralia (2020) modified the two previously used tools (Jones criteria and the WHO criteria) to develop the 2020 Australian guidelines for the diagnosis of ARF. In addition to the history and physical examination, a number of laboratory and diagnostic tests may be ordered for the person with suspected rheumatic fever. For diagnosis guidelines, see Tables 30.5 and 30.6.

- *Full blood count (FBC)* and *erythrocyte sedimentation rate (ESR)* are indicators of the inflammatory process. The WBC count is elevated and the number of RBCs may be low due to the inflammatory inhibition of erythropoiesis. The ESR, a general indicator of inflammation, is elevated.

TABLE 30.5 Diagnostic criteria for acute rheumatic fever (Australia 2020, American Health Association 2015)

MANIFESTATION	HIGH RISK	LOW RISK
Carditis	Major	Major
Subclinical carditis	Major	Major
Prolonged PR interval	Minor	Minor
Polyarthritis	Major	Major
Polyarthralgia	Major	Minor
Aseptic monoarthritis	Major	Minor
Monoarthralgia	Minor	n/a
Subcutaneous nodules	Major	Major
Sydenham's chorea	Major	Major
Erythema marginatum	Major	Major
Fever	Minor Temp ≥ 38°C	Minor Temp ≥ 38.5°C
Raised inflammatory markers	Minor	Minor
Evidence of recent Group A streptococcal infection	Required	Required

Source: RHDAustralia (ARF/RHD Writing Group) (2020). *The 2020 Australian guideline for prevention, diagnosis and management of acute rheumatic fever and rheumatic heart disease* (3rd edition); 2020. Available at https://www.rhdaustralia.org.au/arf-rhd-guideline. Reproduced with permission from Menzies School of Health Research. https://www.rhdaustralia.org.au/.

Medications

As soon as rheumatic fever is diagnosed, antibiotics are started to eliminate the streptococcal infection. Intramuscular benzathine penicillin G (BPG) is the antibiotic of choice to treat group A streptococci. A single dose of intramuscular BPG or a 10-day dose of oral penicillin V is administered. Erythromycin is used if the person is allergic to penicillin (RHDAustralia, 2020).

Joint pain and fever are treated with paracetamol; corticosteroids may be used for severe pain due to inflammation. See the chapter 'Nursing care of people with altered immunity' for information about the use of these anti-inflammatory medications.

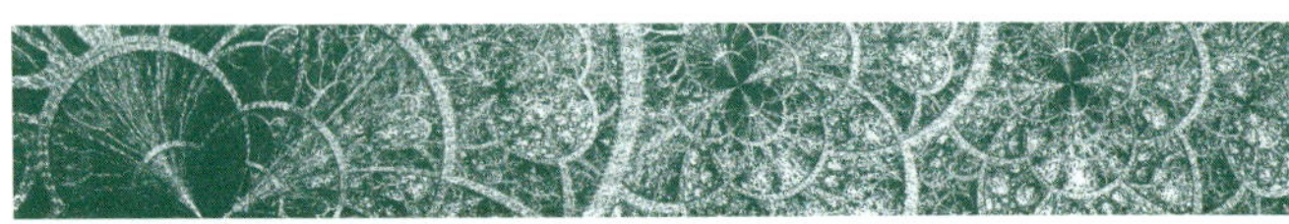

Nursing care

Health promotion

Rheumatic fever is preventable. Prompt identification and treatment of a person's streptococcal throat infection and skin

TABLE 30.6 Updated Australian criteria for acute rheumatic fever diagnosis

	HIGH-RISK GROUPS[†]	LOW-RISK GROUPS
Definite initial episode of ARF	2 major manifestations + evidence of preceding Strep A infection *or* 1 major + 2 minor manifestations + evidence of preceding Strep A infection[‡]	
Definite recurrent[§] episode of ARF in a patient with a documented history of ARF or RHD	2 major manifestations + evidence of preceding Strep A infection *or* 1 major + 2 minor manifestations + evidence of preceding Strep A infection[‡] *or* 3 minor manifestations + evidence of a preceding Strep A infection[‡]	
Probable or possible ARF (first episode or recurrence[§])	A clinical presentation in which ARF is considered a likely diagnosis but falls short in meeting the criteria by either: • one major or one minor manifestation *or* • no evidence of preceding Strep A infection (streptococcal titres within normal limits or titres not measured). Such cases should be further categorised according to the level of confidence with which the diagnosis is made: • probable ARF (previously termed 'probable: highly suspected') • possible ARF (previously termed 'probable: uncertain').	
Major manifestations	Carditis (including subclinical evidence of rheumatic valvulitis on echocardiogram) Polyarthritis[¶] or aseptic monoarthritis or polyarthralgia Sydenham chorea[††] Erythema marginatum[‡‡] Subcutaneous nodules	Carditis (including subclinical evidence of rheumatic valvulitis on echocardiogram) Polyarthritis[¶] Sydenham chorea[††] Erythema marginatum[‡‡] Subcutaneous nodules
Minor manifestations	Fever[§§] ≥ 38°C Monoarthralgia[¶¶] ESR ≥ 30 mm/h or CRP ≥ 30 mg/L Prolonged P-R interval on ECG[†††]	Fever ≥ 38.5°C Polyarthralgia or aseptic monoarthritis[¶¶] ESR ≥ 60 mm/h or CRP ≥ 30 mg/L Prolonged P-R interval on ECG[†††]

[†]High-risk groups are those living in communities with high rates of ARF (incidence > 30/100,000 per year in 5–14-year-olds) or RHD (all-age prevalence > 2/1000). Aboriginal and Torres Strait Islander peoples living in rural or remote settings are known to be at high risk. Data are not available for other populations but Aboriginal and Torres Strait Islander peoples living in urban settings, Māori and Pacific Islanders, and potentially immigrants from developing countries, may also be at high risk.
[‡]Elevated or rising antistreptolysin O or other streptococcal antibody, or a positive throat culture or rapid antigen or nucleic acid test for strep A infection.
[§]Recurrent definite, probable or possible ARF requires a time period of more than 90 days after the onset of symptoms from the previous episode of definite, probable or possible ARF.
[¶]A definite history of arthritis is sufficient to satisfy this manifestation. Note that if polyarthritis is present as a major manifestation, polyarthralgia or aseptic monoarthritis cannot be considered an additional minor manifestation in the same person.
[††]Chorea does not require other manifestations or evidence of preceding Strep A infection, provided other causes of chorea are excluded.
[‡‡]Care should be taken not to label other rashes, particularly non-specific viral exanthems, as erythema marginatum.
[§§]In high-risk groups, fever can be considered a minor manifestation based on a reliable history (in the absence of documented temperature) if anti-inflammatory medication has already been administered.
[¶¶]If polyarthritis is present as a major criterion, monoarthritis or arthralgia cannot be considered an additional minor manifestation.
[†††]If carditis is present as a major manifestation, a prolonged P-R interval cannot be considered an additional minor manifestation.
CRP = C-reactive protein; ECG = electrocardiogram; ESR = erythrocyte sedimentation rate

Source: RHDAustralia (ARF/RHD Writing Group) (2020). *The 2020 Australian guideline for prevention, diagnosis and management of acute rheumatic fever and rheumatic heart disease* (3rd edition); 2020. Available at https://www.rhdaustralia.org.au/arf-rhd-guideline. Reproduced with permission from Menzies School of Health Research. https://www.rhdaustralia.org.au/.

infections helps to decrease spread of the pathogen and the risk of rheumatic fever. Characteristics of streptococcal pharyngitis include a sore throat, odynophagia, headache, fever, tonsillopharyngeal erythema, swollen uvula and lymphadenopathy. The importance of finishing the complete course of medication to eradicate the pathogen must be emphasised. As the route of choice of antibiotic administration is intramuscular, methods to reduce pain at the injection site should be implemented. Simple interventions include: choosing a 23-gauge needle; ensuring the alcowipe is dry before inserting the needle; applying pressure on site (with thumb) for 10 seconds before administration; injecting slowly (over > 2 – 3 minutes); and using distraction techniques to assist with reducing pain.

Assessment

Assess the person at risk of rheumatic fever (prolonged, untreated or recurrent pharyngitis) for possible manifestations.

- *Health history*: complaints of recent sore throat with fever, difficulty swallowing and general malaise; treatment measures; previous history of strep throat or rheumatic fever; history of heart murmur or other cardiac problems; current medications.
- *Physical examination*: vital signs, including temperature; skin colour, presence of rash on trunk or proximal extremities; mental status; evidence of inflamed joints; heart and lung sounds.
- *Diagnostic tests*: full blood count with differential, ESR, CRP results, throat culture, ECG and echocardiogram.

Nursing diagnoses and interventions

The nursing care focus for the person with RHD is on providing supportive care and preventing complications. Teaching to prevent recurrence of rheumatic fever is extremely important. *Pain* and *Activity intolerance* are priority nursing diagnoses for the person with rheumatic fever and RHD.

Acute pain

Joint and chest pain due to acute inflammation is common in rheumatic fever. Pain and inflammation may interfere with rest and healing.

- Administer anti-inflammatory drugs as ordered. Promptly report manifestations of aspirin toxicity, including tinnitus, vomiting and gastrointestinal bleeding. Give aspirin and other NSAIDs with food, milk or antacids to minimise gastric irritation. *Joint pain and fever may be treated with anti-inflammatory agents such as aspirin and NSAIDs. When used for its anti-inflammatory effect, aspirin doses may be high and it is given around the clock (e.g. every 4 hours). Steroids may be prescribed for severe carditis.*
- Provide warm compresses for local pain relief of acutely inflamed joints. *Warmth helps relieve pain associated with inflamed joints by reducing inflammation.*
- Auscultate heart sounds as indicated (every shift or each home visit). Notify the doctor if a pericardial friction rub or a new murmur develops. *A friction rub is produced as inflamed pericardial surfaces rub against each other. This also stimulates pain receptors and may increase discomfort.*

Activity intolerance

The person with acute carditis or RHD may develop heart failure if the heart is unable to supply enough oxygen to meet the body's demand. Manifestations of fatigue, weakness and dyspnoea on exertion may result.

- Explain the importance of activity limitations and reinforce teaching as needed. *Activities are limited during the acute phase of carditis to reduce the workload of the heart. Understanding the rationale improves cooperation with the limitations.*
- Encourage social and diversional activities such as visits with friends and family, reading, playing cards or board games, watching television and listening to music or talking books. *Diversional activities provide a focus for the person whose physical activities must be limited.*
- Encourage gradual increases in activity, monitoring for evidence of intolerance or heart failure. Consult a cardiac rehabilitation specialist to help design an activity progression schedule. *Gradual activity progression is encouraged as the person's condition improves. Activity tolerance is monitored and activities modified as needed.*

Community-based care

Most people with rheumatic fever and carditis do not require hospitalisation. Teaching for home care focuses on both acute care and preventing recurrences and further tissue damage. Include the following topics:

- the importance of completing the full course of antibiotic therapy and continuing antibiotic prophylaxis as prescribed. For the individual with chronic RHD, include the importance of antibiotic prophylaxis for invasive procedures (e.g. dental care, endoscopy or surgery) to prevent bacterial endocarditis. Pamphlets on endocarditis prevention are helpful reminders and are available from the National Heart Foundation of Australia
- preventive dental care and good oral hygiene to maintain oral health and prevent gingival infections, which can lead to recurrence of the disease
- early recognition of streptococcal sore throat and appropriate treatment for both the individual and their family members
- early manifestations of heart failure to report to the doctor
- prescribed medications, including their dosage, route, intended and potential adverse effects, and manifestations to report to the doctor
- dietary sodium restriction if ordered or recommended. A high-carbohydrate, high-protein diet may be recommended to promote healing and combat fatigue.

Refer for home health services or household assistance as indicated.

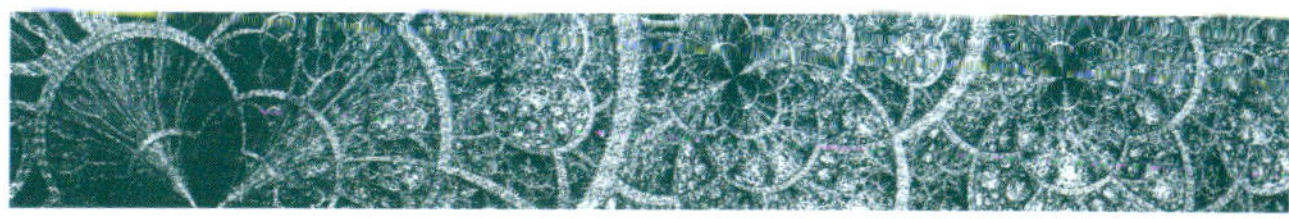

THE PERSON WITH INFECTIVE ENDOCARDITIS

Endocarditis, inflammation of the endocardium, can involve any portion of the endothelial lining of the heart. The valves usually are affected. Endocarditis is usually infectious in nature, characterised by colonisation or invasion of the endocardium and heart valves by a pathogen.

Incidence and risk factors

Endocarditis is relatively uncommon in Australia. In 2016, endocarditis was listed as the cause of death for only 100 people, which equates to 0.24% of all deaths that year (ABS, 2017), and incidence statistics are difficult to locate. Nevertheless, a little over 3,000 people were admitted to hospital with a primary diagnosis of endocarditis in 2020–2021 (AIHW, 2022).

The greatest risk factor for endocarditis is previous heart damage. Lesions develop on deformed valves, on valve prostheses or in areas of tissue damage due to congenital deformities or ischaemic disease. The left side of the heart—the mitral valve, in particular—is usually affected. Intravenous drug use also is a significant risk factor. The right side of the heart usually is affected in these individuals. Other risk factors include invasive catheters (e.g. a central venous catheter, haemodynamic monitoring or an indwelling urinary catheter), dental procedures or poor dental health, and recent heart surgery.

FAST FACTS

- Subacute bacterial endocarditis develops more slowly and usually occurs in people with previous heart valve damage.
- Acute bacterial endocarditis has an abrupt onset and typically affects people with no previous history of heart problems.

Prosthetic valve endocarditis (PVE) may occur in individuals with a mechanical or tissue valve replacement. This infection may develop in the early postoperative period (within 2 months after surgery) or late. Prosthetic valve endocarditis accounts for 10–20% of endocarditis cases (Brusch, 2022). Early PVE occurs within 60 days of valve implantation and is usually due to prosthetic valve contamination during surgery or perioperative bacteraemia. Its course often is rapid and mortality is high. Late-onset PVE occurring after 60 days following surgery more closely resembles subacute endocarditis.

Pathophysiology

Entry of pathogens into the bloodstream is required for infective endocarditis to develop. Bacteria may enter through oral lesions, during dental work or invasive procedures such as intravenous catheter insertion, surgery or urinary catheterisation; during intravenous drug use; or as a result of infectious processes such as urinary tract or upper respiratory infection.

The initial lesion is a sterile platelet–fibrin vegetation formed on damaged endothelium (see Figure 30.4). In acute infective endocarditis, these lesions develop on healthy valve structures, although the mechanism is unknown. In subacute endocarditis, they usually develop on already damaged valves or in endocardial tissue that has been damaged by abnormal pressures or blood flow within the heart.

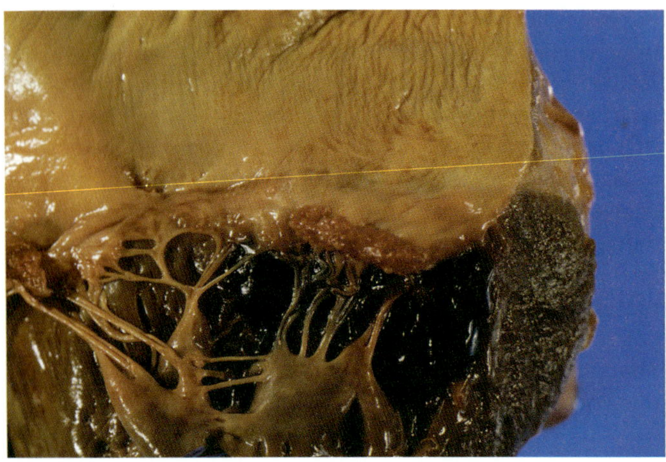

FIGURE 30.4 ***A vegetative lesion of bacterial endocarditis***

Source: Dr E. Walker/Science Photo Library.

Organisms that have invaded the blood colonise these vegetations. The vegetation enlarges as more platelets and fibrin are attracted to the site and cover the infecting organism. This covering 'protects' the bacteria from quick removal by immune defences such as phagocytosis by neutrophils, antibodies and complement. Vegetations may be singular or multiple. They expand while loosely attached to the edges of the valve. Friable vegetations can break or shear off, embolising and travelling through the bloodstream to other organ systems. When they lodge in small vessels, they may cause haemorrhages, infarcts or abscesses. Ultimately, the vegetations scar and deform the valves and cause turbulence of blood flowing through the heart. Heart valve function is affected, either obstructing forward blood flow or closing incompletely.

Endocarditis is classified by its acuity and disease course. *Acute infective endocarditis* (IE) has an abrupt onset and is a rapidly progressive, severe disease. Further classifications can be made as to whether the endocarditis has occurred on a person's native valve (NVE), on a prosthetic valve (PVE) or as a result of intravenous drug abuse (IVDA IE). Although almost any organism can cause infective endocarditis, virulent organisms such as *Staphylococcus aureus* cause a more abrupt onset and destructive course. *S. aureus* is commonly the infective organism in acute endocarditis. In contrast, *subacute infective endocarditis* has a more gradual onset, with predominant systemic manifestations. It is more likely to occur in people with pre-existing heart disease and is commonly caused by alpha-haemolytic streptococci or enterococci. In IVDA infective endocarditis, *S. aureus* is the most common organism with the majority of cases affecting the tricuspid valve (Brusch, 2022).

Manifestations

The manifestations of infective endocarditis often are non-specific (see the 'Manifestations' box). A temperature above 39.4°C and flu-like symptoms develop, accompanied by cough, shortness of breath and joint pain. The presentation of

MANIFESTATIONS Infective endocarditis

- Chills and fever
- General malaise, fatigue
- Arthralgias
- Cough, dyspnoea
- Heart murmur
- Anorexia, abdominal pain
- Petechiae, splinter haemorrhages
- Splenomegaly

acute staphylococcal endocarditis is more severe, with a sudden onset, chills and a high fever. Heart murmurs are heard in 90% of individuals with infective endocarditis. An existing murmur may worsen or a new murmur may develop.

Splenomegaly is common in chronic disease. Peripheral manifestations of infective endocarditis result from microemboli or circulating immune complexes. These manifestations include:

- *Petechiae*: small, purplish-red haemorrhagic spots on the trunk, conjunctiva and mucous membranes.
- *Splinter haemorrhages*: haemorrhagic streaks under the fingernails or toenails.
- *Osler's nodes*: small, reddened, painful raised growths on finger and toe pads.
- *Janeway lesions*: small, non-tender, purplish-red macular lesions on the palms of the hands and soles of the feet.
- *Roth's spots*: small, whitish spots (cottonwool spots) seen on the retina.

Complications

Embolisation of vegetative fragments may affect any organ system, particularly the lungs, brain, kidneys and the skin and mucous membranes, with resulting organ infarction. Other common complications of infective endocarditis include heart failure, abscess and aneurysms due to infiltration of the arterial wall by organisms. Without treatment, endocarditis is almost universally fatal; fortunately, antibiotic therapy is usually effective to treat this disease.

INTERPROFESSIONAL CARE

Eradicating the infecting organism and minimising valve damage and other adverse consequences of infective endocarditis are the priorities of care.

Diagnosis

There are no definitive tests for infective endocarditis, but diagnostic tests help establish the diagnosis.

- *Blood cultures* usually are positive for bacteria or other pathogens. Blood cultures are considered positive when a typical infecting organism is identified from two or more separate blood cultures (drawn from different sites and/or at different times; e.g. 12-hour intervals).
- *Echocardiography* (either transthoracic or transoesophageal) to visualise vegetations can be diagnostic for infective endocarditis when combined with positive blood cultures. See the chapter 'A person-centred approach to assessing the cardiovascular and lymphatic systems' for more information about echocardiography.
- *Serological immune testing* for circulating antigens to typical infective organisms may be done.

Other diagnostic tests may include the FBC, ESR, serum creatinine, chest x-ray and an electrocardiogram.

Medications

Preventing endocarditis in individuals at high risk is important. Antibiotics are commonly prescribed for individuals with pre-existing valve damage or heart disease prior to high-risk procedures.

Antibiotic therapy effectively treats infective endocarditis in most cases. The goal of therapy is to eradicate the infecting organism from the blood and vegetative lesions in the heart. The fibrin covering that protects colonies of organisms from immune defences also protects them from antibiotic therapy. Therefore, an extended course of multiple intravenous antibiotics is required.

Following blood cultures, antibiotic therapy is initiated with drugs known to be effective against the most common infecting organisms: *Staphylococcus*, *Streptococcus* and *Enterococcus* species. The initial regimen will include an antibiotic to which the causative organism is sensitive. See the chapter 'Nursing care of people with infections' for the nursing implications for antibiotic therapy.

Surgery

Some people with infective endocarditis require surgery to:

- replace severely damaged valves
- remove large vegetations at risk of embolisation
- remove a valve that is a continuing source of infection that does not respond to antibiotic therapy.

The most common indication for surgery is valvular regurgitation that causes heart failure and does not respond to medical therapy. When the infection has not responded to antibiotic therapy within 7 to 10 days, the infected valve may be replaced to facilitate eradication of the organism. Individuals with fungal endocarditis usually require surgical intervention. More information on valve replacement surgery is provided in the section on valve disorders.

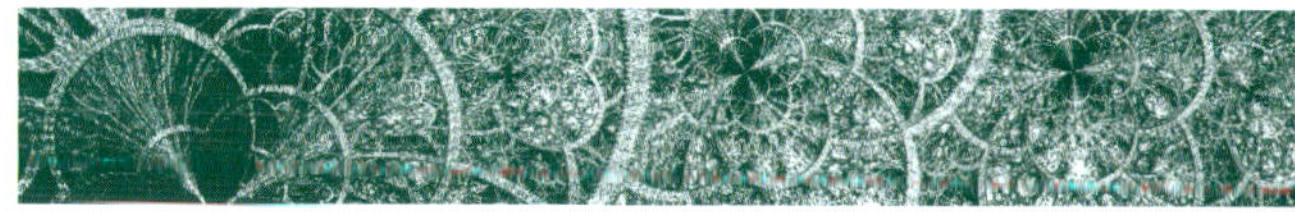

Nursing care

Health promotion

Prevention of endocarditis is vital in susceptible people. Education is a key part of prevention. Use every opportunity to educate individuals and the public about the risks of intravenous drug use, including endocarditis. Discuss preventive measures with all individuals with specific risk factors, such as a heart murmur or known heart disease.

Assessment

Assessment related to infective endocarditis includes identifying risk factors and manifestations of the disease.

- *Health history*: complaints of persistent flu-like symptoms, fatigue, shortness of breath and activity intolerance; history of recent dental work or other invasive procedures; known heart murmur, valve or other heart disorder; recent intravenous drug use.
- *Physical examination*: vital signs, including temperature; apical pulse and heart sounds; rate and ease of respirations, lung sounds; skin colour, temperature and presence of petechiae or splinter haemorrhages.
- *Diagnostic tests*: FBC and differential, ESR; blood culture and sensitivity results; echocardiogram reports.

Nursing diagnoses and interventions

Nursing care focuses on managing the manifestations of endocarditis, administering antibiotics and teaching the person and their family members about the disorder. In addition to the diagnoses identified below, nursing diagnoses and interventions for heart failure also may be appropriate for individuals with infective endocarditis.

Risk of imbalanced body temperature

Fever is common in individuals with infective endocarditis. It may be acutely elevated and accompanied by chills, particularly with acute infective endocarditis. The inflammatory process initiates a cycle of events that affects the regulation of temperature and causes discomfort.

- Record temperature every 2 to 4 hours. Report temperature above 38.5°C. Assess for complaints of discomfort. *Fever is usually low grade (38°C) in infective endocarditis; higher temperatures may cause discomfort. The temperature usually returns to normal within 1 week after initiation of antibiotic therapy. Continued fever may indicate a need to modify the treatment regimen.*
- Obtain blood cultures as ordered, before initial antibiotic dose. *Initial blood cultures are obtained before antibiotic therapy is started to obtain adequate organisms to culture and identify. Follow-up cultures are used to assess the effectiveness of therapy.*
- Provide anti-inflammatory or antipyretic agents as prescribed. *Fever may be treated with anti-inflammatory or antipyretic agents such as aspirin, ibuprofen or paracetamol.*
- Administer antibiotics as ordered; obtain peak and trough drug levels as indicated. Intravenous antibiotics are given to eradicate the pathogen. *Peak and trough levels are used to evaluate the dose effectiveness in maintaining a therapeutic blood level.*

Risk of ineffective tissue perfusion

Embolisation of vegetative lesions can threaten tissue and organ perfusion. Vegetations from the left heart may lodge in arterioles or capillaries of the brain, kidneys or peripheral tissues, causing infarction or abscess. A large embolism can cause manifestations of stroke or transient ischaemic attack, renal failure or tissue ischaemia. Emboli from the right side of the heart become entrapped in pulmonary vasculature, causing manifestations of pulmonary embolism.

- Assess for, document and report manifestations of decreased organ system perfusion:
  a. *Neurological*: changes in level of consciousness, numbness or tingling in extremities, hemiplegia, visual disturbances or manifestations of stroke.
  b. *Renal*: decreased urine output, haematuria, elevated urea or creatinine.
  c. *Pulmonary*: dyspnoea, haemoptysis, diminished breath sounds, restlessness, sudden chest or shoulder pain.
  d. *Cardiovascular*: chest pain radiating to jaw or arms, tachycardia, anxiety, tachypnoea, hypotension.

  All major organs and tissues and the microcirculation may be affected by emboli when vegetations break off due to turbulent blood flow. Emboli may cause manifestations of organ dysfunction. The most devastating effects of emboli are in the brain and the myocardium, with resulting infarctions. Intravenous drug users have a high risk of pulmonary emboli as a result of right-sided endocardial fragments.
- Assess and document skin colour and temperature, quality of peripheral pulses and capillary refill. *Peripheral emboli affect tissue perfusion, with a risk of tissue necrosis and possible extremity loss.*

Ineffective health maintenance

The person with endocarditis is often treated in the community. Teaching about disease management and prevention of possible recurrences of endocarditis is vital.

- Demonstrate intravenous catheter site care and intermittent antibiotic administration if the person and their family will manage therapy. Have the person and/or significant other redemonstrate appropriate techniques. *Intermittent antibiotic infusions may be managed by the person or family members, or the individual may go to an outpatient facility to receive the infusions. Appropriate site care is necessary to reduce the risk of trauma and infection.*
- Explain the actions, doses, administration and desired and adverse effects of prescribed drugs. Identify manifestations to be reported to the doctor. Provide practical information about measures to reduce the risk of superinfection (e.g. the concomitant use of antithrush preparations). *Careful compliance with prescribed drug therapy is vital to eradicate the infecting organism. Antibiotic therapy can, however, cause superinfections such as candidiasis due to elimination of normal body flora.*
- Teach the person about the function of heart valves and the effects of endocarditis on heart function. Include a simple definition of endocarditis and explain the risk of its recurrence. *Information helps the person and their family understand endocarditis, its treatment and its effects. Understanding increases compliance.*
- Describe the manifestations of heart failure to be reported to the doctor. *Evidence of heart failure may necessitate modification of the treatment regimen or replacement of infected valves.*

- Encourage good dental hygiene and mouth care and regular dental check-ups. Teach the person how to prevent bleeding from the gums and avoid developing mouth ulcers (e.g. gentle tooth brushing, ensuring that dentures fit properly and avoiding toothpicks, dental floss and high-flow water devices). *The oropharynx harbours streptococci, which are common causes of endocarditis. Bleeding gums offer an opportunity for bacteria to enter the bloodstream.*
- Encourage the person to avoid people with upper respiratory infections. *Streptococci are normal pathogens in the upper respiratory tract; exposure to people with upper respiratory infections may increase the risk of infection.*
- If anticoagulant therapy is ordered, explain its actions, administration and major side effects. Identify manifestations of bleeding to be promptly reported to the doctor. *Individuals with valve disease or a prosthetic valve following infective endocarditis may require continued anticoagulant therapy to prevent thrombi and emboli. Knowledge is vital for appropriate management of anticoagulant therapy and prevention of complications.*

CONSIDERATION FOR PRACTICE

Stress the importance of notifying all care providers of valve disease, heart murmur or valve replacement before undergoing invasive procedures. Invasive procedures provide a portal of entry for bacteria. A history of valve disease increases the risk of the development or recurrence of endocarditis.

Community-based care

When preparing the person with infective endocarditis for home care, provide teaching as outlined for the nursing diagnosis of *Ineffective health maintenance*. In addition, discuss the following topics:

- Although serious and frightening, infective endocarditis can usually be treated effectively with intravenous antibiotics.
- The importance of promptly reporting any unusual manifestation, such as a change in vision, sudden pain or weakness, so that interventions to control complications can be promptly implemented.
- The rationale for all treatments and procedures.
- Preventing recurrences of infective endocarditis.
- The importance of maintaining contact with the doctor for follow up care and monitoring for long-term effects such as progressive valve damage and dysfunction.
- If appropriate, explain the risks associated with intravenous drug use.

Provide educational materials on infective endocarditis from the National Heart Foundation of Australia. Refer as appropriate to home health or home intravenous therapy services. Refer the person and their family or other significant others as appropriate to a drug or substance abuse treatment program or facility. Provide follow-up care to ensure compliance with the referral and treatment plan.

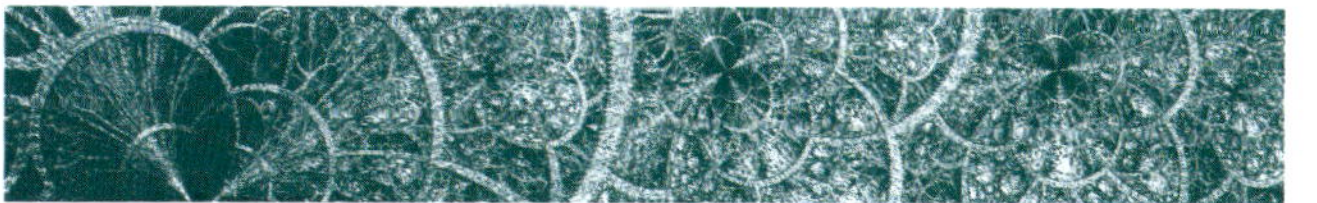

THE PERSON WITH MYOCARDITIS

Myocarditis is inflammation of the heart muscle. It usually results from an infectious process, but also may occur as an immunological response or due to the effects of radiation, toxins or drugs.

Incidence and risk factors

Myocarditis may occur at any age and is more common in men than women. Factors that alter immune response (e.g. malnutrition, alcohol use, immunosuppressive drugs, exposure to radiation, stress and advanced age) increase the risk of myocarditis. It also is a common complication of rheumatic fever and pericarditis. Myocarditis can also be an adverse effect of a common antipsychotic, clozapine.

Pathophysiology

Myocardial cells are damaged by an inflammatory process that causes local or diffuse swelling and damage. Infectious agents infiltrate interstitial tissues, forming abscesses. Autoimmune injury may occur when the immune system destroys not only the invading pathogen but also myocardial cells. The extent of damage to cardiac muscle ultimately determines the long-term outcome of the disease. Viral myocarditis usually is self-limiting; it may progress, however, to become chronic, leading to dilated cardiomyopathy. (See later in this chapter.) Severe myocarditis may lead to heart failure.

Manifestations

The manifestations of myocarditis depend on the degree of myocardial damage. The person may be asymptomatic. Non-specific manifestations of inflammation, such as fever, fatigue, general malaise, dyspnoea, palpitations and arthralgias, may be present. A non-specific febrile illness or upper respiratory infection often precedes the onset of myocarditis symptoms. Abnormal heart sounds such as muffled S_1, an S_3, murmur and pericardial friction rub may be heard. In some cases, manifestations of myocardial infarction, including chest pain, may occur.

COVID-19

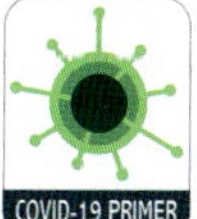

There is a clear risk of cardiovascular complications from some COVID-19 mRNA vaccinations and also from SARS-CoV-2 infection. Males are most at risk (depending on their age). However, it is critical to understand that although the mRNA vaccinations have been attributed to an increased risk of a transient inflammatory response affecting the inside (endocarditis), middle (myocarditis) or outside (pericarditis) of the heart, current evidence suggests that [illegible] risk of heart damage occurs from SARS-CoV-2 infection. Current evidence documents a 2–6 times greater risk of cardiac complications from SARS-CoV-2 infection than from vaccination for boys between 12 and 17 years of age. However, for young men between 18 and 29 years of age, the risk is 7–8 times higher (Block et al., 2022).

INTERPROFESSIONAL CARE

Myocarditis treatment focuses on resolving the inflammatory process to prevent further damage to the myocardium.

Diagnosis

Diagnostic studies may be ordered to help diagnose myocarditis:

- *Electrocardiography* may show transient ST-segment and T-wave changes, as well as arrhythmias and possible heart block.
- *Cardiac markers*, such as creatinine kinase (CK), troponin T (cT_nT) and troponin I (cT_nI), may be elevated, indicating myocardial cell damage.
- *Endomyocardial biopsy* to examine myocardial cells is necessary to establish a definitive diagnosis; patchy cell necrosis and the inflammatory process can be identified.

Medications

If appropriate, antimicrobial therapy is used to eradicate the infecting organism. Antiviral therapy with interferon alpha may be instituted. Immunosuppressive therapy with corticosteroids or other immunosuppressive agents (see the chapter 'Nursing care of people with altered immunity') may be used to minimise the inflammatory response. Heart failure is treated as needed, using ACE inhibitors and other cardiac drugs. Individuals with myocarditis often are particularly sensitive to the effects of digoxin, so it is used with caution. Other medications used in treating myocarditis include anti-arrhythmic agents to control arrhythmias and anticoagulants to prevent emboli.

Bed rest and activity restrictions are ordered during the acute inflammatory process to reduce myocardial work and prevent myocardial damage. While complete recovery occurs for many, some experience a progressive disease that manifests as dilated cardiomyopathy many years later (Banasik & Copstead, 2022).

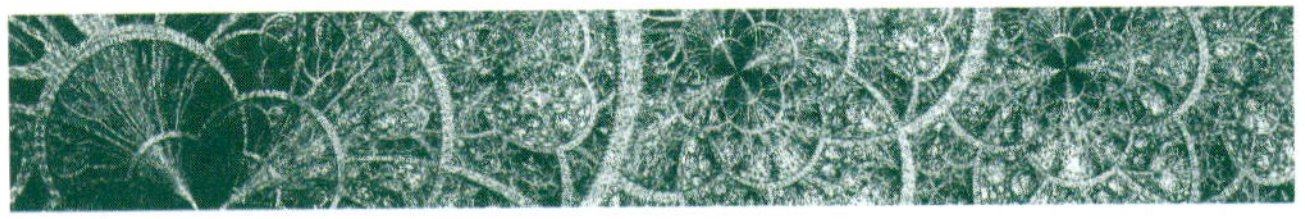

Nursing care

Nursing care is directed at decreasing myocardial work and maintaining cardiac output. Both physical and emotional rest are indicated because anxiety increases myocardial oxygen demand. Haemodynamic parameters and the ECG are monitored closely, especially during the acute phase of the illness. Activity tolerance, urine output and heart and breath sounds are frequently assessed for manifestations of heart failure. Consider the following nursing diagnoses for the person with myocarditis:

- *Risk of activity intolerance* related to impaired cardiac muscle function manifested by inability to undertake activities of daily living independently.
- *Risk of decreased cardiac output* related to myocardial inflammation manifested by hypotension, tachycardia and shortness of breath.
- *Risk of fatigue* related to inflammation and impaired cardiac output manifested by inability to mobilise or perform self-care without resting frequently.
- *Risk of anxiety* related to possible long-term effects of the disorder manifested by verbal statements and behaviour consistent with anxiety.
- *Risk of excess fluid volume* related to compensatory mechanisms for decreased cardiac output manifested by orthopnoea, dyspnoea, oedema and weight gain.

Community-based care

Include the following topics when preparing the person with myocarditis for home care:

- activity restrictions and other prescribed measures to reduce cardiac workload
- early manifestations of heart failure to report to the doctor
- the importance of following the prescribed treatment regimen
- any recommended dietary modifications (such as a low-sodium diet for heart failure)
- prescribed medications, their purpose, doses and possible adverse effects
- the importance of adhering to the treatment plan and recommended follow-up appointments to reduce the risk of long-term consequences such as cardiomyopathy.

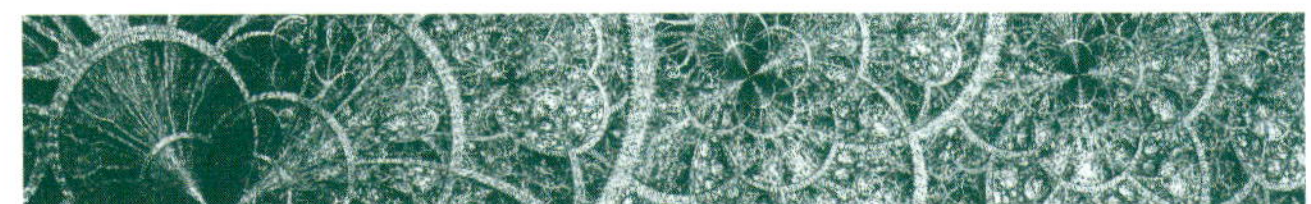

THE PERSON WITH PERICARDITIS

The pericardium is the outermost layer of the heart. It is a two-layered membranous sac with a thin layer of serous fluid (normally no more than 30 to 50 mL) separating the layers. It protects and cushions the heart and the great vessels, provides a barrier to infectious processes in adjacent structures, prevents displacement of the myocardium and blood vessels, and prevents sudden distension of the heart.

Pericarditis is the inflammation of the pericardium. Pericarditis may be a primary disorder or may develop secondarily to another cardiac or systemic disorder. Some possible causes of pericarditis are listed in Box 30.3. Viral infections are more common than bacterial and fungal pericarditis. Other types of pericarditis can develop post myocardial infarction and post cardiotomy (Banasik & Copstead, 2022).

Pathophysiology

Pericardial tissue damage triggers an inflammatory response. Inflammatory mediators released from the injured tissue cause vasodilation, hyperaemia and oedema. Capillary permeability increases, allowing plasma proteins, including fibrinogen, to escape into the pericardial space. White blood cells amass at the

BOX 30.3 Selected causes of pericarditis

Infectious

- Viruses
- Bacteria
- Fungi
- Parasites

Non-infectious

- Myocardial and pericardial injury
- Uraemia
- Neoplasms
- Radiation
- Trauma or surgery
- Myxoedema
- Autoimmune disorders
- Rheumatic fever
- Connective tissue diseases
- Some drugs
- Post-cardiac injury

site of injury to destroy the causative agent. Exudate is formed, usually fibrinous or serofibrinous (a mixture of serous fluid and fibrinous exudate). In some cases, the exudate may contain red blood cells or, if infectious, purulent material. The inflammatory process may resolve without long-term effects or scar tissue and adhesions may form between the pericardial layers.

Fibrosis and scarring of the pericardium may restrict cardiac function. Pericardial effusions may develop as serous or purulent exudate (depending on the causative agent) collects in the pericardial sac. Pericardial effusion may be recurrent. Chronic inflammation causes the pericardium to become rigid.

Manifestations

According to Chiabrando et al. (2020), diagnostically at least two of the following are required: chest pain, pericardial rub, electrocardiogram changes and new or worsening pericardial effusion. Chest pain, the most common symptom, has an abrupt onset. It is caused by inflammation of nerve fibres in the lower parietal pericardium and pleura covering the diaphragm. The pain is usually sharp, may be steady or intermittent and may radiate to the back or neck. The pain can mimic myocardial ischaemia; careful assessment is important to rule out myocardial infarction. Pericardial pain is aggravated by respiratory movements (i.e. deep inspiration and/or coughing), changes in body position or swallowing. Sitting upright and leaning forward reduces the discomfort by moving the heart away from the diaphragmatic side of the lung pleura.

Although not always present, a pericardial friction rub is the characteristic sign of pericarditis. A pericardial friction rub is a leathery, grating sound produced by the inflamed pericardial layers rubbing against the chest wall or pleura. It is heard most clearly at the left lower sternal border with the person sitting up or leaning forward. The rub is usually heard on expiration and may be constant or intermittent.

The person may develop low-grade fever (below 38.4°C) due to the inflammatory process. Dyspnoea and tachycardia are common.

Complications

Pericardial effusion, cardiac tamponade and constrictive pericarditis are possible complications of acute pericarditis.

Pericardial effusion

A *pericardial effusion* is an abnormal collection of fluid between the pericardial layers that threatens normal cardiac function. The fluid may consist of pus, blood, serum, lymph or a combination. The manifestations of a pericardial effusion depend on the rate at which the fluid collects. Although the pericardium normally contains about 30 to 50 mL of fluid, the sac can stretch to accommodate a gradual accumulation of fluid. Over time, the pericardial sac can accommodate up to 2 L of fluid without immediate adverse effects. Conversely, a rapid build-up of pericardial fluid (as little as 100 mL) does not allow the sac to stretch and can compress the heart, interfering with myocardial function. This compression of the heart is known as **cardiac tamponade**. Slowly developing pericardial effusion is often painless and has few manifestations. Heart sounds may be distant or muffled. The person may have a cough or mild dyspnoea.

Cardiac tamponade

Cardiac tamponade is a medical emergency that must be aggressively treated to preserve life. Cardiac tamponade may result from pericardial effusion, trauma, cardiac rupture or haemorrhage. Rapid collection of fluid in the pericardial sac interferes with ventricular filling and pumping, critically reducing cardiac output.

Classic manifestations of cardiac tamponade result from rising intracardiac pressures and decreased diastolic filling and cardiac output. A hallmark of cardiac tamponade is a paradoxical pulse, or *pulsus paradoxus*. A paradoxical pulse markedly decreases in amplitude during inspiration. Intrathoracic pressure normally drops during inspiration, enhancing venous return to the right heart. This draws more blood into the right side of the heart than the left, causing the interventricular septum to bulge slightly into the left ventricle. When ventricular filling is impaired by excess fluid in the pericardial sac, this bulging of the interventricular septum decreases cardiac output during inspiration (see Figure 30.5). On palpation of the carotid or femoral artery, the pulse is diminished or absent during inspiration. A drop in systolic blood pressure of more than 10 mmHg during inspiration also indicates pulsus paradoxus.

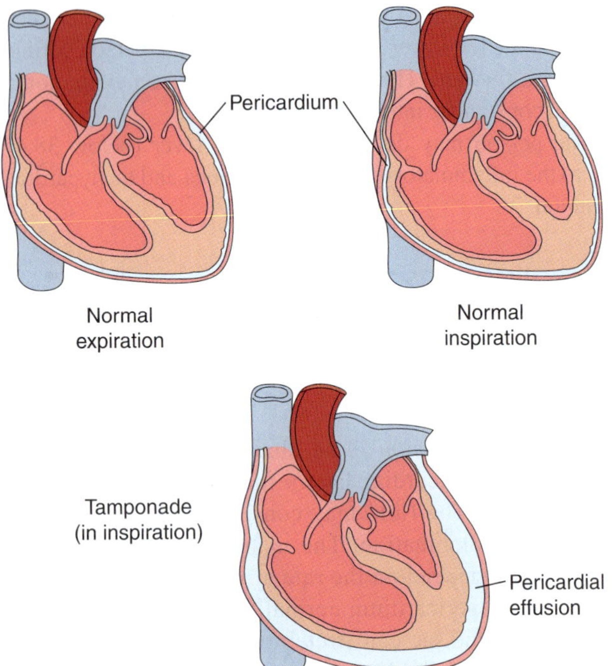

FIGURE 30.5 ***Cardiac tamponade. Note increased volume in the right ventricle during inspiration in both the normal heart and the heart affected by a pericardial effusion. In tamponade, fluid in the pericardial sac and the distended right ventricle restrict filling of the left ventricle and, consequently, cardiac output***

Other manifestations of cardiac tamponade include muffled heart sounds, dyspnoea and tachypnoea, tachycardia, a narrowed pulse pressure and distended neck veins (see the 'Manifestations' box).

Chronic constrictive pericarditis

Chronic pericardial inflammation can lead to scar tissue formation between the pericardial layers. This scar tissue eventually contracts, restricting diastolic filling and elevating venous pressure. Constrictive pericarditis (see Figure 30.6) may follow viral infection, radiation therapy or heart surgery. Its manifestations include progressive dyspnoea, fatigue and weakness. Ascites is common; peripheral oedema may develop. Neck veins are distended and may be particularly noticeable during inspiration (*Kussmaul's sign*). This occurs because the right atrium is unable to dilate to accommodate increased venous return during inspiration.

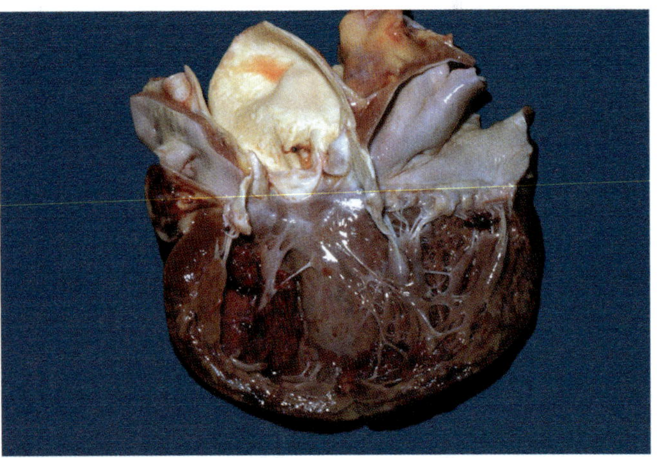

FIGURE 30.6 ***Constrictive pericarditis***

Source: Biophoto Associates/Science Source.

MANIFESTATIONS Cardiac tamponade

- Paradoxical pulse
- Narrowed pulse pressure, hypotension
- Tachycardia
- Weak peripheral pulses
- Distant, muffled heart sounds
- Jugular venous distension
- High central venous pressure
- Decreased level of consciousness
- Low urine output
- Cool, mottled skin

INTERPROFESSIONAL CARE

Care for the person with pericarditis focuses on identifying its cause, if possible, reducing inflammation, relieving symptoms and preventing complications. The person is closely monitored for early manifestations of cardiac tamponade so that it can be treated promptly.

Diagnosis

There are no specific laboratory tests to diagnose pericarditis, but tests are often performed to differentiate pericarditis from myocardial infarction.

- *FBC* shows elevated WBCs and an ESR greater than 20 mm/h, indicating acute inflammation.
- *Cardiac enzymes* may be slightly elevated because the inflammatory process extends to involve the epicardial surface of the heart. Cardiac enzymes are typically much lower in pericarditis than in myocardial infarction.
- *Electrocardiography* shows typical changes associated with pericarditis, such as diffuse ST-segment elevation in all leads. This resolves more quickly than changes of acute MI and is not associated with the QRS-complex and T-wave changes typically seen in MI. With a large pericardial effusion, the QRS amplitude may be decreased. Atrial arrhythmias may occur in acute pericarditis.
- *Echocardiography* is used to assess heart motion, for pericardial effusion and the extent of restriction.
- *Haemodynamic monitoring* may be used in acute pericarditis or pericardial effusion to assess pressures and cardiac output. Elevated pulmonary artery pressures and venous pressures occur with impaired filling due to pericardial effusion or constrictive pericarditis.

- *Chest x-ray* may show cardiac enlargement if a pericardial effusion is present.
- *Computed tomography (CT) scan or magnetic resonance imaging (MRI)* may be used to identify pericardial effusion or constrictive pericarditis.

Medications

Drug treatment for pericarditis addresses its manifestations. Aspirin and paracetamol may be used to reduce fever. NSAIDs are used to reduce inflammation and promote comfort. In severe cases or with recurrent pericarditis, corticosteroids may be given to suppress the inflammatory response.

Pericardiocentesis

Pericardiocentesis may be done to remove fluid from the pericardial sac for diagnostic or therapeutic purposes. The doctor inserts a large (16- to 18-gauge) needle into the pericardial sac and withdraws excess fluid. The needle is attached to an ECG monitoring lead to help determine if the needle is touching the epicardial surface, which helps prevent piercing the myocardium. Pericardiocentesis may be an emergency procedure for the person with cardiac tamponade.

Surgery

For recurrent pericarditis or recurrent pericardial effusion, a rectangular piece of the pericardium, or 'window', may be excised to allow collected fluid to drain into the pleural space. Constrictive pericarditis may necessitate a partial or total *pericardiectomy*, removal of part or all of the pericardium, to relieve the ventricular compression and allow adequate filling.

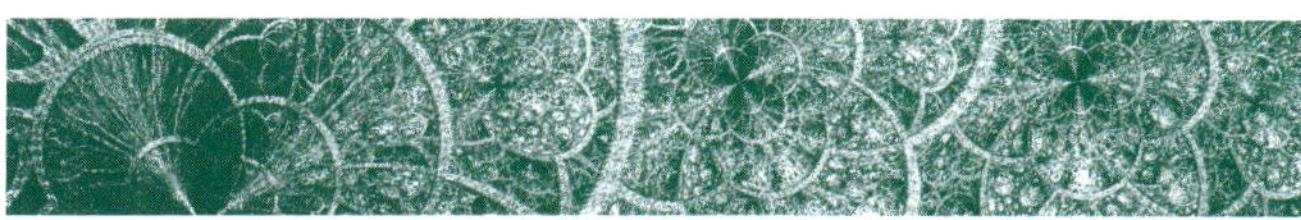

Nursing care

Health promotion

While it may not yet be possible to identify many people at risk and to prevent acute pericarditis, early identification and treatment of the disorder can reduce the risk of complications. Promptly report a pericardial friction rub or other manifestations of pericarditis in individuals with recent acute AMI, cardiac surgery or systemic diseases associated with a risk of pericarditis.

Assessment

Assessment data to collect from the person with suspected pericarditis include:

- *Health history*: complaints of acute substernal or precordial chest pain, effect of movement and breathing on discomfort, pain radiation, associated symptoms; recent acute AMI, heart surgery or other cardiac disorder; current medications, chronic conditions such as renal failure or a connective tissue or autoimmune disorder.
- *Physical examination*: vital signs, including temperature, variation in systolic BP with respirations; strength of peripheral pulses, variations with respiratory movement; apical pulse, clarity, changes with respiratory movement, presence of a friction rub; neck vein distension; level of consciousness, skin colour and other indicators of cardiac output.
- *Diagnostic tests*: FBC and differential, ESR; cardiac enzyme levels; ECG and echocardiogram reports.

Nursing diagnoses and interventions

Nursing care for the person with pericarditis may occur in the acute or community setting. Closely observe for early manifestations of increasing effusion or cardiac tamponade. Priority nursing diagnoses relate to comfort, the risk of tamponade and effects of the acute inflammatory process.

Acute pain

- Inflamed pericardial layers rubbing against each other and the lung pleura stimulate phrenic nerve pain fibres in the lower portion of the parietal pericardium. Pain is usually acute and may be severe until inflammation resolves.
- Assess chest pain using a standard pain scale and noting the quality and radiation of the pain. Note non-verbal cues of pain (grimacing, guarding behaviours) and validate with the person. *Careful assessment helps identify the cause of pain. The pain of pericarditis may radiate to the neck or back and is aggravated by movement, coughing or deep breathing. A pain scale allows evaluation of the effectiveness of interventions.*
- Auscultate heart sounds every 4 hours. *Presence of a pericardial friction rub often correlates with the location and severity of the pain.*
- Administer NSAIDs on a regular basis as prescribed with food. Document effectiveness. NSAIDs reduce fever, inflammation and pericardial pain. *They are most effective when administered around the clock on a consistent basis. Administering the medications with food helps decrease gastric distress.*
- Maintain a quiet, calm environment and position of comfort. Offer back rubs, heat/cold therapy, diversional activity and emotional support. *Supportive interventions enhance the effects of the medication, may decrease pain perception and convey a sense of caring.*

Ineffective breathing pattern

Respiratory movement intensifies pericardial pain. In an effort to decrease pain, the person often breathes shallowly, increasing the risk of pulmonary complications.

- Encourage deep breathing and use of the incentive spirometer. Provide pain medication before respiratory therapy, as needed. *Deep breathing and an incentive spirometer promote alveolar ventilation and prevent atelectasis. Administration of analgesia prior to respiratory treatments improves their effectiveness by decreasing guarding.*
- Administer oxygen as needed. *Supplementary oxygen promotes optimal gas exchange and tissue oxygenation.*
- Place the person in Fowler's or high Fowler's position. Assist the person to a position of comfort. *Appropriate positioning reduces the work of breathing and decreases chest pain due to pericarditis.*

CONSIDERATION FOR PRACTICE

Document respiratory rate, effort and breath sounds every 2 to 4 hours. Report adventitious or diminished breath sounds. Shallow, guarded respirations may lead to increased respiratory rate and effort. Poor ventilation of peripheral alveoli may lead to congestion or atelectasis.

Risk of decreased cardiac output

The acute inflammatory process of pericarditis can lead to significant pericardial effusion and cardiac tamponade. This potentially fatal complication can also occur with chronic pericardial effusion if the amount of fluid exceeds the ability of the pericardial sac to expand. Constrictive pericarditis increases the risk of decreased cardiac output because of restricted cardiac filling.

- Document vital signs hourly during the acute inflammatory processes. *Frequent assessment allows early recognition of manifestations of decreased cardiac output, such as tachycardia, hypotension or changes in pulse pressure.*
- Report significant changes or trends in haemodynamic parameters and arrhythmias. *Compression of the heart interferes with venous return, increasing CVP and right atrial pressures; arrhythmias may also occur.*
- Promptly report other signs of decreased cardiac output: decreased level of consciousness; decreased urine output; cold, clammy, mottled skin; delayed capillary refill; and weak peripheral pulses. *These signs of decreased organ and tissue perfusion indicate a significant drop in cardiac output.*
- Maintain at least one patent intravenous access site. *The person in cardiac tamponade may require rapid intravenous fluid infusion to restore blood volume and administration of emergency drugs to support the circulation.*
- Prepare for emergency pericardiocentesis and/or surgery as necessary. Provide appropriate explanations and reassurance. Observe for adverse responses during pericardiocentesis. *Excess pericardial fluid must be rapidly evacuated to prevent further compromise of cardiac output and death. Emotional support and explanations reduce the person's and their family's anxiety and promote a caring atmosphere.*

Activity intolerance

In chronic constrictive pericarditis, pericardial adhesions and scarring restrict pericardial compliance, restricting heart filling and movement. Restricted filling and ineffective cardiac contraction decrease the cardiac output. The heart cannot compensate for increased metabolic demands by increasing cardiac output and cardiac reserve falls significantly.

- Work with the person and physiotherapist to develop a realistic, progressive activity plan. Monitor response. Encourage independence, but provide assistance as needed. *Involvement in their own planning increases the likelihood of success, as well as the person's self-esteem and sense of control. Promoting self-care provides additional control and independence and enhances self-image. Activity that significantly increases the heart rate (more than 20 bpm over resting) should be stopped and reassessed for intensity.*
- Plan interventions and care activities to allow uninterrupted rest and sleep. *This supports healing and restoration of physical and emotional health.*

Community-based care

Include the following topics when teaching the person and their family in preparation for home care:

- The importance of continuing anti-inflammatory medications as ordered. Advise to take NSAIDs with food, milk or antacids to minimise gastric distress and to notify the doctor if unable to tolerate the drug.
- Prescribed medications, including dose, desired and possible adverse effects, and interactions with other drugs or food.
- Monitoring weight twice weekly because NSAIDs may cause fluid retention.
- Maintaining fluid intake of at least 2,500 mL/day to minimise the risk of renal toxicity due to NSAID use.
- Measures to maintain activity restriction if ordered. Activity will be gradually increased once the inflammatory process has resolved.

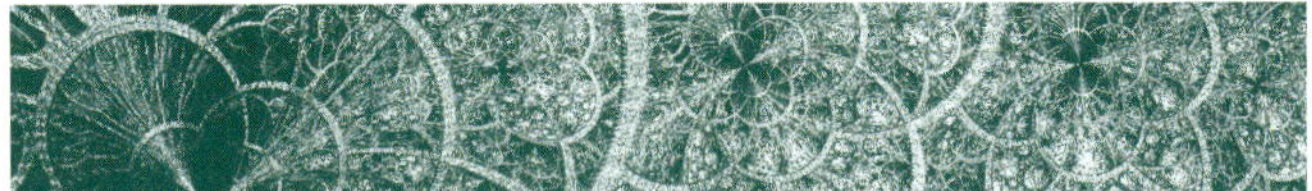

Disorders of cardiac structure

THE PERSON WITH VALVULAR HEART DISEASE

Proper heart valve function ensures one-way blood flow through the heart and vascular system. **Valvular heart disease** interferes with blood flow to and from the heart. Acquired valvular disorders can result from acute conditions, such as infective endocarditis, or from chronic conditions, such as rheumatic heart disease. Rheumatic heart disease is the most common cause of valvular disease (Papadakis, McPhee & Rabow, 2022). Acute myocardial infarction also can damage heart valves, causing tearing, ischaemia or damage to the papillary muscles that affects valve leaflet function. Congenital heart defects may affect the heart valves, often with no manifestations until adulthood.

Physiology review

The heart valves direct blood flow within and out of the heart. The valves are fibroelastic tissue supported by a ring of fibrous tissue (the annulus) that provides support.

The AV valves, the **mitral** (or *bicuspid*) **valve** on the left and the **tricuspid valve** on the right, separate the atria from the ventricles. These valves normally are fully open during diastole, allowing blood to flow freely from the atria into the ventricles. Rising pressure within the ventricles at the onset of systole (contraction) closes the AV valves, creating the S_1 heart sound ('lub'). The leaflets of the AV valves are connected to ventricular papillary muscles by fibrous *chordae tendineae*. The chordae tendineae prevent the valve leaflets from bulging back into the atria during systole.

The semilunar valves, the **aortic** and **pulmonic valves**, separate the ventricles from the great vessels. They open during systole, allowing blood to flow out of the heart with ventricular contraction. As the ventricle relaxes and intraventricular pressure falls at the beginning of diastole, the higher pressure within the great vessels (the aorta and pulmonary artery) closes these valves, creating the S_2 heart sound ('dub').

Pathophysiology

Valvular heart disease occurs as two main types of disorders: stenosis and regurgitation. Stenosis occurs when valve leaflets fuse together and cannot fully open or close. The valve opening narrows and becomes rigid (see Figure 30.7A). Scarring of the valves from endocarditis or infarction and calcium deposits can lead to stenosis. Stenotic valves impede the forward flow of blood, decreasing cardiac output because of impaired ventricular filling or ejection, and stroke volume.

Regurgitant valves (also called *insufficient* or *incompetent* valves) do not close completely (see Figure 30.7B). Regurgitation can result from deformity or erosion of valve cusps caused by the vegetative lesions of bacterial endocarditis, by scarring or tearing from myocardial infarction, or by cardiac dilation. As the heart enlarges, the *valve annulus* (supporting ring of the valve) is stretched and the valve edges no longer meet to allow complete closure.

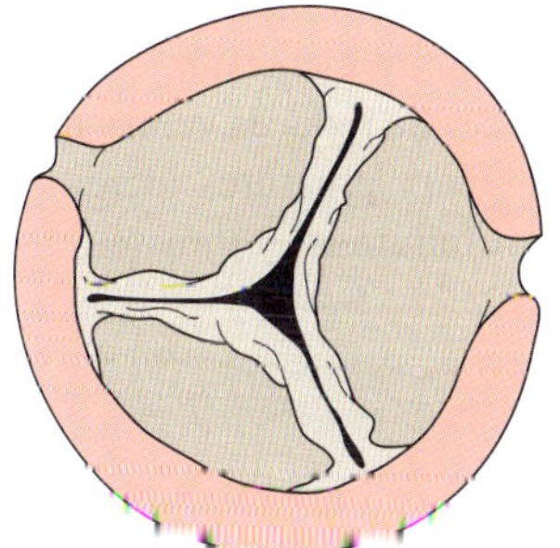

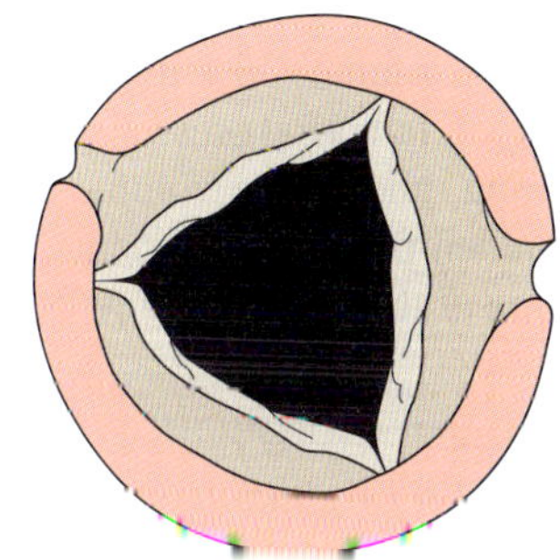

FIGURE 30.7 *Valvular heart disorders. A, Stenosis of a heart valve. B, An incompetent or regurgitant heart valve*

Valvular disease causes haemodynamic changes both in front of and behind the affected valve. Blood volume and pressures are reduced in front of the valve. By contrast, volumes and pressures characteristically increase behind the diseased valve. These haemodynamic changes may lead to pulmonary complications, cardiac remodelling, hypertrophy or heart failure.

Stenosis increases the work of the chamber behind the affected valve as the heart attempts to move blood through the narrowed opening. Excess blood volume behind regurgitant valves causes dilation of the chamber. In mitral stenosis, for example, the left atrium hypertrophies to generate enough pressure to open and deliver its blood through the narrowed mitral valve. Not all of the blood is delivered before the valve closes, leaving blood to accumulate in the left atrium. This chamber dilates to accommodate the excess volume.

Eventually, cardiac output falls as compensatory mechanisms become less effective. The normal balance of oxygen supply and demand is upset and the heart begins to fail. Increased muscle mass and size increase myocardial oxygen consumption. The size and workload of the heart exceed its blood supply, causing ischaemia and chest pain. Eventually, necrosis occurs and functional muscle is lost. Contractile force, stroke volume and cardiac output decrease. High pressures on the left side of the heart are reflected backward into the pulmonary system, causing pulmonary oedema, pulmonary hypertension and, eventually, right ventricular failure.

Valvular disorders interfere with the smooth flow of blood through the heart. The flow becomes turbulent, causing a **murmur**, a characteristic manifestation of valvular disease. Table 30.7 describes the murmurs associated with various types of valvular disorders.

Blood forced through the narrowed opening of a stenotic valve or regurgitated from a higher pressure chamber through an incompetent valve creates a jet stream effect (much like water spurting out of a partially occluded hose opening). The physical force of this jet stream damages the endocardium of the receiving chamber, increasing the risk of infective endocarditis.

The higher pressures on the left side of the heart subject its valves (the mitral and aortic valves) to more stress and damage than those on the right side of the heart (the tricuspid and pulmonic). Pulmonic valve disease is the least common of the valvular disorders.

Mitral stenosis

Mitral stenosis narrows the mitral valve, obstructing blood flow from the left atrium into the left ventricle during diastole. It is usually caused by rheumatic heart disease or bacterial endocarditis; it rarely results from congenital defects. In Australia, the mean age for mitral stenosis is 33 years. However, in the Northern Territory, [illegible] of children aged [illegible] years with rheumatic heart disease have mitral stenosis (RHDAustralia, 2020). Mitral stenosis is chronic and progressive.

In mitral valve stenosis, fibrous tissue replaces normal valve tissue, causing valve leaflets to stiffen and fuse. Resulting changes in blood flow through the valve lead to calcification of

TABLE 30.7 Heart murmur timing and characteristics

MURMUR	CARDIAC CYCLE TIMING	AUSCULTATION SITE	CONFIGURATION OF SOUND	CONTINUITY
Mitral stenosis	Diastole	Apical	S_2 … S_1	Rumble that increases in sound towards the end, continuous
Mitral regurgitation	Systole	Apex	S_1 … S_2	Holosystolic (occurs throughout systole), continuous
Aortic stenosis	Midsystolic	Right sternal border (RSB) 2nd intercostal space (ICS)	S_1 … S_2	Crescendo-decrescendo, continuous
Aortic regurgitation	Diastole (early)	3rd ICS, left sternal border (LSB)	S_2 … S_1	Decrescendo, continuous
Tricuspid stenosis	Diastole	Lower LSB	S_2 … S_1	Rumble that increases in sound towards the end, continuous
Tricuspid regurgitation	Systole	4th ICS, LSB	S_1 … S_2	Holosystolic, continuous

the valve leaflets. As calcium is deposited in and on the valve, the leaflets become more rigid and narrow the opening further (see Figure 30.8). As the valve leaflets become less mobile, the chordae tendineae fuse, thicken and shorten. Thromboemboli may form on the calcified leaflets.

The narrowed mitral opening impairs blood flow into the left ventricle, reducing end-diastolic volume and pressure and decreasing stroke volume. The narrowed opening also forces the left atrium to generate higher pressure to deliver blood to the left ventricle. This leads to left atrial hypertrophy. The left atrium also dilates as obstructed blood flow increases its volume. As the resistance to blood flow increases, high atrial pressures are reflected back into the pulmonary vessels, increasing pulmonary pressures (see Figure 30.8). Pulmonary hypertension increases the workload of the right ventricle, causing it to dilate and hypertrophy. Eventually, heart failure occurs.

MANIFESTATIONS Mitral stenosis may be asymptomatic or cause severe impairment. Its manifestations depend on cardiac output and pulmonary vascular pressures. Dyspnoea on exertion is typically the earliest manifestation. Others include cough, haemoptysis, frequent pulmonary infections such as bronchitis and pneumonia, paroxysmal nocturnal dyspnoea, orthopnoea, weakness, fatigue and palpitations. As the stenosis worsens, manifestations of right heart failure, including jugular venous distension, hepatomegaly, ascites and peripheral oedema, develop. Crackles may be heard in the lung bases. In severe mitral stenosis, cyanosis of the face and extremities may be noted. Chest pain is rare but may occur.

On auscultation, a loud S_1, a split S_2 and a mitral opening snap may be heard. The opening snap reflects high left atrial pressure. The murmur of mitral stenosis occurs during diastole and is typically low pitched, rumbling, crescendo–decrescendo. It is heard best with the bell of the stethoscope in the apical region. It may be accompanied by a palpable thrill (vibration).

COMPLICATIONS Atrial arrhythmias, particularly atrial fibrillation, are common due to chronic atrial distension. Thrombi may form and subsequently embolise to the brain, coronary arteries, kidneys, spleen and extremities—potentially devastating complications.

Women with mitral stenosis may be asymptomatic until pregnancy. As the heart tries to compensate for increased circulating volume (30% more in pregnancy) by increasing cardiac output, left atrial pressures rise, tachycardia reduces ventricular filling, and stroke volume and pulmonary pressures increase. Sudden pulmonary oedema and heart failure may threaten the lives of the mother and fetus.

Mitral regurgitation

Mitral regurgitation or *insufficiency* allows blood to flow back into the left atrium during systole because the valve does not close fully. Rheumatic heart disease is a common cause of mitral regurgitation. Processes that dilate the mitral annulus or affect the supporting structures, papillary muscles or the chordae tendineae may cause mitral regurgitation (e.g. left ventricular hypertrophy and MI). Congenital defects also may cause mitral regurgitation.

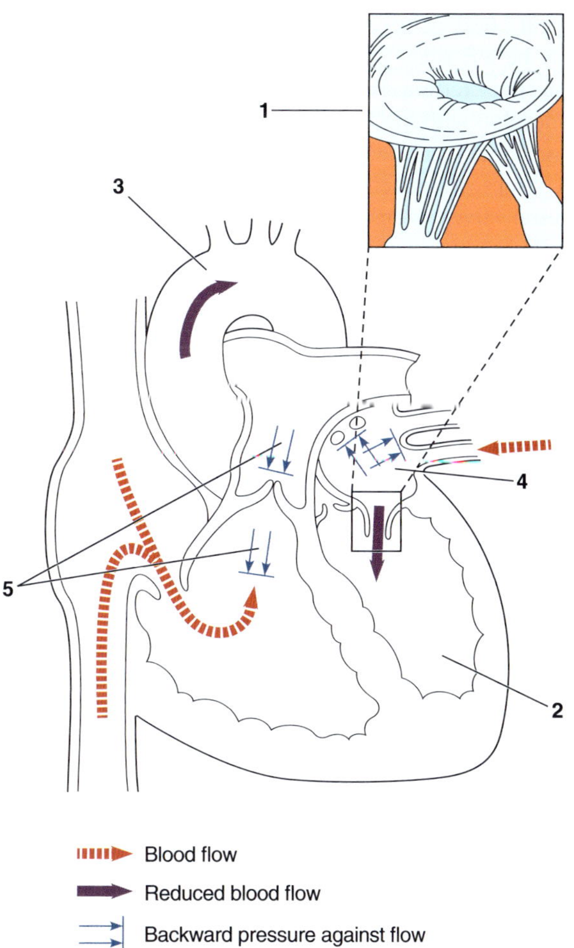

FIGURE 30.8 ***Mitral stenosis. Narrowing of the mitral valve orifice (1) reduces blood volume to left ventricle (2) reducing cardiac output (3). Rising pressure in the left atrium (4) causes left atrial hypertrophy and pulmonary congestion. Increased pressure in pulmonary vessels (5) causes hypertrophy of the right ventricle and right atrium***

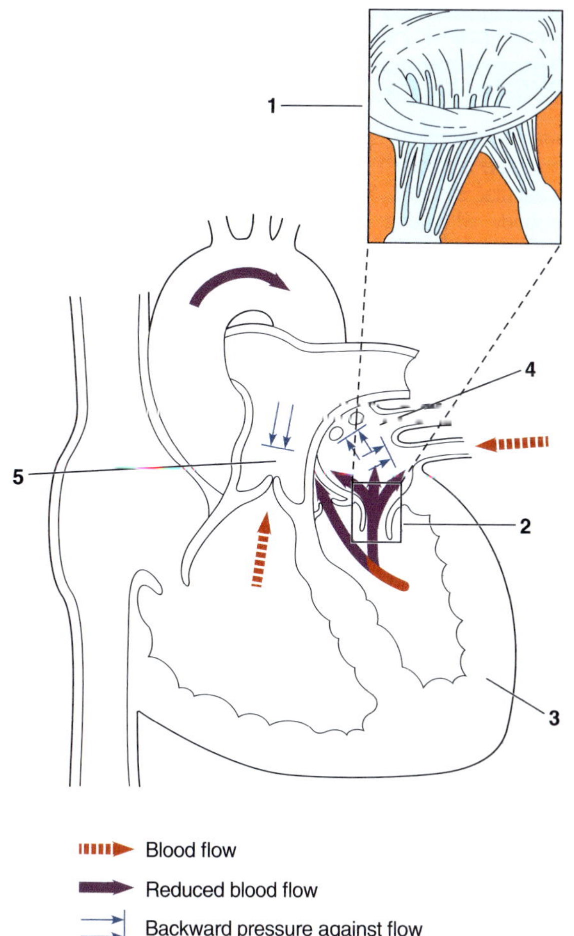

FIGURE 30.9 ***Mitral regurgitation. The mitral valve closes incompletely (1), allowing blood to regurgitate during systole from the left ventricle to the left atrium (2). Cardiac output falls; to compensate, the left ventricle hypertrophies (3). Rising left atrial pressure (4) causes left atrial hypertrophy and pulmonary congestion. Elevated pulmonary artery pressure (5) causes slight enlargement of the right ventricle***

In mitral regurgitation, blood flows into both the systemic circulation and back into the left atrium through the deformed valve during systole. This increases left atrial volume (see Figure 30.9). The left atrium dilates to accommodate its extra volume, pulling the posterior valve leaflet further away from the valve opening and worsening the defect. The left ventricle dilates to accommodate its increased preload and low cardiac output, further aggravating the problem.

MANIFESTATIONS Mitral regurgitation may be asymptomatic or cause symptoms such as fatigue, weakness, exertional dyspnoea and orthopnoea. In severe or acute regurgitation, manifestations of left-sided heart failure develop, including pulmonary congestion and oedema. High pulmonary pressures may lead to manifestations of right-sided heart failure.

The murmur of mitral regurgitation is usually loud, high pitched, rumbling and holosystolic (occurring throughout systole). It is often accompanied by a palpable thrill and is heard most clearly at the cardiac apex.

Mitral valve prolapse

Mitral valve prolapse (MVP) is a type of mitral insufficiency that occurs when one or both mitral valve cusps billow into the atrium during ventricular systole. Its cause often is unclear. However, it can also result from acute or chronic rheumatic damage, ischaemic heart disease or other cardiac disorders. It commonly affects people with inherited connective tissue disorders such as Marfan syndrome (see the 'Genetic considerations' box).

Excess collagen tissue in the valve leaflets and elongated chordae tendineae impair closure of the mitral valve, allowing the leaflets to billow into the left atrium during systole. Some ventricular blood volume regurgitates into the left atrium (see Figure 30.10).

GENETIC CONSIDERATIONS

The person with Marfan syndrome

Marfan syndrome is a genetic (autosomal dominant) connective tissue disorder that affects the skeleton, eyes and cardiovascular system. Skeletal characteristics include a long, thin body, with long extremities and long, tapering fingers, sometimes called *arachnodactyly* (spider fingers). Joints are hyperextensible, and skeletal deformities such as kyphosis, scoliosis, pigeon chest or pectus excavatum are common (Papadakis et al., 2022). The potentially life-threatening cardiovascular effects of Marfan syndrome include mitral valve prolapse, progressive dilation of the aortic valve ring and weakness of arterial walls. People with Marfan syndrome frequently die young, between 30 and 40 years, often due to dissection and rupture of the aorta (Defendi, 2021; Prashanth, 2020).

MANIFESTATIONS AND COMPLICATIONS Mitral valve prolapse is usually asymptomatic. A midsystolic ejection click or murmur may be audible. A high-pitched late systolic murmur, sometimes described as a 'whoop' or 'honk', due to the regurgitation of blood through the valve, may develop in MVP.

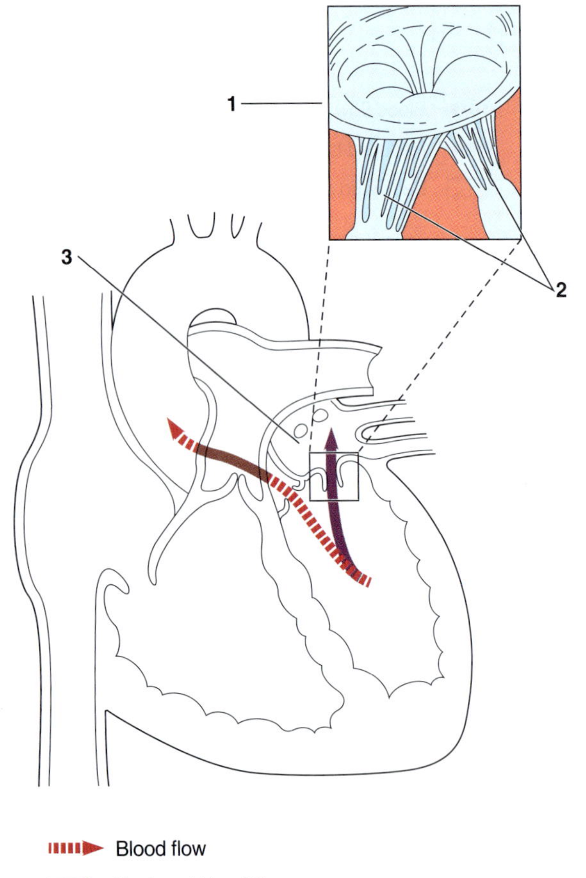

FIGURE 30.10 ***Mitral valve prolapse. Excess tissue in the valve leaflets (1) and elongated chordae tendineae (2) impair mitral valve closure during systole. Some ventricular blood regurgitates into the left atrium (3)***

Atypical chest pain is the most common symptom of MVP. It may be left sided or substernal and is frequently related to fatigue, not exertion (Papadakis et al., 2022). Tachyarrhythmias may develop with MVP, causing palpitations, light-headedness and syncope. Increased sympathetic nervous system tone may cause a sense of anxiety.

Mitral valve prolapse increases the risk of bacterial endocarditis. Progressive worsening of regurgitation can lead to heart failure. Thrombi may form on prolapsed valve leaflets; embolisation may cause transient ischaemic attacks (TIAs).

Aortic stenosis

Aortic stenosis obstructs blood flow from the left ventricle into the aorta during systole. Aortic stenosis may be idiopathic or due to a congenital defect, rheumatic damage or degenerative changes. When rheumatic heart disease is the cause, mitral valve deformity is also often present. RHD destroys aortic valve leaflets, with fibrosis and calcification causing rigidity and scarring. In the older adult, calcific aortic stenosis may result from degenerative changes associated with ageing. Constant wear and tear on this valve can lead to fibrosis and calcification. Idiopathic calcific stenosis generally is mild and does not impair cardiac output.

As aortic stenosis progresses, the valve annulus decreases in size, increasing the work of the left ventricle to eject its volume through the narrowed opening into the aorta. To compensate, the ventricle hypertrophies to maintain an adequate stroke volume and cardiac output (see Figure 30.11). Left ventricular compliance also decreases. The additional workload increases myocardial oxygen consumption, which can precipitate myocardial ischaemia. Coronary blood flow may also decrease in aortic stenosis. As left ventricular end-diastolic pressure increases because of reduced stroke volume, left atrial pressures increase. These pressures also affect the pulmonary vascular system; pulmonary vascular congestion and pulmonary oedema may result.

COURSE AND MANIFESTATIONS Aortic stenosis may be asymptomatic for many years. As the disease progresses and compensation fails, usually between age 50 and 70 years, obstructed cardiac output causes manifestations of left ventricular failure. Dyspnoea on exertion, angina pectoris and exertional syncope are classic manifestations of aortic stenosis. Pulse pressure, an indicator of stroke volume, narrows to 30 mmHg or less.

Aortic stenosis produces a harsh systolic murmur best heard in the second intercostal space to the right of the sternum. This crescendo–decrescendo murmur is produced by turbulence of blood entering the aorta through the stenotic valve. A palpable thrill is often felt. The murmur may radiate to the carotid arteries. Ventricular hypertrophy displaces the cardiac impulse to the left of the midclavicular line. As aortic stenosis progresses, S_3 and S_4 heart sounds may be heard, indicating heart failure and reduced left ventricular compliance.

As cardiac output falls, tissue perfusion decreases. Late in the disease, pulmonary hypertension and right ventricular failure develop. Untreated, symptomatic aortic stenosis has a poor

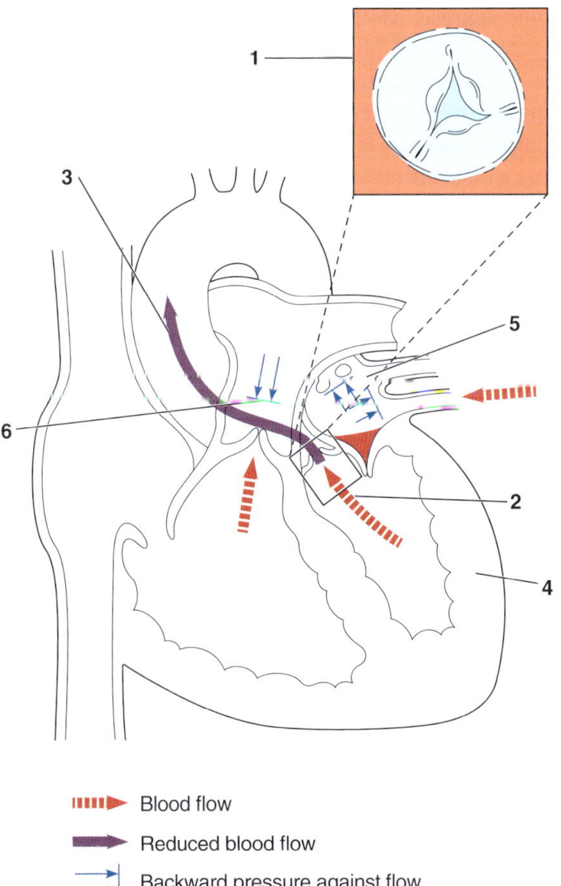

FIGURE 30.11 ***Aortic stenosis. The narrowed aortic valve orifice (1) decreases the left ventricular ejection fraction during systole (2) and cardiac output (3). The left ventricle hypertrophies (4). Incomplete emptying of the left atrium (5) causes backward pressure through pulmonary veins and pulmonary hypertension. Elevated pulmonary artery pressure (6) causes right ventricular strain***

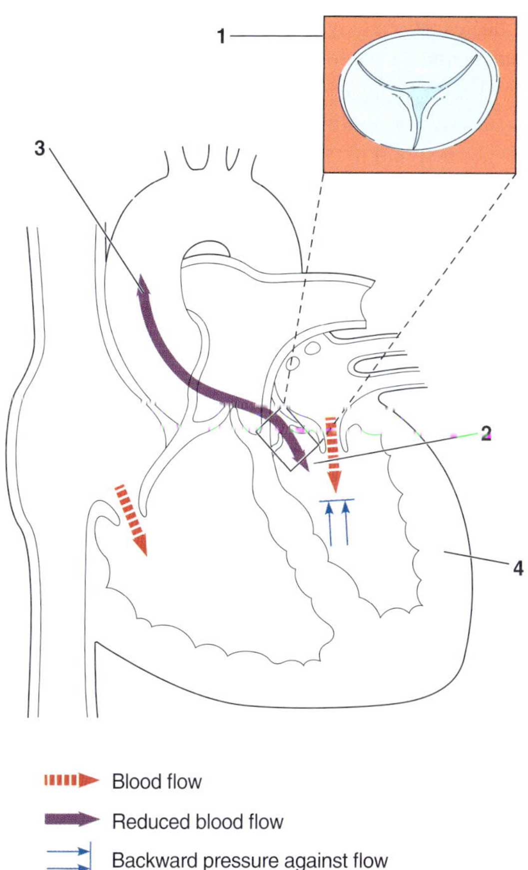

FIGURE 30.12 ***Aortic regurgitation. The cusps of the aortic valve widen and fail to close during diastole (1). Blood regurgitates from the aorta into the left ventricle (2), increasing left ventricular volume and decreasing cardiac output (3). The left ventricle dilates and hypertrophies (4) in response to the increase in blood volume and workload***

prognosis because at 3 years after diagnosis, only approximately 50% of people are still alive (Papadakis et al., 2022).

Aortic regurgitation

Aortic regurgitation, also called *aortic insufficiency*, allows blood to flow back into the left ventricle from the aorta during diastole. Most aortic regurgitation results from rheumatic heart disease. Other causes include congenital disorders, infective endocarditis, blunt chest trauma, aortic aneurysm, syphilis, Marfan syndrome and chronic hypertension.

In aortic regurgitation, thickened and contracted valve cusps, scarring, fibrosis and calcification impede complete valve closure. Chronic hypertension and aortic aneurysm may dilate and stretch the aortic valve opening, increasing the degree of regurgitation.

In aortic regurgitation, volume overload affects the left ventricle as blood from the aorta adds to blood received from the atrium during diastole. This increases diastolic left ventricular pressure. Increased preload causes more forceful contractions and a high stroke volume (see Figure 30.12). With time, muscle cells hypertrophy to compensate for increased cardiac work and afterload; eventually this hypertrophy compromises cardiac output and increases regurgitation.

High left-ventricular pressures increase left atrial workload and pressure. This pressure is transmitted to the pulmonary vessels, causing pulmonary congestion. The workload of the right ventricle increases as a result and right-sided heart failure may develop. Acute aortic regurgitation from traumatic injury or infective endocarditis causes a rapid decline in haemodynamic status from acute heart failure and pulmonary oedema because compensatory mechanisms do not have time to develop.

MANIFESTATIONS Aortic regurgitation may be asymptomatic for many years, even when severe. The increased stroke volume may cause complaints of pounding palpitations, especially when recumbent. A throbbing pulse may be visible in arteries of the neck; the force of contraction may cause a characteristic head bob (Musset's sign) and shake the whole body. Other symptoms include dizziness and exercise intolerance.

Fatigue, exertional dyspnoea, orthopnoea and paroxysmal nocturnal dyspnoea are common in aortic regurgitation. Anginal pain may result from excessive cardiac work and decreased coronary perfusion. Unlike CHD, angina often occurs at night and may not respond to conventional therapy.

The murmur of aortic regurgitation is heard during diastole as blood flows back into the left ventricle from the aorta. It is a 'blowing', high-pitched sound heard most clearly at the third left intercostal space. A palpable thrill and ventricular heave may be noted. An S_3 and S_4 may be heard as the heart fails and ventricular compliance diminishes. The apical impulse is displaced to the left.

High systolic and low diastolic pressures cause a widened pulse pressure. The arterial pressure waveform has a rapid upstroke and quickly collapsing downstroke, known as a *water-hammer pulse*. It is caused by the force of rapid and early delivery of the stroke volume into the aorta.

Tricuspid valve disorders

Tricuspid stenosis obstructs blood flow from the right atrium to the right ventricle. It usually results from rheumatic heart disease; mitral stenosis often occurs concurrently with tricuspid stenosis.

Fibrosed, retracted tricuspid valve cusps and fused leaflets narrow the valve orifice and prevent complete closure. Right ventricular filling is impaired during diastole, and during systole some blood regurgitates back into the right atrium. Pressure in the right atrium increases and enlarges in response to the increased pressure and workload. This increased right atrial pressure is reflected backward into the systemic circulation. Right ventricular stroke volume decreases, reducing the volume delivered to the pulmonary system and left heart. Stroke volume, cardiac output and tissue perfusion fall.

Manifestations of tricuspid stenosis relate to systemic congestion and right-sided heart failure. They include increased CVP, jugular venous distension, ascites, hepatomegaly and peripheral oedema. Low cardiac output causes fatigue and weakness. The low-pitched, rumbling diastolic murmur of tricuspid stenosis is most clearly heard in the fourth intercostal space at the left sternal border or over the xiphoid process.

Tricuspid regurgitation usually occurs secondarily to right ventricular dilation. Stretching distorts the valve and its supporting structures, preventing complete valve closure. Left ventricular failure is the usual cause of right ventricular overload; pulmonary hypertension is another cause. The valve may also be damaged by rheumatic heart disease, infective endocarditis, inferior MI, trauma or other conditions.

Tricuspid regurgitation allows blood to flow back into the right atrium during systole, increasing right atrial pressures. Increased right atrial pressure causes manifestations of right-sided heart failure, including systemic venous congestion and low cardiac output. Atrial fibrillation due to atrial distension is common.

Pulmonic valve disorders

Pulmonic stenosis obstructs blood flow from the right ventricle into the pulmonary system. It usually is a congenital disorder, although rheumatic heart disease or cancer also may cause pulmonic stenosis. Both the right atrium and ventricle hypertrophy to overcome high pressures. Right-sided heart failure occurs when the ventricle can no longer generate adequate pressure to force blood past the narrowed valve opening.

Pulmonic stenosis typically is asymptomatic unless severe. Dyspnoea on exertion and fatigue are early signs. As the condition progresses, right-sided heart failure develops, with peripheral oedema, ascites, hepatomegaly and increased venous pressures. Turbulent blood flow caused by the narrowed valve generates a harsh, systolic crescendo–decrescendo murmur heard in the pulmonic area, the second left intercostal space.

Pulmonic regurgitation is more common than pulmonary stenosis. It is a complication of pulmonary hypertension, which stretches and dilates the pulmonary orifice, causing incomplete valve closure. Infective endocarditis, pulmonary artery aneurysm and syphilis also may cause pulmonic regurgitation.

Incomplete valve closure allows blood to flow back into the right ventricle during diastole, decreasing blood flow to the pulmonary circuit and increasing end-diastolic pressure. When the ventricle can no longer compensate for the increased volume, right-sided heart failure develops.

INTERPROFESSIONAL CARE

A heart murmur identified during routine physical examination often is the initial indication of valvular disease. If no symptoms are present, close observation for disease progression and prophylactic therapy to prevent infection of the diseased heart may be the only treatment. When medical management is no longer effective, surgery is considered.

Diagnosis

The following diagnostic tests help to identify and diagnose valvular disease. See the chapter 'A person-centred approach to assessing the cardiovascular and lymphatic systems' for more information about these tests and related nursing care.

- *Echocardiography* is used routinely to diagnose valvular disease. Thickened valve leaflets, vegetations or growths on valve leaflets, myocardial function and chamber size can be determined, and pressure gradients across valves and pulmonary artery pressures can be estimated. Either transthoracic or transoesophageal echocardiography may be used.
- *Chest x-ray* can identify cardiac hypertrophy, chamber and great vessel enlargement, and dilation of the pulmonary vasculature. Calcification of the valve leaflets and annular openings may also be visible.
- *Electrocardiography* can demonstrate atrial and ventricular hypertrophy, conduction defects and arrhythmias associated with valvular disease.
- *Cardiac catheterisation* may be used to assess contractility and to determine the pressure gradients across the heart valves, in the heart chambers and in the pulmonary system.

Medications

Heart failure resulting from valvular disease is treated with diuretics, ACE inhibitors, vasodilators and possibly digoxin.

Digoxin increases the force of myocardial contraction to maintain cardiac output. Diuretics, ACE inhibitors and vasodilators reduce preload and afterload. (See the 'Medication administration: heart failure' box.)

In individuals with valvular disorders, atrial distension often causes atrial fibrillation. Digoxin or small doses of beta-blockers are given to slow the ventricular response. (See the chapter 'Nursing care of people with coronary heart disease' for more information about atrial fibrillation and its treatment.) Anticoagulant therapy is added to prevent clot and embolus formation, a common complication of atrial fibrillation as blood pools in the non-contracting atria. Anticoagulant therapy also is required following insertion of a mechanical heart valve. See the chapter 'Nursing care of people with vascular and lymphatic disorders' for more information about anticoagulant therapy.

Valvular damage increases the risk of infective endocarditis as altered blood flow allows bacterial colonisation. Antibiotics are prescribed prophylactically prior to any dental work, invasive procedures or surgery to minimise the risk of bacteraemia (bacteria in the blood) and subsequent endocarditis.

Percutaneous balloon valvuloplasty

Percutaneous balloon valvuloplasty is an invasive procedure performed in the cardiac catheterisation laboratory. A balloon catheter similar to that used in coronary angioplasty procedures is inserted into the femoral vein or artery. Guided by fluoroscopy, the catheter is advanced into the heart and positioned with the balloon straddling the stenotic valve. The balloon is then inflated for approximately 90 seconds to divide the fused leaflets and enlarge the valve orifice (see Figure 30.13). Balloon valvuloplasty is the treatment of choice for symptomatic mitral valve stenosis. It is used to treat children and young adults with aortic stenosis. Nursing care of the individual with a balloon valvuloplasty is similar to that of the person having percutaneous coronary revascularisation (see the chapter 'Nursing care of people with coronary heart disease').

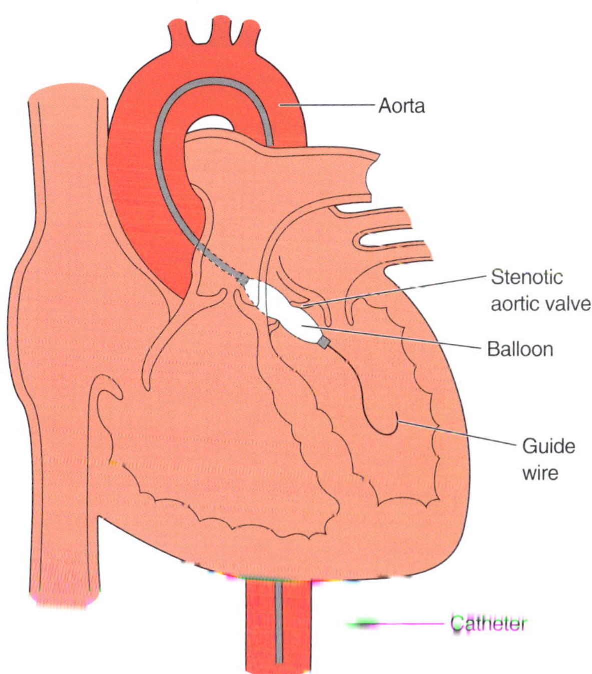

FIGURE 30.13 *Balloon valvuloplasty. The balloon catheter is guided into position straddling the stenosed valve. The balloon is then inflated to increase the size of the valve opening*

Surgery

Surgery to repair or replace the diseased valve may be done to restore valve function, alleviate symptoms and prevent complications and death. The diseased valve is repaired when possible, because the risk of surgical mortality and complications is lower than with valve replacement.

RECONSTRUCTIVE SURGERY *Valvuloplasty* is a general term for reconstruction or repair of a heart valve. Methods include 'patching' the perforated portion of the leaflet, resecting excess tissue, debriding vegetations or calcification, and other techniques. Valvuloplasty may be used for stenotic or regurgitant mitral and tricuspid valves, mitral valve prolapse and aortic stenosis. Common valvuloplasty procedures include the following:

- *open commissurotomy*, surgical division of fused valve leaflets, is done to open stenotic valves
- *annuloplasty*, which repairs a narrowed or an enlarged or dilated valve annulus, the supporting ring of the valve.

VALVE REPLACEMENT Valve replacement is indicated when manifestations of valve dysfunction develop, preferably before left heart function is seriously impaired. In general, three factors determine the outcome of valve replacement surgery: (1) heart function at the time of surgery, (2) intraoperative and postoperative care, and (3) characteristics and durability of the replacement valve.

Many different prosthetic heart valves are available, including mechanical and biological tissue valves. Selection depends on numerous variables, including the valve haemodynamics, resistance to clot formation, ease of insertion, anatomical suitability and the person's acceptance of the procedure. The individual's age, underlying condition and contraindications to anticoagulation (such as a desire to become pregnant) also are considered in selecting the appropriate prosthesis. Table 30.8 lists the advantages and disadvantages of biological and mechanical valves.

Biological tissue valves may be *heterografts*, excised from a pig (see Figure 30.14A), or made of calf pericardium or *homografts* from a human (obtained from a cadaver or during heart transplant). Biological valves allow more normal blood flow and have a low risk of thrombus formation. As a result, long-term anticoagulation rarely is necessary. They are less durable, however, than mechanical valves.

Mechanical prosthetic valves have the major advantage of long-term durability. These valves are frequently used when life expectancy exceeds 10 years. Their major disadvantage is the need for lifetime anticoagulation to prevent the development of clots on the valve.

Most mechanical valves are either a tilting-disk (see Figure 30.14B) or a ball-and-cage design. Both biological and mechanical valves increase the risk of endocarditis, although its incidence is fairly low.

TABLE 30.8 Advantages and disadvantages of prosthetic heart valves

CATEGORY	TYPES	ADVANTAGES	DISADVANTAGES
Mechanical valves	Ball-and-cage Tilting disk	Long-term durability Good haemodynamics	Lifetime anticoagulation Audible click Risk of thromboembolism Infections are harder to treat
Biological tissue valves	Porcine heterograft Bovine heterograft Human aortic homograft	Low incidence of thromboembolism No long-term anticoagulation Good haemodynamics Quiet Infections are easier to treat	Prone to deterioration Frequent replacement is required

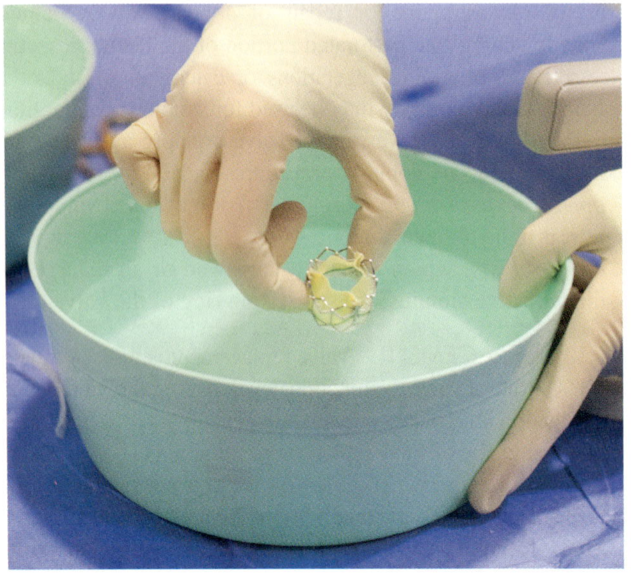

A

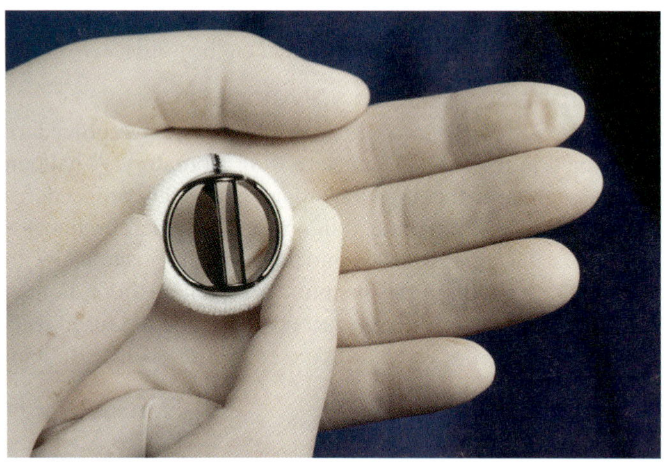

B

FIGURE 30.14 ***Prosthetic heart valves. A, Medtronic Mosaic® bioprosthetic valve. B, St Jude Medical valve***

Sources: *A*, Phanie/Alamy Stock Photo; *B*, Layne Kennedy/Getty Images.

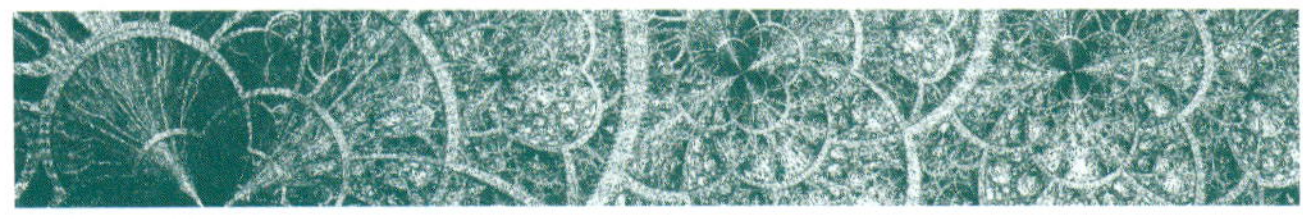

Nursing care

Health promotion

Preventing rheumatic heart disease is a key element in preventing heart valve disorders. Rheumatic heart disease is a consequence of rheumatic fever (see the previous section of this chapter), an immune process that may be a sequela to beta-haemolytic streptococcal infection of the pharynx (strep throat). Early treatment of strep throat prevents rheumatic fever. Teach individuals, families and communities about the importance of timely and effective treatment of strep throat. Emphasise the importance of completing the full prescription of antibiotics to prevent development of resistant bacteria. Prophylactic antibiotic therapy before invasive procedures to prevent infectious endocarditis is an important health promotion measure for individuals with pre-existing heart disease.

Assessment

- Assessment data related to valvular heart disease include the following:
- *Health history*: complaints of decreasing exercise tolerance, dyspnoea on exertion, palpitations; history of frequent respiratory infections; previous history of rheumatic heart disease, endocarditis or a heart murmur.
- *Physical examination*: vital signs; skin colour and temperature, evidence of clubbing or peripheral oedema; neck vein distension; breath sounds; heart sounds and presence of S_3, S_4 or murmur; timing, grade and characteristics of any murmur; palpate for cardiac heave and thrills; abdominal contour, liver and spleen size.
- *Diagnostic tests*: echocardiogram and cardiac catheterisation reports; cardiac index and cardiac output.

Nursing diagnoses and interventions

Nursing priorities include maintaining cardiac output, managing manifestations of the disorder, teaching about the disease process and its management, and preventing complications. Nursing care of the person undergoing valve surgery is similar to that of the person having other types of open-heart surgery, with increased attention to anticoagulation and preventing endocarditis.

Decreased cardiac output

Nearly all valve disorders affect ventricular filling and/or emptying, reducing cardiac output. Stenosis of the AV valves impairs ventricular filling and increases atrial pressures. Regurgitation of these valves reduces cardiac output as a portion of the blood in the ventricle regurgitates into the atria during systole. Stenosis of the semilunar valves obstructs ventricular outflow to the great vessels; regurgitation allows blood to flow back into the ventricles, creating higher filling pressures. When compensatory measures fail, heart failure develops.

- Monitor vital signs and haemodynamic parameters, reporting changes from the baseline. *A fall in systolic blood pressure and tachycardia may indicate decreased cardiac output.*

> **CONSIDERATION FOR PRACTICE**
>
> **Promptly report changes in level of consciousness; distended neck veins; dyspnoea or respiratory crackles; urine output less than 30 mL/h (or 0.5 mL/h in children); cool, clammy or cyanotic skin; diminished peripheral pulses; or slow capillary refill. These findings indicate decreased cardiac output and impaired tissue and organ perfusion.**

- Monitor intake and output; weigh daily. Report weight gain of 1.5 kg within 24 hours. *Fluid retention is a compensatory mechanism that occurs when cardiac output decreases; 1 kg of weight equals 1 L of fluid.*
- Restrict fluids as ordered. *Fluid intake may be restricted to reduce cardiac workload and pressures within the heart and pulmonary circuit.*
- Monitor oxygen saturation continuously and arterial blood gases as ordered. Report oxygen saturation less than 95% (or as specified) and abnormal ABG results. *Oxygen saturation levels and ABGs allow assessment of oxygenation.*
- Elevate the head of the bed. Administer supplemental oxygen as ordered. *These measures improve alveolar ventilation and oxygenation.*
- Provide for physical and emotional rest. *Physical and psychological rest decrease the cardiac workload.*
- Administer prescribed medications as ordered to reduce cardiac workload. *Diuretics, ACE inhibitors and direct vasodilators may be prescribed to reduce fluid volume and afterload, reducing cardiac work*

Activity intolerance

Altered blood flow through the heart impairs delivery of oxygen and nutrients to the tissues. As the heart muscle fails and is unable to compensate for altered blood flow, tissue perfusion is further compromised. Dyspnoea on exertion is often an early symptom of valvular disease.

- Monitor vital signs before and during activities. *A change in heart rate of more than 20 bpm, a change of 20 mmHg or more in systolic BP and complaints of dyspnoea, excessive fatigue, chest pain, diaphoresis, dizziness or syncope may indicate activity intolerance.*
- Encourage self-care and gradually increasing activities as allowed and tolerated. Provide for rest periods, uninterrupted sleep and adequate nutritional intake. *Gradual progression of activities avoids excessive cardiac stress. Encouraging self-care increases the person's self-esteem and sense of power. Adequate rest and nutrition facilitate healing, decrease fatigue and increase energy reserves.*
- Provide assistance as needed. Suggest the person uses a shower chair, sitting while brushing hair or teeth, and other energy-saving measures. *Reducing energy expenditure helps maintain a balance of oxygen supply and demand.*
- Consult with cardiac rehabilitation nurse or physiotherapist for in-bed exercises and an activity plan. *In-bed exercises may help improve strength.*
- Discuss ways to conserve energy at home. *Information provides practical ways to deal with activity limitations and empowers the person to manage these limitations.*

Risk of infection

Damaged and deformed valve leaflets and turbulent blood flow through the heart significantly increase the risk of infective endocarditis. Invasive diagnostic and monitoring lines (e.g. cardiac catheterisation, haemodynamic monitoring) and disrupted skin with surgery also increase the risk of infection.

- Use aseptic technique for all invasive procedures. *Invasive procedures breach the body's protective mechanisms, potentially allowing bacteria to enter. Aseptic technique reduces this risk.*
- Assess wounds and catheter sites for redness, swelling, warmth, pain or evidence of drainage. *These signs of inflammation may signal infection.*
- Administer antibiotics as ordered. Ensure completion of the full course. *Antibiotics are used to prevent and treat infection. Completion of the full course of therapy prevents drug-resistant organisms from multiplying.*
- Monitor FBC and differential. Notify doctor of leucocytosis or leucopenia. *A high WBC count and increased percentage of immature WBCs (bands) may indicate bacterial infection; a low WBC count may indicate an impaired immune response and increased susceptibility to infection.*

Ineffective protection

Anticoagulant therapy commonly is prescribed for people with chronic atrial fibrillation, a history of emboli and following valve replacement surgery. Although chronic anticoagulant therapy decreases the risk of clots and emboli, it increases the risk of bleeding and haemorrhage.

- Test stools and vomitus for occult blood. *Bleeding due to excessive anticoagulation may not be apparent.*
- Instruct to avoid using aspirin or other NSAIDs. Encourage the person to read ingredient labels on over-the-counter drugs; many contain aspirin. *Aspirin and other NSAIDs*

interfere with clotting and may potentiate the effects of the anticoagulant therapy.

- Advise using a soft-bristled toothbrush, electric razor and gentle touch when cleaning fragile skin. *These measures decrease the risk of skin or gum trauma and bleeding.*

CONSIDERATION FOR PRACTICE

Monitor the International Normalized Ratio (INR) or prothrombin time (PT). For anticoagulation in people:

- **with mechanical prosthetic heart valves: INR 2.5–3.5**
- **all other indications such as AF, DVT, PE: INR 2.0–3.0.**

Report an INR > 3.5 or a PT > 2.5 times the normal to the doctor. An excessively high INR or PT indicates excessive anticoagulation and an increased risk of bleeding.

Community-based care

For most individuals, valvular disease is a chronic condition. The person has the primary responsibility for managing effects of the disorder. To prepare the individual and their family for home care, discuss the following topics:

- management of symptoms, including any necessary activity restrictions or lifestyle changes
- the importance of adequate rest to prevent fatigue
- diet restrictions to reduce fluid retention and symptoms of heart failure
- information about prescribed medications, including purpose, desired and possible adverse effects, scheduling, and possible interactions with other drugs
- the importance of keeping follow-up appointments to monitor the disease and its treatment
- notifying all healthcare providers about valve disease or surgery to facilitate prescription of prophylactic antibiotics before invasive procedures or dental work
- reporting increasing severity of symptoms, especially of worsening heart failure or pulmonary oedema; signs of transient ischaemic attacks or other embolic events; evidence of bleeding, such as joint pain, easy bruising, black and tarry stools, bleeding gums or blood in the urine or sputum.

Provide referrals to community resources such as cardiac rehabilitation programs and community support services. Refer the person and their family (especially the primary food preparer) to a dietician or nutritionist for teaching and assistance with menu planning. See the accompanying nursing care plan for additional nursing care and teaching for an individual with mitral valve prolapse.

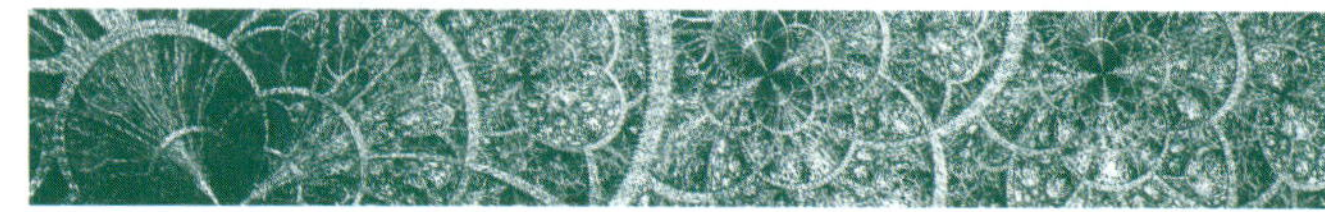

THE PERSON WITH CARDIOMYOPATHY

The **cardiomyopathies** are disorders that affect the heart muscle itself. They are a diverse group of disorders that affect both systolic and diastolic functions. Cardiomyopathies may be either primary or secondary in origin. Primary cardiomyopathies are idiopathic; their cause is unknown. Secondary cardiomyopathies occur as a result of other processes, such as ischaemia, infectious disease, exposure to toxins, connective tissue disorders, metabolic disorders or nutritional deficiencies. In many cases, the cause of cardiomyopathy is unknown. In 2016

NURSING CARE PLAN A person with mitral valve prolapse

Julie Snow, a 22-year-old university student, sees the local medical officer for a physical examination after experiencing palpitations, fatigue and a headache during midterm examinations. Ms Snow stated, 'I'm scared that something is wrong with me.'

Over the past few months, Ms Snow has had occasional palpitations that she describes as 'feeling like my heart is doing flip-flops'. Rarely, these palpitations have been accompanied by a sharp, stabbing pain in her chest that lasts only a few seconds. She initially attributed her symptoms to stress, but she is increasingly concerned because the 'attacks' are becoming more frequent. Ms Snow states that she has 'always been healthy', does not smoke, uses alcohol socially and exercises, albeit intermittently. Ms Snow admits that she has been drinking a lot of coffee and cola and eating a lot of 'junk food' lately.

ASSESSMENT

Ms Snow's assessment revealed the following: height 168 cm, weight 63.6 kg, T 37°C, BP 118/64, P 82 and R 18. She was slightly anxious but in no acute distress. Systolic click and soft crescendo murmur grade II/VI was noted on auscultation. Apical impulse at fifth intercostal space left midclavicular line. Her lungs are clear to auscultation. A review of the remaining systems reveals no apparent abnormalities. An ECG shows sinus rhythm with occasional premature atrial contractions (PACs). Based on the admission history, manifestations and physical assessment, a mitral valve prolapse (MVP) is suspected.

DIAGNOSES

- *Anxiety* related to fear of heart disease and implications for lifestyle manifested by facial expressions and statements consistent with anxiety.
- *Feelings of powerlessness* related to unpredictability of symptoms manifested by anxiety.
- *Risk of infection* (endocarditis) related to altered valve function manifested by chest pain, cardiac dysfunction and fever.

PLANNING

- Consult with and refer the person to a cardiologist for continued monitoring and follow up.
- Discuss symptoms of progressive mitral regurgitation and the need to report these to the cardiologist.

NURSING CARE PLAN — A person with mitral valve prolapse (continued)

- Discuss recommended follow-up care and its rationale.
- Discuss ways to decrease or relieve MVP symptoms.
- Acknowledge the risk of endocarditis and identify precautions to prevent it.
- Discuss the prognosis for MVP, emphasising that most people live normal lives using diet and lifestyle management.
- Discuss lifestyle changes to manage symptoms: aerobic exercise with warm-up and cool-down periods; maintaining adequate fluid intake, especially during hot weather or exercise; relaxation techniques (e.g. meditation, deep-breathing exercises, music therapy, yoga, guided imagery, heat therapy or progressive muscle relaxation) to perform daily; avoiding caffeine and crash diets; forming healthy eating habits.

Expected outcomes

- Verbalises an understanding of MVP and its management.
- Is able to identify signs of deterioration of the condition and the methods by which they will report it.
- Attends follow-up appointments.
- Verbalises methods to prevent endocarditis.
- Demonstrates hopes for future health and management.
- Undertakes lifestyle changes that result in weight loss, increased circulation and improved cardiovascular and musculoskeletal condition.

IMPLEMENTATION

- Teach the person about MVP, including heart valve anatomy, physiology and function, common manifestations of MVP and treatment rationale.
- Provide opportunity for the person to verbalise feelings and share concerns about MVP. Encourage to attend an MVP support group meeting.
- Instruct the person to keep a weekly record of symptoms and their frequency for 1 month.
- Teach the person about infective endocarditis risk and discuss the protocol for prevention with prophylactic antibiotics with the doctor. Encourage notifying dentist and other healthcare providers of MVP before dental or any invasive procedure.

EVALUATION

After several educational sessions Ms Snow verbalises an understanding of MVP by explaining heart valve function, listing common manifestations of MVP and describing indications of deteriorating heart function. She states she will report these manifestations to her cardiologist if they occur. She is given a booklet on MVP for additional reading. She also verbalises understanding of the risk of endocarditis and states that she will notify her doctors of her MVP and the need for antibiotics before invasive procedures. Ms Snow is attending a monthly MVP support group (led by a cardiac rehabilitation nurse) and states, 'I am so glad to know I'm not alone! It really helps to know that others are living well with MVP'. Her weekly symptom log shows her symptoms are associated with late-night studying and drinking large amounts of coffee and cola. Ms Snow has moderated her caffeine intake and increased her fluids, relieving her symptoms. Ms Snow states that she realises that she has 'the ability to control my life through the choices I make'.

CRITICAL THINKING IN THE NURSING PROCESS

1. Develop an action plan for Ms Snow that outlines specific activities she can use to manage symptoms of MVP.
2. Why are people with symptomatic MVP encouraged to include regular exercise in their health habits?
3. How does the support of family, friends and other people with MVP assist individuals in managing their condition?
4. What manifestations would indicate a progressive worsening of Ms Snow's mitral regurgitation?

REFLECTION ON THE NURSING PROCESS

1. Outline what you have learned from this case study that you will apply to your future practice.
2. What techniques would assist you to facilitate communication about lifestyle change principles in an individual with mitral valve prolapse?

in Australia, cardiomyopathy was listed as the cause of death in 972 people, equating to 0.65% of all deaths (ABS, 2017).

Pathophysiology

The cardiomyopathies are categorised by their pathophysiology and presentation into three groups: dilated, hypertrophic and restrictive (Huether & McCance, 2020). Table 30.9 compares the causes, pathophysiology, manifestations and management of the cardiomyopathies.

Dilated cardiomyopathy

Dilated cardiomyopathy is the most common type of cardiomyopathy.

The cause of dilated cardiomyopathy is unknown, although it appears to frequently result from toxins, metabolic conditions or infection. Reversible dilated cardiomyopathy may develop due to alcohol and cocaine abuse, chemotherapeutic drugs, pregnancy and systemic hypertension. In dilated cardiomyopathy, heart chambers dilate and ventricular contraction is impaired. Both end-diastolic and end-systolic volumes increase and the left ventricular ejection fraction is substantially reduced, decreasing cardiac output. Left ventricular dilation is prominent; left ventricular hypertrophy is usually minimal. The right ventricle may also be enlarged and extensive interstitial fibrosis (scarring) may be evident (Goswami, 2018).

MANIFESTATIONS AND COURSE Manifestations of dilated cardiomyopathy develop gradually. Heart failure often presents years after the onset of dilation and pump failure. Both right- and left-sided failure occur, with dyspnoea on exertion, orthopnoea, paroxysmal nocturnal dyspnoea, weakness, fatigue, peripheral oedema and ascites. Both S_3 and S_4 heart

TABLE 30.9 Classifications of cardiomyopathy

	DILATED	HYPERTROPHIC	RESTRICTIVE
Causes	Usually idiopathic; may be secondary to chronic alcoholism or myocarditis	Hereditary; may be secondary to chronic hypertension	Usually secondary to amyloidosis, radiation or myocardial fibrosis
Pathophysiology	Scarring and atrophy of myocardial cells Thickening of ventricular wall Dilation of heart chambers Impaired ventricular pumping Increased end-diastolic and end-systolic volumes Mural thrombi are common	Hypertrophy of ventricular muscle mass Small left ventricular volume Septal hypertrophy may obstruct left ventricular outflow Left atrial dilation	Excess rigidity of ventricular walls restricts filling Myocardial contractility remains relatively normal
Manifestations	Heart failure Cardiomegaly Arrhythmias S_3 and S_4 gallop; murmur of mitral regurgitation	Dyspnoea, anginal pain, syncope Left ventricular hypertrophy Arrhythmias Loud S_4 Sudden death	Dyspnoea, fatigue Right-sided heart failure Mild to moderate cardiomegaly S_3 and S_4 Mitral regurgitation murmur
Management	Management of heart failure Implantable cardioverter-defibrillator (ICD) as needed Cardiac transplantation	Beta-blockers Anti-arrhythmic agents Calcium channel blockers ICD, dual-chamber pacing Surgical excision of part of the ventricular septum	Management of heart failure Exercise restriction

sounds are commonly heard, as well as an AV regurgitation murmur. Arrhythmias are common, including supraventricular tachycardias, atrial fibrillation and complex ventricular tachycardias. Untreated arrhythmias and thromboembolism can lead to sudden death (Goswami, 2018).

The prognosis of dilated cardiomyopathy is grim; most individuals get progressively worse.

Hypertrophic cardiomyopathy

Hypertrophic cardiomyopathy is characterised by decreased compliance of the left ventricle and hypertrophy of the ventricular muscle mass. This impairs ventricular filling, leading to small end-diastolic volumes and low cardiac output. Several people with hypertrophic cardiomyopathy have a family history of the disease. It is genetically transmitted in an autosomal dominant pattern (Banasik & Copstead, 2022).

The pattern of left ventricular hypertrophy is unique in that the muscle may not hypertrophy 'equally'. In a majority of people, the interventricular septal mass, especially the upper portion, increases to a greater extent than the free wall of the ventricle. The enlarged upper septum narrows the passageway of blood into the aorta, impairing ventricular outflow. For this reason, this disorder is also known as *idiopathic hypertrophic subaortic stenosis (IHSS)* or *hypertrophic obstructive cardiomyopathy (HOCM)*.

MANIFESTATIONS AND COURSE Hypertrophic cardiomyopathy may be asymptomatic for many years. Symptoms typically occur when increased oxygen demand causes increased ventricular contractility. They may develop suddenly during or after physical activity; in children and young adults, sudden cardiac death may be the first sign of the disorder. Hypertrophic cardiomyopathy is the probable cause of death in young athletes who die suddenly.

The usual manifestations of hypertrophic cardiomyopathy are dyspnoea, angina and syncope. Angina may result from ischaemia due to overgrowth of the ventricular muscle, coronary artery abnormalities or decreased coronary artery perfusion. Syncope may occur when the outflow tract obstruction severely decreases cardiac output and blood flow to the brain. Ventricular arrhythmias are common; atrial fibrillation also may develop. Other manifestations of hypertrophic cardiomyopathy include fatigue, dizziness and palpitations. A harsh, crescendo–decrescendo systolic murmur of variable intensity heard best at the lower left sternal border and apex is characteristic in hypertrophic cardiomyopathy. An S_4 may also be noted on auscultation.

Restrictive cardiomyopathy

The least common form of cardiomyopathy, *restrictive cardiomyopathy*, is characterised by rigid ventricular walls that impair diastolic filling. Causes of restrictive cardiomyopathy include myocardial fibrosis and infiltrative processes, such as amyloidosis. Fibrosis of the myocardium and endocardium causes excessive stiffness and rigidity of the ventricles. Decreased ventricular compliance impairs filling, with decreased ventricular size, elevated end-diastolic pressures and decreased cardiac output. Contractility is unaffected and the ejection fraction is normal.

MANIFESTATIONS AND COURSE The manifestations of restrictive cardiomyopathy are those of heart failure and decreased tissue perfusion. Dyspnoea on exertion and exercise intolerance are common. Jugular venous pressure is elevated and S_3 and S_4 are common. The prognosis for restrictive cardiomyopathy is poor. Many people die within 3 years as the systemic nature of the underlying disease process precludes effective treatment.

INTERPROFESSIONAL CARE

With the exception of treating an underlying cause, little can be done to treat either dilated or restrictive cardiomyopathies. For these disorders, treatment focuses on managing heart failure and treating arrhythmias. Refer to the section of this chapter on heart failure and the chapter 'Nursing care of people with coronary heart disease' for specific treatment strategies. Treatment of hypertrophic cardiomyopathy focuses on reducing contractility and preventing sudden cardiac death. Strenuous physical exertion is restricted, because it may precipitate arrhythmias or sudden cardiac death. Dietary and sodium restrictions may help diminish the manifestations.

Diagnosis

Diagnosis begins with a history and physical assessment to rule out known causes of heart failure. Other tests may include the following:

- *Echocardiography* is done to assess chamber size and thickness, ventricular wall motion, valvular function and systolic and diastolic function of the heart.
- *Electrocardiography* and *ambulatory ECG monitoring* demonstrate cardiac enlargement and detect arrhythmias.
- *Chest x-ray* shows cardiomegaly, enlargement of the heart and any pulmonary congestion or oedema.
- *Haemodynamic studies* are used to assess cardiac output and pressures in the cardiac chambers and pulmonary vascular system.
- *Radionuclear scans* help identify changes in ventricular volume and mass, as well as perfusion deficits.
- *Cardiac catheterisation* and *coronary angiography* may be done to evaluate coronary perfusion, the cardiac chambers, valves and great vessels for function and structure, pressure relationships and cardiac output.
- *Myocardial biopsy* uses the transvenous route to obtain myocardial tissue for biopsy. The cells are examined for infiltration, fibrosis or inflammation.

Medications

The drug regimen used to treat heart failure also is used for dilated or restrictive cardiomyopathy. This includes ACE inhibitors, vasodilators and digoxin (see the earlier section of this chapter on medications for heart failure). Beta-blockers also may be used with caution in individuals with dilated cardiomyopathy. Anticoagulants are given to reduce the risk of thrombus formation and embolisation. Anti-arrhythmic drugs are avoided if possible due to their tendency to precipitate further arrhythmias (Dumitru, 2022; Papadakis et al., 2022).

Beta-blockers are the drugs of choice to reduce anginal symptoms episodes associated with hypertrophic cardiomyopathy. The negative inotropic effects of beta-blockers and calcium channel blockers decrease the myocardial contractility, decreasing obstruction of the outflow tract. Beta-blockers also decrease heart rate and increase ventricular compliance, increasing diastolic filling time and cardiac output. Vasodilators, digoxin, nitrates and diuretics are contraindicated. Amiodarone may be used to treat ventricular arrhythmias (Dumitru, 2022; Papadakis et al., 2022).

Surgery

Without definitive treatment, individuals with cardiomyopathy develop end-stage heart failure. Cardiac transplant is the definitive treatment for dilated cardiomyopathy. Ventricular assist devices may be used to support cardiac output until a donor heart is available. Transplantation is not a viable option for restrictive cardiomyopathy because transplantation does not eliminate the underlying process causing infiltration or fibrosis and eventually the transplanted organ is affected as well. See the section on heart failure for more information about cardiac transplantation.

An implantable cardioverter-defibrillator (ICD) often is inserted to treat potentially lethal arrhythmias. A dual-chamber pacemaker also may be used to treat hypertrophic cardiomyopathy.

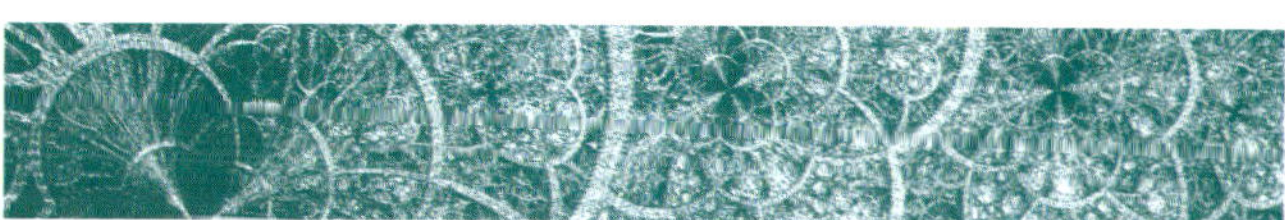

Nursing care

Nursing assessment and care for individuals with dilated and restrictive cardiomyopathy are similar to those for individuals with heart failure. Teaching about the disease process and its management is vital. Some degree of activity restriction is often necessary; assist to conserve energy while encouraging self-care. Support coping skills and adaptation to required

TRANSLATION TO PRACTICE

Nurse-led interventions to manage hypertension in general practice: a systematic review and meta-analysis

ANALYSIS OF NURSE-LED MANAGEMENT OF HYPERTENSION

In a meta-analysis of 11 randomised control trials totalling 4,454 participants by Stephen et al. (2022), clear evidence of nurse-led interventions resulted in significant improvement of cardiovascular risk. It demonstrated a significant reduction in blood pressure and serum lipid levels and an increase in physical activity, general lifestyle measures and medication adherence over 6 months or less. Interestingly, alcohol consumption and smoking rate reduction was inconclusive.

IMPLICATIONS FOR NURSING

Nurses working in primary healthcare settings have the capacity to provide positive influence on a person's cardiovascular health through nurse-led undertakings. With proven success targeted at blood pressure resulting in more far-reaching positive effects, future programs could focus on other chronic health risks, which may result in broader positive personal influence and, subsequently, a further-reaching economic benefit for the already overburdened healthcare system.

CRITICAL THINKING IN PERSON-CENTRED CARE

1 In this study, the findings indicate that practice nurses are capable of positively influencing peoples' cardiovascular health. Given your knowledge of what is required to assist an individual to maintain their cardiovascular health, what components would a nurse-led primary health model contain in the context of heart failure? Consider aspects of education, intervention and monitoring. Make a table outlining these three components with statements to justify each component identified.
2 How will the findings of this study impact on the scope of practice of a practice nurse? What further education requirements would be needed to adequately and safely support a practice-nurse-led model?

Source: Stephen et al. (2022). Nurse-led interventions to manage hypertension in general practice: A systematic review and meta-analysis. *Journal of Advanced Nursing*, 78(5), 1281–1293. https://doi.org/10.1111/jan.15159.

lifestyle changes. Provide information and support for decision making about cardiac transplantation if that is an option. Discuss the toxic and vasodilator effects of alcohol and encourage abstinence. For nursing diagnoses and suggested interventions see the nursing care section for heart failure.

The person with hypertrophic cardiomyopathy requires care similar to that provided for myocardial ischaemia; nitrates and other vasodilators, however, are avoided. If surgery is performed, nursing care is similar to that for any person undergoing open-heart surgery. Discuss the genetic transmission of hypertrophic cardiomyopathy and suggest screening of close relatives (parents and siblings).

Provide pre- and postoperative care and teaching as appropriate for individuals undergoing invasive procedures or surgery for cardiomyopathy.

Nursing diagnoses that may be appropriate for people with cardiomyopathy include:

- *Risk of decreased cardiac output* related to impaired left ventricular filling, contractility or outflow obstruction.
- *Risk of fatigue* related to decreased cardiac output.
- *Risk of ineffective breathing pattern* related to heart failure.
- *Risk of fear* related to risk of sudden cardiac death.
- *Risk of ineffective role performance* related to decreasing cardiac function and activity restrictions.
- *Risk of anticipatory grieving* related to poor prognosis.

Community-based care

Cardiomyopathies are chronic, progressive disorders generally managed in home and community care settings unless surgery or transplant is planned or end-stage heart failure develops. When teaching the person and family for home care, include the following topics:

- activity restrictions and dietary changes to reduce manifestations and prevent complications
- prescribed drug regimen, its rationale, intended and possible adverse effects
- the disease process, its expected ultimate outcome and treatment options
- cardiac transplantation, including the procedure, the need for lifetime immunosuppression to prevent transplant rejection and the risks of postoperative infection and long-term immunosuppression
- symptoms to report to the doctor or for which immediate care is needed
- cardiopulmonary resuscitation procedures and available training sites.

Refer the person and their family for home and social services and counselling as indicated. Provide community resources such as support groups or the National Heart Foundation of Australia.

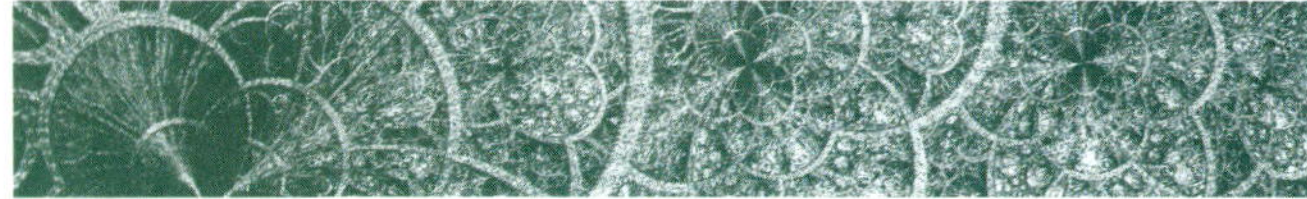

CHAPTER HIGHLIGHTS

- All of the disorders discussed in this chapter can lead to heart failure, a condition in which the heart is unable to pump effectively to meet the body's needs for blood and oxygen to the tissues.
- Coronary heart disease (myocardial ischaemia) and cardiomyopathies are the leading causes of heart failure.
- When the heart starts to fail, compensatory mechanisms are activated to help maintain tissue perfusion. While these mechanisms, including increased contractile force, vasoconstriction, sodium and water retention and remodelling of the heart, effectively maintain cardiac output in the short term, in the long term they hasten deterioration of heart function.
- The goals of heart failure management are to reduce the workload of the heart and improve its function. Medical management includes administration of drugs such as ACE inhibitors, beta-blockers, diuretics and vasodilators to reduce the workload of the heart, and inotropic medications such as digoxin to improve the strength of cardiac muscle contraction.
- Nursing care of the person with heart failure is primarily supportive and educative, providing the individual and their family with necessary knowledge and resources to manage this chronic condition.
- Cardiogenic pulmonary oedema, a manifestation of severe cardiac decompensation, is a medical emergency, requiring immediate and effective treatment to preserve life. The nurse's role in managing pulmonary oedema focuses on supporting respiratory and cardiac function, administering prescribed medications and providing reassurance to the person and their family.
- Inflammatory and infectious processes, such as rheumatic fever, endocarditis, myocarditis and pericarditis, can affect any layer of the heart. While some processes, such as myocarditis and pericarditis, typically are mild and self-limiting, others can have long-term effects on cardiac structure and function.
- Processes such as rheumatic heart disease, endocarditis and congenital conditions can affect the structure and function of the heart valves, resulting in either stenosis (narrowing) of the valve and restricted flow through it, or regurgitation (backflow of blood through a valve that does not fully close). The mitral and aortic valves are commonly affected due to the higher pressures and increased workload of the left side of the heart.
- Valve disorders may be mild, producing a heart murmur but no functional impairment for the individual, or severe, causing symptoms of heart failure even at rest. Repair or replacement of the valve may ultimately be required.
- Cardiomyopathies affect the heart muscle and its ability to stretch during filling and to contract effectively. Dilated cardiomyopathy, the most common type, is progressive, ultimately necessitating heart transplant. Hypertrophic cardiomyopathy affects both ventricular filling and outflow through the aortic valve. Surgical resection of excess tissue may relieve its manifestations.

CONCEPT CHECK

1 In reviewing the doctor's admitting notes for a person with heart failure, the nurse notes that the person has an ejection fraction of 25%. The nurse recognises this as meaning:
1 ventricular function is severely impaired
2 the amount of blood being ejected from the ventricles is within normal limits
3 25% of the blood entering the ventricle remains in the ventricle after systole
4 cardiac output is greater than normal, overtaxing the heart

2 In assessing a person admitted 24 hours previously with heart failure, the nurse notes that the person has lost 1 kg of weight, his heart rate is 88 (HR was 106 on admission) and he now has crackles in the bases of his lung fields only. The nurse correctly interprets these data as indicating:
1 the person's condition is unchanged from admission
2 a need for more aggressive treatment
3 the treatment regimen is achieving the desired effect
4 no further treatment is required at this time as the failure has resolved

3 The nurse assessing a person admitted with left ventricular failure would recognise which of the following findings as consistent with the diagnosis? (Select all that apply.)
1 15 cm jugular vein distension at 30 degrees
2 complaints of shortness of breath with minimal exertion
3 substernal chest pain during exercise
4 bilateral inspiratory crackles to midscapular
5 fatigue

4 Morphine 2–5 mg IV as needed for pain and dyspnoea is ordered for a person in acute pulmonary oedema. The nurse appropriately:
1 questions this order because no time intervals have been specified
2 administers the drug as ordered, monitoring respiratory status
3 withholds the drug until the person's respiratory status improves
4 administers the drug only when the person complains of chest pain

5 An expected assessment finding in a person with mitral stenosis being admitted for a valve replacement would be:
1 muffled heart sounds
2 S_4 and S_4 heart sounds
3 diastolic murmur heard at the apex
4 cardiac heave

6 A person facing heart valve replacement asks the nurse which type of valve is the best, biological or mechanical. Which of the following would be an appropriate response?
1 The need to take drugs to prevent rejection of biological tissue is a major consideration.
2 Clotting is a risk with mechanical valves, necessitating anticoagulant drug therapy after insertion.
3 Biological valves tend to be more durable than mechanical valves.
4 Endocarditis is a risk following valve replacement; it is more easily treated with mechanical valves.

BIBLIOGRAPHY

Aitken, L., Marshall, A. & Chaboyer, W. (2019). *ACCCN's critical care nursing* (4th ed.). Sydney: Elsevier.

American Heart Association (AHA). (2018). *Hypertrophic cardiomyopathy.* Retrieved from https://www.heart.org/

Australian Bureau of Statistics (ABS) (2017). *Causes of death, Australia, 2016.* Retrieved from https://www.abs.gov.au/

Australian Bureau of Statistics (ABS) (2021). *Causes of death, Australia, 2020.* Retrieved from https://www.abs.gov.au/

Australian Institute of Health and Welfare (AIHW) (2021). *Acute rheumatic fever and rheumatic heart disease in Australia: 2015–2019.* Canberra: AIHW. Retrieved from http://aihw.gov.au/

Australian Institute of Health and Welfare (AIHW) (2022). *Separation statistics by principal diagnosis in ICD-10-AM, Australia, 2020–21.* Retrieved from https://www.aihw.gov.au/

Banasik, J. L. & Copstead, L. E. (2022). *Pathophysiology* (7th ed.). New York: Elsevier.

Block, J., Boehmer, T., Forrest, C. et al. (2022). Cardiac complications after SARS-CoV-2 infection and mRNA COVID-19 vaccination—PCORnet, United States, January 2021–January 2022. *Morbidity and Mortality Weekly Report (MMWR), 71*, 517–523. http://dx.doi.org/10.15585/mmwr.mm7114e1

Brusch, J. (2022). Infective endocarditis. *Emedicine*. Retrieved from http://emedicine.medscape.com/

Bullock, S. & Hales, M. (2019). *Principles of pathophysiology* (2nd ed.). Frenchs Forest, NSW: Pearson.

Chiabrando, J. G., Bonaventura, A., Vecchie, A. et al. (2020). Management of acute and recurrent pericarditis JACC state-of-the-art review. *Journal of the American College of Cardiology, 75*(1), 76–92. https://doi.org/10.1016/j.jacc.2019.11.021

Defendi, G. L. (2021). Genetics of Marfan syndrome. *Emedicine*. Retrieved from http://emedicine.medscape.com

Dumitru, I. (2022). Heart failure. *Emedicine*. Retrieved from http://emedicine.medscape.com/

Goswami, V. (2018). Dilated cardiomyopathy. *Emedicine*. Retrieved from http://emedicine.medscape.com/

Huether, S. & McCance, K. L. (2020). *Understanding pathophysiology* (7th ed.). New York: Elsevier.

Levett-Jones, T., Dwyer, T., Reid-Searl, K., Heaton, L., Flenady, T., Applegarth, J., Guinea, S. & Andersen, P. (2017). *Patient Safety Competency Framework (PSCF) for Nursing Students*. Sydney. Retrieved from http://psframework.wpengine.com/

Marieb, E. N. & Hoehn, K. (2019). *Human anatomy and physiology* (11th ed.). San Francisco: Pearson.

McGee, M., Sugito, S., Al-Omary, M. S. et al. (2021). Heart failure outcomes in Aboriginal and Torres Strait Islander peoples in the Hunter New England region of New South Wales. *International Journal of Cardiology, 334*, 65–71. https://doi.org/10.1016/j.ijcard.2021.04.001

National Heart Foundation of Australia (2022). *HEART online: Heart education assessment rehabilitation toolkit*. Retrieved from https://www.heartonline.org.au/

Pandey, A., Kitzman, D., Whellan, D. J. et al. (2019). Frailty among older decompensated heart failure patients: Prevalence, association with patient-centered outcomes, and efficient detection methods. JACC. *Heart Failure, 7*(12), 1079–1088. https://doi.org/10.1016/j.jchf.2019.10.003

Papadakis, M., McPhee, S. & Rabow, M. (2022). *Current medical diagnosis and treatment* (61st ed.). New York: McGraw-Hill Education.

Prashanth, I. (2020). Marfan syndrome. *Emedicine*. Retrieved from http://emedicine.medscape.com/

RHDAustralia (ARF/RHD Writing Group) (2020). *The 2020 Australian guideline for prevention, diagnosis and management of acute rheumatic fever and rheumatic heart disease* (3rd edition). Retrieved from www.rhdaustralia.org.au/arf-rhd-guideline

Stephen, C., Halcomb, E., Fernandez, R., McInnes, S., Batterham, M. & Zwar, N. (2022). Nurse-led interventions to manage hypertension in general practice: A systematic review and meta-analysis. *Journal of Advanced Nursing, 78*(5), 1281–1293. https://doi.org/10.1111/jan.15159

Wallace, M. (2021). Rheumatic fever. *Emedicine*. Retrieved from http://emedicine.medscape.com/

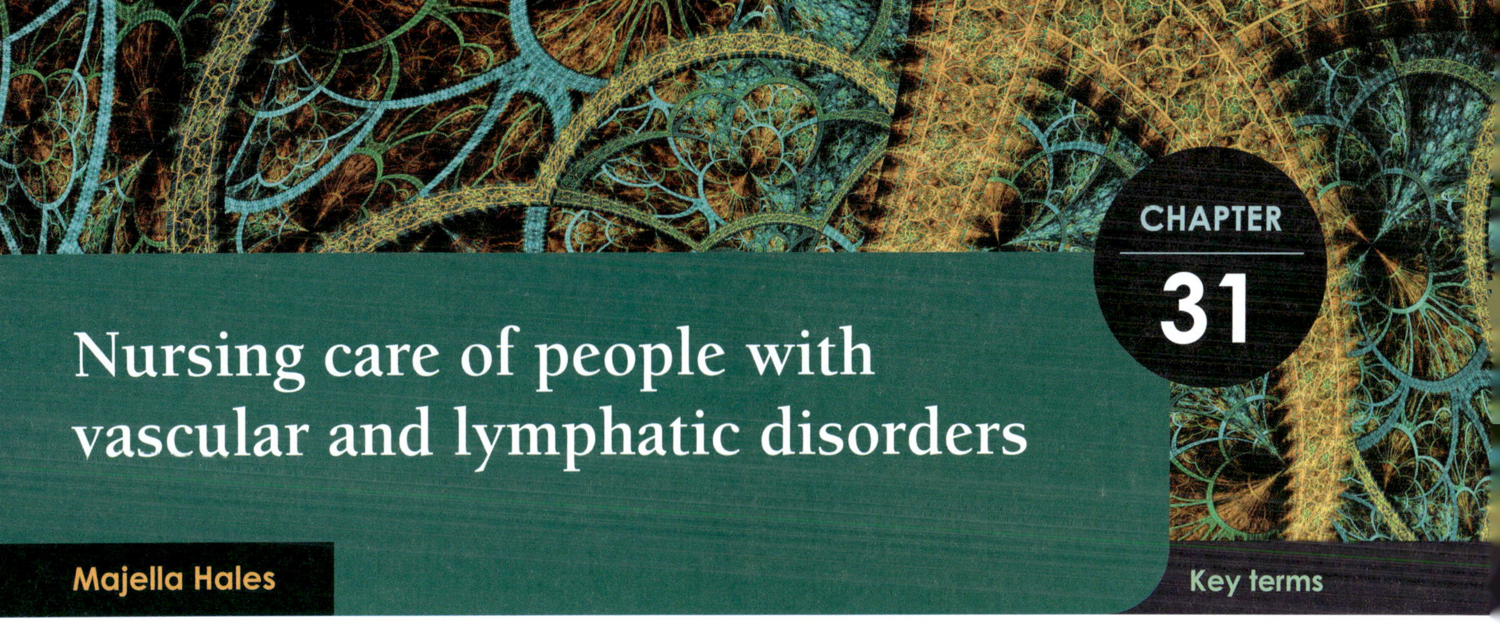

CHAPTER 31

Nursing care of people with vascular and lymphatic disorders

Majella Hales

Learning outcomes

- Discuss the course, implications and health management options for a person with a hypertensive condition.
- Differentiate between various types, implications and management options for an individual with an aneurysm.
- Relate the implications and interventions for a person with peripheral vascular disease to its pathophysiology.
- Compare and contrast the types of arterial occlusive conditions a person may develop.
- Discuss the risks, implications and health management options for a person who has developed a venous thrombosis.
- Differentiate between implications and management options for a person with venous insufficiency or varicose veins.
- Describe the aetiology, pathophysiology and manifestations of lymphadenopathy and lymphoedema.

Clinical competencies

- Perform a comprehensive vascular assessment on people with vascular disorders, using data to select and prioritise appropriate nursing diagnoses, implementation of care and identify desired outcomes of care.
- Identify the effects on the functional health status of people with vascular disorders.
- Use research-informed practice and evidence-based plans to provide individualised care for people with vascular disorders.
- Collaborate with the interprofessional care team in planning and providing care for people with vascular disorders.
- Safely and knowledgeably administer medications and prescribed treatments for people with vascular disorders.
- Provide person and family teaching to promote, maintain and restore health in people with common vascular disorders.

Key terms

aneurysm 1100
atherosclerosis 1107
blood pressure (BP) 1082
chronic venous insufficiency 1125
claudication 1103
deep venous thrombosis (DVT) 1117
diastolic blood pressure 1082
dissection 1103
embolism 1112
hypertension 1082
lymphoedema 1131
mean arterial pressure (MAP) 1082
peripheral vascular disease (PVD) 1107
primary hypertension 1084
pulse pressure 1082
Raynaud's disease 1116
Raynaud's phenomenon 1116
secondary hypertension 1098
systolic blood pressure 1082
thromboangiitis obliterans 1114
thromboembolus 1112
thrombus 1112
varicose veins 1128
vasoconstriction 1107
vasodilation 1107
venous stasis 1125
venous thrombosis 1117

The main processes that interfere with peripheral blood flow and that of lymphatic fluid include constriction, obstruction, inflammation and vasospasm. These conditions lead to disorders of blood pressure regulation, peripheral artery function, aortic structure, venous circulation and lymphatic circulation.

A holistic approach is important when caring for people with disorders of the vascular and lymphatic systems. The focus of care is on teaching long-term care measures, pain relief, improving peripheral blood and lymphatic circulation, preventing tissue damage and promoting healing. The prescribed treatment may have emotional, social and economic effects on the person and family.

Prevalence of cardiovascular conditions such as angina, myocardial infarction, stroke, heart failure, oedema and hypertension are so high that the Australian government considers them to be a National Health Priority. These conditions are not only causing a financial burden, but also a physical and emotional cost for many individuals. See Figure 31.1 for information regarding prevalence of common cardiovascular conditions.

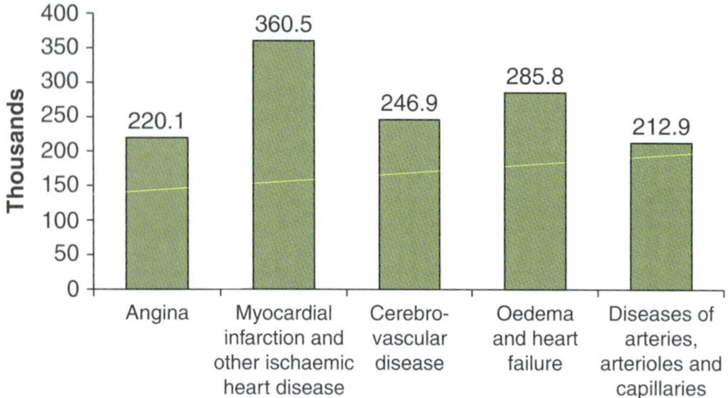

FIGURE 31.1 ***Prevalence of heart, stroke and vascular conditions in Australia, 2020–2021***

Source: Generated using data from Australian Bureau of Statistics (ABS) (2022). *Health conditions prevalence—Table 2: Long-term conditions by age then sex*. Retrieved from https://www.abs.gov.au/statistics/health/health-conditions-and-risks/health-conditions-prevalence/latest-release#data-download.

Disorders of blood pressure regulation

Blood flows through the circulatory system from areas of higher pressure to areas of lower pressure. The amount of pressure in any portion of the vascular system is affected by a number of factors, including blood volume, vascular resistance and cardiac output. The **blood pressure (BP)** is the tension or pressure exerted by blood against arterial walls. A certain amount of pressure within the system is necessary to maintain open vessels, capillary perfusion and oxygenation of all body tissues. Excess pressure, however, has harmful effects, increasing the workload of the heart, altering the structure of the vessels and affecting sensitive body tissues such as the kidneys, eyes and central nervous system (CNS).

This section focuses on **hypertension**, or excess pressure in the arterial portion of systemic circulation. Excessively low blood pressure, *hypotension*, is discussed in the shock section of the chapter 'Nursing care of people experiencing trauma and shock'. Altered pulmonary vascular pressures are discussed in the chapter 'Nursing care of people with gas exchange disorders'.

Physiology review

Blood flow through the circulatory system requires *sufficient blood volume* to fill the blood vessels and *pressure differences* within the system that allow blood to move forward. The arterial, or supply, side of the circulation has relatively high pressures created by the thick elastic walls of the arteries and arterioles. The venous, or return, side of the system, on the other hand, is a low-pressure system of thin-walled, distensible veins. Blood flows through the capillaries linking these two systems from the higher-pressure arterial side to the lower-pressure venous side.

The arterial blood pressure is created by the ejection of blood from the heart during systole (*cardiac output*, or *CO*) and the tension or resistance to blood flow created by the elastic arterial walls (*systemic vascular resistance*, or *SVR*). The blood pressure rises as the heart contracts during systole, ejecting its blood. This pressure wave, or the **systolic blood pressure**, is felt as the peripheral pulse and heard as the Korotkoff's sounds during blood pressure measurement. In healthy adults the average systolic pressure is less than 120 mmHg. During diastole or cardiac relaxation and filling, elastic arterial walls maintain a minimum pressure, the **diastolic blood pressure**, to maintain blood flow through the capillary beds. The average diastolic pressure in a healthy adult is less than 80 mmHg. The difference between the systolic and diastolic pressure, normally about 40 mmHg, is known as the **pulse pressure**. The **mean arterial pressure (MAP)** is the average pressure in the arterial circulation throughout the cardiac cycle. It can be calculated using the formula (systolic BP + diastolic BP + diastolic BP)/3. Diastole counts twice as much as the systole because two-thirds of the cardiac cycle is spent in diastole.

CONSIDERATION FOR PRACTICE

- **Cardiac output and systemic (or peripheral) vascular resistance are the primary factors that determine blood pressure.**
- **A decrease in cardiac output (e.g. due to haemorrhage) or decreased peripheral vascular resistance (e.g. systemic vasodilation) causes the blood pressure to fall.**
- **Increased cardiac output (e.g. during exercise) or increased peripheral vascular resistance (e.g. vasoconstriction due to drug administration) causes the blood pressure to rise.**

Cardiac output is determined by the blood volume and the ability of the ventricles to fill and effectively pump that blood.

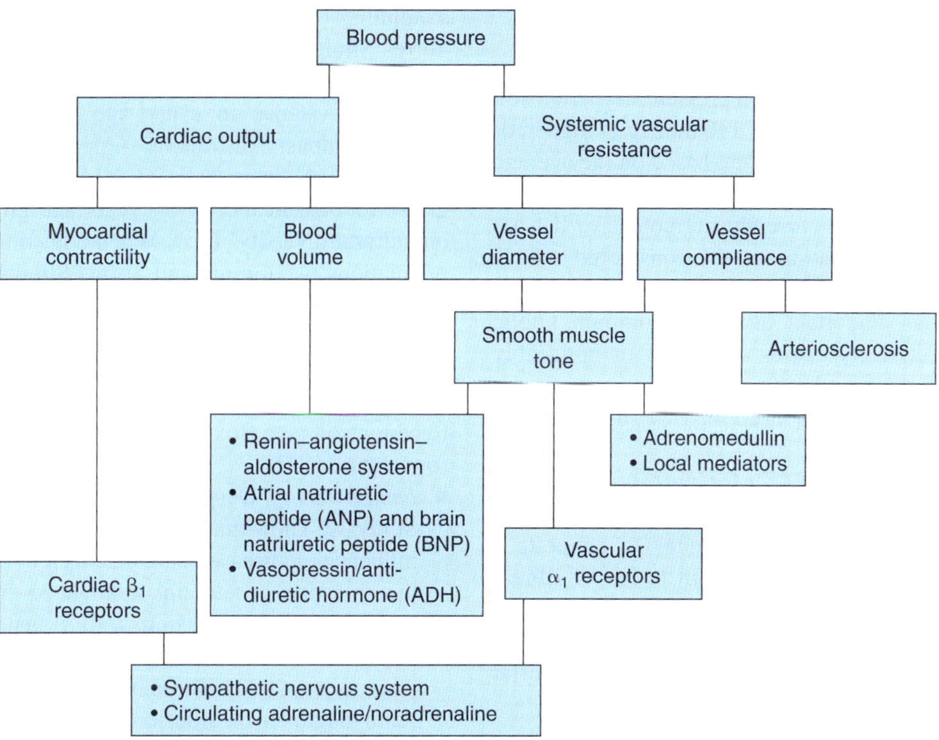

FIGURE 31.2 ***Factors affecting blood pressure***

A number of factors contribute to systemic vascular resistance, including vessel length, blood viscosity and vessel diameter and distensibility (compliance). While vessel length and blood viscosity remain relatively constant, vessel diameter and compliance are subject to normal regulatory activities and disease.

The arterioles normally determine the SVR as their diameter changes in response to a variety of stimuli:

- *Sympathetic nervous system (SNS) stimulation.* Baroreceptors in the aortic arch and carotid sinus signal the SNS via the cardiovascular control centre in the medulla when the MAP changes. A drop in MAP stimulates the SNS, increasing the heart rate and cardiac output and constricting arterioles (except in skeletal muscle). As a result, BP rises. A rise in MAP has the opposite effect, decreasing the heart rate and cardiac output causing arteriolar vasodilation.
- *Circulating adrenaline and noradrenaline* from the adrenal cortex (e.g. the fight-or-flight response) have the same effect as SNS stimulation.
- *Renin–angiotensin–aldosterone system* responds to renal perfusion. A drop in renal perfusion stimulates renin release. Renin converts angiotensinogen to angiotensin I, which is subsequently converted to angiotensin II in the lungs by angiotensin-converting enzyme (ACE). Angiotensin II is a potent vasoconstrictor. It also promotes sodium and water retention both directly and by stimulating the adrenal medulla to release aldosterone. Both SVR and CO increase, resulting in a rise in BP.
- *Atrial natriuretic peptide (ANP)* and *brain natriuretic peptide (BNP)* are released from atrial cells in response to stretching by excess blood volume. These hormones promote vasodilation along with sodium and water excretion, resulting in lowering of BP.
- *Adrenomedullin* is a peptide synthesised and released by endothelial and smooth muscle cells in blood vessels. It is a potent vasodilator.
- *Vasopressin* or *antidiuretic hormone* (from the posterior pituitary gland) promotes water retention and vasoconstriction, resulting in a rise in BP.
- *Local factors* such as inflammatory mediators and various metabolites can promote vasodilation, causing changes in BP.

In addition to the preceding, the primary factor affecting vessel compliance is the extent of arteriosclerosis (hardening of the arteries) and atherosclerosis (plaque accumulation). Figure 31.2 summarises the interrelationships of major factors regulating blood pressure.

CONSIDERATION FOR PRACTICE

- **Sympathetic nervous system stimulation, adrenaline and noradrenaline, and the hormones angiotensin II and vasopressin (antidiuretic hormone or ADH) are *vasoconstrictors*, increasing BP.**
- **Parasympathetic nervous system stimulation and the hormones ANP, BNP and adrenomedullin are *vasodilators*, decreasing BP.**
- **The hormones aldosterone and ADH promote sodium and water retention, increasing BP.**

PRIMARY HYPERTENSION

Primary hypertension, also known as *essential hypertension*, is a persistently elevated systemic blood pressure. Hypertension is defined as systolic blood pressure of 140 mmHg or higher, or diastolic pressure of 90 mmHg or higher, based on the average of three or more readings taken on separate occasions (Unger et al., 2020). People who are currently normotensive but are taking antihypertensive medication are also considered to have hypertension for the sake of statistics.

Hypertension is an important and very common public health issue. While it rarely causes symptoms or noticeably limits the person's functional health patterns, hypertension is a major risk factor for coronary heart disease, heart failure, stroke and kidney failure.

Despite steady improvement over the past three decades, cardiovascular disease (CVD) remains one of the biggest causes of death in Australia and continues to generate a considerable burden on the population in terms of illness and disability. The treatment options for CVD prolong life, but as individuals develop more risk factors such as hypertension, obesity and diabetes, the burden on the health dollar will only increase.

Incidence and risk factors

In Australia, 1 in 14 people have hypertension; however, prevalence increases with age, resulting in more than one-quarter of people over 75 living with hypertension (ABS, 2022). Preventable factors constitute more than one-third of the burden of disease and hypertension is the fourth most common preventable factor contributing to Australia's health liability. Males (36%) are slightly more likely to have hypertension compared to women (31.4%) (AIHW, 2019). Nonetheless, it must be remembered that one elevated reading does not constitute a diagnosis of hypertension, but it should trigger further investigation.

Prevalence of hypertension in Aboriginal and Torres Strait Islander people is very complex. Government statistics examining the prevalence of hypertension in Aboriginal and Torres Strait Islander people report a figure 1.3 times higher than in non-Indigenous Australians. Indigenous Australians exceed prevalence in every age group when compared to non-Indigenous Australians (AIHW: National Indigenous Australians Agency (AIHW: NIAA), 2022). This disparity grows to 14% in the 45–54 years age group (see the 'Focus on cultural diversity' box). When adjusting for age in the two populations, Aboriginal and Torres Strait Islander Australians are twice as likely as non-Indigenous Australians to be hospitalised for a cardiovascular condition directly attributable to their hypertension (AIHW: NIAA, 2022).

A number of risk factors have been identified for primary hypertension (see Box 31.1). Genetics play a role, as do environmental factors.

- *Family history.* Despite completion of the Human Genome Study, we know that there is more data regarding genetic influence on disease being discovered. Currently, it appears that there is a genetic link in about 33–57% of people with primary hypertension, with 21 genes involved in the hormonal control of blood pressure regulation (Alexander, 2019; Silva, 2022). These include genes involved in the renin–angiotensin–aldosterone system, vascular tone, sodium transport, renal function, steroid synthesis, sympathetic nervous system function, endothelial function, obesity and insulin resistance.
- *Age.* The incidence of hypertension rises with increasing age. Ageing affects baroreceptors involved in blood pressure regulation as well as arterial compliance. As the arteries become less compliant, pressure within the vessels increases. This is often most apparent as a gradual increase in the systolic pressure with ageing.
- *Race.* Aboriginal and Torres Strait Islander people are 1.3 times more likely than non-Indigenous Australians to have uncontrolled blood pressure (AIHW: NIAA, 2022).
- *Mineral intake.* High sodium intake is associated with fluid retention and contributes to approximately 30% of hypertension prevalence. Interestingly, hypertension is rare in populations with low sodium consumption

FOCUS ON CULTURAL DIVERSITY

- Aboriginal and Torres Strait Island people are 1.3 times more likely than non-Indigenous Australians to develop hypertension.
- Aboriginal Australians are twice as likely as Torres Strait Islander Australians to develop hypertension.
- Māori people are 1.01 times more likely and Pacific Island people are 1.2 times more likely than European New Zealanders to have hypertension.

Sources: ABS (2022). *Health conditions prevalence—Table 2: Long-term conditions by age then sex.* Retrieved from https://www.abs.gov.au/; New Zealand Ministry of Health (2022). *Cardiovascular health indicators: New Zealand Health Survey 2020-21—Annual Data Explorer.* Retrieved from https://minhealthnz.shinyapps.io/.

BOX 31.1 Factors contributing to hypertension

Modifiable factors

- High sodium intake
- Low potassium, calcium and magnesium intake
- Obesity
- Excess alcohol consumption
- Insulin resistance

Non-modifiable factors

- Genetic factors
- Age
- Family history
- Race

(< 1,000 mg/day) (Campbell et al., 2022). Hypertension related to sodium intake involves a number of different physiological mechanisms, including the renin–angiotensin–aldosterone system, nitric oxide, catecholamines, endothelin and atrial natriuretic peptide. Low potassium, calcium and magnesium intake can contribute to the development of hypertension as it results in renin–angiotensin–aldosterone system activity (Campbell et al., 2022).

- *Obesity.* Central obesity (fat cell deposits in the abdomen), determined by an increased waist-to-hip ratio, has a stronger correlation with hypertension than body mass index or skinfold thickness. Weight gain of 5% is associated with a 20–30% increase in hypertension incidence; weight loss of 4.5 kg maintained for 30 months has been shown to reduce the risk of hypertension by 65% (Shariq & McKenzie, 2020). The pathophysiological mechanism contributing to obesity-related hypertension is a complex interaction between renal, metabolic and neuroendocrine pathways.
- *Insulin resistance.* Insulin resistance with resulting hyperinsulinaemia is linked with hypertension by its effects of excess circulating insulin on the sympathetic nervous system, vascular smooth muscle, renal regulation of sodium and water and ion transport across cell membranes. Insulin resistance may be a genetic or an acquired trait. Although it is more commonly seen in obese individuals, insulin resistance also has been found in people of normal weight.
- *Excess alcohol consumption.* Regular consumption of three or more drinks a day increases the risk of hypertension. Decreasing or discontinuing alcohol consumption reduces the blood pressure, particularly systolic readings. Lifestyle factors associated with excessive alcohol intake (obesity and lack of exercise) may contribute to hypertension as well.
- *Stress.* Physical and emotional stress cause transient elevations of blood pressure, but the role of stress in primary hypertension is less clear. Blood pressure normally fluctuates throughout the day, increasing with activity, discomfort or emotional responses such as anger. Sympathetic nervous system hyperactivity, renin–angiotensin–aldosterone system activation and inflammation-mediated endovascular dysfunction have all been implicated (Shariq & McKenzie, 2020).

Pathophysiology

Primary hypertension is thought to develop from complex interactions among factors that regulate cardiac output and systemic vascular resistance. These interactions may include:

- Excess sympathetic nervous system with overstimulation of alpha and beta-adrenergic receptors, resulting in vasoconstriction and increased cardiac output.
- Altered function of the renin–angiotensin–aldosterone system and its responsiveness to factors such as sodium intake and overall fluid volume. The renin–angiotensin–aldosterone system affects vasomotor tone and salt and water excretion. Chronically high levels of angiotensin II lead to arteriolar remodelling, which permanently increases SVR (Campbell et al., 2022; Harrison, Coffman & Wilcox, 2021; Loscalzo et al., 2022).
- Other chemical mediators of vasomotor tone and blood volume, such as atrial natriuretic peptide, also play a role by affecting vasomotor tone and sodium and water excretion. Vascular endothelium itself produces hormones (*endothelins*) that also affect vasomotor tone. Endothelin-1 is a potent vasoconstrictor (Campbell et al., 2022; Harrison et al., 2021; Loscalzo et al., 2022).
- The interaction between insulin resistance, hyperinsulinaemia and endothelial function may be a primary cause of hypertension. Excess insulin has several effects that potentially contribute to hypertension: (1) sodium retention by the kidneys, (2) increased SNS activity, (3) hypertrophy of vascular smooth muscle, and (4) changes in ion transport across cell membranes (Harrison et al., 2021; Loscalzo et al., 2022).

The result is sustained increases in blood volume and peripheral resistance. The cardiovascular system adapts to increased blood volume by increasing cardiac output. Autoregulatory mechanisms in the systemic arteries react to the increased volume, causing vasoconstriction. The increased systemic vascular resistance causes hypertension.

It appears unlikely that one single cause and pathological process will be found to account for essential hypertension. Increasingly, evidence points to hypertension as a diverse group of pathophysiological mechanisms resulting in the common manifestation of elevated blood pressure.

FAST FACTS

- Major preventable risk factors for CVD include tobacco smoking, hypertensive disease (high blood pressure), high blood cholesterol, inadequate physical activity, overweight and obesity, poor nutrition and diabetes.
- Data from the AIHW report a prevalence of hypertensive disease increases with age, with less than 10% of those aged 25–34 years reporting the disease compared to 44% for those aged 75 years and over (AIHW, 2019).
- The proportion of overweight and obese Australians is increasing. In 1995, 56.3% of people aged 18 years and over were classified as overweight or obese, which increased to an age adjusted 67% by 2020 (AIHW, 2020).

Manifestations

The early stages of primary hypertension typically are asymptomatic, marked only by elevated blood pressure. Blood pressure elevations are initially transient but eventually become permanent. When symptoms do appear, they are usually vague. Headache, usually in the back of the head and neck, may be present on awakening, subsiding during the day. See Box 31.2 for common errors that lead to the undertreatment of hypertension.

Other symptoms result from target-organ damage and may include nocturia, confusion, nausea and vomiting, and visual disturbances. Examination of the retina of the eye may reveal narrowed arterioles, haemorrhages, exudates and *papilloedema* (swelling of the optic nerve).

Complications

Sustained hypertension affects the cardiovascular, neurological and renal systems. The rate of atherosclerosis accelerates, increasing the risk of coronary heart disease and stroke. The workload of the left ventricle increases, leading to ventricular hypertrophy, which then increases the risk of coronary heart disease, arrhythmias and heart failure. The diastolic blood pressure is a significant cardiovascular risk factor until age 50; the systolic pressure then becomes the more important factor contributing to cardiovascular risk. Cardiovascular risk assessment should be performed every 2 years by all Australians 45 years and older who are not already known to be at high risk. Most deaths due to hypertension result from coronary heart disease and acute myocardial infarction or heart failure (Loscalzo et al., 2022; Royal Australian College of General Practitioners, 2021).

Accelerated atherosclerosis associated with hypertension increases the risk of cerebral infarction (stroke). Increased pressure in the cerebral vessels can lead to development of microaneurysms and an increased risk of cerebral haemorrhage. *Hypertensive encephalopathy*, a syndrome characterised by extremely high blood pressure, altered level of consciousness, increased intracranial pressure, papilloedema and seizures, may develop. Its aetiology is unclear.

Hypertension also can lead to nephrosclerosis and renal insufficiency.

BOX 31.2 Common errors in assessing hypertension

The following errors can contribute to undertreatment of hypertension:

- Cuff placed over clothing
- Incorrect cuff size (small cuff overestimates blood pressure and large cuff underestimates blood pressure)
- Poor cuff quality
- Poor cuff position (not level with the heart)
- Poor technique
- Inaccurate/defective sphygmomanometer (e.g. leaky tube, faulty valve, infrequently serviced)
- Arm elevated above heart
- Failure to check that both arms give comparable readings (e.g. at initial visit)
- Person not rested before measurement
- Person talking during measurement
- Failure to palpate radial pulse before auscultatory measurements (results in failure to detect auscultatory gap)
- Rapid cuff deflation (< 2–3 mmHg/beat)
- Re-inflation of cuff (to repeat measurement) before full deflation
- Taking a single measurement
- Observer bias (expectation of expected data)
- Digit preference (rounding a result to an unreasonable value (i.e. > 2 mmHg)
- Patient has not avoided smoking, caffeine and exercise for 30 minutes prior to measurement
- Irregular pulse (especially in automatic sphygmomanometer).

Sources: Jevon (2020). Key principles and types of measuring equipment. *Nursing Times, 116*(7), 37. Retrieved from https://www.nursingtimes.net/; National Heart Foundation of Australia (2016). *Guide to management of hypertension 2016*. Retrieved from https://www.heartfoundation.org.au; Unger et al. (2020). 2020 International Society of Hypertension global hypertension practice guidelines. *Journal of Hypertension, 38*(6), 982–1004. Retrieved from https://www.ahajournals.org/doi/epub/10.1161/hypertensionaha.120.15026.

COVID-19

Hypertension results in the potential for worse COVID-19 outcomes, with an increased risk in intensive care admission and mortality. Although it is difficult to isolate such a risk factor, numerous studies demonstrate that more than 50% of people admitted to the intensive care unit had pre-existing hypertension. This number increased when the affected individual had a second pre-existing factor such as diabetes. As the mechanisms for this association have not yet been elucidated, it is difficult to make concise statements regarding whether it is cause or just correlation. The data is interesting as unadjusted analysis demonstrates strongly worse outcomes. However, after adjusting for age and sex, many studies note the influence is no longer observed (Savoia, Volpe & Kreutz, 2021; Yamazaki & Shibata, 2022).

INTERPROFESSIONAL CARE

Hypertension management focuses on reducing the blood pressure to less than 140 mmHg systolic and 90 mmHg diastolic. The ultimate goal of hypertension management is to reduce cardiovascular and renal morbidity and mortality. The risk of cardiovascular complications (coronary heart disease, heart failure, stroke) decreases when the average blood pressure is less than 140/90; when the person also has diabetes or renal disease, the treatment goal is a blood pressure of less than 130/80. The decision to intervene and the development of a comprehensive management plan (including lifestyle advice and drug treatment) should be based on a thorough clinical investigation to identify associated clinical conditions and/or end-organ damage and assessment of cardiovascular risk (Unger et al., 2020). Although there is no cure for hypertension, it can be controlled. Figure 31.3 shows the recommended algorithm for guidelines as to when to initiate treatment. It is important to note that hypertension management is most successful and cost effective when managing cardiovascular risk rather than just treating blood pressure levels in isolation.

Diagnosis

The person with hypertension is evaluated in the context of a full CVD risk assessment using the Framingham Risk Equation (FRE) (see Table 31.1). The FRE considers several parameters and then provides a heart and stroke score risk which suggests risk of CVD in the next 5 years. This score then drives management decisions.

It is deemed unnecessary for some individuals to have a CVD risk assessment as they are already determined to have a high risk by virtue of a known pre-existing health condition or parameter (see Box 31.3).

If not using the CVD risk calculator such as the one found at https://www.cvdcheck.org.au/calculator, the charts such as those in Figure 31.4 assist in determining risk based on several parameters. Once the appropriate cell is found based on the parameters of the person being investigated, a colour will be identified. Once the colour is identified, the code key can be used to determine risk and the subsequent development of a management plan.

Lifestyle modifications

Lifestyle modifications are recommended for all people whose blood pressure falls within the prehypertension range (120–139/80–89 mmHg) and everyone with intermittent or sustained hypertension. These modifications include weight loss, dietary changes, restricted alcohol use and cigarette smoking, increased physical activity and stress reduction (see Box 31.4).

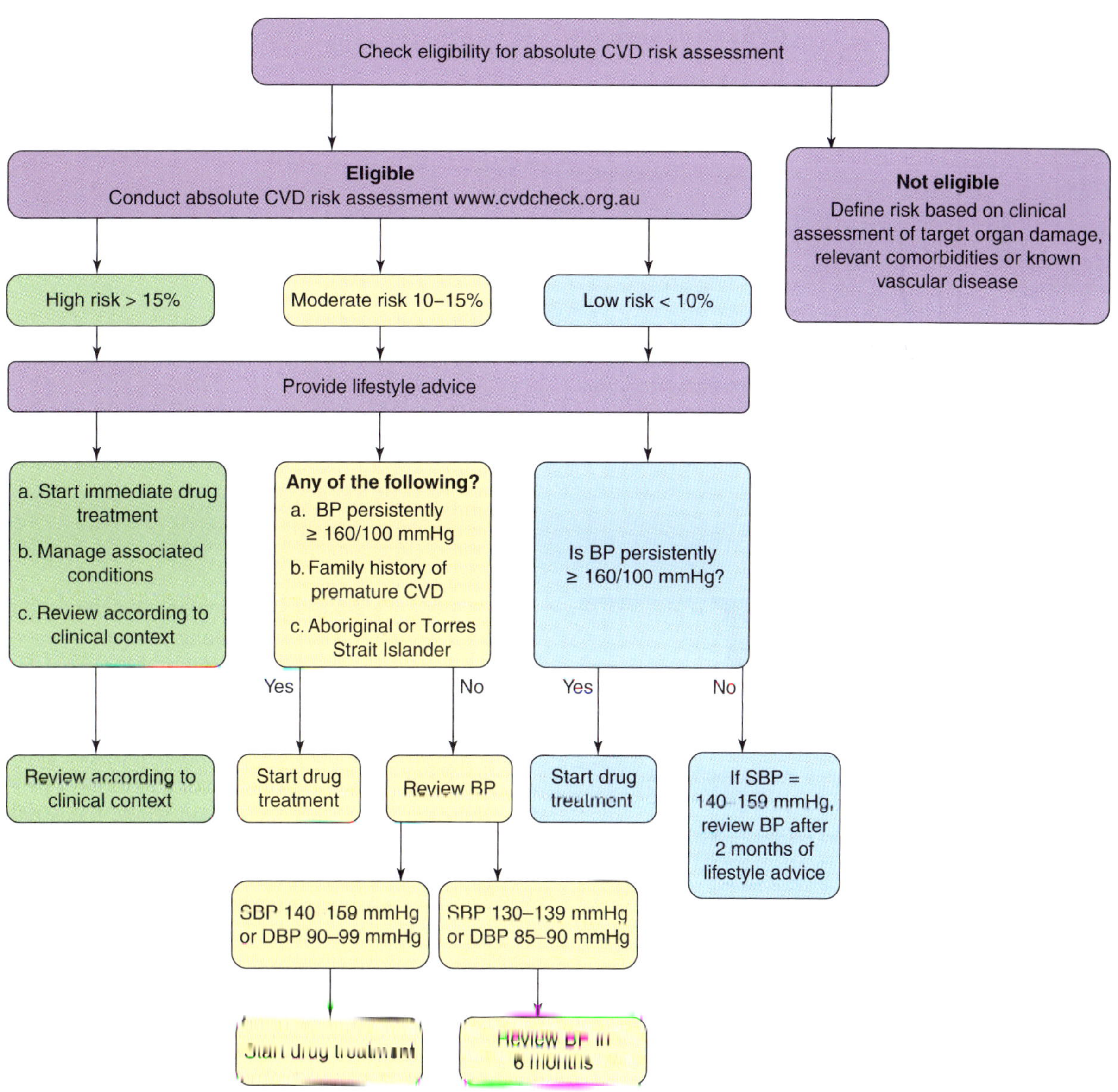

FIGURE 31.3 ***Algorithm for treating hypertension***

Source: National Heart Foundation of Australia (2016). *Guide to management of hypertension 2016*. Retrieved from https://www.heartfoundation.org.au/. Reproduced with permission by National Heart Foundation of Australia.

TABLE 31.1 Absolute cardiovascular risk assessment

PARAMETER	INFLUENCE OF VALUE ON RISK

Gender	• Non-modifiable risk factor
	  • Males develop CVD younger than women and have a higher incidence
	  • Females develop CVD later, with lower incidence, but have higher mortality rates (in older women)
	  • Female-specific factors increasing hypertension include:
	    • pre-eclampsia
	    • gestational hypertension
	    • gestational diabetes mellitus
	    • polycystic ovary syndrome

Age	• Non-modifiable risk factor
	• Differs depending on ethnicity (general population 45–74 years of age)
	  • $>$ 45 years for non-Indigenous Australians
	  • $>$ 35 years for Aboriginal and Torres Strait Islander Australians

Blood pressure	• Modifiable risk factor • Two seated BP measurements over two separate occasions (best practice) • Ambulatory BP measurement is a better predicter of outcomes • See for systolic blood pressure charts
Smoking status	• Modifiable risk factor • Definition of non-smoker also includes a person who has not smoked for $\geq$ 12 months
Total cholesterol	• Modifiable risk factor • $>$ 7.5 mmol/L considered high risk
Diabetes	• Modifiable risk factor • Fasting BGL of $\geq$ 7.0 mmol/L on two separate occasions
BMI and waist circumference	• BMI $\geq$ 30 kg/m^2 increases risk • Waist circumference men: $\geq$ 94 cm increases risk • Waist circumference women: $\geq$ 80 cm increases risk
Left ventricular hypertrophy	• Echocardiography diagnosis is best • ECG diagnosis is acceptable

BGL = blood glucose level; BMI = body mass index; BP = blood pressure; CVD = cardiovascular disease

Sources: Developed using data from Gao et al. (2019); National Heart Foundation of Australia (2016); NPS Medicinewise (2021); National Vascular Disease Prevention Alliance (NVDPA) (2012).

BOX 31.3 Individuals already deemed 'high risk' for CVD

- Systolic BP $\geq$ 180 mmHg or diastolic BP $\geq$ 110 mmHg
- Diabetes 60 years or older
- Diabetes with high protein in urine (microalbuminuria) or poor renal function
- Moderate–severe kidney disease (eGFR $\leq$ 45mL/min/1.73m^2)
- Hypercholesteraemia (serum total cholesterol $>$ 7.5 mmol/L)
- Aboriginal and/or Torres Strait Islander Australian $\geq$ 74 years of age

BP = blood pressure; eGFR = estimated glomerular filtration rate

Source: Based on NPS Medicinewise (2021). *Absolute cardiovascular risk in clinical practice*. Retrieved from https://www.nps.org.au/professionals/blood-pressure/absolute-cardiovascular-risk-in-clinical-practice.

DIET Dietary approaches to managing hypertension focus on reducing sodium intake, maintaining adequate potassium and calcium intakes, and reducing total and saturated fat intake. A mild to moderate sodium restriction (no added salt and reducing high salt-containing foods such as soy sauce and highly processed foods) lowers blood pressure and potentiates the effect of antihypertensive drugs for most people with hypertension. A diet that focuses on whole foods rather than individual nutrients has proven to have beneficial effects in lowering blood pressure (see Box 31.5). Choose a diet rich in fruit and vegetables and whole grains and low in total and saturated fats. The addition of foods high in nitrates (beetroot and leafy vegetables) is also known to assist in blood pressure reduction (Unger et al., 2020).

Managing identifiable lifestyle risk factors is recommended for people with or without hypertension. Weight reduction and use of a non-ethnic-specific measure such as a weight to height ratio of $<$ 0.5 is recommended. Focusing on abdominal obesity is a priority (Unger et al., 2020).

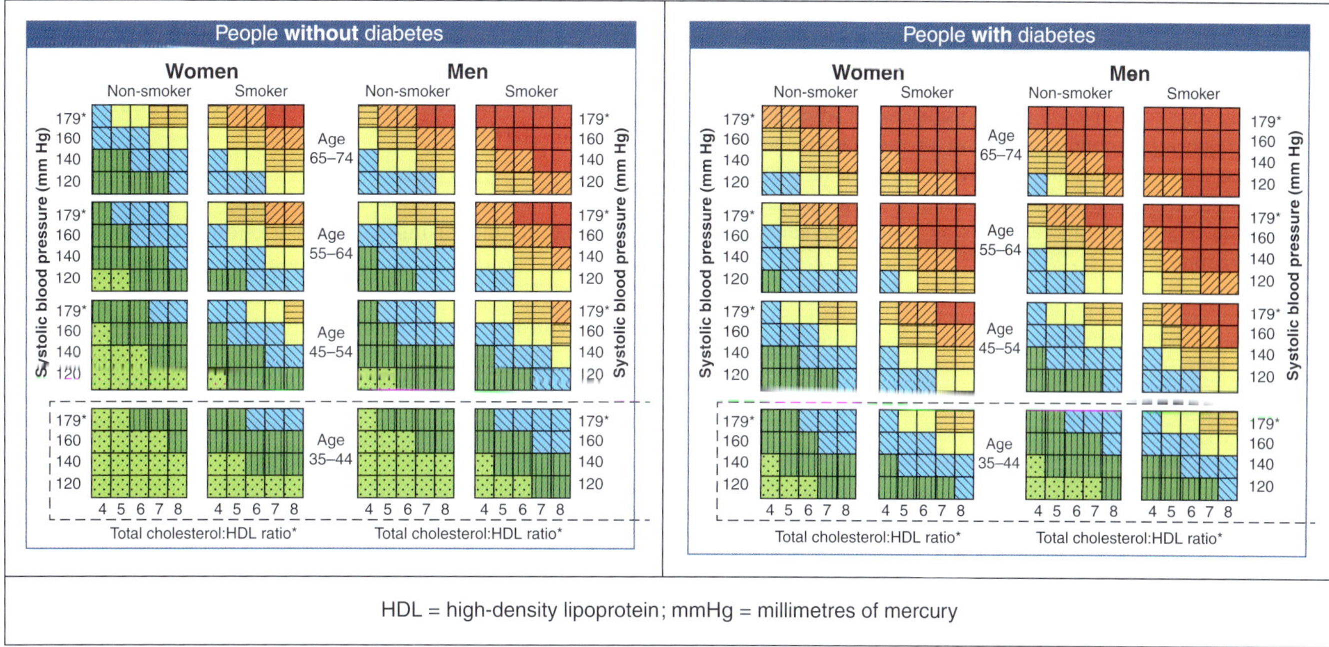

* In accordance with Australian guidelines, patients with systolic blood pressure ≥ 180 mm Hg, or a total cholesterol of > 7.5 mmol/L, should be considered at clinically determined high absolute risk of CVD.

Risk level for 5-year cardiovascular (CVD) risk

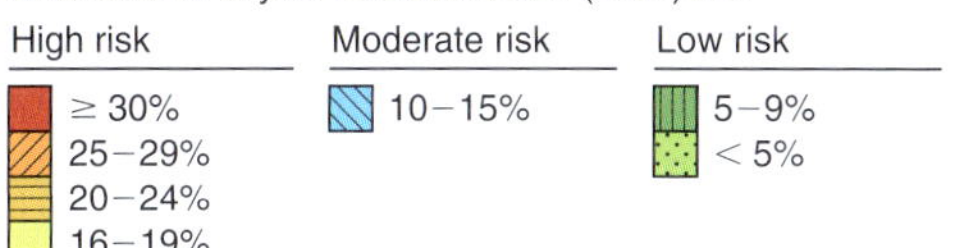

FIGURE 31.4 *Examples of Australian cardiovascular risk charts for people with and without diabetes*

BOX 31.4 Lifestyle modifications for hypertension

The following guidelines need to take into account a person's cultural background and the resources available to them. Further, nurses need to assess a person's readiness for change and tailor recommendations accordingly.

Advise person to aim for healthy targets:

- At least 30 minutes of moderate-intensity physical activity on most, if not all, days of the week (daily total can be accumulated; e.g. three 10-minute sessions). Advise people of all ages to become more active.
- Smoking cessation. Refer the person to Quit Helpline. Consider recommending nicotine replacement therapy and/or prescribing oral therapy (bupropion or varenicline) in people who smoke more than 10 cigarettes per day and have no contraindications.
- Waist measurement < 94 cm for men and < 80 cm for women, and body mass index (BMI) < 25 kg/m². When recommending weight loss, advise the person on reducing kilojoule intake as well as increasing physical activity.
- Dietary salt restriction. There is debate on the value of sodium restriction with evidence suggesting minimal reduction in both systolic and diastolic values. However, it is suggested that reduction of salt intake to ≤ 6 g/day may have general health benefits.
- Recommend low-salt and reduced salt foods as part of a healthy eating pattern.
- Limited alcohol intake: maximum of two standard drinks per day and no more than four on any one occasion.

Source: Based on National Heart Foundation of Australia (2016). *Guide to the management of hypertension 2016*. Retrieved from https://www.heartfoundation.org.au.

PHYSICAL ACTIVITY Regular exercise (such as walking, cycling, jogging, swimming or yoga) reduces blood pressure and contributes to weight loss, stress reduction and feelings of overall wellbeing. Advise all people to become physically active as part of a comprehensive plan to control hypertension, regardless of drug treatment. Aim for 30 minutes of moderate-intensity physical activity 5–7 days per week (National Heart Foundation of Australia, 2016).

ALCOHOL Moderate drinking may increase BP by 38–40 mmHg and binge drinking may increase the risk of hypertension. Reducing alcohol consumption can substantially

BOX 31.5 Dietary recommendations

A healthy eating pattern includes mainly plant-based foods (e.g. fruit, vegetables, pulses); a wide selection of wholegrain foods; moderate amounts of low-fat or reduced-fat dairy products; moderate amounts of lean unprocessed meats, poultry and fish; and moderate amounts of polyunsaturated and monounsaturated fats (e.g. olive oil, canola oil, reduced-salt margarines).

Source: Based on National Heart Foundation of Australia (2016). *Guide to the management of hypertension 2016*. Retrieved from https://www.heartfoundation.org.au.

lower BP in some people. Although alcohol withdrawal may increase blood pressure, this is usually temporary and diminishes as abstinence or restricted intake continues. Advise people with hypertension to limit their intake to a maximum of two standard drinks (a standard drink equals 10 g of alcohol) per day for men, and a maximum of one standard drink per day for women and lighter-weight men. Finally, people should be advised to observe at least two alcohol-free days per week.

SMOKING CESSATION Smoking cessation may not directly reduce BP, but it markedly reduces overall cardiovascular risk. The risk of myocardial infarction is two to six times higher, and the risk of stroke is three times higher, in people who smoke than in non-smokers. Advice from health professionals is effective in increasing quit rates. Even 3–5 minutes taken to encourage smokers to attempt to quit can increase success rates (National Heart Foundation of Australia, 2016).

STRESS REDUCTION Stress stimulates the sympathetic nervous system, increasing vasoconstriction, systemic vascular resistance, cardiac output and blood pressure. Regular, moderate exercise is the treatment of choice for reducing stress in people with hypertension. Relaxation techniques such as biofeedback, therapeutic touch, yoga and meditation to relax both mind and body may also lower blood pressure, although their effect has not been proven in hypertension management (Oza & Garcellano, 2015).

Medications

Current pharmacological treatment of hypertension involves using one or more antihypertensive agent. For most people, two or more antihypertensive drugs selected from different drug classes are necessary to achieve effective control. These drug classes have different sites of action (see Figure 31.5). See the 'Medication administration' box.

The World Health Organization (WHO) (2022) recommendations initiating drug therapy in those with a CVD diagnosis when systolic blood pressure is $\geq$ 130 mmHg, and in those without a CVD diagnosis when systolic blood pressure is $\geq$ 140 mmHg and diastolic blood pressure is $\geq$ 90 mmHg.

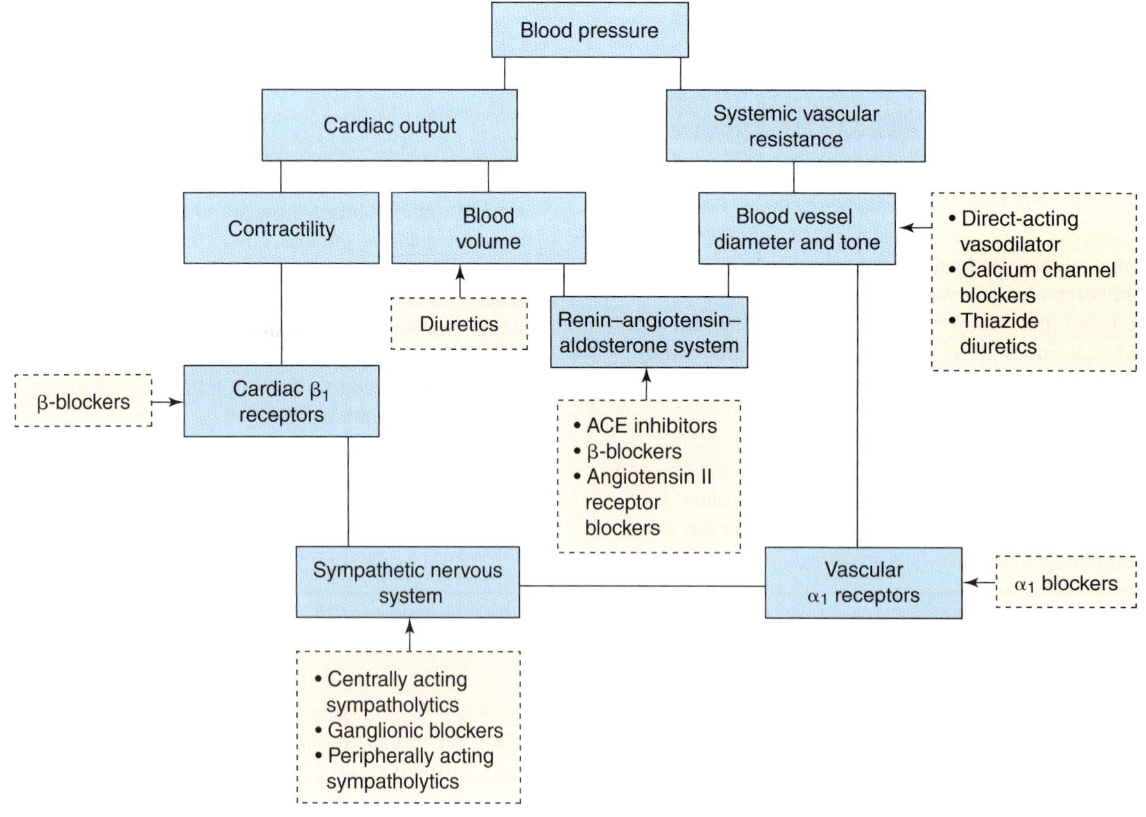

FIGURE 31.5 ***Sites of antihypertensive drug action***

MEDICATION ADMINISTRATION Antihypertensives

ALPHA-ADRENERGIC BLOCKERS

Alpha-adrenergic blocking agents block alpha-receptors in vascular smooth muscle, decreasing vasomotor tone and vasoconstriction. They also reduce serum levels of low-density lipoproteins (LDLs) and very-low-density lipoproteins (VLDLs). However, vasodilation may cause orthostatic hypotension and reflex stimulation of the heart, resulting in tachycardia and palpitations. A beta-blocker may be ordered to minimise this effect.

Nursing responsibilities

- Give the first dose at bedtime to minimise risk of fainting (called 'first-dose syncope'). If the first dose is given in the daytime (or if the dose is increased), instruct to remain in bed for 3 to 4 hours.
- Assess blood pressure and apical pulse before each dose and as indicated thereafter.

Health education for the person and family

- There is a risk of fainting after taking the first dose of this drug. Take the drug at bedtime to reduce this risk and do not drive or engage in other hazardous activities for 12 to 24 hours after the first dose.
- This drug may cause dizziness or light-headedness. Change positions slowly and sit down if you become dizzy or light-headed.
- Notify your primary care provider if you develop nasal congestion or impotence while taking this drug.
- Notify your doctor before discontinuing this medication.

ACE INHIBITORS AND ANGIOTENSIN II RECEPTOR ANTAGONISTS

Angiotensin-converting-enzyme inhibitors (ACEIs) lower blood pressure by preventing conversion of angiotensin I to angiotensin II, which prevents vasoconstriction and sodium and water retention. Angiotensin II receptor blockers (ARBs) stop angiotensin II from binding to its receptor, resulting in the same affects as ACEIs, but working lower down in the renin–angiotensin–aldosterone system. Their primary adverse effects are first-dose hypotension and hyperkalaemia; and for ACEIs, persistent cough.

Nursing responsibilities

- Assess blood pressure before giving the first dose. Monitor blood pressure for 2 hours after the first dose and regularly thereafter.
- Report changes in serum urea or creatinine to the doctor.
- Do not administer to people with renal artery stenosis or who are pregnant.
- Immediately report and treat manifestations of angiooedema (giant wheals and oedema of the tongue, glottis and pharynx). Initiate resuscitation measures as needed. Discontinue drug immediately and do not use in the future.

Health education for the person and family

- Report peripheral oedema, signs of infection or difficulty breathing to your primary care provider.
- Change position (lying to sitting and sitting to standing) slowly to prevent dizziness; sit down if dizziness or light-headedness develops.
- Do not take a potassium supplement or use a potassium-based salt substitute while taking this drug unless prescribed by your doctor.
- Notify your doctor if you become pregnant while taking this drug. Although it is safe early in pregnancy. In late pregnancy, ACEIs may cause renal failure for the mother and (rarely) likely fatal bone deformities in the fetus' skull.

BETA-ADRENERGIC BLOCKERS (BETA-BLOCKERS)

Beta-blockers reduce blood pressure by preventing beta-receptor stimulation in the heart, thereby decreasing heart rate and cardiac output. Beta-blockers also interfere with renin release by the kidneys, decreasing the effects of angiotensin and aldosterone. Potential adverse effects of beta-blockers include bronchospasm, fatigue, sleep disturbances, nightmares, bradycardia, heart block, worsening of heart failure, gastrointestinal disturbances, impotence and increased triglyceride levels.

Nursing responsibilities

- Before giving initial dose, assess for contraindications to beta-blockers, such as asthma, chronic lung disease, bradycardia or heart block.
- Assess blood pressure and apical pulse before giving; notify primary care provider if vital signs are outside established parameters.
- Report adverse effects such as bradycardia, decreased cardiac output (fatigue, dyspnoea with exertion, hypotension, decreased level of consciousness), heart failure, heart block, bronchoconstriction (wheezing, dyspnoea) or altered blood glucose levels (in diabetic people).
- Carefully monitor responses of the older person.

Health education for the person and family

- Monitor blood pressure and pulse daily as instructed.
- Change position (lying to sitting and sitting to standing) slowly to prevent dizziness and possible falls.
- Report effects such as fatigue, lethargy and impotence to your primary care provider.
- Notify your doctor if you become short of breath or develop a cough or swelling of your extremities.
- If you have diabetes, check blood glucose levels more frequently because hypoglycaemia may develop with few symptoms.
- Talk to your primary care provider before taking any over-the-counter medications.
- Carry an adequate supply of the drug when travelling. Do not stop taking this drug without notifying your primary care provider.

CALCIUM CHANNEL BLOCKERS

Calcium channel blockers inhibit the flow of calcium ions across the cell membrane of vascular tissue and cardiac cells. In doing so, they relax arterial smooth muscle, lowering peripheral resistance through vasodilation. Calcium channel blockers can cause reflex tachycardia and some (e.g. verapamil and diltiazem) may impair cardiac function, worsening heart failure.

(continued)

MEDICATION ADMINISTRATION **Antihypertensives (continued)**

Nursing responsibilities

- Assess blood pressure, apical pulse and liver and renal function tests prior to giving these drugs.
- Calcium channel blockers may be given orally or intravenously.
- Do not administer verapamil or diltiazem to people with severe hypotension, sinus or atrioventricular blocks. Administer with caution to people also taking digoxin or a beta-blocker.
- Periodically monitor blood pressure and apical pulse during therapy. Promptly report signs of bradycardia, AV block or heart failure to the doctor.

Health education for the person and family

- Take blood pressure and pulse daily as taught. Notify your doctor if your pulse is less than 60 bpm or your blood pressure is not within the specified range.
- This drug may cause constipation. Drink six to eight glasses of water each day and increase fibre in diet.
- Report shortness of breath, weight gain or swelling in feet or ankles to your primary care provider.

THIAZIDE DIURETICS

These drugs inhibit reabsorption of sodium and chloride in the proximal (diluting) segment of the distal convoluted tubules. They also increase urinary secretion of water, chloride, potassium, magnesium, whereas excretion of uric acid and calcium is decreased. Indications include the treatment of mild to moderate hypertension and oedema associated with heart failure. They should be used with caution for people who have type 1 diabetes, gout, renal or hepatic impairment and in the elderly. These drugs are contraindicated in severe renal impairment, anuria, Addison's disease and in people with thiazide or sulfonamide hypersensitivity (Bullock & Manias, 2022). Loop diuretics (e.g. furosemide) are not recommended as antihypertensive agents unless volume overload is present.

Nursing responsibilities

- Monitor closely if concurrent potassium supplementation or a potassium chloride salt substitute is ordered for people receiving a potassium-sparing diuretic. Hyperkalaemia and death have been reported with this combination.
- Use extreme caution in elderly people. Start with lowest dose possible, titrate slowly to achieve the desired effect.
- Monitor for diuresis and subsequent incontinence.
- Be alert to signs and symptoms of diuretic toxicity, such as anorexia, nausea, vomiting, confusion, increased weakness and paraesthesia of the extremities.
- When diuretic is to be discontinued, reduce the drug gradually to avoid the development of fluid retention and oedema.
- If plasma potassium concentration drops below the laboratory reference range during thiazide diuretic therapy, a potassium-sparing diuretic may be prescribed in combination with the thiazide.

Health education for the person and family

- Fluid intake should be discussed with the individual as many people refer to diuretics as 'water pills' and mistakenly believe they should restrict their fluid intake.
- Report any anorexia, nausea, vomiting, confusion or increased weakness of arms and legs to your health care provider.
- Do not decrease or discontinue medication without talking to your healthcare provider.
- Advise person their urinary output will be increased and they may experience incontinence. Provide education on managing same.

OTHER

Most of the drugs in this category are adjunctive therapies to those listed in the above categories. Please refer to pharmacology texts for guidance on the use of these additional drugs.

Source: Selected data in this box is adapted from MIMS Australia (2022). Retrieved from http://www.mimsonline.com.au/; National Heart Foundation of Australia (2016). *Guide to the management of hypertension 2016.* https://www.heartfoundation.org.au/images/uploads/publications/PRO-167_Hypertension-guideline-2016_WEB.pdf. © National Heart Foundation of Australia.

The WHO also recommends undertaking a complete cardiovascular assessment before commencing treatment (if it does not delay treatment). When requiring more than one antihypertensive agent, the WHO recommends that combination therapy provided in one pill increases adherence.

DRUG CLASSES Initial pharmacological intervention could include drug diuretics, medications acting on the renin–angiotensin–aldosterone system or calcium channel blockers.

In uncomplicated hypertension, the following classes of antihypertensive agents are equally effective for first-line use, both in initial and maintenance therapy:

- low-dose thiazide diuretics
- ACEIs
- ARBs
- calcium channel blockers (CCBs).

Thiazide diuretics have been associated with increased risk of new-onset diabetes and should be used with caution in people with glucose intolerance and/or metabolic syndrome. The use of thiazide diuretics as first-line therapy should be limited to older people, in whom the benefits of managing isolated systolic hypertension and preventing stroke with these agents are likely to outweigh the risk of diabetes onset. Beta-blockers are no longer recommended as first-line therapy in uncomplicated hypertension because of the increased risk of developing diabetes and the recently described trend towards worse outcomes in people treated with beta-blockers compared to those treated with other classes of antihypertensive drugs.

For people with stable, well-controlled hypertension who are already taking a beta-blocker, it is reasonable to continue the regimen unchanged.

The initial drug choice should be based on:

- age
- presence of associated clinical conditions or end-organ damage
- presence of other coexisting conditions that either favour or limit the use of particular drug classes
- potential interactions with other drugs
- implications for adherence
- cost.

Most classes of antihypertensive agents used as monotherapy lower BP by a similar average amount. However, the individual response to each agent is unpredictable.

People with heart failure, coronary heart disease (CHD) or diabetes may initially be treated with a beta-blocker. These drugs lower blood pressure, apparently by reducing peripheral vascular resistance. They may also reduce the amount of renin released by the kidneys by blocking beta$_1$-receptors in the kidney. Beta-blockers reduce the risk of complications such as heart failure and stroke. They are, however, relatively contraindicated for people with asthma or chronic obstructive pulmonary disease, because they promote bronchial constriction.

ACE inhibitors and ARBs also are commonly used in initial treatment of hypertension, particularly for people who are diabetic or have heart failure, a history of myocardial infarction (MI) or chronic kidney disease. ACE inhibitors block formation of angiotensin II by inhibiting the action of angiotensin-converting enzyme. Angiotensin II is a potent vasoconstrictor that also stimulates aldosterone release from the adrenal gland; blocking its action prevents vasoconstriction and sodium and water retention resulting from aldosterone release. ARBs have a very similar effect, although their action is to block angiotensin II receptors, thus preventing its vasoconstrictive and volume expansion effects.

Several drug classes work through their ability to promote vasodilation and reduce peripheral vascular resistance. Alpha-blockers such as prazosin and terazosin block stimulation of alpha$_1$-receptors on arterioles and veins, preventing vasoconstriction. Because of their ability to dilate both arterioles and veins, alpha-blockers can cause significant orthostatic hypotension, particularly following the initial dose. Calcium channel blockers promote dilation of arterioles, the primary regulators of peripheral vascular resistance. These drugs can cause reflex tachycardia. Some calcium channel blockers, verapamil and diltiazem in particular, also suppress heart function, reducing stroke volume and cardiac output. Reflex tachycardia is minimal with these calcium channel blockers. Direct-acting vasodilators such as hydralazine and minoxidil also directly affect the arterioles, reducing peripheral vascular resistance. These drugs have little effect on veins, so the risk of orthostatic hypotension is minimal. They are, however, associated with reflex tachycardia and fluid retention, so rarely are administered as in single-drug treatment regimens.

Other factors considered in selecting drugs for treating hypertension include demographic characteristics of the person, concurrent conditions, quality of life, cost and possible interactions among prescribed drugs. In general, diuretics and calcium channel blockers are more effective for treating hypertension than beta-blockers or ACE inhibitors. Beta-blockers are preferred to treat hypertension with concurrent coronary heart disease and angina but are contraindicated for those who have asthma or depression. Beta-blockers also reduce exercise tolerance and may adversely affect lifestyle for some people.

DRUG REGIMENS Treatment usually is initiated using a single antihypertensive drug at a low dose. Unless otherwise indicated, a diuretic is recommended as the initial drug of choice. The dose is slowly increased until optimal blood pressure control is achieved. If the drug does not effectively lower the blood pressure or has troubling side effects, a different drug from another class of antihypertensive medications is substituted. If, on the other hand, the drug is tolerated well but has not lowered blood pressure to the desired level, a second drug from another class may be added to the treatment regimen.

Treatment of people with stage 2 hypertension generally is more aggressive to minimise the risk of MI, heart failure or stroke. When the average blood pressure is greater than 200/120 mmHg, immediate therapy and possible hospitalisation is vital.

After a year of effective hypertension control, an effort may be made to reduce the dosage and number of drugs. This is known as step-down therapy. It is more successful in people who have made lifestyle modifications. Careful blood pressure monitoring is necessary during and after step-down therapy because the blood pressure often rises again to hypertensive levels.

Complementary therapies

Behavioural and mind–body therapies may be helpful for some people in lowering blood pressure. Blood pressure increases in response to physiological and psychological stress and anxiety. Mind–body therapies such as yoga and tai chi, meditation and guided imagery are designed to modify both physiological and cognitive aspects of the stress response. However, it is critical to understand that alternative medicines and foods can negatively influence conventional treatments.

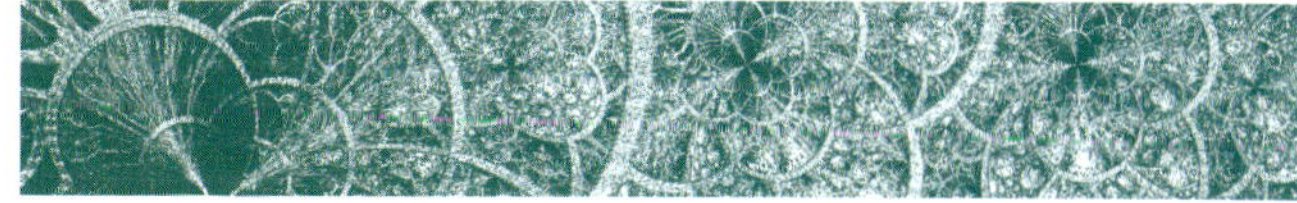

Nursing care

Health promotion

Health promotion teaching and activities focus on the modifiable risk factors for hypertension. Advise and support all people (including children and adolescents) to stop or never start smoking. Discuss the risks of obesity, excess alcohol intake and a sedentary lifestyle. Encourage everyone to eat a diet rich in fruit and vegetables and low in total and saturated fat. Discuss the potential benefits of following a healthy diet.

TRANSLATION TO PRACTICE Evidence-based practice: monopill versus quadpill in patients with hypertension

In an Australian research project comparing the efficiency of a quarter dose of four different classes of antihypertensive medications (in one tablet) (quadpill) to a single drug (monopill), the quadpill was found to be more effective (Chow et al., 2021). Safety data for typical for antihypertensive medications did not differ statistically between the quadpill versus the monopill. Not only does this research potentially demonstrate that reduced dosing of multiple drugs simultaneously is effective, the formulation into one tablet (instead of four different tablets) most likely improved medication adherence related to the ease of following the prescription.

IMPLICATIONS FOR NURSING

Understanding new possible antihypertensive formulations which may reduce high blood pressure will be beneficial in clinical practice. Nurses not only are responsible for administration of medications in both acute and community care situations, they are often the healthcare professional tasked with ensuring that individuals understand medication that they are prescribed.

CRITICAL THINKING IN PERSON-CENTRED CARE

1 Review the four concepts of pharmacokinetics: absorption, distribution, metabolism and excretion. Consider how each of these parameters may be influenced and what result this would have on an antihypertensive medication.
2 Consider the possible adverse effects for bisoprolol, irbesartan, indapamide and amlodipine. Given combination medications such as this quadpill have all of these drugs in the one formulation, for which adverse effects might you be observing after administration?
3 How will this research influence your future practice?

Links to National Patient Safety Standards

NSQHS: Medication Safety Standard

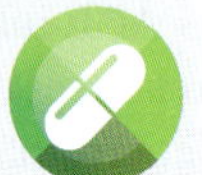

'Leaders of a health service organisation describe, implement and monitor systems to reduce the occurrence of medication incidents, and improve the safety and quality of medication use. The workforce uses these systems.' (Australian Commission on Safety and Quality in Health Care (ACSQHC) 2021, p. 36)

Implementing this standard is achieved by ensuring organisation-wide systems to control, distribute and follow-up on matters of medication safety. Mechanisms capable of assisting this mission include that factors surrounding legal and appropriate documentation, continuity of medication management and procedures embracing safe storage, authorisation, supply, prescription, dispensing, monitoring and disposal exist and are adhered to.

As the provision of medications constitutes the single most common treatment an individual will receive in hospital, errors anywhere in the process may result in significant and widespread adverse events. Not only is this problematic (or potentially catastrophic) for the person experiencing the adverse incident, it is also costly to the facility, as financial burden resulting from the adverse event will tax the already stressed healthcare dollar further.

Source: ACSQHC (2021). *National Safety and Quality Health Service Standards* (2nd ed.). Sydney: ACSQHC. © Australian Commission on Safety and Quality in Health Care.

Advise all people to remain active and engage in aerobic exercise 5 or more days a week. Discuss the stress-reducing benefits of exercise.

Offer blood pressure screening and refer individuals for follow-up as indicated.

Assessment

Absolute cardiovascular risk

The management plan for a person with hypertension should take into consideration the individual's absolute risk of CVD. Absolute cardiovascular risk is the probability (expressed as a percentage) of an individual experiencing a cardiovascular event (e.g. myocardial infarction or stroke) during a predefined period of time (e.g. the next 5 years). Blood pressure is a major determinant of absolute cardiovascular risk. People at highest absolute risk include those with existing CVD or those with multiple risk factors (e.g. diabetes, older age, overweight/obesity and dyslipidaemia).

The purposes of assessing absolute cardiovascular risk are to:

- identify other modifiable risk factors that require management
- predict who will benefit most from intervention and determine the appropriate management plan to reduce BP
- enable the person to understand the degree of urgency for reducing BP and correcting other risk factors.

Risk analysis in Aboriginal and Torres Strait Islander people is complex for numerous reasons, including the increased prevalence of comorbidity at a younger age than non-Indigenous Australians. Indigenous Australians also have an exceedingly high mortality, which has not reduced in the past 40 years despite targeted actions. Therefore, the National Vascular Disease Prevention Alliance recommends screening of Aboriginal and Torres Strait Islander people from 35 years of age (instead of 45 years as for non-Indigenous Australians) and the use of specifically designed absolute risk charts.

Absolute cardiovascular risk assessment is now recommended for all Australians aged 45–74 who are not already known to be at high risk, whether or not they have hypertension.

The management of hypertension should be based on a thorough clinical assessment that includes an estimate of the person's absolute risk of CVD, as well as BP levels and other clinical investigations.

Assessment of absolute cardiovascular risk helps both the healthcare practitioners and the person understand the individual's overall risk profile and the potential benefit of preventive interventions.

People who need immediate antihypertensive drug treatment include (but are not restricted to) those at high absolute cardiovascular risk (> 15% probability of a cardiovascular event within the next 5 years).

Focused assessment of the person with hypertension includes:

- *Health history*: complaints of morning headache, cervical pain; cardiovascular or central nervous system manifestations; history of hypertension, renal disease, diabetes; family history of high blood pressure, heart failure or kidney disease; current medications.
- *Physical examination*: pulse rate, rhythm and character, jugular venous pulse and pressure, evidence of cardiac enlargement (displaced apex, extra heart sounds) or evidence of decompensation (basal crackles or wheeze on lung auscultation, peripheral oedema, abdominal signs; e.g. pulsatile liver).
- *Diagnostic tests*: blood analysis (sodium, potassium, chloride, bicarbonate, urea, creatinine, uric acid, haemoglobin, fasting glucose, total cholesterol, LDL-cholesterol, HDL-cholesterol, triglycerides, liver function tests).
  - *Electrocardiogram (ECG)* to detect conduction disturbances, arrhythmias, coronary heart disease or left ventricular hypertrophy. The presence of strain pattern (ST depression and T-wave inversion) is associated with increased cardiovascular risk in people with hypertension.
  - *Dipstick testing of urine* for blood and protein. If abnormal, proceed to urine microscopy. If proteinuria detected (≥ 1 + on dipstick), measure 24-hour urinary protein excretion.

Nursing diagnoses and interventions

All people with primary hypertension and their families need significant teaching to manage this chronic condition. Health maintenance is a high-priority problem. Depending on the stage of hypertension and concurrent illnesses, other appropriate nursing diagnoses may include *Imbalanced nutrition*, *Excess fluid volume* and *Risk of non-compliance*.

Ineffective health maintenance

Unhealthy lifestyle and behaviours can contribute to health problems such as hypertension. When hypertension has been identified, knowledge of the disease and its management is vital for the person. Willingness to take responsibility for hypertension management is central to effective blood pressure control. Adopting healthy lifestyle changes enhances drug therapy; in some cases, the need for medications may be eliminated or reduced. Because hypertension is often an asymptomatic disease and many antihypertensive drugs have unpleasant side effects, it is vital that the person understand the chronic progressive nature of the disease and its long-term consequences.

- Assist with identifying current behaviours that contribute to hypertension. The person must first identify contributory behaviours before they can change them. *Using knowledge of hypertension risk factors, the nurse can help identify behaviours and factors contributing to hypertension that can be changed. Including the family in this process is important to reduce potential sabotage of the person's efforts to adopt healthier behaviours.*
- Assist in developing a realistic health maintenance plan. *Preparing a health maintenance plan for the person does little to encourage personal responsibility for health. However, nurses can guide people in developing realistic goals and expectations for the treatment plan and modifying risk factors such as smoking, exercise, diet and stress.*
- Help the person and family identify strengths and weaknesses in maintaining health. *Discussing areas of the health maintenance plan that are working well and those that present difficulties can help to identify necessary changes in the plan and additional strategies for implementing it.*

Risk of non-compliance

Non-compliance, or failure to follow the identified treatment plan, is a continuing risk of any person with a chronic disease. Recommended lifestyle changes such as diet, exercise, restricted alcohol intake, stress reduction and smoking cessation often are difficult to maintain on a continuing basis. In addition, prescribed medications may have undesirable effects, whereas hypertension itself often has no symptoms or noticeable effects.

- Inquire about reasons for non-compliance with recommended treatment plan. Listen openly and without judging. *Non-threatening discussion of factors contributing to non-compliance validates the person's self-esteem and partnership in the treatment plan.*

CONSIDERATION FOR PRACTICE

Assess factors contributing to non-compliance, such as adverse drug effects. Suggest measures to manage adverse effects or, if indicated, contact the primary care provider about possible alternative drugs. Some adverse effects of antihypertensive drugs, such as gastric upset, light-headedness or nocturia, may be easily managed by changing the timing of the drug dose. Others, such as fatigue, decreased exercise tolerance or impotence, may interfere with lifestyle and life roles to the extent that the person finds them intolerable.

- Evaluate knowledge of hypertension, its long-term effects and treatment. *Provide additional information and reinforce teaching as needed. Knowledge increases the sense of control, which also increases the likelihood of compliance with treatment.*
- Assist to develop realistic short-term goals for lifestyle changes. *Attempting to lose weight, exercise daily, stop smoking and dramatically change the diet all at the same time may be overwhelming, leading to a sense of failure. Smaller, gradual changes are more easily incorporated into lifestyle and daily activities, improving compliance.*

CONSIDERATION FOR PRACTICE

Work with the person to develop mutual outcomes for the treatment plan. Discuss measures to improve compliance. The person has absolute control over compliance with the treatment plan. Demonstrating respect and involving the person in decision making and planning can improve compliance.

- Help the person identify cues and develop reminders (e.g. written notes, a medication box filled weekly) to assist with maintaining a schedule for exercise and medications. *Cues and other devices provide helpful reminders of activities and schedules until they are incorporated into habits.*
- Reassure the person that relapse into old habits and behaviours is common. Encourage avoiding feelings of guilt associated with relapse and use the circumstance to renew efforts to comply with treatment. *Guilt and feelings of failure can lead to further non-compliance unless the event is used to identify reasons for non-compliance and ways to prevent it from recurring in the future.*

Imbalanced nutrition: more than body requirements

The relationship between obesity, excess alcohol intake and hypertension is well documented. Hypertension is particularly associated with central obesity, identified by waist circumference greater than hip circumference. Although weight loss is difficult and takes commitment to changing eating and exercise habits, it is possible for most people to achieve.

- Assess usual daily food intake and discuss possible contributing factors to excess weight, such as sedentary lifestyle or using food as a reward or stress reliever. Inquire about diversional activities, exercise patterns and previous weight reduction efforts (e.g. participation in weight reduction programs or using fad or crash diets). *Assessment data provide clues about contributing factors to obesity, the person's knowledge base about the relationship between eating and exercise habits and weight, and safe weight loss strategies. This provides direction for further teaching and for developing a realistic weight reduction plan.*
- Mutually determine with the person a realistic target weight (e.g. loss of 10% of current body weight over a 6-month period). Regularly monitor weight. Encourage a system of non-food rewards for achieving small, incremental goals. *Setting weight loss goals helps formalise the process and provides motivation for continued progress. Developing realistic goals may be difficult; unrealistic goals, however, set the person up for failure. Continuous incremental weight loss provides reassurance that it can be achieved and promotes permanent weight reduction.*
- Refer to a dietitian for information about low-fat, low-kilojoule foods and eating plans. Focus on changing eating habits as opposed to 'following a diet'. *Focusing on changing eating habits promotes the sense that low-fat, low-kilojoule eating patterns should become a part of lifestyle, rather than a short-term measure to be endured until the weight loss goal is achieved.*
- Recommend participating in an approved weight loss program such as Weight Watchers. *Organised weight loss programs provide structure for a balanced weight reduction program, as well as mutual support from others trying to lose weight.*

Excess fluid volume

Excess fluid volume often contributes to hypertension by increasing the cardiac output. A number of factors associated with hypertension can cause excess fluid volume, including sodium retention and disruption of the renin–angiotensin–aldosterone system. In addition, some antihypertensive drugs, such as calcium channel blockers and vasodilators, can contribute to excess fluid in the interstitial spaces and peripheral oedema.

- Monitor intake and output and weigh daily (if in an acute or long-term care facility) or weekly (in the community). *Rapid weight changes (over days) more accurately reflect fluid balance than intake and output records. 1 L of fluid weighs 1 kg. Weight changes and intake and output records help monitor the effects of therapy.*
- Monitor for peripheral oedema (sacral oedema in the bedridden person). *Drugs such as vasodilators can cause fluid accumulation in interstitial tissues, leading to peripheral or dependent oedema. Adding a diuretic to the treatment plan may be necessary.*

CONSIDERATION FOR PRACTICE

Monitor blood pressure and other vital signs as indicated: every 1 to 2 hours or more frequently during acute hypertensive states; once a week or more frequently during initial treatment in the community. Vital signs are an indicator of fluid balance and the effectiveness of treatment. An elevated blood pressure, pulse and respiratory rate may indicate fluid retention, whereas orthostatic hypotension and tachycardia may indicate fluid volume deficit.

- Refer to a dietitian for teaching about a restricted sodium diet. Discuss the relationship between sodium intake and fluid retention. Provide opportunities to choose low-sodium foods from simulated menus. Support efforts and reassure that lifestyle changes such as consuming less sodium take time. *Knowledge provides the power to take control of sodium intake. Patience and perseverance are needed to succeed; positive reinforcement of efforts to change long-standing dietary patterns is important.*

CONSIDERATION FOR PRACTICE

Monitor laboratory values, such as urine-specific gravity, urea and creatinine, electrolytes and haematocrit and haemoglobin. Hypertension can alter renal perfusion and function, leading to fluid retention and altered laboratory values. Changes in urea and creatinine indicate impaired renal function, whereas changes in haematocrit and haemoglobin often reflect changes in fluid volume.

- Discuss the importance of adhering to treatment plans such as dietary restrictions and medication schedules. *Understanding the rationale for treatment measures promotes the person's sense of control and encourages compliance with the treatment regimen.*

Community-based care

Effective control of hypertension requires the person not only to participate in the plan of care, but also to take an active role in managing the disease. Treatment is managed in community settings, with regular visits to a clinic or office to monitor blood pressure and effects of treatment measures. Include the following topics in teachings about hypertension:

- Specific lifestyle changes recommended for the person and suggestions for implementing them. For example:
  - Increase activity gradually. Develop a realistic exercise program that is enjoyable and fits into lifestyle. Identify an exercise buddy for additional motivation. Activity and exercise, through a gradual conditioning of muscles and blood vessels, lower blood pressure by reducing peripheral vascular resistance. As the heart becomes conditioned and pumps more efficiently, kidney perfusion improves and intravascular volume falls, further reducing blood pressure. Exercise also reduces stress and contributes to weight loss and maintenance. Aerobic exercise, such as walking, jogging, swimming and cycling, are appropriate; isometric activities (such as weight lifting) should be avoided without doctor's approval.
  - Adopt healthy eating patterns, following a low-fat, low-cholesterol, moderate-sodium diet that also is rich in fruit and vegetables and includes at least two servings of low-fat milk or milk products daily. Do not give up if you slip into old eating habits on occasion; use such occasions to identify ways to avoid future lapses.
  - Stop smoking. Participating in organised smoking cessation programs or using aids such as nicotine patches can help.
  - Use alcohol in moderation if at all, consuming no more than 10–20 g of alcohol per day.
  - Use stress-reducing techniques such as meditation, relaxation, deep breathing and exercise to manage stress. Anger and hostility intensify vasoconstriction; channelling these emotions into more positive responses such as using a change process to modify factors that provoke these emotions can reduce their harmful effects on blood pressure.
- Prescribed medications, their intended effect, dose and timing, interactions and possible adverse effects. Discuss effects that should be reported to the doctor and those that can be managed by the person or that will diminish over time.
- The importance of monitoring blood pressure and regular visits to the primary care provider or hypertension clinic to monitor treatment. During follow-up visits, assess the blood pressure and specific laboratory work (such as serum urea, creatinine and electrolytes) to evaluate the disease and the effects of antihypertensive medications.

Refer the person to community blood pressure clinics and to home health services as needed for regular follow-up and reinforcement of teaching. Refer to a dietitian or to an organised weight loss program as indicated for further teaching and weight loss support. The 'Nursing care plan' provides additional information about community-based care for the person with high blood pressure.

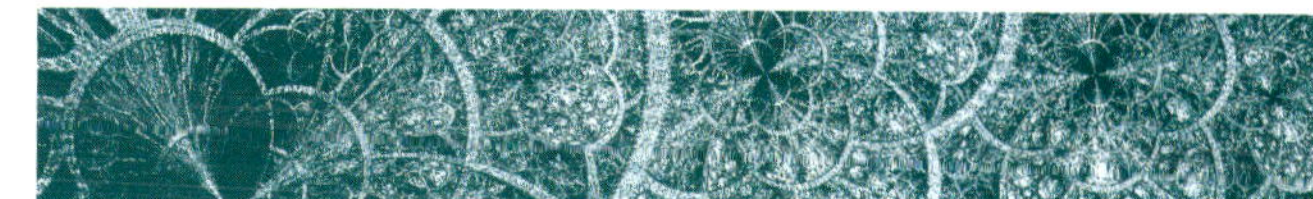

NURSING CARE PLAN **A person with hypertension**

Margaret Simpson is a married, 49-year-old Anglo-Australian with six children whose ages range from 6 to 16 years. For the past 2 months, Mrs Simpson has had frequent morning headaches and occasional dizziness and blurred vision. At her annual health check 1 month ago, her blood pressure was 168/104 mmHg and 150/94 mmHg. She was instructed to reduce her fat and cholesterol intake, to avoid using salt at the table and to start walking for 30 to 45 minutes daily. Mrs Simpson returns to the clinic for follow up.

ASSESSMENT

While escorting Mrs Simpson to the exam room and obtaining her weight, blood pressure and history, Lisa Christos, RN, notices that Mrs Simpson seems restless and upset. Ms Christos says, 'You look upset about something. Is everything OK?' Mrs Simpson responds, 'Well, my head is throbbing and I'm sort of dizzy. I think I'm just overdoing it and not getting enough rest. You know, raising six children is a lot of work and expense. I just started working part time so we wouldn't get behind in our bills. I thought the extra money might relieve some of my stress, but I'm not so sure that's really happening. I'm not getting any better and I'm worried that I'll lose my job or become disabled and that my husband won't be able to manage the children by himself. I really need to go home, but first, I want to get rid of this awful headache. Would you please get me a couple of aspirin or something?'

(continued)

NURSING CARE PLAN A person with hypertension (continued)

Mrs Simpson's history shows a steady weight gain during the past 18 years. She has no known family history of hypertension. Physical findings include height 160 cm, weight 102 kg, T 37.2°C, P 100 regular, R 16, BP 180/115 mmHg (lying), 170/110 mmHg (sitting), 165/105mmHg (standing), average 10 point difference in readings between right and left arm (lower on left). Skin cool and dry, capillary refill 4 seconds right hand, 3 seconds left hand. Mrs Simpson's total serum cholesterol is 6.33 mmol/L (normal < 5.2 mmol/L). All other blood and urine studies are within normal limits. Based on analysis of the data, Mrs Simpson is started on enalapril 5 mg and placed on a low-fat, low-cholesterol, no-added-salt diet.

DIAGNOSES

- *Fatigue* related to effects of hypertension and stresses of daily life.
- *Imbalanced nutrition: more than body requirements* related to excessive food intake.
- *Ineffective health maintenance* related to inability to modify lifestyle.
- *Deficient knowledge* related to effects of prescribed treatment.

PLANNING

- Discuss strategies for achieving a realistic weight loss goal.
- Refer for a dietary consultation for further teaching about fat and sodium restrictions.
- Discuss stress-reducing techniques, helping identify possible choices.

Expected outcomes

- Reduce blood pressure readings to less than 150 systolic and 90 diastolic by return visit next week.
- Incorporate low-sodium and low-fat foods from a list provided into her diet.
- Develop a plan for regular exercise.
- Verbalise understanding of the effects of prescribed drug, dietary restrictions, exercise and follow-up visits to help control hypertension.

IMPLEMENTATION

- Teach to take own blood pressure daily and record it, bringing the record to scheduled clinic visits.
- Teach name, dose, action and side effects of antihypertensive medication.
- Instruct to walk for 15 minutes each day this week and to investigate swimming classes at the local pool.

EVALUATION

Mrs Simpson returns to the clinic 1 week later. Her average blood pressure is now 148/88 mmHg. She has lost 1 kg and states that her oldest daughter has suggested that they join a weight reduction program together. Mrs Simpson is walking for an average of 20 minutes each day. She verbalises an understanding of her medication and is taking it in the morning and before dinner each day. She met with the dietitian and discussed ways to reduce the sodium and fat in her diet. The dietitian provided a list of low-fat, low-sodium foods and recommended cookbooks to help Mrs Simpson modify her cooking. Mrs Simpson tells Ms Christos, 'I just can't believe how much better I feel already. My headaches are gone and I've actually lost some weight—and I feel motivated to keep going. If I had only known how much better I could feel! I don't expect I'll ever go back to my old habits again; it's just not worth it!'

CRITICAL THINKING IN THE NURSING PROCESS

1 Identify the factors that contributed to Mrs Simpson's hypertension. Which were modifiable and which were not?
2 What is the rationale for reducing sodium and fat in Mrs Simpson's diet?
3 Suppose that a hypertensive person is homeless and has no source of income. How could you help ensure that this person would follow the treatment plan? What would you do if the person did not follow it?
4 Discuss the role of stress in hypertension. What factors in Mrs Simpson's life contribute to her stress level?
5 Develop a plan of care for the nursing diagnosis *Low self-esteem* related to obesity.

REFLECTION ON THE NURSING PROCESS

1 Listening to people is an essential quality and skill. Discuss which essential cues in Mrs Simpson's presentation lead the nurse to question her further.
2 What health promotion strategies/programs could be advised for Mrs Simpson to engage in and how are they relevant to her presenting condition?

SECONDARY HYPERTENSION

Secondary hypertension is elevated blood pressure resulting from an identifiable underlying process. In the adult population, secondary hypertension is considered to occur in less than 10% of identified cases of hypertension; however, it is suggested to be the cause in up to 97% of hypertension in children (Nugent et al., 2022). Kidney disease is the most common identifiable cause of high blood pressure in both adults and children. Other common identifiable causes of hypertension in adults include renovascular disease (reduced blood flow to the kidneys), disorders of the adrenal cortex, pheochromocytoma, coarctation of the aorta and sleep apnoea (Alexander, 2019). The pathophysiology of selected causes of high blood pressure are summarised here:

- *Kidney disease.* Any disease that affects renal blood flow (e.g. renal artery stenosis) or renal function (e.g. glomerulonephritis, renal failure) can lead to hypertension. Disruption of the blood supply stimulates the renin–angiotensin–aldosterone system, with resulting vasoconstriction and sodium and water retention. Altered kidney function affects the elimination of water and electrolytes, leading to hypertension.
- *Coarctation of the aorta.* Coarctation of the aorta is narrowing of the aorta, usually just distal to the subclavian arteries. Reduced renal and peripheral blood flow stimulates the renin–angiotensin–aldosterone system and local vasoconstrictive responses, raising the blood pressure.

A marked difference between pressures in the upper and lower extremities is common, with weak pulses and poor capillary refill in the lower extremities.

- *Endocrine disorders.* Adrenal gland disorders such as Cushing's syndrome and primary aldosteronism can cause hypertension. A rare tumour of the adrenal medulla, *pheochromocytoma*, causes persistent or intermittent hypertension. Other endocrine disorders such as hyperthyroidism and pituitary disorders also can lead to hypertension.
- *Neurological disorders.* Increased intracranial pressure causes an elevated blood pressure as the body attempts to maintain cerebral blood flow. Disorders that interfere with autonomic nervous system regulation (such as high spinal cord injury) may allow the sympathetic nervous system to predominate, increasing systemic vascular resistance and blood pressure.
- *Drug use.* Oestrogen and oral contraceptive use may lead to hypertension, possibly by prompting sodium and water retention and affecting the renin–angiotensin–aldosterone system. Stimulant drugs, such as cocaine and methamphetamines, increase systemic vascular resistance and cardiac output, resulting in hypertension.
- *Pregnancy.* About 10% of all pregnant women are hypertensive. Hypertension may pre-date pregnancy or occur as a direct response to the pregnancy. The mechanism of pregnancy-induced hypertension (PIH) is unclear. It is a significant cause of maternal and foetal morbidity and mortality and requires careful perinatal management.

The pattern of secondary hypertension varies, depending on its cause. Pheochromocytoma may cause attacks of hypertension that last for minutes to hours, accompanied by anxiety, palpitations, diaphoresis, pallor and nausea and vomiting. Primary aldosteronism may cause hypertension, weakness, paraesthesias, polyuria and nocturia (see the chapter 'A person-centred approach to assessing the endocrine system'). Symptoms of kidney disease accompany hypertension when a renal disorder is the cause.

The following diagnostic tests may be ordered to differentiate primary from secondary hypertension:

- *Renal function studies* and *urinalysis* to identify renal causes of hypertension. Elevated serum urea and creatinine, haematuria, proteinuria and casts often indicate kidney disease.
- *Serum potassium* is decreased in hyperaldosteronism.
- *Blood chemistries*, including serum electrolytes, glucose and lipid studies, are done to detect abnormalities indicative of endocrine or CVD.
- *Intravenous pyelography (IVP), renal ultrasonography, renal arteriography and CT or MRI* may be done when secondary hypertension is suspected.

Interprofessional and nursing care for the person with secondary hypertension is the same as that for primary hypertension, discussed in the previous section. In addition, the underlying process is treated. See chapters covering specific disorders for more information about treatment measures.

HYPERTENSIVE CRISIS

Some people with hypertension may, for reasons not clearly understood, develop rapid, significant elevations in systolic and/or diastolic pressures. See Figure 31.6 for management considerations. Prolonged severe hypertension damages the walls of the arterioles and renal blood vessels and may lead to intravascular coagulation and acute renal failure.

People presenting with a hypertensive emergency may have manifestations such as headache, confusion, swelling of the optic nerve (papilloedema), blurred vision, restlessness and motor and sensory deficits. Manifestations of hypertensive emergencies are listed in the 'Manifestations' box.

MANIFESTATIONS Hypertensive emergencies

- Rapid onset
- Blurred vision, papilloedema
- Systolic pressure > 180 mmHg
- Diastolic pressure > 120 mmHg
- Headache
- Confusion
- Motor and sensory deficits
- Other vasodilating agents that may be used are outlined in Table 31.2. Management also focuses on treating any underlying or coexisting heart, kidney and CNS disorders.

TABLE 31.2 Intravenous drugs used to treat hypertensive emergencies

DRUG	ONSET	DURATION	NURSING IMPLICATIONS
Sodium nitroprusside dihydrate	Seconds	1 to 2 min	• Effective, easy to titrate • May cause nausea, vomiting, muscle twitching, sweating • Use with caution in increased intracranial pressure
Glyceryl trinitrate	2 to 5 min	5 to 10 min	• Used when coronary ischaemia accompanies hypertension • May cause headache, vomiting • Tolerance may develop with prolonged use
Diazoxide	1 to 2 min	4 to 24 h	• Avoided in people with coronary artery disease • Used with beta-blockers and diuretics • Painful if it enters tissues
Hydralazine	10 to 30 min	2 to 6 h	• May be used for hypertension associated with eclampsia • Avoided in people with CHD • May cause tachycardia, flushing, headache, vomiting, angina

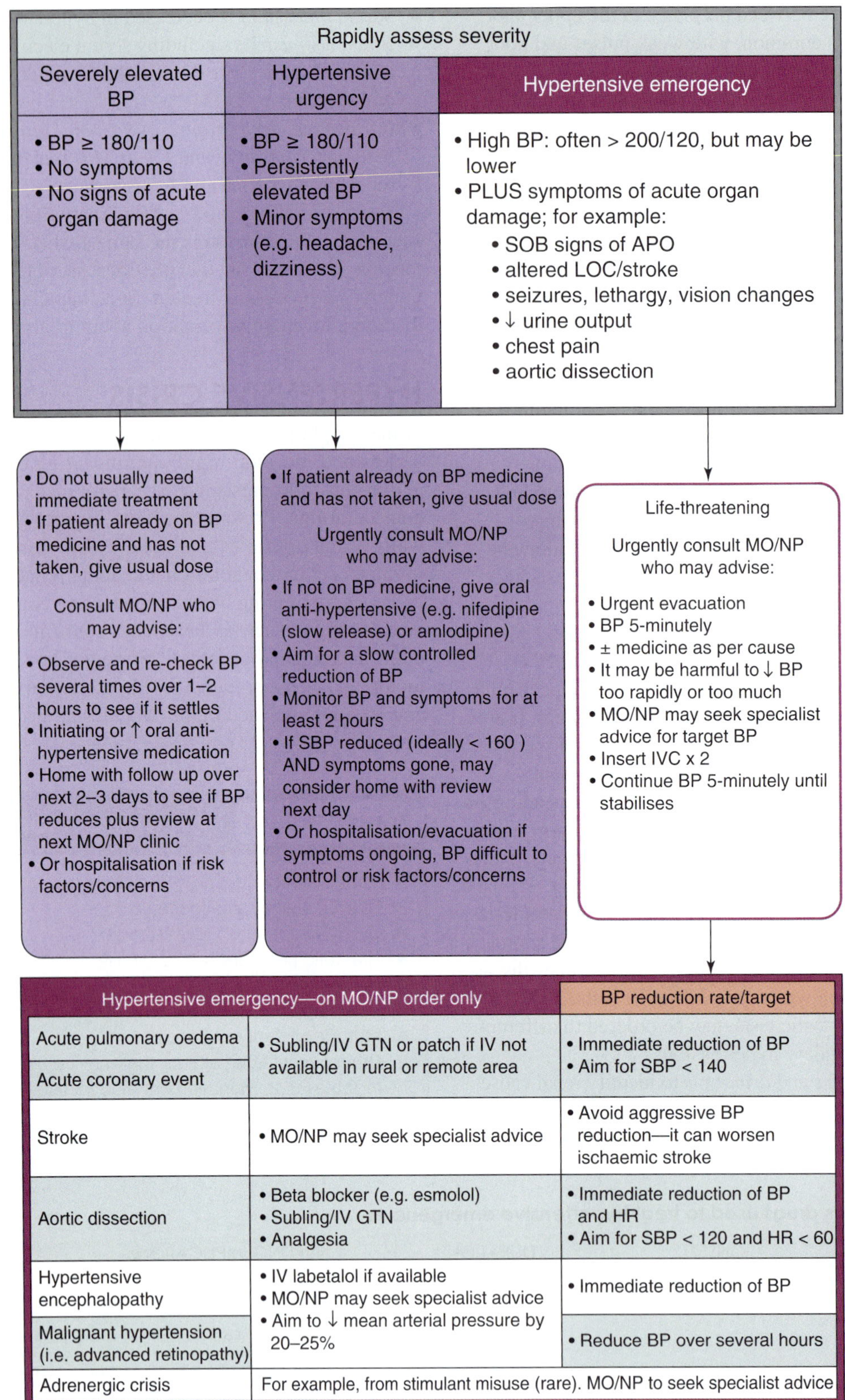

FIGURE 31.6 ***Hypertensive crisis definitions, characteristics and management***

APO - acute pulmonary oedema; BP = blood pressure; GTN = glyceryl trinitrate; HR = heart rate; IV = intravenous; IVC = intravenous cannula; LOC = loss of consciousness; MO = medical officer; NP = Nurse Practitioner; SOB = shortness of breath; SBP = systolic blood pressure

Source: Queensland Health, Royal Flying Doctor Service (Queensland Section) (2022) *Primary clinical care manual* (11th ed.). Cairns: Office of Rural and Remote Health, Queensland Government, p. 117. Retrieved from https://www.health.qld.gov.au/__data/assets/pdf_file/0011/1160003/PCCM_11th_ed.pdf.

Nursing care for people with a hypertensive emergency focuses on continuous monitoring of the blood pressure and titrating drugs as ordered to achieve desired blood pressure. Reassure the person and family of the rapid effect of prescribed drugs. Provide psychological and emotional support as needed. Maintain an attitude of confidence that the treatment will achieve the desired effect. Following resolution of the hypertensive crisis, review causes of the crisis. Educate the person and family on measures to effectively manage hypertension and prevent future hypertensive emergencies.

Disorders of the aorta and its branches

The aorta and its branches may be affected by occlusions, aneurysms and inflammations. These disorders may be chronic or acute and life threatening (e.g. a thoracic dissection). This section focuses on aneurysms of the aorta and its branches.

THE PERSON WITH AN ANEURYSM

An **aneurysm** is an abnormal dilation of a blood vessel, commonly at a site of a weakness or tear in the vessel wall. Aneurysms commonly affect the aorta and peripheral arteries because of the high pressure in these vessels. An aneurysm also may develop in the ventricular wall, usually affecting the left ventricle. Most arterial aneurysms are caused by arteriosclerosis or atherosclerosis; trauma also may lead to aneurysm formation.

Arterial aneurysms are most common in men over age 50, most of whom are asymptomatic at the time of diagnosis. Hypertension is a major contributing factor in the development of some types of aortic aneurysms.

FAST FACTS

- The incidence of aortic-aneurysm-related deaths for males in Australia in 2020 was 595.
- The incidence of aortic-aneurysm-related deaths for females in Australia in 2020 was 592.
- Aortic aneurysm and dissection in 2020 accounted for 0.67% of all deaths in Australia (ABS, 2021)

Pathophysiology and manifestations

Aneurysms form due to weakness of the arterial wall. The main structural proteins of the aorta are collagen and elastin. Collagen provides tensile strength of the vessel, preventing excessive dilation. Elastin allows vessel recoil, during which the vessel returns to its original size following systole. This recoil provides continued propulsion of the bolus of blood expelled from the ventricle. Elastin is a primary component of internal elastic lamina, which separates the intimal and medial layers of the aorta and of the media, the smooth muscle layer of the aorta. Destruction of elastin can lead to abnormal dilation of the vessel; collagen destruction can allow the vessel to rupture (Tseng, 2021).

True aneurysms are caused by slow weakening of the arterial wall due to the long-term, eroding effects of atherosclerosis and hypertension. True aneurysms affect all three layers of the vessel wall and most are fusiform and circumferential. *Fusiform aneurysms* are spindle shaped and taper at both ends. Circumferential aneurysms involve the entire diameter of the vessel (see Figure 31.7). They generally grow slowly but progressively. Their length and diameter vary considerably among people. A large fusiform aneurysm may affect most of the ascending aorta as well as a large portion of the abdominal aorta.

False aneurysms, also known as traumatic aneurysms, are caused by a traumatic break in the vessel wall rather than weakening of the vessel. They often are *saccular*, shaped like small outpouchings (sacs) on a portion of the vessel wall (see Figure 31.8). A *berry aneurysm* is a type of saccular aneurysm. They are often small (less than 2 cm in diameter), caused by congenital weakness in the tunica media of the artery. Berry aneurysms are commonly found in the circle of Willis in the brain.

Dissecting aneurysms are unique, developing when a break or tear in the tunica intima and media allows blood to invade or *dissect* the layers of the vessel wall. The blood usually is contained by the adventitia, forming a saccular or longitudinal aneurysm.

Aneurysms affect different segments of the aorta and its branches. Their manifestations generally are due to pressure

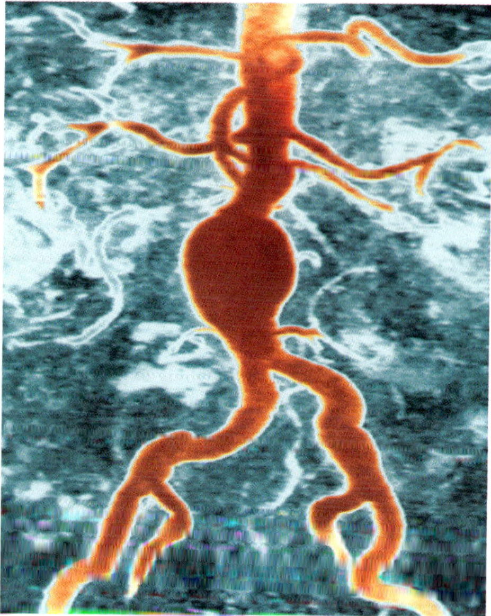

FIGURE 31.7 *A magnetic resonance angiogram (MRA) showing a circumferential aneurysm of the lower abdominal aorta*

Source: Zephyr/Science Photo Library.

TABLE 31.3 Manifestations and complications of aortic aneurysms

TYPE OR LOCATION	MANIFESTATIONS	COMPLICATIONS
Thoracic	• May be asymptomatic • Back, neck or substernal pain • Dyspnoea, stridor or brassy cough if pressing on trachea • Hoarseness and dysphagia if pressing on oesophagus or laryngeal nerve • Oedema of the face and neck • Distended neck veins	• Rupture and haemorrhage
Abdominal	• Pulsating abdominal mass • Aortic calcification noted on x-ray • Mild to severe midabdominal or lumbar back pain • Cool, cyanotic extremities if iliac arteries are involved • Claudication (ischaemic pain with exercise, relieved by rest)	• Peripheral emboli to lower extremities • Rupture and haemorrhage
Aortic dissection	• Abrupt, severe, ripping or tearing pain in area of aneurysm • Mild or marked hypertension early • Weak or absent pulses and blood pressure in upper extremities • Syncope	• Haemorrhage • Kidney failure • MI, heart failure, cardiac tamponade • Sepsis • Weakness or paralysis of lower extremities

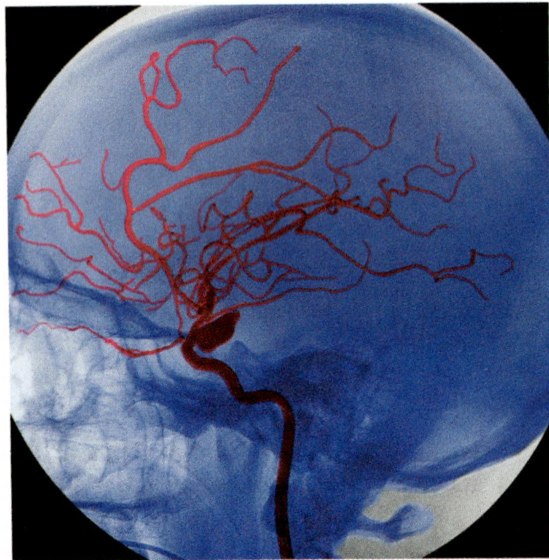

FIGURE 31.8 ***An angiogram showing a saccular (berry) aneurysm in the carotid artery of a 50-year-old man***

Source: Simon Fraser/RNC, Newcastle/Science Photo Library.

of the aneurysm on adjacent structures. Table 31.3 summarises the manifestations and complications of various types of aortic aneurysms.

Thoracic aortic aneurysms

In Australia, *thoracic aortic aneurysms* (see Figure 31.9) accounted for approximately 15.5% of all aortic aneurysm admissions. Thoracic aortic aneurysms usually result from weakening of the aortic wall by arteriosclerosis and hypertension. Other causes include trauma, coarctation of the aorta, tertiary syphilis, fungal infections and Marfan syndrome. The syphilis spirochete can invade and weaken aortic smooth muscle, causing an aneurysm to develop as long as 20 years after the primary infection. Marfan syndrome fragments elastic fibres of the aortic media, weakening the vessel wall. The 'Genetic considerations' box discusses genetic links associated with thoracic aortic aneurysms.

Thoracic aneurysms frequently are asymptomatic. When present, manifestations are caused by the effects of the aneurysm on blood flow (to the coronary arteries and great vessels of the head and upper body) and pressure placed by distended aorta on surrounding structures. Consequently, manifestations vary by the location, size and growth rate of the aneurysm. Substernal, neck or back pain may occur. Pressure on the trachea, oesophagus, laryngeal nerve or superior vena cava may cause dyspnoea, stridor, cough, difficult or painful swallowing, hoarseness, oedema of the face and neck, and distended neck veins.

Aneurysms of the ascending aorta typically cause angina due to disruption of blood flow into the coronary arteries. Heart failure may develop as a result of disruption of the aortic valve and regurgitation of blood back into the left ventricle. Aneurysms of the aortic arch often cause dysphagia, dyspnoea, hoarseness, confusion and dizziness (due to disrupted cerebral blood flow). Thrombi that form within a thoracic aneurysm can embolise, causing a stroke, renal or mesenteric ischaemia, or ischaemia of the lower extremities. Aneurysms of the thoracic aorta tend to enlarge progressively and may rupture, causing death (Tseng, 2021).

GENETIC CONSIDERATIONS
THORACIC AORTIC ANEURYSMS

About 30% of people with aortic aneurysms have a family history of the disorder (Luyckx et al., 2022). There are now 40 genes known to be associated with thoracic aneurysm risk. Regrettably, mortality rates can be as high as 70%. Therefore, timely identification and management is critical. Prophylactic surgery, which in itself carries significant risks, is currently the only curative intervention available.

Abdominal aortic aneurysms

Abdominal aortic aneurysms are associated with arteriosclerosis and hypertension. Increasing age and smoking are believed to contribute as well. Most abdominal aortic aneurysms are found in adults over age 70. The vast majority (over 90%) develop below the renal arteries, usually where the abdominal aorta branches to form the iliac arteries (Rahimi, 2021). In Australia in 2020, a little over 3,220 people were admitted with an abdominal aneurysm (AIHW, 2021).

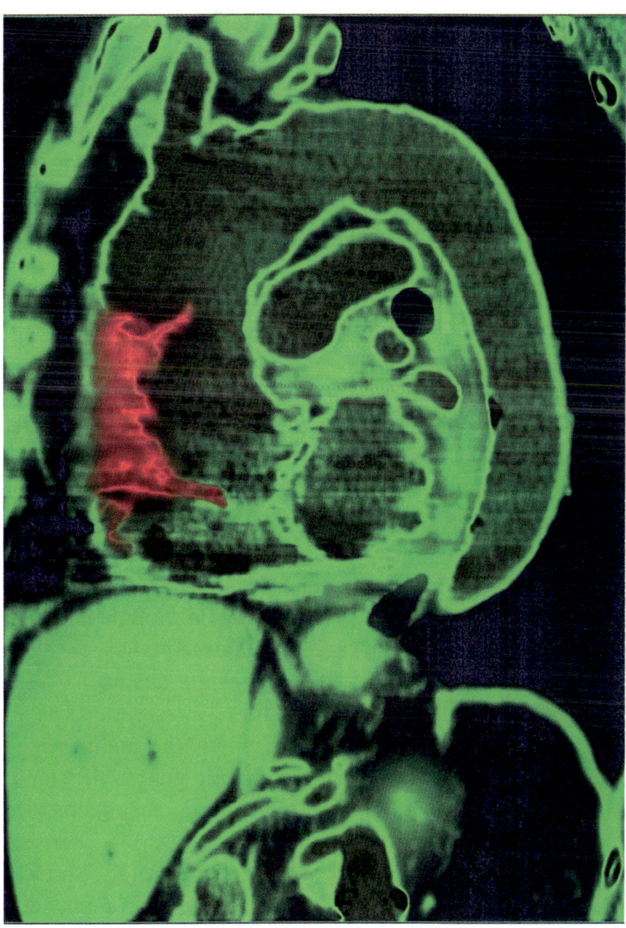

FIGURE 31.9 ***In an aortic dissection, a tear in the intima and media of the artery allows blood to invade and dissect the wall of the aorta***

Source: Cavallini James/BSIP/Science Photo Library.

Most abdominal aneurysms are asymptomatic, but a pulsating mass in the mid and upper abdomen and a bruit over the mass are found on exam. When pain is present, it may be constant or intermittent, usually felt in the midabdominal region or lower back. Its intensity may range from mild discomfort to severe pain. Pain intensity often correlates with the size and severity of the aneurysm. Severe pain may indicate impending rupture.

Sluggish blood flow within the aneurysm may cause thrombi (blood clots) to form. These can become emboli (circulating clots), travelling to the lower extremities and occluding peripheral arteries. Aneurysms generally enlarge by approximately 0.2–0.8 mm/year; eventually they may rupture, resulting in haemorrhage and hypovolaemic shock (Rahimi, 2021).

Popliteal and femoral aneurysms

Most popliteal and femoral aneurysms are due to arteriosclerosis. They are often bilateral and usually affect men.

Popliteal aneurysms (see Figure 31.10) may be asymptomatic. Manifestations, if any, are due to decreased blood flow to the lower extremity and include intermittent **claudication** (cramping or pain in the leg muscles brought on by exercise and relieved by rest), rest pain and numbness. A pulsating

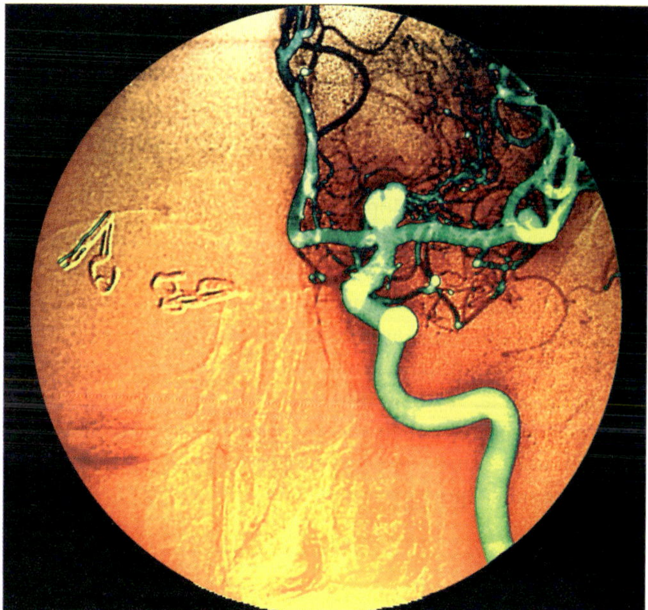

FIGURE 31.10 ***An angiogram showing several popliteal aneurysms***

Source: Zephyr/Science Photo Library.

mass may be palpable in the popliteal fossa (behind the knee). Thrombosis and embolism are complications; gangrene may result, often necessitating amputation.

A *femoral aneurysm* usually is detected as a pulsating mass in the femoral area. The manifestations are similar to those of popliteal aneurysms, resulting from impaired blood flow. Femoral aneurysms may rupture.

Aortic dissections

Dissection is a life-threatening emergency caused by a tear in the intima of the aorta with haemorrhage into the media. The haemorrhage dissects or splits the vessel wall, forming a blood-filled channel between its layers. Dissection can occur anywhere along the aorta. *Type A dissection* (also called *proximal dissection*) affects the ascending aorta; *type B dissection* (*distal dissection*) is limited to the descending aorta.

Hypertension is a major predisposing factor for aortic dissection, accounting for 70% of aortic dissections. Cystic medial necrosis also is a major risk factor. Other risk factors include male gender, advancing age, pregnancy, congenital defects of the aortic valve, coarctation of the aorta, deceleration chest injury, cocaine use and inflammatory aortitis. Important, but less common, are iatrogenic causes (caused by healthcare intervention), which include aortic and mitral valve replacements, coronary artery bypass graft surgery and cardiac catheterisation (Mancini, 2022).

Dissection of the thoracic aortic walls progresses along the length of the vessel, moving both proximally and distally. As the aneurysm expands, pressure may prevent the aortic valve from closing or may occlude the branches of the aorta. Descending aortic dissection may extend into the renal, iliac or femoral arteries.

The primary symptom of an aortic dissection is sudden, excruciating pain. The pain, often described as a ripping or tearing sensation, is usually over the area of dissection. Thoracic dissections cause chest or back pain. Other symptoms may include syncope, dyspnoea and weakness. The blood pressure may initially be increased, but rapidly falls and is often inaudible as the dissection occludes blood flow. Peripheral pulses are absent for the same reason.

Complications develop if major arteries are affected. Obstruction of the carotid artery causes neurological symptoms such as weakness or paralysis. The myocardium, kidneys or bowel may become ischaemic or infarct if blood flow to the coronary arteries, renal arteries or mesenteric artery is affected. Acute aortic regurgitation may develop with dissection of the ascending aorta. With treatment, the long-term prognosis is generally good, although the in-hospital mortality rate with medical management is approximately 60% and following surgery remains quite high at 30% (Mancini, 2022).

INTERPROFESSIONAL CARE

Most aneurysms are asymptomatic, detected through a routine physical examination. Treatment depends on the size of the aneurysm. Small, asymptomatic aneurysms may not be treated or are medically managed; large aneurysms (> 5 cm) at risk of rupture require surgery.

Diagnosis

Diagnostic studies done to establish the diagnosis and determine the size and location of the aneurysm may include:

- *chest x-ray* to visualise thoracic aortic aneurysms
- *abdominal ultrasonography* to diagnose abdominal aortic aneurysms
- *transoesophageal echocardiography* to identify the specific location and extent of a thoracic aneurysm and to visualise a dissecting aneurysm
- *contrast-enhanced CT* or *MRI* allows precise measurements of aneurysm size
- *angiography*uses contrast solution injected into the aorta or involved vessel to visualise the precise size and location of the aneurysm.

Medications

Thoracic aortic aneurysms may be treated with long-term beta-blocker therapy and additional antihypertensive drugs as needed to control heart rate and blood pressure.

People with aortic dissection are initially treated with intravenous beta-blockers to reduce the heart rate to about 60 bpm. Sodium nitroprusside infusion is started concurrently to reduce the systolic pressure to 120 mmHg or less. Calcium channel blockers also may be used. Constant monitoring of vital signs, haemodynamic pressures and urine output is vital to ensure adequate perfusion of vital organs.

Following surgical correction of an aneurysm, anticoagulant therapy may be initiated. Heparin therapy is used initially, with conversion to oral anticoagulation prior to discharge. Many people are maintained indefinitely on anticoagulant therapy; others may use lifelong, low-dose aspirin therapy to reduce the risk of clot formation.

Surgery

Operative repair of aortic aneurysms is indicated when the aneurysm is symptomatic or expanding rapidly. Ascending thoracic aneurysms of more than 5.5 cm and descending thoracic aneurysms of 6.5cm or more should be surgically repaired; asymptomatic abdominal aneurysms greater than 5 cm in diameter may be repaired, depending on the person's operative risk factors. It is recommended that individuals with Marfan syndrome or familial aneurysms should be repaired at 0.5 cm or sooner (Tseng, 2021).

Endovascular aneurysm repair (EVAR) utilising a minimally invasive approach is increasingly used to treat abdominal and thoracic aortic aneurysms. Multiple factors will be considered when surgical approach is planned. It is interesting to note a review by Yei et al. (2022) found that although an open approach is associated with higher 30-day mortality rates and more perioperative complications, it results in lower 6-year mortality rates, rupture and the need for re-intervention.

An open surgical procedure in which the aneurysm is excised and replaced with a synthetic fabric graft is the standard treatment for expanding abdominal aortic aneurysms (see Figure 31.11). Although the aneurysm walls may be excised, they usually are left intact and used to cover the graft. Surgical repair of thoracic aneurysms is similar but more complex due to major vessels exiting at the aortic arch. Cardiopulmonary bypass is required if the ascending aorta is involved. The aortic valve also may be replaced during surgery.

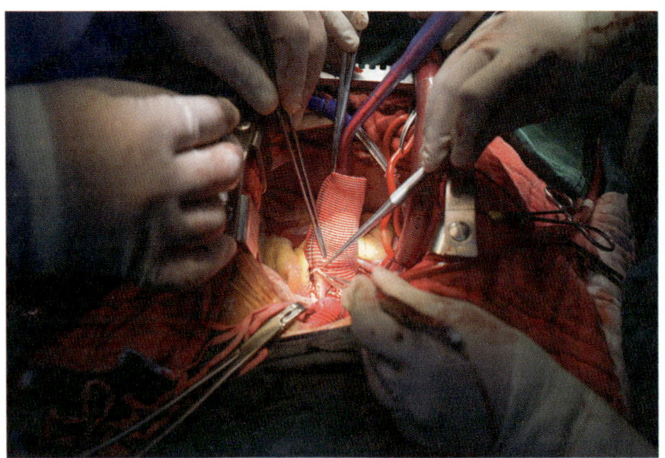

FIGURE 31.11 ***Repair of an abdominal aortic aneurysm. The aorta is exposed and clamped between the renal and iliac arteries. Atherosclerotic plaque and thrombotic material are removed. A synthetic graft is used to replace the aneurysm. The aneurysm walls are then sutured around the graft***

Source: Chanawit Sitthisombat/123RF.

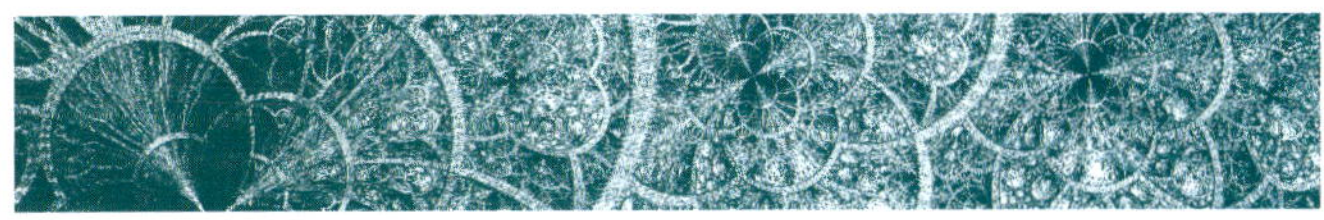

Nursing care

Assessment

Focused assessment for the person with a suspected aortic aneurysm includes:

- *Health history*: complaints of chest, back or abdominal pain; extremity weakness; shortness of breath, cough, difficult or painful swallowing, hoarseness; history of hypertension, coronary heart disease, heart failure or peripheral vascular disease.
- *Physical examination*: vital signs, including blood pressure in upper and lower extremities; peripheral pulses; skin colour and temperature; neck veins; abdominal exam, including gentle palpation for masses and auscultation for bruits; neurological exam, including level of consciousness (LOC), sensation and movement of extremities.

Nursing diagnoses and interventions

Nursing care for people with an aneurysm of the aorta or its branches focuses on monitoring and maintaining tissue perfusion, relieving pain and reducing anxiety. Nursing care usually is acute, precipitated by a complication or surgical repair of the aneurysm.

Risk of ineffective tissue perfusion

People with aortic aneurysms are at risk of impaired tissue perfusion due to aneurysm rupture with resulting haemorrhage and lack of blood flow to tissues distal to the rupture. In addition, thrombi often form within the aneurysm and may become emboli, obstructing distal arterial blood flow.

NURSING CARE OF THE PERSON **having surgery of the aorta**

PREOPERATIVE CARE

- As time permits, provide routine preoperative care and teaching as outlined in the chapter 'Nursing care of people having surgery'. *People having vascular surgery have similar preoperative nursing care needs to other people having major abdominal or thoracic surgery. If emergency surgery is required, time for preoperative care and teaching may be limited.*
- Implement measures to reduce fear and anxiety:
  a. Orient to the intensive care unit, if appropriate.
  b. Describe and explain the reason for all equipment and tubes, such as cardiac monitors, ventilators, nasogastric tubes, urinary catheters, intravenous lines and fluids, and intra-arterial lines.
  c. Explain what to expect following surgery (sights, sounds, frequency of taking vital signs, dressings, pain relief measures, communication strategies).
  d. Allow time for questions and expression of fears and concerns.

  These explanations provide a sense of control for the person and family.
- Monitor for and implement care to reduce the risk of aneurysm rupture (see the following section). *People with a rapidly expanding or symptomatic aneurysm are at risk of rupture prior to surgical repair.*

POSTOPERATIVE CARE

- Provide routine postoperative care and specific measures as ordered by the doctor. *People undergoing aneurysm repair require nursing care similar to that provided to all people with major thoracic or abdominal surgery, in addition to specific measures related to vascular surgery.*
- Maintain fluid replacement and blood or volume expanders as ordered. Promptly report changes in vital signs, level of consciousness and urine output. *Hypovolaemic shock may develop due to blood loss during surgery, third spacing, inadequate fluid replacement and/or haemorrhage if graft separation or leakage occurs.*

CONSIDERATION FOR PRACTICE

Monitor for and report manifestations of graft leakage:

a. ecchymoses of the scrotum, perineum or penis; a new or expanding haematoma
b. increased abdominal girth
c. weak or absent peripheral pulses; tachycardia; hypotension
d. decreased motor function or sensation in the extremities
e. fall in haemoglobin and haematocrit
f. increasing abdominal, pelvic, back or groin pain
g. decreasing urinary output (less than 30 mL/h in adults)
h. decreasing CVP, pulmonary artery pressure or pulmonary artery wedge pressure.

These manifestations may signal graft leakage and possible haemorrhage. Pain may be due to pressure from an expanding haematoma or bowel ischaemia. Decreased renal perfusion causes the glomerular filtration rate and urine output to fall.

- Report manifestations of lower extremity embolism: pain and numbness in lower extremities, decreasing pulses and pale, cool or cyanotic skin. *Pulses may be absent for 4 to 12 hours postoperatively due to vasospasm; however, absent pulses with pain, changes in sensation and a pale, cool extremity are indicative of arterial occlusion.*
- Report manifestations of bowel ischaemia or gangrene: abdominal pain and distension, occult or fresh blood in stools, and diarrhoea. *Bowel ischaemia may result from an embolism or occur as a complication of surgery.*
- Report manifestations of impaired renal function: urine output less than 30 mL/h, fixed specific gravity, increasing serum urea and creatinine levels. *Hypovolaemia or clamping of the aorta during surgery may impair renal perfusion, leading to acute renal failure.*
- Report manifestations of spinal cord ischaemia: lower extremity weakness or paraplegia. *Impaired spinal cord perfusion may lead to ischaemia and impaired function.*

> **CONSIDERATION FOR PRACTICE**
> **Immediately report manifestations of impending rupture, expansion or dissection of the aneurysm: increased pain; discrepancy between upper and lower extremity blood pressures and peripheral pulses; increased mass size; change in LOC or motor or sensory function; laboratory results. Rapid expansion may indicate increased risk of rupture, with resulting haemorrhage, shock and possible death. Elective or planned surgery may rapidly become emergency surgery to prevent complications.**

- Implement interventions to reduce the risk of aneurysm rupture:
  a. Maintain bed rest with legs flat.
  b. Maintain a calm environment, implementing measures to reduce psychological stress.
  c. Prevent straining during defecation and instruct to avoid holding the breath while moving.
  d. Administer beta-blockers and antihypertensives as prescribed.

  Activity, stress and the Valsalva manoeuvre increase blood pressure, increasing the risk of rupture. Elevating or crossing the legs restricts peripheral blood flow and increases pressure in the aorta or iliac arteries. Beta-blockers and antihypertensives often are ordered to reduce pressure in the dilated vessel.

> **CONSIDERATION FOR PRACTICE**
> **Report manifestations of arterial thrombosis or embolism: absent peripheral pulses; a pale or cyanotic, cool extremity; severe, diffuse abdominal pain with guarding; or increased groin, lumbar or lower extremity pain. Sluggish blood flow within the aneurysm often causes thrombi to form. These thrombi can break loose, becoming emboli that can occlude peripheral arteries or arteries to the kidneys or mesentery. Arterial occlusion may necessitate emergency surgery to restore blood flow and prevent tissue infarct or gangrene.**

- Continuously monitor cardiac rhythm. Report complaints of chest pain or changes in ECG tracing. Administer oxygen as indicated. *Aortic dissection and repair place the person at significant risk of MI, a major cause of postoperative mortality and morbidity (Mancini, 2022). Rapid identification and treatment of this complication can reduce the risk of death or long-term adverse effects of MI.*

> **CONSIDERATION FOR PRACTICE**
> **Immediately report changes in mental status or symptoms of peripheral neurological impairment (weakness, paraesthesias, paralysis). The expanding aneurysm or dissection can affect carotid and cerebral blood flow or spinal cord perfusion, leading to neurological symptoms. Immediate restoration of blood flow is vital to prevent permanent neurological deficits.**

Risk of injury

Potent antihypertensive drugs often are given intravenously to reduce the pressure on an expanding or dissecting aneurysm. Continuous monitoring of infusions and haemodynamic parameters such as arterial pressure, pulmonary pressures and cardiac output is vital to ensure that adequate tissue perfusion is maintained during infusions of these potent drugs.

- Continuously monitor arterial pressure and haemodynamic parameters as indicated. Promptly report results outside the specified parameters to the doctor. *Many of the drugs used are effective within minutes. Responses vary among individuals, particularly in the older adult, necessitating continuous monitoring.*
- Monitor urine output hourly. Report output less than 30 mL/h. *The kidneys are very sensitive to reduced perfusion pressure; inadequate renal blood flow can lead to acute kidney failure.*

> **CONSIDERATION FOR PRACTICE**
> **Use an infusion control device for all drug infusions. These devices prevent accidental or inadvertent changes in the rate of the infusion and dose of the drug.**

Anxiety

People with aortic aneurysms often are highly anxious because of the urgent nature of the disorder. The nurse must manage the anxiety levels of both the person and family members to effectively address physiological care needs. Stress reduction also is necessary to help maintain the blood pressure within desired limits.

- Explain all procedures and treatments, using simple and understandable terms. *Simplified explanations are necessary when anxiety levels interfere with learning and understanding.*
- Respond to all questions honestly, using a calm, empathetic but matter-of-fact manner. *Honesty with the person and family promotes trust and provides reassurance that the true nature of the situation is not being 'hidden' from them.*
- Provide care in a calm, efficient manner. *Using a calm manner, even during preparations for emergency surgery, reassures the person and family that although the situation is critical, the staff is prepared to handle things effectively.*
- Spend as much time as possible with the person. Allow supportive family members to remain with the person when possible. *The presence of a health professional and supportive family member reassures the person that they are not alone in facing this crisis.*

Community-based care

Topics to discuss when preparing people and their families for home care or care in a community-based setting depend on the treatment plan. Discuss the following topics when surgical repair is not immediately planned and the aneurysm will be monitored:

- measures to control hypertension, including lifestyle and prescribed drugs
- the benefits of smoking cessation
- manifestations of increasing aneurysm size or complications to report to the doctor.

Following surgery, discuss the following topics in preparing the person and family for home care:

- wound care and preventing infection; manifestations of impaired healing or infection to be reported
- prescribed antihypertensive and anticoagulant medications and their expected and unintended effects
- the importance of adequate rest and nutrition for healing
- measures to prevent constipation and straining at stool (such as increasing fluid and fibre in the diet)
- the importance of avoiding prolonged sitting, lifting heavy objects, engaging in strenuous exercise and having sexual intercourse until approved by the doctor (usually 6 to 12 weeks)
- signs and symptoms of complications to report to the doctor.

Provide referrals to a home health agency or community health service as necessary. Referrals are especially important for older adults and their caregivers, who may require additional assistance with the complex care needs.

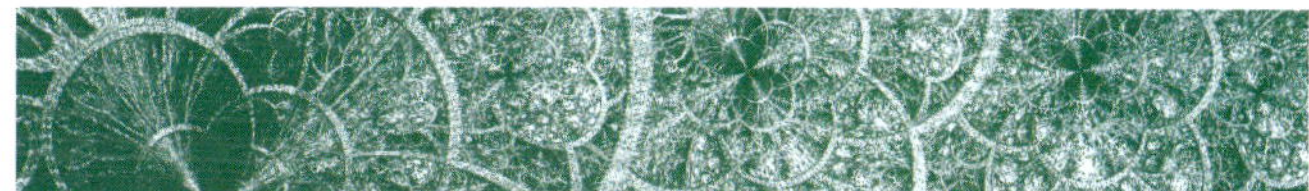

Disorders of the peripheral arteries

Disorders that impair peripheral arterial blood flow may be acute (e.g. arterial thrombosis) or chronic (e.g. peripheral arteriosclerosis). Chronic occlusive disorders may be due to structural defects of the arterial walls or spasm of affected arteries. Impaired peripheral arterial circulation limits the availability of oxygen and nutrients to the tissues and can have significant adverse effects. This section focuses on acute and chronic disorders affecting peripheral arteries. The nurse's role in caring for people with peripheral arterial disorders focuses on maintaining tissue perfusion and educating the person and family about the disorder and its management.

Physiology review

Peripheral arteries are the part of the systemic circulation that delivers oxygen and nutrients to the skin and the extremities. Arterial walls have three layers: the intima, which includes the endothelium and a layer of connective tissue and the basement membrane; the media, composed of smooth muscle and elastic fibres; and the adventitia, a thin layer of connective tissue that contains collagen and elastic fibres. The smooth muscle of peripheral arteries controls blood flow as it contracts and relaxes. Contraction narrows the vessel lumen (**vasoconstriction**), whereas smooth muscle relaxation expands the vessel (**vasodilation**). Peripheral arteries become progressively smaller; arterioles are less than 0.5 mm in diameter and are composed primarily of smooth muscle. The arterioles control blood flow through the capillary beds where gas, nutrient and waste product exchange occurs. Capillary walls are very thin, consisting of a single layer of endothelial cells surrounded by a thin basement membrane.

Blood flows from an area of higher pressure to an area of lower pressure. *Resistance* opposes blood flow. Resistance is created by friction of the blood itself, although the primary determinants of vascular resistance are the diameter and length of the blood vessel. See the physiology review section earlier in this chapter under 'Disorders of blood pressure regulation' for more information about factors that determine vessel resistance.

THE PERSON WITH PERIPHERAL VASCULAR DISEASE

Arteriosclerosis is the most common chronic arterial disorder, characterised by thickening, loss of elasticity and calcification of arterial walls. **Atherosclerosis** is a form of arteriosclerosis in which deposits of fat and fibrin obstruct and harden the arteries. In the peripheral circulation, these pathological changes impair the blood supply to peripheral tissues, particularly the lower extremities. This is known as **peripheral vascular disease (PVD)** or peripheral artery disease (PAD).

Incidence and risk factors

PVD usually affects people over 65; men are more often affected than women. Approximately 15% of Australians are affected. Rates of PVD are more than two times higher among Indigenous Australians than among non-Indigenous Australians (AIHW, 2022; Chuter et al., 2022).

Risk factors for PVD are similar to those for atherosclerosis and CHD (see the chapter 'Nursing care of people with coronary heart disease'). The main preventable risk factors for peripheral

FAST FACTS

- PVD is a common manifestation of atherosclerosis, particularly in older men.
- Peripheral vascular disease refers to diseases of arteries outside the heart and brain. It occurs when fatty deposits build up in the inner walls of these arteries and affect blood circulation, mainly in the arteries leading to the legs and feet. It ranges from asymptomatic disease, through to pain on walking, to pain at rest and limb-threatening reduced blood supply that can lead to amputation.
- Regular daily exercise is a primary intervention for all types of peripheral arterial disease to promote development of collateral circulation and maintain tissue perfusion.
- Individuals with PVD have a 3–4 times increased risk of myocardial infarction (Aitken, 2020).

vascular disease are diabetes, cigarette smoking, hypertension, hyperviscosity, hypercholesterolaemia and obesity (Stephens, 2022).

Pathophysiology

The pathophysiology of atherosclerosis is detailed in the chapter 'Nursing care of people with coronary heart disease'. Atherosclerotic lesions involve both the intima and the media of the involved arteries. Lesions typically develop in large and midsized arteries, particularly the abdominal aorta, iliac, femoral popliteal, tibial peroneal arteries.

Plaque tends to form at arterial bifurcations. The vessel lumen is progressively obstructed, decreasing blood flow to the lower extremities. Tissue hypoxia or anoxia results. With gradual obstruction of the vessel, collateral circulation often develops. However, it is usually not adequate to supply tissue needs, especially when metabolic demand increases (e.g. during exercise). Manifestations typically develop only when the vessel is occluded by 60% or more.

Manifestations and complications

Pain is the primary symptom of peripheral atherosclerosis. Intermittent claudication—a cramping or aching pain in the calves of the legs, the thighs and the buttocks that occurs with a predictable level of activity—is characteristic of PVD. The pain is often accompanied by weakness and is relieved by rest.

Rest pain, in contrast, occurs during periods of inactivity. It is often described as a burning sensation in the lower legs. Rest pain increases when the legs are elevated and decreases when the legs are dependent (e.g. hanging over the side of the bed). The legs also may feel cold or numb along with the pain. Sensation is diminished and the muscles may atrophy.

Peripheral pulses may be decreased or absent. A bruit may be heard over large affected arteries, such as the femoral artery and the abdominal aorta. The legs are pale when elevated, but often are dark red when dependent (*dependent rubor*). The skin often is thin, shiny and hairless, with discoloured areas. Toenails may be thickened. Areas of skin breakdown and ulceration may be evident. Oedema may develop with severe PVD. See the 'Manifestations' box for manifestations of peripheral atherosclerosis.

Complications of peripheral atherosclerosis include gangrene and extremity amputation, rupture of abdominal aortic aneurysms and possible infection and sepsis.

MANIFESTATIONS Peripheral atherosclerosis

- Intermittent claudication
- Rest pain
- Paraesthesias (numbness, decreased sensation)
- Diminished or absent peripheral pulses
- Pallor with extremity elevation, dependent rubor when dependent
- Thin, shiny, hairless skin; thickened toenails
- Areas of discolouration or skin breakdown

INTERPROFESSIONAL CARE

Management of peripheral vascular disease focuses on slowing the atherosclerotic process and maintaining tissue perfusion.

Diagnosis

Although PVD often can be diagnosed by the history and physical examination, some diagnostic tests may be ordered to evaluate its extent. Non-invasive studies are often sufficient.

- *Doppler ultrasound (DUS)* uses sound waves reflected off moving red blood cells within a vessel to evaluate blood flow velocity and volume. The impulses may be translated into an audible signal or a graphic waveform. With significant PVD, the waveform becomes progressively flatter as the transducer is moved distally along the affected vessel.
- *Systolic ankle brachial index* or *toe brachial index* uses a sphygmomanometer cuff and Doppler to assess maximal pressure on the artery (systolic pressure) at the various sites measurements are required. The ratio of the two pressures provides insight into presence and severity of disease (Chang, 2022).
- *Duplex Doppler ultrasound* combines the audible or graphic Doppler ultrasound with ultrasound imaging to identify arterial or venous abnormalities. Ultrasonic imaging provides views of the affected vessel, while Doppler ultrasound evaluates blood flow. *Colour-flow Doppler ultrasound (CDU)* provides colour images of the vessel and blood flow.
- *Angiography* or *magnetic resonance angiography (MRA)* is done before revascularisation procedures to locate and evaluate the extent of arterial obstruction. For angiography, a contrast medium is injected and vessels are visualised using fluoroscopy and x-rays. MRA does not require injection of a contrast medium and may replace angiography.

See the chapter 'A person-centred approach to assessing the cardiovascular and lymphatic systems' for more information on diagnostic testing for PVD.

Medications

Drug treatment of peripheral atherosclerosis is less effective than it is for coronary heart disease. Medications to inhibit platelet aggregation, such as aspirin or clopidogrel, are ordered to reduce the risk of arterial thrombosis. Pentoxifylline decreases blood viscosity and increases red blood cell flexibility, increasing blood flow to the microcirculation and tissues of the extremities. Parenteral vasodilator prostaglandins may be given on a long-term basis to decrease pain and facilitate healing in people with severe limb ischaemia (Chuter et al., 2022).

Treatments

Smoking cessation is vital. Nicotine not only promotes atherosclerosis but also causes vasospasm, further reducing blood flow to the extremities.

Meticulous foot care is vital to prevent ulceration and infection (see Box 31.6). Elastic compression stockings, which reduce circulation to the skin, are avoided. Elevating the head of the bed on blocks may help relieve rest pain. Regular, progressively strenuous exercise, such as 30 to 45 minutes of walking daily, is important. The person is taught to rest at the onset of claudication, resuming activity when the pain resolves.

BOX 31.6 Foot care for the person with peripheral atherosclerosis

1. Keep legs and feet clean, dry and comfortable.
   - Wash legs and feet daily in warm water, using mild soap.
   - Pat dry using a soft towel; be sure to dry between the toes.
   - Apply moisturising cream to prevent drying.
   - Use powder on the feet and between the toes.
   - Buy shoes in the afternoon (when feet are largest); never buy shoes that are uncomfortable. Be sure toes have adequate room.
   - Wear a clean pair of cotton socks each day
2. Prevent accidents and injuries to the feet.
   - Always wear shoes or slippers when getting out of bed.
   - Walk on level ground and avoid crowds, if possible.
   - Do not go barefoot.
   - Inspect legs and feet daily; use a mirror to examine backs of legs and bottoms of feet.
   - Have a professional foot care provider trim toenails and care for corns, calluses, ingrown toenails or athlete's foot.
   - Always check the temperature of the water before stepping into the tub.
   - Do not get the legs or tops of the feet sunburned.
   - Report leg or foot problems (increased pain, cuts, bruises, blistering, redness or open areas) to your healthcare provider.
3. Improve blood supply to the legs and feet.
   - Do not cross legs.
   - Do not wear garters or knee stockings.
   - Do not swim or wade in cold water.

NURSING CARE OF THE OLDER ADULT Peripheral vascular disease

With ageing, blood vessels thicken and become less compliant. These changes reduce oxygen delivery to the tissues and impair carbon dioxide and waste product removal from the tissues. When normal effects of ageing combine with an increased risk of atherosclerosis, the risk of peripheral vascular disease is high.

HEALTH EDUCATION FOR THE PERSON AND FAMILY

The older adult with peripheral vascular disease requires the same care and teaching as other people. However, visual deficits and osteoarthritis may make foot care more difficult. Long-standing smoking habits are difficult to break. Mobility may be impaired by arthritis or the effects of neurological disorders. The person who lives alone may resist walking. Periodic visits by a community or home health nurse may be helpful, as may be encouraging the person to join a support group for stopping smoking, changing eating habits and taking part in regular activity.

Other measures to slow the process of atherosclerosis, such as controlling diabetes and hypertension, lowering cholesterol levels and weight loss, also are recommended. See the 'Nursing care of the older adult' box for care of the older adult.

See the chapter 'Nursing care of people with coronary heart disease' for more information about revascularisation procedures.

Revascularisation

Revascularisation may be performed if symptoms are progressive, severe or disabling. More than 70% of surgery for PVD in Australia is via an endovascular approach including balloon angioplasty or stent placement. However, open surgeries are still more appropriate approaches in some individuals. An open surgery does provide superior long-term patency compared to endovascular approaches (Aitken, 2020).

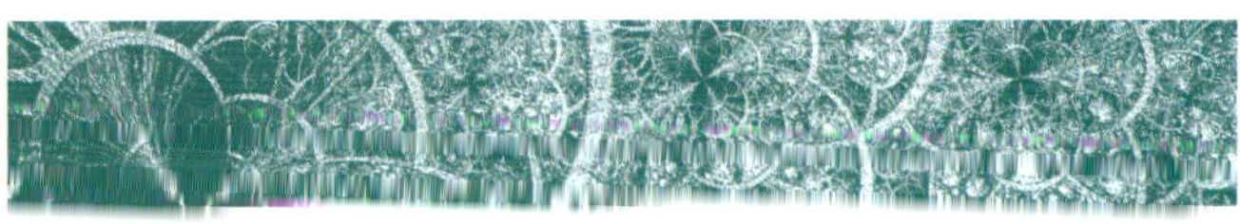

Nursing care

Health promotion

Discuss healthy lifestyle habits with community and religious groups, schoolchildren and through the print media to reduce the incidence and slow the progression of atherosclerosis.

Strongly encourage all people to avoid smoking in the first place and to stop all forms of tobacco use. Discuss the adverse effects of smoking and the benefits of quitting. Provide information about dietary recommendations to maintain a healthy weight and optimal cholesterol levels. Discuss the benefits and importance of regular exercise. Finally, encourage people with cardiovascular risk factors to undergo regular screening for hypertension, diabetes and hyperlipidaemia.

Assessment

Focused assessment related to peripheral atherosclerosis includes the following:

- *Health history*: complaints of pain, its relationship to exercise or rest, timing, associated symptoms and relief measures; history of coronary heart disease, peripheral vascular disease, hyperlipidaemia, hypertension or diabetes; current medications; smoking history; usual diet and activity patterns.
- *Physical examination*: vital signs; strength and equality of peripheral pulses of all extremities; capillary refill; skin colour, temperature, hair distribution, presence of any discolourations or lesions; movement and sensation of lower extremities.

Nursing diagnoses and interventions

Impaired tissue perfusion is an obvious problem in peripheral atherosclerosis. Acute and chronic pain may interfere with ADLs, and ambulation may be limited. The possibility of losing a lower extremity is frightening.

Ineffective tissue perfusion: peripheral

Impaired blood flow to the lower extremities affects gas, nutrient and waste product exchange between the capillaries and cells. Oxygen and nutrient deprivation impairs cell function and tissue integrity, causing pain and impaired healing. Pain develops with exercise and when extremities are elevated.

- Assess peripheral pulses, pain, colour, temperature and capillary refill every 4 hours and as needed. Use a Doppler device if pulses are not palpable. Mark pulse locations with an indelible marker. *Assessment data provide a baseline for evaluating the effectiveness of interventions and identifies changes in arterial blood flow.*
- Position with extremities dependent. *Gravity promotes arterial flow to the dependent extremity, increasing tissue perfusion and relieving pain.*
- Discuss the benefits of regular exercise. *Exercise promotes development of collateral circulation to ischaemic tissues and slows the process of atherosclerosis.*
- Use a foot cradle and lightweight blankets, socks and slippers to keep extremities warm. Avoid electric heating pads or hot water bottles. *Keeping extremities warm conserves heat, prevents vasospasm and promotes arterial flow. External heating devices are avoided to reduce the risk of burns in the person with impaired sensation. A foot cradle protects tissues from compression by bed linen.*
- Encourage frequent position changes. Instruct to avoid crossing legs or using a pillow under the knees. Position changes promote blood flow and reduce damage caused by pressure. *Leg crossing and excessive flexion of the hip or knee joints can compress partially obstructed arteries and impair blood flow to distal tissues.*

> **CONSIDERATION FOR PRACTICE**
>
> **Instruct to avoid smoking. If necessary, obtain an order for a nicotine patch or gum from the doctor. Refer to Quit Helpline for practical and ongoing support. Nicotine is a potent vasoconstrictor that further impairs arterial blood flow. Smoking cessation is a vital component of care. Nicotine patches and gum contain less nicotine than cigarettes and can help reduce the stress of smoking cessation.**

Pain

Impaired blood flow results in tissue ischaemia. Metabolism shifts from an efficient aerobic process to an anaerobic process. Lactic acid and metabolic waste products accumulate in tissues, causing pain. Severe and cramping pain generally occurs with exercise early in the disease. Rest initially produces relief, similar to the process used to treat angina (see the chapter 'Nursing care of people with coronary heart disease'). As the disease progresses, pain develops with less exercise and often occurs even at rest. Rest pain disrupts sleep, the sense of wellbeing and has significant disruptive effects on life roles.

- Assess pain at least every 4 hours, using a standard pain scale. Pain is a subjective experience. *Using a standard pain scale allows evaluation of treatment measures in relieving pain and restoring blood flow.*
- Keep extremities warm. *Cooling leads to vasoconstriction, increasing pain. Warming the extremities promotes vasodilation and improves arterial flow, reducing pain.*
- Teach pain relief and stress reduction techniques such as relaxation, meditation and guided imagery. *Pain increases stress. The stress response leads to vasoconstriction, increasing pain. Stress reduction techniques, when combined with other measures to promote blood flow, can help reduce pain.*

Impaired skin integrity

People with PVD are at risk of impaired skin integrity as a result of oxygen and nutrient deprivation. Chronic tissue ischaemia leads to dry, scaly and atrophied skin. Pruritus can lead to scratching; minor injuries may go unnoticed due to impaired sensation. Impaired tissue healing can lead to ulceration, infection and potential gangrene.

- Provide meticulous daily skin care, keeping the skin clean and dry. Apply a moisturising cream to dry or scaly areas. *Intact skin is the body's first defence against bacterial invasion. Ischaemic tissues of the injured extremity provide an excellent medium for microorganism growth. Clean, dry, supple skin decreases the risk of breakdown.*

> **CONSIDERATION FOR PRACTICE**
>
> **Assess and document skin condition at least every 8 hours or with each home visit; or more frequently as indicated. Tissue ischaemia increases the risk of damage, even with minor trauma such as pressure from poorly fitting shoes or bed linens. Frequent inspection and documentation of skin condition is vital to identify early indicators of impaired skin integrity and reduce the risk of complications such as infection.**

- Apply a bed cradle. *The bed cradle suspends bed linen over the legs, preventing them from placing pressure on extremities and injured tissues. Minimising pressure on the tissues promotes capillary blood flow.*
- Provide an egg-crate mattress, flotation pad, sheepskin or heel protectors. *Ischaemic tissues may be damaged by minor trauma such as that created by the shearing forces of skin against bed linen.*

Activity intolerance

Pain and impaired perfusion of peripheral tissues may limit the person's ability to engage in desired activities, even impairing self-care.

- Assist with care activities as needed. Severe claudication or rest pain may limit activities. Muscle atrophy of affected extremities is common, leading to fatigue and weakness.
- Unless contraindicated, encourage gradual increases in duration and intensity of exercise. Teach to rest with extremities dependent when claudication develops, resuming activity after pain has abated. *Gradual increases in the duration and intensity of exercise promote development of collateral circulation, improve exercise tolerance, provide a sense of wellbeing and support self-esteem.*

NURSING CARE PLAN A person with peripheral vascular disease

William Duffy, aged 69, is retired. His wife convinces him to see his doctor about his increasing leg pain with walking and other exercise.

ASSESSMENT

Katie Kotson, RN, obtains Mr Duffy's history before he sees his doctor. He states that he can only walk about a block before the pain in his calves gets so bad that he has to stop and rest. As a result, he has been less and less active, spending most of his time the past few months watching sports on television. He denies rest pain. He was diagnosed with type 2 diabetes about 15 years ago, which he manages with daily metformin and glibenclamide. He also has stable angina, for which he takes atenolol and an occasional glyceryl trinitrate tablet. His alcohol intake is moderate, averaging one to two beers per day, and he smokes about a packet of cigarettes per day. He states he tried to quit smoking after developing angina, but 'after nearly 50 years of smoking, I think that's impossible!'.

Physical exam findings include height 173 cm, weight 107 kg, BP 168/78, P 66, R 16, T 36.5°C; upper extremities warm and pink, normal hair distribution, pulses strong and equal; lower extremities below knees cool and ruddy when dependent, pale to pink when elevated, skin shiny, scant hair; posterior tibial pulses weak bilaterally; weak pedal pulse on R, unable to palpate on L; 1+ to 2+ oedema both feet and ankles.

The doctor finds that Mr Duffy's systolic blood pressure in his legs is an average of 28 mmHg lower than in his arms. He makes the diagnosis of peripheral atherosclerosis and schedules Mr Duffy for an exercise stress test with ankle pressure measurements before and after exercise and a colour-flow Doppler ultrasound. Mr Duffy is to return in 3 weeks after these studies have been completed.

DIAGNOSES

- *Activity intolerance* related to poor blood flow to lower extremities.
- *Ineffective health maintenance* related to smoking and lack of information about disease management.
- *Risk of impaired skin integrity* related to ischaemic tissues of legs and feet.
- *Risk of peripheral neurovascular dysfunction* related to impaired peripheral blood flow to lower extremities.

PLANNING

- With Mr and Mrs Duffy, plan strategies to start and maintain a program of regular exercise.
- Schedule an appointment with the dietitian to develop a low-kilojoule, low-fat and low-cholesterol diet that includes preferred foods and considers usual eating patterns.
- Plan meeting times with Mr Duffy to discuss prevention and risk factors including modifiable factors.

Expected outcomes

- Walk for at least 15 minutes three to four times per day, gradually increasing his pace and duration of exercise.
- Relate the benefits of smoking cessation.
- Identify strategies to improve chances for success in stopping smoking.
- Meet with dietitian before next visit to discuss dietary measures to promote weight loss and slow atherosclerosis.
- Verbalise an understanding of appropriate foot care measures.
- Identify measures to prevent inadvertent injury of feet and legs.

IMPLEMENTATION

- Teach about peripheral atherosclerosis and its relationship to Mr Duffy's symptoms.
- Instruct to warm up slowly and to stop exercise and rest for 3 minutes (or until pain is relieved) when claudication develops, then resume exercising.
- Discuss the effects of smoking on blood vessels.
- Help Mr Duffy identify smoking cessation strategies such as support groups, clinics and nicotine patches.
- Reinforce and supplement previous foot care teaching.
- Discuss effects of impaired circulation on sensation in feet and legs and measures to prevent injury.

EVALUATION

When Mr Duffy returns 3 weeks later, his diagnosis has been confirmed by the diagnostic studies. The doctor decides to continue conservative therapy, now prescribing atorvastatin to lower Mr Duffy's serum cholesterol level and cilostazol to reduce the risk of thrombosis and improve symptoms of claudication. Mr Duffy also asks his doctor for a prescription for nicotine patches, saying he is ready to quit smoking, but thinks he needs help to be successful. Mr and Mrs Duffy tell Nurse Kotson that they are walking before every meal and really enjoying being outside more. They plan to walk in the local shopping centre whenever the weather is poor. Mrs Duffy has bought an Australian Heart Foundation cookbook (*The Deliciously Healthy Cookbook*) and is carefully planning their meals. Mr and Mrs Duffy have both lost between 0.5 and 1 kg a week since the previous visit. Mr Duffy's skin on his legs and feet remains intact and he identifies the measures he is using to protect his lower extremities from injury.

CRITICAL THINKING IN THE NURSING PROCESS

1. What additional lifestyle changes related to peripheral atherosclerosis might be appropriate to suggest to Mr Duffy at this time? Why?
2. Explain the relationship between physical exercise and pain in the person with peripheral atherosclerosis. Compare this relationship to that between exercise and angina.
3. Mr Duffy uses a beta-blocker, atenolol, to prevent angina. Why is this drug not effective in preventing claudication?
4. What is the relationship between Mr Duffy's diabetes and his cardiovascular disease?

REFLECTION ON THE NURSING PROCESS

1. What strategies can be initiated to ensure Mr Duffy remains on track with improving his health?
2. Mr Duffy stated he tried to quit smoking after developing angina, but 'after nearly 50 years of smoking, I think that's impossible!'. What would the nurse assess to ensure he is compliant with improving his health?

- Provide diversional activities during periods of prescribed bed rest. Encourage relaxation techniques to reduce muscle tension. *Diversional activities help prevent boredom and stress associated with enforced rest. Relaxation techniques reduce vasoconstriction induced by stress, improving peripheral circulation.*
- Encourage frequent position changes and active range-of-motion exercises. Encourage self-care to the extent possible. *Position changes relieve pressure on tissues, improving capillary circulation and reducing tissue ischaemia. Range-of-motion exercises help prevent muscle atrophy and joint contractures. Self-care supports self-esteem.*

Community-based care

Discuss the following topics when preparing the person and family for home and community-based care (see the accompanying nursing care plan for additional community-based nursing interventions):

- smoking cessation strategies and ways to avoid second-hand smoke
- prescribed medications and anticoagulants, their purpose, doses, desired and adverse effects
- signs of excess bleeding to report to the doctor
- skin surveillance and foot care (see Box 31.6)
- recommended diet and exercise
- weight loss strategies if appropriate.

If revascularisation or surgery has been performed, include the following topics as appropriate:

- incision care
- manifestations of complications (e.g. infection, graft leakage or thrombosis) to be reported to the doctor
- activity limitations.

Provide referrals to home health services, physical or occupational therapy and home maintenance assistance services as indicated. Consider resources such as Meals on Wheels for people who are severely limited by their disease.

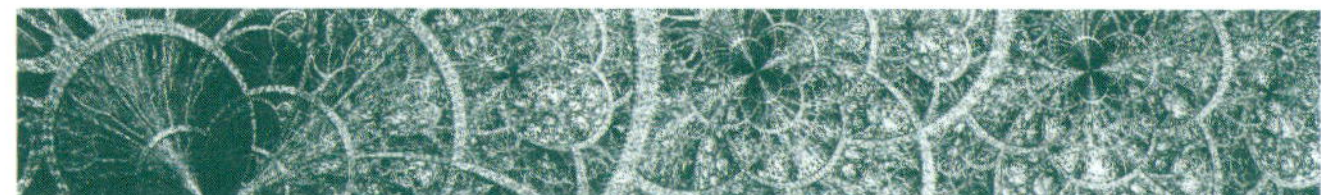

The person with selected peripheral arterial conditions

ACUTE ARTERIAL OCCLUSION

A peripheral artery may be acutely occluded by development of a thrombus (blood clot) or by an embolism. Blood flow to tissues supplied by the artery is impaired, resulting in acute tissue ischaemia and a risk of necrosis and gangrene.

Pathophysiology

Arterial thrombosis

A **thrombus** is a blood clot that adheres to the vessel wall. Thrombi tend to develop in areas where intravascular factors stimulate coagulation (e.g. where a vessel lumen is partially obstructed and its wall is damaged and roughened by atherosclerosis). Other disorders, such as infection or inflammation of the vessel wall or pooling of blood (e.g. in an aneurysm), also can prompt coagulation and thrombus formation (Dominguez, 2022). A developing thrombus can occlude arterial blood flow through the vessel, leading to ischaemia of tissues supplied by that artery. The extent of ischaemia depends on the size of the affected artery and the degree of collateral circulation. In gradual processes of arterial occlusion such as atherosclerosis, collateral vessels often develop to compensate for impaired arterial flow. The extent of collateral circulation affects the degree of tissue ischaemia distal to the thrombus.

Arterial embolism

An **embolism** is the sudden obstruction of a blood vessel by debris. A thrombus can break loose from the arterial wall to become a **thromboembolus**. Other substances also can become emboli: atherosclerotic plaque, masses of bacteria, cancer cells, amniotic fluid, bone marrow fat and foreign objects (e.g. air bubbles or broken intravenous catheters). Regardless of cause, an embolus eventually lodges in a vessel that is too small to allow it to pass.

Arterial emboli often originate in the left side of the heart. They are associated with myocardial infarction, valvular heart disease, left-sided heart failure, atrial fibrillation or infectious heart diseases. Emboli from the left heart often enter the carotid arteries and become trapped in the cerebral circulation, causing neurological deficits. Thromboemboli that develop in the aorta or peripheral arterial circulation tend to lodge in areas where the arterial lumen is narrowed by atherosclerotic plaque and at arterial bifurcations.

Manifestations

The manifestations of arterial thrombosis and embolism are those of tissue ischaemia. Ischaemic tissues are painful, pale and cool or cold. Distal pulses are absent. Paraesthesias (numbness and tingling) develop in the extremity. Cyanosis and mottling are common. Paralysis and muscle spasms may develop in the affected extremity. A line of demarcation between normal and ischaemic tissue may be seen, particularly with embolism. Tissue below the line is cool or cold and pale, cyanotic or mottled. See the 'Manifestations' box.

MANIFESTATIONS Acute arterial occlusion

- Pain
- Pallor or mottling
- Paraesthesias (numbness and tingling)
- Cool or cold skin
- Pulselessness distal to the blockage
- Possible paralysis, weakness or muscle spasms
- Possible line of demarcation; with pallor, cyanosis and cooler skin distal to the blockage (especially with arterial embolism)

Arterial occlusion can result in permanent vessel and limb damage. Complete arterial occlusion leads to tissue necrosis and gangrene unless blood flow is promptly restored.

INTERPROFESSIONAL CARE

Acute arterial occlusions may require emergency treatment to preserve the limb if the obstructed vessel is large or collateral circulation is minimal. If the limb is not in jeopardy, more conservative management may be initiated.

Diagnosis

The diagnosis of acute arterial occlusion often is apparent by the signs and symptoms. *Arteriography* is used to confirm the diagnosis, locate the occlusion and determine its extent.

Medications

Anticoagulation with intravenous heparin is initiated to prevent further clot propagation and recurrent embolism. Anticoagulation is continued with oral anticoagulants after discharge. See the section on venous thrombosis later in this chapter for more information about anticoagulant therapy.

Arterial thrombosis may be treated with intra-arterial fibrinolytic therapy using streptokinase, urokinase or tissue plasminogen activator (t-PA) (see the chapter 'Nursing care of people with coronary heart disease').

Local intra-arterial injection of the fibrinolytic drug allows use of lower doses and reduces the bleeding risk associated with fibrinolytic drugs.

Surgery

Immediate embolectomy (within 4 to 6 hours) is the treatment of choice for acute arterial occlusion by an embolus to prevent tissue necrosis and gangrene. When the involved vessel is in an extremity, local anaesthesia and a special balloon-tipped catheter known as a Fogarty catheter may be used for people with a high surgical risk (Papadakis, McPhee & Rabow, 2022).

An embolus in the mesenteric circulation necessitates emergency laparotomy. The risk of complications and limb loss increases significantly if surgery is delayed by 12 or more hours. Potential major complications include compartment syndrome (see the chapter 'Nursing care of people with musculoskeletal trauma'), acute respiratory distress syndrome (the chapter 'Nursing care of people with gas exchange disorders') or acute kidney failure (the chapter 'Nursing care of people with kidney disorders').

Arterial thrombosis also may be treated surgically, although the required surgery may be more extensive due to the length of the vessel involved. *Thromboendarterectomy* is done to remove the thrombus and plaque in the artery. An arterial graft may be required. Nursing care for people who have undergone embolectomy or thrombus removal is discussed in the nursing care section that follows.

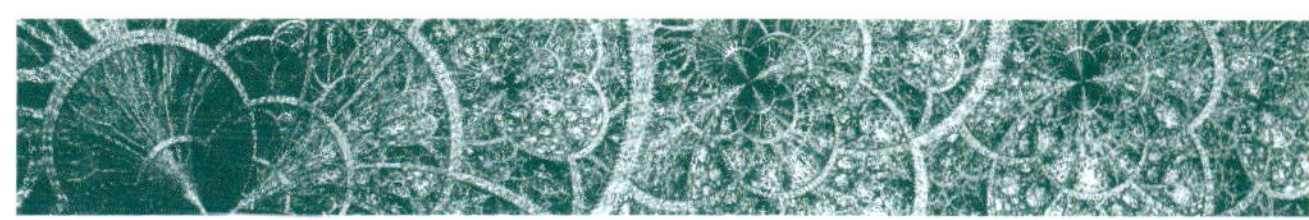

Nursing care

Assessment

Nursing assessment for the person with an acute arterial occlusion is highly focused due to the emergency nature of the problem.

- *Health history*: complaints of pain, numbness, tingling or weakness in the involved extremity; history of atherosclerotic vessel disease, heart disease or recent invasive procedure (e.g. angiography, percutaneous revascularisation procedure).
- *Physical examination*: vital signs; peripheral pulses in both extremities; colour, temperature, sensation and movement of involved extremity; skin condition; presence of a line of demarcation.

Nursing diagnoses and interventions

Nursing care related to acute arterial occlusion focuses on protecting the affected extremity, managing anxiety and reducing the risk of complications related to anticoagulant therapy.

Ineffective tissue perfusion: peripheral

Protecting ischaemic tissue from injury prior to surgery or medical thrombolysis is vital. Following surgery, there is a risk of thrombosis at the graft site or impaired perfusion due to oedema of the surgical site.

> **CONSIDERATION FOR PRACTICE**
>
> **Monitor extremity perfusion, comparing affected and unaffected extremities. Assess peripheral pulses (using the Doppler stethoscope as needed), skin temperature and colour, capillary refill, movement and sensation every 1 to 4 hours. Promptly report changes or complaints of increased or unrelieved pain. Propagation of a thrombus can further obstruct arterial flow, increasing tissue ischaemia. Following surgery, arterial spasms may cause a cyanotic, pulseless extremity; normal colour and pulses should return within 12 hours. A thrombus may form at the surgical site or within a graft, causing tissue ischaemia with pain and other manifestations of arterial occlusion. Further measures to restore circulation may be necessary.**

- Maintain intravenous fluids as ordered. *Adequate circulating blood volume is necessary to maintain cardiac output and tissue perfusion.*
- Protect the extremity, keeping it horizontal or lower than the heart. Use a cradle to keep bedclothes off the extremity and a sheepskin or foam pad to protect it from hard or abrasive surfaces. Do not apply heat or cold. *Keeping the extremity lower than the heart promotes collateral blood flow. Ischaemic tissue is easily damaged by minimal trauma such as shearing by bed linen or heat or cold application.*

- Following surgery, avoid raising the knees, placing pillows under the knees or sitting with 90-degree hip flexion. *These activities may impair blood flow through the affected vessel.*

Anxiety

People with an acute arterial occlusion often are very anxious. The rapid and intense nature of preoperative activities can be overwhelming, increasing anxiety about the disorder and its outcome. Manifestations of anxiety may include trembling, palpitations, restlessness, dry mouth, helplessness, inability to relax, irritability, forgetfulness and lack of awareness of surroundings. Nursing measures focus on establishing trust and minimising the effects of anxiety to decrease surgical risk and improve recovery.

- Spend as much time as possible with the person. Provide opportunities to verbalise anxiety; offer reassurance and support. Support adaptive coping mechanisms. *The presence of a caring nurse provides a safe environment for expressing fears and anxieties. Coping mechanisms reduce the immediate perceived threat and increase the ability to deal with the situational crisis.*
- Perform required measures in an expedient but calm manner. *Calm, confident performance of treatment measures reassures the person and family that appropriate care is being given to treat the problem at hand.*
- Assess anxiety level at least every 8 hours; more often as needed. Intervene as indicated to reduce anxiety. *Assessment helps determine the intensity of anxiety, the person's ability to control it and directs interventions to reduce it.*
- Decrease sensory stimuli as much as possible. *Reducing environmental stimuli provides the person with a degree of control over anxiety.*
- Speak slowly and clearly and avoid unnecessary interruptions when listening. Give concise directions, focusing on the present. Involve the person in simple tasks and decisions to the extent possible. *High levels of anxiety interfere with learning. Keeping interactions focused on the present situation directs the person's focus and provides reassurance that it is the most important focus for the nurse as well. Providing opportunities for self-care and decision making reinforces the person's importance and power to control the situation.*

Altered protection

Fibrinolytic and/or anticoagulant therapy used to dissolve existing clots and prevent further clot formation increases the risk of bleeding. Close monitoring of physical status and laboratory data is vital, as are measures to reduce the risk of injury and bleeding.

- Monitor activated partial thromboplastin time (APTT) during heparin therapy and prothrombin time (PT) or International Normalized Ratio (INR) during oral anticoagulant therapy. Report values outside desired range. *The APTT, PT and INR are prolonged by anticoagulant therapy. Values higher than the desired range may indicate an increased risk of bleeding; values below the target may indicate inadequate anticoagulation.*
- Protect from injury: use side rails or other measures as needed to prevent falls; avoid parenteral injections and other invasive procedures as much as possible; hold firm pressure over injection and intravenous sites for 5 minutes and over arterial punctures for 20 minutes; use a soft toothbrush or sponge for oral care; use an electric razor for shaving. *Minor trauma can lead to extensive bleeding, particularly in the person who has received a fibrinolytic drug.*

CONSIDERATION FOR PRACTICE

Assess for and report manifestations of impaired clotting, including excessive incisional bleeding; prolonged oozing from injection sites; bleeding gums, nosebleed or haematuria; petechiae, bruising or purpura. Anticoagulants and fibrinolytics interfere with the clotting cascade and may cause abnormal bleeding.

Community-based care

When preparing the person and family for home or community-based care related to an acute arterial occlusion, discuss the following topics as indicated:

- care of the incision
- manifestations of complications to be reported, including symptoms of infection or occlusion of the graft or artery
- long-term anticoagulant therapy, including the reason, prescribed dose, follow-up laboratory testing and appointments, interactions with other drugs and manifestations of excessive bleeding
- any activity restrictions or dietary modifications
- lifestyle modifications to slow atherosclerosis and control hypertension
- measures to promote peripheral circulation and maintain tissue integrity (see the discussion of peripheral atherosclerosis earlier in the chapter).

Refer for home care services (nursing care, physical therapy, housekeeping services) as indicated.

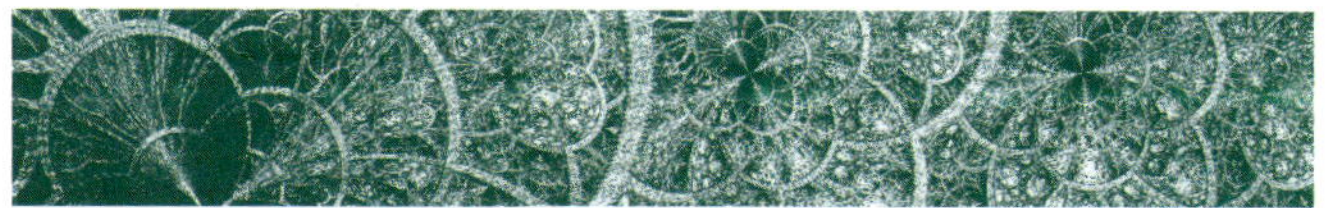

THE PERSON WITH THROMBOANGIITIS OBLITERANS

Thromboangiitis obliterans (also called *Buerger's disease*) is an occlusive vascular disease in which small and medium-sized peripheral arteries become inflamed and spastic, causing clots to form. This disease may affect either the upper or lower extremities; it often affects a leg or foot. Its exact aetiology is unknown.

Incidence and risk factors

Thromboangiitis obliterans primarily affects men under age 40 who smoke. Cigarette smoking is the single most significant cause of the disease. The disease is more prevalent in Asians and people of Eastern European descent. The incidence of HLA-B5 and 2A9 antigens is higher in people with thromboangiitis obliterans, suggesting a genetic link.

Pathophysiology and course

Inflammatory cells infiltrate the wall of small and midsized arteries in the feet and possibly the hands. This inflammatory process is accompanied by thrombus formation and vasospasms of arterial segments that impair blood flow. Adjacent veins and nerves also may be affected. As the disease progresses, affected vessels become scarred and fibrotic.

The course of the disease is intermittent with dramatic exacerbations and marked remissions. The disease may remain dormant for periods of weeks, months or years. As the disease progresses, collateral vessels are more extensively involved. Consequently, subsequent episodes are more intense and prolonged. Prolonged periods of tissue hypoxia increase the risk of tissue ulceration and gangrene.

Manifestations and complications

Pain in the affected extremities is the primary manifestation of thromboangiitis obliterans. Both claudication, cramping pain in the calves and feet or the forearms and hands, and rest pain in the fingers and toes may occur. Sensation is diminished. Eventually, the skin becomes thin and shiny and the nails are thickened and malformed. On examination, the involved digits and/or extremities are pale, cyanotic or ruddy, and cool or cold to touch. Distal pulses (e.g. the dorsalis pedis, posterior tibial, ulnar or radial) are either difficult to locate or absent, even with a Doppler device.

Painful ulcers and gangrene may develop in the fingers and toes as a result of severely impaired blood flow. Amputation may be necessary to remove necrotic tissue.

INTERPROFESSIONAL CARE

Diagnosis

Thromboangiitis obliterans usually is diagnosed by the history and physical examination. Doppler studies may be used to locate and determine the extent of the disease. Angiography and magnetic resonance imaging may also be used to evaluate the extent of the disease, but usually are unnecessary.

Lifestyle modifications

The one most important component in managing this disease is smoking cessation. While stopping smoking does not cure the disease, it may slow its extension to other vessels. With continued smoking, attacks become increasingly intense and last much longer, significantly increasing the risk of ulcerations and gangrene.

Additional conservative measures are used to prevent vasoconstriction, improve peripheral blood flow and prevent complications of chronic ischaemia. These measures include keeping extremities warm, managing stress, keeping affected extremities in a dependent position, preventing injury to affected tissues and regular exercise. Walking for 20 or more minutes several times a day is recommended.

Medications

There are no specific drugs for thromboangiitis obliterans. Calcium channel blockers, such as diltiazem or verapamil and/or oxpentifylline, which decrease blood viscosity and increase red blood cell flexibility to improve peripheral blood flow, may provide some symptom relief.

Surgery

Surgical approaches for thromboangiitis obliterans include sympathectomy or arterial bypass graft. Sympathectomy interrupts sympathetic nervous system input to affected vessels, reducing vasoconstriction and spasm. Arterial bypass grafts may be useful when larger vessels are affected by the disease. Amputation of an affected digit or extremity may be necessary if gangrene develops (see the chapter 'Nursing care of people with musculoskeletal trauma' for more information about amputation). Only portions of digits or of limbs (e.g. below the knee) are usually amputated, to preserve as much healthy tissue as possible.

The prognosis for thromboangiitis obliterans depends significantly on the person's ability and willingness to stop smoking. With smoking cessation and good foot care, the prognosis for saving the extremities is good, even though no cure is available.

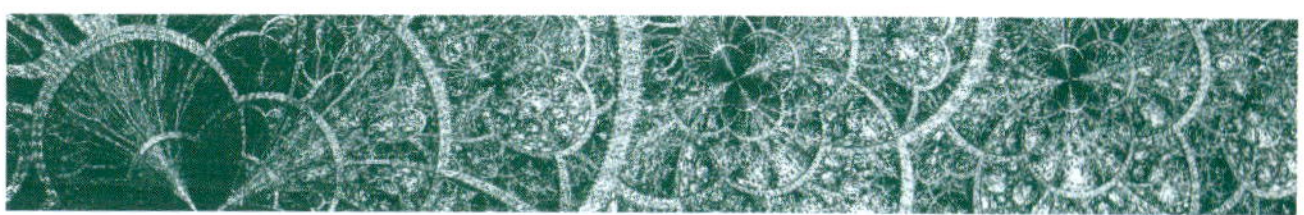

Nursing care

Health promotion

Health promotion activities to prevent thromboangiitis obliterans focus on preventing smoking, especially in high-risk populations.

Assessment

Nursing assessment and care for people with this disease are similar to those provided for people with other arterial occlusive diseases. Nursing care focuses on promoting arterial circulation and preventing prolonged tissue hypoxia. Due to inflammation, spastic episodes may be unpredictable; care focuses on smoking cessation and relieving acute manifestations. In addition, postsurgical care is necessary if surgery has been performed. See the nursing care section for peripheral atherosclerosis, as well as nursing care of the postsurgical person (the chapter 'Nursing care of people having surgery') and following amputation (the chapter 'Nursing care of people with musculoskeletal trauma').

Community-based care

Discuss the following topics when preparing people with thromboangiitis obliterans and their families for home or community-based care:

- absolute necessity of smoking cessation
- foot care
- protecting affected extremities from injury
- purpose, dose, desired and adverse effects, interactions and any precautions associated with prescribed medications
- signs and symptoms to report to the doctor.

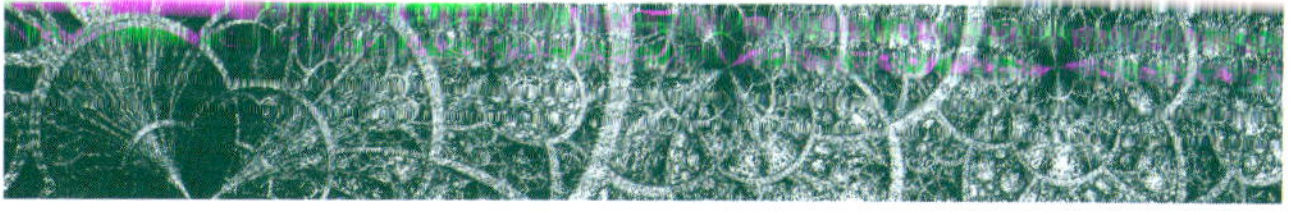

THE PERSON WITH RAYNAUD'S DISEASE

Raynaud's disease and **Raynaud's phenomenon** are characterised by episodes of intense vasospasm in the small arteries and arterioles of the fingers and sometimes the toes (Hansen-Dispenza, 2022). Raynaud's disease and Raynaud's phenomenon differ only in terms of cause. Raynaud's disease has no identifiable cause; Raynaud's phenomenon occurs secondarily to another disease (such as collagen vascular diseases such as scleroderma and rheumatoid arthritis), other known causes of vasospasm or long-term exposure to cold or machinery (Hansen-Dispenza, 2022).

Raynaud's disease primarily affects young women between the ages of 20 and 40. Genetic predisposition may play a role in its development, but the actual cause is unknown. Table 31.4 compares Raynaud's disease and thromboangiitis obliterans.

Pathophysiology and manifestations

Raynaud's disease and Raynaud's phenomenon are characterised by spasms of the small arteries in the digits. The arterial spasms limit arterial blood flow to the fingers and possibly the toes. Initial attacks may involve only the tips of one or two fingers; with disease progression, the entire finger and all fingers may be affected.

The manifestations of Raynaud's occur intermittently when spasms develop. Raynaud's disease has been called the 'blue-white-red disease', because affected digits initially turn blue as blood flow is reduced due to vasospasm, then white as circulation is more severely limited and, finally, very red as the fingers are warmed and the spasm resolves (see Figure 31.12). Sensory changes may occur during attacks, including numbness, stiffness, decreased sensation and aching pain.

The attacks tend to become more frequent and prolonged over time. With repeated attacks (and resultant decrease in oxygenation), the fingertips thicken and the nails become brittle. Ulceration and gangrene are serious complications that rarely occur.

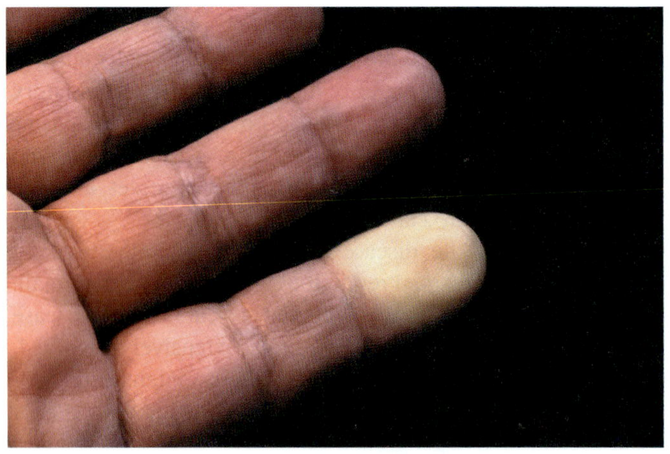

FIGURE 31.12 *Fingers of a patient with Raynaud's phenomenon. Note the extreme pallor of the fifth digit in response to exposure to cold*

Source: Custom Medical Stock Photo/Alamy Stock Photo.

INTERPROFESSIONAL CARE

Diagnosis

Raynaud's disease and Raynaud's phenomenon are primarily diagnosed by the history and physical examination. There are no specific diagnostic tests for these disorders.

TABLE 31.4 Comparison of Raynaud's disease and thromboangiitis obliterans

TOPIC	RAYNAUD'S DISEASE	THROMBOANGIITIS OBLITERANS
Aetiology	• Unknown • Possible genetic predisposition	• Cigarette smoking most probable single cause • Possible autoimmune response
Incidence/course of the disease	• Onset commonly between 15 and 45 years of age • Usually affects young women • Becomes progressively worse over time	• Occurs predominantly in men under age 40 • More common in people of Asian or European heritage • Intermittent course with exacerbations and remissions • Increased severity and duration of attacks over time
Triggering stimuli	• Emotional stress • Exposure to cold	• Cigarette smoking
Assessment findings	• Usually affects hands, sometimes toes • Pain becomes more severe and prolonged as disease progresses • 'Blue-white-red' changes in colour of hands with accompanying changes in skin temperature	• Claudication and pain • Numbness or diminished sensation • Cool, pale or cyanotic skin • Shiny, thin skin and white, malformed nails in affected extremities • Distal pulses difficult to find or absent • Trophic changes to nail beds • Ulceration and gangrene in later stages • Small, red, tender vascular cords in affected extremities
Management	• Avoid unnecessary cold exposure • Emphasise smoking cessation • Medications such as calcium channel or alpha-adrenergic blockers as indicated • Teach stress management	• Stop smoking (crucial) • Regular exercise • Protect extremities from cold injury • Teach stress management

Medications

Vasodilators may be prescribed to provide symptomatic relief. Low doses of a sustained-release calcium channel blocker such as nifedipine or diltiazem may be prescribed. The alpha-adrenergic blocker prazosin also may reduce the frequency and severity of attacks. Transdermal glyceryl trinitrate (or longer-acting oral nitrates) helps some people by decreasing the amount of time necessary for the hands to return to normal following an attack (Papadakis et al., 2022).

Lifestyle modifications

Conservative measures are a mainstay of treatment. People are instructed to keep their hands warm, wearing gloves when outside in cold weather and kitchen gloves when handling cold items (e.g. when preparing and serving cold foods and cleaning the refrigerator). Measures to avoid injury to the hands are taught. Sometimes attacks can be stopped by swinging the arms back and forth, increasing perfusion pressure in the small arteries by centrifugal force.

Smoking cessation is important. Stress reduction measures such as exercise, relaxation techniques, massage therapy, hobbies, aromatherapy and counselling are taught or suggested. Additional lifestyle habits that contribute to vascular health are encouraged, such as reducing dietary fat, increasing activity level and maintaining normal body weight.

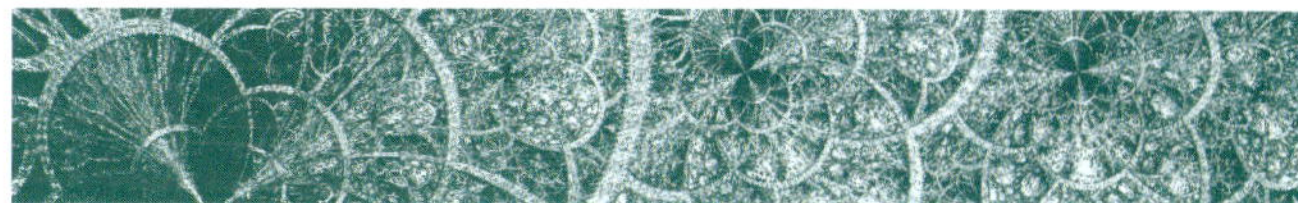

Nursing care

Nursing care for the person with Raynaud's disease or Raynaud's phenomenon is primarily educative and supportive. Protecting the hands and feet from exposure to cold and trauma is the main teaching topic. Nursing diagnoses and interventions previously outlined for peripheral atherosclerosis also are appropriate for people with Raynaud's disease.

Community-based care

Reassure people with Raynaud's phenomenon that most people with the disorder experience only mild, infrequent episodes. Discuss the following topics in preparing the person for managing the disorder:

- Dress warmly, keeping the trunk and hands warm.
- Avoid unnecessary exposure to cold.
- Stop smoking or do not start.
- The use, purpose, desired and potential adverse effects of prescribed medications, if any.

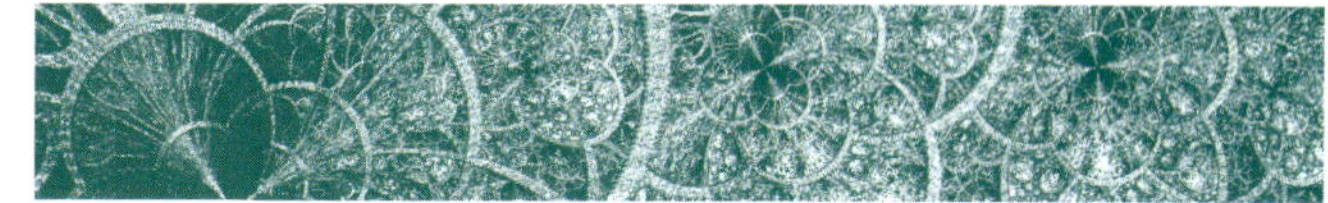

Disorders of venous circulation

The two primary categories of venous system disorders are occlusive disorders and those related to ineffective venous blood flow. Impaired venous blood flow can lead to stasis and clotting, as well as tissue changes associated with venous congestion.

Physiology review

The venous system is a low-pressure system compared with arterial circulation. Veins and venules are thin-walled, distensible vessels. While they contain smooth muscle that allows them to contract or expand, the media (muscle layer) of veins is significantly thinner than that of arteries. The low pressures in the venous system allow it to serve as a reservoir for blood. Stimulation by the sympathetic nervous system causes veins to contract, helping maintain vascular volume. The low-pressure venous system relies on skeletal muscle contractions and pressure changes in the abdomen and thorax to facilitate blood return to the heart. Unlike arteries, veins of the extremities contain valves to prevent retrograde blood flow.

THE PERSON WITH VENOUS THROMBOSIS

Venous thrombosis (also known as *thrombophlebitis*) is a condition in which a blood clot (thrombus) forms on the wall of a vein, accompanied by inflammation of the vein wall and some degree of obstructed venous blood flow.

Venous thrombi are more common than arterial thrombi because of lower pressures and flow within the venous system (Patel, 2019). Thrombi can form in either superficial or deep veins. **Deep venous thrombosis (DVT)** is a common complication of hospitalisation, surgery and immobilisation. Obstetric and orthopaedic procedures carry a higher risk of venous thrombosis; it may develop in more than 50% of people having orthopaedic surgery, particularly surgeries involving the hip or knee (Patel, 2019). Other significant risk factors for venous thrombosis include abdominal or thoracic surgery, certain cancers, trauma, pregnancy and use of oral contraceptives or hormone replacement therapy (see Box 31.7).

Pathophysiology

Three pathological factors, called *Virchow's triad*, are associated with thrombophlebitis: stasis of blood, vessel damage and increased blood coagulability. Vessel trauma stimulates the clotting cascade. Platelets aggregate at the site, particularly when venous stasis is present. Platelets and fibrin form the initial clot. Red blood cells are trapped in the fibrin meshwork and the thrombus propagates (grows) in the direction of blood flow. The inflammatory response is triggered, causing tenderness, swelling and erythema in the area of the thrombus. Initially the thrombus floats within the vein.

BOX 31.7 Factors associated with venous thrombosis

- Immobilisation: myocardial infarction, heart failure, stroke, postoperative
- Surgery: orthopaedic, thoracic, abdominal, genitourinary
- Cancer: pancreatic, lung, ovary, testes, urinary tract, breast, stomach
- Trauma: fractures of the spine, pelvis, femur, tibia; spinal cord injury
- Pregnancy and delivery
- Hormone therapy: oral contraceptives, hormone replacement therapy
- Coagulation disorders

Pieces of the thrombus may break loose and travel through the circulation as emboli. Fibroblasts eventually invade the thrombus, scarring the vein wall and destroying venous valves. Although patency of the vein may be restored, valve damage is permanent. Approximately 80% of deep venous thromboses begin in the deep veins of the calf, often propagating into the popliteal and femoral veins (see Figure 31.13) (Baur & Lip, 2022).

FAST FACTS

- DVT is a common complication of surgery and immobility. It usually develops in the deep veins of the calf (80%).
- Venous stasis (sluggish blood flow), altered blood coagulation and damage (e.g. inflammation) to blood vessels are precipitating factors for DVT.
- A thrombus or a portion of a thrombus may break loose, travelling through the venous system to the right side of the heart and into the pulmonary circulation, where it ultimately becomes lodged (pulmonary embolus).

Deep venous thrombosis

The deep veins of the legs, primarily in the calf and the pelvis, provide the most hospitable environment for venous DVT usually is asymptomatic; in some people, a pulmonary embolism may be the first indication.

MANIFESTATIONS When present, the manifestations of DVT are primarily due to the inflammatory process accompanying the thrombus. Calf pain, which may be described as tightness or a dull, aching pain in the affected extremity,

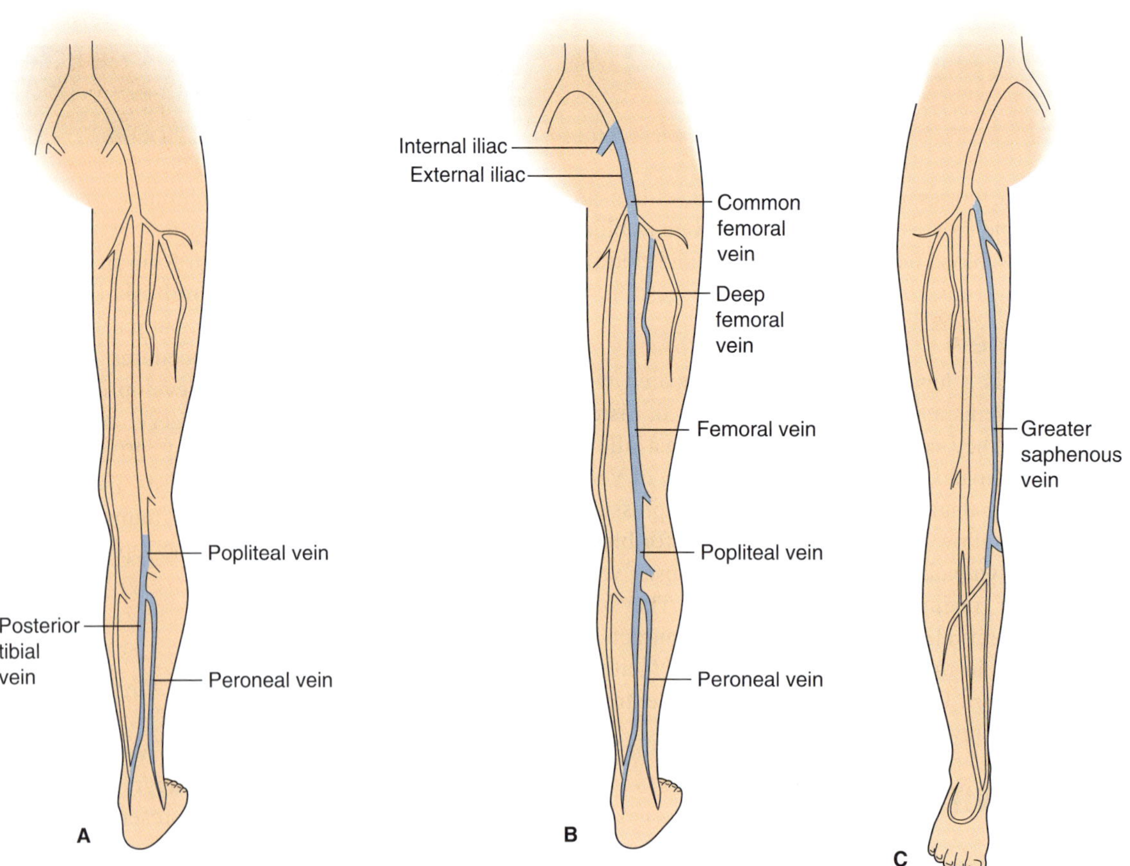

FIGURE 31.13 *Common locations of venous thrombosis. A, The most common sites of DVT. B, DVT extending from the calf to the iliac veins. C, Superficial venous thrombosis*

> MANIFESTATIONS **Venous thrombosis**
>
> **DEEP VENOUS THROMBOSIS**
> - Usually asymptomatic
> - Dull, aching pain in affected extremity, especially when walking
> - Possible tenderness, warmth, erythema along affected vein
> - Cyanosis of affected extremity
> - Oedema of affected extremity
>
> **SUPERFICIAL VENOUS THROMBOSIS**
> - Localised pain and tenderness over the affected vein
> - Redness and warmth along the course of the vein
> - Palpable cordlike structure along the affected vein
> - Swelling and redness of surrounding tissue

particularly upon walking, is the most common symptom. Tenderness, swelling, warmth and erythema may be noted along the course of involved veins. The affected extremity may be cyanotic and often is oedematous. Rarely, a cord may be palpated over the affected vein. A positive Homans' sign (pain in the calf when the foot is dorsiflexed) is an unreliable indicator of DVT. See the 'Manifestations' box.

COMPLICATIONS The major complications of DVT are chronic venous insufficiency (see below) and pulmonary embolism. Pulmonary embolism occurs when the clot fragments or breaks loose from the vein wall. As the clot travels, it moves through progressively larger veins and into the right side of the heart. From there it enters the pulmonary circulation, where it eventually occludes arterial flow to a portion of the lungs. The result is a mismatch between ventilation (air flow) and perfusion (blood flow) in a portion of the lungs. The effect on gas exchange depends on the size of the embolism and the vessel it occludes. See the chapter 'Nursing care of people with gas exchange disorders' for more information about pulmonary emboli.

Superficial venous thrombosis

Venous catheters and infusions are the primary risk factors for superficial venous thrombosis. Superficial venous thrombosis also may develop in conjunction with thromboangiitis obliterans, varicose veins or DVT. It may develop spontaneously in pregnant women or following delivery. In some cases, superficial venous thrombosis of the long saphenous vein is the earliest sign of an abdominal cancer such as pancreatic cancer (Baur & Lip, 2022).

Superficial venous thrombosis is marked by pain and tenderness at the site of the thrombus. A reddened, warm, tender cord extending along the affected vein can be palpated. The area surrounding the vein may be swollen and red (see the 'Manifestations' box).

INTERPROFESSIONAL CARE

It is important to differentiate venous thrombosis from other causes of extremity pain, such as cellulitis, muscle strain, contusion and lymphoedema. The history, physical examination and diagnostic tests are used to establish the diagnosis. Treatment focuses on preventing further clotting or extension of the clot and addressing underlying causes.

Diagnosis

- *Duplex venous ultrasonography* is a non-invasive test used to visualise the vein and measure the velocity of blood flow in the veins. Although the clot often cannot be visualised directly, its presence can be inferred by an inability to compress the vein during the examination.
- *Plethysmography* is a non-invasive test that measures changes in blood flow through the veins. It is often used in conjunction with Doppler ultrasonography. Plethysmography is most valuable in diagnosing thromboses of larger or more superficial veins.
- *Magnetic resonance imaging (MRI)* is another non-invasive means of detecting DVT. It is particularly useful when thrombosis of the venae cavae or pelvic veins is suspected.
- *Ascending contrast venography* uses an injected contrast medium to assess the location and extent of venous thrombosis. Although invasive, expensive and uncomfortable, contrast venography is the most accurate diagnostic tool for venous thrombosis. It is used when the results of less invasive tests leave the diagnosis unclear (Baur & Lip, 2022).

Prophylaxis

Medications and other measures are used to prevent venous thrombosis when the risk is high. Low-molecular-weight (LMW) heparins prevent DVT in people who are undergoing general or orthopaedic surgery, experiencing acute medical illness or are on prolonged bed rest. Oral anticoagulation also may be used as a prophylactic measure in people with fractures or who are undergoing orthopaedic surgery.

Elevating the foot of the bed with the knees slightly flexed promotes venous return. Early mobilisation and leg exercises such as ankle flexion and extension assist venous flow by muscle compression. Intermittent pneumatic compression devices applied to the legs are effective to prevent DVT. They also are used when anticoagulation is contraindicated due to the increased risk of bleeding (Loscalzo et al., 2022). Elastic stockings are also used to prevent venous thrombosis in people at risk.

Medications

Anticoagulants to prevent clot propagation and enable the body's own lytic system to dissolve the clot are the mainstay of treatment for venous thrombosis.

Non-steroidal anti-inflammatory agents (NSAIDs) such as indomethacin or naproxen may be ordered to reduce inflammation in the veins and provide symptomatic relief, particularly for people with superficial venous thrombosis.

ANTICOAGULANTS Anticoagulants are given to prevent clot extension and reduce the risk of subsequent pulmonary embolism. See the 'Medication administration' box for the nursing implications for anticoagulant therapy.

Anticoagulation is initiated with unfractionated heparin or low-molecular-weight (LMW) heparin. Following an initial intravenous bolus of 7,500 to 10,000 units of unfractionated heparin, a continuous heparin infusion of 1,000 to 1,500 international units per hour (IU/h) is started. The dosage is calculated to maintain the activated partial thromboplastin time (APTT) at approximately twice the control or normal value. An infusion pump is used to deliver the prescribed dosage. Frequent monitoring of the infusion is an important nursing responsibility. Subcutaneous heparin injections may be used as an alternative to intravenous infusion in some instances.

LMW heparins are increasingly used to prevent and treat venous thrombosis. They do not require the close laboratory monitoring of unfractionated heparins. LMW heparin is administered subcutaneously in fixed doses once or twice daily, allowing for the option of community-based treatment. LMW heparins have additional advantages, in that they are more effective and carry lower risks for bleeding and thrombocytopenia than conventional, unfractionated heparins.

Oral anticoagulation with warfarin may be initiated concurrently with heparin therapy. Overlapping heparin and warfarin therapy for 4 to 5 days is important because the full anticoagulant effect of warfarin is delayed and it may actually promote clotting during the first few days of therapy (Baur & Lip, 2022). Warfarin doses are adjusted to maintain the INR at 2.0 to 3.0 (Solano, 2022). Once this level is achieved, the heparin is discontinued and a maintenance dose of warfarin is prescribed to prevent recurrent thrombosis.

MEDICATION ADMINISTRATION Anticoagulant therapy

HEPARIN

Heparin interferes with the clotting cascade by inhibiting the effects of thrombin and preventing the conversion of fibrinogen to fibrin. This prevents the formation of a stable fibrin clot. At therapeutic levels, heparin prolongs the thrombin time, clotting time and activated partial thromboplastin time. When given intravenously, its effect is immediate. Given subcutaneously, its onset of action is within 1 hour. *Heparin-induced thrombocytopenia (HIT)* is a potential complication of therapy with unfractionated heparin. See the chapter 'Nursing care of people with haematological disorders' for more information about HIT and nursing responsibilities in monitoring for this dangerous potential complication.

Nursing responsibilities

- Assess for history of unexplained or active bleeding. Assess laboratory results for abnormal clotting profile or evidence of active bleeding.
- Give a test dose as indicated to people with a history of multiple allergies or a history of asthma.
- Administer by deep subcutaneous injection; abdominal sites are preferred. Avoid injecting within 5 cm of the umbilicus. Rotate sites. Do not aspirate prior to injecting or massage after the injection.
- Intravenous solutions may be diluted with dextrose, normal saline or Ringer's solution. Use an infusion pump.
- Keep protamine sulfate, a heparin antagonist, available to treat excessive bleeding.
- Monitor and report abnormal laboratory results and APTT values outside the desired range.
- Promptly report evidence of bleeding such as haematemesis, haematuria, bleeding gums or unexplained abdominal or back pain.

Health education for the person and family

- Report unusual bleeding or excessive menstrual flow.
- Use an electric razor and a soft-bristle toothbrush; prevent injury by clearing pathways, using a night light and other measures. Do not consume alcohol.
- Avoid contact sports while on anticoagulant therapy.
- Do not consume large amounts of food rich in vitamin K (yellow and dark green vegetables).
- Do not use aspirin or NSAIDs while on heparin therapy unless advised to do so by your doctor.
- Wear a MedicAlert® tag and advise all healthcare providers (including dentists and podiatrists) of therapy.

LOW-MOLECULAR-WEIGHT HEPARINS

Enoxaparin
Dalteparin
Sapropterin
Danaparoid

LMW heparins are the most bioavailable fraction of heparin. They provide a more precise and predictable anticoagulant effect than unfractionated heparins. Like unfractionated heparin, LMW heparin prevents conversion of prothrombin to thrombin, liberation of thromboplastin from platelets and formation of a stable clot. LMW heparins cannot be used interchangeably with each other or with unfractionated heparin. Although the risk of heparin-induced thrombocytopenia is significantly lower with LMW heparin, people who were previously treated with unfractionated heparin may develop HIT when treated with LMW heparin.

Nursing responsibilities

- Assess for evidence of active bleeding, a history of bleeding disorders or thrombocytopenia, or sensitivity to heparin, sulfites or pork products.
- Monitor for unusual or masked bleeding. PT and APTT levels may be within normal levels even in the presence of haemorrhage.
- Administer by deep subcutaneous injection into abdominal wall, thigh or buttocks. Rotate sites. Do not aspirate or massage.

Health education for the person and family

- Subcutaneous self-administration technique, timing of doses and site rotation. To minimise bruising, do not rub site after administering.
- Do not take aspirin, NSAIDs or other over-the-counter drugs unless recommended by your doctor.
- Promptly report excessive bruising or bleeding, chest pain, difficulty breathing, itching, rash or swelling to your healthcare provider.
- Keep follow-up appointments as scheduled.

ORAL ANTICOAGULANT

Direct oral anticoagulants (DOACs)

Traditionally, warfarin (a high-risk-use drug) has been used in the management of venous thrombosis prevention following a recent thrombosis event. DOACs work by directly interfering with the coagulation cascade through direct inhibition of specific clotting factors: either Factor Xa (apixavan and rivaroxaban)

MEDICATION ADMINISTRATION **Anticoagulant therapy (continued)**

or Factor IIa (dabigatran). With the advent of DOACs such as the factor Xa inhibitors (rivaroxaban and apixaban) and the direct thrombin inhibitor (dabigatran), anticoagulation has become safer. DOACs are established as being equally as effective as warfarin, have significantly reduced risk of bleeding, do not require laboratory monitoring and have fewer food and drug interactions (Stevens, Tran & Gibbs, 2019). However, individuals who weigh less than 50 kg or more than 120 kg, have severe chronic kidney disease or have antiphospholipid syndrome would be more appropriately managed on warfarin.

Warfarin

Warfarin interferes with synthesis of vitamin-K-dependent clotting factors by the liver, leading to depletion of these factors. It has no effect on already circulating clotting factors or on existing clots. Warfarin inhibits extension of existing thrombi and the formation of new clots. Its action is cumulative and more prolonged than that of heparin.

Nursing responsibilities

- Assess laboratory results and history for evidence of abnormal bleeding.
- Multiple drugs affect the metabolism and protein binding of warfarin; note all medications and assess for interactions with warfarin.
- Do not give during pregnancy because warfarin may cause congenital malformations.
- Oral tablets may be crushed and given without regard to meals.
- Dilute intravenous warfarin with supplied dilutant; administer within 4 hours by direct intravenous injection at a rate of 25 mg/min.
- Keep vitamin K available to reverse effects of warfarin in the event of excessive bleeding or haemorrhage.
- Monitor PT or INR; report values outside the desired range.

Health education for the person and family

- If bleeding occurs (haematemesis, bright red or black tarry faeces, haematuria, bleeding gums, excessive bruising, etc.), do not take your prescribed dose and notify your doctor immediately. Report rash or manifestations of hepatitis (dark urine, malaise, yellow skin or sclera).
- Take your warfarin at the same time every day; do not change brands because their effects may differ.
- Menstrual bleeding may be slightly increased; contact your healthcare provider if it increases significantly. Use reliable birth control to prevent pregnancy while taking warfarin. Immediately contact your doctor if you think you may be pregnant.
- Take precautions to prevent injury and bleeding: use a soft-bristle toothbrush and electric razor, wear shoes and use a night light. Avoid participating in contact sports.
- Do not smoke, use alcohol or take any over-the-counter drugs unless specifically recommended by your doctor. Notify all healthcare providers, including dentists and podiatrists, of therapy. Wear a MedicAlert® tag.
- Obtain lab tests as scheduled and keep all scheduled follow-up appointments.

Anticoagulation generally is continued for at least 3 months. When DVT is recurrent or risk factors such as altered coagulability or cancer are present, anticoagulant therapy may be prolonged. Regular follow up is necessary to be sure prothrombin times (INR) remain within the desirable range for anticoagulation.

Treatments

Treatment of venous thrombosis also includes measures to relieve symptoms and reduce inflammation. With superficial venous thrombosis, applying warm, moist compresses over the affected vein, extremity rest and anti-inflammatory agents usually provide relief of symptoms.

Bed rest may be ordered for deep venous thrombosis. The duration of bed rest typically is determined by the extent of leg oedema. The legs are elevated 15 to 20 degrees, with the knees slightly flexed, above the level of the heart to promote venous return and discourage venous pooling. Elastic anti-embolism stockings (TEDS) or pneumatic compression devices are also frequently ordered to stimulate the muscle-pumping mechanism that promotes the return of blood to the heart. When permitted, walking is encouraged while avoiding prolonged standing or sitting. Crossing the legs also is avoided, as are tight-fitting garments or stockings that bind.

Surgery

Venous thrombosis usually is effectively treated with conservative measures and anticoagulation. In some cases, however, surgery is required to remove the thrombus, prevent its extension into deep veins or prevent the effects of embolisation.

Venous thrombectomy is done when thrombi lodge in the femoral vein and their removal is necessary to prevent pulmonary embolism or gangrene. Successful thrombus removal rapidly improves venous circulation. The duration of this effect varies.

When venous thrombosis is recurrent and anticoagulant therapy is contraindicated, a filter may be inserted into the vena cava to capture emboli from the pelvis and lower extremities, preventing pulmonary embolism. Several different filters are available (see Figure 31.14). The Greenfield filter is widely

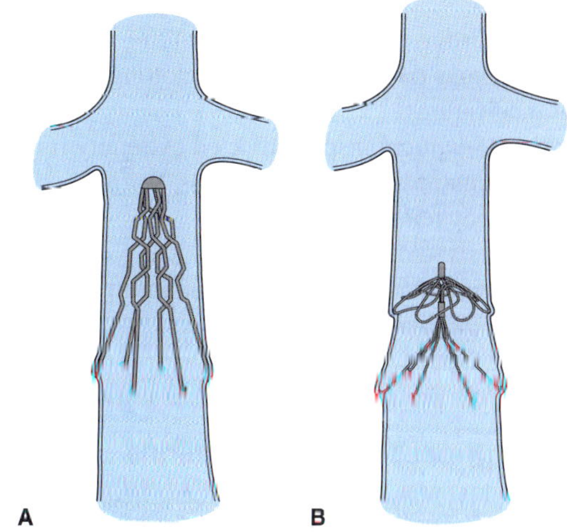

FIGURE 31.14 *Venal caval filters. A, Greenfield filter. B, Nitinol filter*

used for its ability to trap emboli within its apex while maintaining patency of the vena cava. The filter can be inserted under fluoroscopy with local anaesthesia. Mortality and morbidity associated with the filter are very low.

Extensive thrombosis of the saphenous vein may necessitate ligation and division of the saphenous vein where it joins the femoral vein to prevent clot extension into the deep venous system. A vein affected by septic venous thrombosis is excised to control the infection. Antibiotic therapy also is initiated.

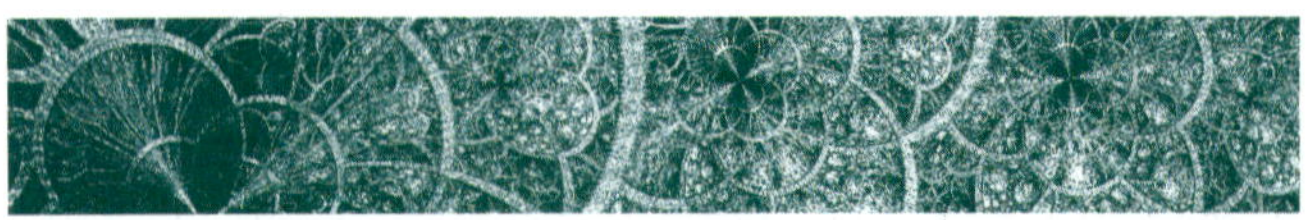

Nursing care

Health promotion

Prevention of venous thrombosis is an important component of nursing care for all at-risk people. Position people to promote venous blood flow from the lower extremities, with the feet elevated and the knees slightly bent. Avoid placing pillows under the knees and positions in which the hips and knees are sharply flexed. Use a recliner chair or footstool when sitting. Ambulation should be encouraged as soon as possible and a regular schedule of ambulation maintained throughout the day. Teach ankle flexion and extension exercises and remind people to frequently perform them. Apply elastic compression stockings and pneumatic compression devices when appropriate. Instruct to avoid crossing legs when in bed or sitting. Inquire about possible prophylactic heparin or warfarin therapy for people undergoing orthopaedic surgery or other high-risk procedures. Frequently assess intravenous sites. Change the site and catheter as dictated by agency protocol and if evidence of local inflammation is noted.

Assessment

Assess people at risk of venous thrombosis for manifestations and risk factors.

- *Health history*: complaints of leg or calf pain, its duration and characteristics, and the effect of walking on the pain; history of venous thrombosis or other clotting disorders; current medications.
- *Physical examination*: inspect affected extremity for redness, oedema; palpate for tenderness, warmth, cordlike structures; body temperature.
- *Diagnostic tests*: clotting studies (activated partial thromboplastin time (APTT), prothrombin time (PT), International Normalized Ratio (INR)).

See the accompanying nursing care plan for an example of an assessment of a person with deep venous thrombosis.

Nursing diagnoses and interventions

In addition to the preventive measures identified earlier, priority nursing diagnoses for the person with venous thrombosis relate to pain, maintenance of tissue perfusion and integrity, and the potential adverse effects of prescribed treatments.

Pain

The pain associated with venous thrombosis results from inflammation of the involved vein. It may be aggravated by use of the involved extremity. Associated oedema and swelling may contribute to discomfort. Measures to reduce the inflammation often help relieve the pain.

- Regularly assess pain location, characteristics and level using a standardised pain scale. Report increasing pain or changes in its location or characteristics. *Tissue substances released during the inflammatory process can stimulate pain receptors. In addition, localised swelling presses on pain-sensitive structures in the area of the inflammation, contributing to discomfort. As inflammation and swelling are reduced, pain should abate. Continued or increasing pain may indicate extension of the thrombosis. Sudden chest pain may indicate a pulmonary embolism, necessitating immediate intervention.*
- Measure calf and thigh diameter of the affected extremity on admission and daily thereafter. Report increases promptly. *The inflammatory process causes vasodilation and increases vessel permeability, causing oedema of the affected extremity. Baseline and subsequent measurements provide a measure of treatment effectiveness.*
- Apply warm, moist heat to affected extremity at least four times daily, using warm, moist compresses or an aqua-K pad. *Moist heat penetrates tissues to a greater depth. Warmth promotes vasodilation, allowing reabsorption of excess fluid into the circulation. Vasodilation also reduces resistance within the affected vessel, reducing pain. As oedema subsides, pressure on surrounding tissues is relieved, thereby reducing pain.*
- Maintain bed rest as ordered. *Using leg muscles during walking exacerbates the inflammatory process and increases oedema. This, in turn, increases venous compression and pain.*

Ineffective tissue perfusion: peripheral

As thrombi develop, they occlude the lumen of the vein and obstruct blood flow. In addition, the accompanying inflammatory response may precipitate vessel spasms, further impairing arterial and venous blood flow and tissue perfusion. Impaired tissue perfusion, in turn, deprives tissues of nutrients and oxygen. As a result, distal tissues of the affected extremity are at risk of ulceration and infection.

> **CONSIDERATION FOR PRACTICE**
>
> **Assess peripheral pulses, skin integrity, capillary refill times and colour of extremities at least every 8 hours. Report changes promptly. Assessment of both extremities allows comparison of the affected and unaffected limbs. Weak or absent pulses, impaired capillary refill or significant colour changes in the affected extremity may indicate extension of the thrombus or a possible complication.**

- Assess skin of the affected lower leg and foot at least every 8 hours; more often as indicated. *Frequent assessment is important to rapidly detect early signs of tissue breakdown*

NURSING CARE PLAN A person with deep venous thrombosis

Mrs Opal Hipps, aged 75, lives alone with her dog, Roxy, in her family home in the western suburbs of Melbourne. She retired from her job at the post office 10 years ago and now spends a lot of time reading and watching television. Over the past week she has developed a vague aching pain in her right leg. She ignored the pain until last night when it developed into a much more severe pain in her right calf. She noticed that her right lower leg seemed larger than the left and it was very tender to the touch. After seeing her doctor and undergoing Doppler ultrasound studies, Mrs Hipps is admitted to the hospital with the diagnosis of deep venous thrombosis in the right leg. She is placed on bed rest and intravenous heparin. Michael Cookson, RN, is assigned to admit and care for Mrs Hipps.

ASSESSMENT

RN Cookson notices that Mrs Hipps was admitted 14 months ago for repair of a fractured femur. Mrs Hipps says, 'This business about a blood clot really has me worried.' She also tells Mr Cookson that she is worried about who will care for her dog while she is in the hospital. Physical findings include height 157 cm, weight 68 kg, T 37.3°C; vital signs within normal limits otherwise. Her left leg is warm and pink, with strong peripheral pulses and good capillary refill. Her right calf is dark red, very warm and dry to touch. It is tender to palpation. The right femoral and popliteal pulses are strong, but the pedal and posterior tibial pulses are difficult to locate. The right calf diameter is 1.27 cm larger than the left.

DIAGNOSES

- *Pain* related to inflammatory response in affected vein.
- *Anxiety* related to unexpected hospitalisation and uncertainty about the seriousness of her illness.
- *Ineffective tissue perfusion: peripheral* related to decreased venous circulation in the right leg.
- *Risk of impaired skin integrity* related to pooling of venous blood in the right leg.

PLANNING

- Plan time with Mrs Hipps to explain venous thrombosis and its treatment.
- Discuss arrangements for a friend or neighbour to care for Mrs Hipps' dog.
- Plan time to liaise with interprofessional team for assessment and interventions.

Expected outcomes

- Verbalise relief of right leg pain by day of discharge.
- Verbalise reduced anxiety by the second day of her hospitalisation.
- Demonstrate reduced right leg diameter by 0.65 cm by the fifth day of hospitalisation.
- Maintain intact skin in the right foot throughout the hospital stay

IMPLEMENTATION

- Elevate legs, maintaining slight knee flexion, while in bed.
- Apply warm, moist compresses to right leg using a 2-hour-on, 2-hour-off schedule around the clock.
- Administer prescribed analgesics and evaluate effectiveness.
- Spend time with Mrs Hipps to explain venous thrombosis and its treatment.
- Arrange for a friend or neighbour to care for Mrs Hipps' dog.
- Apply anti-embolism stockings as ordered; remove for 30 minutes every 8 hours.
- Monitor laboratory values to assess effect of anticoagulant therapy; report values outside desired range.
- Assist with progressive ambulation when allowed.
- Inspect legs and feet and record findings every 8 hours.

EVALUATION

Seven days after admission, the pain in Mrs Hipps' right leg has subsided and the diameter of her right calf is equal to that of her left calf. Mrs Hipps admits to RN Cookson that her fears really relate to a cousin who was hospitalised for a similar problem and had his leg amputated. After talking about her condition and the steps she can take to prevent its recurrence, she is much less anxious. Before discharge, Mr Cookson reviews instructions for anti-embolism stockings, daily walking, warfarin schedule and scheduled follow-up appointment. Mrs Hipps' neighbour, Kate, has come to pick her up. As Mr Cookson is helping Mrs Hipps into the car, Kate hands her a small brown dog and says, 'I took good care of Roxy for you, but he's missed you.' Mrs Hipps smiles and assures Mr Cookson that she will call the number he provided if she has any questions.

CRITICAL THINKING IN THE NURSING PROCESS

1. Describe the pathophysiological reasons for the pain in Mrs Hipps' right leg.
2. How would you respond if Mrs Hipps tells you she does not have the money to buy the prescribed anticoagulant when she goes home?
3. How would you change your teaching and discharge planning if Mrs Hipps had difficulty caring for herself?
4. Design a plan of care for Mrs Hipps for the nursing diagnosis *Activity intolerance*.

REFLECTION ON THE NURSING PROCESS

1. Focusing on the elements of listening to the person, what in Mrs Hipps' case would be important when obtaining a patient history?
2. Discuss four priorities of education pertinent to Mrs Hipps' presentation.

and implementation of measures to protect vulnerable tissues. Early intervention allows healing and restoration of tissue integrity; allowed to continue, the process can lead to necrosis and potential gangrene.

- Elevate extremities at all times, keeping knees slightly flexed and legs above the level of the heart. *Elevation of the extremities promotes venous return and reduces peripheral oedema. Knee flexion promotes muscle relaxation.*
- Use mild soaps, solutions and lotions to clean the affected leg and foot daily. Pat dry after washing and apply a non-alcohol-based lotion or moisturising cream. *Daily hygiene with non-drying soaps and solutions removes potential*

pathogens from the skin surface and maintains skin integrity and the first line of defence against infection. Caustic or harsh soaps or solutions can dry and crack the skin. Dry, cracked skin permits bacteria and other microorganisms to enter and infect the tissue, potentially leading to ulceration and venous gangrene.

CONSIDERATION FOR PRACTICE

Remove anti-embolic stockings or pneumatic compression device for 30 to 60 minutes during daily hygiene. Anti-embolic stockings and pneumatic compression devices exert pressure on the extremity and promote venous return. They can, however, impair perfusion of the dermis. Removing them periodically allows assessment of the underlying tissue and restores perfusion of the dermis, reducing the risk of skin breakdown. Their use may be continued following discharge to reduce the risk of recurrent venous thrombosis.

- Use an egg-crate mattress or sheepskin on the bed as needed. *Egg-crate mattresses and sheepskins distribute weight more evenly, preventing excess pressure on affected tissues.*
- Encourage frequent position changes, at least every 2 hours while awake. *Frequent position changes reduce pressure on bony prominences and oedematous tissue, reducing the risk of tissue breakdown.*

Ineffective protection

Anticoagulant therapy interferes with the body's normal clotting mechanisms, increasing the risk of bleeding and haemorrhage.

- Monitor laboratory results, including the INR (prothrombin time), APTT, haemoglobin and haematocrit, as indicated. Report values outside the normal or desired range. *Coagulation studies are used to monitor the effect of anticoagulant medications. Values within the desired range prevent further clot development while carrying a low risk of bleeding and haemorrhage. A fall in the haemoglobin and haematocrit may indicate undetected bleeding.*

CONSIDERATION FOR PRACTICE

Assess for and promptly report evidence of bleeding, such as petechiae, bruising, bleeding gums, obvious or occult blood in vomitus, stool or urine, unexplained back or abdominal pain. Anticoagulants interfere with the ability to form a stable clot and prevent excessive bleeding. Even minor trauma such as tooth brushing or bumping into furniture can result in bleeding.

Impaired physical mobility

Although prolonged bed rest rarely is required, it is associated with many problems, including constipation, joint contractures, muscle atrophy and boredom. Nursing care goals include maintaining joint range of motion, minimising muscle atrophy and reducing boredom.

- Encourage active range-of-motion (ROM) exercises at least every 8 hours. Provide passive range of motion as needed. *ROM exercises maintain joint mobility and prevent contractures. Active range of motion (performed by the person) also helps prevent muscle atrophy and preserve function. While passive ROM exercises do not prevent muscle atrophy, they do maintain joint mobility.*
- Encourage frequent position changes, deep breathing and coughing. *Prolonged immobility can lead to impaired airway clearance and respiratory complications, such as atelectasis or pneumonia. Turning, coughing and deep breathing facilitate expulsion of secretions from the respiratory tract, airway clearance and alveolar ventilation.*
- Encourage increased fluid and dietary fibre intake. *Constipation is a frequent complication of immobility due to decreased gastrointestinal motility and loss of abdominal muscle strength. Increasing fluid and fibre intake helps maintain soft, easily expelled stools.*
- Assist with and encourage ambulation as allowed. *Ambulation promotes venous blood flow, helps maintain muscle tone and joint mobility, and increases the sense of wellbeing.*
- Encourage diversional activities such as reading, handiwork or other hobbies, television or video games, and socialising. *Boredom may lead to dozing and inertia, with little physical movement or mental stimulation, increasing the risk of complications of immobility.*

Risk of ineffective tissue perfusion: cardiopulmonary

A thrombus that forms in the deep veins of the legs or pelvis may break loose or fragment, becoming an embolism. Emboli that originate in the venous system usually become trapped in the pulmonary circulation (pulmonary embolism). Gas exchange in the affected area is impaired as blood flow ceases or is reduced to an area of the lungs that is well ventilated (see the chapter 'Nursing care of people with ventilation disorders').

- Frequently assess respiratory status, including rate, depth, ease and oxygen saturation levels. *A mismatch of ventilation and perfusion can significantly affect gas exchange, leading to rapid, shallow respirations, dyspnoea and air hunger, and a fall in oxygen saturation levels.*
- Initiate oxygen therapy, elevate the head of the bed and reassure the person who is experiencing manifestations of pulmonary embolism. *Oxygen therapy and elevating the head of the bed promote ventilation and gas exchange in those alveoli that are well perfused, helping maintain tissue oxygenation. Reassurance helps reduce anxiety and slow the respiratory rate, promoting greater respiratory depth and alveolar ventilation.*

CONSIDERATION FOR PRACTICE

Immediately report complaints of chest pain and shortness of breath, anxiety or a sense of impending doom. The manifestations of pulmonary embolism are similar to those of myocardial infarction. Prompt intervention to restore pulmonary blood flow can reduce the risk of significant adverse effects.

Community-based care

Treatment measures for venous thrombosis may be initiated and carried out on an outpatient basis or continued for an extended period of time following hospital discharge. Include the following topics when teaching for home care:

- explanation of the disease process
- treatment measures, including laboratory tests and their purposes, medications and adverse effects that should be reported
- appropriate methods of heat application
- prescribed activity restrictions
- measures to prevent future episodes of venous thrombosis
- the importance of follow-up visits and laboratory tests as scheduled.

Refer people for community nursing services for continued assessment and reinforcement of teaching. Provide referrals for assistance with ADLs and home maintenance services as indicated. Consider referral for physical therapy if needed.

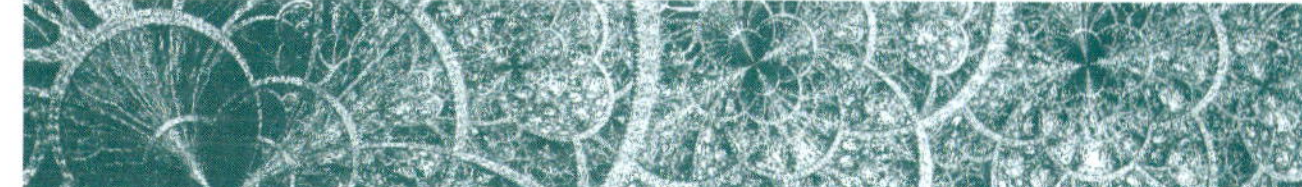

Selected peripheral venous conditions

THE PERSON WITH CHRONIC VENOUS INSUFFICIENCY

Chronic venous insufficiency is a disorder of inadequate venous return over a prolonged period. Deep venous thrombosis (DVT) is the most frequent cause of chronic venous insufficiency. Other conditions, such as varicose veins or leg trauma, may contribute; in some instances, it develops without an identified precipitating cause (Weiss, 2020).

Pathophysiology

Following DVT, large veins may remain occluded, increasing the pressure in other veins of the extremity. This increased pressure distends the veins, separating valve leaflets and impairing their ability to close. DVT also damages valve leaflets, causing them to thicken and contract. The result is impaired unidirectional blood flow and deep vein emptying (Weiss, 2020).

When venous valves are incompetent, the muscle-pumping action produced during activity cannot propel blood back to the heart. Venous blood collects and stagnates in the lower leg (**venous stasis**). Venous pressures in the calf and lower leg increase, particularly during ambulation. This increased pressure impairs arterial circulation to the lower extremities as well. The body's ability to provide sufficient oxygen and nutrients to the cells and remove metabolic waste products diminishes. Eventually, there is so little oxygen and nutrients that cells begin to die. The skin atrophies and subcutaneous fat deposits necrose. Breakdown of red blood cells in the congested tissues causes brown skin pigmentation (Flugman, 2020). Venous stasis ulcers develop. Congested tissues impair the body's ability to increase the supply of oxygen, nutrients and metabolic energy to heal the ulcer. As a result, the condition worsens and, over time, the ulcers enlarge. The congested venous circulation also prevents the blood from mounting effective inflammatory and immune responses, significantly increasing the risk of infection in the ulcerated tissue (Flugman, 2020).

Manifestations

Manifestations of chronic venous insufficiency include lower leg oedema, itching and discomfort of the affected extremity that increase with prolonged standing. The extremity is cyanotic. Recurrent stasis ulcers develop (see Figure 31.15), usually forming just above the ankle, on the medial or anterior aspect of the leg. They heal poorly, forming scar tissue that breaks down easily. Tissue surrounding the ulcer is shiny, atrophic and cyanotic, and there is a brownish pigmentation to the skin. Other skin changes may develop as well, such as eczema or stasis dermatitis. Necrosis and fibrosis of subcutaneous tissue cause the affected area of the leg to feel hard and somewhat leathery to the touch, but even the slightest trauma to the area can produce serious tissue breakdown. See the 'Manifestations' box for the manifestations of chronic venous insufficiency. Table 31.5 compares venous and arterial ulcers.

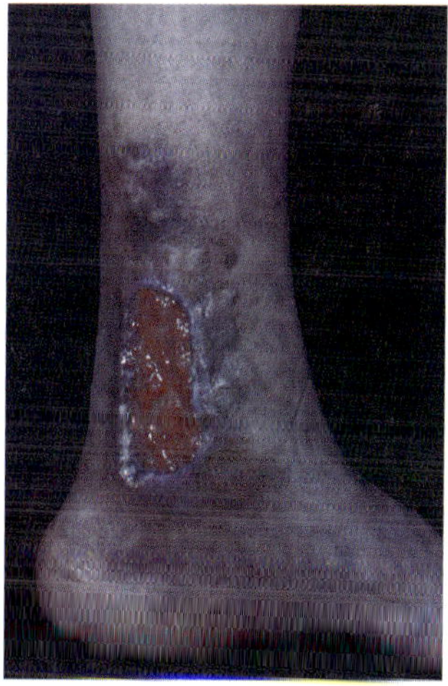

FIGURE 31.15 *Chronic venous insufficiency. Note the discolouration of the ankle and the stasis ulcer*

Source: Biophoto Associates/Science Source.

TABLE 31.5 Comparison of arterial and venous leg ulcers

FACTOR	ARTERIAL ULCERS	VENOUS ULCERS
Location	Toes, feet, shin	Over medial or anterior ankle
Ulcer appearance	Deep, pale	Superficial, pink
Skin appearance	Normal to atrophic Pallor on elevation Rubor on dependency	Brown discolouration Stasis dermatitis Cyanosis on dependency
Skin temperature	Cool	Normal
Oedema	Absent or mild	May be significant
Pain	Usually worse when legs elevated Usually severe Intermittent claudication Rest pain	Usually worse when legs dependent Usually mild
Gangrene	May occur	Does not occur
Pulses	Decreased or absent	Normal

MANIFESTATIONS Chronic venous insufficiency

- Lower extremity oedema that worsens with standing
- Itching, dull leg discomfort or pain that increases with standing
- Thin, shiny, atrophic skin
- Cyanosis and brown skin pigmentation of lower leg and foot
- Possible weeping dermatitis
- Thick, fibrous (hard) subcutaneous tissue
- Recurrent ulcerations of medial or anterior ankle

INTERPROFESSIONAL CARE

Collaborative care for the person with venous insufficiency focuses on relieving symptoms, promoting adequate circulation and healing and preventing tissue damage.

Diagnosis

The history and physical examination often establish the diagnosis of chronic venous insufficiency. Because a history of DVT is a major risk factor, careful evaluation of the past medical history and questioning of the person is important. There are no specific diagnostic tests to confirm the diagnosis of chronic venous insufficiency.

Lifestyle modifications

Conservative management of venous insufficiency focuses on reducing oedema and treating ulcerations. Prolonged standing or sitting is discouraged. Graduated compression hosiery is ordered for daytime use and frequent elevation of the legs and feet during the day is recommended. At night, the legs and feet should be elevated above the level of the heart by raising the foot of the mattress.

Treatment

Treatment of associated stasis dermatitis revolves around managing the chronic venous insufficiency through promoting measures to reduce venous hypertension, including continuous compression therapy, leg elevation when sitting, daily walking and weight reduction as needed.

Other interventions include patient education regarding causes, prevention measures and treatment. Provide assistance with dry skin, pruritus and inflammation and education about the use of mild liquid cleansers to clear scale, bacteria and crusts, and the use of bland emollients or white petroleum jelly as needed, and application of topical corticosteroids to reduce the inflammatory process (Fransway, 2022).

Wet dressing may be required if the person is experiencing exudative eczema and it may reduce pruritus. A number of solutions may be used including saline or potassium permanganate, Burow's solution or a zinc and copper sulphate solution applied to soft cotton roll gauze covered with light dry cotton which is air permeable. This process may be undertaken a couple of times a day for 2–3 hours, for short periods of time if necessary. If the site is impetiginised (affected by impetigo—a skin infection), topical antibiotics may be necessary. Severe infection resulting in cellulitis will require systemic antibiotics following wound MCS (microscopy, culture and sensitivity testing) to direct antibiotic choice (Fransway, 2022).

Surgery

A very large, chronic ulcer may require surgery. In this case, the incompetent veins are ligated, the ulcer is excised and the area is covered with a skin graft (see the chapter 'Nursing care of people wth burns').

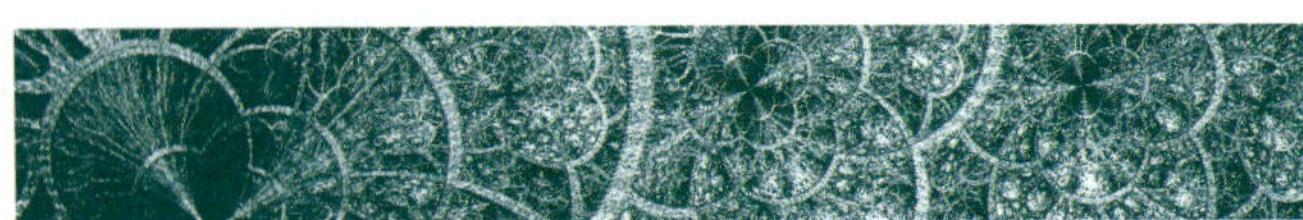

Nursing care

Education

Nursing care for the person with chronic venous insufficiency is primarily educative and supportive. Teaching includes the following recommendations:

- Elevate the legs while resting and during sleep.

- Walk as much as possible but avoid sitting or standing for long periods of time.
- When sitting, do not cross your legs or allow pressure on the back of the knees (such as sitting on the side of the bed).
- Do not wear anything that pinches your legs (such as knee-high stockings, garters).
- Wear elastic compression stockings as prescribed. They should be tighter over the feet than at the top of the leg. Be sure the tops of the stockings do not cut into your legs. Put them on after your legs have been elevated.
- Keep the skin on your feet and legs clean, soft and dry. Follow guidelines in Box 31.6 for care of the legs and feet.

The following nursing diagnoses may apply to the person with chronic venous insufficiency.

- *Disturbed body image* related to oedema and stasis ulcers on lower leg.
- *Ineffective health maintenance* related to lack of knowledge about disorder and prescribed treatments.
- *Risk of infection* related to ulcerations.
- *Impaired physical mobility* related to pain and oedema in lower legs.
- *Impaired skin integrity* related to presence of stasis ulcers.
- *Ineffective tissue perfusion: peripheral* related to incompetent venous valves.

See other sections of this chapter for specific nursing interventions related to many of these diagnoses. See the 'Nursing care of the older adult' box for nursing care of the older adult with chronic venous stasis.

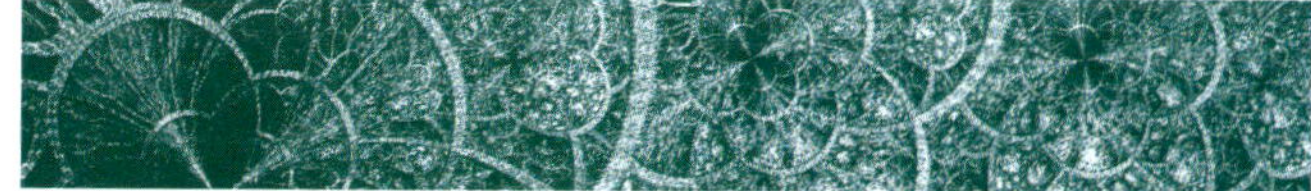

NURSING CARE OF THE OLDER ADULT Chronic venous stasis

Disorders of venous stasis are common after the fifth decade of life. Ageing affects vessels and tissues, increasing the risk of venous insufficiency and varicose veins. In addition, mobility frequently declines with ageing, reducing the effect of the muscle pump in promoting venous return.

HEALTH EDUCATION FOR THE PERSON AND FAMILY

Regular exercise—walking, in particular—is an important part of the treatment plan. Safety when walking is an important issue for older people. Assess the person's mobility and stability during ambulation. If appropriate, suggest using a walker and quad-cane as needed. Assist older people holding jobs that require prolonged standing to identify strategies to minimise standing and incorporate periods of activity into their work.

HOME CARE

Following surgery or during treatment for stasis ulcers, older people may need additional assistance with home care and maintenance. Initiate referral to social services as needed to arrange for home nursing care, meals, assistance with ADLs and home maintenance services as indicated. In some instances, temporary placement in an extended care facility is necessary until the person and family can assume care.

TRANSLATION TO PRACTICE Patient explanation of adherence and non-adherence to venous leg ulcer treatment: a qualitative study

A study by Weller et al. (2021) undertook a qualitative investigation with 31 people experiencing venous leg ulcers to identify barriers and enablers to wound dressing adherence.

The group identified many factors across several domains including knowledge, beliefs, behaviour, social influence, and environmental contexts and resources. They were able to determine various important reasons that contributed to adherence and also to non-adherence in the management of the individuals' leg ulcer wound. Although the study included only 31 people within a geographical area within Melbourne, the information gleaned can inform further research into factors influencing adherence to leg ulcer management plans in primary care.

IMPLICATIONS FOR NURSING

The results of this study are important for nurses to understand factors that may promote or reduce success in managing a venous leg ulcer. This knowledge can be used in education sessions, primary community healthcare situations and further planning of research into adherence to wound care plans. Ultimately, the information may lead to strategies to assist in reducing morbidity or predicting the individuals who would most benefit from further support and information.

CRITICAL THINKING IN PERSON-CENTRED CARE

1. When designing an education session on venous leg ulcer recurrence, which identified factors are modifiable and which are non-modifiable? How will these considerations influence the information provided?
2. How can the results of this research project help a nurse to develop strategies to increase the likelihood of success and adherence to a wound care management plan? Can a nurse influence a person's self efficacy? Explain.
3. How will this information influence your future practice when caring for individuals with current or previous venous ulcers?

THE PERSON WITH VARICOSE VEINS

Varicose veins are irregular, tortuous veins with incompetent valves. Varicosities may develop in any vein and be called other names (e.g. haemorrhoids in the rectum and varices in the oesophagus). They usually affect the veins of the lower extremities; the long saphenous vein is often affected and they also may develop in the short saphenous vein.

Incidence and risk factors

Varicose veins affect about approximately 30% of Western populations (Ahmed et al., 2022). They are more common in women over age 35. Studies also suggest that the increased risk of varicose veins in women may relate to venous stasis during pregnancy. Ageing is a risk factor, possibly related to decreased exercise and other factors that contribute to venous stasis. People in occupations that involve prolonged standing (such as beauticians, salespeople and nurses) also have an increased incidence of varicose veins. Race is a risk factor: white-skinned people are more frequently affected than dark. Many people with primary varicose veins (those affecting superficial veins) have a family history of the disorder, suggesting a genetic link. A large study of over 800,000 people has resulted in the mapping of 237 possible genes at 46 possible loci (Ahmed et al., 2022). A person is twice as likely to develop varicose veins if a parent has a similar condition. Prevalence in a person with an affected female relative is 43%; with a male relative, it is approximately 19%. Yet, there is 75% prevalence in monozygotic twins if one is affected (Weiss, 2020).

Most varicosities occur in the deep veins of the legs. Contributing causes include obesity, venous thrombosis, congenital arteriovenous malformations or sustained pressure on abdominal veins (as in pregnancy and/or the presence of abdominal tumours). The effects of gravity, produced by long periods of standing, are a major causative factor.

Pathophysiology

Varicose veins are classified as primary (with no involvement of deep veins) or secondary (caused by the obstruction of deep veins). In both cases, long-standing increased venous pressure stretches the vessel wall. This sustained stretching impairs the ability of the venous valves to close, causing them to become incompetent.

The erect position produces a twofold negative effect on the veins. When standing, the leg veins resemble vertical columns and must withstand the full force of venous blood pressure. Prolonged standing, the force of gravity, lack of leg exercise and incompetent venous valves all weaken the muscle-pumping mechanism, reducing venous blood return to the heart. As standing continues, the amount of blood pooled in the veins increases, further stretching the vessel wall. The venous valves become increasingly incompetent.

Manifestations

Although varicose veins may be asymptomatic, most cause manifestations such as severe aching leg pain, leg fatigue, leg heaviness, itching or feelings of heat in the legs. The degree of valvular incompetence does not seem to correlate well with the extent of symptoms. The menstrual cycle tends to worsen symptoms, suggesting a possible correlation with hormonal factors in women. Assessment reveals obvious dilated, tortuous veins beneath the skin of the upper and lower leg. If varicose veins are long standing, the skin above the ankles may be thin and discoloured, with a brown pigmentation. (See the 'Manifestations' box.)

MANIFESTATIONS Varicose veins

- Severe, aching pain in the leg
- Leg fatigue, heaviness
- Itching of the affected leg (stasis dermatitis)
- Feelings of warmth in the leg
- Visibly dilated veins
- Thin, discoloured skin above the ankles
- Stasis ulcers

Complications

Complications of varicose veins include venous insufficiency and stasis ulcers. Chronic stasis dermatitis may also develop. Superficial venous thrombosis may develop in varicose veins, especially during and after pregnancy, following surgery and in people on oestrogen therapy (oral contraceptives or hormone replacement therapy).

INTERPROFESSIONAL CARE

Varicose veins usually can be managed using conservative measures, although surgery may be required if symptoms are severe, when complications develop or for cosmetic reasons.

Diagnosis

While varicose veins often are diagnosed by the history and physical examination, diagnostic tests may be ordered.

- *Doppler ultrasonography* or *duplex Doppler ultrasound* may be performed to identify specific locations of incompetent valves. This test is particularly useful before surgery to identify valves that allow reflux of blood from the femoral, popliteal or peripheral deep veins into the superficial veins.
- *Trendelenburg test* may be performed to determine the underlying cause of superficial venous insufficiency. The leg is elevated, then an elastic tourniquet is placed around the distal thigh. The varicosities then are observed as the person stands. When valves of the deep veins are incompetent, the veins remain flat on standing; they rapidly distend when the superficial venous valves are the underlying cause.

Treatments

Although there is no real cure, conservative measures are the core of treatment for most people with uncomplicated varicose veins. These measures often relieve symptoms and prevent complications by improving venous circulation and relieving pressure on venous tissues. Properly fitted graduated compression stockings are commonly prescribed. They compress the veins, propelling blood back to the heart.

Compression stockings augment the muscle pumping action of the legs. When worn during times of prolonged standing and in combination with frequent leg elevation, compression stockings often prevent progression of the condition and development of complications.

Regular, daily walking also is important. Prolonged sitting and standing are discouraged, although elevating the legs for specified periods during the day is beneficial. Leg elevation promotes venous return, prevents venous stasis and decreases leg heaviness and fatigue.

COMPRESSION SCLEROTHERAPY In compression sclerotherapy, a sclerosing solution is injected into the varicose vein and a compression bandage is applied for a period of time. This obliterates the vein. Venous blood is rerouted through healthy vessels whose valves are not compromised. Compression sclerotherapy may be used to treat small, symptomatic varicosities. It may be the primary treatment or it may be used in conjunction with varicose vein surgery. While compression sclerotherapy may be done for cosmetic reasons, complications such as phlebitis, tissue necrosis or infection may occur and need to be considered prior to the procedures.

Surgery

Surgical treatment options for varicose veins have improved, with advances in technique and technology. There are several possible approaches depending on the reason for the intervention. Surgery may reduce symptoms and improve quality of life for those who experience recurrent superficial venous thrombosis and/or develop stasis ulcers. For others, it may be considered for cosmetic reasons. Options now include:

- *Endovenous laser therapy*, where ablation follows the insertion of a laser fibre placed inside the target vessel. Firing the laser causes irreversible thermal damage to the endothelial tissues to collapse the vessel. This process is repeated after each pulse and the catheter is withdrawn approximately 2 mm for the length of the target vessel needing treatment.
- *Radiofrequency ablation*, where ablation is achieved with a radiofrequency catheter placed inside the target vessel. Firing the laser causes irreversible thermal damage of 120ºC using radiofrequency energy in sections of 7 cm for the length of the target vessel needing treatment.
- *Stab-avulsion technique*, where a phlebectomy hook is inserted through a microincision, and after traction is applied, the vessel is pulled out of the body (tearing it from its tributary vessels).
- *Saphenectomy* is the old technique where the section to be removed is ligated and divided from its associated tributary vessels. It has been almost entirely replaced with the newer techniques described above.

Unlike the extensive ligation and stripping techniques of the past, the newer interventions require less post-intervention care as they can be completed in under an hour, and not necessarily in a theatre environment. A different post-therapy requirement includes the need to walk for approximately 5–10 minutes every hour (during the day) or for between 20 and 60 minutes for the radiofrequency ablation. A compressive stocking will be applied and needs to be left on for at least 48 hours following the surgery, then during waking hours for the next 6 weeks. Cool compresses may be used to assist with pain. Non-steroidal medications including aspirin should be avoided. However, the interventions are generally well tolerated.

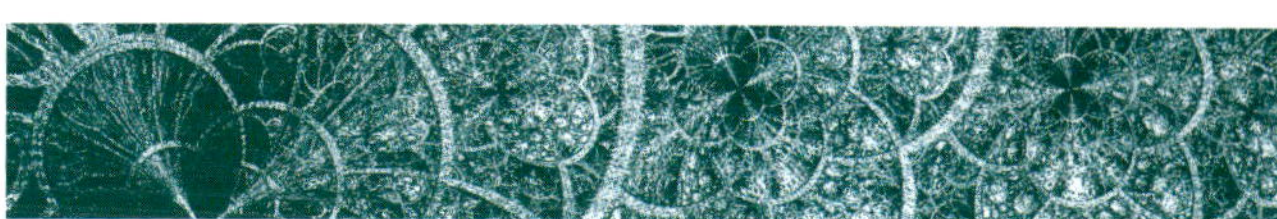

Nursing care

Health promotion

Health promotion activities to reduce the incidence of varicose veins include teaching all people, particularly young women, the benefits of regular exercise continued over the lifetime. Discuss the effect of prolonged sitting or standing on the legs and encourage the person whose occupation involves these activities to periodically get up and move or to sit with the legs elevated. Encourage everyone to maintain normal weight for his or her height.

Assessment

Focused assessment of the person with varicose veins includes the following:

- *Health history*: complaints of leg pain, aching, heaviness or fatigue; ankle swelling; history of venous thrombosis.
- *Physical examination*: visible, dilated, tortuous superficial veins in lower extremities.

Nursing diagnoses and interventions

In planning and providing nursing care for people with varicose veins, emphasis is placed on the importance of health teaching to manage the symptoms of varicose veins, particularly because there is no cure for the disease. Nursing care for people who have undergone surgical treatment for varicose veins focuses on assessing and promoting wound healing and preventing infection. Nursing diagnoses may include those related to pain, impaired tissue perfusion and skin integrity, and a risk of impaired neurovascular function.

Chronic pain

Varicose veins can lead to pooling of venous blood in the lower extremities. Venous congestion can cause a dull ache or feeling of pressure in the legs, particularly after prolonged standing. As venous pressure rises, arterial circulation and delivery of oxygen and nutrients to tissues is impaired. Tissue ischaemia contributes to the pain. The pain associated with varicose veins tends to be chronic, developing and progressing gradually over a long period of time.

- Assess pain, including its intensity, duration and aggravating and relieving factors. *Pain assessment allows collaborative planning with the person to identify appropriate interventions.*
- Inquire about current measures being used by the person to manage pain and its effects. Ask about the

effectiveness of current management strategies and the desire to change. *Chronic pain management ultimately falls to the person. Strategies to address the pain must meet the person's needs.*

CONSIDERATION FOR PRACTICE

Suggest keeping a diary of pain intensity, timing, precipitating events and effectiveness of relief measures. Systematic tracking of pain is an important measure in improving its management.

- Teach and reinforce non-pharmacological pain management strategies such as progressive relaxation, imagery, deep breathing, distraction and meditation. *The effectiveness of such strategies is well documented. Non-pharmacological measures provide a variety of options for controlling pain while maintaining independence. These measures also can reduce reliance on analgesics.*
- Collaborate with the person to establish a pain control plan. *Collaborative planning for pain management increases the person's sense of control and reduces powerlessness. This, in turn, enhances the ability to cope with pain and its effects.*
- Regularly evaluate the effectiveness of planned interventions and pain management strategies. *Regular evaluation allows modification of the care plan as needed, as well as providing a measure of disease progression. Increasing or poorly controlled pain may necessitate additional collaborative interventions to manage the disorder.*

Ineffective tissue perfusion: peripheral

Varicose veins and venous stasis impair delivery of nutrients and oxygen to peripheral tissues as elevated venous pressures interfere with blood flow through the capillary beds. Improving venous blood flow reduces venous pressures and promotes arterial flow to peripheral tissues.

- Assess peripheral pulses, capillary refill, skin colour and temperature, and extent of oedema. *Assessment of arterial flow and tissue perfusion provides baseline and continuing data for evaluating the effectiveness of interventions.*
- Teach application and use of properly fitted elastic graduated compression stockings. *Elastic compression stockings compress the veins, promoting venous return from the lower extremities. During ambulation, the stockings enhance the blood-pumping action of the muscles. Because elastic stockings inhibit blood flow through small superficial vessels, they should be removed at least once each day for at least 30 minutes.*

CONSIDERATION FOR PRACTICE

Instruct to maintain a program of regular exercise, such as walking for 20 to 30 minutes several times a day. Exercise stimulates circulation and promotes blood flow through the vascular system. When ambulation is restricted, active ROM exercises help maintain muscle tone, joint mobility and venous return.

- Advise to elevate the legs for 15 to 20 minutes several times a day and to sleep with the legs elevated above the level of the heart. *Elevating the legs promotes venous return, reducing tissue congestion and improving arterial circulation. Improved venous return also increases the cardiac output and renal perfusion, promoting elimination of excess fluid and decreasing peripheral oedema.*

Risk of impaired skin integrity

Ineffective venous valve function impairs venous return and increases venous pressures. These increased pressures oppose arterial blood flow and the delivery of oxygen and nutrients to the cells. As a result, tissues are vulnerable to any additional insult and may break down.

- Assess lower extremity colour, temperature and moisture, and for evidence of pressure or breakdown, on admission and at each visit. *Initial and continuing assessment allows timely detection of early signs of skin and tissue breakdown. This, in turn, allows early institution of measures to prevent further tissue damage and promote healing.*
- Teach foot and skin care measures such as daily cleansing with non-drying soap, gentle drying and lotions to prevent skin dryness and cracking. *Cleansing removes potentially harmful microorganisms and stimulates circulation. Care is taken to keep the skin moist and supple, promoting its function as the first line of defence against infection.*
- Discuss the importance of adequate nutrition and fluid intake. *Adequate nutrients are necessary to maintain tissue integrity and promote healing. A diet high in protein, carbohydrates and vitamins and minerals promotes growth and maintenance of skin cells, provides energy and helps prevent skin breakdown. Adequate hydration helps maintain the moisture and turgor of skin, reducing the risk of drying and breakdown.*

Risk of peripheral neurovascular dysfunction

Severe varicose veins can lead to chronic venous insufficiency, impaired arterial circulation and, ultimately, disrupted sensation in the affected extremity. Impaired neurological function increases the person's risk of injury and infection of the extremity, because minor trauma may go unnoticed.

- Assess circulation, sensation and movement of the lower extremities. *Disrupted circulation and venous congestion may interfere with sensory and motor function of the affected extremity. The potential for nerve and muscle involvement is especially high in people with venous stasis ulcers.*
- Teach measures to protect the extremities from injury, such as always wearing shoes or firm slippers, cotton socks to absorb moisture and testing the temperature of bath water with a thermometer or the upper extremities before stepping in. *Sensation in the lower extremities*

may be affected by poor circulation, necessitating additional measures to protect the legs and feet from injury.

CONSIDERATION FOR PRACTICE

Instruct to report signs of neurovascular dysfunction, such as numbness, coldness, pain or tingling of an extremity. Early recognition of neurovascular dysfunction facilitates institution of interventions to prevent complications. Because the postoperative hospital stay following varicose vein surgery or venous stasis ulcer repair is brief, manifestations of neurovascular dysfunction may initially be detected by the person. Careful assessment and prompt reporting help prevent potential complications such as skin breakdown, infection and nerve damage.

Community-based care

Most people with varicose veins provide self-care at home. Include the following topics when preparing the person and family for home care:

- leg elevation and exercise program
- application and use of graduated elastic compression stockings
- foot and leg care (see Box 31.6 earlier in this chapter)
- measures to avoid injury and skin breakdown
- symptoms or potential complications to report to the doctor.

Provide information about suppliers of elastic stockings and any other required supplies. If venous stasis ulcers have developed, consider referral to home health services for regular assessment of healing and additional teaching.

Disorders of the lymphatic system

The lymphatic system, which includes the lymphatic vessels and the lymph nodes, is a unique part of the circulatory system. The lymphatic system returns plasma and plasma proteins filtered out of the capillaries from interstitial tissues to the bloodstream. This fluid is called *lymph*. The lymphatic system consists of closed capillaries leading to larger lymphatic venules and lymphatic veins. These vessels contain smooth muscle and one-way valves that help move fluid towards the heart. Lymphatic vessels share the same sheath as arteries and veins; arterial pulsations and skeletal muscle contractions compress the lymphatic vessels to assist in maintaining lymph flow. As lymph moves through the lymphatic system, it is filtered through thousands of bean-shaped lymph nodes clustered along the vessels. Within these nodes, phagocytes remove foreign material from the lymph, preventing it from entering the bloodstream.

THE PERSON WITH LYMPHATIC SYSTEM COMPROMISE

Lymphadenopathy

Lymphadenopathy, enlarged lymph nodes, may be localised or generalised. Localised lymphadenopathy usually results from an inflammatory process (e.g. streptococcal pharyngitis or an infected wound). The node enlarges as lymphocytes and monocytes proliferate within the node to destroy infectious material. Palpable lymph nodes often develop in response to minor trauma or a localised infection. Generalised lymphadenopathy usually is associated with malignancy or disease. Malignant cells or other abnormal cells invade the node, causing it to enlarge.

Lymphangitis, inflammation of the lymph vessels draining an infected area of the body, is characterised by a red streak along the inflamed vessels, pain, heat and swelling. Fever and chills also may be present. Local lymph nodes are swollen and tender.

Treatment for lymphadenopathy and lymphangitis focuses on identifying and treating the underlying condition. Elevating the body part and applying heat to inflamed lymphatic vessels help reduce swelling and promote blood flow to the affected area.

Lymphoedema

Lymphoedema may be a primary or a secondary disorder resulting from inflammation, obstruction or removal of lymphatic vessels. It is characterised by extremity oedema due to accumulation of lymph. *Primary lymphoedema* is uncommon, affecting about 1 in every 6 people (Australasian Lymphology Association, 2022). It affects females more frequently than males and may be associated with a genetic disorder such as Turner's syndrome or Klinefelter's syndrome. (See the 'Genetic considerations' box.)

Secondary lymphoedema is an acquired condition, resulting from damage, obstruction or removal of lymphatic vessels. The most common worldwide cause of secondary lymphoedema is *filariasis*, infestation of the lymphatic vessels by filaria, a nematode worm. Other important causes of secondary lymphoedema include recurrent episodes of bacterial lymphangitis, obstruction of lymph vessels by tumours and surgical or radiation treatment for breast cancer (Schwartz, 2021).

GENETIC CONSIDERATIONS
Primary Lymphoedema

- Primary lymphoedema develops as a result of agenesis, hypoplasia or obstruction of lymphatic vessels.
- *Congenital lymphoedema* appears shortly after birth; two other forms of lymphoedema develop later, one at the time of puberty (*lymphoedema praecox*), the other usually after age 35 (*lymphoedema tarda*)
- Congenital lymphoedema and lymphoedema praecox may be inherited as an autosomal dominant trait with variable penetrance.

Pathophysiology and manifestations

Obstruction of lymph drainage prevents fluid and protein molecules from interstitial tissues from returning to the circulation. The protein molecules increase the osmotic pressure in interstitial tissues, drawing in additional fluid that causes oedema in the soft tissues. One or both extremities may be affected.

The oedema begins distally, progressing up the limb to involve the entire extremity. Initial oedema is soft and pitting; with chronic congestion, subcutaneous tissues become fibrotic, causing thick, rough skin and a woody texture of the limb (*brawny oedema*). In contrast, the oedema associated with venous disorders is softer and the skin often is hyperpigmented with evidence of stasis dermatitis. Lymphoedema generally is painless, although the limb may feel heavy.

INTERPROFESSIONAL CARE

Interprofessional care for the person with lymphoedema focuses on relieving oedema and preventing or treating infection. The disorder may be difficult to treat effectively and can lead to progressive disability due to the weight and awkwardness of the affected extremity.

Diagnosis

Abdominal or pelvic ultrasound and CT scans are used to detect obstructing lesions. MRI can show oedema and identify lymph nodes and enlarged lymphatic vessels. More invasive procedures such as lymphangiography and radioactive isotope studies may occasionally be necessary to identify the lymphatic defect causing lymphoedema.

- *Lymphangiography* uses injected contrast media to illustrate lymphatic vessels on x-rays. Organic dyes are used to identify a distal lymphatic vessel and then a contrast medium is injected into the vessel for visualisation of the lymphatic system of the limb. In primary lymphoedema, lymph vessels are absent or hypoplastic (underdeveloped). In secondary lymphoedema, lymph channels often are dilated; it may be possible to determine the level of obstruction (Schwartz, 2021).
- *Lymphoscintigraphy* involves injecting a radioactively tagged substance into distal subcutaneous tissues of the extremity, then mapping its flow through the lymphatic system. The pattern of lymph fluid distribution and transport is abnormal in people with lymphoedema.

Treatments

Meticulous skin and foot care is vital to prevent infection in the affected extremity. Shoes should always be worn to reduce the risk of injury. Careful cleansing and use of emollient lotions are recommended to prevent drying of the skin. Exercise is encouraged, as are frequent periods of leg elevation. The foot of the bed is raised by 15 to 20 degrees at night to promote lymph flow. Elastic graduated compression stockings may be ordered for use during the day. In some cases, an intermittent pneumatic compression device to reduce oedema may be prescribed for home use.

Antibiotics are given to prevent and treat infection, which can be recurrent and difficult to eradicate. Diuretic therapy may be used intermittently, particularly when primary lymphoedema is exacerbated by the menstrual cycle or seasonal variability (Morfoisse et al., 2021).

People who do not respond to conservative treatment measures or who experience recurrent episodes of cellulitis and lymphangitis may require surgical treatment. Microvascular techniques may be used to create anastomoses between obstructed lymphatic vessels and adjacent veins, providing channels to redirect lymph into the venous system. Successful surgery may improve both extremity function and its cosmetic appearance (Schwartz, 2021).

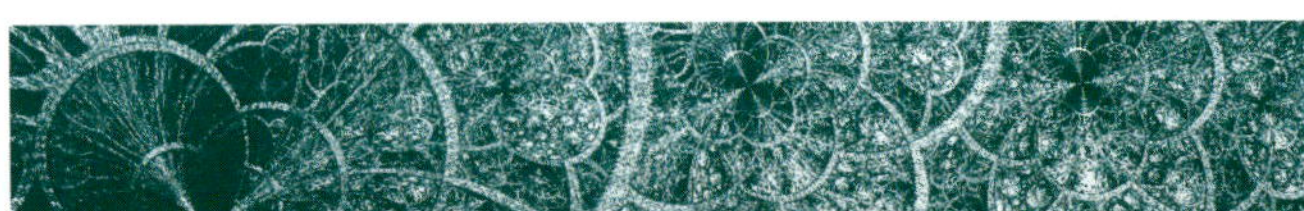

Nursing care

Nursing care for people with lymphatic disorders focuses on reducing oedema, preventing tissue damage related to the oedema and promoting effective coping with the impact of the disorder on body image and function.

Nursing diagnoses and interventions

Nursing diagnoses for the person with lymphoedema may include *Impaired tissue integrity*, *Excess fluid volume* and *Disturbed body image*.

Impaired tissue integrity

Obstructed lymphatic flow leads to fluid congestion of the interstitial spaces of subcutaneous tissue. The resulting oedema compresses and damages tissues of the affected extremity. Subcutaneous tissues become fibrotic, reducing their protective functions of shock absorption and insulation. In addition, obstructed lymphatic flow reduces the effectiveness of lymph nodes in filtering and removing foreign material and pathogens from the body. This increases the risk of local tissue infection such as *cellulitis*, a diffuse bacterial infection of the skin. Cellulitis increases the risk of skin and tissue breakdown and, if not effectively treated, can lead to sepsis.

CONSIDERATION FOR PRACTICE

Frequently inspect the skin of the affected extremity, documenting condition with each assessment. Promptly report areas of pallor, redness or apparent inflammation. Breaks in the skin surface allow microbial invasion and increase the risk of infection. Prompt identification and treatment of any lesions is vital to prevent further tissue breakdown and infection.

- Apply well-fitting elastic graduated compression stockings or intermittent pneumatic pressure devices as ordered. *Elastic stockings and/or pneumatic pressure devices oppose the movement of fluid out of capillaries and improve its reabsorption into vascular spaces for transportation back to the heart.*

- Instruct to elevate the extremities while seated and during sleep. *Elevation of the extremities diminishes venous congestion, promotes venous return, facilitates arterial circulation and tissue perfusion and helps reduce the accumulation of excess fluids in interstitial spaces of the affected extremity.*

CONSIDERATION FOR PRACTICE

Remove elastic stockings and intermittent pressure devices every 8 hours or at each home visit to inspect the underlying skin for evidence of redness, irritation, dryness or breakdown. Elastic graduated compression stockings, anti-embolic stockings and pneumatic compression devices compress small vessels nourishing the skin and subcutaneous tissue. Periodic removal not only allows inspection of the underlying skin, but also allows restoration of blood flow to these small vessels and the tissues.

CONSIDERATION FOR PRACTICE

Use preventive skin care devices as indicated. Collected fluid in the affected extremity increases its weight and interferes with regular movement. The increased weight places greater pressure on surfaces of the limb that come in contact with furniture. Protective devices such as egg-crate foam, sheepskin, pillows or padding help prevent tissue compression, promoting circulation and reducing the risk of skin and tissue breakdown.

- Keep skin clean and dry, especially in interdigital spaces. Teach skin and foot care to the person and family. *Clean, dry skin provides the first line of defence against infection. Significant limb oedema can interfere with reaching the distal extremity and cleaning interdigital spaces. The dark, moist spaces between the toes are an excellent environment for bacterial growth. Teaching fosters self-care and independence, as well as preparing the person and family to manage this often chronic condition.*
- Discuss the importance of adhering to the therapeutic regimen. *Lymphoedema generally is a chronic condition; effective management requires active person participation in planning and implementing care to reduce oedema and maintain tissue integrity.*

Excess fluid volume

In lymphoedema, obstruction, destruction or congenital malformation of lymphatic vessels interferes with the normal circulation of lymphatic fluid. As a result, lymph collects in the subcutaneous tissues of the affected extremity, causing excess fluid volume of that extremity. Some people may benefit from intermittent diuretic therapy and dietary sodium restriction.

- Discuss the rationale for restricted sodium intake if ordered. Teach ways to maintain the recommended sodium restriction and assist to choose foods that are low in sodium. *Sodium causes retention of extracellular water; restricting dietary sodium may help prevent additional fluid accumulation in interstitial spaces.*
- During acute periods, assess the affected extremity daily for increased oedema; measure girth of the extremity using consistent technique. *The size of the affected extremity provides a measure of the effectiveness of ordered interventions and progression of the disorder.*

CONSIDERATION FOR PRACTICE

Monitor intake and output and/or weight (daily or weekly). Use consistent scales, timing and clothing for accurate weight measurements. Intake and output records and short-term changes in weight reflect fluid balance. Measures of fluid balance permit evaluation of the effectiveness of interventions such as restricted sodium intake and diuretic therapy.

Disturbed body image

The disproportionate size of an extremity or extremities due to lymphoedema can profoundly affect body image. During early stages of the disease, conservative measures may effectively reduce the oedema and size of the affected limb. However, as the disease progresses, conservative measures may become less effective, leading to more permanent disfigurement. Mobility may be impaired and the person may develop an increasingly negative self-perception.

- Encourage discussions about usual coping patterns and perception of self. *Knowledge of existing coping patterns and behaviours helps the nurse assess the person's ability to cope with the current situation. This knowledge is then used to reinforce effective coping mechanisms and help develop more effective coping strategies. This exchange also allows the person to voice feelings related to actual or perceived changes in body image.*
- Accept the person's perception of self and of the impact of the changes in appearance. *Non-judgmental acceptance of the person's view of self and of the effects of changes in appearance builds trust and promotes rapport. A trusting relationship promotes the person's ability to take an active role in managing the disorder, participate in healthcare decisions and adhere to the plan of care. Non-judgmental listening also promotes mutual respect and demonstrates caring and compassion.*
- Encourage active participation in self-care. Assist with identifying alternative self-care strategies when the extent of oedema interferes with performing some aspects of self-care such as trimming toenails or washing feet. *The person initially may have difficulty viewing or touching the affected body part. Gentle encouragement and support from the nurse help the person assume self-care and accept the affected body part. Brainstorming to identify alternative care strategies promotes the person's independence even when total self-care is not feasible.*

Community-based care

When preparing the person with chronic lymphoedema and family to manage the disorder, include the following teaching topics:

- recommended program of exercise and elevation of the extremity
- foot and skin care

- use of elastic graduated compression stockings and/or intermittent pressure devices
- importance of wearing elastic stockings during the majority of waking hours, removing them once during the daytime and while sleeping
- measures to prevent infection in the affected extremity, such as wearing gloves while gardening
- signs and symptoms to report to the healthcare provider (e.g. manifestations of tissue breakdown or infection, increasing oedema or evidence of compromised circulation)
- use and precautions associated with any prescribed medications
- sodium-restricted diet if ordered.

Provide information about contacts for questions and make referrals as needed. Evaluate the need for home health, home maintenance assistance and other services such as physical or occupational therapy.

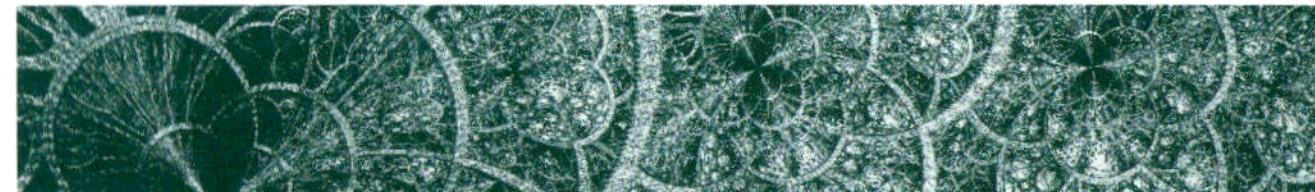

CHAPTER HIGHLIGHTS

- Essential hypertension, blood pressure of 140/90 mmHg or higher with no clearly identified cause, rarely causes symptoms but is a major risk factor for coronary heart disease, heart failure, stroke and renal insufficiency.
- Prehypertension, a newly identified category, is an average blood pressure of 120–139/80–89 mmHg. People with prehypertension are advised to make lifestyle changes indicated for hypertension (weight loss, exercise, dietary changes, limited alcohol intake and stress reduction), but generally are not treated with medications unless other risk factors such as diabetes or kidney disease are present.
- Systolic hypertension, an elevated systolic blood pressure without elevation of the diastolic pressure, is common in older adults and contributes to complications such as coronary heart disease and stroke.
- Cardiovascular disease in Indigenous Australians is 30% more common than in non-Indigenous Australians.
- Risk factors for CVD are more common in Indigenous Australians than in non-Indigenous Australians: diabetes is four times as common, smoking daily and obesity are twice as common.
- Medications to treat hypertension include diuretics, alpha- and beta-adrenergic blockers, ACE inhibitors and angiotensin II blockers, calcium channel blockers and vasodilators. A combination of two or more drugs often is required for effective blood pressure control.
- Aneurysms, abnormal dilation of a blood vessel, commonly affect the aorta and the iliac arteries, particularly in older men. A slowly expanding abdominal aortic aneurysm that does not produce symptoms or impair flow through the renal arteries may not be repaired, particularly in an older person. Percutaneously inserted endovascular splints provide an alternative to surgery for abdominal aortic aneurysms.
- Peripheral vascular disease, obstruction or occlusion of peripheral arteries by atherosclerotic plaque, is common and a leading cause of disability and amputation.
- Smoking cessation and regular daily exercise are key components of treatment for peripheral vascular disorders such as atherosclerosis, thromboangiitis obliterans and Raynaud's disease.
- Venous thrombosis, particularly of the deep veins of the legs and pelvis, develops as a result of venous stasis, blood vessel damage and increased coagulability of the blood. The developing clot may fragment or break loose, becoming an embolus that typically lodges in the pulmonary circulation (pulmonary embolus). Chronic venous insufficiency and venous stasis may develop as a result of deep venous thrombosis.
- Prophylactic anticoagulation and mobilisation of the person are the primary preventive measures for venous thrombosis. Monitoring coagulation studies and assessing for evidence of bleeding (overt or covert) are important nursing measures for the person on anticoagulant therapy.
- Lymphadenopathy (enlarged lymph nodes), lymphangitis (inflammation of the lymph vessels) and lymphoedema are the most common disorders affecting the lymph system.

CONCEPT CHECK

1 A potential blood donor whose blood pressure is found to average 180/106 mmHg on two different readings tells the nurse, 'I don't understand how it could be so high—I feel just fine.' The appropriate response by the nurse is:

1. 'This is probably just a false reading due to "white coat syndrome". Don't worry about it.'
2. 'It is unusual that you are not having some symptoms such as severe headaches and nosebleeds.'
3. 'High blood pressure often has few or no symptoms; that's why it is called the "silent killer".'
4. 'You probably should have your blood pressure rechecked in 3 months or so and then follow up with your primary care provider if it is still high.'

2 The nurse teaching a person about a healthy diet determines that additional teaching is necessary when the person states:

1. 'I'm glad I can still eat as much pasta as usual; I was afraid I would have to give up my weekly lasagne.'
2. 'It will be a challenge to incorporate all those servings of fruit and vegetables into my diet.'
3. 'Having a handful of nuts when the pre-dinner "munchies" hit is a good idea.'
4. 'I will enjoy having frozen yogurt as my bedtime snack on occasion.'

3 The nurse teaching a person about his new prescription for Co-Diovan, a combination angiotensin II receptor blocker and thiazide diuretic, includes which of the following in his instructions? (Select all that apply.)

1. Use a potassium-based salt substitute to prevent hypokalaemia while taking this drug.
2. Use caution when rising from bed or a chair to prevent dizziness.
3. Take the drug at bedtime to reduce the risk of falling due to light-headedness.
4. Report a persistent disruptive cough to your doctor.
5. You may stop taking this drug once your blood pressure is within the normal range for 2 months.

4 A person is complaining of new-onset calf and foot pain. The nurse notes that the leg below the knee is cool and pale and that dorsalis pedis and posterior tibial pulses are absent. The priority nursing intervention is to:
1 notify the doctor
2 place a cradle over the leg to prevent pressure from bedding
3 position the leg flat, supported in anatomical position
4 prepare to initiate heparin therapy

5 An 86-year-old person with a newly diagnosed abdominal aortic aneurysm wonders if he will need surgery to repair the aneurysm, even though he feels fine. The nurse's response is based on the knowledge that:
1 the risk of surgical repair is lower than the risk that the aneurysm will rupture
2 opening the abdomen for the surgical procedure greatly increases the risk of rupture
3 surgery is indicated for type A aneurysms
4 a percutaneously inserted endovascular stent may be considered because of his age

6 An expected assessment finding in a person with peripheral atherosclerosis would be:
1 pallor of the legs and feet when dependent
2 increased hair growth on the affected extremity
3 higher blood pressure readings in the affected extremity
4 impaired sensation in the affected extremity

7 All of the following are appropriate home care measures for the person with peripheral vascular disease. Place them in order of priority.
1 foot and leg care
2 smoking cessation
3 daily inspection of feet and legs
4 regular daily exercise
5 weight loss strategies

8 The nurse evaluates her teaching of a person admitted with deep venous thrombosis as effective when the person states:
1 'I'll use a hard-backed, upright chair when sitting instead of my recliner.'
2 'I'll get my blood drawn as scheduled and notify the doctor if I have any unusual bleeding or bruising.'
3 'I understand why I am not allowed to exercise for the next 6 weeks and will take it easy.'
4 'I'll have my wife buy a low-cholesterol cookbook and we'll make an appointment with the dietitian to learn about a low-fat, low-cholesterol diet.'

9 A person with visible varicose veins tells the nurse that she wants to have surgery to remove them, because 'my legs ache every evening and they are really ugly!'. The most appropriate response would be:
1 'Often measures such as elevating your legs and elastic stockings can relieve the discomfort associated with varicose veins.'
2 'Surgery will have a good cosmetic effect, but will not relieve the discomfort associated with varicose veins.'
3 'All varicose veins should be surgically removed to restore adequate blood flow to your legs and prevent gangrene.'
4 'Surgery is never indicated unless the varicose veins are interfering with circulation. Have you tried cosmetic measures to cover them up?'

10 Which of the following nursing interventions is of highest priority for the person with lymphoedema?
1 Elevate affected extremities at night.
2 Assist to don elastic compression stockings during the day.
3 Carefully dry and apply emollient lotion to affected extremities after bathing.
4 Reinforce the importance of taking prescribed diuretics.

BIBLIOGRAPHY

Ahmad, W., Kleeman, S., Ng, M. et al. (2022). Genome-wide association analysis and replication in 810,625 individuals with varicose veins. *Nature Communications, 13*, 3065. https://doi.org/10.1038/s41467-022-30765-y

Aitken, S. (2020). Peripheral artery disease in the lower limbs: The importance of secondary risk prevention for improved long-term prognosis. *Australian Journal of General Practice, 49*(5), 239–244. https://doi.org/10.31128/AJGP-11-19-5160

Alexander, M. (2019). Hypertension. *Emedicine*. Retrieved from http://emedicine.medscape.com/

Australasian Lymphology Association (2022). *Lymphoedema*. Retrieved from https://www.lymphoedema.org.au/

Australian Bureau of Statistics (ABS) (2021). *Causes of death, Australia, 2020*. (Cat. no. 3303.) Retrieved from https://www.abs.gov.au/

Australian Bureau of Statistics (ABS) ([illegible]). *Health conditions prevalence—Table 2: Long-term conditions by age then sex*. Retrieved from https://www.abs.gov.au/

Australian Commission on Safety and Quality in Health Care (ACSQHC) (2021). *National Safety and Quality Health Service Standards* (2nd ed.). Sydney: ACSQHC.

Australian Institute of Health and Welfare (AIHW) (2019). *High blood pressure*. Canberra: AIHW. Retrieved from www.aihw.gov.au

Australian Institute of Health and Welfare (AIHW) (2020). *Overweight and obesity: An interactive insight*. Canberra: AIHW. Retrieved from www.aihw.gov.au/

Australian Institute of Health and Welfare (AIHW) (2021). *Separation statistics by principal diagnosis in ICD-10-AM 11th edition, Australia, 2020–21*. Retrieved from www.aihw.gov.au/

Australian Institute of Health and Welfare (AIHW) (2022). Australian Burden of Disease Study: Impact and causes of illness and death in Aboriginal and Torres Strait Islander people 2018. *Australian Burden of Disease Study Series, 26*. Cat. no. BOD 32. Canberra: AIHW. Retrieved from https://www.aihw.gov.au/

Australian Institute of Health and Welfare: National Indigenous Australians Agency (AIHW: NIAA) (2022). *Tier 1 – Health status and outcomes 1.07. High blood pressure*. Canberra: AIHW. Retrieved from https://www.aihw.gov.au/

[illegible] (2022). Overview of the causes of venous thrombosis. *Uptodate*. Retrieved from https://www.uptodate.com

Bullock, S. & Manias, E. (2022). *Fundamentals of pharmacology* (9th ed.). Sydney: Pearson.

Campbell, N., Whelton, P. K., Orias, M. et al. (2022). 2022 World Hypertension League, resolve to save lives and international society of hypertension dietary sodium (salt) global call to action. *Journal of Human Hypertension*. https://doi.org/10.1038/s41371-022-00690-0

Chang, W. (2022). Ankle-brachial Index (ABI) measurement technique. *Emedicine*. Retrieved from http://emedicine.medscape.com

Chow, C. K., Atkins, E. R., Hillis, G. S. et al. (2021). Initial treatment with a single pill containing quadruple combination of quarter doses of blood pressure medicines versus standard dose monotherapy in patients with hypertension (QUARTET): A phase 3, randomised, double-blind, active-controlled trial. *The Lancet, 398*(10305), 1043–1052. https://doi.org/10.1016/S0140-6736(21)01922-X

Chuter, V., Quigley, F., Tosenovsky, P., Ritter, J. C., Charles, J., Cheney, J., Fitridge, R. & Australian Diabetes-related Foot Disease Guidelines & Pathways Project (2022). Australian guideline on diagnosis and management of peripheral artery disease: Part of the 2021 Australian evidence based guidelines for diabetes-related foot disease. *Journal of Foot and Ankle Research, 15*(1), 51. https://doi.org/10.1186/[illegible]

Dominguez, J. ([illegible]). Peripheral arterial occlusive disease. *Emedicine*. Retrieved from http://emedicine.medscape.com/

Flugman, S. (2020). Stasis dermatitis. *Emedicine*. Retrieved from http://emedicine.medscape.com/

Fransway, A. (2022). Stasis dermatitis. *UpToDate*. Retrieved from https://www.uptodate.com/

Gao, Z. Chen, Z., Sun, A. & Deng, X. (2019). Gender differences in cardiovascular disease. *Medicine in Novel Technology and Devices*, *4*, 100025. https://doi.org/10.1016/j.medntd.2019.100025

Hansen-Dispenza, H. (2022). Raynaud phenomenon. *Emedicine*. Retrieved from http://emedicine.medscape.com/

Harrison, D., Coffman, T. M. & Wilcox, C. S. (2021). Pathophysiology of hypertension: The mosaic theory and beyond. *Circulation Research*, *128*(7), 847–863. https://doi.org/10.1161/CIRCRESAHA.121.318082

Jevon, P. (2020). Blood pressure 1: Key principles and types of measuring equipment. *Nursing Times*, *116*(7), 37. Retrieved from https://www.nursingtimes.net/

Loscalzo, J., Fauci, A. S., Kasper, D. L., Hauser, S. L. & Longo, D. (2022). *Harrison's principles of internal medicine* (21st ed.). New York: McGraw Hill Medical.

Luyckx, I., Callejon, I., Buccioli, L. & Loeys, B. (2022). Update on the molecular landscape of thoracic aortic aneurysmal disease. *Current Opinion in Cardiology*, *37*(3), 201–211. doi: 10.1097/HCO.0000000000000954

Mancini, M. (2022). Aortic dissection. *Emedicine*. Retrieved from http://emedicine.medscape.com/

MIMS Australia (2022). Retrieved from http://www.mimsonline.com.au/

Morfoisse, F., Zamora, A., Marchaud, E. et al. (2021). Sex hormones in lymphedema. *Cancers*, *13*(3), 530. https://doi.org/10.3390/cancers13030530

National Heart Foundation of Australia (2016). *Guide to management of hypertension 2016*. Retrieved from https://www.heartfoundation.org.au/

National Vascular Disease Prevention Alliance (NVDPA) (2012). *Guidelines for the management of absolute cardiovascular disease risk*. Canberra: National Stroke Foundation. Retrieved from https://www.heartfoundation.org.au/

New Zealand Ministry of Health (2022). *Cardiovascular health indicators: New Zealand Health Survey 2020–21—Annual Data Explorer*. Retrieved from https://minhealthnz.shinyapps.io/

NPS Medicinewise (2021). *Absolute cardiovascular risk in clinical practice*. Retrieved from https://www.nps.org.au

Nugent, J., Young, C., Funaro, M. et al. (2022). Prevalence of secondary hypertension in otherwise healthy youths with a new diagnosis of hypertension: A meta-analysis. *The Journal of Pediatrics*, *244*, 30–37.e10. https://doi.org/10.1016/j.jpeds.2022.01.047

Oza, R. & Garcellano, M. (2015). Nonpharmacologic management of hypertension: What works? *American Family Physician*, *91*(11), 772–776.

Papadakis, M. A., McPhee, S. J. & Rabow, M. W. (2022). *Current medical diagnosis and treatment* (61st ed.). New York: McGraw-Hill Education.

Patel, K. (2019). Deep venous thrombosis. *Emedicine*. Retrieved from http://emedicine.medscape.com/

Queensland Health, Royal Flying Doctor Service (Queensland Section) (2022). *Primary clinical care manual* (11th ed.). Cairns: Office of Rural and Remote Health, Queensland Government. Retrieved from https://www.health.qld.gov.au/

Rahimi, S. (2021). Abdominal aortic aneurysm. *Emedicine*. Retrieved from http://emedicine.medscape.com/

Royal Australian College of General Practitioners (RACGP) (2021). *Guidelines for preventive activities in general practice*. Retrieved from https://www.racgp.org.au/

Savoia, C., Volpe, M. & Kreutz, R. (2021). Hypertension, a moving target in COVID-19. *Circulation Research*, *128*, 1062–1079. doi: 10.1161/CIRCRESAHA.121.318054

Schwartz, R. (2021). Lymphedema. *Emedicine*. Retrieved from http://emedicine.medscape.com/

Shariq, O. & McKenzie, T. J. (2020). Obesity-related hypertension: A review of pathophysiology, management, and the role of metabolic surgery. *Gland Surgery*, *9*(1), 80–93. https://doi.org/10.21037/gs.2019.12.03

Silva, A. (2022). Practical applicability of genetics for the prevention and treatment of hypertension. *The Journal of Clinical Hypertension*, *24*(2), 119–121. https://doi.org/10.1111/jch.14400

Solano, J. (2022). International Normalized Ratio (INR) targets: Venous thromboembolism. *Emedicine*. Retrieved from http://emedicine.medscape.com/

Stephens, E. (2022). Peripheral vascular disease. *Emedicine*. Retrieved from http://emedicine.medscape.com/

Stevens, H., Tran, H. & Gibbs, H. (2019). *Venous thromboembolism: Current management*. Retrieved from https://www.nps.org.au/

Tseng, E. (2021). Thoracic aortic aneurysm. *Emedicine*. Retrieved from http://emedicine.medscape.com/

Unger, T., Borghi, C., Charchar, F. et al. (2020). 2020 International Society of Hypertension global hypertension practice guidelines. *Journal of Hypertension*, *38*(6), 982–1004. https://doi.org/10.1097/HJH.0000000000002453

Weiss, R. (2020). Varicose veins and spider veins. *Emedicine*. Retrieved from http://emedicine.medscape.com/

Weller, C. D., Richards, C., Turnour, L. & Team, V. (2021). Patient explanation of adherence and non-adherence to venous leg ulcer treatment: A qualitative study. *Frontiers in Pharmacology*, *12*, 663570. https://doi.org/10.3389/fphar.2021.663570

World Health Organization (WHO) (2022). *Guideline for the pharmacological treatment of hypertension in adults: Summary*. Retrieved from https://www.who.int/

Yamazaki, O. & Shibata, S. (2022). Severe COVID-19 and pre-existing hypertension: A matter of age? *Hypertension Research*, *45*, 1523–1525. https://doi.org/10.1038/s41440-022-00978-1

Yei, K., Mathlouthi, A., Naazie, I., Elsayed, N., Clary, B. & Malas, M. (2022). Long-term outcomes associated with open vs endovascular abdominal aortic aneurysm repair in a medicare-matched database. *JAMA Network Open*, *5*(5), e2212081. https://doi.org/10.1001/jamanetworkopen.2022.12081

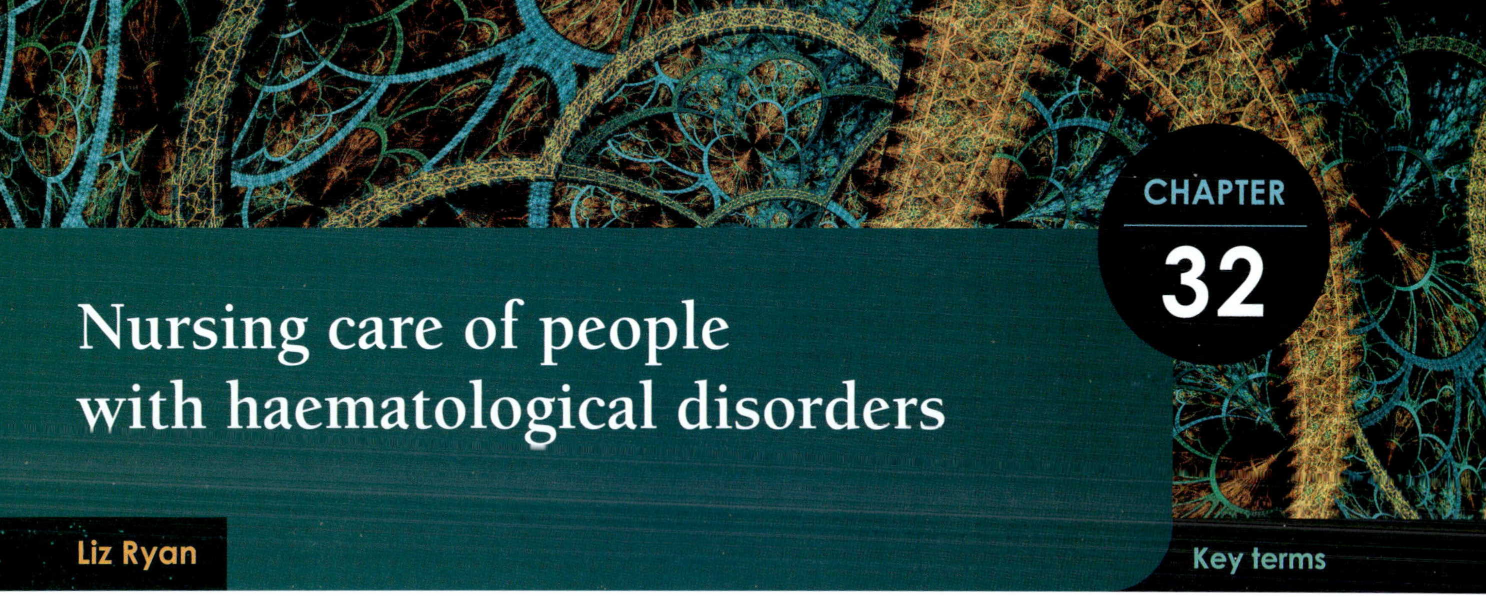

CHAPTER 32

Nursing care of people with haematological disorders

Liz Ryan

Learning outcomes

- Relate changes in erythrocyte morphology to the pathophysiological effects resulting in red blood cell disorders.
- Identify the care and health management principles for individuals experiencing red blood cell disorders.
- Describe the main types of leukaemia and examine their major health management principles.
- Discuss indications, complications and management practices for a person receiving bone marrow and stem cell transplant.
- Differentiate between Hodgkin's disease and non-Hodgkin's lymphoma.
- Compare and contrast the pathophysiology, manifestations and management for people experiencing bleeding disorders.

Clinical competencies

- Assess effects of haematological disorders and prescribed treatments on a person's functional health status.
- Monitor and document continuing assessment data, including laboratory test results, subjective and objective information, and reporting data outside the normal or expected range.
- Based on knowledge of pathophysiology, prescribed treatment and assessed data, identify and prioritise nursing diagnoses for people with haematological disorders.
- Use nursing research and evidence-based practice to identify and implement individualised nursing interventions for the person with a haematological disorder.
- Safely and knowledgeably administer prescribed medications and treatments for people with haematological disorders.
- Collaborate with the interprofessional care team to plan and provide coordinated, effective care for people with haematological disorders.
- Provide appropriate teaching for people with haematological disorders, evaluating learning and the need for continued reinforcement of information.
- Use continuing assessment data to revise the plan of care as needed to restore, maintain or promote functional health in the person with a haematological disorder.

Key terms

Disorders affecting blood and blood-forming organs have effects that range from minor disruptions in daily activities to major life-threatening crises. People with haematological disorders need holistic nursing care, including emotional support and care for problems involving major body systems.

This chapter focuses on health changes resulting from changes in red cells, white cells, platelets and clotting factors. Before proceeding with this chapter, read the chapter 'A person-centred approach to assessing the cardiovascular and lymphatic systems', which provides a review of the physiology of blood and its formation as well as important information about assessing those with haematological disorders.

Red blood cell disorders

Red blood cells (RBCs) transport oxygen to body tissues and help return carbon dioxide to the lungs for excretion. Alterations in the number, size, shape or composition of RBCs affect their ability to effectively carry out these functions. Anaemia, the most common RBC disorder, is an abnormally low RBC count or reduced haemoglobin content. Polycythaemia is an abnormally high RBC count.

THE PERSON WITH ANAEMIA

Anaemia is an abnormally low number of circulating RBCs, low haemoglobin concentration, or both. Decreased numbers of circulating RBCs is the usual cause of anaemia. This may result from blood loss, inadequate RBC production or increased RBC destruction. Insufficient or defective haemoglobin within RBCs contributes to anaemia. Depending on its severity, anaemia may affect all major organ systems.

FAST FACTS

- Iron deficiency anaemia, a nutritional anaemia, is the most common type of anaemia.
- Blood loss anaemia may be acute, resulting from haemorrhage, or chronic, resulting from chronic blood loss (e.g. menstrual flow, slow GI bleeding).

Physiology review

As blood flows through the pulmonary vascular system, oxygen diffuses from alveoli into capillary blood. The majority of the oxygen binds reversibly with the haemoglobin in RBCS; only about 3% of the oxygen remains in solution in the blood. When the blood reaches the capillaries serving body tissues, oxygen is released from the haemoglobin molecule and diffuses out of the capillary to reach the cells. The amount of oxygen that reaches the tissues depends on a number of factors, including:

- available oxygen in the alveoli
- diffusing surface and capacity of the lungs
- number of RBCs and the amount and type of haemoglobin they contain
- ability of the cardiovascular system to transport blood and oxygen to the tissues.

For more information about RBCs and haemoglobin, and their production and function, see the chapter 'A person-centred approach to assessing the cardiovascular and lymphatic systems'.

Pathophysiology and manifestations

A number of different pathological mechanisms can lead to anaemia (see Box 32.1). Regardless of the cause, every type of anaemia reduces the oxygen-carrying capacity of the blood due to a deficiency of RBCs or haemoglobin, leading to tissue

BOX 32.1 Pathophysiological mechanisms of anaemia

Decreased RBC production

- Altered haemoglobin synthesis
- Iron deficiency
- Thalassaemia
- Chronic inflammation
- Altered DNA synthesis
- Vitamin B_{12} or folic acid malabsorption or deficiency
- Bone marrow failure
- Aplastic anaemia (stem cell dysfunction)
- Red cell aplasia
- Myeloproliferative leukaemia
- Cancer metastasis, lymphoma
- Chronic infection or inflammation, physical and emotional fatigue

Increased RBC loss or destruction

- Acute or chronic blood loss
- Haemorrhage or trauma
- Chronic gastrointestinal bleeding, menorrhagia
- Increased haemolysis
- Hereditary cell membrane disorders
- Defective haemoglobin—sickle cell anaemia or trait
- Pyruvate kinase (PK) or glucose-6-phosphate dehydrogenase (G6PD) deficiency affecting glycolysis or cell oxidation
- Immune mechanisms and disorders (e.g. blood reaction, hypersensitivity responses, autoimmune disorders)
- Splenomegaly and hypersplenism
- Infection
- Erythrocyte trauma (e.g. due to cardiopulmonary bypass, haemolytic uraemic syndrome)

hypoxia. The resulting effects on a person depend on the severity of the anaemia, how quickly it develops and other factors such as age and health status.

When anaemia develops gradually and the RBC reduction is moderate, successful compensatory mechanisms may result in few symptoms except when the oxygen needs of the body increase due to exercise or infection. Symptoms develop as RBCs and haemoglobin levels are further reduced. Pallor of the skin, mucous membranes, conjunctiva and nail beds develops as a result of blood redistribution to vital organs and lack of haemoglobin (see Figure 32.1). As tissue oxygenation decreases, the heart and respiratory rates rise in an attempt to increase cardiac output and tissue perfusion. Tissue hypoxia may cause angina, fatigue, dyspnoea on exertion and night cramps. It also stimulates erythropoietin release; increased erythropoietin activity stimulates RBC production in the bone marrow and may lead to bone pain. Cerebral hypoxia can lead to headache, dizziness and dim vision. Heart failure may develop in severe anaemia.

With rapid blood loss, blood volume is decreased as well as the oxygen-carrying capacity of the blood. Initial manifestations include tachycardia and tachypnoea; the skin may be pale, cool and clammy as peripheral vessels constrict to maintain blood flow to the heart and brain. With significant blood loss, signs of circulatory shock may occur, including hypotension, tachycardia, decreased level of consciousness and oliguria. With chronic bleeding, fluid shifts from the interstitial spaces into the vessels, in an effort to maintain blood volume. Blood viscosity is reduced, which may result in a systolic heart murmur. See 'Multisystem effects of anaemia'.

Anaemia is categorised by cause: blood loss, nutritional, haemolytic and bone marrow suppression. The pathophysiology and specific manifestations of these types of anaemias follow.

Blood loss anaemia

When anaemia results from acute or chronic bleeding, RBCs and other blood components (such as iron) are lost from the body. With acute blood loss, circulating volume decreases. As a result, cardiac output falls. Compensatory mechanisms are activated to maintain the cardiac output: the heart rate increases and peripheral blood vessels constrict. Vessels in the liver, a blood storage organ, also constrict, increasing circulating volume. Fluid shifts from the interstitial spaces into the vascular compartment to maintain blood volume, diluting the cellular components of the blood and reducing its viscosity. If haemorrhage continues, compensatory mechanisms become less effective, increasing the risk of shock and circulatory failure (see the chapter 'Nursing care of people experiencing trauma and shock').

In acute blood loss, circulating RBCs are of normal size and shape (*normocytic*). Early in the haemorrhage, the RBC count, haemoglobin and haematocrit may be normal; as fluid shifts from the interstitial space into the vascular space to maintain circulating volume, the RBC count, haemoglobin and haematocrit fall. If sufficient iron is available, haemoglobin levels and the number of circulating RBCs return to normal within 3 to 4 weeks after the bleeding episode. Chronic blood loss, on the other hand, depletes iron stores as RBC production attempts to maintain the RBC supply. The resulting RBCs are *microcytic* (small) and *hypochromic* (pale).

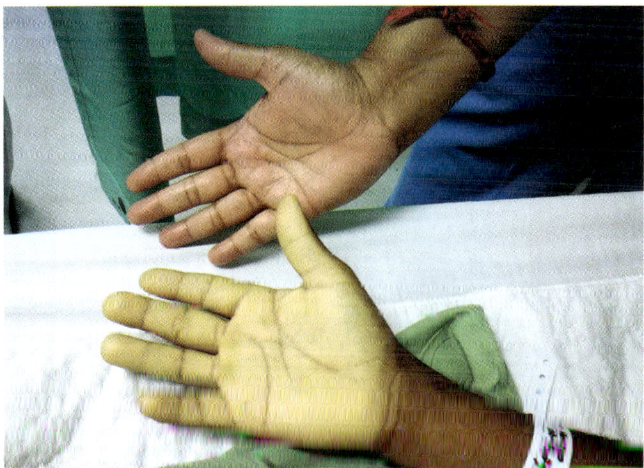

FIGURE 32.1 ***The skin of the person with anaemia appears pale beside that of a person with a normal haemoglobin and haematocrit***

Source: Casa nayafana/Shutterstock.

Nutritional anaemias

Many different nutrients are required for normal RBC development (erythropoiesis). Iron is a key nutrient necessary for haemoglobin synthesis. In addition, adequate supplies of protein (and its building blocks, amino acids), vitamins and other minerals are required. The B group vitamins, particularly B_{12} (cobalamin) and folate (B_9), play a key role in RBC development. Vitamins C and E are also necessary. Nutritional anaemias result from nutrient deficits that affect RBC formation or haemoglobin synthesis. The nutrient deficit may be caused by inadequate diet, malabsorption of the nutrient, or an increased need for the nutrient. The most common types of nutritional anaemias are iron deficiency anaemia, vitamin B_{12} anaemia and folic acid deficiency anaemia. Vitamin B_{12} and folic acid anaemias are sometimes called *megaloblastic* anaemias, because enlarged nucleated RBCs called megaloblasts are seen in these anaemias.

IRON DEFICIENCY ANAEMIA **Iron deficiency anaemia** is the most common type of anaemia. It develops when the supply of iron is inadequate for optimal RBC formation, as the body cannot synthesise haemoglobin without iron. Normally, the body efficiently recycles and stores iron, reusing much of the iron contained in RBCs that are removed from circulation due to age or damage. However, small amounts of iron are continually lost in the faeces; therefore, adequate iron intake is necessary for normal haemoglobin synthesis and RBC production. Iron deficiency anaemia results in fewer numbers of RBCs, microcytic and hypochromic RBCs, as well as malformed RBCs (*poikilocytosis*) (see Figure 32.2).

Excessive iron loss due to chronic bleeding is the usual cause of iron deficiency anaemia in adults. Menstrual blood loss is the most common cause in adult females. Iron deficiency anaemia also may result from inadequate dietary iron intake (less than 1 mg/day), malabsorption syndromes or the increased iron requirements associated with pregnancy and lactation. Box 32.2 summarises common causes of iron deficiency anaemia.

Multisystem effects of anaemia

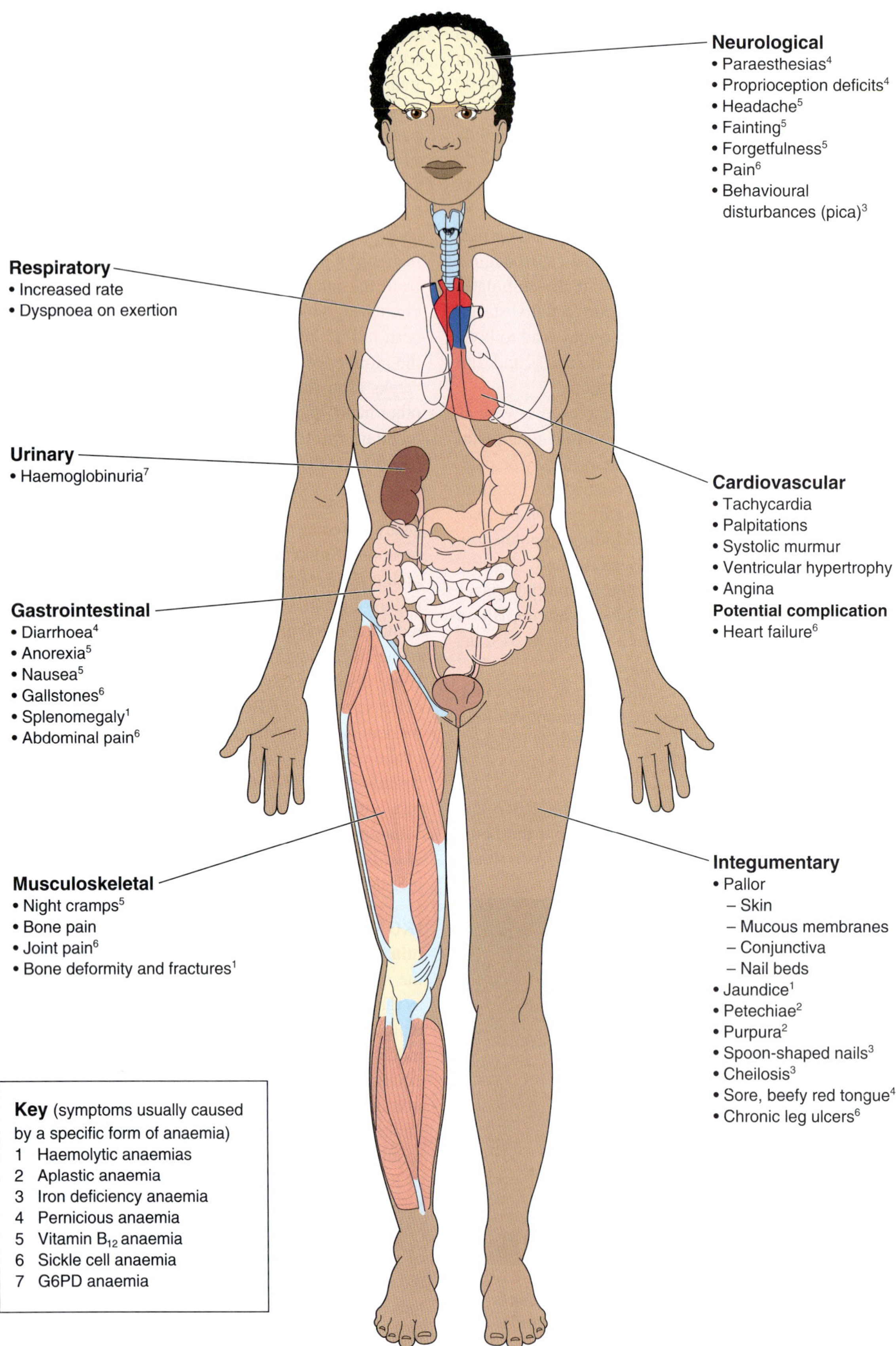

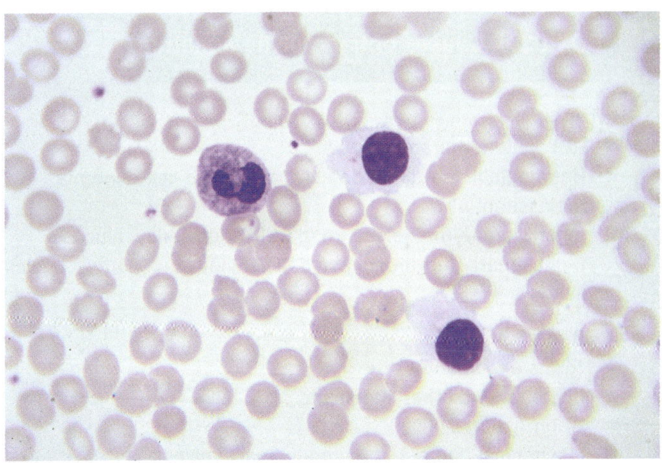

FIGURE 32.2 ***A blood smear showing RBCs characteristically seen in iron deficiency anaemia. Note the pale colour of the RBCs (hypochromic). Many of the cells also are smaller than normal (microcytic) and misshapen, reducing their oxygen-carrying capacity***

Source: Jarun Ontakrai/Shutterstock.

BOX 32.2 Causes of iron deficiency anaemia

- Dietary deficiencies
- Vegetarian diet
- Inadequate protein intake
- Decreased absorption
- Partial or total gastrectomy
- Chronic diarrhoea
- Malabsorption syndromes
- Increased metabolic requirements
- Pregnancy
- Lactation
- Blood loss
- Gastrointestinal bleeding (often related to ulcers or chronic aspirin use)
- Menstrual losses
- Chronic haemoglobinuria

Iron deficiency anaemia is particularly common in older adults. Chronic, occult (hidden) blood loss may occur from slowly bleeding peptic ulcers, gastrointestinal inflammation, haemorrhoids and cancer. Inadequate dietary iron intake also contributes to anaemia. Access to transportation may limit fresh food consumption, a factor contributing to poor iron intake among all adults, especially people with limited or fixed incomes.

Manifestations In addition to the general manifestations of anaemia described earlier, chronic iron deficiency may lead to brittle, spoon-shaped nails, cheilosis (cracks at the corners of the mouth), a smooth, sore tongue; and *pica* (a craving for unusual substances, such as clay or starch).

VITAMIN B_{12} DEFICIENCY ANAEMIA Vitamin B_{12} is necessary for DNA synthesis and is almost exclusively found in foods derived from animals. *Vitamin B_{12} deficiency anaemia* occurs when inadequate vitamin B_{12} is consumed or, more commonly, when it is poorly absorbed from the gastrointestinal tract. Deficiency of this vitamin impairs cell division and maturation of the cell nucleus, especially in rapidly proliferating RBCs. As a result, macrocytic (large), misshapen (oval rather than concave) RBCs with thin membranes are produced. Great numbers of these large, immature RBCs enter the circulation. These cells are fragile, incapable of carrying adequate amounts of oxygen and have a shortened lifespan.

Failure to absorb dietary vitamin B_{12} is called **pernicious anaemia**. It develops due to lack of intrinsic factor, a substance secreted by the gastric mucosa. Intrinsic factor binds with vitamin B_{12} and travels with it to the ileum, where the vitamin is absorbed. In the absence of intrinsic factor, vitamin B_{12} cannot be absorbed into the body, most commonly seen in elderly people.

Vitamin B_{12} deficiency may also result from other malabsorption disorders and dietary factors. Resection of the stomach or ileum, loss of pancreatic secretions and chronic gastritis can affect vitamin B_{12} absorption. Dietary deficiencies of vitamin B_{12} are rare, usually occurring only among strict vegetarians. Parasites, such as fish tapeworm, and some medications, such as metformin, proton pump inhibitors and H_2 receptor antagonists, can also contribute to the loss or compromise of vitamin B_{12} in humans. Chronic excess alcohol intake can also cause significant B_{12} deficiency.

Manifestations Manifestations of vitamin B_{12} deficiency anaemia develop gradually as bodily stores of the vitamin are depleted. Pallor or slight jaundice and weakness develop. In pernicious anaemia, a smooth, sore, beefy red tongue and diarrhoea may occur. Because vitamin B_{12} is important for neurological function, paraesthesia (altered sensations, such as numbness or tingling) in the extremities and problems with proprioception (the sense of one's position in space) develop. These manifestations may progress to difficulty maintaining balance due to spinal cord damage. Central nervous system (CNS) manifestations of relatively short duration (a few months) are reversible with treatment but may be permanent if treatment is delayed.

FOLIC ACID DEFICIENCY ANAEMIA Like vitamin B_{12}, folic acid is required for DNA synthesis and normal maturation of RBCs. *Folic acid deficiency anaemia* is characterised by fragile, megaloblastic (large and immature) cells. Folic acid is found in green leafy vegetables, fruit, cereals and meats, and is absorbed from the intestines.

Folic acid deficiency anaemia due to inadequate intake is more common among people who are chronically undernourished. This includes older adults, alcoholics and the drug addicted. Alcoholics are especially at risk because alcohol suppresses folate metabolism, which forms folic acid. Increased folic acid requirements also may lead to anaemia, with pregnant women at greatest risk. Infants and teenagers can also develop temporary folic acid deficiencies during periods of rapid growth. Impaired folic acid absorption and metabolism can cause folic acid deficiency anaemia. Malabsorption disorders, such as coeliac sprue (a hereditary gastrointestinal disorder characterised by inability to metabolise amino acids found in gluten), and certain medications, such as methotrexate and some chemotherapeutic agents, may be contributing factors. Causes of folic acid deficiency anaemia are summarised in Box 32.3.

BOX 32.3 Causes of folic acid deficiency anaemia

- Inadequate dietary intake
  At risk:
  a. Older adults
  b. Chronic excessive alcohol consumers
  c. People receiving total parenteral nutrition (TPN)
- Increased metabolic requirements
  At risk:
  a. Pregnant women
  b. Infants and teenagers
  c. People undergoing haemodialysis
  d. People with forms of haemolytic anaemia
- Folic acid malabsorption and impaired metabolism
  a. Coeliac sprue
  b. Chemotherapeutic agents, folate antagonists (methotrexate, pentamidine) or anticonvulsants
  c. Alcoholism

Manifestations The manifestations develop gradually as folic acid stores are depleted. Signs and symptoms may include pallor, progressive weakness and fatigue, shortness of breath and heart palpitations. Manifestations similar to those associated with vitamin B_{12} anaemia, such as glossitis, cheilosis and diarrhoea, are common. No neurological symptoms occur with folic acid deficiency anaemia, thus helping to differentiate it from vitamin B_{12} deficiency anaemia. These two nutritional anaemias do, however, sometimes coexist.

Maternal levels of folic acid are strongly associated with the prevention of neural tube defects (NTD). NTDs, including spina bifida, encephalocoele and anencephaly, result from the failure of the spinal cord or brain to develop normally during early fetal development, often before pregnancy is recognised. The seriousness of these abnormalities is reflected by the fact that fewer than 40% of babies affected survive to birth. People born with an NTD, especially those with spina bifida, will experience lifelong disability. Hence, the Royal Australian and New Zealand College of Obstetricians and Gynaecologists (2019) recommends folic acid supplements of at least 500 micrograms daily. If there is a known risk of NTD, 5 mg per day is recommended. Folic acid should be taken for at least 1 month pre-conception and during the first 12 weeks of pregnancy.

Haemolytic anaemias

Haemolytic anaemias are characterised by premature destruction (*lysis*) of RBCs. When RBCs break down, iron and other by-products of their destruction remain in the plasma. RBC lysis (haemolysis) may occur within the circulatory system or due to phagocytosis by white blood cells (WBCs) such as circulating monocytes and macrophages in the spleen. In response to haemolysis, the haematopoietic activity of bone marrow increases, leading to increased reticulocytes (immature RBCs) in circulating blood. Most types of haemolytic anaemia are characterised by normocytic and normochromic RBCs.

There are many different causes of haemolytic anaemia (see Box 32.4). The cause may be *intrinsic*, arising from disorders within the RBC itself, or *extrinsic*, originating outside the RBC. Intrinsic disorders include cell membrane defects, defects in haemoglobin structure and function, and inherited enzyme deficiencies. See the accompanying 'Focus on cultural diversity' box for more information about inherited intrinsic RBC disorders associated with haemolytic anaemia. Extrinsic causes of haemolytic anaemia include drugs, bacterial and other toxins, and trauma. This section discusses sickle cell anaemia, thalassaemia, acquired haemolytic anaemia and glucose-6-phosphate dehydrogenase (G6PD) anaemia.

BOX 32.4 Causes of haemolytic anaemia

Intrinsic
- RBC cell-membrane defects
- Haemoglobin structure defects (e.g. sickle cell anaemia, thalassaemia)
- Inherited enzyme defects (e.g. G6PD deficiency (glucose-6-phosphate dehydrogenase deficiency))

Extrinsic
- Drugs, chemicals
- Toxins and venoms
- Bacterial and other infections
- Trauma, burns
- Mechanical damage (prosthetic heart valves)

SICKLE CELL ANAEMIA **Sickle cell anaemia** is a hereditary, chronic haemolytic anaemia. It is characterised by episodes of *sickling*, during which RBCs become abnormally crescent shaped. The disorder is transmitted as an autosomal recessive genetic defect (see Figure 32.3). This defect causes synthesis of an abnormal form of haemoglobin (HbS) within RBCs. Sickle cell anaemia can significantly shorten lifespan,

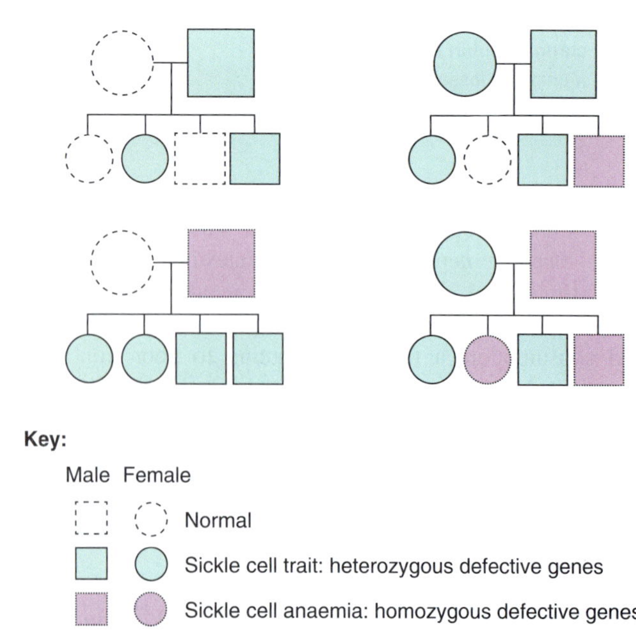

FIGURE 32.3 *Inheritance pattern for sickle cell anaemia*

with complications such as infections, stroke, acute chest syndrome through blocked blood vessels of the lung, pulmonary hypertension and organ damage, to name a few.

Sickle cell disease is one of the most common inherited conditions worldwide and is most common among people from African, Middle Eastern and Southern Europe populations, as well as from India, Pakistan, South America and the Caribbean (see the 'Focus on cultural diversity' box). However, in Australia this disease is quite rare, with the majority of cases originating from New South Wales. Of the children born in Australia with sickle cell anaemia, more than half were from South-East Asia and the Middle East (Argent et al., 2012). Australian Sickle Cell Advocacy Inc. estimates that around 1,000 people currently have this condition in Australia (ASCA, 2022). It is most commonly seen in Lebanese residents, many of whom live in Greater Sydney (Australian Bureau of Statistics, 2022; Department of Health and Aged Care, 2022).

The HbS gene changes the structure of the beta chain of the haemoglobin molecule. When hypoxaemia develops and HbS is deoxygenated, it crystallises into rod-like structures. Clusters of these rods form long chains that deform the erythrocyte into a crescent or sickle shape (see Figure 32.4). The sickled cells tend to clump together and obstruct capillary blood flow, causing ischaemia and possible infarction of surrounding tissue. See 'Pathophysiology illustrated: sickle cell anaemia'.

When normal oxygen tension is restored, the sickled RBCs resume their normal shape; that is, they 'unsickle'. Repeated episodes of sickling and unsickling weaken RBC cell membranes. The weakened RBCs are haemolysed and removed. Consequently, the normal lifespan of RBCs is greatly reduced in sickle cell anaemia, increasing the demand for RBC production. Conditions likely to trigger sickling include hypoxia, low environmental or body temperature, excessive exercise, anaesthesia, dehydration, infections or acidosis.

Manifestations and complications The acute and chronic manifestations of sickle cell anaemia arise from episodes of RBC sickling. Sickling causes general manifestations of haemolytic anaemia, including pallor, fatigue, jaundice and irritability. Extensive sickling can precipitate a crisis due to

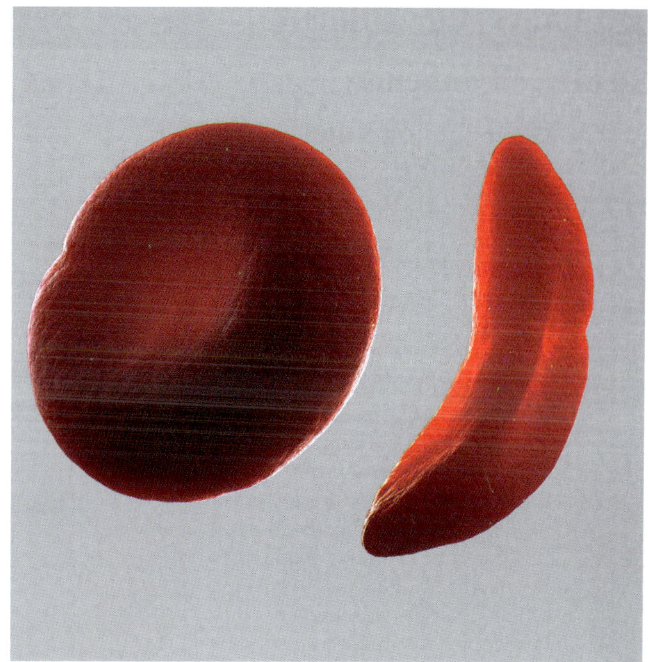

FIGURE 32.4 ***Blood smear containing normal red blood cells and sickle cells***

Source: SCIEPRO/Science Photo Library/Getty Images.

occluded circulation, impaired erythropoiesis or sequestration of large amounts of blood in the liver or spleen.

A vaso-occlusive or thrombotic crisis occurs when sickling develops in the microcirculation. Obstruction of blood flow triggers vasospasm that halts all blood flow in the vessel. Lack of blood flow leads to tissue ischaemia and infarction. Vaso-occlusive crises are painful and last an average of 4 to 6 days. Infarction of small vessels in the extremities causes painful swelling of the hands and feet; large joints also may be affected. Priapism (persistent, painful erection of the penis) may develop. Abdominal pain may signal infarction of abdominal organs and structures. Infarction may affect bone marrow or lead to aseptic necrosis of affected bones. Stroke may result from cerebral vessel occlusion. Skin ulcers may develop as

FOCUS ON CULTURAL DIVERSITY **Inherited haemolytic anaemias**

- Sickle cell disease is one of the most common inherited conditions of haemoglobin in the world.
- It is estimated that over 300,000–400,000 neonates born yearly worldwide have sickle cell disease, with most found in sub-Saharan Africa. Almost 90% of all people with sickle cell disease live in only three countries – Nigeria, India and the Democratic Republic of Congo (DeBaun & Galadanci, 2022; Dua et al., 2022).
- In Australia, people of Southern European and Middle Eastern origin are more commonly affected. However, in 2021, there were only just under 5,000 hospital admissions nationally (in public hospitals) directly relating to thalassaemia (Australian Institute of Health and Welfare (AIHW), 2022).
- Alpha thalassaemia primarily affects people of South-East Asian, Indian, Chinese or Filipino ancestry. However, the disorder also occurs in other groups, including people from the Pacific Islands and New Zealand. It has also been identified in some Aboriginal and Torres Strait Islander communities (Department of Health and Aged Care, 2022).
- Beta-thalassaemia primarily affects people from the Middle East, Southern Europe and India, and is said to be carried by 0.4% of the population in Australia (Department of Health and Aged Care, 2022; Halim-Fikri et al., 2022).

Pathophysiology illustrated

Sickle cell anaemia

Haemoglobin S and red blood cell sickling

Sickle cell anaemia is caused by an inherited autosomal recessive defect in Hb synthesis. Sickle cell haemoglobin (HbS) differs from normal haemoglobin only in the substitution of the amino acid valine for glutamine in both beta chains of the haemoglobin molecule.

When HbS is oxygenated, it has the same globular shape as normal haemoglobin. However, when HbS off loads oxygen, it becomes insoluble in intracellular fluid and crystallises into rodlike structures. Clusters of rods form polymers (long chains) that bend the erythrocyte into the characteristic crescent shape of the sickle cell.

Incorrect amino acids
β chains
Haemoglobin S molecule
α chains
Polymerised deoxyhaemoglobin S
Oxyhaemoglobin S
O_2
Deoxyhaemoglobin S
Oxygenated erythrocyte
Deoxygenated erythrocyte
Sickled erythrocyte

The shortened RBC lifespan and compromised erythropoiesis can lead to profound *aplastic anaemia* in sickle cell disease. *Sequestration crises* are marked by pooling of large amounts of blood in the liver and spleen. This sickle cell crisis only occurs in children and is thought to be the cause of deaths in early childhood related to sickle cell disease.

The sickle cell disease process

Sickle cell disease is characterised by episodes of acute painful crises. Sickling crises are triggered by conditions causing high tissue oxygen demands or that affect cellular pH. As the crisis begins, sickled erythrocytes adhere to capillary walls and to each other, obstructing blood flow and causing cellular hypoxia. The crisis accelerates as tissue hypoxia and acidic metabolic waste products cause further sickling and cell damage.

Sickle cell crises cause microinfarcts in joints and organs, and repeated crises slowly destroy organs and tissues. The spleen and kidneys are especially prone to sickling damage.

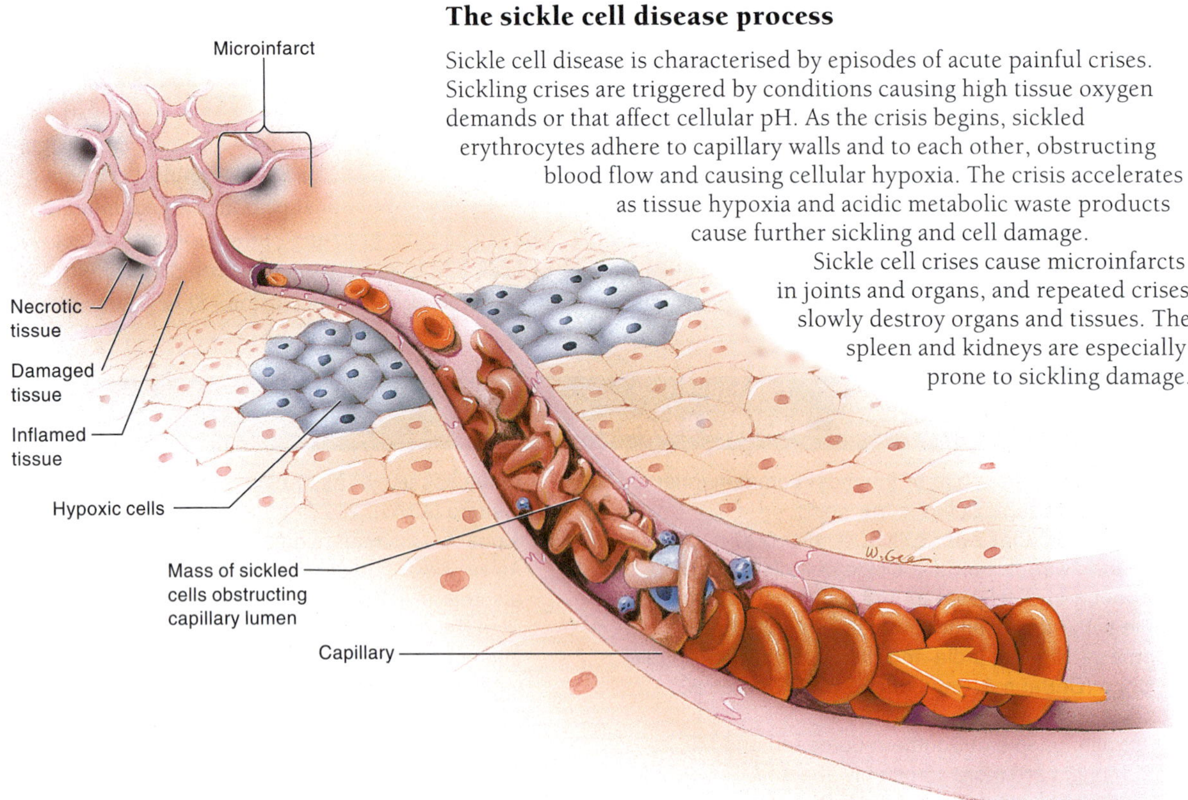

the result of occluded vessels supplying the dermis. Repeated infarcts associated with sickling can affect the structure and function of nearly every organ system. People with sickle cell disease may develop an enlarged spleen and liver, renal insufficiency, gallstones and other manifestations of organ dysfunction. *Acute chest syndrome*, a symptom complex that includes fever, chest pain, an increasing WBC count and pulmonary infiltrates, may develop, as well as other pulmonary complications such as pneumonia, pulmonary infarction and pulmonary embolism. Treatment for sickle cell crisis is still predominately blood transfusion, but there have been recent advances in the use of nitric oxide inhalation for its vasodilatory properties, and the option of haematopoietic cell transplantation (HCT) (Marieb & Hoehn, 2019; Stallings et al., 2020).

THALASSAEMIA The **thalassaemias** are inherited disorders of haemoglobin synthesis in which either the alpha or the beta chains of the haemoglobin molecule are missing or defective. This leads to deficient haemoglobin production and fragile hypochromic, microcytic RBCs called *target cells* because of their distinctive bull's-eye appearance.

Thalassaemia usually affects certain populations. People of Mediterranean descent (southern Italy and Greece) are more likely to have beta-defect thalassaemias (often called *Cooley's anaemia* or Mediterranean anaemia). People of Asian ancestry, especially from Thailand, the Philippines and China, more often have alpha-defect thalassaemia. As with sickle cell anaemia, only one defective beta-chain forming gene may be present (*beta-thalassaemia minor*), causing mild symptoms; or both may be defective (*beta-thalassaemia major*), leading to more severe symptoms. Children with thalassaemia major rarely reach adulthood, although repeated blood transfusions may extend their lifespan. Four genes are responsible for alpha chain formation; one, two, three or all four may be defective. In the last case (*alpha-thalassaemia major*), death is inevitable and usually occurs in utero. Genetic studies and counselling are recommended for people at risk of this illness.

Manifestations and complications People with thalassaemia minor are often asymptomatic. When manifestations do occur, they include mild to moderate anaemia, mild splenomegaly, bronze skin colouring and bone marrow hyperplasia. The major form of the disease causes severe anaemia, heart failure and liver and spleen enlargement from increased red cell destruction. Fractures of the long bones, ribs and vertebrae may result from bone marrow expansion and thinning due to increased haematopoiesis. Jaundice may develop due to haemolysis, as well as hepatomegaly and splenomegaly. Accumulation of iron in the heart, liver and pancreas following repeated transfusions for treatment may eventually cause failure of these organs.

ACQUIRED HAEMOLYTIC ANAEMIA *Acquired haemolytic anaemia* results from haemolysis due to factors outside of the RBC. Causes of acquired haemolytic anaemias include:

- mechanical trauma to RBCs produced by prosthetic heart valves, severe burns, haemodialysis or radiation
- autoimmune disorders
- bacterial or protozoal infection
- immune-system-mediated responses, such as transfusion reactions
- drugs, toxins, chemical agents or venoms.

The manifestations of acquired haemolytic anaemia depend on the extent of haemolysis and the body's ability to replace destroyed RBCs. The anaemia itself often is mild to moderate as erythropoiesis increases to replace the destroyed RBCs. The spleen enlarges as it removes damaged or destroyed RBCs. If the breakdown of haem units exceeds the liver's ability to conjugate and excrete bilirubin, jaundice develops. When the condition is severe, bone marrow expands and bones may be deformed or may develop pathological fractures. The severity of generalised manifestations of anaemia (tachycardia, pallor, etc.) depends on the degree of anaemia and deficiency of tissue oxygenation.

GLUCOSE-6-PHOSPHATE DEHYDROGENASE (G6PD) ANAEMIA *Glucose-6-phosphate dehydrogenase (G6PD) anaemia* is caused by a hereditary defect in RBC metabolism. It is relatively common in people of African and Mediterranean descent. The defective gene is located on the X chromosome and therefore affects more males than females. There are many variations of this genetic defect.

G6PD is an enzyme that catalyses glycolysis, the process in which an RBC derives cellular energy. A defect in G6PD action causes direct oxidation of haemoglobin, damaging the RBC. Haemolysis usually occurs only when the affected person is exposed to stressors (e.g. drugs such as aspirin, sulfonamides or vitamin K derivatives) that increase the metabolic demands on RBCs. The G6PD deficiency impairs the necessary compensatory increase in glucose metabolism and causes cellular damage. Damaged RBCs are destroyed over a period of 7 to 12 days.

When exposed to a stressor triggering G6PD anaemia, symptoms develop within several days. These may include pallor, jaundice, haemoglobinuria (haemoglobin in the urine) and an elevated reticulocyte count. As new RBCs develop, counts return to normal.

Aplastic anaemia

In **aplastic anaemia**, the bone marrow fails to produce all three types of blood cells, leading to *pancytopenia*. Normal bone marrow is replaced by fat. Fortunately, aplastic anaemia is rare. *Fanconi anaemia* is a rare aplastic anaemia caused by defects of DNA repair. The underlying cause of about 50% of acquired aplastic anaemia is unknown (*idiopathic aplastic anaemia*). Other cases follow stem cell damage caused by exposure to radiation or certain chemical substances such as benzene, arsenic, nitrogen mustard, certain antibiotics (especially chloramphenicol) and chemotherapeutic drugs (Huether & McCance, 2020; Marieb & Hoehn, 2019). Aplastic anaemia also may occur with viral infections such as mononucleosis, hepatitis C and HIV disease.

In aplastic anaemia, the number of stem cells in the bone marrow is significantly reduced. The stem cell pool may be less than 1% of normal when the disease is recognised. Anaemia develops as the bone marrow fails to replace RBCs that have reached the end of their lifespan. Remaining RBCs may be normochromic and normocytic, or may be large with increased mean corpuscular volume.

MANIFESTATIONS Manifestations of aplastic anaemia vary with the severity of the pancytopenia. Its onset usually is insidious but it may be sudden. Manifestations include fatigue, pallor, progressive weakness, exertional dyspnoea, headache and, ultimately, tachycardia and heart failure. Platelet deficiency leads to bleeding problems; bleeding gums, excessive bruising and nosebleeds may be the initial symptoms. A deficiency of WBCs increases the risk of infection, causing manifestations such as sore throat and fever.

INTERPROFESSIONAL CARE

Ensuring adequate tissue oxygenation is the priority of care in treating anaemia. Specific therapy is determined by the underlying cause of the disorder. Usual treatments include medications, dietary modifications, blood replacement or supportive interventions. Table 32.1 outlines interprofessional care measures for selected types of anaemia.

Diagnosis

When anaemia is suspected, the following laboratory and diagnostic tests may be ordered:

- *Full blood count (FBC)* is done to determine blood cell counts, haemoglobin, haematocrit and RBC indices. The severity of the anaemia and the shape, volume and iron content of the RBCs can help determine the cause of anaemia.
- *Iron levels* and *total iron-binding capacity* are performed to detect iron deficiency anaemia. A low serum iron concentration and elevated total iron-binding capacity are indicative of iron deficiency anaemia.
- *Serum ferritin* is low due to depletion of the total iron reserves available for haemoglobin synthesis. Ferritin is an iron-storage protein produced by the liver, spleen and bone marrow. Ferritin mobilises stored iron when metabolic needs are higher than dietary intake.
- *Sickle cell test* is a screening test to evaluate haemolytic anaemia and detect HbS.
- *Haemoglobin electrophoresis* separates normal haemoglobin from abnormal forms. It is used to evaluate haemolytic anaemia, diagnose thalassaemia and differentiate sickle cell trait from sickle cell disease.
- *Schilling test* measures vitamin B_{12} absorption before and after intrinsic factor administration to differentiate between pernicious anaemia and intestinal malabsorption of the vitamin. A 24-hour urine sample is collected following administration of radioactive vitamin B_{12}. Lower than normal levels of the tagged B_{12} when intrinsic factor is given concurrently indicate malabsorption rather than pernicious anaemia.
- *Bone marrow examination* is done to diagnose aplastic anaemia. In aplastic anaemia, normal marrow elements are significantly decreased as they are replaced by fat cells. Nursing implications for bone marrow collection are described in the 'Nursing care of the person having bone marrow studies' box in the chapter 'A person-centred approach to assessing the cardiovascular and lymphatic systems'.
- *Quantitative assay of G6PD* may be performed to confirm a diagnosis of glucose-6-phosphate dehydrogenase deficiency.

Medications

Medications used to treat anaemia depend on its cause. Iron replacement therapy is ordered for iron deficiency anaemia. Supplemental iron may be given by mouth or parenterally. Intravenous administration of iron is becoming more common, particularly in those with an acute deficiency and in anaemia associated with chronic GI blood loss, chronic renal failure and other chronic conditions that increase the need for blood cell production (e.g. cancers). The safest and currently most

Links to National Patient Safety Standards

NSQHS: Blood Management Standard

The blood management standard aims to improve outcomes for patients by identifying risks and using strategies that optimise and conserve a patient's own blood, as well as ensuring that any blood and blood products patients receive are safe and appropriate (Australian Commission on Safety and Quality in Health Care (ACSQHC), 2021).

Implementing this standard is achieved by the establishment of systems to ensure safe and appropriate prescription and administration of blood and blood products, including autologous transfusions. These systems include processes facilitating accurate documentation, storage, transport, use and disposal. Effective communication regarding risks, benefits and use should exist between all individuals involved in a person's care, including the person, significant others and clinicians.

Caring for individuals experiencing haematological conditions will often result in the need to administer blood or blood products in order to manage the person's condition. As with any biological material, various risks are involved in all facets of this treatment. Efficient and appropriate systems are imperative to ensure the safety of not only the person receiving the product, but also any other individual involved in their care.

Source: ACSQHC (2021). *National Safety and Quality Health Service Standards* (2nd ed.). Sydney: ACSQHC. © Australian Commission on Safety and Quality in Health Care.

TABLE 32.1 Interprofessional care focus for major anaemias

TYPE OF ANAEMIA	INTERPROFESSIONAL CARE
Iron deficiency anaemia	• Increased dietary intake of iron-rich foods • Oral or parenteral iron supplements
Vitamin B_{12} deficiency	• Increased dietary intake of foods containing vitamin B_{12} (e.g. meats, eggs and dairy products) • Oral or parenteral vitamin B_{12} supplements • Parenteral vitamin B_{12} for deficiency due to malabsorption or lack of intrinsic factor
Folic acid deficiency	• Increased dietary intake of foods rich in folic acid (folate) • Oral folic acid supplements • Folic acid supplements recommended for women who are pregnant or may become pregnant to prevent neural tube defects

Sickle cell anaemia	• Treatment is primarily supportive
	• Hydroxyurea 10–30 mg/kg per day
	• Sickle cell crisis:
	  • Rest
	  • Oxygen therapy to maintain SaO_2
	  • Narcotic analgesia
	  • Vigorous hydration
	  • Treatment of precipitating factors
	  • Nitric oxide inhalation
	  • Adakveo (arizanlizumab)
	• Acute chest syndrome:
	  • Careful hydration; haemodynamic monitoring
	  • Oxygen therapy
	  • Transfusion
	• Folic acid supplements
	• Blood transfusions during surgery or pregnancy as necessary
	• Genetic counselling recommended

Thalassaemia	• Regular blood transfusions • Folic acid supplements • Possible splenectomy • Genetic counselling
Aplastic anaemia	• Withdrawal of the causative agent, if known • Blood transfusions • Bone marrow transplant as indicated • Stem cell transplant–donor blood, umbilical cord blood, bone marrow sources

frequently used parenteral iron is ferric carboxymaltose. The risk of anaphylaxis is a major concern when iron dextran is given intravenously, and administration needs to be diluted in normal saline and infused slowly to reduce the risk. Other parenteral iron solutions, including intravenous sodium ferric gluconate and iron sucrose (Venofer), carry a much lower risk of adverse and allergic reactions. For any intramuscular administration of iron, a large deep muscle such as the ventrogluteal muscle is the preferred site. Utilising the Z track method of injection is recommended for the intramuscular administration of iron because it decreases irritation and staining and assists with sealing the medication in muscle tissue.

Parenteral vitamin B_{12} is given when malabsorption or lack of intrinsic factor leads to vitamin B_{12} deficiency anaemia. Folic acid is ordered for women of childbearing age, pregnant women and those with folic acid deficiency or sickle cell anaemia to meet the increased demands of the bone marrow. Hydroxyurea, a drug that promotes fetal haemoglobin production, may be prescribed for people with sickle cell disease, particularly those with frequent crises or severe disease. Resulting increased levels of fetal haemoglobin interfere with the sickling process and reduce the incidence of painful crises. Nursing implications for people receiving iron, vitamin B_{12} and folic acid are found in the 'Medication administration' box.

Erythropoietin may be ordered for people with low erythropoietin levels (e.g. those with chronic renal failure) and anaemia associated with other chronic diseases. Erythropoietin (Aranesp) is given subcutaneously or intravenously and may be given as often as three times a week in chronic renal failure. Because erythropoietin stimulates RBC production, adequate iron must be present. People receiving erythropoietin may require regular intravenous iron therapy as well.

Immunosuppressive therapy with antithymocyte globulin (ATG), corticosteroids and cyclosporine may be used to treat aplastic anaemia. Androgens may stimulate blood cell production in some people with aplastic anaemia. See the chapter 'Nursing care of people with altered immunity' for more information about immunosuppression.

Nutrition

Dietary modifications are recommended for nutritional deficiency anaemias, such as iron deficiency anaemia, vitamin B_{12} deficiency anaemia or folic acid deficiency anaemia. Box 32.5 identifies good sources of dietary iron, folic acid and vitamin B_{12}.

MEDICATION ADMINISTRATION Drugs to treat anaemia

IRON SOURCES

Ferric carboxymaltose (Ferinject)
Ferrous sulfate (Ferro-Gradumet, Fefol, FGF)
Ferro fumerate (Ferro-tab)
Iron polymaltose (Ferrosig)
Iron sucrose (Venofer)

Iron preparations are normally taken by mouth and are absorbed from the gastrointestinal tract. They are given to treat anaemias resulting from iron deficiency or blood loss. When absorbed, iron combines with transferrin. This complex then is transported to the bone marrow and incorporated into haemoglobin.

Nursing responsibilities

- Prior to giving the drug, assess for use of drugs that might interact with iron (e.g. antacids, allopurinol, chloramphenicol, tetracyclines, vitamin E), gastrointestinal bleeding and manifestations of anaemia.
- Administer iron preparations with orange juice to enhance absorption.
- If using an elixir, give it through a straw to prevent staining the teeth.
- Monitor for manifestations of iron toxicity: nausea, diarrhoea or constipation; symptoms of anaphylactic shock (extreme cases).
- Monitor haemoglobin and reticulocyte counts.
- If the person is also taking tetracyclines, schedule the dose of iron 2 hours before the tetracycline (iron reduces the absorption of tetracyclines).
- When administering IM or IV, monitor closely for anaphylaxis.

Health education for the person and family

- Gastrointestinal side effects may be reduced by taking iron with food (but not milk, which decreases absorption).
- Stools may be dark green or black; this is harmless.
- Increase fluids and fibre in diet to decrease constipation.

VITAMIN B_{12} SOURCES

Cyanocobalamin oral, parenteral

Cyanocobalamin is used to treat vitamin B_{12} deficiencies or malabsorption and pernicious anaemia. It is rapidly absorbed when administered orally or by injection and it is stored in the liver. Intrinsic factor is necessary for absorption from the gastrointestinal tract.

Nursing responsibilities

- Do not expose crystalline injection to light.
- Assess for other drugs that might interfere with the therapeutic response: chloramphenicol, cimetidine, colchicine and timed-release potassium decrease its effectiveness.
- Do not mix cyanocobalamin in a syringe with other medications.
- Administer parenteral doses intramuscularly or deep subcutaneously to decrease local irritation.
- Monitor haemoglobin, RBC counts, reticulocyte counts and potassium levels.

Health education for the person and family

- A burning sensation with injection is temporary.
- Avoid alcohol, which interferes with absorption.
- If used to treat pernicious anaemia, the medication must be taken for life.

FOLIC ACID SOURCES

Folic acid (folate)

Synthetic folic acid is used to treat folic acid deficiency and megaloblastic or macrocytic anaemia. It is absorbed from the gastrointestinal tract and stored in the liver.

Nursing responsibilities

- Prior to giving the medication, assess for use of drugs that alter its effect: corticosteroids, methotrexate, oral contraceptives, phenytoin, sulfonamides.
- Do not mix folic acid with other medications in the same syringe.
- Monitor for possible hypersensitivity response of skin rash.

Health education for the person and family

- Large doses of folic acid may cause the urine to become darker yellow.
- Excess alcohol intake increases folic acid requirements.

Blood transfusion

Blood transfusions may be indicated to treat anaemias resulting from major blood loss, such as from trauma or major surgery and severe anaemia regardless of cause. In acute haemorrhage, whole blood may be given to replace both blood cells and volume. A unit of packed RBCs may be given when anaemia is severe and the person demonstrates cardiovascular instability or compromise. Blood transfusions are fully discussed in the chapter 'Nursing care of people experiencing trauma and shock'.

Complementary therapies

Complementary healthcare practitioners may recommend specific plant enzymes to treat nutritional anaemias. There is limited quality evidence that complementary therapies can assist with the pathology or symptoms of anaemia.

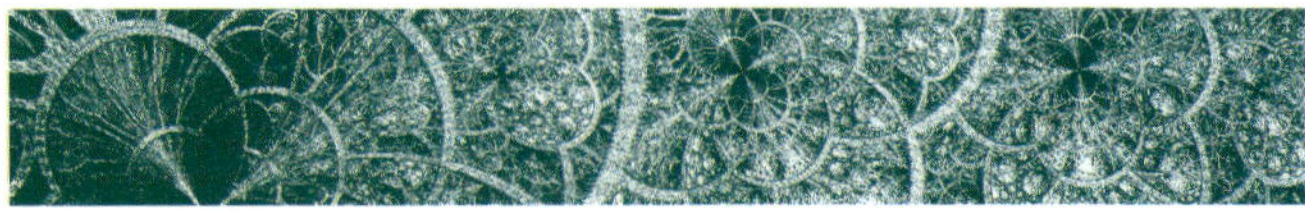

Nursing care

For nursing care specific for a person with folic acid deficiency anaemia, see the nursing care plan.

Health promotion

Nursing measures to prevent anaemia focus on teaching good dietary habits to everyone, regardless of age. Stress the importance of consuming adequate amounts of iron, folate and the B vitamins. Provide a list of dietary sources of these nutrients. Discuss alternate iron sources with those with vegetarian diets

BOX 32.5 Dietary sources of iron, folic acid and vitamin B_{12}

Iron

Iron in the diet comes from two sources. *Haem iron* makes up about one-half of the iron from animal sources. *Non-haem iron* includes the remaining iron from animal sources and all the iron from plants, legumes and nuts. Haem iron promotes absorption of non-haem iron from other foods when both forms are consumed at the same time. Absorption of non-haem iron is also enhanced by vitamin C and inhibited by tea and coffee.

Sources of haem iron

- Beef
- Chicken
- Egg yolk
- Oysters
- Pork loin
- Turkey
- Veal

Sources of non-haem iron

- Bran flakes
- Brown rice
- Wholegrain breads
- Oatmeal
- Dried fruits
- Leafy green vegetables
- Dried beans

Sources of folic acid

- Green leafy vegetables
- Broccoli
- Organ meats
- Eggs
- Wheat germ
- Asparagus
- Liver
- Milk
- Yeast
- Kidney beans

Sources of vitamin B_{12}

- Liver
- Prawns and oysters
- Eggs
- Milk
- Kidney
- Meats (muscle)
- Cheese

and teach them that foods high in vitamin C enhance the absorption of iron from grains, legumes and other sources. Emphasise the importance of adequate iron intake in women of childbearing age and older adults. Stress the increased need for these nutrients during pregnancy and discuss strategies to ensure an adequate intake.

Assessment

Assessment data to collect for people with suspected anaemia include:

- *Health history*: complaints of shortness of breath with activity, fatigue, weakness, dizziness or fainting, palpitations; history of previous anaemia, bleeding episodes; menstrual history (if appropriate); medications, chronic diseases; usual diet and patterns of alcohol intake or cigarette smoking.
- *Physical examination*: general appearance, skin colour; vital signs, including temperature, heart and lung sounds; peripheral pulses, capillary refill; abdominal tenderness; obvious bleeding or bruising.
- *Diagnostic tests*: FBC, haemoglobin and haematocrit; bone marrow studies; specialised tests (e.g. haemoglobin electrophoresis, Schilling test).

Nursing diagnoses and interventions

Anaemia affects circulating oxygen levels and tissue oxygenation. Priority nursing diagnoses include activity intolerance, altered oral mucous membranes and self-care deficits. With acute blood-loss anaemia, risk of insufficient cardiac output also is a priority. People with sickle cell disease have specific needs related to the effects of the disease on tissue perfusion. See the section on disseminated intravascular coagulation later in this chapter for nursing interventions appropriate to ineffective tissue perfusion, associated pain and maintaining oxygenation.

Activity intolerance

Anaemia causes weakness and shortness of breath on exertion. These symptoms are due to decreased circulating oxygen levels secondary to low haemoglobin levels. Weakness, fatigue and/or vertigo may occur even during activities of daily living, including those associated with self-care, home life, job performance and social roles.

- Help identify ways to conserve energy when performing necessary or desired activities. *Modifying the approach to a particular activity may reduce cardiorespiratory symptoms and activity-related fatigue. Alternative ways of performing tasks (e.g. sitting when performing hygiene care and kitchen tasks) may reduce oxygen demands. In some cases, assistance from others is necessary to conserve energy and reduce symptoms.*
- Help the person and family establish priorities for tasks and activities. *Because family members may need to assume responsibility for additional tasks, the plan's success depends on mutually established goals.*
- Assist to develop a schedule of alternating activity and rest periods throughout the day. *Rest periods decrease oxygen needs, reducing strain on the heart and lungs and allowing restoration of homeostasis before further activities.*
- Encourage 8 to 10 hours of sleep at night. *Rest decreases oxygen demands and increases available energy for morning activities.*
- Monitor vital signs before and after activity. *Vital signs provide a measure of activity tolerance. Increased heart and respiratory rates or a change in blood pressure may indicate intolerance of the activity.*
- Discontinue activity if any of the following occurs:
  a. complaints of chest pain, breathlessness or vertigo
  b. palpitations or tachycardia that does not return to normal within 4 minutes of resting
  c. bradycardia
  d. tachypnoea or dyspnoea
  e. decreased systolic blood pressure.

  These changes may signify cardiac decompensation due to insufficient oxygenation. The intensity, duration or frequency of the activity needs to be reduced.

- Instruct the person not to smoke. *Smoking causes vasoconstriction and increases carbon monoxide levels in the blood, interfering with tissue oxygenation.*

Impaired oral mucous membrane

Glossitis and cheilosis may occur with nutritional deficiencies of iron, folate and vitamin B_{12}. The tongue and lips become very red and fissures or cracks may form at the corners of the mouth.

- Monitor condition of lips and tongue daily. *Glossitis and cheilosis increase the risk of bleeding and infection and may require medical treatment. Pain and discomfort may interfere with oral intake, further worsening the nutritional deficiency.*
- Use a mouthwash of saline, saltwater or half-strength peroxide and water to rinse the mouth every 2 to 4 hours. Avoid alcohol-based mouthwashes. *This cleanses and soothes oral mucous membranes. Alcohol-based mouthwashes further irritate and dry oral tissues.*
- Provide frequent oral hygiene (after each meal and at bedtime) with a soft-bristle toothbrush or sponge. *Removing food debris from painful fissures promotes comfort. A soft toothbrush reduces irritation or bleeding of oral mucosa. Keeping the oral cavity clean also reduces the risk of infection.*
- Apply a petroleum-based lubricating jelly or ointment to the lips after oral care. *Lubricating ointment helps to retain moisture, facilitate healing and protect the lips from other drying agents.*
- Instruct to avoid hot, spicy or acidic foods. *Such foods may further irritate and dry mucous membranes.*
- Encourage soft, cool, bland foods. Foods that are soothing to the mucous membranes promote comfort and help maintain adequate food and fluid intake. Minimising oral pain may also promote compliance with oral care routines.

NURSING CARE PLAN A person with folic acid deficiency anaemia

Iris Matthews is a 76-year-old widow who lives alone. She tells Lisa Kennedy RN, the practice nurse in the general practice surgery, that she liked to cook when her husband was alive but preparing an entire meal just for herself seems senseless. She relates that her typical day's menu includes tea for breakfast, a ham sandwich and tea for lunch, a cup of soup, a few biscuits and a glass of milk for dinner.

ASSESSMENT

Mrs Matthews' nursing history includes a 9 kg weight loss since her husband died 8 months ago. She states that she sometimes has heart palpitations and always feels weak. Physical assessment shows: 37.1°C, P 110, R 22, BP 90/52. Skin warm, pale and dry. Diagnostic tests indicate folic acid deficiency anaemia. Mrs Matthews is started on an oral folic acid supplement and instructed about foods containing folic acid.

DIAGNOSES

- *Activity intolerance* related to weakness secondary to decreased tissue oxygenation.
- *Imbalanced nutrition: less than body requirements* related to lack of motivation to cook and understanding of nutritional needs, as manifested by weight loss of 9 kg and folic acid deficiency.
- *Deficient knowledge* related to lack of information about a well-balanced diet and foods containing folic acid.

PLANNING

- Discuss foods required for a well-balanced diet, as well as dietary sources of folic acid.
- Discuss the importance of taking the folic acid supplement. Advise to continue taking it even after she begins to feel better.

Expected outcomes

- Verbalise and understand the importance of taking folic acid supplements and eating a balanced diet.
- Gain at least 0.45 kg per week.
- Return to previous level of physical energy.
- Consume a balanced diet, including foods containing folic acid.

IMPLEMENTATION

- Develop a balanced dietary plan with Mrs Matthews that includes food preferences and foods that are easy and quick to prepare.
- Include foods that contain folic acid or assist her in organising supplements.
- Help Mrs Matthews develop a schedule of activities that provides adequate rest and energy for cooking.

EVALUATION

Mrs Matthews gained 0.5 kg during the first week of treatment. She has met with a dietitian and has a better understanding of nutritional needs. She states that she can prepare hot meals when she schedules a rest period before and after lunch. She has provided written and verbal information about the folic acid supplement and diet. Mrs Matthews verbalises understanding, stating, 'I will continue to take the folic acid until the doctor tells me to stop. I'm beginning to enjoy cooking again, now that I have a reason to cook!' Ms Kennedy contacts the local seniors group to determine if Mrs Matthews is able to participate in the local Meals on Wheels program.

CRITICAL THINKING IN THE NURSING PROCESS

1. What is the pathophysiological basis for Mrs Matthews' abnormal vital signs during her initial assessment?
2. Design a week's menu that includes foods high in folic acid.
3. Why was Mrs Matthews placed on a folic acid supplement in addition to dietary modifications?
4. Why is the older adult at increased risk of developing folic acid deficiency anaemia? Consider physiological, economic and social factors.

REFLECTION ON THE NURSING PROCESS

1. Outline the most important communication and education points you have learned from this case study.
2. How can you use this information in your practice?

- Encourage eating four to six small meals daily with high protein and vitamin content. Small, frequent meals may be better tolerated, increasing intake. Nutrient-rich meals promote healing of the mucous membranes.

Risk of decreased cardiac output

Cardiac output may be affected by acute bleeding and volume loss or by heart failure resulting from severe anaemia. In addition, impaired tissue oxygenation leads to an increased respiratory rate and dyspnoea.

- Monitor vital signs, breath sounds and apical pulse. *Increased cardiac workload can affect the blood pressure, heart and respiratory rates. Increased blood flow can lead to heart murmur or abnormal heart sounds such as S_3 or S_4. Tachypnoea and dyspnoea may affect the depth of respirations, alveolar ventilation and blood and tissue oxygenation.*
- Assess for pallor, cyanosis and dependent oedema. *Blood is shunted to the vital organs, causing vasoconstriction of skin vessels. This, in addition to lower levels of haemoglobin, causes pallor. Cyanosis, especially of the lips and nail beds, indicates inadequate oxygenation of blood. Dependent oedema occurs in response to right ventricular failure.*

CONSIDERATION FOR PRACTICE

Report signs of decreased cardiac output to the medical officer. Severe anaemia can lead to heart failure, necessitating additional treatment.

- Closely monitor for manifestations of anaphylaxis (urticaria, erythema or flushing, oedema, wheezing, dyspnoea, nausea and vomiting, anxiety) when administering parenteral iron preparations, particularly iron dextran. Immediately notify the doctor and prepare to administer prescribed drugs such as adrenaline as ordered. Institute cardiopulmonary resuscitation measures as necessary. *Anaphylaxis, a systemic type I hypersensitivity (allergic) reaction, is a risk when administering parenteral iron preparations—iron dextran, in particular. Anaphylaxis can lead to severe cardiopulmonary compromise, necessitating emergency measures to preserve life.*

Self-care deficit

Energy expenditures for activities of daily living (ADLs) may cause oxygen demands to exceed supply in the person with severe anaemia.

- Assist with ADLs, such as bathing, grooming and eating, as needed. *Assistance decreases energy expenditures and tissue requirements for oxygen, reducing cardiac workload.*
- Discuss the importance of rest periods prior to such activities as dressing. *Rest reduces oxygen demand and cardiac workload. The person who is able to perform self-care in ADLs maintains independence, self-esteem and morale.*

Community-based care

With the exception of anaemia resulting from acute haemorrhage, most people with anaemia are treated in the home and community setting. Include the following topics when preparing the person and family for home care:

- nutritional strategies to address deficiencies
- prescribed medications, vitamins or mineral supplements, and their appropriate use, intended effect, possible adverse effects, and interactions with food or other medications
- energy conservation strategies
- other recommended treatment measures and follow up
- if the anaemia is genetically transmitted, such as sickle cell anaemia, include inheritance patterns of the disorder, symptoms of crisis and manifestations to report to the doctor.

Provide referrals for counselling to facilitate decisions about pregnancy as indicated. Also refer for nutritional assistance and teaching, home healthcare or assistance with self-care and home maintenance activities as indicated. Older adults with nutritional anaemias may benefit from community services such as Meals on Wheels.

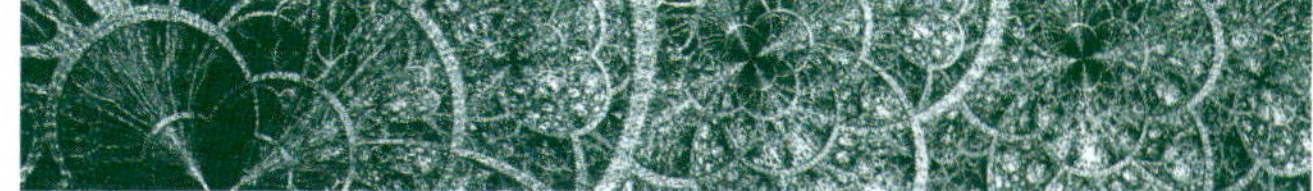

THE PERSON WITH MYELODYSPLASTIC SYNDROME

Myelodysplastic syndrome (MDS) is a group of blood disorders characterised by abnormal-appearing bone marrow and cytopenia (low numbers of circulating blood cells). MDS is not a single disease; at least eight variations of the disorder have been identified. Anaemia that does not respond to treatment (*refractory anaemia*) is a characteristic of most forms of myelodysplasia.

Idiopathic MDS primarily affects older adults; men have a slightly higher incidence of the disorder than women. Risk factors for secondary MDS include exposure to environmental toxins such as cigarette smoke, benzene, radiation, radiation therapy or chemotherapy for cancer treatment, and other anaemias such as aplastic anaemia or, more rarely, Fanconi's anaemia (Leukaemia Foundation, 2022a).

FAST FACTS

- In Australia, 5 in 100,000 people have MDS, but this increases with age, up to 20 to 50 in 100,000 over 60 years of age.
- Of MDS cases, 90% occur in people over 60 years of age. Other factors that can contribute include smoking or exposure to environmental toxins, radiation, chemotherapy or other risk factors (Leukaemia Foundation, 2022a).

Pathophysiology

MDS is a stem cell disorder in which stem cells fail to reproduce and differentiate into the various types of blood cells. The genetic components of stem cells (nuclear DNA and/or mitochondrial DNA) are altered, the bone marrow loses its ability to produce normal blood cells, instead producing abnormal (*dysplastic*) cells, and ineffective haematopoiesis results. With significant alterations, leukaemia (proliferation of abnormal WBCs) may develop in people with MDS.

Manifestations

Anaemia is the predominant early manifestation of MDS. The person may develop symptoms of the anaemia with increasing fatigue, weakness, dyspnoea and pallor, and susceptibility to frequent infections. In many cases, the disorder is asymptomatic, identified when a routine blood test shows anaemia. Splenomegaly may develop, leading to discomfort and a feeling of fullness in the left upper quadrant of the abdomen. Hepatomegaly also may develop, leading to right upper quadrant discomfort. Thrombocytopenia can lead to abnormal bleeding tendencies and petechiae, and neutropenia increases the risk of infection (Aster & Stone, 2022; Besa, 2022a).

INTERPROFESSIONAL CARE

People with MDS require long-term supportive care and therapy to maintain their quality of life. Stem cell transplant offers the only real hope for cure in MDS. See the 'Interprofessional care' section of 'The person with leukaemia' later in this chapter for more information about stem cell transplant and associated nursing care.

Diagnosis

- The *FBC* reveals anaemia. Although anaemia may be the only abnormality of the blood count, the WBC count also may be low, as may the platelet count. Abnormalities of size and shape may be noted in all blood cells.
- The *bone marrow* often appears normal, although precursor cells may have an abnormal appearance. Increased numbers of myeloblasts (granulocyte precursor cells) may be present in the bone marrow.
- *Serum erythropoietin, vitamin B_{12}, serum iron, total iron-binding capacity, ferritin levels* and *RBC folate levels* are drawn to help guide supportive therapy. X-rays, ECGs, immunophenotyping and cytogenetic testing are also undertaken.

Treatment

Management of MDS is based on the severity of the disease. Several classification systems are available, the most common being the revised International Prognostic Scoring System (IPSS-R) (Garcia-Manero, Chien & Montalban-Bravo, 2020). These systems are used to guide therapy for the person with MDS. Early diagnosis increases the likelihood of remaining well and may include 'watchful waiting' depending on the progression of symptoms. Late diagnosis often results in poor prognosis, albeit improving with more medical developments. Management of MDS is primarily supportive therapy such as blood transfusions, bone marrow stimulation and/or cytotoxic chemotherapy (Besa, 2022a). Bone marrow transplant is appropriate in fewer than 5% of people with MDS.

All those with MDS require monitoring, with regular GP visits and pathology evaluations. Psychosocial support is provided to assist the person and their family in dealing with a chronic, progressive and ultimately fatal disease.

People with MDS may require frequent RBC transfusions to treat the predominant anaemia. Each unit of packed RBCs contains 250 to 300 mg of iron. The body is unable to excrete this excess iron, so it accumulates, leading to problems such as endocrine dysfunction, cirrhosis, pericarditis and heart failure. *Iron chelation therapy* is used to remove excess iron from the body. Desferrioxamine (Desferal) can be administered by slow intravenous infusion or continuous subcutaneous infusion using an infusion pump to maintain a normal or negative iron balance. This drug is relatively safe, although local skin reactions such as rash and urticaria may develop. Oral options, such as deferiprone and deferasirox, have also recently expanded.

Blood cell growth factors may be administered to stimulate stem cell development in MDS, although the response rate is low. Platelet transfusions are given when bleeding occurs due to low platelet levels. Antibiotic therapy is initiated for bacterial infections (Leukaemia Foundation, 2022a). Chemotherapy regimens similar to those employed to treat leukaemia may be used, but rarely are effective in treating MDS. Azacitidine (Vidaza), an antileukaemic agent that acts on abnormal blood-forming cells in the bone marrow, is more effective in treating MDS than standard chemotherapy regimens, and is now one of the first-line treatments for high-risk MDS patients (Garcia-Manero et al., 2020).

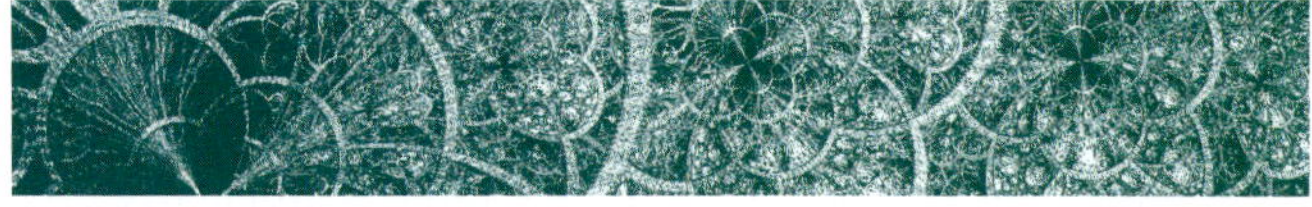

Nursing care

Nursing diagnoses and interventions

Activity intolerance and the need for education about this disorder are the priorities of nursing care for the person with MDS being managed in a community-based setting. Although neutropenia and thrombocytopenia may accompany the anaemia of MDS, these problems are less common. See the section of this chapter on leukaemia for additional potential nursing diagnoses and interventions for the person with MDS.

Activity intolerance

The person with MDS experiences fatigue, weakness and shortness of breath on exertion related to the lack of RBCs and ineffective oxygen transport. These symptoms may affect the person's ability to maintain self-care, home life, job performance and social roles.

- Monitor vital signs, breath sounds and apical pulse. *Increased cardiac workload due to anaemia and impaired oxygen transport can affect the blood pressure, heart and respiratory rates. Increased blood flow can lead to heart murmur or abnormal heart sounds such as S_3 or S_4. Accumulated iron can lead to pericarditis and a pericardial friction rub.*

- Help identify energy-conserving ways of performing necessary or desired activities. *Alternative ways of performing tasks (e.g. sitting while performing hygiene measures) may reduce oxygen demands and fatigue.*
- Help the person and family establish priorities for tasks and activities. *Because family members may need to assume responsibility for additional tasks, the plan's success depends on mutually established goals.*
- Suggest planning recreational activities following a transfusion and adjusting activity level between transfusions to match energy and minimise fatigue. *The person with MDS will have more energy and activity tolerance following a transfusion when RBC counts, haemoglobin and haematocrit approach normal levels and oxygen transport is optimal.*
- Encourage 8 to 10 hours of sleep at night. *Rest decreases oxygen demands and increases available energy for morning activities.*
- Discontinue activity if any of the following occurs:
  a. complaints of chest pain, breathlessness or vertigo
  b. palpitations or tachycardia that does not return to normal within 4 minutes of resting
  c. bradycardia
  d. tachypnoea or dyspnoea
  e. decreased systolic blood pressure.

  These changes may signify cardiac decompensation due to insufficient oxygenation. The intensity, duration or frequency of the activity needs to be reduced.
- Instruct the person not to smoke. *Smoking causes vasoconstriction and increases carbon monoxide levels in the blood, interfering with tissue oxygenation.*

Risk of ineffective health maintenance

MDS is a chronic, usually progressive disorder, requiring active management to maintain functional status and quality of life. Regular visits to the doctor may be necessary. In addition, the person or family members may need to learn to administer iron chelation therapy or chemotherapy drugs and measures to prevent complications. The chronic nature of the disorder, and the often advanced age of the person and family caregivers, may interfere with effective management of the disorder.

- Assess knowledge of the disorder and the related treatments. *Assessment allows identification of knowledge gaps and provides a basis on which to provide additional information. Impaired disease management may be due to lack of knowledge or an inability to learn and perform psychomotor skills (e.g. administration of parenteral drug therapy).*
- Provide information about the disorder, its effects and prescribed medications and treatments. *Individualised instruction is more effective than general, possibly irrelevant information. The person and caregivers need to be able to identify and manage possible adverse effects of drug therapy, as well as recognise potential complications to be reported to the doctor.*
- Provide emotional support, expressing confidence in the person's and caregivers' abilities to manage care. *Emotional support helps the person and family caregivers incorporate the care regimen into their lifestyle.*
- Provide supervised learning and practice opportunities for administering parenteral medications if ordered. *Successful practice sessions instil confidence in the ability to manage care and provide an opportunity for questions and exploring alternatives.*

Community-based care

The person with myelodysplastic syndrome needs information about this chronic and ultimately fatal disease. Provide information about the various treatment options available, including management of any infusion device if ordered. Discuss the timing of and options for stem cell transplant and assist the person to evaluate the potential benefits and risks of this treatment option.

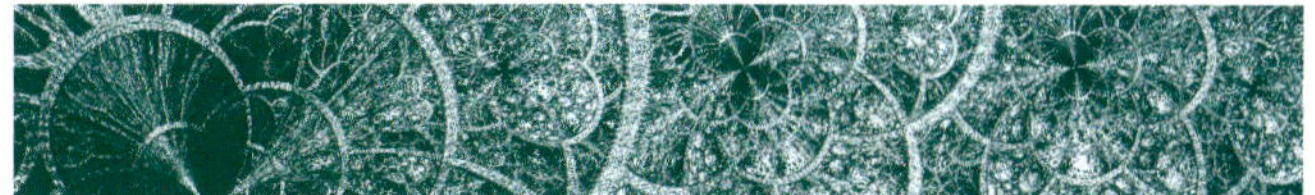

THE PERSON WITH POLYCYTHAEMIA

Polycythaemia, or *erythrocytosis*, is an excess of RBCs characterised by a haematocrit higher than 55%. The two main types of polycythaemia are primary and secondary. A third type of polycythaemia, relative polycythaemia, results from a fluid volume deficit, not excess RBCs.

FAST FACTS

- *Primary polycythaemia* (*polycythaemia vera*) is uncommon.
  - In primary polycythaemia, RBC production is increased.
  - Primary polycythaemia is most commonly diagnosed in men over the age of 55.
- *Secondary polycythaemia* (*erythrocytosis*) is the most common form of polycythaemia.
  - Secondary polycythaemia occurs when erythropoietin levels are elevated.
  - It may affect people of any age or origin.
  - It usually develops in response to hypoxia (living at a high altitude, smoking or chronic lung disease).
- *Relative polycythaemia* occurs due to fluid deficit, not excess RBCs.
  - In relative polycythaemia the total RBC count is normal.
  - The haematocrit is elevated because of increased cell concentration.
  - It is corrected by rehydration.

Pathophysiology

Primary polycythaemia

Primary polycythaemia, or *polycythaemia vera* (PV), is a neoplastic stem cell disorder characterised by overproduction of RBCs and, to a lesser extent, WBCs and platelets. It is classified as a myeloproliferative disorder. Its cause is unknown. In PV, colonies of endogenous erythroid stem cells develop. These colonies produce RBCs in the absence of erythropoietin, leading to excess RBC production (Nagalla, 2022).

MANIFESTATIONS Initially, PV is asymptomatic and the diagnosis may be made during routine blood tests. Its manifestations are caused by increased blood volume and viscosity. Hypertension is common and may lead to complaints of headaches, dizziness and vision and hearing disruptions. Venous stasis causes *plethora*, a red colour of the face, hands, feet and mucous membranes. This often is accompanied by severe, painful itching of the fingers and toes, and gout. Retinal and cerebral vessels may be engorged. Hypermetabolism develops, causing weight loss and night sweats. Mental status may be altered, leading to drowsiness or delirium, and spenomegaly may occur.

Thrombosis and haemorrhage are potential complications of PV. Thrombosis may cause transient ischaemic attacks, angina or manifestations of peripheral vascular disease. Gastrointestinal bleeding may occur and portal hypertension may develop.

Secondary polycythaemia

Secondary polycythaemia, or erythrocytosis, is increased numbers of RBCs in response to excess erythropoietin secretion or prolonged hypoxia. Secondary polycythaemia is the most common form of polycythaemia.

Abnormally high erythropoietin levels can result from kidney disease or erythropoietin-secreting tumours (e.g. renal cell carcinoma). Chronic hypoxia that stimulates erythropoietin release is a more common cause of secondary polycythaemia. People living at high altitudes where the atmospheric oxygen pressure is lower develop a degree of polycythaemia, as do people with chronic heart or lung disease and smokers. Abnormal haemoglobin that forms tighter bonds with oxygen also may lead to secondary polycythaemia. Blood doping in sport causes a purposeful artificial polycythaemia. RBCs are drawn off and stored, and the body responds by producing erythropoietin and increasing RBC production. The stored cells are reinfused, thus producing excess RBC or polycythaemia. This was done to increase the oxygen-carrying capacity for the athlete but has since been banned (Seeger & Grau, 2020).

MANIFESTATIONS The manifestations of secondary polycythaemia are similar to those of primary polycythaemia. Splenomegaly, however, does not develop. Early symptoms often are overshadowed by the manifestations of the underlying disorder. For the manifestations of polycythaemia, see the 'Manifestations' box.

MANIFESTATIONS Polycythaemia

- Hypertension
- Headache, tinnitus, blurred vision
- Plethora: dark redness of the lips, feet, ears, fingernails and mucous membranes
- Splenomegaly (polycythaemia vera)
- Severe pruritus, extremity pain
- Weight loss, night sweats
- Gastrointestinal bleeding
- Intermittent claudication
- Symptoms from thrombosis within various organs

INTERPROFESSIONAL CARE

Diagnosis

In polycythaemia vera, serum erythropoietin levels are low. Bone marrow studies show hyperplasia of all haematopoietic elements. With secondary polycythaemia, serum erythropoietin levels usually are high and bone marrow studies show only red stem cell hyperplasia.

Treatments

For secondary polycythaemia, treatment focuses on the underlying cause of the disorder. It is a physiological response in people living at high altitudes and, unless the haematocrit is too high or oxygen saturation levels are low, no treatment is usually necessary. Smokers are urged to quit. Measures to raise oxygen saturation levels and reduce tissue hypoxia often will relieve the polycythaemia. People with both primary and secondary polycythaemia benefit from periodic phlebotomy or venesection, removing 300 to 500 mL of blood, to keep blood volume and viscosity within normal levels. For PV, chemotherapeutic agents or myelosuppressive drugs such as hydroxyurea may be used to suppress marrow function but may increase the risk of developing leukaemia (discussed later in this chapter). Interferon may also be used to control RBC production. Anagrelide may be used to reduce platelet production. Pruritus may be relieved by antihistamines or may require more aggressive treatment with interferon alpha or other treatments. Aspirin may be prescribed daily to control thrombosis without increasing the risk of bleeding.

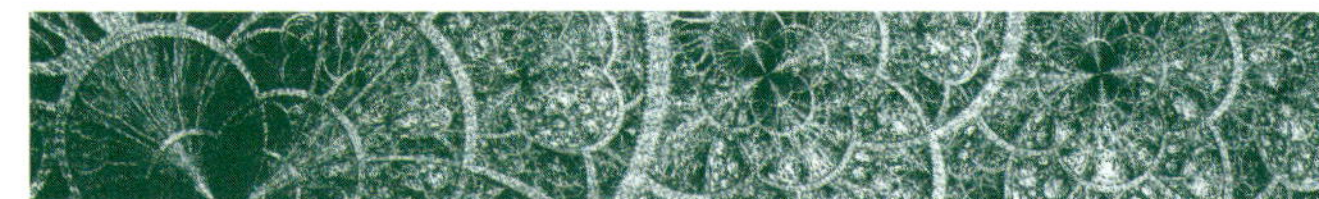

Nursing care

Preventing polycythaemia begins with educating children and adults about the dangers of smoking. Measures to reduce risk factors for cardiovascular disease also may be beneficial.

This chronic condition is managed in community-based settings unless a complication develops. Teach the person and family the importance of maintaining adequate hydration and increasing fluid intake during hot weather and when exercising. Discuss measures to prevent blood stasis: elevating legs and feet when sitting, using support stockings and continuing treatment measures. Instruct to report manifestations of thrombosis (leg or calf pain, chest pain, neurological symptoms) or bleeding (black, tarry stools, vomiting of blood or coffee-grounds emesis) immediately. Monitor the haematocrit and cell counts throughout treatment.

Examples of nursing diagnoses appropriate for the person with polycythaemia follow:

- *Pain* related to effects of altered blood flow in distal extremities.
- *Risk of ineffective tissue perfusion* related to sluggish blood flow and increased risk of thrombosis.

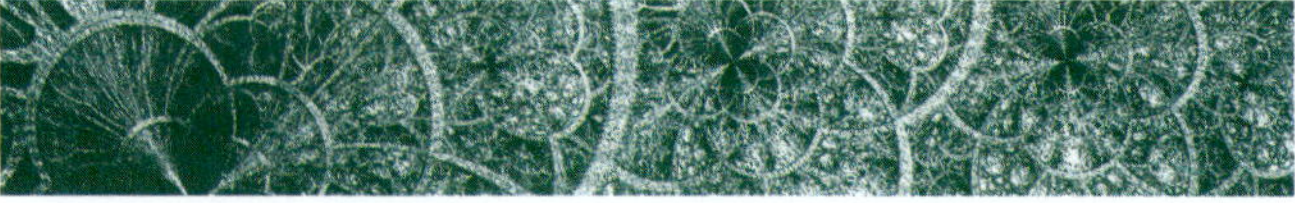

White blood cell and lymphoid tissue disorders

Important disorders of the WBCs and lymphoid tissue include the leukaemias, multiple myeloma and malignant lymphomas (Hodgkin's disease and non-Hodgkin's lymphoma). Review the physiology of WBCs and lymphoid tissues and assessment of their function in the chapter 'A person-centred approach to assessing the cardiovascular and lymphatic systems' before proceeding with this section.

THE PERSON WITH LEUKAEMIA

Leukaemia (literally, 'white blood') is a group of chronic malignant disorders of WBCs and WBC precursors. Precursor cells are stem cells that have developed to the stage where they are committed to forming a particular kind of new blood cell. All leukaemias start in the bone marrow where developing blood cells, usually developing white cells, undergo a malignant change.

In leukaemia, the usual ratio of red to WBCs is reversed. Leukaemias are characterised by replacement of bone marrow by malignant immature WBCs, abnormal immature circulating WBCs and infiltration of these cells into the liver, spleen and lymph nodes throughout the body. There are four main types of leukaemia. They are discussed later in this section.

Incidence and risk factors

Although leukaemia is often thought of as a childhood disease, it is diagnosed 10 times more often in adults than in children; the majority over 50 years old. It is estimated that just over 5,200 people were diagnosed with leukaemia in 2022, making it the 11th most common type of cancer (AIHW, 2022; Cancer Australia, 2022a).

Although the cause of most leukaemia is unknown, certain risk factors have been identified. Men are affected more frequently than women. People with certain genetic disorders such as Down syndrome have a higher incidence of leukaemia. Environmental risk factors play a role as well. Risk factors for myeloid leukaemia include cigarette smoking and chemicals such as benzene (present in cigarette smoke and petrol). Exposure to ionising radiation increases the risk of several types of leukaemia. People who have undergone treatment for cancer have an increased risk. The human T-cell leukaemia/lymphoma virus-1, a retrovirus, is known to cause certain leukaemias and lymphomas.

Physiology review

WBCs are the most diverse of the cellular components of the blood. WBCs arise from three different precursor cells: myeloblasts, which further differentiate into the granular leucocytes (granulocytes), neutrophils, eosinophils and basophils; monoblasts, which mature into circulating monocytes and ultimately into macrophages; and lymphoblasts, which become lymphocytes and mature in lymphoid tissue to B cells and T cells.

As a whole, the primary function of WBCs is to help maintain the body's immune defences. Neutrophils, the most numerous WBC in circulation, are active phagocytes, the first cells to arrive to injured tissue. Monocytes and macrophages also are phagocytic cells that dispose of foreign and waste material from tissues. Eosinophils and basophils are more specialised. Eosinophils are primarily involved in allergic responses and parasitic infections. Basophils are actively involved in the inflammatory response, releasing substances such as histamine and heparin into inflamed tissues. Lymphocytes, the smallest of the WBCs, are an integral part of the immune system. B cells are part of the humoral immune response, producing antibodies to specific antigens. T cells are part of the cell-mediated immune response. For more information about the inflammatory and immune responses, see the chapter 'Nursing care of people with altered immunity'. The normal WBC count and differential are presented in Table 32.2.

Pathophysiology

Leukaemia begins with malignant transformation of a single stem cell. Leukaemic cells proliferate slowly, but do not differentiate normally. They have a prolonged lifespan and accumulate in the bone marrow. As they accumulate, they compete with the proliferation of normal cells. Leukaemic cells do not function as mature WBCs and are ineffective in the inflammatory and immune processes. Leukaemic cells replace normal haematopoietic elements in the marrow. Because erythrocyte- and platelet-producing cells are crowded out, severe anaemia, splenomegaly and bleeding difficulties result.

Leukaemic cells leave the bone marrow and travel through the circulatory system, infiltrating other body tissues such as the central nervous system, testes, skin, gastrointestinal tract and the lymph nodes, liver and spleen. Death usually is due to internal haemorrhage and infections.

Manifestations

The general manifestations of leukaemia (regardless of type) result from anaemia, infection and bleeding. These include pallor, fatigue, tachycardia, malaise, lethargy and dyspnoea

TABLE 32.2 Normal white blood cell count and differential

LABORATORY TEST	VALUE
WBC count	3.7–11.0 × 10^9/L
Differential WBC count	
Neutrophils	2.0–7.5 × 10^9/L
Eosinophils	0.05–0.5 × 10^9/L
Basophils	< 0.1 × 10^9/L
Lymphocytes	1.5–3.7 × 10^9/L
Monocytes	0.2–0.4 × 10^9/L

on exertion. Infection may cause fever, night sweats, oral ulcerations and frequent or recurrent respiratory, urinary, integumentary or other infections. Increased bleeding due to thrombocytopenia leads to bruising, petechiae, bleeding gums and bleeding within specific organs and tissues. See 'Multisystem effects of leukaemia'.

Other manifestations result from leukaemic cell infiltration, increased metabolism and increased leucocyte destruction. Infiltration of the liver, spleen, lymph nodes and bone marrow causes pain and tissue swelling in the involved areas. Meningeal infiltration may cause manifestations of increased intracranial pressure, such as headache, altered level of consciousness, cranial nerve impairment, nausea and vomiting. Infiltration of the kidneys may affect renal function, with decreased urine output and increased blood urea nitrogen and creatinine. Increased metabolism causes heat intolerance, weight loss, dyspnoea on exertion and tachycardia. Destruction of large numbers of WBCs releases substantial amounts of uric acid into the circulation; uric acid crystals may obstruct renal tubules, causing renal insufficiency.

Without treatment, leukaemia is invariably fatal, usually due to complications of leukaemic cell infiltration of bone marrow or vital organs. With treatment, prognosis varies. The overall 5-year survival rate is 63% (Cancer Australia, 2022a). Survival rates differ by type of leukaemia: people with acute myeloid leukaemia can have a 10–30% 5-year survival rate, with a mean of 24%, favouring the younger generation in response to treatment. Those with chronic lymphocytic leukaemia may not even require treatment or may need it only after 10 years or more, as their 5-year survival rate is around 73% (Cancer Council, 2022; Leukaemia Foundation, 2022b). This has increased significantly from previous years (Cancer Australia, 2022a). The types, pathology, manifestations and treatment for the major leukaemias are outlined in Table 32.3.

Classifications

Leukaemias are classified by their acuity and by the predominant cell type involved. The *acute* leukaemias are characterised by an acute onset, rapid disease progression and immature or undifferentiated blast cells. *Chronic* leukaemias, on the other hand, have a gradual onset, prolonged course and abnormal, mature-appearing cells. *Lymphocytic* (or *lymphoblastic*) leukaemias involve immature lymphocytes and their precursor cells in the bone marrow. Lymphocytic leukaemias infiltrate the spleen, lymph nodes, CNS and other tissues. *Myeloid* (also called *myelogenous, myelocytic* or *myeloblastic*) leukaemias involve myeloid stem cells in the bone marrow, interfering with the maturation of all types of blood cells, including granulocytes, RBCs and thrombocytes. Acute lymphoblastic leukaemia is the most common type of leukaemia in children. In adults, acute myeloid leukaemia and chronic lymphocytic leukaemia are the most common types (Leukaemia Foundation, 2022b). In summary, the general types of leukaemia are as follows:

- acute myeloid (myeloblastic) leukaemia (AML)
- chronic myeloid (myelogenous) leukaemia (CML)
- acute lymphocytic (lymphoblastic) leukaemia (ALL)
- chronic lymphocytic leukaemia (CLL).

This general system of classifying leukaemias does not differentiate subtypes of acute leukaemias. The FAB system for classifying acute leukaemias further differentiates acute leukaemias by the predominant cell involved and the degree of cell differentiation (see Table 32.4).

Acute myeloid leukaemia

Acute myeloid leukaemia (AML) is characterised by uncontrolled proliferation of myeloblasts (the precursors of granulocytes) and hyperplasia of the bone marrow and spleen (see Figure 32.5). Treatment induces complete remission in around two-thirds of people, although only about 30–40% achieve cure or long-term remission.

The manifestations of AML result from neutropenia and thrombocytopenia. Decreased neutrophils lead to recurrent severe infections, such as pneumonia, septicaemia, abscesses and mucous membrane ulceration. The manifestations of thrombocytopenia include petechiae, purpura, ecchymoses (bruising), epistaxis (nosebleeds), haematomas, haematuria and gastrointestinal bleeding. Bone infarctions or subperiosteal infiltrates of leukaemic cells may cause bone pain. Anaemia is a late manifestation, causing fatigue, headaches, pallor and dyspnoea on exertion. Death usually results from infection or haemorrhage.

TABLE 32.3 Major types of leukaemia

CLASSIFICATION	CHARACTERISTICS	MANIFESTATIONS	TREATMENT
Acute lymphoblastic leukaemia (ALL)	Primarily affects children and young adults; leukaemic cells may infiltrate CNS	Recurrent infections; bleeding; pallor, bone pain, weight loss, sore throat, fatigue, night sweats, weakness	Chemotherapy; bone marrow transplant (BMT) or stem cell transplant (SCT)
Chronic lymphocytic leukaemia (CLL)	Primarily affects older adults; insidious onset and slow, chronic course	Fatigue; exercise intolerance; lymphadenopathy and splenomegaly; recurrent infections, pallor, oedema, thrombophlebitis	Often requires no treatment; chemotherapy; BMT
Acute myeloid leukaemia (AML)	Common in older adults, may affect children and young adults. Strongly associated with toxins, genetic disorders and treatment of other cancers	Fatigue, weakness, fever; anaemia; headache; bone and joint pain; abnormal bleeding and bruising; recurrent infection; lymphadenopathy, splenomegaly and hepatomegaly	Chemotherapy; SCT
Chronic myeloid leukaemia (CML)	Primarily affects adults; early course slow and stable, progressing to aggressive phase in 3-4 years	Early: weakness, fatigue, dyspnoea on exertion; possible splenomegaly Later: fever, weight loss, night sweats	Interferon alpha; chemotherapy with imatinib, hydroxyurea and combination chemotherapy

Multisystem effects of leukaemia

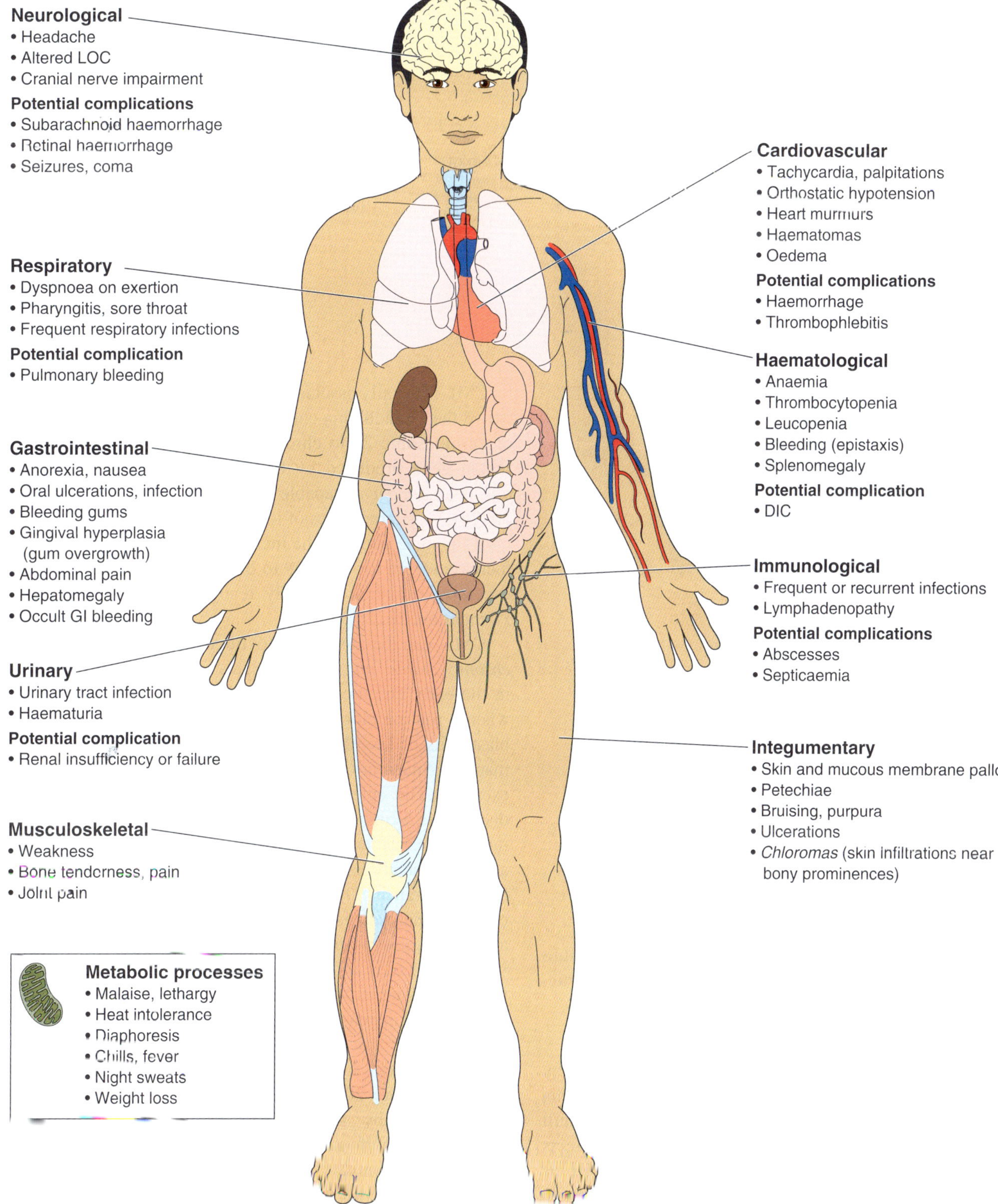

TABLE 32.4 FAB classification of acute leukaemia

TYPE	CLASS	PREDOMINANT CELLS	PROGNOSIS
Acute lymphocytic leukaemia	L_1	Immature lymphoblasts	> 90% remission rate in children
	L_2	Mature lymphoblasts	Relapse common after 2 or more years of remission
Acute myeloid leukaemia	M_0	Undifferentiated cells	Poor
	M_1	Immature myeloblasts	Good; complete response in 65% or more
	M_2	Mature myeloblasts	Good for 2 or more years of remission
	M_3	Promyelocytes	Good in adults
	M_4	Myelocytes and monocytes	Poorest in adults
	M_5	Poorly or well-differentiated monocytes	Poor
	M_6	Predominant erythroblasts	Variable
	M_7	Megakaryocytes	Poor

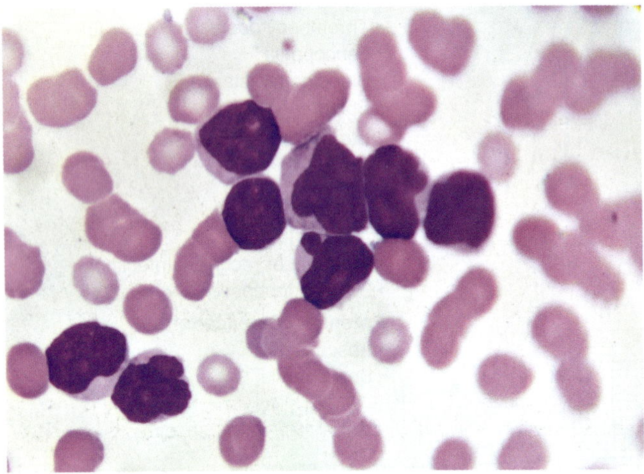

FIGURE 32.5 ***A blood smear from the bone marrow of a person with acute myeloid leukaemia. Note the abnormally large number of myelocyte WBCs (stained purple) among the small RBCs***

Source: Jarun Ontakrai/123RF.

Bone marrow aspiration shows a proliferation of immature WBCs. The FBC shows thrombocytopenia and normocytic, normochromic anaemia.

Chronic myeloid leukaemia

Chronic myeloid leukaemia (CML) is characterised by abnormal proliferation of all bone marrow elements. This type of leukaemia constitutes approximately 15% of adult leukaemias, and 0.03% of all diagnosed cancers. It affects men more frequently than women. The onset of CML is most common after the age of 40, although it is seen in children and adolescents as well (Leukaemia Foundation, 2022b).

CML is usually associated with a chromosome abnormality called the Philadelphia chromosome, a balanced translocation of chromosome 22 to chromosome 9 (see Figure 32.6). The fusion gene produced by this translocation, known as *bcr/abl*, is an *oncogene* capable of initiating a malignancy (Besa, 2022b). Very large doses of ionising radiation also may induce CML in some people. The incidence of CML in Australia has increased from around 200 to 330 new cases each year, with excessive radiation the only recognised cause (Leukaemia Foundation, 2022b).

CML can be divided into three distinct phases. In the *chronic stable phase*, individuals are often asymptomatic in the early chronic stages and, in fact, are often diagnosed when a routine blood test reveals abnormal cell counts, with blast cells of less than 10% in peripheral blood and in bone marrow. Anaemia causes weakness, fatigue and dyspnoea on exertion. The spleen often is enlarged, causing abdominal discomfort. Within 3 to 4 years, the disease can progress to a more aggressive or *accelerated phase*. Rapid cell proliferation and hypermetabolism cause fatigue, weight loss, sweating and heat intolerance. The spleen enlarges, leading to a sensation of abdominal fullness and discomfort. Blast cells increase to approximately 10–19% of the sampled blood, with increasing white blood cells and an enlarging spleen that is unresponsive to therapy. Platelet function is affected in this stage, leading to bleeding and increased bruising. Finally, the disease evolves to acute leukaemia or a blast phase, with blast cell proliferation. At the last stage, known as the *blast crisis*, blast cell counts increase to over 20% of the peripheral blood. This phase is characterised by significant constitutional manifestations including splenomegaly and infiltration of leukaemic cells into the skin, lymph nodes, bones and CNS. Survival is calculated according to well-tested scoring calculators which take into account age, spleen size, platelet count and percentage of blast cells in peripheral blood (Kotiah, 2020).

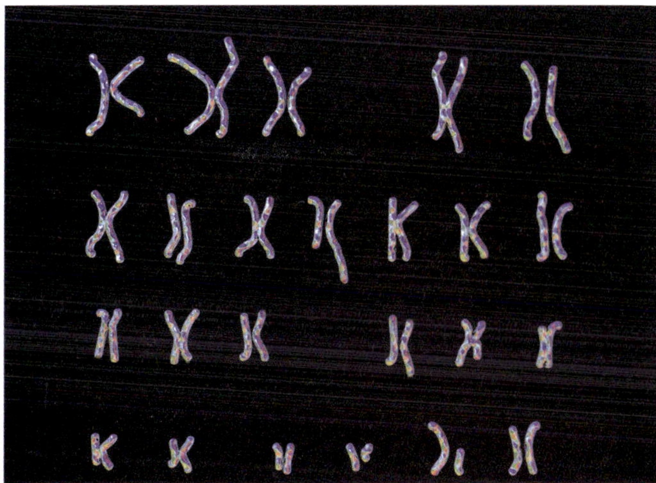

FIGURE 32.6 ***The Philadelphia chromosome. Note the chromosomes of pairs 9 and 22. In each instance, the left-hand chromosome of the pair is normal, whereas an exchange of material between chromosomes has made the right-hand chromosome 9 larger and the right-hand chromosome 22 smaller. In stem cells within the bone marrow, the chromosome 22 defect leads to chronic myeloid leukaemia***

Source: Kateryna Kon/Shutterstock.

Acute lymphocytic leukaemia

Acute lymphocytic leukaemia (ALL) is the most common type of leukaemia in children and young adults. In adults, ALL is rarely seen until late middle age and then its incidence increases with ageing. Genetic factors may play a role in its development, particularly the *bcr/abl* translocation also implicated in CML.

Most (85%) cases of ALL result from malignant transformation of B cells, with the remaining 10–15% arising from T cells and less than 1% from NK cells (Horton, Steuber & Aster, 2022). The malignant cells resemble immature lymphocytes (*lymphoblasts*); however, they do not mature or function effectively to maintain immunity. These lymphoblasts accumulate in the bone marrow, lymph nodes and spleen, as well as in circulating blood. Some types of lymphoma (discussed later in this chapter) are thought to represent a later stage of the same disease.

The onset of ALL is usually rapid. Lymphoblasts proliferating in bone marrow and peripheral tissues crowd the growth of normal cells (see Figure 32.7). Normal haematopoiesis is suppressed, leading to thrombocytopenia, leucopenia and anaemia. Manifestations of infections, bleeding and anaemia develop. Bone pain resulting from rapid generation of marrow elements, lymphadenopathy and liver enlargement are also common. Infiltration of the CNS causes headaches, visual disturbances, vomiting and seizures.

The FBC shows an elevated WBC count with increased lymphocytes on the differential. RBC and platelet counts are decreased. Bone marrow studies reveal a hypercellular marrow with growth of lymphoblasts. Combination chemotherapy produces complete remission in 80–90% of adults with ALL, and even higher rates in children.

Chronic lymphocytic leukaemia

Chronic lymphocytic leukaemia (CLL) is characterised by proliferation and accumulation of small, abnormal, mature lymphocytes in the bone marrow, peripheral blood and body tissues (Rai & Stilgenbauer, 2022). The abnormal cells are usually B lymphocytes that are unable to produce adequate antibodies to maintain normal immune function. CLL occurs more commonly in adults, especially in older adults (median age 65). CLL is the least common type of the major leukaemias, with about 1,000 people diagnosed in Australia yearly, and is thought to have possible familial tendencies in some patients (Leukaemia Foundation, 2022c).

CLL has a slow onset and is often diagnosed during a routine physical examination. If symptoms are present, they usually include vague complaints of weakness or malaise. Possible clinical findings include anaemia, infection and enlarged lymph nodes, spleen and liver. As in other leukaemias, bone marrow hyperplasia is present. Erythrocyte and platelet counts are reduced. Leucocyte counts may either be elevated or reduced, but abnormal cells are always present. In CLL, years may elapse before treatment is required. Survival of this disease averages approximately 7 years.

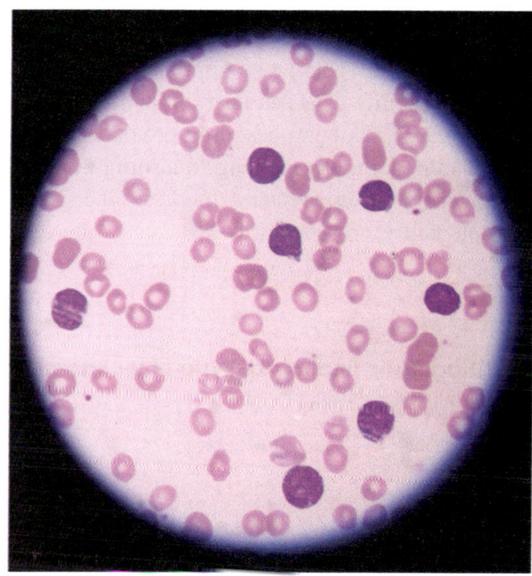

FIGURE 32.7 ***A blood smear from the bone marrow of a person with acute lymphocytic leukaemia. Note the abnormally large number of lymphocytes (stained purple) crowding the bone marrow. As a result, normal production of RBCs, functional WBCs and platelets is suppressed***

Source: [illegible]/123RF

INTERPROFESSIONAL CARE

Treatment for leukaemia focuses on achieving remission or cure and relieving symptoms. The methods of treatment may include chemotherapy, radiation therapy and bone marrow or stem cell transplantation. Cure is more often achieved in children with acute leukaemia than in adults, although long-term remissions (disease-free periods with no signs or symptoms) often can be achieved.

Diagnosis

The following diagnostic tests are ordered when leukaemia is suspected:

- *FBC* with differential is done to evaluate cell counts, haemoglobin and haematocrit levels, and the number, distribution and morphology (size and shape) of WBCs.
- *Platelets* are measured to identify possible thrombocytopenia secondary to the leukaemia and the risk of bleeding.
- *Bone marrow examination* provides information about cells within the marrow, the type of erythropoiesis and the maturity of erythropoietic and leucopoietic cells.

Table 32.5 outlines usual diagnostic test results in the various forms of leukaemia.

Chemotherapy

With the rapid advances in cancer knowledge and chemotherapeutic manufacture, the protocols for management of leukaemia are changing as new drugs become available. The goal of chemotherapy is to inhibit cellular proliferation and prevent tumour multiplication. These two approaches are targeted at reducing the possibility of tissue invasion and metastasis. Prolific cancer research involving best drug protocols are resulting in rapidly changing choices of drugs and drug combinations. Combination chemotherapy reduces drug resistance and toxicity and interrupts cell growth at various stages of the cell cycle, producing a complementary effect of the drugs used. Cancer treatment with chemotherapy is discussed in detail in the chapter 'Nursing care of people with cancer'.

Chemotherapy for leukaemia generally is divided into the induction phase and post-remission therapy. During *induction*, drug doses are high to eradicate leukaemic cells from the bone marrow. These high doses often also damage stem cells and interfere with production of normal blood cells. Circulating mature blood cells are not affected because they are no longer dividing. The degree of bone marrow suppression is influenced by a number of factors, including age, nutritional status, concurrent chronic diseases such as impaired liver or renal function, the drug and drug dose, and prior treatment.

Colony-stimulating factors (CSFs), also called haematopoietic growth factors, often are administered to 'rescue' the bone marrow following induction chemotherapy. CSFs are cytokines that regulate the growth and differentiation of blood cells. Factors that support neutrophil maturation, *granulocyte-macrophage CSF (GM-CSF)* and *granulocyte CSF (G-CSF)*, are commonly used. Bone pain is a common side effect of therapy with these agents. People may also experience fevers, chills, anorexia, muscle aches and lethargy.

Once remission has been achieved, post-remission chemotherapy is continued to eradicate any additional leukaemic cells, prevent relapse and prolong survival. A single chemotherapeutic agent, combination therapy or bone marrow transplant may be used for post-remission treatment.

Radiation therapy

Radiation therapy damages cellular DNA. While the cell continues to function, it cannot divide and multiply. Cells that divide rapidly, such as bone marrow and cancer cells (radiosensitive cells), respond quickly to radiation therapy. Although normal cells are affected, they are better able to recover from the damage caused by the radiation than are cancer cells. The types of delivery, effects and toxicities of radiation are discussed in greater detail in the chapter 'Nursing care of people with cancer'.

TABLE 32.5 Diagnostic findings by type of leukaemia

TEST	AML	CML	ALL	CLL
RBC count	Low	Low	Low	Low
Haemoglobin	Low	Low	Low	Low
Haematocrit	Low	Low	Low	Low
Platelet count	Very low	High early, low late	Low	Low
WBC count	Varies	Increased	Varies	Increased
Myeloblasts	Present			
Neutrophils	Decreased	Increased	Decreased	Normal
Lymphocytes		Normal		Increased
Monocytes		Normal/low		
Bone marrow	Hypercellular		Hypercellular	
Myeloblasts	Present			
Lymphoblasts			Present	
Lymphocytes				Present

Bone marrow transplant

Bone marrow transplant (BMT) is the treatment of choice for some types of leukaemia (see Table 32.3). BMT often is used in conjunction with or following chemotherapy or radiation. There are two main categories of BMT: in allogeneic BMT, the bone marrow of a healthy donor is infused into the person with the illness; in autologous BMT, the person is infused with their own bone marrow.

ALLOGENEIC BMT *Allogeneic BMT* uses bone marrow cells from a donor (often from a sibling with closely matched tissue antigens; closely matched unrelated donors also may be used). Prior to allogeneic BMT, high doses of chemotherapy and/or total body irradiation are used to destroy leukaemic cells in the bone marrow. The donor's bone marrow is aspirated (see Figure 32.8) and infused through a central venous line into the recipient. Prior to BMT and re-establishment of bone marrow function, the person is critically ill and at significant risk of infection and bleeding due to depletion of WBCs and platelets.

AUTOLOGOUS BMT *Autologous BMT* uses the person's own bone marrow to restore bone marrow function after chemotherapy or radiation. This procedure is often called *bone marrow rescue*. In autologous BMT, about 1 L of bone marrow is aspirated (usually from the iliac crests) during a period of disease remission. The bone marrow is then frozen and stored for use after treatment. If relapse occurs, lethal doses of chemotherapy or radiation are given to destroy the immune system and malignant cells and to prepare space in the bone marrow for new cells. The filtered bone marrow is then thawed and infused intravenously through a central line. The infused marrow cells slowly become a part of the person's bone marrow, the neutrophil count increases and normal haematopoiesis takes place.

As in allogeneic BMT, the person is critically ill during the period of bone marrow destruction and immunosuppression. The person is hospitalised in a private room for 6 to 8 weeks or more. Potential complications include malnutrition, infection and bleeding.

Stem cell transplant

Allogeneic **stem cell transplant (SCT)** is an alternative to bone marrow transplant. SCT results in complete and sustained replacement of the recipient's blood cell lines (WBCs, RBCs and platelets) with cells derived from the donor stem cells.

Donors must have tissue that is closely matched with that of the recipient. Prior to harvesting, haematopoietic growth factors, including G-CSF and GM-CSF, are administered to the donor for 4 to 5 days. This increases the concentration of stem cells in peripheral blood, allowing it to be used for the transplant instead of bone marrow. Peripheral blood is removed and white cells are separated from the plasma, then administered via a large central venous catheter. Large concentrations of stem cells also are present in umbilical cord blood. This may be stored in cord blood banks and used for treatment.

The recipient undergoes similar treatment prior to SCT as for BMT. The risks of infection and other complications, as well as graft-versus-host disease, are similar.

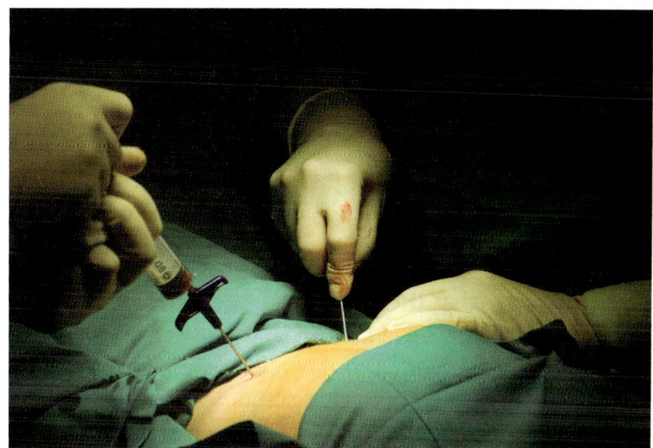

FIGURE 32.8 ***Allogeneic bone marrow transplant. Bone marrow from the donor is aspirated, then filtered and infused into the recipient***

Source: Tino Soriano/National Geographic Creative/Alamy Stock Photo.

Graft-versus-host disease

Allogeneic BMT or SCT may precipitate *graft-versus-host disease (GVHD)*, which develops in between 10% and 60% of all people receiving an allogeneic BMT or SCT, depending on their risk factors, with age being a major factor. The average incidence in the paediatric population is approximately 20%, but up to 70% in those over 50 years of age. The incidence also increases when there is more than one antigen mismatch between the donor and the recipient, and can be as high as 90% when there are 2–3 antigen mismatches (Ruiz, 2021). In GVHD, immune cells of the donated bone marrow identify the recipient's body tissue as foreign. Consequently, T lymphocytes in the donated marrow attack the liver, skin and GI tract, causing skin rashes progressing to desquamation (loss of skin), diarrhoea, GI bleeding and liver damage. *Acute GVHD* develops within the first 100 days of the transplant and is usually marked by a pruritic, maculopapular rash that begins on the palms and soles of the feet and may extend over the entire body. Vaso-occlusive disease of the liver affects many allogeneic bone marrow transplant recipients, with jaundice and elevated liver function tests. *Chronic GVHD* develops later, 100 or more days after the transplant. The survival rate in chronic GVHD is approximately 40%, provided there are not more complicating factors such as extensive disease or thrombocytopenia (Ruiz, 2021). It may follow acute GVHD or develop in people with no prior symptoms. GVHD is treated with antihistamines, calcineurin inhibitors, antibiotics and steroids. Primarily, corticosteroids are the first-line management. However, many new targeted therapies are being trialled and adopted for the management of GVHD. Such agents include extracorporeal photopheresis, anti TNF antibodies and interleukin-2 receptor antibodies, and numerous other advances are being achieved (Mandanas, 2021; Yang, Ning & Tang, 2022; Zeiser, 2022).

Biological therapy

Cytokines such as interferons and interleukins are biological agents that may be used to treat some leukaemias. These agents modify the body's response to cancer cells; in some cases, they are cytotoxic as well. Interferons are a complex group of messenger proteins normally produced in response to antigens such as viruses (see the chapter 'Nursing care of people with infections'). They have multiple effects, including moderating immune function and inhibiting abnormal cell proliferation and growth. Side effects commonly associated with interferon therapy include flu-like symptoms, persistent fatigue and lethargy, weight loss and muscle and joint pain.

Complementary therapies

Although many complementary and alternative medicine therapies have been purported to treat cancer in general, at this time none has been shown to have sustained benefit in treating leukaemia. Clinical trials have demonstrated the efficacy of both coping skills training (relaxation and imagery) and hypnosis to significantly reduce oral discomfort associated with leukaemia and its treatment.

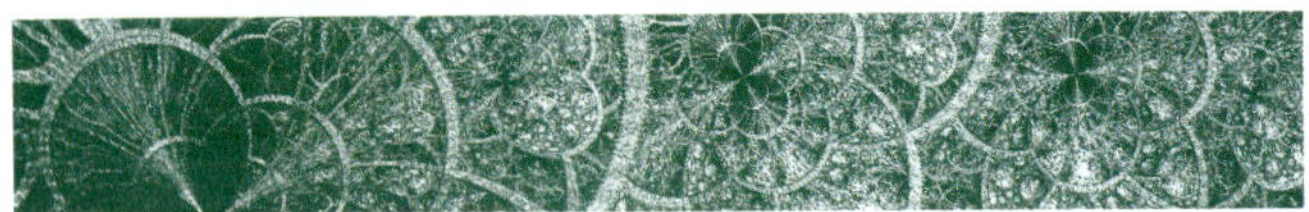

Nursing care

For nursing care specific to the person undergoing diagnostic testing for leukaemia, see the accompanying nursing care plan.

Health promotion

Health promotion activities related to leukaemia include teaching about leukaemia risk factors, particularly those that can be controlled. Discuss the potential dangers of exposure to ionising radiation and certain chemicals such as benzene. Encourage all people to avoid smoking cigarettes. Discuss genetic counselling with people at high risk of having a child with Down syndrome (women over age 35).

Assessment

Focused assessment data related to leukaemia include:

- *Health history*: complaints of fatigue, weakness, dyspnoea on exertion, frequent infections, sore throat, night sweats, bleeding gums or nosebleeds; recent weight loss; exposure to ionising radiation (multiple x-rays, residence near a site of radiation or atomic testing) or chemicals (occupational); prior treatment for cancer; history of an immune disorder.
- *Physical examination*: skin and mucous membranes for bruising, purpura, petechiae, ulcers or lesions; pallor; vital signs, including orthostatic vitals; heart and lung sounds; abdominal examination; stool for occult blood.
- *Diagnostic tests*: blood count with differential; bone marrow studies.

Nursing diagnoses and interventions

When caring for the person with leukaemia, the nurse considers the chronic and life-threatening nature of the disease as well as the effects of treatment. See the 'Translation to practice' box. Priority nursing problems may include *Risk of infection*, *Imbalanced nutrition: less than body requirements*, *Impaired oral mucous membranes*, *Ineffective protection (bleeding)* and *Anticipatory grieving*.

Risk of infection

Changes in WBC function impair the immune and inflammatory responses in leukaemia, increasing the risk of infection. WBCs may be immature and ineffective or, in some cases, deficient. Chemotherapy or radiation therapy further depresses bone marrow function and increases the risk of infection.

- Promptly report manifestations of infection: fever, chills, throat pain, cough, chest pain, burning on urination, purulent drainage and itching and burning in vaginal or rectal areas. *Prompt reporting allows timely intervention to prevent overwhelming infection and sepsis.*
- Institute infection protection measures:
  a. Maintain protective isolation as indicated.
  b. Ensure meticulous hand hygiene among all people in contact with the person.
  c. Assist as needed with appropriate hygiene measures.
  d. Restrict visitors with colds, flu or infections.
  e. Provide oral hygiene after every meal.
  f. Avoid invasive procedures when possible, including injections, intravenous catheters, catheterisations and rectal and vaginal procedures. When necessary, use strict aseptic technique for all invasive procedures and monitor carefully for infection.

  These precautions minimise exposure to bacterial, viral and fungal pathogens. Infection is the main cause of death in people with leukaemia. Mucous membranes are especially susceptible to breakdown and infection as a result of tissue damage from chemotherapy or radiation.
- Monitor vital signs, including temperature and oxygen saturation, every 4 hours. Report temperature spikes with chilling, tachypnoea, tachycardia, restlessness, change in PaO_2 and hypotension. *The inflammatory response may be impaired in leukaemia, masking signs of infection until sepsis develops, indicated by manifestations such as those above.*
- Monitor neutrophil levels (measured in cubic millimetres) for relative risk of infection:

  2.0 to 2.5 × 10^9/L: no risk
  1.0 to 2.0 × 10^9/L: minimal risk
  0.5 to 1.0 × 10^9/L: moderate risk
  Below 0.5 × 10^9/L: severe risk.
  - Neutrophils are the first line of defence against infection. As levels decrease, the risk of infection increases.
- Explain infection precautions and restrictions and their rationale; explain that these measures are usually temporary. *Understanding of these aspects by the person and family increases compliance and lowers the risk of infection.*

Imbalanced nutrition: less than body requirements

The person with leukaemia may have difficulty meeting nutritional needs due to increased metabolism, fatigue, loss of

TRANSLATION TO PRACTICE Evidence-based practice for people with acute leukaemia and lymphoma

People with acute leukaemia and malignant lymphoma experience a number of distressing manifestations of their disease, including malaise and fatigue, fever, night sweats, infections and possible haemorrhage. Treatments such as radiation therapy and chemotherapy often have numerous adverse effects as well, including anorexia and nausea, stomatitis, lethargy, malaise and fatigue. There are other psychological effects and stressors that people in remission from acute leukaemia or malignant lymphoma have to deal with; for example, emotional and economic stress as well as physical stress. The younger the person, the greater these stressors impact on their quality of life (Jones et al., 2015; Raphael, Frey & Gott, 2017).

IMPLICATIONS FOR NURSING

Nurses need to actively focus their care on the physical problems experienced during treatment, especially energy loss and nutritional problems. Overwhelming fatigue interferes with the person's ability to provide self-care, but its effects may not be readily apparent to nurses. However, it is important to also remember the psychological and emotional impact of treatment and remission. People need to become equipped to deal with the remission phase as well as the treatment phase and to feel safe and supported when home from treatment. The long-term effects physically, emotionally and financially indicate a need for continued follow-up care, teaching, resource availability and ongoing access to support, with possible referral to counselling services as required.

CRITICAL THINKING IN PERSON-CENTRED CARE

1 Explain the physiological responses to malignancies and cancer treatments that cause fatigue, malaise and nutritional problems.
2 People undergoing treatment for leukaemia, malignant lymphoma and other cancers may have few outward manifestations of their disease or responses to treatment. Discuss how this apparent wellbeing may affect nurses' perceptions of care needs.
3 How may continued physical and emotional problems of fatigue and lack of psychological and sexual energy affect family relations?
4 Develop a nursing care plan for a person with acute leukaemia to address the nursing diagnosis of *Ineffective sexuality patterns* related to fatigue and lack of energy.
5 Appreciate the experiences of people who live with these diseases. Everyone's experience is different. Read the stories of people who are living with leukaemias, lymphomas, myeloma or a related blood disorder. Available from Leukaemia Australia: https://www.leukaemia.org.au/disease-information/blood-cancer-resources/inspiring-stories/.

appetite from radiation, nausea and vomiting from chemotherapy, or painful oral mucous membranes that make chewing and swallowing difficult and/or painful.

- Weigh regularly and evaluate weight loss over time to determine degree of malnutrition. *A weight loss of 10–20% may indicate malnutrition. A minimum intake of nutrients is necessary for health and tissue repair; cancer increases metabolic needs over this basal requirement. Weight loss occurs when metabolic requirements are not met. Both the disease process and its treatment can interfere with nutrient intake.*
- Address causative or contributing factors to inadequate food and fluid intake:
  a. Provide mouth care before and after meals; use a soft toothbrush or sponges as necessary.
  b. Provide liquids with different textures and tastes.
  c. Increase liquid intake with meals.
  d. Reduce intake of milk and milk products, which makes mucus more tenacious.
  e. Assist to a sitting position for eating.
  f. Ensure that the environment is clean and odour free.
  g. Provide medications for pain or nausea 30 minutes before meals, if prescribed.
  h. Provide rest periods before meals.
  i. Offer small, frequent meals including low fat, high-kilojoule foods throughout the day.
  j. Provide commercial supplements, such as Ensure.
  k. Avoid painful or unpleasant procedures immediately before or after meals.
  l. Suggest measures to improve food tolerance, such as eating dry foods when arising, consuming salty foods if allowed and avoiding very sweet, rich or greasy foods.

Anorexia, nausea and vomiting, diarrhoea, stomatitis, taste changes and dysphagia often make eating difficult during cancer treatment when good nutrition is most important. Maintaining nutritional status decreases morbidity and mortality by preventing weight loss, improving the response to treatment, minimising adverse effects and improving quality of life. Small, frequent meals are often better tolerated, especially highprotein, high-kilojoule foods.

Impaired oral mucous membrane

Stomatitis, inflammation and ulceration of the oral mucous membrane, is common in leukaemia. Chemotherapy can further impair the integrity of constantly dividing oral tissues.

- Inspect the buccal region, gums, sublingual area and the throat daily for swelling or lesions. Ask about oral pain or burning. *Breakdown of the oral mucous membrane increases the risk of infection and bleeding, causes pain and discomfort with eating and swallowing, and may cause swelling that interferes with the airway.*
- Culture any oral lesions. *Herpes simplex virus and* Candida *(yeast) are more common in those with neutropenia. Herpes lesions are usually red, raised, fluid-filled blisters;* Candida *causes a white coating and patches of white plaque.*

NURSING CARE PLAN A person with acute myelocytic leukaemia

Catherine Cole is a 37-year-old secretary who lives with her husband, Ray, and teenage daughter, Amy, in an apartment in a large metropolitan area. About 2 months ago, Mrs Cole began to tire easily and experience night sweats several times a week. She also noted that she was pale, bruised easily and was having heavier menstrual periods. Blood tests ordered by her local general practitioner (GP) are abnormal. She is admitted for a bone marrow biopsy.

ASSESSMENT

Mary Grant, RN, obtains a nursing history and physical assessment for Mrs Cole. Catherine tells her, 'I'm so tired and I have these bruises all over me. I'm so afraid of the results of the bone marrow examination. I don't know what we will do if I have cancer.' Mrs Cole clutches her husband's hand and begins to cry. Physical assessment data include height 156 cm; weight, 48.1 kg; vital signs: T 36.5°C, P 102, R 22, BP 130/82. Numerous petechiae scattered over trunk and arms; ecchymoses noted on lower right arm and right calf. Oral mucosa is red, with several small ulcerations in buccal areas.

Blood count shows reduced RBCs, haemoglobin and haematocrit levels. The WBC is high, with myeloblasts seen on differential. The platelet count is very low. A tentative diagnosis of acute myelogenous leukaemia is made.

DIAGNOSES

- *Risk of infection* related to altered WBC production and immune function.
- *Ineffective protection* related to reduced platelet count and risk of bleeding.
- *Impaired oral mucous membrane* secondary to anaemia and reduced platelets.
- *Fatigue related to anaemia.*
- *Anxiety* related to fear of leukaemia diagnosis.

PLANNING

- Monitor and reduce the risk of infection and bleeding.
- Assist with management of self-care issues.
- Assist with management of emotional state.

Expected outcomes

- Remain free of infection.
- Experience no significant bleeding.
- Have intact oral mucous membranes.
- Manage self-care activities despite fatigue.
- Develop strategies for managing anxiety.

IMPLEMENTATION

- Place in a private room, if available.
- Limit visitors to immediate family/significant others for the present (consider cultural implications around family, illness and hospitalisation).
- Instruct all staff, the family and Mrs Cole to carefully wash hands. Post a sign on the door and over the washbasin in the room as a reminder.
- Record vital signs every 4 hours.
- Avoid invasive procedures unless absolutely necessary.
- Monitor for bleeding every 4 hours, including skin, oral mucosa, abdominal assessment, body fluids and menstrual pad count.
- Instruct to perform oral hygiene every 2 to 4 hours, using a soft-bristle toothbrush.
- Ask the dietitian to work with Mrs Cole to identify preferred foods. Instruct to avoid foods that may damage oral mucosa, such as very hot, very cold or highly acidic or spicy foods.
- Provide for periods of rest alternating with activity.
- Teach about the bone marrow biopsy. Allow time for questions and to talk through fears.
- Refer to the oncology nurse specialist for further teaching and support.
- Refer to an oncology social worker where economic or social challenges are pressing.
- Provide written and/or online links to further information and support services for people living with a diagnosis of acute myelocytic leukaemia.

EVALUATION

The bone marrow biopsy confirms the diagnosis of acute myelogenous leukaemia. Mrs Cole is very upset, but calms as the doctor and the oncology nurse discuss treatment plans and the possibility of remission. She decides to have outpatient chemotherapy. During her hospital stay, Mrs Cole remained free of infection or further bleeding. She tells RN Grant that her mouth feels better, although it is still painful. During routine assessment, Mrs Cole remarks, 'You know, I was so scared when I came here, but I think I am a little less so now. Sometimes not knowing what is wrong is worse than knowing.'

CRITICAL THINKING IN THE NURSING PROCESS

1. Describe how alterations in WBCs can increase a person's susceptibility to infection.
2. List sources of potential infection for the hospitalised person.
3. What is the rationale for having the person do her own oral and physical hygiene?
4. Outline a teaching plan for this person and her family for home care to prevent infection.
5. Develop a care plan for Mrs Cole for the nursing diagnosis *Activity intolerance*.

REFLECTION ON THE NURSING PROCESS

1. What are the take-home points that you have learned from this case study?
2. How can you use them in your daily practice area? Where will you find further information about this disease and its effects on people who live with it?

- Assist with mouth care and oral rinses with saline or a bicarbonate of soda solution. Apply lip balm to the lips to prevent dryness and cracking. *These measures help prevent infection and increase comfort.*
- Encourage use of soft-bristle toothbrush or sponge to clean teeth and gums. *Toothbrushes with hard bristles may abrade inflamed mucosa, causing bleeding and increasing the risk of infection.*

- Administer medications as ordered to treat infection or relieve pain. *Topical antifungal agents such as nystatin may be prescribed to treat* Candida *infections. Topical anaesthetics such as lignocaine may be prescribed to relieve discomfort and facilitate good oral care.*
- Instruct to avoid alcohol-based mouthwashes, citrus fruit juices, spicy foods, very hot or very cold foods, alcohol and crusty foods. Suggest bland, cool foods and cool liquids at least every 2 hours. *Avoiding mucosa-traumatising foods and liquids increases comfort; bland, cool foods and liquids cause the least pain. Intake of adequate fluids is necessary to prevent dehydration.*
- If the patient is undergoing treatments such as haematopoetic stem cell transplant they may benefit from palifermin—a recombinant human keratinocyte growth factor-1, which decreases the duration and incidence of mucositis.

Ineffective protection

Bleeding is the second most common cause of leukaemia deaths. As platelet counts decrease, the risk of bleeding increases (see the section later in this chapter on thrombocytopenia). Tumour lysis syndrome also is a risk in people with leukaemia who are undergoing their initial treatment with chemotherapy. Tumour lysis syndrome develops when a large number of malignant cells are destroyed by treatment with chemotherapy or radiation. The resultant by-products of cell lysis can overwhelm the body's ability to effectively eliminate them, leading to hyperkalaemia, hyperphosphataemia with secondary hypocalcaemia and hyperuricaemia.

- Assess vital signs every 4 hours and body systems every shift for bleeding:
  a. skin and mucous membranes for petechiae, ecchymoses and purpura
  b. gums, nasal membranes and conjunctiva for bleeding
  c. vomitus, stool and urine for visible or occult blood
  d. vaginal bleeding
  e. prolonged bleeding from puncture sites
  f. neurological changes such as headache, visual changes, altered mentation, decreased level of consciousness, seizures
  g. abdomen for complaints of epigastric pain, diminished bowel sounds, increasing abdominal girth, rigidity or guarding.

  Early identification of bleeding helps prevent significant blood loss and potential shock. Internal haemorrhage may lead to tachycardia, hypotension, pallor and diaphoresis Bleeding into the lungs may cause dyspnoea; bleeding into the abdomen causes increased girth, pain and guarding. Intracranial bleeding affects mental status and level of consciousness.
- Avoid invasive procedures such as rectal temperatures and suppositories, vaginal douches, suppositories, tampons, urinary catheterisation and parenteral injections if possible. *Diagnostic procedures such as biopsy or lumbar puncture should not be done if the platelet count is low and there is risk of bleeding. Invasive procedures can cause tissue trauma and bleeding. Procedures that use large-bore needles should be delayed until the platelet count is increased.*
- Apply pressure to injection sites for 3 to 5 minutes and to arterial punctures for 15 to 20 minutes. *Pressure prevents prolonged bleeding by prompting haemostasis and clot formation.*
- Instruct to avoid forcefully blowing or picking the nose, forceful coughing or sneezing, and straining to have a bowel movement. *These activities can damage mucous membranes, increasing the risk of bleeding.*
- Monitor and promptly report abnormal blood levels of electrolytes, uric acid, urea nitrogen and creatinine, or manifestations of tumour lysis syndrome. *Significant alterations in electrolyte levels can lead to complications such as cardiac arrhythmias, muscle weakness or tetany, paraesthesias and mental status changes. Excess uric acid can compromise renal function and lead to metabolic acidosis and gout.*
- Maintain adequate hydration and administer prescribed medications such as allopurinol and diuretics as ordered. *Hydration is vital to maintain renal function and promote elimination of tumour lysis by-products. Allopurinol reduces the risk of uric acid crystallisation in the kidneys and other tissues.*

Anticipatory grieving

The diagnosis of cancer and a potentially life-threatening illness causes actual or perceived losses, such as loss of function, independence, normal appearance, friends, self-esteem and self. Grieving is the emotional response to those losses. The adaptive process of mourning a loss and resolving grief is called grief work; grief work cannot begin until a loss is acknowledged. See the chapter 'Nursing care of people experiencing loss, grief and death' for a detailed discussion of grief and loss.

- Discuss roles of the person and family and ways in which they managed stressful situations in the past. Assess coping strategies and their effectiveness. Help identify sources of strength and support. Discuss changing roles resulting from leukaemia diagnosis and its effect on spiritual, social and economic status and usual lifestyle. Evaluate cultural or ethnic factors that affect grief reactions. *Grieving is a normal response to a real or potential loss that begins at the time of diagnosis. The timing, duration and intensity of grief and responses to grief may differ among family members. Share information on diagnosis, role change and physical loss among all family members to build the foundation for mutual understanding and trust.*
- Use therapeutic communication skills to facilitate open discussion of losses and provide permission to grieve. *Encouraging discussion of the meaning of the loss helps decrease some of the anxiety associated with loss. This in turn allows the person and their family to examine the current situation and compare it with past situations that they have coped with successfully.*

- Provide information about agencies that may help in resolving grief and make referrals as indicated. Consider self-help groups, cancer support groups and bereavement groups. *Participating in support groups with others who are anticipating or experiencing a similar loss can decrease feelings of isolation.*

Community-based care

Person and family teaching for home care after treatment for leukaemia focuses on encouraging self-care, providing information about the disease and the treatment, preventing infection and injury, and promoting nutrition. Teaching topics for each of these areas are as follows.

Encouraging self-care

- Hygiene measures and energy conservation during self-care activities.
- Oral hygiene, including using a soft-bristle toothbrush several times daily; avoiding flossing.
- Reporting lesions, bleeding or signs of infection promptly.
- Maintaining a balance of rest and activity.

Information about leukaemia and treatment

- Bone marrow function, the pathophysiology of leukaemia and potential complications of leukaemia.
- Prognosis for the specific type of leukaemia.
- Treatment measures such as chemotherapy, radiation, bone marrow or stem cell transplant, their purpose and effects, where treatment is available, and potential adverse effects or risks.
- Community, regional and national resources for people with leukaemia.

Preventing infection and injury

- Handwashing and other measures to reduce exposure to pathogens, such as avoiding people who are ill and avoiding crowds.
- Avoiding food-borne illnesses by washing fruits and vegetables and storing food properly.
- Dental hygiene measures.
- Avoiding immunisations.
- Manifestations to report: fever, chills, burning on urination, foul-smelling urine, vaginal or rectal discharge, skin lesions.
- Avoiding contact sports or strenuous exercise if platelet count is low.
- Using an electric razor for shaving, avoiding rectal or vaginal suppositories, vaginal tampons or enemas.
- Increasing dietary fibre and using a bulk-forming laxative as needed to prevent straining.
- Avoiding over-the-counter or prescription drugs that interfere with platelet function (see Box 32.6).
- The importance of reporting any bleeding (nosebleeds, rectal bleeding, vomiting blood, excessive menstrual periods, blood in the urine, bleeding gums, bruises or collections of blood under the skin) or changes in behaviour to the healthcare provider.

BOX 32.6 Medications that may interfere with platelet function

Over-the-counter medications

- Aspirin and salicylates, including:
  - Ecotrin
  - Aspalgin
  - Astrix
  - Cartier
  - Cardiprin
- NSAIDs such as:
  - Naproxen
  - Ibuprofen

Prescription medications

- Aspirin-containing analgesics
- Chemotherapy drugs
- Antibiotics such as penicillin
- Carbamazepine (Tegretol)
- Colchicine
- Dipyridamole (Persantin)
- Heparin
- Quinine derivatives
- Sulfonamides
- Thiazide diuretics

Promoting nutrition

- Eating several small, low-fat, high-kilojoule meals and drinking five to eight glasses of water daily; ensure culturally appropriate food choices are available.
- Reporting continued weight loss, loss of appetite or inability to eat for 24 hours.
- Discussing dietary needs with the dietitian.

Assistance with physical care, finances and transportation may be required following discharge, especially for people who live in rural and remote locations. Refer the person and family to social services, support groups, home-care services as needed and other agencies that can provide needed services.

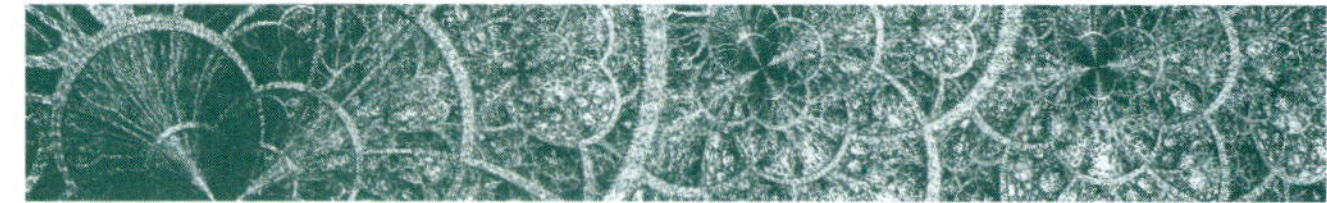

THE PERSON WITH MALIGNANT LYMPHOMA

Lymphomas are malignancies of lymphoid tissue. They are characterised by the proliferation of lymphocytes, histiocytes (resident monocytes or macrophages) and their precursors or derivatives. Lymphomas are closely related to lymphocytic leukaemias. Some experts consider them to be different forms or stages of the same disease processes.

Although there are many types of malignant lymphoid cells, at this time lymphomas commonly are identified as Hodgkin's disease or non-Hodgkin's lymphoma.

Incidence and risk factors

In Australia, it is estimated that 7,397 people were diagnosed with lymphoma in 2022; lymphoma is the sixth most common cancer for both men and women (AIHW, 2022; Cancer Australia, 2022b). The incidence of non-Hodgkin's lymphoma has nearly doubled since 1970, but currently has stabilised, primarily due to a fall in its incidence related to HIV infection and AIDS. The incidence of Hodgkin's disease has significantly declined since 1990.

While the cause of lymphoma is unknown, some risk factors have been identified. Immunosuppression due to drug therapy following organ transplant or to HIV disease increases the risk of non-Hodgkin's lymphoma. Infectious agents such as HTLV-1 and Epstein–Barr virus (EBV) also have been identified as risk factors. Others may include occupational herbicide or chemical exposure (Cancer Australia, 2022b).

Pathophysiology

Hodgkin's disease

Hodgkin's disease is a rare lymphatic cancer, occurring most often in people between the ages of 15 and 35. Approximately 600 new cases of Hodgkin's disease are diagnosed each year in Australia (Leukaemia Foundation, 2022d). The exact cause of Hodgkin's disease is unknown, but both EBV infection and genetic factors appear to play a role in its development. Hodgkin's disease is one of the most curable cancers and most people with Hodgkin's lymphoma can be cured. While many people with localised disease achieve cure with a normal lifespan, there may be an increased risk of a second cancer occurrence throughout life.

Hodgkin's disease develops in a single lymph node or chain of nodes, spreading to adjoining nodes. Involved lymph nodes contain *Reed–Sternberg cells* (malignant cells) surrounded by host inflammatory cells. These malignant cells secrete inflammatory mediator substances, attracting inflammatory cells to the tumour site. They may invade almost any tissue in the body. The spleen often is involved; as the disease progresses, the liver, lungs, digestive tract and CNS may be affected. Rapid proliferation of abnormal lymphocytes impairs the immune response, especially cell-mediated immune responses. Infections are common.

Hodgkin's disease is classified as classic Hodgkin's disease or as nodular-lymphocyte-predominant Hodgkin's disease. The classic form of the disease accounts for 95% of all cases; nodular-lymphocyte-predominant Hodgkin's is rare. Classic Hodgkin's can be further divided into other subtypes by cells identified within the tumour, but the subtype does not affect the prognosis.

MANIFESTATIONS The most common symptom of Hodgkin's disease is one or more painlessly enlarged lymph nodes, usually in the cervical or subclavicular region. Systemic manifestations such as persistent fever, night sweats, fatigue and weight loss are associated with a poorer prognosis for the disease. Late symptoms such as malaise, pruritus and anaemia can indicate spread of the disease. The spleen may be enlarged and other organ systems such as the lungs and gastrointestinal tract are occasionally involved, causing difficulty breathing or bloating symptoms.

Non-Hodgkin's lymphoma

Non-Hodgkin's lymphoma is a diverse group of lymphoid tissue malignancies that do not contain Reed–Sternberg cells. **Non-Hodgkin's lymphomas** tend to arise in peripheral lymph nodes and spread early to tissues throughout the body. Non-Hodgkin's lymphoma is more common than Hodgkin's disease, affecting around 90% of all lymphoma cases in Australia (Cancer Australia, 2022b). Older adults are more often affected and it occurs more frequently in men than in women. Like Hodgkin's disease its cause is unknown, although both genetic and environmental factors (e.g. viral infections such as EBV, human T-cell leukaemia/lymphoma virus-1 or -2 and HIV) are thought to play a role.

As in most malignancies, non-Hodgkin's lymphoma begins as a single transformed cell; it may arise from T cells, B cells or tissue macrophages (histocytes). The primary types of non-Hodgkin's lymphomas are identified in Table 32.6. Although non-Hodgkin's lymphoma usually arises in a lymph node, it can originate in any lymphoid tissue. It tends to spread early and unpredictably to other lymphoid tissues and organs. Extranodal spread may involve the nasopharynx, GI tract, bone, CNS, thyroid, testes and soft tissue.

The prognosis for non-Hodgkin's lymphoma ranges from excellent to poor, depending on the identified cell type and grade of differentiation. Low-grade tumours (better differentiated) tend to be less aggressive and more curable. Higher-grade tumours often are disseminated at the time of diagnosis and have a poorer prognosis.

MANIFESTATIONS The early manifestations of non-Hodgkin's lymphoma are similar to those for Hodgkin's disease. Painless lymphadenopathy may be localised or widespread (see Figure 32.9). Systemic manifestations such as fever, night sweats, fatigue and weight loss may be present, but are less common in non-Hodgkin's lymphoma. Organ system involvement

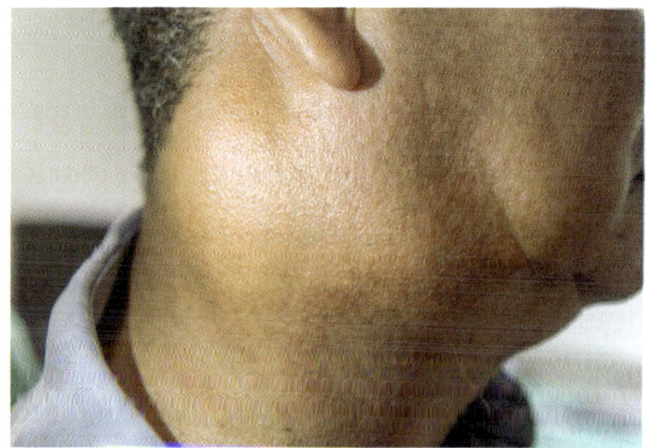

FIGURE 32.9 ***Cervical lymphadenopathy in a person with lymphoma of the neck***

Source: Karan Bunjean/Shutterstock.

TABLE 32.6 Subtypes of non-Hodgkin's lymphoma

SUBTYPE	INCIDENCE	COURSE AND PROGNOSIS
B-cell lymphomas		
Diffuse large B-cell lymphomas	Most common adult type (40–50% of adult lymphomas) More common in males Incidence increases with ageing	Aggressive tumour 45–50% cure rate
Follicular lymphoma	Accounts for 40% of adult lymphomas, rare in children Incidence increases with ageing	Bone marrow frequently involved, course slow, indolent 72% 5-year survival
Extranodal marginal zone lymphoma (MALT lymphoma)	Accounts for about 5% of adult lymphomas, rare in children Incidence increases with ageing More common in Italy	Presents with tumours outside lymphatic system: GI tract, lung, thyroid, urinary tract, skin, CNS. Slow, indolent course 74% 5-year survival
Mantle cell lymphoma	Accounts for 3–4% of adult lymphomas, rare in children Predominantly affects older men (74%)	Aggressive, difficult to cure 27% 5-year survival
Burkitt lymphoma	Rare in adults ($<1\%$ of lymphomas), more common in children (~30% NHL)	Rapidly progressive but responds well to therapy 45% 5-year survival
T-cell lymphomas		
Precursor T-cell lymphoblastic leukaemia/lymphoma	More common in children and young adults More common in males than females	Can present either as ALL or lymphoma Aggressive disease 26% 5-year survival
Peripheral T-cell lymphoma	Most common T-cell lymphoma in adults	Often presents as disseminated disease 25% 5-year survival
Mycosis fungoides/cutaneous T-cell lymphoma	Onset typically during mid-fifties; more common in African Americans	Cutaneous lymphoma Slow course, progressing from patchy skin lesions to plaque to cutaneous tumours

may cause symptoms such as abdominal pain, nausea and vomiting. Headaches, peripheral or cranial nerve symptoms, altered mental status or seizures may signal CNS involvement.

The manifestations and clinical features of Hodgkin's disease and non-Hodgkin's lymphoma are compared in Table 32.7.

Course

In both Hodgkin's disease and non-Hodgkin's lymphoma, the stage of the disease, the presence of systemic manifestations and factors such as age help determine the prognosis. The prognosis is good when the disease is localised to one or two node regions. Factors such as anaemia, thrombocytopenia and older age reduce the likelihood of disease cure.

INTERPROFESSIONAL CARE

Chemotherapy and radiation therapy, either alone or in combination, are the primary treatments for Hodgkin's and non-Hodgkin's lymphomas. Use of monoclonal antibodies to target lymphoma cells and bone marrow and peripheral stem cell transplants are under investigation for treating lymphomas as well. See the previous section on treatment of leukaemia for more information about these transplants.

Diagnosis

The following diagnostic tests may be ordered for lymphomas:

- *FBC* often shows a mild normochromic, normocytic anaemia in Hodgkin's disease; other findings in Hodgkin's disease may include leucocytosis with high neutrophil and eosinophil counts and an elevated erythrocyte sedimentation rate (ESR). In non-Hodgkin's lymphoma, the FBC typically remains normal until late in the disease, when pancytopenia may develop.
- An *ESR* is done to identify possible inflammatory causes of lymph node enlargement.
- *Blood studies* of major organ function (including liver function tests and renal function studies) are performed to identify possible organ involvement. Serum LDH levels and protein electrophoresis also may be done when Hodgkin's disease is suspected.

TABLE 32.7 Features and manifestations of Hodgkin's disease and non-Hodgkin's lymphoma

FEATURE OR MANIFESTATION	HODGKIN'S DISEASE	NON-HODGKIN'S LYMPHOMA
Lymphadenopathy	Localised to a single node or chain, often cervical, subclavicular or mediastinal	Multiple peripheral nodes, nodes of the mesentery often involved
Spread	Orderly and continuous	Diffuse and unpredictable
Extranodal involvement	Rare	Early and common
Bone marrow involvement	Uncommon	Common
Fever, night sweats, weight loss	Common	Uncommon until disease is extensive
Other manifestations	Fatigue, pruritus, splenomegaly; anaemia, neutrophilia	Abdominal pain, nausea, vomiting; dyspnoea, cough; CNS symptoms; lymphocytopenia

- *Chest x-ray* is done to identify possible enlarged mediastinal lymph nodes and pulmonary involvement.
- *CT scans* of the chest, abdomen and pelvis are performed to identify abnormal or enlarged nodes.
- *Positron emission tomography (PET or gallium scans)* may be performed in diagnosing the disease, as well as to evaluate the effectiveness of treatment.
- *Biopsy* of the largest, most central enlarged lymph node and of the bone marrow is done to establish the diagnosis for both Hodgkin's disease and non-Hodgkin's lymphoma. The presence of Reed–Sternberg cells confirms the diagnosis of Hodgkin's disease.

Staging

Staging is used to determine the extent of the disease and appropriate treatment. The staging systems used in Australia are the Ann Arbor Staging System or the Lugano Staging System (Lymphoma Australia, 2022), which assess the extent and severity of lymphomas. The stages are:

- Stage I: involvement of a single lymph node region or lymphoid structure (above or below the diaphragm).
- Stage II: involvement of two or more lymph node regions on the same side of the diaphragm.
- Stage III: involvement of at least one lymph node regions or structures on both sides of the diaphragm.
- Stage IV: involvement of an extranodal site (not proximal or contiguous with an involved node) such as the liver, lung or pleura, bone or bone marrow, or skin.

The presence or absence of systemic symptoms is indicated by either an 'A' (no systemic symptoms) or 'B' (systemic symptoms of fever, night sweats, weight loss). 'E' is used when lymphoma has spread to an area or organ outside the lymph nodes. 'X' is used when the tumour is larger than 10 cm in size. 'S' is used when there is a lymphoma lesion in the spleen. The letter is always placed after the stage; for example, 2A or 4E (Leukaemia Foundation, 2022d).

Chemotherapy

Combination chemotherapy is used to treat both Hodgkin's disease and non-Hodgkin's lymphoma. In both cases, chemotherapy often is followed by radiation therapy to involved lymph node regions. The choice of drug combination depends on the stage of the disease as well as the person's age and general condition. Combination regimens may also be used and, with the range of new drugs continually coming onto the market for management of lymphoma, protocols are evolving rapidly. Drugs such as monoclonal antibodies and other immunotherapy agents are changing the treatment landscape by helping the immune system to recognise and fight the cancer rather than the drug targeting the lymphoma itself (such as CAR T-cell therapy). There are also other medications which target markers specific to lymphoma cells. These regimens also may be combined in alternating months to reduce the adverse effects and improve tumour cell kill. Finally, antibiotics may be beneficial for lymphomas caused by infections such as *Helicobacter pylori (H. pylori)*, as in MALT lymphomas. More than 75% of people with Hodgkin's disease who do not have systemic symptoms may achieve complete remission with treatment. The prognosis for those with non-Hodgkin's lymphoma varies by the type and stage of the disease (Leukaemia Foundation, 2022d). For more information about nursing care of the person receiving combination chemotherapy, see the chapter 'Nursing care of people with cancer'.

Radiation therapy

Radiation therapy may be the primary treatment for early-stage Hodgkin's disease, although early chemotherapy is becoming more common. In later stages and in non-Hodgkin's lymphoma, it is usually combined with chemotherapy. Many lymphomas are highly responsive to radiation. The involved lymph node region is treated, with careful shielding to protect unaffected areas and minimise the extent of radiation burn and normal cell destruction (see Figure 32.10). If the disease is advanced, total nodal irradiation may be done. See the chapter 'Nursing care of people with cancer' for nursing care of the person receiving radiation therapy.

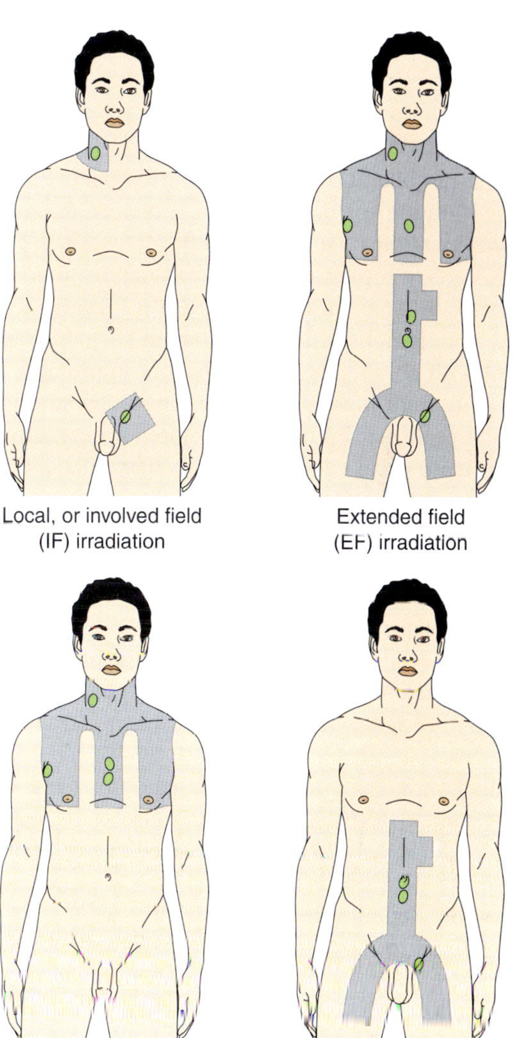

FIGURE 32.10 ***Patterns of radiation therapy used to treat lymphoma based on the location and extent of the disease***

TRANSLATION TO PRACTICE Evidence-based practice: sleep disruption, depression and fatigue among haematopoietic cell transplant (HCT) recipients

Fatigue and depression are common adverse effects of chemotherapy and radiation therapy in people undergoing cancer treatment. Fatigue is prevalent, affecting 80–100% of people undergoing standard chemotherapy and often leading to lost work time and difficulty maintaining functional roles within the family and society. Ongoing depression, fatigue and sleep disruption can be risk factors for relapse and mortality (Rentscher et al., 2021).

IMPLICATIONS FOR NURSING

These data suggest that nurses should assess for fatigue and depression in people following stem cell transplant (SCT). Nursing measures to help conserve the person's energy are appropriate to manage fatigue. Early screening, referral and intervention for fatigue may actually reduce the intensity of fatigue at its peak. Nurses can use this information to prepare people for common symptom patterns following SCT, thus reducing anxiety and concern that their condition may be declining rather than improving after SCT. Families and caregivers are also at risk of depression and psychological distress and should be screened accordingly. Assessment tools to measure fatigue and depression in people undergoing SCT can be incorporated into nursing care, with ongoing screening recommended.

CRITICAL THINKING IN PERSON-CENTRED CARE

1. The average age of participants ($N = 241$) in this study was 51 years; 60% were male, 40% female. Does this sample reflect your local demographic of people undergoing haematopoietic cell transplant?
2. In this study, there was a higher association between fatigue interference and mortality in men prior to HCT, and women post HCT. How would understanding this result improve your care for individuals who have received haematopoietic stem cell transplant?
3. Interestingly, biobehavioural symptoms did not seem to affect the likelihood of chronic graft-versus-host disease (cGVHD). What might be the significance of this finding?

Stem cell transplant

Autologous peripheral blood stem cell transplant (PBSCT) is a treatment option for people who experience remission of malignant lymphoma. Autologous PBSCT uses the person's own stem cells to restore bone marrow function after chemotherapy or radiation. In autologous PBSCT, stem cells are obtained from peripheral blood following chemotherapy and treatment with colony-stimulating factors to promote development of normal blood cells. The blood containing these normal stem cells is then frozen and stored for use after treatment. If relapse occurs, lethal doses of chemotherapy or radiation are given to destroy the immune system and malignant cells. The frozen blood is then thawed and infused intravenously through a peripheral line. The infused stem cells become a part of the person's bone marrow and normal haematopoiesis takes place.

The person is critically ill during the period of bone marrow destruction and immunosuppression and is hospitalised in a private room for 6 to 8 weeks or more. See the 'Translation to practice' box.

For clarity, it is important to understand that there are several terms used to describe stem cell transplants. Haematopoietic stem cell transplant (HSCT), haematopoietic cell transplant (HCT), stem cell transplant (SCT) and bone marrow transplant (BMT) are all used interchangeably.

Complications of treatment

Both chemotherapy and radiation therapy may have long-term effects. Permanent sterility is common, especially in older adults. Bone marrow depression can lead to immunosuppression, anaemia and bleeding. Secondary cancers and cardiac injury are the most serious late adverse effects of treatment. Some chemotherapy regimens may risk causing acute leukaemia. Cancers such as breast or lung cancer may develop 10 or more years after thoracic radiation. Thoracic radiation can increase the risk of coronary heart disease and hypothyroidism.

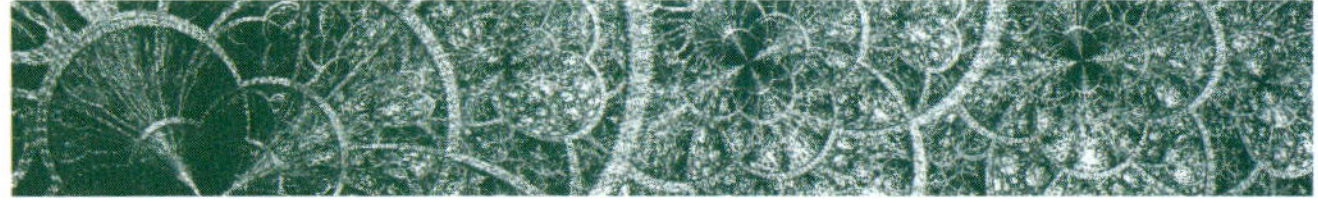

Nursing care

Assessment and priority nursing care for the person with lymphoma follows. See also the nursing care plan later in this section for application of nursing care strategies for a person with Hodgkin's disease.

Assessment

Focused assessment of the person with Hodgkin's disease or non-Hodgkin's lymphoma includes:

- *Health history*: complaints of enlarged lymph node(s), fever, night sweats, weight loss, fatigue or general malaise, abdominal pain, respiratory symptoms, numbness or tingling of extremities, visual changes or changes in mentation; history of infectious mononucleosis, HIV disease or other immunosuppressive disorders.
- *Physical examination*: mental status exam; inspect and palpate lymph nodes (cervical, subclavicular, axillary and inguinal) for enlargement, tenderness; heart and lung sounds; abdominal examination for tenderness, masses, liver or spleen enlargement.
- *Diagnostic tests*: FBC, haemoglobin and haematocrit, ESR; serum blood results; x-ray, scan and biopsy results.

Nursing diagnoses and interventions

Nursing care of the person with malignant lymphoma involves both physical and emotional support during diagnosis and treatment. Common nursing care problems include impaired protection due to bone marrow suppression, fatigue, nausea and altered body image. See the nursing care section for leukaemia for specific nursing interventions for *Ineffective protection*.

Fatigue

General malaise and fatigue may accompany malignant lymphoma and are side effects of chemotherapy. In addition, the physical and psychological stress of dealing with a chronic, debilitating disease and its treatment may cause fatigue.

- Inquire about feelings of malaise (a vague feeling of body weakness or discomfort) and fatigue (a pervasive, drained feeling that cannot be eliminated). *Both malaise and fatigue are subjective experiences with physiological, situational and psychological components.*
- Encourage verbalisation of feelings about the impact of the disease and fatigue on lifestyle. *Discussion of feelings helps the person clarify values and may assist in identifying priorities.*
- Encourage enjoyable but quiet activities, such as reading, listening to music or hobbies. Enjoyable activities help decrease feelings of fatigue. *Quiet activities conserve energy while yielding a sense of accomplishment.*
- Encourage establishing priorities and including rest periods or naps when scheduling daily activities. *This provides a sense of control over activities and helps maintain self-esteem. Scheduled rest periods help restore energy and decrease fatigue.*
- Encourage delegation of some responsibilities to family members. *Delegation helps maintain the person's involvement and role in family decisions and responsibilities, while conserving energy for those activities identified as high priority by the person.*
- Identify and encourage the person to use energy-saving equipment. *Performing tasks with less exertion and in less time helps conserve energy.*
- Encourage a diet high in carbohydrates and fluids. *A high-carbohydrate diet helps maintain muscle glycogen stores. A liberal fluid intake promotes excretion of metabolic by-products that may contribute to malaise and fatigue.*

Nausea

The effects of malignant lymphoma and its treatment with chemotherapy and/or radiation therapy can contribute to nausea and interfere with nutritional status. Nausea, a sensation of abdominal fullness and fear of vomiting often limit food intake. See also the nursing diagnosis of *Imbalanced nutrition* in the section on leukaemia for additional interventions.

- Assess precipitating factors for nausea and/or vomiting, the frequency of vomiting and relief measures used by the person. *Careful assessment allows development of interventions tailored to the person's situation and needs.*

> **CONSIDERATION FOR PRACTICE**
>
> **Provide ordered anti-emetics before chemotherapy is started. Administering prescribed anti-emetics before chemotherapy helps prevent nausea and the psychological association of nausea with chemotherapy.**

- Teach measures to prevent or relieve nausea and vomiting:
  a. Eat cracker biscuits and suck on hard lollies.
  b. Eat soft, bland foods that are cold or at room temperature.
  c. Avoid unpleasant odours and get fresh air.
  d. Eat prior to but not immediately before chemotherapy.
  e. Use distraction or progressive muscle relaxation when nauseated.
  f. If vomiting occurs, gradually resume oral intake with frequent sips of clear liquids or ice, progressing to bland foods.

  Cracker biscuits and lollies often relieve queasiness, whereas hot, spicy, sweet or strong-smelling foods may increase nausea. Alternative nausea relief measures may be effective.
- Provide small feedings of high-kilojoule, high-protein foods and fluids. *This increases nutritional intake.*
- Assist with oral care, general hygiene and environmental control of temperature, appearance and odours. *These measures enhance appetite.*
- Identify and provide preferred foods. *This promotes nutritional intake.*
- Assist to a sitting position during and immediately after meals. *The sitting position helps decrease early feelings of fullness.*

Disturbed body image

The diagnosis of cancer is often devastating to the sense of trust in and the perception of one's body. Radiation and chemotherapy lead to changes in appearance and body function (e.g. hair loss, reduced libido and infertility), further altering body image. Reactions to this diagnosis vary and may include refusal to look in a mirror or discuss the effects of the disease or treatment, unwillingness to participate in rehabilitation, inappropriate treatment decisions, increasing dependence on others or refusal to provide self-care, hostility, withdrawal and signs of grieving.

- Assess perception of body image through subjective information such as:
  a. what the person likes most and least about their body
  b. pre-illness perception of people who are sick or have a disability
  c. current understanding of health and limitations imposed by illness or treatment
  d. feelings about the illness and its effect on perception of self and others

  Body image is one's mental idea or picture of the body. It is based on past and present experiences and includes components of one's actual body and emotional responses to that body. Body image changes constantly. There is often a time lag between an actual body change and the changed body image; during this time, the diagnosis, teaching and treatment may be rejected.

- Discuss the risk of and measures to cope with alopecia. Suggest wearing wigs, scarves, hats or caps. Teach proper scalp care using baby shampoo or mild soap, a soft brush, sunscreen and mineral oil to reduce itching. If eyelashes and eyebrows are lost, teach eye protection, such as wearing eyeglasses and caps with wide brims. *Chemotherapeutic agents attack rapidly dividing cells such as those responsible for hair growth. Hair loss usually begins 1 to 2 weeks after initiation of chemotherapy, with maximum loss 1 to 2 months later. Alopecia may range from thinning to total hair loss. Regrowth depends on the treatment schedule and doses; however, it usually begins 2 to 3 months after treatment ends. New hair may be softer, more curly and slightly different in colour. Teaching and emotional support help the person anticipate hair loss, discuss its potential effect on body image and learn self-care techniques.*
- Discuss available resources for financial assistance with purchase of wigs, including assistance from the Australian Cancer Council. *A well-matched wig (or one the colour the person has always wished for!) can help maintain a positive body image.*

Sexual dysfunction

Sexual dysfunction may result from the malignancy and the effects of radiation and chemotherapy. Reproductive tissues are made of rapidly dividing cells and cancer treatment may cause

NURSING CARE PLAN A person with Hodgkin's disease

Max Patterson, RN, aged 28, is the nurse manager of a thoracic critical care unit in a large teaching hospital. Lately he has been more tired than usual, often wakes up at night covered with sweat and just does not feel well. He had thought that his symptoms were due to a viral illness and his busy work schedule. However, yesterday morning Max noticed a large swollen area on the right side of his neck. He made an appointment with his general practitioner who found a large cervical lymph node. A biopsy of the node and a CT scan of the chest were scheduled.

ASSESSMENT

David Smart, RN, the practice nurse at the medical centre, obtains a nursing history and assessment of Mr Patterson. His physical examination is essentially normal, with the exception of the enlarged node, which is not tender to palpation. When Mr Patterson is weighed, he tells RN Smart that he has lost 3.2 kg in the past 2 months. In reviewing the results of the blood studies, RN Smart notes mild anaemia and an increased neutrophil count. The lymph node biopsy shows Reed–Sternberg cells. The doctor and RN Smart tell Mr Patterson that the findings indicate stage 1B Hodgkin's disease but that the prognosis is very good. The doctor recommends a short course of combination chemotherapy followed by radiation therapy to involved sites.

DIAGNOSES

- *Anxiety* related to the diagnosis of Hodgkin's disease and effects of treatment on job performance.
- *Risk of infection* related to potential bone marrow depression due to chemotherapy.
- *Fatigue* related to effects of cancer, chemotherapy and radiation therapy.

PLANNING

- Reduce anxiety through discussion and education.
- Improve and extend energy levels.
- Monitor and reduce risk of infection.

Expected outcomes

- Verbalise reduced anxiety.
- Remain free of infection.
- Identify and use methods to preserve energy.

IMPLEMENTATION

- Encourage Mr Patterson to consider a leave of absence from work during course of treatment.
- Discuss joining a support group for people with cancer.
- Provide information about the illness, combination chemotherapy and radiation therapy.
- Reinforce knowledge of actions to decrease the risk of infection.
- Discuss ways to decrease fatigue and maintain energy:
- Take a 1- to 2-hour nap once or twice a day.
- Avoid overexertion during weekends and time off.
- Maintain a well-balanced diet.

EVALUATION

When Mr Patterson returns the following week to begin chemotherapy, he brings his friend Nina to meet RN Smart and asks him to discuss his treatment with her. Mr Patterson says, 'I am still really scared, but being able to talk about this with Nina will help a lot.' Mr Patterson has made arrangements to take 4 months' leave from work, with the understanding that his job will be held for him. He states that he will have some problems with money but is working them out. He also says he feels that taking a daytime sleep is silly but that he will rest to maintain his energy level. Mr Patterson and Nina express confidence that he will be cured and say they plan to be active members of the cancer support group—even after recovery.

CRITICAL THINKING IN THE NURSING PROCESS

1 Discuss the rationale for treating Hodgkin's disease with chemotherapy and radiation.
2 Design a teaching plan to help Mr Patterson prevent infection while he is at home.
3 What effect does the diagnosis of cancer have on the developmental tasks of a young adult?
4 Develop a care plan for Mr Patterson for the nursing diagnosis of *Ineffective role performance*.

REFLECTION ON THE NURSING PROCESS

1 What are the take-home points that you have learned from this case study?
2 How can you use them within your daily practice?
3 Where would you find good-quality information for a person in Mr Patterson's situation?

temporary or permanent sterility, changes in menstruation and changes in libido.

- Encourage discussion of actual or potential sexual dysfunction or sterility with the person and significant other. *People may be reluctant to discuss this unintended effect of treatment unless encouraged.*
- Assess knowledge, provide information and clarify misconceptions. Discuss realistic measures for coping (e.g. sperm banking prior to chemotherapy or radiation therapy). *People and their partners may be unclear about expected effects on sexuality, reproduction and the permanency of these effects.*
- Refer for counselling as indicated. *Sexual counselling can help the person and partner develop alternative strategies for expressing their sexuality.*

Risk of impaired skin integrity

Malignant lymphomas may cause significant pruritus and drenching night sweats. As a result, skin integrity may be impaired. In addition, radiation therapy can cause superficial burns, which also may affect skin integrity.

- Frequently assess skin, especially in areas undergoing radiation. *Early identification of lesions allows timely treatment and can prevent further disruption of this important line of defence against infection.*
- Provide and teach measures to promote comfort and relieve itching: use cool water and a mild soap to bathe; blot (rather than rub) dry skin; apply plain cornflour or non-perfumed lotion or powder to the skin unless contraindicated, being careful not to clog pores; use lightweight blankets and clothing; maintain adequate humidity and a cool room temperature; wash bedding and clothes in mild detergent and put them through a second rinse cycle. *Pruritus is aggravated by excessive warmth, excessive dryness, rough fabrics, fatigue and stress. Lotions and some powders may be contraindicated during radiation therapy.*

Community-based care

When teaching the person and family for home care, include the following topics in addition to those previously identified for specific nursing diagnoses:

- information about the illness, planned treatment and anticipated side effects of treatment
- skin care and measures to relieve itching and protect areas of radiation
- symptoms to report to the doctor, including those of vertebral compression (decreased sensation or strength in lower extremities)
- use of analgesics and alternative relief strategies for abdominal pain and peripheral neuropathies
- respiratory care if mediastinal nodes are enlarged or lungs or pleurae are involved
- planning activities of daily living to ensure adequate rest and exercise
- measures to relieve nausea and maintain adequate nutrition.

Refer the person and their family members to the local oncology clinic, cancer support group or Cancer Council for information, assistance and counselling. A list of state and local agencies that offer information about malignant lymphoma and financial assistance can be obtained from the Leukaemia Foundation: https://www.leukaemia.org.au.

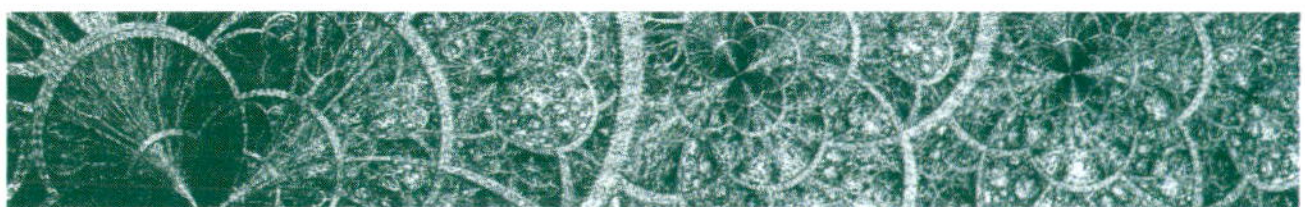

THE PERSON WITH MULTIPLE MYELOMA

Multiple myeloma is a malignancy in which plasma cells multiply uncontrollably and infiltrate the bone marrow, lymph nodes, spleen and other tissues. *Plasma cells* are B-cell lymphocytes that develop to produce antibodies (immunoglobins).

Incidence and risk factors

The incidence of multiple myeloma is increasing slightly, with an estimated 2,625 diagnosed in 2022 (Cancer Australia, 2022c). The incidence of multiple myeloma increases with age, rarely occurring before age 40, with most new cases occurring after 70. It occurs more frequently in men than in women (Cancer Australia, 2022c). Its cause is unknown. Possible contributing factors include genetic alterations, radiation exposure, oncogenic virus, inflammatory stimuli and chronic antigenic stimulation. The risk of developing multiple myeloma is higher in people of lower socioeconomic status. This increased risk may relate to environmental factors such as poor housing, occupational hazards, poor nutritional status and other physical and psychosocial stressors such as exposure to infectious agents.

Pathophysiology

Malignant plasma cells arise from one clone (*monoclonal*) of B cells that produce abnormally large amounts of a particular immunoglobin called the *M protein*. This abnormal protein interferes with normal antibody production and impairs the humoral immune response. It also increases blood viscosity and may damage kidney tubules. As myeloma cells proliferate, they replace the bone marrow and infiltrate the bone itself. Cortical bone is progressively destroyed by tumour growth and enzymes produced by myeloma cells. These enzymes facilitate bone destruction, its infiltration by tumour cells, development of new blood vessels to sustain the tumour and growth of myeloma cells (Shah, 2022). Affected bones (primarily the vertebrae, ribs, skull, pelvis, femur, clavicle and scapula) are weakened and may break without trauma (*pathological fracture*). With disease progression, malignant cells spread via the bloodstream to invade other organs (see Figure 32.11).

Manifestations

The disease develops slowly, with many people diagnosed during evaluation for unrelated problems. Manifestations of multiple myeloma are due to its effects on the bone and the

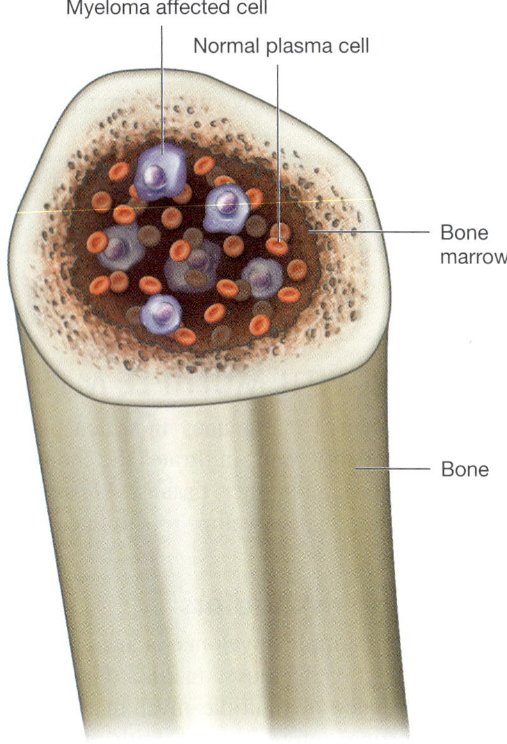

FIGURE 32.11 ***An illustration of the progress of multiple myeloma in a male. Abnormal plasma cells proliferate uncontrollably, gradually replacing bone marrow and infiltrating bone itself. As the disease progresses, these cells spread to other organs via the bloodstream***

impaired immune response due to M-protein production. The most common presenting problem is bone pain that is usually felt in the back or ribs and is increased with movement (Cancer Australia, 2022c; Shah, 2022). With progression of the disease, the pain may increase in severity and become more localised. Rapid bone destruction releases calcium from the bone, leading to hypercalcaemia and manifestations of neurological dysfunction, such as lethargy, confusion and weakness.

As functional antibody formation decreases and the humoral immune response is suppressed, recurrent infections develop. Cell-mediated immunity remains intact. Bence Jones proteins are found in the urine in multiple myeloma. These proteins are toxic to the renal tubules and may lead to renal failure with azotaemia and uraemia. (See the chapter 'Nursing care of people with kidney disorders' for more information about renal failure.)

As treatment options improve, now approximately 55% of people experiencing multiple myeloma have a survival rate of at least 5 years (Cancer Australia, 2022c). More frequently, the disease course is chronic, progressing more rapidly with each relapse after remission. The acute terminal stage of the disease is marked by pancytopenia and widespread organ infiltration by myeloma cells.

INTERPROFESSIONAL CARE

Diagnosis and staging

Diagnostic tests for multiple myeloma include the following:

- *X-rays* and other radiological studies of the bone may reveal multiple punched-out lesions.
- *Bone marrow examination* shows an abnormal number of immature plasma cells.
- *FBC* shows moderate to severe anaemia and the *ESR* usually is elevated.
- *Protein electrophoresis* shows a spike of one type of antibody, usually immunoglobulin G (IgG).
- *Serum calcium, creatinine, uric acid* and *blood urea nitrogen (BUN)* levels often are elevated.
- *Urinalysis* shows Bence Jones protein in the urine.
- *Biopsy* of myeloma lesions confirms the diagnosis of multiple myeloma.

Staging of multiple myeloma is based on the haemoglobin and serum calcium levels, the amount of abnormal protein present and the degree of bone involvement.

Treatment

There is no cure for multiple myeloma. In some people, active observation is indicated, as the disease may continue with a slow, *indolent* (sluggish, not developing or progressing) course for many years. When indicated by disease stage or progression, standard treatment includes induction chemotherapy followed by stem cell transplant and maintenance chemotherapy to control progression of the disease. Supportive care is provided to reduce complications of the disease and their effects.

Combination chemotherapy with an alkylating agent melphalan (Alkeran), cyclophosphamide (Cytoxan) or chlorambucil (Chloromycetin) and corticosteroids such as prednisone administered for 4 to 7 days every 4 to 6 weeks is commonly used. Chemotherapy typically reduces bone pain, hypercalcaemia, anaemia and the number of infections. Other therapies include immunomodulatory drugs, alkylating agents, bisphosphonates and protease inhibitors which can contribute to improved survival rates and better response rates when compared to conventional chemotherapy. Localised radiation therapy may be used to treat painful bone lesions. High-dose chemotherapy followed by peripheral allogeneic stem cell transplant (SCT) may be more effective in achieving a cure but is associated with a high mortality rate. When autologous SCT is used, granulocyte colony-stimulating factor is administered prior to harvesting and preserving peripheral stem cells for transplant.

Supportive care may include treatment of hypercalcaemia with hydration, possible bisphosphonate therapy to reduce bone loss (see the chapter 'Nursing care of people with musculoskeletal disorders') and calcium, vitamin D and fluoride supplements to support bone structure. Plasma exchange therapy (plasmapheresis) to remove circulating M proteins is used as needed to treat acute renal failure. Infections are treated promptly when they develop.

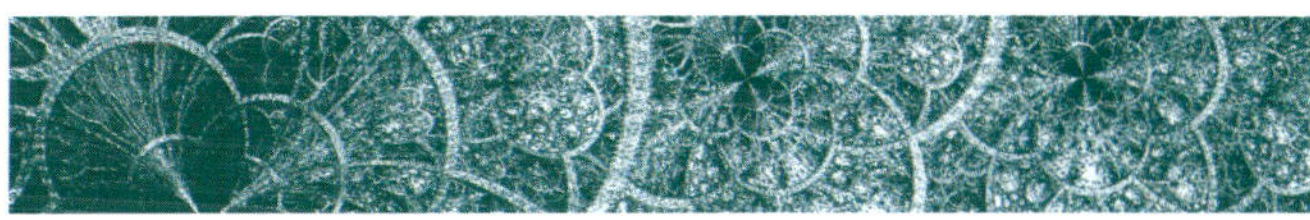

Nursing care

Assessment

Focused assessment data for the person with multiple myeloma include the following:

- *Health history*: complaints of back or bone pain, onset, duration and intensity; complaints of weakness, fatigue, anorexia; history of frequent or recurrent infections; neurological symptoms such as numbness and tingling or clumsiness.
- *Physical examination*: level of consciousness and mental status; mobility, gait; localised tenderness or pain, bony crepitus with movement or palpation; movement and sensation in extremities.

Nursing diagnoses and interventions

Nursing care of the person with multiple myeloma focuses on problems of chronic pain, impaired mobility and the risk of injury. Risk of infection is a major nursing care focus; see the previous section on leukaemia for specific interventions to reduce this risk. Other nursing care needs are similar to those of people with other cancers and chronic pain. See the chapters 'Nursing care of people in pain' and 'Nursing care of people with cancer' for additional specific nursing interventions for these problems.

Chronic pain

People with multiple myeloma typically experience chronic back pain and deep bone pain as myeloma cells saturate the bone marrow and invade the bone structure. Pathological fractures are a common and reoccurring problem.

- Assess pain, including intensity (use a standard pain scale), onset, duration, precipitating factors and effective relief measures. *Identifying the intensity, causes and precipitating factors of pain helps determine and evaluate effective pain relief measures.*
- Determine position of greatest comfort and assist as needed into this position. *The person is best able to identify positions that minimise pain but may need assistance with repositioning.*
- Support position with pillows. *Bony prominences may be painful due to infiltrates. Pillows can help relieve pressure on these prominences, thus reducing pain.*
- Provide uninterrupted rest periods. *Adequate rest facilitates pain relief and improves pain tolerance.*
- Teach adjunctive pain relief strategies such as relaxation or guided imagery. *A combination of pharmacological and non-pharmacological methods provides better management of chronic pain, especially bone pain.*
- Teach effective analgesic use, including the family in instruction. *Analgesics are most effective when taken before pain becomes severe. People and their families may be reluctant to use prescription analgesics on a regular basis.*
- Report unrelieved pain to the doctor. *A different analgesic or addition of an adjunctive medication such as a non-steroidal anti-inflammatory drug (NSAID) may be needed to effectively control pain.*

Impaired physical mobility

Painful bony infiltrates and pathological fractures may limit mobility. A brace or splint may be used to protect extremities or support the back. In addition, persistent weakness associated with the cancer and anaemia may limit the person's ability to participate in usual activities.

- Assist to change position at least every 2 hours. *Assistance with repositioning is necessary due to weakness. Frequent repositioning improves comfort and reduces the risk of impaired skin and tissue integrity.*

> **CONSIDERATION FOR PRACTICE**
>
> **Gently support extremities during repositioning. Weakened extremities due to infiltration of bone by myeloma cells and muscle atrophy from lack of use increase the risk of pathological fractures.**

- Provide a trapeze to assist with repositioning. *A trapeze provides better leverage, allowing the person to assist with repositioning and providing a degree of independence. The ability to participate in self-care improves self-esteem.*

Risk of injury

The bone involvement of multiple myeloma places the person at high risk of pathological and traumatic fractures. Pathological fractures can occur with simple activities such as turning or reaching for an item. The spine usually is affected; the ribs and bones of the extremities also may be at risk of fracture.

- Place needed items close at hand. *Straining to reach objects increases the risk of falling or sustaining other injury.*
- Provide safety measures to prevent falls from bed: place the bed in a low position, use side rails as indicated and place the call bell within reach. *Safety measures help prevent accidental injury. A secure environment minimises risk and helps prevent falls.*
- Provide shoes with non-skid soles, a clear pathway, adequate lighting and a level surface free of scatter rugs or other hazards when ambulating. Provide a walker as needed for support and security. *Weight-bearing exercise promotes bone repair. Safety measures, such as an unobstructed pathway and a firm walking surface, help prevent falls.*

Community-based care

When teaching people and their families for home care, include the following topics:

- strategies for home maintenance management
- signs and symptoms of complications to be reported to the doctor (e.g. symptoms of vertebral and extremity fractures)

- manifestations of infection to report: fever and chills; increased malaise, fatigue or weakness; cough with or without sputum; sore throat; dysuria, nocturia, frequency, urgency or malodourous urine.

Provide referrals for home health and home maintenance services, physical or occupational therapy, social services and hospice care as appropriate.

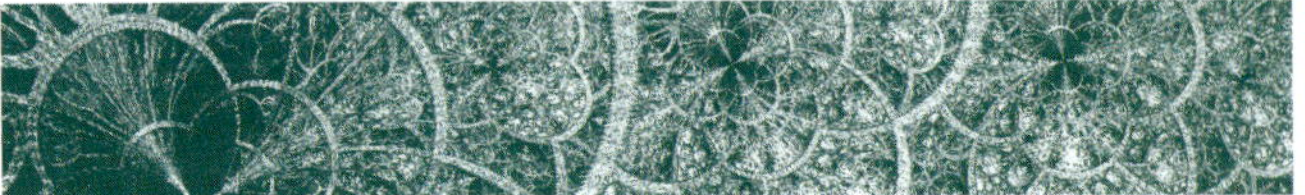

THE PERSON WITH NEUTROPENIA

Leucopenia is a decrease in the total circulating WBC count. Although any type of WBC may be affected, neutrophils, which make up the majority of WBCs, are affected most often. *Neutropenia* is a decrease in circulating neutrophils, usually less than 1×10^9/L to 1.5×10^9/L. Neutropenia may be either congenital or acquired, developing secondarily to prolonged infection, haematological disorders, starvation or autoimmune disorders (such as rheumatoid arthritis). Chemotherapy and other drugs can suppress the bone marrow. Neutropenia develops in approximately half of people undergoing chemotherapy to treat cancer. *Agranulocytosis* is severe neutropenia, with less than 0.5×10^9/L. Numbers of other granulocytes also are reduced. It is usually due to impaired leucocyte formation in the bone marrow or increased cell destruction in circulating blood. Agranulocytosis significantly increases the risk of infection (DeFaria, 2021). *Aplastic anaemia* affects production of all blood cells, resulting in anaemia, thrombocytopenia and agranulocytosis.

Pathophysiology and manifestations

Neutrophils are an integral component of the immune response. They are phagocytes, drawn to and activated by infection and inflammation to engulf and degrade invading microorganisms. Their lifespan in peripheral blood is short, less than 1 day. When *granulopoiesis* (the development and maturation of granulocytes) in the bone marrow is suppressed, the number of circulating neutrophils falls rapidly. As a result, the body's ability to defend itself against infection is significantly reduced.

The manifestations of neutropenia reflect the resulting impaired immunity and inflammatory response. Opportunistic bacterial, fungal and protozoal infections develop, commonly affecting the respiratory tract and mucosa of the mouth, GI tract and vagina. Malaise, chills and fever with extreme weakness and fatigue are common manifestations (Berliner, 2022; DeFaria, 2021).

INTERPROFESSIONAL CARE

The diagnosis of neutropenia is made based on the person's manifestations, risk factors and the FBC. The total white blood count is low, 4×10^9/L.

Haematopoietic growth factors such as granulocyte-macrophage colony-stimulating factor are administered to stimulate granulocyte maturation and differentiation. Infections are treated with antibiotic therapy. Protective isolation procedures may be initiated to prevent exposure to pathogens. When neutropenia is related to chemotherapy, cancer treatment often must be halted, at least temporarily, to allow the bone marrow to recover.

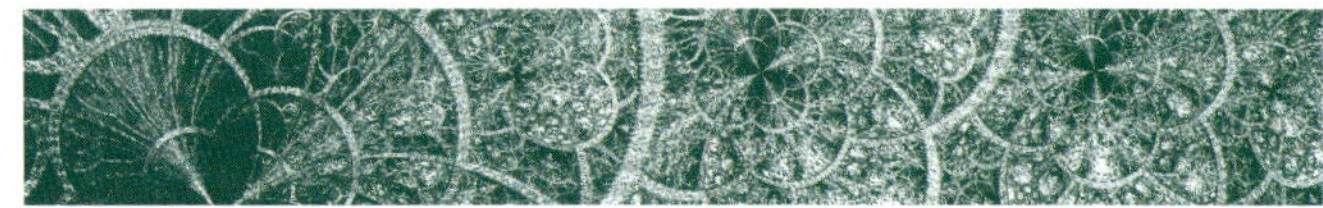

Nursing care

The primary nursing care focus is early identification of neutropenia and protecting the person from infection. The WBC count is monitored on a regular basis and any decline reported to the doctor. Protective isolation may be indicated, including restricting the number of visitors and people with apparent illness. See *Risk of infection* in the earlier section on leukaemia for specific nursing interventions for the person with neutropenia.

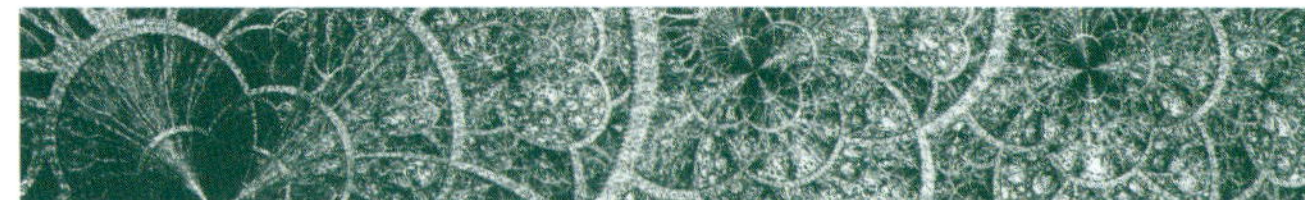

Platelet and coagulation disorders

Platelet and coagulation disorders affect **haemostasis**, control of bleeding. Haemostasis maintains a relatively steady state of blood volume, blood pressure and blood flow through injured vessels. Bleeding disorders result from deficient platelets, disruption of the clotting cascade or a combination of factors.

THE PERSON WITH THROMBOCYTOPENIA

Thrombocytopenia is a platelet count of less than 150×10^9/L of blood. It can lead to abnormal bleeding. A continuing decline in circulating platelets can lead to spontaneous bleeding and

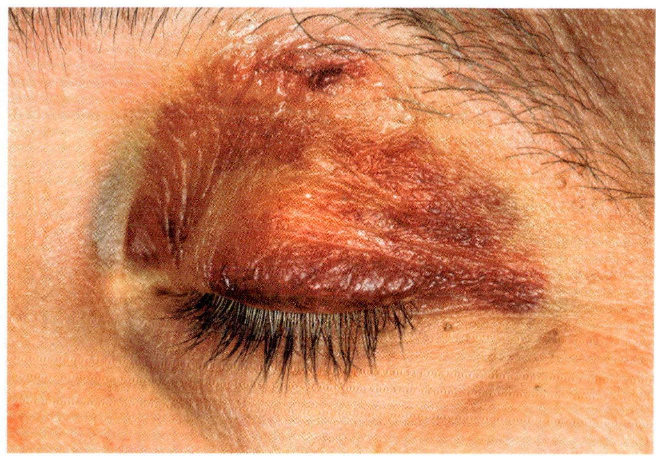

FIGURE 32.12 ***Significant ecchymosis of the eyelid associated with minor trauma in a person with thrombocytopenia***

Source: © Scott Camazine/Science Source.

haemorrhage from minor trauma (see Figure 32.12). Bleeding due to platelet deficiency usually occurs in small vessels, causing manifestations such as *petechiae* and *purpura* (Arnold & Cuker, 2022). The mucous membranes of the nose, mouth, GI tract and vagina often bleed. Serious and potentially fatal bleeding may occur when the platelet count is less than 150×10^9/L.

Thrombocytopenia results from one of three mechanisms: decreased production, increased sequestration in the spleen or accelerated destruction. Primary thrombocytopenia that leads to increased platelet destruction is discussed below. Secondary thrombocytopenia may be caused by aplastic anaemia, bone marrow malignancy, infection, radiation therapy or drug therapy. It may also be pregnancy related (see Box 32.7). Heparin therapy is the most common drug-induced thrombocytopenia; it is included in the discussion that follows. Platelet sequestration usually is due to an enlarged spleen. Up to 80% of platelets may be removed from circulation with significant splenomegaly. Finally, thrombocytopenia may result from premature platelet destruction associated with disseminated intravascular coagulation (DIC).

Physiology review

Effective control of bleeding requires a series of complex interactions between the damaged tissue and blood vessel, platelets, clotting factors and processes to dissolve clots once bleeding has been controlled. Platelets are formed in the bone marrow under control of thrombopoietin, a protein produced by the liver, kidney, smooth muscle and bone marrow. Platelets are attracted to the damaged vessel wall, where they aggregate and release mediators that activate the clotting process. See the chapter 'A person-centred approach to assessing the cardiovascular and lymphatic systems' for a more complete discussion about platelets, clotting and haemostasis.

Pathophysiology

The two types of primary thrombocytopenia are immune thrombocytopenic purpura and thrombotic thrombocytopenic purpura.

BOX 32.7 Selected causes of secondary thrombocytopenia

Diseases

- Vitamin B_{12} anaemia
- Folic acid anaemia
- Aplastic anaemia
- Leukaemia
- Alcoholism
- DIC
- Infectious mononucleosis
- Viral infections
- HIV disease
- Pregnancy

Drugs

- Thiazide diuretics
- Aspirin
- Ibuprofen
- Indomethacin
- Naproxen
- Sulfonamides
- Phenytoin
- Cimetidine
- Digoxin
- Frusemide
- Heparin
- Morphine

Treatments

- Radiation therapy
- Chemotherapy
- Massive transfusion of stored blood

Immune thrombocytopenic purpura

Immune thrombocytopenic purpura (ITP), also known as *idiopathic thrombocytopenic purpura*, is an autoimmune disorder in which platelet destruction is accelerated. In ITP, proteins on the platelet cell membrane stimulate autoantibody production, usually IgG antibodies. These autoantibodies adhere to the platelet membrane. Although the platelets function normally, the spleen reacts to them as being foreign and destroys the altered platelets after only 1 to 3 days of circulation.

MANIFESTATIONS The manifestations of ITP are due to bleeding from small vessels and mucous membranes. Petechiae and purpura develop, often on the anterior chest, arms, neck and oral mucous membranes. Bruising also may be apparent. As bleeding progresses, epistaxis (nosebleed), haematuria, excess menstrual bleeding and bleeding gums occur. Spontaneous intracranial bleeding is rare but does occur. Associated symptoms include weight loss, fever and headache.

INCIDENCE AND COURSE Acute ITP affects people of any age following a viral illness. Acute ITP typically lasts only 1 to 2 months, resolving without long-term consequences. In its chronic form, ITP typically affects adults between ages 20 and 50; women are affected more often than men. Its onset is insidious. Chronic (or adult) ITP often occurs in people with other immune-associated disorders such as systemic lupus erythematosus or HIV disease.

Thrombotic thrombocytopenic purpura

Thrombotic thrombocytopenic purpura (TTP) is a rare disorder in which thrombi occlude arterioles and capillaries of the microcirculation. Many organs are affected, including the heart, kidneys and brain. The incidence of TTP is increasing. Its cause is unknown. Platelet aggregation is a key feature of the disorder. As RBCs circulate through partially occluded vessels, they fragment, leading to haemolytic anaemia.

MANIFESTATIONS TTP may be acute, the more common and severe form, or chronic. Acute idiopathic TTP may be fatal within months if untreated. The manifestations of TTP include purpura and petechiae and neurological symptoms such as headache, seizures and altered consciousness.

Heparin-induced thrombocytopenia

Heparin-induced thrombocytopenia (HIT) develops as a result of an abnormal response to heparin therapy. Unfractionated heparin carries a greater potential to precipitate HIT; it can, however, develop in people receiving low-molecular-weight heparin who have previously been treated with unfractionated heparin. See the chapter 'Nursing care of people with vascular and lymphatic disorders' for further discussion of heparin therapy and the forms of heparin.

Heparin is a protein that occurs naturally in human tissues and inflammatory cells. It can react directly with platelets, causing them to agglutinate (clump) and be removed from circulation by phagocytosis. This form of HIT, called type I HIT, typically causes mild thrombocytopenia. The more severe form, type II HIT, results from an immune reaction to heparin. In type II HIT, heparin forms an immune complex with a platelet protein known as platelet factor 4 (PF4). This complex acts as a foreign antigen in some people, stimulating antibody production. The antibody binds with the heparin–PF4 complex and these heparin–PF4–antibody complexes subsequently bind with circulating platelets, causing them to aggregate. As affected platelets aggregate, they are removed from circulation, leading to thrombocytopenia. In addition, small pieces of platelets can break loose, stimulating the clotting cascade and the development of thrombosis (clotting). The thrombocytopenia and thrombosis can be reversed by prompt withdrawal of heparin therapy, and an alternative replacement commenced (Arepally, 2017).

MANIFESTATIONS Despite thrombocytopenia, bleeding is usually a manifestation of HIT, probably because of the increased tendency to form clots that deplete clotting factors. The person may develop manifestations of an arterial thrombosis (severe pain, paraesthesias, pallor and cool skin temperature, and pulselessness distal to the arterial occlusion) or of venous thrombosis (oedema, redness and warmth of the affected area). On rare occasions, an intravenous bolus of unfractionated heparin can precipitate an acute inflammatory response with manifestations that may mimic an acute pulmonary embolism: fever, chills, hypertension, tachycardia, dyspnoea, chest pain and cardiopulmonary arrest.

INTERPROFESSIONAL CARE

The diagnosis of thrombocytopenia is based on history, manifestations and diagnostic test results. Management focuses on treating or removing any causative factors and treating the platelet deficiency.

Diagnosis

The following diagnostic tests are used to identify thrombocytopenia:

- *FBC with platelet count* is done to evaluate blood cell counts, haemoglobin and haematocrit.
- *Antinuclear antibodies (ANA)* are measured to assess for autoantibodies and identify possible contributing disorders such as systemic lupus erythematosus.
- *Serological studies* for hepatitis viruses, cytomegalovirus (CMV), EBV, toxoplasma and HIV may be done. Serological testing also may be performed when HIT is suspected.
- *Bone marrow examination* evaluates for aplastic anaemia and megakaryocyte production.

Medications

Oral glucocorticoids, such as prednisone, are prescribed to suppress the autoimmune response. Many people who respond to glucocorticoid treatment relapse when the drug is withdrawn, however. Immunosuppressive drugs such as azathioprine, cyclophosphamide and cyclosporin may be used.

Prompt withdrawal of heparin therapy is vital when HIT is the cause of thrombocytopenia. All sources of heparin are removed, including heparin used to flush intravenous or other catheters and heparin-coated catheters.

Treatments

Platelet transfusions may be required to treat acute bleeding due to thrombocytopenia. Platelets are prepared from fresh whole blood; one unit contains 30 to 60 mL of platelet concentrate. The expected increase in platelets after one unit is infused is 10,000/mL. *Plasmapheresis*, or *plasma exchange therapy*, is the primary treatment for acute thrombotic thrombocytopenic purpura. The person's plasma is removed and replaced with fresh frozen plasma to remove autoantibodies, immune complexes and toxins.

Surgery

A *splenectomy* (surgical removal of the spleen) is the treatment of choice if the person with ITP relapses when glucocorticoids are discontinued. The spleen is the site of platelet destruction and antibody production. This surgery often cures the disorder, although relapse may occur years after splenectomy.

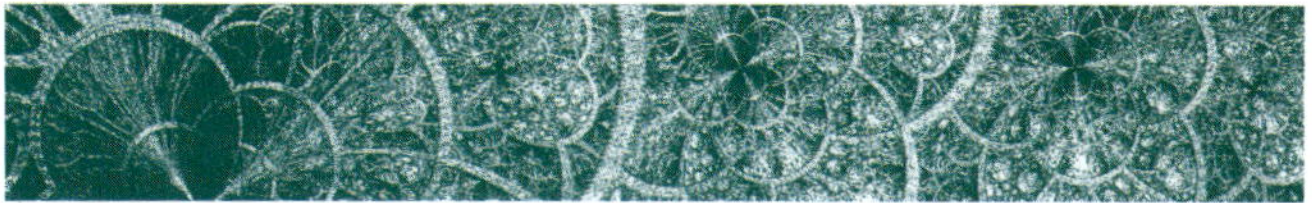

Nursing care

Assessment

- *Health history*: complaints of bruising with minor or no trauma, bleeding gums, nosebleed, heavy or prolonged menstrual periods, black, tarry or bloody stools, haematemesis, headache, fever or neurological symptoms; recent weight loss; recent viral or other illness; current and recent medications; exposure to toxins; previous exposure to heparin.
- *Physical examination*: skin and mucous membranes for colour, temperature, petechiae, purpura or bruises; vital signs; weight; mental status and level of consciousness;

heart and breath sounds; abdominal exam; body fluids for occult blood.

- *Diagnostic tests*: FBC, haemoglobin and haematocrit, platelet count; serological and ANA test results; bone marrow examination results.

Nursing diagnoses and interventions

Inadequate platelets impair haemostasis, placing the person at risk of bleeding. Bleeding gums, an early sign of the disorder, affect oral mucous membrane integrity as well.

Ineffective protection

Bleeding is a serious complication associated with thrombocytopenia. As platelet counts decrease, the risk of bleeding increases. The risk is minimal with counts greater than 100×10^9/L, moderate when the count is around 50×10^9/L and significant when the count falls below 20×10^9/L.

- Monitor vital signs, heart and breath sounds every 4 hours. Frequently assess for other manifestations of bleeding:
  a. skin and mucous membranes for petechiae, ecchymoses and haematoma formation
  b. gums, nasal membranes and conjunctiva for bleeding
  c. overt or occult blood in emesis, urine or stool
  d. vaginal bleeding
  e. prolonged bleeding from puncture sites
  f. neurological changes: headache, visual changes, altered mental status, decreasing level of consciousness, seizures
  g. abdominal: epigastric pain, absence of bowel sounds, increasing abdominal girth, abdominal guarding or rigidity.

  Early identification of bleeding is important to prevent serious blood loss and shock.

> **CONSIDERATION FOR PRACTICE**
>
> **Avoid invasive procedures such as rectal temperatures, urinary catheterisation and parenteral injections to the extent possible. Diagnostic procedures such as biopsy or lumbar puncture should be avoided if the platelet count is less than 150×10^9/L. Invasive procedures can cause tissue trauma and bleeding. Procedures that use large-bore needles should be delayed until the platelet count is increased.**

- Apply pressure to puncture sites for 3 to 5 minutes; apply pressure to arterial puncture sites for 15 to 20 minutes. *Pressure promotes haemostasis and clot formation.*
- Instruct to avoid forcefully blowing the nose or picking crusts from the nose, straining to have a bowel movement and forceful coughing or sneezing. *These activities increase the risk of external and internal bleeding.*

Impaired oral mucous membranes

Thrombocytopenia frequently leads to bleeding of the gums and oral mucosa. As a result, risk of infection and impaired nutrition increases.

- Frequently assess the mouth for bleeding. Inquire about oral pain or tenderness. *Breakdown of oral mucous membranes increases the risk of infection and bleeding and causes discomfort with eating.*
- Encourage use of a soft-bristle toothbrush or sponge to clean teeth and gums. *Hard bristles may abrade oral mucosa, causing bleeding and increasing the risk of infection.*
- Instruct to rinse the mouth with saline every 2 to 4 hours. Apply petroleum jelly to lips as needed to prevent dryness and cracking. *Saline mouth rinses and petroleum jelly help maintain oral tissue integrity and promote cleansing and healing.*
- Instruct to avoid alcohol-based mouthwashes, very hot foods, alcohol and crusty foods. Teach to drink cool liquids at least every 2 hours. *Avoiding foods and liquids that traumatise oral mucosa increases comfort; fluid intake prevents dehydration and helps maintain mucous membrane integrity.*

Community-based care

In the adult, ITP often is a chronic disorder that the person and their family must learn to manage. Secondary thrombocytopenia may be either acute or chronic. Discuss the following topics when preparing the person and family for home care:

- nature of the disorder, its usual course and the treatment plan
- use of and desired and potential adverse effects of prescribed medications
- risks and benefits of surgery or treatments such as plasma replacement therapy
- the importance of follow-up tests and visits for care
- measures to reduce the risk of bleeding: safety measures such as a soft-bristle toothbrush, electric razor, avoidance of contact sports and hazardous activities, and avoiding medications that further interfere with platelet function (see Box 32.6).

Refer for home health or other community services (e.g. housekeeping, shopping) as indicated.

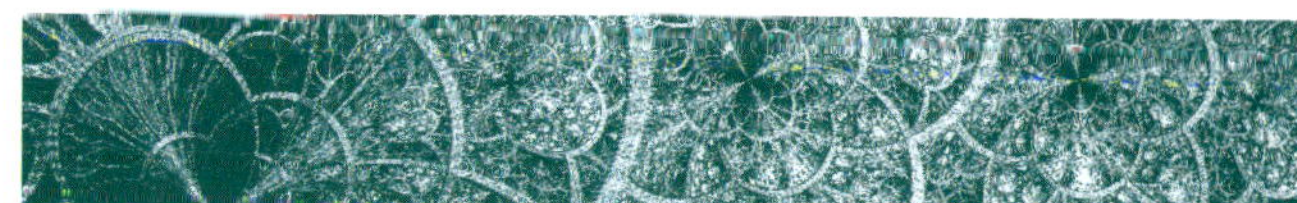

THE PERSON WITH HAEMOPHILIA

Haemophilia is a group of hereditary clotting factor disorders that lead to persistent and sometimes severe bleeding, with a 40% reduction in normal clotting factor (see the 'Genetic considerations' box). Although often considered a disease of children, haemophilia may be diagnosed in adults. There are over 3,000 people in Australia diagnosed with haemophilia and it is estimated that 2,300 people may have von Willebrand disease alone, with many more undiagnosed (Haemophilia Foundation Australia, 2022). Deficiencies of three clotting factors—VIII, IX and XI—account for 90–95% of the bleeding disorders collectively called haemophilia.

GENETIC CONSIDERATIONS
Focus on haemophilia

The incidence and pattern of inheritance for the forms of haemophilia differ:

- Haemophilia A occurs in about 1 in 10,000 male births, transmitted on the X chromosome: each male offspring has a 50% risk of inheriting the defective gene; each female offspring has a 50% risk of becoming a carrier.
- Haemophilia B occurs in about 1 in 100,000 male births, transmitted on the X chromosome.
- Von Willebrand's disease is usually inherited as an autosomal trait: offspring of an affected person have a 50% risk of inheriting the trait and the disorder.
- Factor XI deficiency inherited as an autosomal recessive trait: each offspring of a carrier and an unaffected individual has a 50% risk of inheriting the trait; each offspring of two carriers has a 50% risk of being a carrier and a 25% risk of having the disorder.

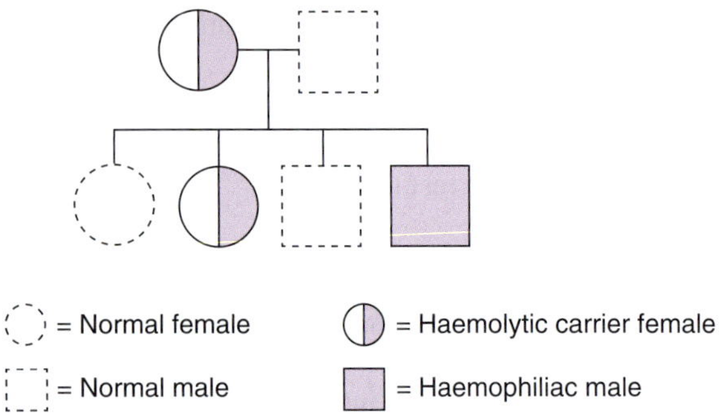

FIGURE 32.13 ***The inheritance pattern of haemophilia A and B. Both are transmitted as X-linked recessive disorders. Females may be carriers, but males develop these disorders***

Physiology review

When tissue injury occurs, platelets collect at the site, adhering to the damaged vessel wall (the platelet plug). Activation of the clotting cascade, a sequential process of interactive reactions of clotting factors, is vital to form a stable clot. Clotting factors are plasma proteins primarily produced by the liver. A number of these factors require the presence of vitamin K for synthesis and activation. Once the clot has been formed and stabilised, it begins to retract, pulling together the edges of the damaged blood vessel to initiate the healing process.

Pathophysiology

Haemophilia A (or *classic haemophilia*) is the most common type of haemophilia, caused by deficiency or dysfunction of clotting factor VIII. It is transmitted as an X-linked recessive disorder from mothers to sons (see Figure 32.13). The genetic defect of haemophilia A on the X chromosome may cause deficient factor VIII production or a defective form of the protein. When the concentration of the clotting factor is 5–35% of normal, the disease is *mild*. Bleeding is infrequent and usually associated with trauma. Concentrations of 1–5% of normal result in *moderate* disease. Again, bleeding usually occurs secondarily to trauma. *Severe* haemophilia occurs when concentrations are less than 1% of normal. Bleeding is frequent, often occurring without trauma.

Haemophilia B (also called *Christmas disease*) accounts for about 15% of cases and is caused by a deficiency in factor IX. Despite the difference in clotting factor deficits, haemophilia A and B are clinically identical.

Von Willebrand's disease, often considered a type of haemophilia, is the most common hereditary bleeding disorder (Haemophilia Foundation Australia, 2022). It is caused by a deficit of or defective von Willebrand (vW) factor, a protein that mediates platelet adhesion. Reduced levels of factor VIII often also are present because vW factor carries factor VIII. This clotting disorder affects men and women equally. Bleeding associated with von Willebrand's disease rarely is severe. It often is diagnosed when prolonged bleeding follows surgery or a dental extraction.

Factor XI deficiency (or *haemophilia C*) is usually a mild disorder, identified when postoperative bleeding is prolonged. A comparison of the types of haemophilia is found in Table 32.8.

People with haemophilia form a platelet plug at the site of bleeding, but the clotting factor deficit impairs formation of a stable fibrin clot. The effect of vW factor deficiency is somewhat different, in that platelet aggregation at the site of injury is impaired. In either case, prolonged or extensive bleeding may result. Often bleeding occurs in response to injury or as a result of surgery. However, a severe clotting factor deficit can lead to spontaneous bleeding into the joints (*haemarthrosis*), deep tissues and CNS. Haemarthrosis often causes joint deformity and disability, usually of the elbows, hips, knees and ankles (Hoots & Shapiro, 2022).

Manifestations

The following are manifestations of haemophilia:

- haemarthrosis
- easy bruising and cutaneous haematoma formation with minor trauma (e.g. an injection)

TABLE 32.8 Types of haemophilia

TYPE/NAME	DEFICIENCY	CHARACTERISTICS	TREATMENT
Haemophilia A (classic haemophilia)	Factor VIII	Transmitted by females; occurs primarily in males; bleeding time normal; coagulation time prolonged	Factor VIII concentrate or cryoprecipitate
Haemophilia B	Factor IX	Transmitted by females; occurs primarily in males; bleeding time normal; coagulation time prolonged	Factor IX (Christmas disease concentrate)
Von Willebrand's disease	vW factor Factor VIII	Occurs in both females and males; bleeding time and coagulation time are both prolonged	Cryoprecipitate and desmopressin acetate (DDAVP)
Factor XI deficiency	Factor XI	Occurs in both males and females; the activated partial thromboplastin time is prolonged	Fresh frozen plasma

- bleeding from the gums and prolonged bleeding following minor injuries or cuts
- gastrointestinal bleeding, with haematemesis (vomiting blood), occult blood in the stools, gastric pain or abdominal pain
- spontaneous haematuria or epistaxis (nosebleed)
- pain or paralysis due to the pressure of haematomas on nerves
- intracranial haemorrhage is a potentially life-threatening manifestation of haemophilia.

INTERPROFESSIONAL CARE

Treatment of haemophilia focuses on preventing and/or treating bleeding, primarily by replacing deficient clotting factors. Specific treatment depends on the severity of the disorder and the specific factor deficiency. Care may be complicated by hepatitis or HIV disease in people with haemophilia treated with clotting factor concentrates prepared from multiple units of donated blood. Today, routine testing of all blood, improved blood donor screening and current methods of treating haemophilia have significantly reduced the risk of these blood-borne diseases.

Diagnosis

The following laboratory tests may be ordered:

- *Serum platelet levels* are measured and are usually normal.
- *Coagulation studies* such as APTT, bleeding time and prothrombin time are used to screen for haemophilia when abnormal bleeding occurs. APTT is increased in all types of haemophilia. Prothrombin time is unaffected in these disorders but may be measured to rule out other disorders. Bleeding time is prolonged in von Willebrand's disease but normal in haemophilia A and B.
- *Factor assays* are performed; factor VIII is decreased in haemophilia A and often in von Willebrand's disease, factor IX is decreased in haemophilia B and factor XI in haemophilia C.
- *Amniocentesis* or *chorionic villus sampling* is used to identify the genetic defect of haemophilia when there is a known family history of the disease.

Medications

Deficient clotting factors are replaced regularly, as a prophylactic measure before surgery and dental procedures, and to control bleeding. Clotting factors may be given as fresh frozen plasma, cryoprecipitates or concentrates. Factor levels are measured on a regular basis to determine whether the treatment is adequate. Clotting factors are often self administered and may be taken on either a regular or intermittent schedule.

Fresh frozen plasma replaces all clotting factors (including both factor VIII and factor IX) except platelets. When the cause of bleeding is not yet determined, fresh frozen plasma may be administered intravenously until a definitive diagnosis is made.

Haemophilia A is usually treated with either heat-treated factor VIII concentrate (heat treating reduces the risk of transmitting disease) or recombinant factor VIII. Although recombinant factor VIII, produced using recombinant DNA technology, eliminates the risk of viral disease transmission, its use is limited by cost. The dose of factor VIII is determined by the severity of the deficit and the presence or prospect of active bleeding (e.g. planned surgery).

Desmopressin acetate (DDAVP) may be given to people with mild haemophilia A or von Willebrand's disease prior to minor surgeries. This drug causes release of factor VIII and will raise blood levels two- or threefold for several hours, reducing the risk of bleeding and the need for clotting factor concentrate (Haemophilia Foundation Australia, 2022).

Factor IX concentrate (administered intravenously) is used to treat haemophilia B. Because factor IX concentrates also contain a number of other proteins, there is risk of thrombosis with recurrent use. They are used judiciously, only when needed. Products produced by recombinant technology or that are monoclonally purified carry a lower risk of stimulating thrombus formation (Loscalzo et al., 2022). Fresh frozen plasma replaces factor XI and is used when necessary. It may be given daily until the risk of bleeding decreases.

Factor VIII concentrates contain functional vW factor and may be used to treat von Willebrand's disease. Aspirin is avoided in all types of haemophilia.

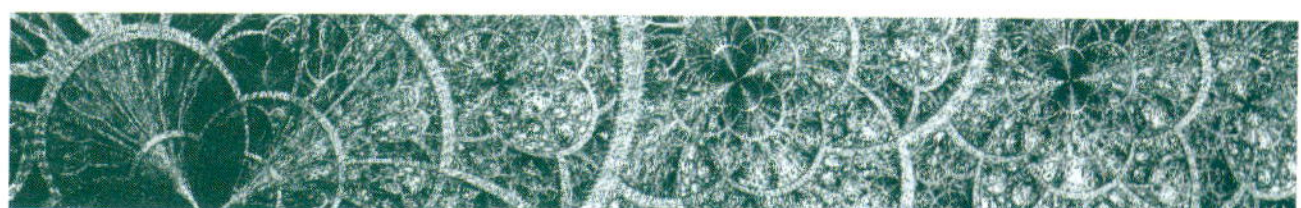

Nursing care

Although primary responsibility for care falls to the person and family, nursing care presents challenges. For additional assessment and nursing care strategies for a person with haemophilia, see the accompanying nursing care plan.

Health promotion

Encourage people with a family history of haemophilia or bleeding disorders to seek genetic counselling during their family planning process. Although tests are available for the haemophilia gene, the technology to correct the disorder in utero does not yet exist. See the chapter 'Genetic implications of adult health nursing'.

Assessment

While severe haemophilia usually is diagnosed in childhood, milder cases may not be identified until surgery, invasive dental work or a traumatic injury causes extensive or prolonged bleeding. Focused assessment related to haemophilia includes the following:

- *Health history*: previous bleeding episodes with or without trauma; history of easy bruising, haematomas, epistaxis, bleeding gums, haematuria, vomiting blood or joint pain; aspirin use; family history of haemophilia or bleeding disorders.

- *Physical examination*: vital signs; bruising or bleeding of skin or mucous membranes; mental status; abdominal assessment; presence of joint deformity, decreased range of motion.
- *Diagnostic tests*: FBC including haemoglobin, haematocrit and platelet count; clotting factor assays; tests for occult blood (urine, stool, emesis); x-ray and scan results for evidence of bleeding.

Nursing diagnoses and interventions

Impaired blood clotting, the need for continuing care and disease management, and the risk of genetic transmission of haemophilia are priority problems for the person with haemophilia.

Ineffective protection

The inability to form stable clots and stem bleeding from injured blood vessels creates a significant risk for the person with haemophilia. Nursing care measures focus on preventing injury and protecting the skin from damage.

- Monitor for signs of bleeding, including haematomas, ecchymoses and purpura, as well as surface oozing or bleeding. Check emesis and stool for occult blood. *Bleeding may occur in cutaneous tissues as well as internal organs. Bleeding in the upper gastrointestinal tract may not be readily apparent in the stool.*
- Notify the doctor of any apparent bleeding. *Prompt intervention with administration of clotting factor concentrate decreases the risk of haemorrhage and subsequent hypovolaemia.*
- Avoid intramuscular injections, rectal temperatures and enemas. *These can pose a risk of tissue and vascular trauma, which can precipitate bleeding.*
- Use safety measures in personal care. For example, use an electric razor rather than a razor blade to shave. *Use of an electric razor minimises the opportunity to develop superficial cuts that may result in bleeding.*
- If bleeding occurs, control blood loss using gentle pressure, ice or a topical haemostatic agent, such as topical thrombin. *Direct pressure occludes bleeding vessels. Ice, a vasoconstrictor, may facilitate bleeding control, as do topical haemostatic agents.*

NURSING CARE PLAN A person with haemophilia

John Cruise is a 20-year-old TAFE student. He is admitted to the emergency department with a nosebleed that began when he fell during a touch football game. It has continued to bleed for over an hour.

ASSESSMENT

Mr Cruise states that he has haemophilia and realises that playing contact sport 'is probably a dumb thing to do'. He adds that he has not had any recent bleeding episodes. An icebag and manual pressure are applied in the emergency department. The doctor orders factor VIII concentrate to be administered. Physical assessment findings are 36.2°C, BP 118/64, R 18. Skin pale but warm. Laboratory tests reveal a prolonged APTT and a normal bleeding time and PT. Following treatment, Mr Cruise's bleeding subsides.

DIAGNOSES

- *Risk of aspiration* related to uncontrolled nosebleed.
- *Non-compliance* with activity recommendations.
- *Ineffective protection* related to lack of clotting factor VIII.

PLANNING

- Monitoring and reduction of potential complications required.
- Education required regarding disease risks and how to treat symptoms.

Expected outcomes

- Maintain an open airway.
- Maintain vital signs within his usual range.
- Exhibit no further signs of bleeding.
- Identify sports and recreation activities in which he can safely participate.
- Verbalise self-care measures to control bleeding.

IMPLEMENTATION

- Monitor vital signs and for further signs of bleeding.
- Assess airway and auscultate breath sounds.
- Review emergency measures to help stop bleeding.
- Reiterate the importance of seeking prompt medical attention if bleeding should occur.
- Advise regarding the importance of wearing a Medic-Alert® bracelet identifying him as a haemophiliac.
- Discuss alternative non-contact sports and recreational activities.

EVALUATION

On discharge, Mr Cruise has no further signs of bleeding, shock or aspiration. He is able to verbalise methods to help stop local bleeding and the importance of seeking medical attention promptly when bleeding continues. Mr Cruise agrees to stop at a local chemist on the way home to order a MedicAlert® bracelet. In addition, Mr Cruise verbalises an understanding of the importance of avoiding contact sports and has identified swimming and golf as alternative leisure activities that he might enjoy.

CRITICAL THINKING IN THE NURSING PROCESS

1. What is the pathophysiological basis for the bleeding that occurs in haemophilia A and B?
2. What was Mr Cruise's priority nursing diagnosis? Why?
3. Why is family planning a special consideration with a person who has haemophilia?
4. Outline a plan to teach the family of a person diagnosed with haemophilia how to administer an intravenous infusion.
5. Develop a care plan for Mr Cruise for the nursing diagnosis of *Impaired social interaction*. Consider Mr Cruise's age and developmental level in creating the plan.

REFLECTION ON THE NURSING PROCESS

1. What are the take-home messages you have learned in this case study?
2. How can they be used within your daily practice?

- Instruct to avoid activities that increase the risk of trauma, including contact sports and physical exertion associated with job performance, and to eliminate safety hazards in the home. *Depending on the severity of the clotting factor deficit, even minor trauma can lead to serious bleeding episodes. Safer activities such as non-contact sports (e.g. swimming, golf) and occupations that do not require physical labour may be substituted.*

Risk of ineffective health maintenance

Haemophilia is a chronic disorder, requiring active management to prevent and control bleeding and complications. Frequent visits to the doctor or clinic may be necessary. In addition, the person may need to learn to self-administer clotting factors and measures to prevent complications. The lifelong nature of the disorder may interfere with compliance, especially during early adulthood.

- Assess knowledge of disorder and the related treatments. Assessment allows identification of knowledge gaps and provides a basis on which to provide additional information. *Impaired disease management may be due to lack of knowledge or a conscious decision not to follow the recommendations of the healthcare provider.*
- Provide information about the bleeding disorder and prescribed medications and treatments. *Individualised instruction is more effective than general, possibly irrelevant information.*
- Provide emotional support, expressing confidence in the person's self-care abilities. *Emotional support helps the person incorporate the care regimen into their lifestyle.*
- Provide supervised learning and practice opportunities for administering clotting factors and topical haemostatic agents. *Successful practice sessions instil confidence in the ability to manage care and provide an opportunity for questions and exploring alternatives.*

Community-based care

Discuss the following topics when preparing the person with a bleeding disorder and the family for home care:

- Recognising the manifestations of internal bleeding: pallor, weakness, restlessness, headache, disorientation, pain, swelling. These manifestations require emergency medical care and should be reported immediately.
- Applying cold packs and immobilising the joint for 24 to 48 hours if haemarthrosis occurs.
- Using analgesics for pain; avoiding prescription and over-the-counter drugs containing aspirin.
- Ensuring a safe home environment (e.g. padding sharp edges of furniture, using transition lighting or a night light, avoiding scatter rugs and wearing protective gloves when working in the house or garden).
- Using safe grooming practices such as electric razors.
- Wearing a MedicAlert® bracelet in case of accident.
- Practising good dental hygiene to decrease potential tooth decay and extractions. If dental procedures are necessary, discuss the need for prophylactic factor administration with the dentist and doctor
- Following safer sex practices.
- Preparing and administering intravenous medications.

Refer the person and family to a local haemophilia or bleeding disorders support group. Provide contact information for national organisations and support services, such as the Australian Haemophilia Foundation https://www.haemophilia.org.au.

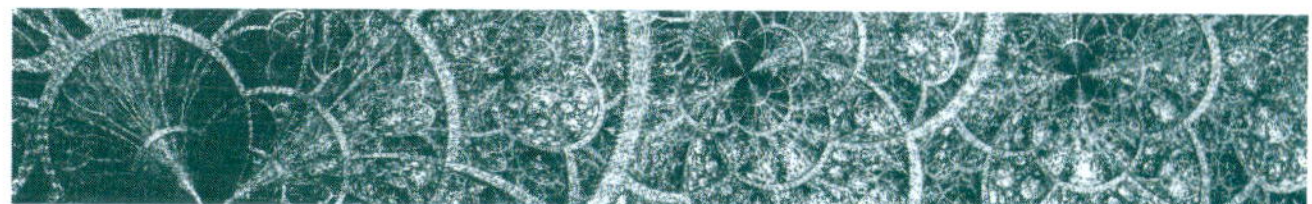

THE PERSON WITH DISSEMINATED INTRAVASCULAR COAGULATION

Disseminated intravascular coagulation (DIC) is a disruption of haemostasis characterised by widespread intravascular clotting and bleeding. It may be acute and life threatening or relatively mild. DIC is a clinical syndrome that develops as a complication of a wide variety of other disorders (see Box 32.8). Sepsis is the most common cause of DIC, as well as trauma, cancer, childbirth and pregnancy complications, and less commonly snake bites (Levi, 2022).

Pathophysiology

DIC is triggered by endothelial damage, release of tissue factors into the circulation or inappropriate activation of the clotting cascade by an endotoxin. Both the intrinsic and the extrinsic clotting cascade may be activated, although the extrinsic cascade usually is the one activated. Extensive thrombin entering the systemic circulation overwhelms natural anticoagulants, leading to unrestricted clot formation. Clotting may be localised to an individual organ or widespread with deposition of small thrombi and emboli throughout the microvasculature. The widespread clotting consumes clotting factors (prothrombin, platelets, factor V and factor VIII, in particular) and activates fibrinolytic processes with anticoagulant production (Levi, 2022). As a result, haemorrhage occurs (see Figure 32.14).

The sequence of DIC follows:

1. Endothelial damage, tissue factors or toxins stimulate the clotting cascade.
2. Excess thrombin within the circulation overwhelms naturally occurring anticoagulants.

BOX 32.8 Conditions that may precipitate disseminated intravascular coagulation

Tissue damage

- Trauma: burns, gunshot wounds, frostbite, head injury
- Obstetric complications: septic abortion, abruptio placentae, amniotic fluid embolus, retained dead fetus
- Neoplasms: acute leukaemia, adenocarcinomas
- Haemolysis
- Fat embolism

Vessel damage

- Aortic aneurysm
- Acute glomerulonephritis
- Haemolytic uraemic syndrome

Infections

- Bacterial infection or sepsis
- Viral or mycotic infections
- Parasitic or rickettsial infection

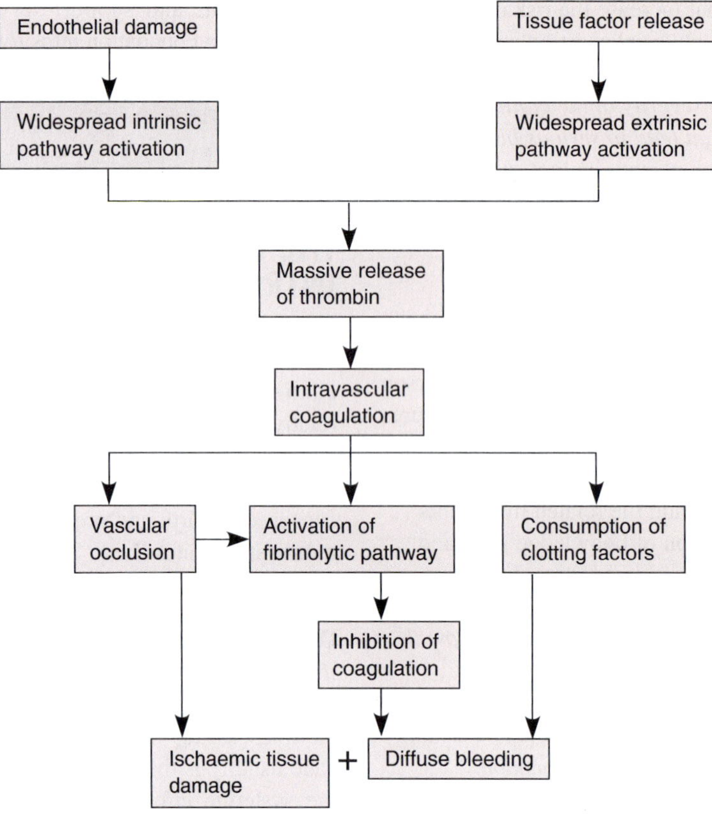

FIGURE 32.14 ***Disseminated intravascular coagulation (DIC). Endothelial cell injury or release of tissue factors activates the intrinsic or extrinsic clotting pathway (or both). As a result, numerous microthrombi form throughout the vasculature, causing ischaemic tissue damage. Simultaneously, rapid consumption of clotting factors and activation of fibrinolytic mechanisms trigger widespread bleeding***

3. Widespread clotting occurs within the microvasculature.
4. Thrombi and emboli impair tissue perfusion, leading to ischaemia, infarction and necrosis.
5. Clotting factors and platelets are consumed faster than they can be replaced.
6. Clotting activates fibrinolytic processes, which begin to break down clots.
7. Fibrin degradation products (FDPs, potent anticoagulants) are released, contributing to bleeding.
8. Clotting factors are depleted, the ability to form clots is lost and haemorrhage occurs.

Manifestations

The manifestations of DIC result from both clotting and bleeding, although bleeding is more obvious, especially in acute DIC. Bleeding ranges from oozing blood following an injection to frank haemorrhage from every body orifice (see the 'Manifestations' box). Chronic DIC may be asymptomatic or may present with peripheral cyanosis, thrombosis and pre-gangrenous changes in the fingers and toes, nose and genitalia with superficial thrombophlebitis, as well as deep venous thrombosis.

MANIFESTATIONS **DIC**

- Frank haemorrhage from incisions
- Oozing of blood from punctures, intravenous catheter sites
- Purpura, petechiae, bruising
- Cyanosis of extremities
- Gastrointestinal bleeding or haemorrhage
- Dyspnoea, tachypnoea, bloody sputum
- Tachycardia, hypotension
- Haematuria, oliguria, acute renal failure
- Manifestations of increased intracranial pressure: decreased level of consciousness, pupillary, motor and sensory changes
- Mental status changes

INTERPROFESSIONAL CARE

Treatment of DIC is directed towards treating the underlying disorder and preventing further bleeding or massive thrombosis. Prompt treatment stabilises the person, reduces complications and allows recovery to occur; it does not cure DIC.

Diagnosis

Diagnostic tests are used to confirm the diagnosis of DIC and evaluate the risk of haemorrhage.

- *FBC* and *platelet count* are used to evaluate the haemoglobin, haematocrit and number of circulating platelets. *Schistocytes*, fragmented RBCs, may be noted due to cell trapping and damage within fibrin thrombi. The platelet count is decreased.
- *Coagulation studies* show prolonged prothrombin time (PT), *partial thromboplastin time (PTT)* and thrombin time, and a *low fibrinogen level* due to depletion of clotting factors. The fibrinogen level helps predict bleeding in DIC: as it falls, the risk of bleeding increases.
- *Fibrin degradation products (FDPs)* or *fibrin split products (FSPs)*, and plasma D-dimers are increased due to the fibrinolysis that occurs with DIC.

Treatment

When bleeding is the major manifestation of DIC, fresh frozen plasma and platelet concentrates are given to restore clotting factors and platelets. Heparin, although controversial, may be administered. Heparin interferes with the clotting cascade and may prevent further clotting factor consumption due to uncontrolled thrombosis. It is used when bleeding is not controlled by plasma and platelets, as well as when the person has manifestations of thrombotic problems such as acrocyanosis and possible gangrene. Long-term heparin therapy (administered by injection or continuous infusion using a portable pump) may be necessary for people with chronic DIC.

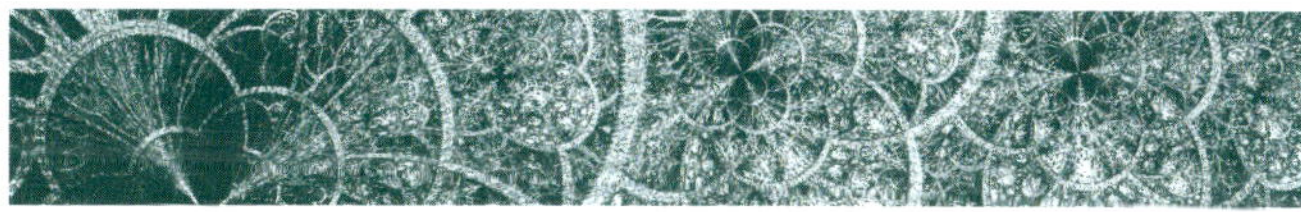

Nursing care

Assessment

Nurses can be instrumental in identifying early manifestations of DIC, facilitating timely intervention. Focused nursing assessment for DIC includes:

- *Health history*: recent abortion (spontaneous or therapeutic) or current pregnancy; presence of a known malignant tumour; history of abnormal bleeding episodes or a haematological disorder.
- *Physical examination*: bleeding from puncture wounds (e.g. injections), IV sites, incisions, haematuria, obvious or occult blood in emesis or stool, epistaxis, other abnormal bleeding; vital signs; heart and breath sounds; abdominal assessment, including girth, contour, bowel sounds, tenderness or guarding to palpation; colour, temperature, skin condition of hands, feet and digits; petechiae or purpura of skin, mucous membranes.
- *Diagnostic tests*: FBC with haemoglobin, haematocrit; platelet count; coagulation studies; evaluations of organ system function (e.g. liver and renal function tests); CT scans of the head and abdomen.

Nursing diagnoses and interventions

People with acute DIC often are critically ill, with multiple nursing care needs. Priority nursing diagnoses discussed in this section focus on impaired tissue perfusion and gas exchange, pain and fear. Septic shock may precipitate DIC; haemorrhagic shock may occur as a complication of DIC. See the chapter 'Nursing care of people experiencing trauma and shock' for nursing diagnoses and interventions related to these problems.

Ineffective tissue perfusion

Thrombi and emboli forming throughout the microcirculation affect the perfusion of multiple organs and tissues. Additionally, bleeding due to clotting factor consumption affects cardiac output and blood flow to these tissues.

- Assess extremity pulses, warmth and capillary refill. Monitor level of consciousness (LOC) and mental status. *Monitoring central and peripheral tissue perfusion facilitates early treatment of impaired perfusion.*
- Carefully reposition person at least every 2 hours. *Position changes facilitate circulation and tissue perfusion and also provide an opportunity to assess for purpura, pallor and bleeding.*
- Discourage crossing the legs and do not elevate the knees on the bed or with a pillow. *These positions may impair arterial and venous flow to the lower legs and feet, increasing vascular stasis and the risk of thrombosis.*
- Minimise use of tape on the skin, using binders, non-adhesive dressings and other devices as needed. *Preventing skin trauma reduces the risk of bleeding and potential infection.*

> **CONSIDERATION FOR PRACTICE**
>
> **Promptly report complaints of chest pain, changes in mental status, LOC, tissue perfusion, respirations, gastrointestinal function and urinary output. Chest pain or respiratory changes (tachypnoea, dyspnoea, orthopnoea) may be due to angina, pulmonary embolism or bleeding into lung tissue. Changes in mentation or LOC can indicate cerebral ischaemia. A painful, pale and cold extremity with no or diminished pulses indicates arterial occlusion. Prompt intervention is critical to save the extremity. Acute abdominal pain, decreased bowel sounds and GI bleeding may indicate mesenteric occlusion, a surgical emergency. Decreased urine output may signify renal artery thrombosis; renal failure may develop.**

Impaired gas exchange

Microclots in the pulmonary vasculature are likely to interfere with gas exchange in the person with DIC.

- Monitor oxygen saturation continuously. Administer oxygen as required/ordered. Oxygen saturation levels are a non-invasive means of assessing gas exchange. *Supplemental oxygen promotes gas exchange and reduces cardiac work, relieving dyspnoea.*

> **CONSIDERATION FOR PRACTICE**
> **Monitor arterial blood gas results; report abnormal results to the doctor. Low PaO_2 and rising $PaCO_2$ levels indicate impaired gas exchange and may signify the need for additional treatment.**

- Place in Fowler's or high-Fowler's position as tolerated. *Elevating the head of the bed improves diaphragmatic excursion and alveolar ventilation.*
- Maintain bed rest. *Bed rest reduces oxygen demands and cardiac work.*
- Encourage deep breathing and effective coughing. *Increased respiratory depth and clearance of secretions from airways improves alveolar ventilation and oxygenation.*
- Cautious nasotracheal suctioning may be instituted if cough is ineffective or an endotracheal tube is in place. *Removal of secretions facilitates ventilation and oxygenation. However, care must be used to minimise suction-induced hypoxia and airway trauma.*
- Administer analgesics and anti-anxiety drugs as needed to control pain and anxiety. Provide reassurance and comfort measures. *Pain and anxiety increase the respiratory rate and decrease the depth of respirations, reducing effective ventilation and gas exchange.*

Pain

Both the underlying cause of DIC and tissue ischaemia from microvascular clots can cause pain. Identifying the aetiology of pain is important to identify potential complications or harmful effects of DIC and to institute effective treatment.

- Use a standard pain scale to evaluate and monitor pain and analgesic effectiveness. *Monitoring pain and response to medication facilitates development of an appropriate and effective treatment plan.*
- Handle extremities gently. *Gentle handling reduces the risk of further injury to, and pain in, ischaemic tissues.*
- Apply cool compresses to painful joints. *Application of cold decreases pain through the gate-control mechanism, inhibiting the dorsal horn of the spinal cord and reducing the sensation of pain.*

> **CONSIDERATION FOR PRACTICE**
> **Notify the doctor promptly of new or a sudden increase in pain, especially when accompanied by changes in assessment findings. New or increased complaints of pain may signify increased circulatory impairment and ischaemic changes in tissues such as the heart, bowel or extremities. Circulation to a painful, pale or cyanotic, or cold extremity may be occluded by an arterial clot. Prompt intervention is necessary to save the extremity. Acute abdominal pain may signify mesenteric occlusion, a surgical emergency. Anginal pain may indicate occlusion of coronary arteries.**

> **CONSIDERATION FOR PRACTICE**
> **Continuously monitor effects of analgesics and mental and respiratory status. Analgesics may mask manifestations of neurological impairment due to thromboembolism and may depress the respiratory centre, further impairing gas exchange. Judicious analgesic administration with careful monitoring is vital to safely provide effective pain relief.**

Fear

The underlying serious illness and a complication such as DIC result in an uncertain prognosis, often accompanied by fear.

- Encourage the person and family to verbalise concerns. *This helps the person and family identify their concerns and frame questions.*
- Answer questions truthfully. Providing honest answers is vital to developing a therapeutic nurse–individual relationship. *Accurate responses allow the person and their family to set priorities as they plan for an uncertain future.*
- Help the person and family identify coping strategies to manage this significant situational stressor. *Implementing past effective coping methods may provide the skills to manage the current crisis.*
- Provide emotional support. *The presence of a caring nurse helps reduce the fear and anxiety associated with a crisis.*
- Maintain a calm environment. *A calm environment provides reassurance that the situation is in control, reduces anxiety and promotes rest.*
- Respond promptly when the person calls for help. *Prompt response to expressed needs helps develop a trusting relationship and a sense of security that assistance is readily available.*
- Teach relaxation techniques. *Relaxation techniques can reduce muscle tension and other signs of anxiety. Gaining control over physical responses can help the person gain a sense of control over the situation.*

Community-based care

Although the immediate crisis of acute DIC is resolved prior to discharge, the person may have some continuing effects of the disorder, such as impaired tissue integrity of distal extremities. Teach the person and family about specific care needs, such as foot care (see Box 31.6) or dressing changes. Provide instruction about any continuing medications and follow-up care.

People with chronic DIC may require continuing heparin therapy, using either intermittent subcutaneous injections or a portable infusion pump. Teach the person and family members how to administer the injection or manage the infusion pump. Provide a referral to home healthcare or a home intravenous management service for assistance. Discuss the manifestations of excessive bleeding or recurrent clotting that need to be reported to the doctor.

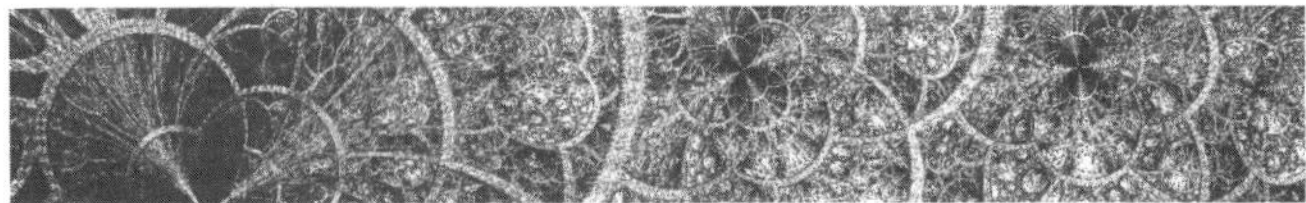

CHAPTER HIGHLIGHTS

- Anaemia is the most common disorder of the red blood cells; nutritional deficiencies are the most common causes of anaemia. Its manifestations relate to the function of red blood cells and haemoglobin, transporting oxygen to the cells: fatigue, increased respiratory and heart rates, shortness of breath with activity and pallor.
- Genetically transmitted disorders such as sickle cell disease and thalassaemia can cause significant anaemia and associated problems in affected populations. These people require teaching and episodic acute care for crises such as vaso-occlusive crisis in sickle cell disease.
- Nursing care related to anaemia is primarily educational to prepare the person for effective self-care, including diet, prescribed medications and measures to prevent sickling episodes (for those with sickle cell disease).
- Leukaemia and lymphomas are the primary disorders of white blood cells and lymphoid tissues.
- Manifestations of the leukaemias reflect the altered ability of abnormal white blood cells to perform effective immune surveillance and crowding of the bone marrow and other organs by rapidly proliferating cells. Frequent sore throats, increased risk of infection and manifestations of anaemia and thrombocytopenia are seen, as well as an enlarged spleen and abdominal pain.
- Four major subgroups of leukaemia are identified: acute and chronic myeloid leukaemias, and acute and chronic lymphocytic (or lymphoblastic) leukaemias. The primary population affected differs for each of these leukaemias, as does their course.
- Genetic alterations and certain viruses are linked to the development of leukaemia, as are exposure to chemotherapy drugs, environmental toxins and ionising radiation.
- Lymphocytic leukaemias and lymphomas are closely related disorders.
- Nursing care for people with leukaemia and lymphoma focuses on reducing the risk of infection and bleeding, managing the effects of chemotherapy and radiation therapy and, in some cases, caring for people before and after bone marrow or stem cell transplant.
- The major risks associated with bone marrow and stem cell transplant are infection prior to, and immediately following, the transplant; and graft-versus-host disease, a potentially fatal condition. A pruritic rash and desquamation of the palms and soles; abdominal pain, nausea and diarrhoea; and jaundice and elevated liver enzymes are common early manifestations of GVHD.
- The treatment of and nursing care for people with lymphomas (including Hodgkin's disease and non-Hodgkin's lymphoma) is similar to that provided for people with leukaemia.
- Multiple myeloma is a malignancy of plasma cells, which are B lymphocytes that produce antibodies. Circulating M proteins and Bence Jones proteins in the urine are seen in multiple myeloma. The usual presenting manifestation is bone pain. Pathological fractures and hypercalcaemia are common complications of multiple myeloma as bone is destroyed.
- Bleeding and clotting disorders can result from either inadequate platelets (thrombocytopenia) or disruption of the clotting mechanisms (haemophilia, DIC). Petechiae and purpura are common manifestations of bleeding/clotting disorders.
- Haemophilias are genetically transmitted disorders. Haemophilia A and B are transmitted on the X chromosome (sex-linked) from mother to son. Von Willebrand's disease, the most common bleeding disorder, is transmitted as an autosomal dominant disorder and affects men and women equally.
- Haemophilias are treated by replacement of the missing clotting factor and measures to prevent injury and bleeding.
- Disseminated intravascular coagulation is a disorder of widespread microvascular clotting. It commonly is precipitated by sepsis, but also may occur with conditions such as major trauma, malignancy or as an obstetric emergency.
- In DIC, platelets and clotting factors are consumed by the abnormal clotting processes, leading to the manifestations of bleeding, including frank haemorrhage, haematuria, oozing blood from parenteral and intravenous injection sites, and GI bleeding. Blood flow to organs and tissues is compromised by clot formation, leading to manifestations such as cyanosis of extremities, abdominal pain, kidney failure and changes in mental status and level of consciousness. Nursing care is supportive, focusing on administering prescribed treatments and monitoring and supporting cardiovascular, respiratory and kidney function.

CONCEPT CHECK

1 In assessing a woman with moderate anaemia, the nurse would expect to find which of the following?

1 haematocrit 45%
2 pulse rate 140
3 complaints of shortness of breath with exercise
4 WCC 150 $\times$ 10^9/L

2 The nurse caring for a person after gastric resection observes carefully for evidence of nutritional deficiency anaemia related to malabsorption, including:

1 numbness and tingling of extremities
2 steatorrhoea
3 dark yellow or bronze skin colour
4 bone pain

3 The nurse caring for a person with acute myeloid leukaemia plans which of the following nursing interventions during hospitalisation? (Select all that apply.)

1 Place in a private room.
2 Implement airborne infection control precautions.
3 Assist with oral hygiene after meals.
4 Monitor rectal temperature q4h.
5 Request soft, bland diet.

4 The nurse caring for a person with lymphoma who is being started on chemotherapy regimens understands that chemotherapy drugs are used in combination to:

1 target malignant cells in different organs
2 prevent the development of adverse effects
3 target different phases of the cell cycle
4 support growth and development of normal cells

5 A person with multiple myeloma calls the home health nurse complaining of new-onset severe back pain. The appropriate response by the nurse is to:

1 reassure the person that bone pain is expected with this disease
2 inquire about the person's use of NSAIDs and analgesics to manage pain
3 suggest use of a back brace to reduce pain
4 notify the doctor of the onset of new pain

6 The nurse observes reddish-purple spots and areas of purple bruising on a newly admitted person. Which laboratory results support this assessment finding?

1 haematocrit 28%
2 platelets 100×10^9/L
3 INR 4.0
4 WCC 150×10^9/L

7 A person whose husband has haemophilia asks if her newborn baby girl could have the disease. The nurse's response is based on the knowledge that:

1 the most common forms of haemophilia are transmitted as sex-linked recessive disorders; her daughter is at risk of carrying the defective gene
2 because haemophilia is a sex-linked recessive disorder carried on the Y chromosome, her daughter has no risk of having or carrying the disease
3 haemophilia is an autosomal dominant disorder; therefore, her daughter has a 50% chance of having the disorder
4 although haemophilia is genetically transmitted, its pattern of inheritance is unknown and her daughter will need to be tested for the defective gene

8 The nurse administering platelets to a person with disseminated intravascular coagulation (DIC) understands that the intended effect of this treatment is to:

1 replace specific clotting factors
2 promote intravascular clotting
3 restore tissue oxygenation
4 replace depleted platelets

BIBLIOGRAPHY

Arepally, G. M. (2017). Heparin-induced thrombocytopenia. *Blood, 129*, 2864–2872. https://doi.org/10.1182/blood-2016-11-709873

Argent, E., Emdur, P., Monagle, P. et al. (2012). Australian paediatric surveillance unit study of haemoglobinopathies in Australian children. *Journal of Paediatrics and Child Health*, *48*(4), 356–360. doi: 10.1111/j.1440-1754.2011.02236.x

Arnold, D. & Cuker, A. (2022). Diagnostic approach to the adult with unexplained thrombocytopenia. *UpToDate*. Retrieved from https://www.uptodate.com/

Aster, J. & Stone, R. (2022). Clinical manifestations and diagnosis of myelodysplastic syndromes (MDS). *UpToDate*. Retrieved from https://www.uptodate.com/

Australian Bureau of Statistics (2022). *Census of population and housing: Cultural diversity data summary, 2021*. Retrieved from https://www.abs.gov.au/statistics/

Australian Commission on Safety and Quality in Health Care (ACSQHC) (2021). *National Safety and Quality Health Service Standards* (2nd ed.). Sydney: ACSQHC.

Australian Institute of Health and Welfare (AIHW) (2022). *Principal diagnosis data cube under ICD-10-AM Edition 11, 2020–21*. Canberra: AIHW.

Australian Sickle Cell Advocacy Inc. (2022). Retrieved from https://aussicklecelladvocacy.org/

Berliner, N. (2022). Approach to the adult with unexplained neutropenia. *UpToDate*. Retrieved from https://www.uptodate.com/

Besa, E. (2022a). Myelodysplastic syndrome (MDS). *Emedicine*. Retrieved from https://emedicine.medscape.com/

Besa, E. (2022b). Chronic myelogenous leukemia (CML). *Emedicine*. Retrieved from https://emedicine.medscape.com/

Cancer Australia (2022a). *Leukaemia statistics*. Retrieved from https://canceraustralia.gov.au/

Cancer Australia (2022b). *Lymphoma statistics*. Retrieved from https://canceraustralia.gov.au/

Cancer Australia (2022c). *Multiple myeloma statistics*. Retrieved from https://canceraustralia.gov.au/

Cancer Council (2022). *Leukaemia*. Retrieved from https://www.cancer.org.au/

DeBaun, M. & Galadanci, N. (2022). Sickle cell disease in sub-Saharan Africa. *UpToDate*. Retrieved from https://www.uptodate.com/

DeFaria, C. (2021). Neutropenia. *Emedicine*. Retrieved from https://emedicine.medscape.com/

Department of Health and Aged Care (2022). Retrieved from https://www.health.gov.au/

Dua, M., Bello-Manga, H., Carroll, Y. M., Galadanci, A., Ibrahim, U., King, A., Olanrewaju, A. & Estepp, J. (2022). Strategies to increase access to basic sickle cell disease care in low- and middle-income countries. *Expert Review of Hematology, 15*(4), 333–344. https://doi.org/10.1080/17474086.2022.2063116

Garcia-Manero, G., Chien, K. & Montalban-Bravo, G. (2020). Myelodysplastic syndromes: 2021 update on diagnosis, risk-stratification and management. *American Journal of Haematology, 95*(11), 1399–1420. https://doi.org/10.1002/ajh.25950

Haemophilia Foundation Australia (2022). *Haemophilia*. Retrieved from https://www.haemophilia.org.au

Halim-Fikri, B. H., Lederer, C. W., Baig, A. A. et al. (2022). Global Globin Network consensus paper: Classification and stratified roadmaps for improved thalassaemia care and prevention in 32 countries. *Journal of Personalised Medicine*, *12*, 552. https://doi.org/10.3390/jpm12040552

Hoots, K. & Shapiro, A. (2022). Clinical manifestations and diagnosis of hemophilia. *UpToDate*. Retrieved from https://www.uptodate.com/

Horton, T., Steuber, C. & Aster, J. (2022). Overview of the clinical presentation and diagnosis of acute lymphoblastic leukemia/lymphoma in children. *UpToDate*. Retrieved from https://www.uptodate.com/

Huether, S. & McCance, K. L. (2020). *Understanding pathophysiology* (7th ed.). New York: Elsevier.

Jones, W. C., Parry, C., Devine, S., Main, D. S. & Okuyama, S. (2015). Understanding distress in posttreatment adult leukemia and lymphoma survivors: A lifespan perspective. *Journal of Psychosocial Oncology*, *33*(2), 142–162.

Kotiah, S. (2020). Chronic myelogenous leukemia (CML) staging. *Emedicine*. Retrieved from https://emedicine.medscape.com/

Leukaemia Foundation (2022a). *Myelodysplastic syndromes (MDS)*. Retrieved from https://www.leukaemia.org.au/

Leukaemia Foundation (2022b). *Understanding chronic myeloid leukaemia (CML)*. Retrieved from https://www.leukaemia.org.au

Leukaemia Foundation (2022c). *Understanding chronic lymphocytic leukaemia* (CLL). Retrieved from https://www.leukaemia.org.au

Leukaemia Foundation (2022d). *Understanding Hodgkin lymphoma*. Retrieved from https://www.leukaemia.org.au

Levi, M. (2022). Disseminated intravascular coagulation (DIC). *Emedicine*. Retrieved from https://emedicine.medscape.com/

Loscalzo, J., Fauci, A. S., Kasper, D. L., Hauser, S. L. & Longo, D. (2022). *Harrison's principles of internal medicine* (21st ed.). New York: McGraw Hill Medical.

Lymphoma Australia (2022). *Hodgkin lymphoma—Subtypes*. Retrieved from https://www.lymphoma.org.au/

Mandanas, R. (2021). Graft versus host disease (GVHD). *Emedicine*. Retrieved from https://emedicine.medscape.com/

Marieb, E. N. & Hoehn, K. N. (2019). *Human anatomy and physiology* (11th ed.). Upper Saddle River, NJ: Pearson Education.

Nagalla, S. (2022). Polycythemia vera. *Emedicine*. Retrieved from https://emedicine.medscape.com/

Rai, K. & Stilgenbauer, S. (2022). Overview of the treatment of chronic lymphocytic leukemia. *UpToDate*. Retrieved from https://www.uptodate.com/

Raphael, D., Frey, R. & Gott, M. A. (2017). Psychological distress in haematological cancer survivors: An integrative review. *European Journal of Cancer Care, 26*(6), e12640.

Rentscher, K. E., Carroll, J. E., Juckett, M. B., Coe, C. L., Broman, A. T., Rathouz, P. J., Hematti, P. & Costanzo, E. S. (2021). Sleep disruption, fatigue, and depression as predictors of 6-year clinical outcomes following allogeneic hematopoietic cell transplantation. *Journal of the National Cancer Institute, 113*(10), 1405–1414.

Royal Australian and New Zealand College of Obstetricians and Gynaecologists (2019). *Vitamin and mineral supplementation and pregnancy*. Retrieved from https://www.ranzcog.edu.au/

Ruiz, P. (2021). Pediatric graft versus host disease. *Emedicine*. Retrieved from https://emedicine.medscape.com/

Seeger, B. & Grau, M. (2020). Relation between exercise performance and blood storage condition and storage time in autologous blood doping. *Biology*, *10*(1), 14. https://doi.org/10.3390/biology10010014

Shah, D. (2022). Multiple myeloma. *Emedicine*. Retrieved from https://emedicine.medscape.com/

Stallings, A. M., Majhail, N. S., Nowacki, A. S., Ominoe, G. I., Hanna, R. & Piccone, C. M. (2020). Paediatric haematologists' attitudes regarding haematopoietic cell transplantation as treatment for sickle cell disease. *British Journal of Haematology*, *188*(6), 976–984.

Yang, L., Ning, Q. & Tang, S. (2022). Recent advances and next breakthrough in immunotherapy for cancer treatment. *Journal of Immunology Research*, *2022*, 8052212–8052219. https://doi.org/10.1155/2022/8052212

Zeiser, R. (2022). Prevention of graft-versus-host disease. *UpToDate*. Retrieved from https://www.uptodate.com/

UNIT 8 BUILDING CLINICAL COMPETENCE

Responses to altered cardiovascular function

Clinical scenario

You have been assigned to work with the following four people for the 0700 shift on a cardiac telemetry unit. Significant data obtained during report are as follows:

- Betty Williams, aged 62, was admitted with acute anterior MI and had successful fibrinolytic therapy 3 days ago. Significant history includes type 2 diabetes, angina, hypertension and a history of smoking (1.5 to 2 packets per day for 45 years). Her CCU course was uneventful. Current vital signs are T 37.2°C, P 76, R 16, BP 148/88. Cardiac monitor shows normal sinus rhythm with no ectopy. She has been pain free since her glyceryl trinitrate infusion was titrated off in the CCU 2 days ago. Lung sounds are clear.
- Arnold Markus, aged 71, was admitted with acute heart failure 2 days ago, treated and stabilised in the CCU, and transferred to the cardiac telemetry unit. Current vital signs are T 36.9°C, P 88, R 18, BP 112/74. Cardiac monitor shows normal sinus rhythm with new isolated premature ventricular contractions (PVCs). Lung sounds are clear in upper lobes with crackles in the left base and he was able to sleep intermittently during the night using two pillows.
- Theresa Cartwright is a 34-year-old female admitted for anticoagulant therapy after developing a deep venous thrombosis after a fall down the steps and hitting her calf. She was started on heparin yesterday and needs blood drawn for an activated partial thromboplastin time (APTT) to determine her morning dose of heparin.
- Scott Jacoby is a 25-year-old with Down syndrome. He was admitted yesterday with an upper respiratory infection. On assessment he was pale, T 38.3°C, P 100, R 30 with dyspnoea on exertion, BP of 118/86 and multiple bruises and petechiae on his arms and legs. He is scheduled for a bone marrow examination this morning.

Critical-thinking questions

1 In what order would you visit these people after report?

1. ________
2. ________
3. ________
4. ________

2 What top two priority nursing diagnoses would you choose for each of the people presented above? Can you explain, if asked, the rationale for your choices?

	Priority Nursing Diagnosis #1	Priority Nursing Diagnosis #2
Betty Williams		
Arnold Markus		
Theresa Cartwright		
Scott Jacoby		

3 You are completing a beginning-of-shift assessment with Mr Markus. Which of the following items would take priority?

1. rhythm strip analysis
2. lung sounds
3. oxygen saturation
4. heart sounds

4 The charge nurse tells you that the monitor at the nursing station shows that Mr Markus is having an increase in PVCs. You would be most concerned after reviewing a rhythm strip if the PVCs had which of the following characteristics?

1. a frequency of 4 per minute
2. could be felt by the person
3. were unifocal in morphology
4. fell on the T wave of the preceding beat

5 Ms Williams rings the call bell and tells you that she is having pressure in her chest. On assessment, she rates it as a 5. Which of the following nursing actions should take priority?

1. Obtain a full symptom assessment.
2. Administer a prn glyceryl trinitrate tablet SL.
3. Call for an electrocardiogram.
4. Notify the doctor.

6 Which is the most important for you to report when caring for Mr Jacoby?

1. constipation and straining with bowel movements
2. fever and burning on urination
3. weight loss and decreased appetite
4. dyspnoea and shortness of breath with exercising

7 When a person is placed on warfarin therapy, which laboratory studies would you expect to draw? (Select all that apply.)

1. activated partial thromboplastin time (APTT)
2. International Normalized Ratio (INR)
3. partial thromboplastin time (PTT)
4. full blood cell count (FBC)
5. white blood cell count (WBC)
6. prothrombin time (PT)

8 Mrs Cartwright needs further teaching regarding anticoagulant therapy when she makes which statement?

1. 'The heparin will be continued for four to five days for the Coumadin to reach a good effect.'
2. 'I need to continue to have blood drawn to watch my drug levels as long as I am taking these drugs.'
3. 'I cannot continue to take birth control pills while I am taking these drugs.'
4. 'I need to take the medication at the same time every day for the drug to be effective.'

9 After a person has undergone mitral valve replacement surgery, the nurse would be most concerned about possible risks to medication therapy if the person had a history of which of the following disorders listed in the medical record?

1. glaucoma
2. gout
3. duodenal ulcer
4. osteoarthritis

10 Which nursing diagnosis has the highest priority for the person with varicose veins?

1. *Body image disturbance*
2. *Impaired tissue perfusion*
3. *Activity intolerance*
4. *Risk of infection*

11 Which is a priority teaching instruction for the person with a history of Raynaud's disease?

1. Enter a smoking cessation program.
2. Reduce dietary fats and carbohydrates.
3. Wear gloves and socks in cold weather.
4. Begin an exercise program.

12 A prescription for the calcium channel blocker diltiazem is ordered for a person with hypertension. What will the nurse instruct the person regarding medication administration?

1. Limit fluids to decrease the development of peripheral oedema.
2. Notify the doctor for a pulse of less than 60 bpm.
3. Increase fibre in the diet as diarrhoea may be a side effect.
4. Report tachycardia and an increase in blood pressure.

13 A person with history of haemophilia fell and cut his leg while bushwalking. Which intervention should the person perform until help arrives?

1. Apply a tourniquet above the cut.
2. Splint the leg to prevent movement.
3. Apply pressure to the femoral artery.
4. Apply gentle pressure over the cut.

Case study

Grace Schmidt is a 49-year-old female who works as a teacher at a high school. She comes to the medical centre complaining of a throbbing headache and dizziness. Her height and weight are 162 cm and 111 kg. Upon assessment her vital signs are P 100, R 16, BP lying is 180/115, sitting is 170/110 and standing is 165/105. Her skin is cool and dry. Her capillary refill is 4 seconds. She denies smoking, drinks an occasional glass of wine and does not participate in a regular exercise program. She states that her job can be stressful at times. Nutrition assessment indicates a diet high in fats and sodium. She denies any family history of hypertension or heart disease. She is married and has a daughter and son who live in the same town. A medical diagnosis of hypertension is determined.

Based on Mrs Schmidt's assessment, blood pressure readings and weight, the priority nursing diagnosis of *Ineffective health maintenance* is identified for planning nursing care.

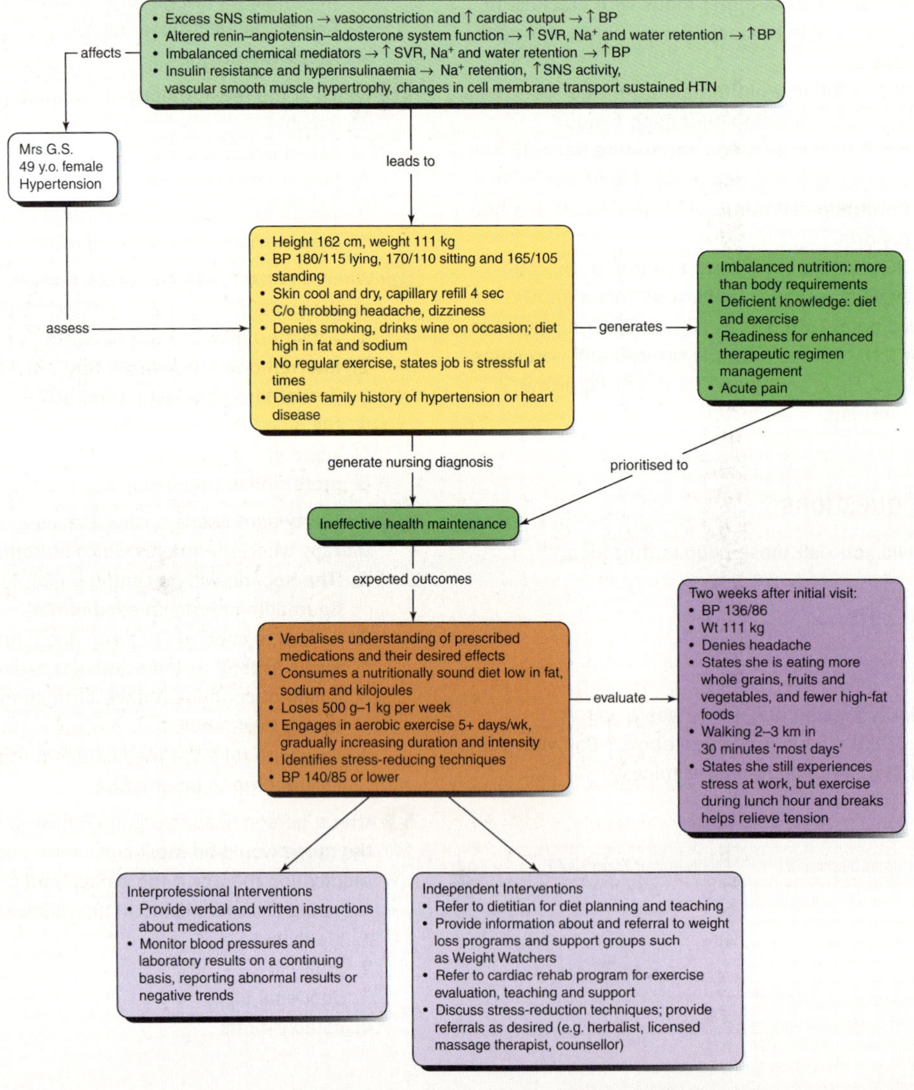

Essentials for nurses: COVID-19

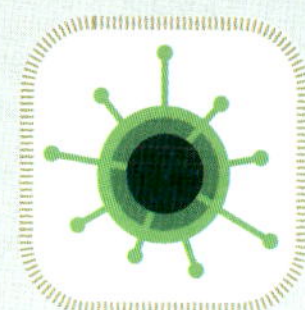

Stay current: knowledge about COVID-19 is changing daily. Check the following sources regularly for the latest information:

- **Australian Commission on Safety and Quality in Health Care:** https://www.safetyandquality.gov.au/covid-19-resources
- **Australian Government:** refer to relevant state or territory health departments for further details.
- **Australian Government:** refer to relevant state or territory health departments for further details on long COVID clinics.
- **Centers for Disease Control and Prevention (CDC):** https://www.cdc.gov/coronavirus/2019-ncov/index.html
- **Children and COVID-19:** refer to relevant state or territory children's hospitals for further details
- **Department of Health and Aged Care:** https://www.health.gov.au
- **Healthdirect:** https://www.healthdirect.gov.au/covid-19
- **Palliative Care Australia**: https://palliativecare.org.au/covid-19-updates/
- **Therapeutics Goods Administration (TGA):** https://www.tga.gov.au/
- **World Health Organization (WHO):** https://www.who.int/health-topics/coronavirus

PATHOPHYSIOLOGY AND TRANSMISSION

COVID-19 is a novel coronavirus, which means that it is a new virus not previously seen in humans. It is considered infectious and is caused by the SARS-CoV-2 virus (WHO, 2022a). The full name of this disease is coronavirus disease 2019. In the abbreviation COVID-19, *CO* represents *corona*, *VI* is *virus*, *D* is *disease* and *19* is *the year* it was identified (CDC, 2021a).

In the asymptomatic phase of COVID-19, the virus enters the nose and starts to replicate. In this stage, the person is infectious even though the viral burden is low. The virus is covered with spiked surface proteins that attach to receptors on cells, particularly in the lungs. It enters healthy cells through ACE2 receptors and destroys the cells. Over the next few days, the virus moves down the respiratory tract, which has a greater concentration of ACE2 receptors, and triggers an inflammatory response and respiratory symptoms. About 80% of individuals have mild symptoms. In the other 20% of individuals, shortness of breath develops in 5–8 days, followed by acute respiratory distress syndrome (ARDS) (Jackson et al., 2022; Mason, 2020).

Older adults and individuals with chronic illness are at greatest risk of developing symptoms and complications of COVID-19. At the time of writing, people aged 65 years and older and those who reside in aged care homes or long-term care facilities have had the greatest risk of mortality (National Institutes of Health (NIH), 2021). In Australia, the highest number of COVID-19 deaths was among those aged 80–89 years (85.2 years for males, 88.4 years for females).

Children may have asymptomatic infection or tend to experience similar, but milder, clinical manifestations that resemble a cold or flu (CDC, 2021a; Department of Health and Aged Care, 2022a). Some children develop a rare condition known as multisystem inflammatory syndrome that affects the heart, lungs, brain, skin, eyes and gastrointestinal tract (CDC, 2021b).

COVID-19 can be transmitted by both asymptomatic and symptomatic individuals. The incubation period for this virus (time from exposure to virus to onset of symptoms) is between 1 and 14 days, with a median onset of symptoms 5–6 days after exposure to a person with COVID-19 (CDC, 2021a; Healthdirect, 2022a).

COVID-19 spreads from the infected individual to another person primarily through respiratory droplets sprayed from the infected individual during coughing, sneezing, speaking, singing and breathing. The droplets range from large particles to smaller aerosols that may be inhaled into the lungs or land on another person's face, eyes, nose or mouth. The disease may also be transmitted by touching the face, mouth, nose or eyes with infected hands. The likelihood of transmission by droplets is greater when people are within 1.5–2 metres of each other (CDC, 2021c; Department of Health and Aged Care, 2022a; WHO, 2022a).

Viral shedding occurs when someone 'sheds' COVID-19 by breathing, sneezing, coughing or through their faeces and urine. It may occur up to several weeks after symptoms resolve. Some people continue to have non-infectious fragments which may still return a positive result when tested (CDC, 2021d; Department of Health and Aged Care, 2022a). The immune response and duration of immunity of individuals who have been infected with COVID-19 is not clearly understood and continues to be researched (CDC, 2021e).

At the time of writing, 13 variants of SARS-CoV-2 have been identified as causing COVID-19; however, only five (and their sub-variants such as XBB) continue to be classified as variants of concern—Alpha, Beta, Delta, Gamma and Omicron (Department of Health and Aged Care, 2022a; WHO, 2022a). Since 2019, the number of cases have risen significantly and continue to fluctuate due to these variants, which have caused severe illness in both vaccinated and unvaccinated people. It is thought that vaccinated people can carry and spread these variants to others. Although vaccinated people who contract one of these variants seem to have the same high amount of the virus, in most cases, they appear to have a milder case.

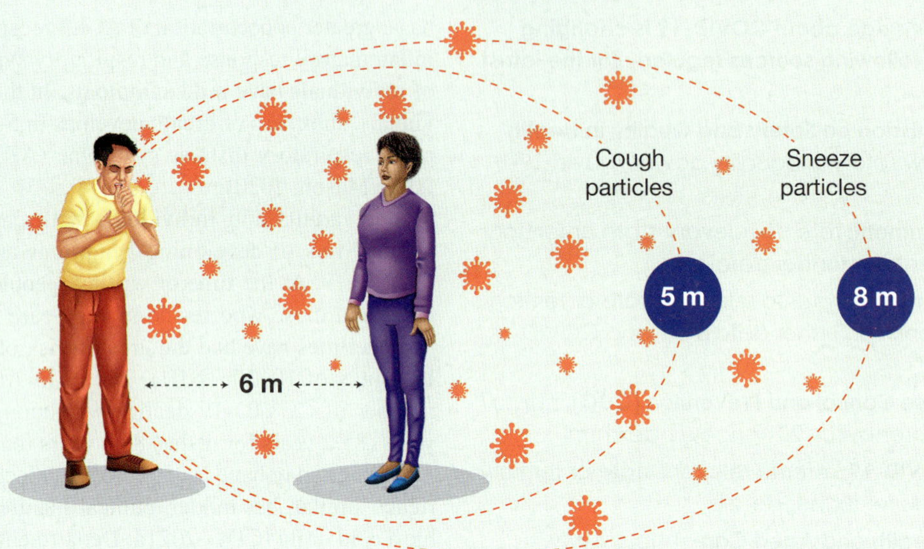

REDUCING AND PREVENTING SPREAD OF INFECTION

In the community: community spread of COVID-19 can be reduced or prevented by doing the following:

- placing at least 1.5 metres distance between people
- washing hands regularly with soap and water or hand sanitiser 70% + alcohol for a minimum of 20 seconds
- wearing a facemask in areas where it is a requirement, including healthcare settings, aged care facilities, doctors' surgeries and allied health clinics, public transport etc.
- sneezing or coughing into the elbow or a tissue if a mask is not being worn
- avoiding touching the face, eyes, nose and mouth
- receiving a vaccination against COVID-19
- disinfecting commonly touched surfaces and items.

In healthcare settings: spread of COVID-19 in healthcare settings can be reduced or prevented by:

- following policy for donning, doffing and disposing of PPE
- performing hand hygiene before entering a patient's room and/or donning PPE (gown, face shield or goggles and mask)
- correctly removing and disposing of PPE when leaving a patient's room followed by hand hygiene. (The Department of Health and Aged Care (2022b) and the Australian Commission on Safety and Quality in Health Care (ACSQHC) (2020) provide guidelines and resources about donning and doffing PPE in various healthcare settings.)
- avoiding touching the face and eyes
- washing hands frequently with soap and water for 20 seconds and/or using approved antimicrobial solutions
- taking breaks and eating food in designated areas away from the patient care unit.

In the home: nurses can reduce transmission of COVID-19 to family and others who share their living space by (American Nurses Association Enterprise, 2020):

- changing clothes and shoes before leaving work, if possible
- always washing hands before leaving work
- cleaning objects that are used at home and work, such as mobile phones, before leaving work
- removing shoes and clothing worn at work before entering the house and placing in a plastic bag or box
- washing hands before entering or immediately after entering the home
- washing scrubs/work clothes in hot soapy water and avoid mixing them with other clothing; discarding the plastic bag that held the contaminated items and washing hands
- leaving items such as stethoscope and pens at work.

SIGNS AND SYMPTOMS

Individuals with COVID-19 can present with various signs and symptoms; the most common are similar to cold and flu (CDC, 2021a; Department of Health and Aged Care, 2022a) including:

- fever
- coughing
- sore throat
- shortness of breath.

Other symptoms experienced include:

- runny nose or congestion
- headache or fatigue
- muscle or joint pains
- nausea or loss of appetite
- diarrhoea or vomiting
- temporary loss of smell or altered sense of taste.

TRIAGE, TELEHEALTH AND TESTING

Nurses are using telehealth (providing health services and information through the use of technology) to assess which patients need urgent care requiring hospitalisation and those who can be treated at home. Nurses may also be involved in triaging patients in the emergency department or other facilities set up to care for patients with COVID-19.

As of January 2022, the MBS telehealth national arrangements are permanent. Services include:

- a wide range of telephone and video services across a number of healthcare professionals (e.g. GPs, NPs, allied health, mental health, specialists)
- longer phone consultations for patients who have received a positive COVID-19 test (introduced in July 2022)
- electronic prescriptions.

All MBS telehealth services are informed by the relevant MBS Review Taskforce Principles in order to support safe and equitable services (Department of Health and Aged Care, 2022c). When using telehealth, it is important to:

- ***Prioritise!*** If the patient is experiencing a life-threatening emergency, advise the individual to call **000** and tell the operator if they have been in contact with or are experiencing symptoms of COVID-19 (Department of Health and Aged Care, 2022a).
- Ask patients if they have travelled to a place with a COVID-19 outbreak.
- Ask about vaccination status, signs and symptoms of the virus and any medical conditions that place individuals at high risk, such as chronic obstructive pulmonary disease (COPD), asthma, heart failure, diabetes, compromised/impaired immunity, liver disease, chronic kidney disease, obesity, neurological conditions and pregnancy.

The nurse will then direct patients to the appropriate level of care based on the severity of symptoms, other medical conditions and exposure. If patients are recommended to go to the hospital emergency department and/or a healthcare provider, they must review the relevant website and/or call to confirm any additional requirements prior to attending (e.g. face mask, RAT etc.).

A *polymerase chain reaction* (PCR) or *rapid antigen test* (RAT) may be performed to determine whether an individual currently has a COVID-19 infection. There are a variety of RATs available; their accuracy varies as they may not detect COVID-19 immediately. A PCR is recommended for confirmation (Department of Health and Aged Care, 2022c).

A number of laboratory-based serology immunoassay tests and point-of-care serology tests have also been approved by the TGA for use in Australia (TGA, 2022a).

An *antibody test* determines whether an individual has previously had a COVID-19 infection, which can take up to 2 weeks or more to be detectable. However, these tests do not detect active viral shedding and therefore cannot detect if the person is actually infectious (CDC, 2021f; TGA, 2022a).

A *point-of-care* serology test detects IgG and/or IgM antibodies for COVID-19. The test is performed from venous or finger prick blood samples placed on a test strip, with results obtained within 15–30 minutes. A positive test along with a clinical picture may be used as a possible positive diagnosis to determine subsequent patient management (TGA, 2022a).

It is important to note that these tests may produce false-positive results and/or fail to detect COVID-19 if they are performed during the acute phase prior to the development of detectable antibodies. Although these tests provide information on a person's past exposure to COVID-19, there is no evidence to date that detection of antibodies provides protective immunity (TGA, 2022a).

HOME CARE FOR PATIENTS WITH COVID-19

Individuals who are experiencing severe symptoms of COVID-19 should call **000**. Those who are experiencing mild symptoms should ideally speak to their healthcare professional and have either a telehealth or an in-person assessment (NIH, 2021). Suggested care for the patient with mild symptoms of COVID-19 includes the following:

- Stay home, even if no symptoms are present.
- Drink plenty of fluids to stay hydrated.
- Cough medicine may provide relief for dry and productive cough—take as per manufacturer recommendations.
- Take paracetamol for fever and/or pain as per manufacturer recommendations.
- Non-steroidal anti-inflammatory drugs (NSAIDs) such as ibuprofen (Nurofen) have also been reported to decrease signs and symptoms—take as per manufacturer recommendations.
- Continue to monitor for signs and symptoms that require calling **000**, including breathing difficulties, shortness of breath, pain or pressure in the chest that persists, confusion, inability to awaken and cyanosis (blue lips or face) (Department of Health and Aged Care, 2022a; CDC, 2021a).

- Monitor oxygen saturation (SpO_2) at home if a pulse oximeter is available. Advise the patient to use a warm finger and to notify their healthcare professional or **000** if the value is repeatedly (not one time) below 95% (NIH, 2021).
- Try resting in the prone (face-down) position if feeling short of breath (NIH, 2021).
- Stay away from other people as much as possible and wear a face mask when around others both in and outside the home.
- Wash hands often using soap and water or antimicrobial gel and disinfect common surfaces regularly.
- Do not share dishes and utensils.
- If possible, use a separate bathroom and bedroom. If this is not possible, improve ventilation such as by opening windows and disinfecting after use.

Nurses should educate patients staying at home about the signs and symptoms that require calling **000** and should provide or refer patients to the relevant federal, state or territory health department site for additional information.

HOSPITAL CARE FOR PATIENTS WITH COVID-19

The pandemic has and continues to have a profound impact on all private and public hospital activities including emergency departments, elective surgery and overall patient admissions (Australian Institute of Health and Welfare (AIHW), 2022).

The majority of people with COVID-19 will not require hospitalisation or any additional treatments, particularly if they have been vaccinated (AIHW, 2022). Individuals who are at high risk for serious COVID-19 and those with moderate to severe symptoms require close monitoring since there is a risk of them becoming critically ill and being admitted to ICU as soon as 1 week following the onset of symptoms (CDC, 2021d). However, where appropriate and available, individuals will be cared for on the ward in rooms with negative pressure or airflow that will lower the risk of transmission (Healthdirect, 2022b).

COVID-19 is a respiratory illness that weakens the immune system, causing inflammation, and leads to poor respiratory outcomes including pneumonia and secondary infections (Australian Bureau of Statistics (ABS), 2022).

The time taken to develop severe symptoms, such as dyspnoea and ARDS, and to be admitted to ICU varies among individuals depending on their current health, co-morbidities, vaccination status and other factors. At the time of writing, Australia had over 11 million total reported cases of COVID-19 and almost 18,000 deaths due to COVID-19, most of which had laboratory confirmation that they had died *with or from* the virus (ABS, 2022).

The Australian and New Zealand Intensive Care Society (ANZICS) has developed COVID-19 guidelines providing recommendations and suggestions to ensure the continued delivery of high-quality care in the ICU (adults and paediatric patients) and to its workforce (ANZICS, 2021).

LONG COVID OR POST-COVID CONDITIONS

The majority of people who contract COVID-19 will have symptoms for a short period of time and usually recover within a few weeks. However, some may continue to experience symptoms for weeks, months or sometimes years after diagnosis (WHO, 2022a).

A person is considered to have long COVID if symptoms have continued for more than 12 weeks after their initial infection (Healthdirect, 2022c). Although many long-term side effects remain unknown, common symptoms (Department of Health and Aged Care, 2022d, 2022e) include:

- extreme fatigue
- persistent cough, hoarse voice
- shortness of breath, heart palpitations, chest pains
- numbness, 'pins and needles' and joint or muscle pain
- issues with sleeping
- change in sense of taste or smell, reduced appetite and weight loss
- changes in mood such as anxiety, stress and depression
- cognitive dysfunction
- low-grade fever and rash
- headaches.

Research to date has identified that those who are at greater risk of long COVID varies and includes:

- those with underlying conditions (e.g. respiratory disease, diabetes, hypertension, chronic cardiovascular disease, chronic kidney disease, active cancer etc.)
- those who initially had mild illness which was managed at home
- those who suffered a severe illness during the initial phase of COVID-19
- those who were admitted to ICU
- those over 35 years of age
- females.

A Global Technical Network for Clinical Management of COVID-19 has been established by the WHO to undertake studies of patients in order to understand the proportion of patients experiencing long-term effects, how long they persist and why they occur in order to develop further guidance for patient care for both adults and children (WHO, 2022a).

At the time of writing, no specific treatment has been identified for long COVID. States and territories have opened long COVID clinics to specifically support those with ongoing symptoms, including personalised treatment plans requiring support from a range of healthcare professionals (Department of Health and Aged Care, 2022b, 2022c, 2022f; Healthdirect, 2022c).

DRUG THERAPY FOR COVID-19

According to the *Australian Guidelines for the Clinical Care of People with COVID-19*, treatment for patients is based on illness severity and monitoring of clinical progression markers (e.g. SpO_2, respiratory failure, sepsis etc.), particularly during days 5–10 of symptom onset (Department of Health and Aged Care, 2022g).

Patients with hypoxaemia despite increasing levels of oxygen supplementation may benefit from a trial of awake prone positioning. Careful positioning and protection are needed to avoid peripheral nerve and skin injury in the prone position (NIH, 2021). This position should not be used in patients who are haemodynamically unstable, in respiratory distress and who require imminent intubation (NIH, 2021).

In 2020 and 2021, the TGA provisionally approved the following drugs for the use in COVID-19 treatment:

- tixagevimab and cilgavimab (Evusheld)
- sotrovimab (Xevudy)
- remdesivir (Veklury).

In January 2022, the TGA also provided provisional approval for the first oral drug treatments—molnupiravir (Lagevrio®) and nirmatrelvir + ritonavir (Paxlovid®).

The Australian Guidelines provide a list of drug treatments recommended for use and those that are not recommended—detailed information is provided in the guidelines found at https://www.health.gov.au/health-alerts/covid-19/treatments/about.

The WHO continues to update and release new versions related to therapeutics and the role of medication management in COVID-19 patient treatment (Department of Health and Aged Care, 2022g; WHO, 2022b).

INDEPENDENT NURSING INTERVENTIONS

Nursing care for patients with COVID-19 focuses on supportive care, such as:

- monitoring vital signs, capillary refill and oxygen saturation levels (SpO_2)
- monitoring cardiac, respiratory, neurological, renal and other body systems for complications such as pneumonia, hypoxia, sepsis and septic shock, arrhythmias, cardiomyopathy, acute renal failure, thromboembolism and ARDS
- teaching patients to use a face mask when in contact with healthcare professionals
- turning and positioning patients, including the prone position
- providing psychosocial support to the patient and family
- providing care for patients requiring endotracheal intubation and mechanical ventilation.

Nurses are advocates for patients who are unable to express their own wishes and for family members who cannot be present with their loved ones. Nurses often create the technological connection between patients and families to say their goodbyes, explain care to families and provide both patients and families with end-of-life support. Nurses can also call on team members, such as chaplains and social workers, to provide patient and family support (Delgado, 2020; Palliative Care Australia, 2020).

Nurses who work with or need help having difficult conversations with patients and families may find the following resources useful:

- Palliative Care Australia, COVID-19 resources: https://palliativecare.org.au/covid-19-updates/
- VitalTalk, COVID-19 Ready Communication Playbook: https://www.vitaltalk.org/covid-resources/.

COLLABORATIVE CARE

Successfully dealing with any pandemic requires a multifaceted approach and strategies. This includes both clinical and non-clinical support as well as personal, cultural and socioeconomic mitigation measures (Lim et al., 2022; NIH, 2021) such as:

- administering supplemental oxygen, such as high-flow nasal cannula or non-invasive positive pressure ventilation
- administering medications, as prescribed, such as:
    - paracetamol for fever control
    - NSAIDs for pain relief
    - anticoagulants for thromboembolic prophylaxis
    - antibiotics for bacterial pulmonary infection
    - (See *Australian Guidelines for the Clinical Care of People with COVID-19* (Department of Health and Aged Care, 2022g) for recommended drug treatments: https://www.health.gov.au/health-alerts/covid-19/treatments/about.)
- consulting with healthcare providers and pharmacists before administering medications and treatments that are not yet TGA approved or are investigational/experimental to learn about factors such as indications, side effects and criteria to monitor
- assessing and managing fluid volume
- using prone position in patients with dyspnoea and mechanically ventilated patients with refractory hypoxaemia (NIH, 2021)
- using collaborative models and pathways of care that are supported by primary care and community organisations to alleviate pressure on hospitals so they can provide care for those with more severe illness or with risk factors for disease progression (Lim et al., 2022).

COVID-19 VACCINATIONS

There are currently four COVID-19 vaccines that are authorised by the TGA in Australia and recommended by the Australian Technical Advisory Group on Immunisation (ATAGI) for use (TGA, 2022b). See https://www.health.gov.au/our-work/covid-19-vaccines/advice-for-providers/clinical-guidance/doses-and-administration.

Viral vector, protein-based and mRNA vaccines work in different ways to protect against COVID-19. The *viral vector* vaccine uses recombinant viral vectors that do not replicate in the host but do induce an immune response. The *protein-based vaccine* contains part of the coronavirus spike protein. The immune system cells recognise the spike protein as a threat and begin building an immune response against it. The *mRNA* vaccine works by inserting fragments into the cells of the body to reprogram them to make antigens against the pathogen. The antigen then triggers an immune response (Department of Health and Aged Care, 2022h).

Common side effects that may occur following vaccination include pain, redness or swelling around the injection site. The person may also report fatigue, headache, muscle pain, chills, fever and nausea.

Side effects from the second dose may be more intense than following the first dose or there may be none at all (CDC, 2021g). The third booster dose and forth dose are recommended for those in high-risk categories—see ATAGI recommendations (TGA, 2022b).

Blood clots have been reported following viral vector vaccination (AstraZeneca). Severe allergic reaction (anaphylaxis) and myocarditis and pericarditis have been reported following protein-based vaccination (Novavax) (Department of Health and Aged Care, 2022i). Myocarditis and pericarditis have also been reported following mRNA vaccinations (Pfizer and Moderna), especially in adolescents and young adults (CDC, 2021h). These cases were predominantly in males aged 16 and older, within several days of being vaccinated, and often after the second dose. Be alert to shortness of breath, chest pain and palpitations in this age group following vaccination.

Children infected with the COVID-19 virus can become sick and can spread the virus to others. Please refer to ATAGI recommendations for further information regarding children and vaccine recommendations.

VACCINE HESITANCY

Many people have been hesitant to receive the COVID-19 vaccine and boosters. Reasons for this hesitancy include being against vaccines in general, believing the vaccines are not safe due to rushed production and lack of trust of authorities, government and science (Kaufman, Tuckerman & Danchin, 2022; Troiano & Nardi, 2021).

Other factors that may affect decisions about accepting the vaccine include cultural, social and political considerations (CDC, 2021c), along with potential allergic reactions (e.g. anaphylaxis) to any components or contraindications to the vaccines.

The first step in overcoming vaccine hesitancy is to listen to understand the person's concerns. Talk to the person who has vaccine concerns in an objective manner. Provide accurate and honest information to dispel the myths about the vaccines (CDC, 2021i; Department of Health and Aged Care, 2022j). There is a lot of misinformation in the media and online about the vaccines. Always choose a reliable source of information.

SELF-CARE FOR NURSES

This is an especially tough time for nurses and other healthcare professionals as they navigate the numerous stresses and detrimental impacts of the pandemic. Frontline healthcare workers have and continue to experience increased personal and professional challenges (Lewis et al., 2022; US Department of Veterans Affairs (DVA), 2020), including:

- risk in relation to the uncertainty and vulnerability of becoming infected and transmitting the virus to family and friends
- managing the strain of donning and doffing PPE over long periods of time
- managing the stress of restrictions and lockdowns
- mental and physical health issues such as anxiety, emotional distress and exhaustion, moral distress, palpitations, fatigue, burnout, feelings of anger and guilt, disruptions in usual self-care and coping strategies
- working with limited resources, both human and equipment, to ensure the delivery of safe, quality patient care.

Healthcare professionals have been faced with making difficult ethical decisions about who received care and who did not. Using an *egalitarian* approach, each patient has an equal chance to receive care. The *utilitarian* approach looks at who will benefit the most from receiving care. The *prioritarian* approach selects the sickest person first. These difficult and controversial decisions contribute to moral distress (Australian College of Nursing (ACN), 2020; Lewis, et al., 2022; US DVA, 2020).

There are significant challenges for healthcare organisations in recognising and supporting the wellbeing of frontline staff. Self-care actions that nurses who are engaged in patient care can take to manage stress and work demands (ACN, 2020; Lewis, et al., 2022) include:

- taking breaks, going outside and practising relaxation techniques (e.g. breathing exercises, meditation, short walks, listening to music)
- paying attention to bodily needs, such as using the bathroom, keeping hydrated and eating healthy food at regular intervals
- recognising strengths and maintaining strong boundaries to be more effective
- resting, engaging in regular exercise and enjoyable relaxation activities
- working as a team and supporting co-workers
- checking in regularly with colleagues (e.g. R U OK).

The following actions may be helpful to reduce the negative effects of moral distress (ACN, 2020; American Psychiatric Nurses Association, 2020; Greenberg et al., 2020):

- Engage in debriefing sessions to provide support and to help team members cope with the physical and emotional stress they are experiencing.
- Seek peer support and communicate with colleagues who can validate feelings.
- Engage in self-care activities such as journalling, meditating, breathing exercises and walking outside.
- Seek professional assistance to develop healthy coping mechanisms and process experiences.
- Check in regularly with colleagues on their mental wellbeing.

Discussion questions for nursing students

After you have read the news report and journal article, consider the following questions:

- Bernstein, L. & Gerberg, J. (2020). *A Brooklyn ICU amid a pandemic: Patients alone, comforted by nurses and doctors.* https://www.washingtonpost.com/national/health-science/in-the-icu-health-care-workers-with-little-to-offer-covid-19-

patients-soldier-on/2020/04/04/16face9e-74f3-11ea-a9bd-9f8b593300d0_story.html

- Raper, R. (2021). The implications of living with COVID-19 for intensive care in Australia. *Medical Journal of Australia, 215*(11), 511–512. doi: 10.5694/mja2.51332
- ***Discussion 1***: There are seven patients with COVID-19 in the emergency department who need a ventilator, but the hospital has only four available ventilators. Taking into consideration severity of COVID-19 symptoms, age, health, family role (e.g. mother of three young children), quality of life and other variables, how do you decide who receives ventilatory treatment?
- ***Discussion 2***: Think of the conversations you might have with patients and family members of those who will not receive ventilatory treatment due to lack of availability. Role-play these conversations with other group members.
- ***Discussion 3***: The intensive care unit at Best Hospital only has a 10-bed ICU capacity. Discuss ways to expand ICU capacity. What education and training will be necessary to make this change? Consider the changes that affect nurses as well as the interprofessional team.
- ***Discussion 4***: The nurses on a COVID unit are concerned about bringing the virus home to their families. Discuss measures that nurses can take to reduce virus spreading. Consider both your workplace and home resources and environment in your response.
- ***Discussion 5***: Experts are talking about a possible resurgence of COVID-19 infections in the next 1–2 years. Consider the resources in your workplace, community and at state/territory and federal levels and develop three changes that could be implemented as part of an overall plan to meet the predicted surge.
- ***Discussion 6***: You hear friends or family discussing their reluctance to be vaccinated against COVID-19 or hear them spreading misinformation about the disease. Think about how you will respond to these individuals. Practise role-playing your conversation with another student and have them give you feedback on your ability to listen and be objective.

Bibliography

American Nurses Association Enterprise (2020). *Keeping yourself and your family safe*. Retrieved from https://www.nursingworld.org/

American Psychiatric Nurses Association (2020). *Managing stress & self-care during COVID-19: Information for nurses*. Retrieved from https://www.apna.org/

Australian and New Zealand Intensive Care Society (ANZICS) (2021). *COVID-19 guidelines* (4th ed.). Retrieved from https://www.anzics.com.au

Australian Bureau of Statistics (ABS) (2022). *COVID-19 mortality in Australia, deaths registered to 31 January 2022*. Retrieved from https://www.abs.gov.au/

Australian College of Nursing (ACN) (2020). *Self-care resources*. Retrieved from https://www.acn.edu.au/

Australian Commission on Safety and Quality in Health Care (2020). Retrieved from https://www.safetyandquality.gov.au/

Australian Institute of Health and Welfare (AIHW) (2022). *Australia's hospitals at a glance*. Retrieved from https://aihw.gov.au/

Bernstein, L. & Gerberg, J. (2020). *A Brooklyn ICU amid a pandemic: Patients alone, comforted by nurses and doctors*. Retrieved from https://www.washingtonpost.com/

Centers for Disease Control and Prevention (CDC) (2021a). *Coronavirus disease 2019 (COVID-19). Frequently asked questions*. Retrieved from https://www.cdc.gov/

Centers for Disease Control and Prevention (CDC) (2021b). *For parents: Multisystem inflammatory syndrome in children (MIS-C) associated with COVID-19*. Retrieved from https://www.cdc.gov/

Centers for Disease Control and Prevention (CDC) (2021c). *Building confidence in COVID-19 vaccines*. Retrieved from https://www.cdc.gov/

Centers for Disease Control and Prevention (CDC) (2021d). *Interim clinical guidance for management of patients with confirmed coronavirus disease (COVID-19)*. Retrieved from https://www.cdc.gov/

Centers for Disease Control and Prevention (CDC) (2021e). *Clinical questions about COVID-19: Questions and answers*. Retrieved from https://www.cdc.gov/

Centers for Disease Control and Prevention (CDC) (2021f). *Testing for COVID-19*. Retrieved from https://www.cdc.gov/

Centers for Disease Control and Prevention (CDC) (2021g). *Possible side effects after getting a COVID-19 vaccine*. Retrieved from https://www.cdc.gov/

Centers for Disease Control and Prevention (CDC) (2021h). *Myocarditis and pericarditis following mRNA COVID-19 vaccination*. Retrieved from https://www.cdc.gov/

Centers for Disease Control and Prevention (CDC) (2021i). *How to talk to your patients about COVID-19 vaccination*. Retrieved from https://www.cdc.gov/

Delgado, S. (2020). End-of-life care during the COVID-19 pandemic. *AACN blog*. Retrieved from https://www.aacn.org/

Department of Health and Aged Care (2022a). *COVID-19 signs and symptoms*. Retrieved from https://www.health.gov.au/

Department of Health and Aged Care (2022b). *COVID-19—Donning and doffing personal protective equipment in primary care*. Retrieved from https://www.health.gov.au/

Department of Health and Aged Care (2022c). *Providing health care remotely during the COVID-19 pandemic*. Retrieved from https://www.health.gov.au/

Department of Health and Aged Care (2022d). *Getting help for long COVID*. Retrieved from https://www.health.gov.au/

Department of Health and Aged Care (2022e). *Long-term effects of COVID-19*. Retrieved from https://www.health.gov.au/

Department of Health and Aged Care (2022f). *Protect yourself and others from COVID-19*. Retrieved from https://www.health.gov.au/

Department of Health and Aged Care (2022g). *Treatments. Australian guidelines* ([illegible]). Retrieved from https://www.health.gov.au/

Department of Health and Aged Care (2022h). *Approved COVID-19 vaccines*. Retrieved from [illegible]

Department of Health and Aged Care (2022i). *Nuvaxovid (Novavax)*. Retrieved from https://www.health.gov.au/

Department of Health and Aged Care (2022j). *Is it true? Get the facts on COVID-19 vaccines*. Retrieved from https://www.health.gov.au/

Greenberg, N., Docherty, M., Gnanaoragasam, S. & Wessely, S. (2020). Managing mental health challenges faced by healthcare workers during COVID-19 pandemic. *British Medical Journal*, *368*, m1211.

Healthdirect (2022a). *Symptoms of COVID-19 and when to seek medical advice*. Retrieved from https://www.healthdirect.gov.au/

Healthdirect (2022b). *Hospital and intensive care for COVID-19*. Retrieved from https://www.healthdirect.gov.au/

Healthdirect (2022c). *Understanding post COVID-19 symptoms and long COVID*. Retrieved from https://www.healthdirect.gov.au/

Jackson, C. B., Farzan, M., Chen, B. & Choe, H. (2022). Mechanisms of SARS-CoV-2 entry into cells. *Natural Review Molecular Cell Biology*, *23*, 3–20. https://doi.org/10.1038/s41580-021-00418-x

Kaufman, J., Tuckerman, J. & Danchin, M. (2022). Overcoming COVID-19 vaccine hesitancy: Can Australia reach the last 20 percent? *Expert Review of Vaccines*, *21*(2), 159–161. https://doi.Org/10.1080/14760584.2022.2013819

Lewis, S., Wills, K., Bismark, M. & Smallwood, N. (2022). A time for self-care? Frontline health workers' strategies for managing mental health during the COVID-19 pandemic. *SSM Mental Health*, *2*, 100053. doi: 10.1016/j.ssmmh.2021.100053

Lim, S. M., Allard, N. L., Devereux, J. et al. (2022). The COVID Positive Pathway: A collaboration between public health agencies, primary care and metropolitan hospitals in Melbourne. *The Medical Journal of Australia*, *216*(8), 413–419.

Mason, R. (2020). Pathogenesis of COVID-19 from a cell biology perspective. *European Respiratory Journal*, *55*. Retrieved from https://erj.ers-journals.com/

National Institutes of Health (NIH) (2021). *Coronavirus disease (COVID-19) treatment guidelines*. Retrieved from https://www.covid19treatmentguidelines.nih.gov/

Palliative Care Australia (2020). *Palliative care and COVID-19: Grief, bereavement and mental health*. Retrieved from https://palliativecare.org.au/

Raper, R. (2021). The implications of living with COVID-19 for intensive care in Australia. *Medical Journal of Australia*, *215*(11), 511–512. doi: 10.5694/mja2.51332

Therapeutic Goods Administration (TGA) (2022a). *COVID-19 testing in Australia—Information for health professionals*. Retrieved from https://www.tga.gov.au/

Therapeutic Goods Administration (TGA) (2022b). *Approved COVID-19 vaccines*. Retrieved from https://www.health.gov.au

Troiano, G. & Nardi, A. (2021). Vaccine hesitancy in the era of COVID-19. *Public Health*, *194*, 245–251.

US Department of Veterans Affairs (DVA) (2020). *Managing healthcare workers' stress associated with the COVID-19 virus outbreak*. Retrieved from https://www.ptsd.va.gov/

VitalTalk (2020). *COVID-19 Ready Communication Playbook*. Retrieved from https://www.vitaltalk.org/

World Health Organization (WHO) (2022a). *Coronavirus disease (COVID-19)*. Retrieved from https://www.who.int/

World Health Organization (WHO) (2022b). *Therapeutics and COVID-19: Living guideline*. Retrieved from https://www.who.int/

Glossary

abrasion Partial-thickness denudation of an area of integument, generally resulting from falls or scrapes.

accommodation The ability of the eye to adjust to variations in distance.

achalasia Absence of peristalsis of the oesophagus and high gastro-oesophageal sphincter pressure resulting in dilation and loss of tone in the oesophagus.

acidosis The condition in which the hydrogen ion concentration increases above normal (reflected in a pH below 7.35).

acid A substance that releases hydrogen ions in solution.

acne Disorder of the pilosebaceous (hair and sebaceous gland) structure, resulting in eruption of papules or pustules.

acoustic neuroma (schwannoma) Benign tumour of cranial nerve VIII.

acquired immune deficiency syndrome (AIDS) A specific group of diseases or conditions that are indicative of severe immunosuppression related to infection with the human immunodeficiency virus.

acromegaly Meaning literally 'enlarged extremities', this is a condition resulting from excessive growth hormone secretion during adulthood.

actinic keratosis Also called senile or solar keratosis, this is an epidermal skin lesion directly related to chronic sun exposure and photo damage.

active immunity Production of antibodies or development of immune lymphocytes against specific antigens.

active sense of self The development of meaning, purpose and direction in one's life.

active transport Movement of molecules across cell membranes and epithelial membranes against a concentration gradient; requires energy.

acute coronary syndrome (ACS) A general term used to describe the effects of coronary heart disease, including angina and myocardial infarction.

acute gastritis A benign, self-limiting disorder associated with ingestion of gastric irritants such as aspirin, alcohol, caffeine or foods contaminated with certain bacteria.

acute illness An illness that occurs rapidly, lasts for a relatively short time and is self-limiting.

acute inpatient unit A ward in a mental health facility that admits people who are generally very mentally unwell.

acute kidney injury (AKI) Kidney injury characterised by a rapid onset of symptoms that are potentially reversible with prompt intervention that addresses the initial cause of the injury.

acute myocardial infarction (AMI) Necrosis (death) of myocardial cells.

acute pain Usually temporary, localised and of sudden onset; it lasts for less than 6 months and has an identifiable cause, such as trauma, surgery or inflammation.

acute respiratory distress syndrome (ARDS) Non-cardiac pulmonary oedema and progressive refractory hypoxaemia.

acute tubular necrosis (ATN) A syndrome of abrupt and progressive decline in tubular and glomerular function.

adaptive immune response A specific and systemic immune response initiated by and directed against particular antigens.

addiction Dependency on a drug, which can be either physical or psychological.

Addisonian crisis A rare, life-threatening response to acute adrenal insufficiency, occurs in about [illegible] of patients.

Addison's disease A rare endocrine disorder whereby the adrenal glands produce insufficient steroid hormones.

adrenal crisis A constellation of symptoms that indicate severe adrenal insufficiency caused by insufficient levels of the hormone cortisol.

advance directive Also called a *living will*, this is a document in which a person formally states preferences for healthcare in the event that he or she later becomes mentally incapacitated, and names a person who has durable power of attorney to serve as a substitute decision maker to implement the patient's stated preferences.

afterload The resistance the ventricles must overcome to eject their blood volume; the pressure in the arterial system ahead of the ventricles.

agnosia The inability to recognise one or more subjects that were previously familiar; agnosia may be visual, tactile or auditory.

albuminuria Albumin (protein) in the urine.

alcohol An organic compound obtained by substituting a hydroxyl group for a hydrogen on a hydrocarbon.

alcoholic cirrhosis (Laënnec's cirrhosis) The end result of alcoholic liver disease.

alkalis Substances that accept hydrogen ions in solution.

alkalosis The condition where the hydrogen ion concentration decreases below normal (reflected in a pH above 7.45).

alleles Different forms of a gene or DNA occupying the same place on a pair of chromosomes; an allele for each gene is inherited from each parent.

allergy A hypersensitivity response to environmental or exogenous antigens.

allografts Grafts between members of the same species but who have different genotypes and HLA antigens. See also *homograft*.

alopecia Loss of hair; baldness.

Alzheimer's disease (AD) A form of dementia characterised by progressive, irreversible deterioration of the general intellectual functioning.

amenorrhoea Absence of menstruation.

amputation Partial or total removal of a body part.

anaemia An abnormally low number of circulating red blood cells, haemoglobin concentration or both.

anaesthesia State produced by medications given intravenously, intraspinally, subcutaneously or by inhalation to create temporary partial or total loss of sensation and consciousness in a person for invasive procedures such as surgery or painful diagnostic tests.

analgesic A medication that reduces or eliminates the perception of pain.

anaphylactic shock Shock resulting from a widespread hypersensitivity reaction (called *anaphylaxis*). The pathophysiology in this type of shock includes vasodilation, pooling of blood in the periphery and hypovolaemia with altered cellular metabolism.

anaphylaxis An acute systemic type I response that occurs in highly sensitive people following injection of a specific antigen.

anaplasia The regression of a cell to an immature or undifferentiated cell type.

anasarca Severe, generalised oedema.

androgens Hormones synthesised in the testes, ovaries and adrenal cortex that promote expression of male sex characteristics.

anergy Inability to react to specific antigens.

aneurysm Abnormal dilation of a blood vessel, commonly at a site of a weakness or tear in the vessel wall.

angina pectoris (angina) Chest pain resulting from reduced coronary blood flow that causes a temporary imbalance between myocardial blood supply and demand.

angioma (haemangioma) Benign vascular tumour.

anion gap The difference between the sum of two measured anions, chloride and bicarbonate, and the principal measured cation, sodium.

ankylosing spondylitis (AS) A chronic inflammatory arthritis that primarily affects the axial skeleton, leading to pain and progressive stiffening and fusion of the spine.

anorexia Loss of appetite.

anorexia nervosa An eating disorder characterised by a body weight less than 85% of expected for age and height, and an intense fear of gaining weight.

anorgasmia Absence of orgasm.

anosmia Inability to smell.

antibodies Immunoglobulin molecules that bind with an antigen to inactivate it.

antibody-mediated (humoral) immune response Activation of B cells to produce antibodies to respond to antigens such as bacteria, bacterial toxins and free viruses.

anticipatory grieving A combination of intellectual and emotional responses and behaviours by which people adjust their self-concept in the face of a potential loss.

antigen A substance capable of evoking a specific immune response; usually a protein, which the body recognises as foreign, causing an immune response to be stimulated.

anxiety An unpleasant feeling that is typically associated with uneasiness, apprehension, fear or worry.

aortic valve The semilunar valve between the left ventricle of the heart and the aorta in the heart. It prevents blood from flowing backwards into the ventricle.

aphasia Defective or absent language function.

apical impulse A normal, visible pulsation (thrust) in the area of the midclavicular line in the left fifth intercostal space. It can be seen on inspection in about half of the adult population.

aplastic anaemia A condition manifested by failure of the bone marrow to produce all three types of blood cells.

apnoea Cessation of breathing lasting from a few seconds to a few minutes.

appendicitis Inflammation of the vermiform appendix.

apraxia The inability to carry out a motor pattern (such as drawing a figure) even when strength and coordination are adequate.

arrhythmia Abnormal heart rate or rhythm.

arterial blood gas (ABG) A laboratory test used to evaluate acid-base balance and gas exchange.

arthritis Joint inflammation.

ascites Excess fluid in the peritoneal cavity.

asphyxiation Oxygen deprivation.

asthma Chronic inflammatory disorder of the airways that is characterised by recurrent episodes of wheezing, breathlessness, chest tightness and coughing.

astigmatism A condition that develops with abnormal curvature of the cornea or eyeball, causing the image to focus at multiple points on the retina.

ataxia Uncoordinated, irregular gait and muscle movement; weakness.

atelectasis Collapse of lung tissue following obstruction of the bronchus or bronchioles.

atherosclerosis A form of arteriosclerosis in which deposits of fat and fibrin obstruct and harden the arteries.

atrial natriuretic peptide (ANP) A hormone released by atrial muscle cells in response to distension from fluid overload.

atrioventricular block A block in the normal conduction pathways.

Australian College of Mental Health Nurses (ACMHN) Peak professional college for mental health nurses in Australia.

autograft Transplant of the person's own tissue; the most successful type of tissue transplant.

autoimmune disorder Failure of the immune system to recognise itself, resulting in normal host tissue being targeted by immune defences.

autonomic dysreflexia Exaggerated sympathetic response that occurs in people with spinal cord injuries at or above the T6 level.

autosome A single chromosome from any one of the 22 pairs of chromosomes not involved in sex determination (X or Y); humans have 22 pairs of autosomes.

B lymphocytes (B cells) Bursa-equivalent lymphocytes responsible for synthesising humoral antibody.

bacterial vaginosis Non-specific vaginitis.

bactericidal agent Capable of killing an organism without immune system intervention. These include the penicillins, cephalosporins and aminoglycoside antibiotics.

bacteriostatic agent Inhibits the growth of a microorganism, leaving its destruction to the host's immune system.

balloon tamponade The application of pressure to stop oesophageal bleeding using an inflatable balloon.

bariatric care The branch of healthcare that deals with the causes, prevention and treatment of obesity. The term *bariatrics* was created around 1965, from the Greek root *bar-* ('weight' as in barometer), suffix *-iatr* ('treatment' as in paediatrics) and suffix *-ic* ('pertaining to'). The field encompasses dieting, exercise and behavioural therapy approaches to weight loss, as well as psychotherapy, pharmacotherapy and surgery.

basal cell carcinoma (BCC) Epithelial tumour that is believed to originate either from the basal layer of the epidermis or from cells in the surrounding dermal structures. These tumours are characterised by an impaired ability of the basal cells of the epidermis to mature into keratinocytes, with mitotic division beyond the basal layer.

basal metabolic rate (BMR) The energy used when the body is at rest.

base excess (BE) A calculated value also known as buffer base capacity. Base excess reflects the degree of acid-base imbalance by indicating the status of the body's total buffering capacity.

bases (or alkalis) Substances that accept hydrogen ions in solution.

Bell's palsy (facial paralysis) Disorder of the facial nerve (seventh cranial nerve), characterised by unilateral paralysis of the facial muscles.

benign prostatic hyperplasia (BPH) Enlargement of the prostate gland.

benzodiazepines Minor tranquillisers belonging to the sedative-hypnotic group of drugs that have a CNS depressant effect through action at the gamma-aminobutyric acid (GABA) receptor sites.

bile A greenish, watery solution containing bile salts, cholesterol, bilirubin, electrolytes, water and phospholipids.

biliary colic A severe, steady pain in the epigastric region or upper right quadrant of the abdomen.

binge-eating disorder An eating disorder characterised by recurrent episodes of eating an excessive amount of food during a defined period of time, and a sense of lack of control over eating during binge episodes.

biofilms Polymicrobial microbial communities that proliferate and are encased in a protective glycocalax matrix.

biomedical model of health A model of health that mainly focuses on biological health determinants and broadly views health as the absence of disease. This model is also known as the medical model.

biopsychosocial model of health The biopsychosocial model of health broadly views health as individual holistic wellbeing.

biotherapy Treatment that modifies the biological processes that result in malignant cells, primarily through enhancing the person's own immune responses.

bitemporal homonymous hemianopia Loss of vision in each temporal visual field (outer half of vision) resulting from compression of the optic chiasm.

blood flow The volume of blood transported in a vessel, in an organ or throughout the entire circulation over a given period of time.

blood glucose levels (BGLs) The amount of glucose present in blood.

blood pressure The tension or pressure exerted by blood against arterial walls.

blunt trauma The type of trauma that occurs when there is no communication from the damaged tissues to the outside environment.

body mass index (BMI) Used to identify excess adipose tissue, BMI is calculated by dividing the weight (in kilograms) by the height (in metres squared, m^2).

bone marrow transplant (BMT) Infusion of bone marrow cells to restore bone marrow function after chemotherapy or radiation; allogeneic BMT uses donor bone marrow cells from a donor; autologous BMT uses the person's own bone marrow.

borborygmus Hyperactive high-pitched, tinkling, rushing or growling bowel sound.

botulism A severe, life-threatening form of food poisoning caused by *Clostridium botulinum*.

bradypnoea Abnormally low respiratory rate.

brain death The cessation of cerebral blood flow with global brain infarction and permanent loss of all brain function.

brain death criteria Clinical signs used to determine whether a comatose person is brain dead.

breakthrough pain A sudden flare or increase in pain despite comfort with or without baseline analgesia.

bronchiectasis Permanent abnormal dilation of one or more large bronchi and destruction of bronchial walls, usually accompanied by infection.

bronchitis Inflammation of the bronchi.

bruit An adventitious sound heard during auscultation; of venous or arterial origin.

buffer A substance that prevents major changes in pH by removing or releasing hydrogen ions.

bulimia nervosa An eating disorder characterised by recurring episodes of binge eating followed by purge behaviours such as self-induced vomiting, use of laxatives or diuretics, fasting or excessive exercise.

burn An injury resulting from exposure to heat, chemicals, radiation, cold injuries or electric current.

burn shock Hypovolaemic shock resulting from the shift of a massive amount of fluid from the intracellular and intravascular compartments into the interstitium following burn injury.

bursitis Inflammation of the bursa.

cachectic The state of very poor health and malnourishment in a person.

cachexia The wasted physical appearance characteristic of cancer and other chronic illnesses. It is characterised by rapid depletion of the body's protein, particularly in skeletal muscle, with less rapid loss of fat.

caffeine A bitter, white crystalline xanthine alkaloid that is a psychoactive stimulant drug.

calculi An abnormal concentration in the body, commonly called a stone; occur in the kidneys, ureters, bladder or urethra.

cancer A family of complex diseases with manifestations that vary according to body system and type of tumour cells involved; marked by uncontrolled growth and the spread of abnormal cells.

cancer pain A common condition of people suffering with advanced cancer, it is often persistent and arises from a number of factors.

candidiasis Infection of mucous membranes caused by *Candida albicans*, a yeast-like fungus.

cannabis The general name given to the psychoactive substances found in the marijuana plant, Cannabis sativa, the main active constituent being delta 9-tetra-hydrocannabinol (THC).

carbuncle A group of infected hair follicles.

carcinogen Cancer-causing agent.

carcinogenesis The production or origin of cancer.

cardiac arrest Sudden failure of the heart to pump.

cardiac index Cardiac output adjusted for body size.

cardiac output (CO) The amount of blood pumped by the ventricles into the pulmonary and systemic circulations in 1 minute.

cardiac rehabilitation A long-term program of medical evaluation, exercise, risk factor modification, education and counselling designed to limit the physical and psychological effects of cardiac illness and improve the person's quality of life.

cardiac reserve The ability of the heart to respond to the body's changing need for cardiac output.

cardiac tamponade Compression of the heart due to pericardial effusion, trauma, cardiac rupture or haemorrhage.

cardiogenic shock Shock that occurs when the heart's pumping ability is compromised to the point that it cannot maintain cardiac output and adequate tissue perfusion.

cardiomyopathy Primary abnormality of the heart muscle that affects its structural or functional characteristics.

cardiovascular disease (CVD) Generic term for disorders of the heart and blood vessels.

carpopedal spasm Involuntary flexion and contraction of the wrist and ankle joints.

carrier Any individual who carries a single copy of an altered gene or mutation for a recessive condition on one chromosome of a chromosome pair and an unaltered form of that gene on the other chromosome; a carrier generally is not affected by the gene alteration; on average, each person in the general population is a carrier of five or six gene mutations for recessive disorders.

catabolism Biochemical process involving the breakdown of complex structures into simpler forms.

cataract Opacification (clouding) of the lens of the eye.

cell cycle The four phases that occur during growth and development of a cell.

cell-mediated (cellular) immune response Direct or indirect inactivation of antigen by lymphocytes.

cellulitis A localised infection of the dermis and subcutaneous tissue.

central nervous system (CNS) depressants Drugs that can be used to slow down brain activity.

central obesity Obesity characterised by a waist-to-hip ratio of greater than 1 in men or 0.8 in women.

central pain Related to a lesion in the brain that may spontaneously produce high-frequency bursts of impulses that are perceived as pain.

cerebral oedema An increase in the volume of brain tissue due to abnormal accumulation of fluid.

cerumen Earwax.

chalazion Granulomatous cyst or nodule of the eyelid.

chancre Hard, syphilitic primary ulcer.

cheilosis Painful lesions at corners of mouth.

chemotherapy Cancer treatment involving the use of cytotoxic medications to decrease tumour size, adjunctive to surgery or radiation therapy, or to prevent or treat suspected metastases.

chlamydia A group of syndromes caused by *Chlamydia trachomatis*, a bacterium that behaves like a virus spreading within a host cell; spread by sexual contact and to the neonate by passage through the birth canal of an infected mother.

cholecystitis Inflammation of the gallbladder, usually associated with stones in the cystic or common bile duct.

cholelithiasis Formation of stones (calculi) within the gallbladder or biliary duct system.

chromosome Genetic material carried by each cell; found in the cell nucleus.

chronic bronchitis Excessive secretion of bronchial mucus characterised by a productive cough lasting 3 or more months in 2 consecutive years.

chronic condition A disease involving a long course in its development or its symptoms.

chronic gastritis Disorders characterised by progressive and irreversible changes in the gastric mucosa.

chronic hepatitis Chronic infection of the liver.

chronic kidney disease The presence of impaired or reduced kidney function that lasts longer than 3 months.

chronic obstructive pulmonary disease (COPD) Chronic airflow obstruction due to chronic bronchitis and/or emphysema.

chronic sorrow A cyclical, recurring and potentially progressive pattern of pervasive sadness experienced in response to continual loss, throughout the trajectory of an illness or disability.

chronic venous insufficiency A chronic disorder of inadequate venous return.

Chvostek's sign Contraction of the lateral facial muscles in response to tapping the face in front of the ear; caused by decreased blood calcium levels.

circulating nurse Assists scrub nurses and surgeons during surgery.

cirrhosis A progressive, irreversible disorder, eventually leading to liver failure; the end stage of chronic liver disease.

claudication Cramping, aching pain in the calves, thighs and buttocks that occurs with a predictable level of activity and is relieved by rest.

clinical governance A system of policies, processes and accountabilities that is directed at improving patient safety and the quality and effectiveness of patient care within a health service.

clinical pathway A healthcare plan designed to provide care with a multidisciplinary, managed-action focus; developed for specific diagnoses, usually those that are high volume, high risk and high cost.

clinical reasoning The process by which nurses (and other clinicians) collect cues, process the information, come to an understanding of a person's problem or situation, plan and implement interventions, evaluate outcomes, and reflect on and learn from the process.

cocaine An illegal drug extracted from a cocoa leaf that is white, odourless, and takes the form of a crystalline powder.

cognition The ability to process information and apply knowledge.

cold sore See *herpes simplex*.

colectomy Surgical removal of the colon.

collateral vessels Accessory pathways connected to the smaller arteries in the coronary system.

colostomy Ostomy made in the colon.

comedones Non-inflammatory acne lesions.

communication The exchange of information between two or more people, groups or entities. It involves verbal and written exchanges, as well as body language, attitude and tone.

community A collection of people who share some attribute of their lives.

community mental health nurse A nurse in mental health nursing who works with consumers who are living in the community. They are often involved in case management.

compartment syndrome Condition in which excess pressure constricts the structures within a compartment and reduces circulation to muscles and nerves.

concussion Injury resulting from a violent jar, shake or impact with an object.

conjunctivitis Inflammation of the conjunctiva.

consciousness A condition in which a person is aware of self and environment and is able to respond appropriately to stimuli; full consciousness requires both normal rousal and full cognition.

constipation The infrequent (two or fewer bowel movements weekly) or difficult passage of stools.

consultation liaison (CL) A specialist mental health nurse who is the interface between medicine and psychiatry.

consumer-directed care A model of service delivery designed to give more care choice and flexibility to consumers. This model provides consumers with more control over the types of care and services they access, and the delivery of those services, including who delivers the services and when they are delivered.

continuum of care The provision of ongoing quality healthcare in acute and community settings to optimise quality of life for people, underpinned by an interprofessional consultative team approach.

contractility The inherent capability of the cardiac muscle fibres to shorten.

contracture Permanent shortening of connective tissue.

contralateral deficit Manifestations of a stroke on the side of the body opposite the side of the brain that is damaged.

contusion Superficial tissue injury resulting from blunt trauma, such as a kick or blow from an object, that causes the breakage of small blood vessels and bleeding into the surrounding tissue.

convergence Moving inward of the eyes to see an object close to the face.

cor pulmonale Condition of right ventricular hypertrophy and failure that results from longstanding pulmonary hypertension.

corneal reflex Closure of eyelids (blinking) due to corneal irritation.

corneal ulcer Local necrosis of the cornea, may be caused by infection, exposure trauma or the misuse/overuse of contact lenses.

coronary heart disease (CHD) Heart disease caused by impaired blood flow to the myocardium.

coryza (rhinorrhoea) Profuse nasal discharge.

COVID-19 COVID-19 is a novel coronavirus, which means that it is a new virus not previously seen in humans. It is considered infectious and is caused by the SARS-CoV-2 virus.

crackles Discontinuous lung sound heard by auscultation; can be fine or coarse. Produced by air passing over airway secretions or the opening of collapsed airways.

creatinine The end product from the breakdown of creatine phosphate in muscles.

crepitation A grating sound heard on movement of a joint.

Creutzfeldt–Jakob disease (CJD, spongiform encephalopathy) Rare, progressive neurological disease that causes brain degeneration without inflammation.

critical thinking Self-directed thinking that is focused on what to believe or do in a specific situation.

Crohn's disease (regional enteritis) Chronic, relapsing inflammatory disorder affecting the gastrointestinal tract.

cultural competence Practising in a way that demonstrates the importance of social and cultural influences on patients' health beliefs and behaviours, and devising interventions that take these issues into account.

cultural safety The effective nursing practice of a person or family from another culture, as determined by that person or family.

culture A learned world viewpoint or paradigm shared by a population or group and transmitted socially. It influences values, beliefs, customs and behaviours, and is reflected in the language, dress, food, materials and social interactions of a group.

Curling's ulcers Acute ulcerations of the stomach or duodenum that form following a burn injury.

Cushing's disease One form of Cushing's syndrome caused by a functioning pituitary adenoma, leading to increased secretion of adrenocorticotropic hormone (ACTH), causing excessive cortisol levels.

Cushing's syndrome A chronic disorder in which hyperfunction of the adrenal cortex produces excessive amounts of circulating cortisol or adrenocorticotropic hormone (ACTH).

Cushing's ulcers Stress ulcers occurring as sequelae of head injury or central nervous system surgery.

cyanosis A bluish discolouration of the skin and mucous membranes due to oxygen deficiency.

cyst A sac containing fluid or semisolid fluid.

cystectomy Complete surgical removal of the urinary bladder and adjacent muscles and tissues.

cystic fibrosis (CF) Inherited disorder of the exocrine glands that results in the secretion of abnormal amounts of mucus.

cystitis Inflammation of the urinary bladder.

cytokines Hormone-like polypeptides produced primarily by monocytes, macrophages and T cells. Cytokines act as messengers of the immune system, facilitating communication between the cells to adjust or vary the inflammatory reaction or to initiate immune cell proliferation and differentiation.

dawn phenomenon A rise in blood glucose between 4 am and 8 am that is not a response to hypoglycaemia.

day surgery units/centres Facilities where surgery is performed and the person is discharged on the same day.

death Irreversible cessation of circulatory and respiratory functions or irreversible cessation of all functions of the entire brain, including the brainstem.

death anxiety Worry or fear related to death or dying.

debridement Process of removing dead tissue from a wound.

decerebrate posturing Abnormal posture with the neck extended; the jaw clenched; arms pronated, extended and close to the sides; legs extended and feet plantar flexed. Results from lesions of the midbrain, pons or diencephalons.

decorticate posturing Abnormal posture with the upper arms close to the sides; the elbows, wrists and fingers flexed; the legs extended and internally rotated; and the feet plantar flexed. Results from lesions of the corticospinal tracts.

deep venous thrombosis (DVT) Blood clot (thrombus) formation and inflammation within a deep vein, usually in the pelvis or lower extremities; a common complication of hospitalisation, surgery and immobilisation.

dehiscence An unintended separation of wound margins due to incomplete healing.

dehydration Loss of water.

delegation Assigning appropriate work activities to other members of the healthcare team. When the nurse delegates nursing care activities to another person, that person is authorised to act in the place of the nurse, while the nurse retains the accountability for the activities performed.

delusion A fixed false belief that is firmly sustained despite what constitutes incontrovertible and obvious proof or evidence to the contrary. The belief is not one ordinarily accepted by other members of the person's culture or subculture.

dementia A global impairment of cognitive function that usually is progressive and may be permanent; interferes with normal social and occupational activities.

dermatitis Acute or chronic inflammation of the skin characterised by erythema and pain or pruritus.

dermatophytoses Superficial fungal infection of the skin; also called *ringworm*.

determinants of health Factors that influence health in either a positive or a negative way. Some of these function on an individual level (e.g. health behaviours such as smoking or exercise, or our genetic make-up). Others function at a broader societal level, such as the availability of health services, vaccination programs or clean drinking water and healthy food.

diabetes insipidus (DI) The result of antidiuretic hormone insufficiency.

diabetes mellitus (DM) Group of chronic disorders of the endocrine pancreas, all categorised under a broad diagnostic label. The condition is characterised by inappropriate hyperglycaemia caused by a relative or absolute deficiency of insulin or by a cellular resistance to the action of insulin.

diabetic ketoacidosis (DKA) A form of metabolic acidosis induced by stress in a person with type 1 diabetes mellitus.

diabetic nephropathy A disease of the kidneys characterised by the presence of albumin in the urine, hypertension, oedema and progressive renal insufficiency.

diabetic neuropathies Disorders of the peripheral nerves and the autonomic nervous system manifesting one or more of the following: sensory and motor impairment, muscle weakness and pain, cranial nerve disorders, impaired vasomotor function, impaired gastrointestinal function and impaired genitourinary function.

diabetic retinopathy The collective name for the changes in the retina that occur in the person with diabetes. The retinal capillary structure undergoes alterations in blood flow, leading to retinal ischaemia and a breakdown in the blood retinal barrier.

***Diagnostic and Statistical Manual of Mental Disorders* (DSM)** A manual that is published by the American Psychiatric Association that provides common language and standard criteria for the classification of mental disorders.

dialysate Dialysis solution.

dialysis The diffusion of solute molecules across a semipermeable membrane from an area of higher concentration to one of lower concentration.

diaphoresis Copious production of sweat.

diarrhoea An increase in the frequency, volume and fluid content of the stool.

diastolic blood pressure The minimum pressure maintained by elastic arterial walls during diastole (cardiac relaxation) to maintain blood flow through capillary beds; averages 80 mmHg in a healthy adult.

differentiation A process occurring over many cell cycles that allows cells to specialise in certain tasks.

'differentness' Being different from another person or group of people.

diffuse oesophageal spasm Non-peristaltic contraction of oesophageal smooth muscle.

diffusion The process by which solute molecules move from an area of high solute concentration to an area of low solute concentration to become evenly distributed.

digital health A broad range of technologies that can be used to treat patients and collect and share a person's health information.

dilemma A choice between two unpleasant, ethically troubling alternatives.

diplopia Double vision.

disaster Event that requires extraordinary efforts beyond those needed to respond to everyday emergencies.

discharge planning A planned process beginning with the person's initial presentation, considering the needs of the unique individual, based upon the availability of, and access to, support and resources. This process ensures that these needs are met through ongoing assessment and consultation involving the relevant healthcare professionals, patient, family, carers and community services.

discovery Encompasses equality and respect. Equality is the belief that all people ought to be treated equally. Respect is esteem for, or a sense of the worth or excellence of, a person, a personal quality, ability or a manifestation of a personal quality or ability.

disease Literally meaning 'without ease', this term describes alterations in structure and function of the body or mind. Diseases may have mechanical, biological or normative causes.

dislocation Separation of contact between two bones of a joint.

dissection (aortic) A life-threatening emergency caused by a tear in the intima of the aorta with haemorrhage into the media.

disseminated intravascular coagulation (DIC) A disruption of haemostasis characterised by widespread intravascular clotting and bleeding; a syndrome that develops as a complication of many other disorders.

distal determinants Determinants of health that tend to be stable and concern historical, national, institutional, political, legal and cultural factors.

distributive shock Also called *vasogenic shock*, this includes several types of shock that result from widespread vasodilation and decreased peripheral resistance.

diverticulitis Inflammation in and around the diverticular sac; typically affects only one diverticulum, usually in the sigmoid colon.

diverticulosis Indicates the presence of diverticula.

DNA-based tests Tests that incorporate new, sophisticated technology that permits the examination of the DNA itself, obtained from blood, bone marrow, amniotic fluid, fibroblast cells of the skin or buccal cells from the mouth.

do-not-resuscitate (DNR) directive Usually written by the doctor for the person who has a terminal illness or is near death, this order is usually based on the wishes of the person and family that no cardiopulmonary resuscitation be performed for respiratory or cardiac arrest.

Down syndrome A human genetic disease caused by the presence of an extra chromosome 21; characterised by mental retardation and heart and respiratory defects.

dumping syndrome Complication of partial gastrectomy characterised by nausea, weakness, sweating, palpitation, syncope, sensation of warmth and occasionally diarrhoea.

duodenal ulcers Peptic ulcer disease affecting the duodenum.

dwarfism A medical disorder, the term being used to describe a person of short stature.

dysarthria Difficulty speaking.

dysfunctional uterine bleeding (DUB) Vaginal bleeding that is usually painless but abnormal in amount, duration or time of occurrence.

dysmenorrhoea Pain associated with menstruation.

dyspareunia Painful intercourse.

dysphagia Difficulty swallowing.

dysphonia Change in the tone of voice.

dysplasia The loss of DNA control over differentiation occurring in response to adverse conditions.

dyspnoea Difficult or laboured breathing.

dysuria Painful urination.

ecchymosis A flat, irregularly shaped lesion of varying size with no pulsation; caused by blood collecting under the skin.

ectopic beats Impulses originating outside normal conduction pathways of the heart.

ejection fraction (EF) The percentage of total blood remaining in the ventricle at the end of diastole (relaxation); normal is 50–70%.

electrolytes Substances that dissociate in solution to form charged particles called ions.

electronic medical records (EMRs) Electronic (digital) collections of medical information about a person that are stored on a computer. An electronic medical record includes information about a patient's health history, such as diagnoses, medicines, tests, allergies, immunisations and treatment plans. It can be seen by all healthcare providers who are taking care of a patient and can be used by them to help make recommendations about the patient's care. Also called EHR and electronic health record.

embolism Sudden obstruction of a blood vessel by debris.

emphysema Destruction of the walls of the alveoli, with resulting enlargement of abnormal air spaces.

empowerment Developing confidence in one's own capacities.

empyema Accumulation of purulent exudate in the pleural cavity.

encephalitis An acute inflammation of the parenchyma of the brain or spinal cord.

end-of-life care Care provided in the final weeks of life when death is imminent.

endocarditis Inflammation of the endocardium.

endogenous insulin The insulin the pancreas makes.

endometriosis A condition in which multiple, small implants of endometrial tissue develop throughout the pelvic cavity.

endotoxins Found in the cell wall of Gram-negative bacteria, endotoxins are released only when the cell is disrupted. They act as activators of many human regulatory systems, producing fever, inflammation and potentially clotting, bleeding or hypotension when released in large quantities.

end-stage kidney disease (ESKD) The final stage of chronic kidney failure in which the kidneys are unable to excrete metabolic wastes and regulate fluid and electrolyte balance adequately; characterised by a glomerular filtration rate of less than 5% of normal.

enduring power of attorney A document that can delegate the authority to make health, financial and/or legal decisions on a person's behalf. It must be provided in writing and state that the designated person is authorised to make healthcare decisions.

enophthalmos Sunken appearance of the eyes.

enteral nutrition Administration of liquid nutritional formulas to meet kilojoule and protein needs in people unable to consume adequate food; also called *tube feeding*.

enucleation Surgical removal of an eye.

epidemic A widespread occurrence of an infectious disease (biological), localised to a particular community, region or population.

epididymitis Infection or inflammation of the epididymis.

epidural haematoma (extradural haematoma) A collection of blood between the dura and the skull.

epilepsy Chronic seizure activity.

epistaxis Nosebleed.

erectile dysfunction Inability of the male to attain and maintain an erection sufficient to permit satisfactory sexual intercourse.

erosive gastritis Inflammation and superficial erosions of the gastric mucosa that may occur as a complication of other life-threatening conditions such as shock, severe trauma, major surgery, sepsis, burns or head injury.

erysipelas Infection of the skin most often caused by group A streptococci.

erythema A reddening of the skin.

erythropoiesis Red blood cell production.

eschar Hard, leathery crust that covers a burn wound and harbours necrotic tissue.

escharotomy Surgical removal of eschar from the torso or extremity to prevent circumferential constriction.

euthyroid The state of having normal thyroid gland function.

evisceration Protrusion of body contents through a surgical wound.

exogenous insulin The insulin people inject or infuse via an insulin pump.

exophthalmos Protrusion of the eyeballs.

exotoxins Soluble proteins secreted into surrounding tissue by the microorganism. Exotoxins are highly poisonous, causing cell death or dysfunction.

extracorporeal shock wave lithotripsy (ESWL, transcutaneous shock wave lithotripsy) Non-invasive technique for fragmenting kidney stones using shock waves generated outside the body.

faecal impaction A rock-hard or putty-like mass of faeces in the rectum.

family Two or more people who are emotionally involved with each other.

fascial excision (fasciectomy) Process of excising the wound to the level of fascia.

fasciculations Involuntary twitching.

fat embolism syndrome (FES) Characterised by neurological dysfunction, pulmonary insufficiency and a petechial rash on the chest, axilla and upper arms due to fat globules lodged in the pulmonary vascular bed or peripheral circulation.

fibrocystic changes (FCCs) Physiological nodularity and breast tenderness that increase and decrease with the menstrual cycle.

fibroid tumours (uterine leiomyomas) See *leiomyomas*.

fibromyalgia A common rheumatic syndrome characterised by musculoskeletal pain, stiffness and tenderness.

filtration The process by which water and dissolved substances (solutes) move from an area of higher hydrostatic pressure to an area of lower hydrostatic pressure.

flaccidity Decreased muscle tone in disease or trauma of the lower motor neurons.

flail chest Free-floating segment of the chest wall, resulting from two or more consecutive ribs fractured in multiple places.

flatus Gas in the digestive tract.

fluid resuscitation Replacement of the extensive fluid and electrolyte losses associated with major burn injuries.

fluid volume deficit (FVD) A decrease in intravascular, interstitial and/or intracellular fluid in the body.

fluid volume excess (FVE) Excess extracellular fluid resulting from retention of both water and sodium in the body.

focused assessment A physical assessment that concentrates on the part of the body that may be affected by disease or injury.

folliculitis Bacterial infection of the hair follicle, most commonly caused by *Staphylococcus aureus*.

forensic mental health A subspecialty of mental health in which scientific and clinical expertise is applied in legal contexts, combining civil, criminal, correctional and legislative matters.

fracture A break in a bone, usually due to trauma.

friction rub The sound heard when two dry surfaces are rubbed together.

full-thickness avulsion injuries Injuries that result in loss of all of the layers of the skin, causing fat and muscle to be exposed.

full-thickness burn A burn that involves all layers of the skin, including the epidermis, dermis and epidermal appendages.

fulminant hepatitis Hepatitis with a rapid and severe onset and course.

furuncle Often called a boil; an inflammation of the hair follicle.

gamma hydroxybutyrate (GHB) A dissociative anaesthetic agent; another of the newer drugs diverted to illicit use.

gastric mucosal barrier A protective barrier consisting of lipids, bicarbonate ions and mucous gel that protects the stomach lining from the damaging effects of gastric juices.

gastric outlet obstruction Obstruction of the pyloric region of the stomach and duodenum that impairs gastric outflow; a potential complication of peptic ulcer disease.

gastric ulcers Ulcers of the stomach lining, usually in the lesser curvature and antrum; more common in older adults.

gastritis Inflammation of the stomach lining.

gastroduodenostomy (Billroth I) Excision of the pylorus of the stomach with the anastomosis of the upper stomach to the duodenum; commonly used partial gastrectomy procedure.

gastroenteritis Inflammation of the gastrointestinal tract; not a specific disease, but a group of syndromes or a collection of related manifestations.

gastrojejunostomy (Billroth II) Subtotal excision of the stomach with closure of the duodenum and side-to-side anastomosis of the jejunum to the stomach; commonly used partial gastrectomy procedure.

gastro-oesophageal reflux Backward flow of gastric contents into the oesophagus.

gastro-oesophageal reflux disease (GORD) Causes heartburn, usually after meals, when bending over or reclining.

gene A sequence of DNA on a chromosome that represents a fundamental unit of heredity; occupies a specific spot on a chromosome (gene locus).

gene expression When the protein product of a gene is visible (e.g. through the presence of a body structure or identifiable through biochemical tests such as insulin or phenylalanine levels).

general anaesthesia Deep sedation, which includes analgesia and muscle paralysis. This type of anaesthesia requires respiratory maintenance without the aid of the person's respiratory musculature.

genetic locus The term used to describe a gene's location on a specific chromosome.

genetics The scientific study of heredity and hereditary variation.

genital herpes (herpes simplex genitalis) An infection of the external genitalia caused by herpes simplex genitalis; transmitted by vaginal, anal or oral–genital contact.

genital warts (*condyloma acuminatum*, venereal warts) A sexually transmitted condition caused by the human papillomavirus.

genomics The study of whole sets of genes and their interactions.

genotype The genes and the variations therein that a person inherits from his or her parents.

gigantism Occurs when growth hormone hypersecretion begins before puberty and the closure of the epiphyseal plates, leading the person to become abnormally tall.

gingivitis Inflammation of the gums, characterised by inflammation, redness and bleeding.

glaucoma Condition characterised by increased intraocular pressure of the eye and a gradual loss of vision.

glomerular filtration rate (GFR) The rate at which plasma is filtered through the glomeruli of the kidney.

glomerulonephritis Inflammation of the capillary loops of the glomeruli

glossitis Inflammation of the tongue.

glucagon Hormone that stimulates the liver to breakdown glycogen into glucose and to synthesise glucose from lactic acid and non-carbohydrate molecules.

gluconeogenesis Formation of glucose from fats and proteins.

glucosuria Excessive glucose in urine.

glycogenolysis Breakdown of liver glycogen to glucose.

goitre An enlarged thyroid gland. Enlargement results from both inadequate and excessive synthesis of thyroid hormones.

gonorrhoea (GC, clap) An infection caused by *Neisseria gonorrhoeae* that is transmitted by direct sexual contact or by delivery of a neonate by an infected mother.

gout A syndrome that occurs from an inflammatory response to the production or excretion of uric acid resulting in high levels of uric acid in the blood (hyperuricaemia) and in other body fluids, including synovial fluid.

Graves' disease Caused by a defect in immunoregulation in genetically predisposed individuals, leading to production of thyroid-stimulating antibodies.

grief The emotional response to loss and its accompanying changes.

grieving The internal process the person uses to work through the response to loss.

Guillain–Barré syndrome (GBS) Acute demyelinating disorder of the peripheral nervous system characterised by progressive, usually rapid muscle weakness and paralysis.

gynaecomastia Breast enlargement in men.

haemangioma See *angioma*.

haematemesis Blood in the vomit.

haematochezia Blood in the stool.

haematopoiesis Blood cell formation.

haematuria Blood in the urine.

haemodialysis A procedure in which electrolytes, waste products and excess water are removed from the body by diffusion and ultrafiltration as blood passes by an artificial semipermeable membrane outside the body.

haemolysis The process of red blood cell destruction.

haemolytic anaemia Premature destruction (lysis) of red blood cells.

haemophilia A group of hereditary clotting factor disorders that lead to persistent and potentially severe bleeding.

haemoptysis Bloody sputum.

haemorrhage Rapid or excessive bleeding.

haemorrhagic stroke (intracranial haemorrhage) Cerebrovascular accident (CVA) occurring when a cerebral blood vessel ruptures.

haemorrhoids (piles) Clusters of dilated veins in swollen anal tissue.

haemostasis Control of bleeding.

haemothorax Blood in the pleural space.

halitosis (bad breath) A common condition caused by an increase in sulfur-producing bacteria in the oral cavity.

hallucination An alteration of sensory perception in the absence of a stimulus.

hallucinogens Drugs that produce hallucinations.

harm reduction A way of reducing the impact of drug- and/or alcohol-related harm to individuals and the community through a range of cost-effective public health policies, strategies and practices.

Hashimoto's thyroiditis An autoimmune disorder caused by the development of antibodies that destroy thyroid tissue.

health As defined by the World Health Organization, 'a state of complete physical, mental and social well-being, and not merely the absence of disease or infirmity'.

Health Care Home (HCH) A general practice that coordinates care for people with chronic and complex conditions.

health determinants Factors that affect the health of people.

health education Individualistic strategies to improve health, often by increasing knowledge or influencing attitudes to alter behaviours and lifestyle. Health education is often used interchangeably with health promotion although they are not the same.

health promotion Any activity undertaken for the purpose of achieving a higher level of health and wellbeing.

healthcare-associated infection (HAI) An infection contracted during residence in a hospital or extended care facility.

heart failure Inability of the heart to pump adequate blood to meet the metabolic demands of the body.

hemianopia The loss of half of the visual field of one or both eyes.

hemiparesis Weakness of the left or right half of the body.

hemiplegia Paralysis of the left or right half of the body.

hepatitis Inflammation of the liver, usually caused by a virus; may be acute or chronic.

hepatorenal syndrome Renal failure accompanied by azotaemia, sodium retention, oliguria and hypotension in people with cirrhosis and ascites.

hernia A defect in the abdominal wall that allows abdominal contents to protrude out of the abdominal cavity.

herpes simplex (fever blister, cold sore) Acute viral infections of the skin and mucous membranes caused by two types of herpes virus: HSV I and HSV II.

herpes zoster (shingles) Viral infection of a dermatome section of the skin caused by varicella zoster, the same herpes virus that causes chickenpox.

heterograft (xenograft) Skin obtained from an animal, usually a pig.

heterozygous Non-identical copies of a particular gene (different alleles) on the paired chromosomes.

hiatal hernia Protrusion of part of the stomach through the oesophageal hiatus of the diaphragm into the mediastinal cavity.

hirsutism Increased growth of coarse hair, usually on the face and trunk.

histocompatibility The ability of cells and tissues to survive transplantation without immunological interference by the recipient.

Hodgkin's disease Develops in a single lymph node or chain of nodes and spreads to adjoining nodes. Involved lymph nodes contain *Reed–Sternberg cells* (malignant cells) surrounded by host inflammatory cells. These malignant cells secrete inflammatory mediator substances, attracting inflammatory cells to the tumour site. They may invade almost any tissue in the body.

holistic healthcare Care in which all aspects of a person (physical, psychosocial, cultural, spiritual and intellectual) are considered as essential components of individualised care.

homeostasis The body's tendency to maintain a state of physiological balance in the presence of constantly changing conditions.

homograft (allograft) Human skin that has been harvested from cadavers.

homologous chromosomes Chromosomes that are members of the same pair and normally have the same number and arrangement of genes; usually one copy is from the mother and the other copy is from the father.

homozygous Identical copies of a particular gene (same alleles) on both paired chromosomes.

hope A belief in a positive outcome related to events and circumstances in one's life; the foundation of recovery from mental illness.

hordeolum (sty) Staphylococcal abscess that may occur on either the external or internal margin of the lid.

hospice care The delivery of care for terminally ill people either in healthcare facilities or in the person's home.

human genome The total amount of the DNA (genes) in an individual's cells.

human immunodeficiency virus (HIV) Virus responsible for AIDS.

Huntington's disease Progressive, degenerative, inherited neurological disease characterised by increasing dementia and chorea.

hydrocephalus An abnormal accumulation of cerebrospinal fluid within the cranial vault and dilation of the ventricles.

hydrocoele Fluid-filled mass within the scrotum.

hydronephrosis Distension of the urinary tract with urine behind an obstruction.

hyperglycaemia Elevated blood glucose levels (above 126 mg/dL), which causes osmotic diuresis and, if chronic, damages vessel epithelium and renal glomeruli.

hyperopia (farsightedness) The condition in which the eyeball is short, causing the image to focus behind the retina.

hyperosmolar hyperglycaemic state (HHS) A condition of very high blood glucose with adequate insulin to prevent ketosis, but which does cause diuresis.

hyperparathyroidism Results from an increase in the secretion of parathyroid hormone, which regulates normal serum levels of calcium and phosphate.

hyperplasia An increase in the number or density of normal cells.

hypersensitivity Exaggerated response of the immune system to an antigen.

hypertension Excess pressure in the arterial portion of systemic circulation.

hyperthyroidism A disorder caused by excessive delivery of thyroid hormone to the peripheral tissues. Also called thyrotoxicosis.

hypertrophic scar Overgrowth of dermal tissue that remains within the boundaries of the wound.

hyphaema Bleeding into the anterior chamber of the eye, possibly as the result of blunt eye trauma.

hypoglycaemia Low blood glucose levels; deficiency of blood sugar.

hypoparathyroidism A condition that results from abnormally low parathyroid hormone levels, causing hypocalcaemia and an elevated blood phosphate level.

hypothyroidism A disorder that results when the thyroid gland produces an insufficient amount of thyroid hormone.

hypovolaemic shock Shock caused by a decrease in intravascular volume of 15% or more. This form of shock is caused by the loss of whole blood, blood plasma or extracellular fluid.

hypoxaemia Decreased oxygen concentration in the blood, measured by PaO_2.

ileostomy An ostomy made in the ileum of the small intestine.

illness–wellness continuum A continuum representing health as a dynamic process, with high-level wellness at one extreme of the continuum and death at the opposite extreme.

illusion A distortion of the senses.

immunity The protection of the body from disease.

immunocompetent Possessing an immune system that can identify antigens and effectively destroy or remove them.

immunoglobulin (Ig) A protein that functions as an antibody.

immunosuppression Inability of the immune system to respond to an antigen. Occurs in response to disease or medications; may be intentional to prevent rejection of transplants or a side effect of some medications.

impetigo Infection of the skin caused by either *Staphylococcus aureus* or beta-haemolytic streptococci.

impotence Inability to achieve or maintain an erection.

impulse control The ability to control behavioural impetuosity.

increased intracranial pressure (IICP, intracranial hypertension) Sustained elevated pressure (10 mmHg or higher) within the cranial cavity.

Indigenous health A broad term which generally refers to the health status and health outcomes of the Aboriginal and Torres Strait Islander population of Australia.

infection Colonisation by and multiplication of an organism within a host. The host can be any organism capable of supporting the nutritional and physical growth requirements of the microorganism—for example, humans.

inflammation A complex, non-specific, adaptive response to injury that brings fluid, dissolved substances and blood cells into the interstitial tissues where the invasion or damage has occurred.

inflammatory bowel disease (IBD) Chronic inflammation of the bowel common to a group of conditions that includes Crohn's disease and ulcerative colitis.

influenza Highly contagious viral respiratory disease characterised by coryza, fever, cough and constitutional manifestations such as headache and malaise.

informed consent Disclosure of risks associated with the intended procedure or operation to the patient. The language of the document varies according to statutory and common law of each state.

innate immunity Specific and non-specific responses that prevent or limit the entry of invaders into the body, thereby limiting the extent of tissue damage and reducing the workload of the adaptive immune system.

insight The degree to which a person has an understanding of their illness or disorder.

instrument nurse The nurse primarily responsible for manual dexterity and in-depth knowledge of the anatomical and mechanical aspects of a particular surgery. The instrument nurse handles sutures, instruments and other equipment immediately adjacent to the sterile field.

insulin A hormone that facilitates entry of glucose into fat and muscle cells for energy.

insulin reaction Hypoglycaemia in people with type 1 diabetes mellitus.

intermediate determinants Determinants of health that concern community infrastructure, personal wealth or access to resources, natural, physical and built environments. This level also includes access to healthcare and health systems.

International Classification of Diseases (ICD) Classification of diseases, functioning and disability.

interprofessional care Care provided by an interprofessional team where two or more professions work together as a team with a common purpose, commitment and mutual respect (Freeth et al. 2005, cited in Dunston et al., 2009, p. 6).

intersectoral Working with more than one sector of society to take action on an area of shared interest, such as health.

intracerebral haematomas A collection of blood in the brain tissue, most often located in the frontal or temporal lobes.

intracranial aneurysm Saccular outpouching of a cerebral artery that occurs at the site of a weakness in the vessel wall.

intraoperative phase The time during surgery, from beginning to end.

iron deficiency anaemia The most common type of anaemia; results from inadequate iron for optimal red blood cell formation.

irritable bowel syndrome (IBS) A motility disorder of the gastrointestinal tract characterised by alternating periods of constipation and diarrhoea.

ischaemia Deficient blood flow to tissue.

ischaemic Deprived of oxygen.

isograft Tissue transplant where the donor and recipient are identical twins.

jaundice Yellow-to-orange colour visible in the skin and mucous membranes; most often the result of a hepatic disorder.

Kaposi's sarcoma (KS) A vascular malignancy (a tumour of the endothelial cells lining small blood vessels) that presents as vascular macules, papules or violet lesions affecting the skin and viscera. It is often the presenting symptom of AIDS.

keloid Elevated, irregularly shaped, progressively enlarging scar arising from excessive amounts of collagen in the stratum corneum during scar formation in connective tissue repair.

keratin A fibrous, water-repellent protein that gives the epidermis its tough, protective quality.

keratitis Inflammation of the cornea.

keratosis Any skin condition in which there is a benign overgrowth and thickening of the cornified epithelium.

ketamine A central nervous system depressant, best described as a dissociative anaesthetic agent.

ketonuria The presence of ketones in the urine.

ketosis An accumulation of ketone bodies produced during the oxidation of fatty acids.

kidney replacement therapy Therapy provided through haemodialysis, peritoneal dialysis or kidney transplantation.

kinaesthaesia The ability to perceive movement and sense of position.

Klinefelter's syndrome A syndrome in which males have an extra X chromosome in most of their cells (also known as the XXY condition).

knowledge resource base Ways in which knowledge is developed.

Korotkoff's sounds Sounds heard during auscultation of blood pressure.

kyphosis Exaggerated thoracic curvature of the spine common in older adults.

labyrinthitis Inflammation of the inner ear.

laceration Open wound that results from sharp cutting or tearing. Injuries to the integument are at risk of contamination from dirt, debris or foreign objects.

laminectomy Removal of the lamina of the vertebrae.

laparoscopic cholecystectomy Removal of the gallbladder using an endoscope.

laryngectomy Removal of the larynx.

laryngitis Inflammation of the larynx.

leiomyomas Solid, pedunculated benign tumours.

leucocytes Also called white blood cells, these are the primary cells involved in both non-specific and specific immune system responses. These cells isolate the infecting organism or injury, destroy pathogens and promote healing.

leucocytosis An increase in the number of leucocytes in the blood (above 10,000/mm^3), usually caused by infection.

leucopenia Abnormal decrease of circulating leucocytes, usually below 5,000/mm^3; occurs when bone marrow activity is suppressed, or when leucocyte destruction increases.

leucoplakia Formation of white patches or spots on the mucous membranes or tongue; these lesions may become malignant.

leukaemia ('white blood') A group of chronic malignant disorders of white blood cells (WBCs) and WBC precursors; characterised by replacement of bone marrow by malignant immature WBCs, abnormal immature circulating WBCs and infiltration of malignant cells into other tissues.

libido Instinctive drive associated with sexual desire.

life-limiting illness An illness where it is expected that death will be a direct consequence of the specified illness.

lipoatrophy Atrophy of subcutaneous tissue.

lipodystrophy Hypertrophy of subcutaneous tissue that may result if the same injection sites are used repeatedly, especially with porcine and bovine insulins.

lithiasis Stone formation.

lithotripsy Crushing of renal calculi.

liver transplantation Surgery to remove a diseased liver and transplant a healthy liver (whole or segment) from another person.

locked-in syndrome Person is alert and fully aware of the environment, but is unable to communicate through speech or movement as a result of blocked efferent pathways to the brain.

lordosis Increased lumbar curve.

loss An actual or potential situation in which a valued object, person, relationship, body part or emotion that was formerly present is lost or changed and can no longer be seen, felt, heard, known or experienced.

lung abscess Localised area of lung destruction or necrosis and pus formation.

lung compliance Distensibility of the lungs.

lymphadenopathy The enlargement of lymph nodes (over 1 cm) with or without tenderness. It may be caused by inflammation, infection or malignancy of the nodes or the regions drained by the nodes.

lymphocytes Account for 20–40% of circulating leucocytes. Lymphocytes are the principal effector and regulator cells of specific immune responses.

lymphoedema Extremity oedema due to accumulated lymph; may be primary or secondary, resulting from inflammation, obstruction or removal of lymphatic vessels.

lymphomas Malignancy of lymphoid tissue.

macrophages Monocytes mature into macrophages after settling into tissue. Macrophages are large phagocytes. They are important in the body's defence against chronic infections.

macular degeneration Destructive changes in the macula due to injury or gradual failure of the outer pigmented layer of the retina (the retinal layer adjacent to the choroid), which removes cellular waste products and keeps the retina attached to the choroid.

major trauma Serious single-system injury (such as the traumatic amputation of a leg) or multiple-system injuries. Also known as multiple trauma.

malabsorption A condition in which nutrients are ineffectively absorbed by the intestinal mucosa, resulting in their excretion in the stool.

malignant melanoma Skin cancer that arises from melanocytes.

malnutrition Inadequate nutrient intake to meet body needs; may include deficiency of major nutrients (kilojoules, carbohydrates, proteins and fats) or micronutrients such as vitamins and minerals.

man-made disasters Either accidental or intentional, they are complex emergencies, technological disasters, material shortages and other disasters not caused by natural hazards.

mass casualty incident (MCI) An event that generates more patients at one time than locally available resources can manage using routine procedures.

mastoiditis Bacterial infection of the mastoid process.

mean arterial pressure (MAP) The average pressure in the arterial circulation throughout the cardiac cycle; the product of cardiac output and systemic vascular resistance (SVR).

medical–surgical nursing The health promotion, healthcare and illness care of adults, based on knowledge derived from the arts and sciences and shaped by knowledge (the science) of nursing.

meiosis A modified type of cell division in sexually reproducing organisms consisting of two rounds of cell division but only one round of DNA replication. It results in cells with half the number of chromosome sets as the original cell.

melaena Black, tarry stool that contains blood.

melanin Skin pigment that forms a protective shield to protect keratinocytes and nerve endings in the dermis from the damaging effects of ultraviolet light.

memory The ability to store, retain and recall information.

Ménière's disease Chronic disorder of unknown cause characterised by recurrent attacks of vertigo with tinnitus and a progressive unilateral hearing loss.

meningitis Inflammation of the meninges of the brain and spinal cord.

menopause Permanent cessation of menses.

menorrhagia Excessive or prolonged menstruation.

menstrual cycle Cyclic build up of the uterine lining, ovulation and sloughing of the lining occurring approximately every 28 days in non-pregnant females.

menstruation Periodic shedding of the uterine lining in a woman of childbearing age who is not pregnant.

Mental Health Act Mental health legislation.

Mental Health Nurse Practitioner (MHNP) A specialist mental health nurse with qualifications at master's degree level.

mental state examination (MSE) A clinical assessment that describes the sum total of the examiner's observations at the time of the interview or interaction.

metabolic syndrome A cluster of manifestations often associated with type 2 diabetes. Includes insulin resistance, hypertension, low high-density lipoprotein cholesterol and high triglycerides.

metabolism The breakdown of complex structures into simpler forms to produce energy (catabolism) and the combination of simpler molecules to produce and maintain more complex structures necessary to living organisms (anabolism).

metaplasia A change in the normal pattern of differentiation such that dividing cells differentiate into cell types not normally found in that location in the body.

metastasis Secondary tumour; the process by which spreading of malignant neoplasms occurs; the transfer of disease from one organ or part to another not directly connected with it.

metrorrhagia Bleeding between menstrual periods; may be caused by hormonal imbalances, pelvic inflammatory disease, cervical or uterine polyps, uterine fibroids or cervical or uterine cancer.

microalbuminuria Protein in the urine.

micturition Releasing urine from the urinary bladder (voiding).

minor trauma Injury to a single part or system of the body, usually treated in the hospital or emergency department.

mitigation The action taken to prevent or reduce the harmful effects of a disaster on human health or property; it involves future-oriented activities to prevent subsequent disasters or to minimise their effects.

mitochondria Provide the energy a cell needs to move, divide, produce secretory products and contract.

mitosis A process of nuclear division in eukaryotic cells conventionally divided into five stages: prophase, prometaphase, metaphase, anaphase and telophase. Mitosis conserves chromosome numbers by allocating replicated chromosomes equally to each of the daughter nuclei.

mitral valve (bicuspid valve) Valve between the left atrium and ventricle in the heart; prevents blood from flowing backwards into the atrium.

monosomy (monosomic) When one member of the chromosome pair is missing—for example, in Turner syndrome (45, XO).

mood The way in which a person describes their feelings at a particular time.

morbid obesity Weight greater than 100% over ideal body weight.

motor neurone disease (MND) Progressive, degenerative neurological disease characterised by weakness and wasting of the involved muscles, without any accompanying sensory or cognitive changes; also called *Lou Gehrig's disease*.

mourning The actions or expressions of the bereaved, including the symbols, clothing and ceremonies that make up the outward manifestations of grief.

multifactorial Health conditions determined by multiple factors, including genetic and environmental factors, each having an additive effect.

multiple myeloma A malignancy in which plasma cells multiply uncontrollably and infiltrate the bone marrow, lymph nodes, spleen and other tissues.

multiple sclerosis (MS) A chronic demyelinating neurological disease of the CNS (brain, optic nerves and spinal cord), associated with an abnormal immune response to an environmental factor.

multiple trauma Most often the result of a motor vehicle crash, this type of trauma requires immediate intervention specifically focused on ensuring survival.

murmurs Sounds made by turbulent blood flow through the heart.

muscular dystrophy (MD) A group of inherited muscle diseases that cause progressive muscle degeneration and wasting.

myasthenia gravis Chronic, progressive neuromuscular disorder characterised by fatigue and severe weakness of skeletal muscles.

myocarditis Inflammatory disorder of the heart muscle.

myopia (nearsightedness) A condition in which the eyeball is elongated, causing the image to focus in front of the retina instead of on it.

myringotomy Incision of the tympanic membrane.

myxoedema An alternative term for severe or advanced hypothyroidism.

myxoedema coma A life-threatening complication of longstanding, untreated hypothyroidism usually triggered by an acute illness or trauma.

naevi (moles) Flat or raised macules or papules with rounded, well-defined borders.

natural disasters Disasters caused by acts of nature or emerging diseases. Some are unexpected, and some are predictable through advanced meteorological technologies.

natural killer cells (NK cells) Large, granular lymphocytes (found in the spleen, lymph nodes, bone marrow and blood) that provide immune surveillance and resistance to infection, and play an important role in the destruction of early malignant cells.

nausea An unpleasant sensation usually followed by vomiting.

neglect syndrome (unilateral neglect) A disorder of attention. In this syndrome, the person cannot integrate and use perceptions from the affected side of the body or from the environment on the affected side and, hence, ignores that part.

neoplasm A mass of new tissue (a collection of cells) that grows independently of its surrounding structures and has no physiological purpose.

nephrectomy Removal of the kidney.

nephrotic syndrome A condition marked by massive proteinuria, hypoalbuminaemia, hyperlipidaemia and oedema.

neurogenic bladder Dysfunctional urinary bladder due to lesion of central or peripheral nervous system.

neurogenic shock Shock resulting from an imbalance between parasympathetic and sympathetic stimulation of vascular smooth muscle. If parasympathetic overstimulation or sympathetic understimulation persists, sustained vasodilation occurs and blood pools in the venous and capillary beds.

neuropathic pain Pain caused by a lesion or dysfunction in the nervous system from the primary afferent conducting mechanism to the central nervous system.

nicotine An alkaloid found in the nightshade family of plants (*Solanaceae*) which constitutes approximately 0.6–3.0% of the dry weight of tobacco, with biosynthesis taking place in the roots and accumulating in the leaves.

nociception The physiological processes related to pain perception.

nociceptors Sensory nerve fibres that conduct pain impulses from the periphery to the central nervous system.

nocturia Voiding two or more times at night.

nondisjunction An error in meiosis or mitosis in which members of a pair of homologous chromosomes or a pair of sister chromatids fail to separate properly from each other.

non-Hodgkin's lymphoma (NHL) Lymphoid tissue malignancies that do not contain Reed–Sternberg cells.

non-union A state that exists when the ends of a fracture fail to heal together.

normal sinus rhythm (NSR) Normal heart rhythm, in which impulses originate in the sinus node and travel through normal conduction pathways without delay.

nursing process The series of critical-thinking activities nurses use as they provide care to patients; this logical approach to care ensures that patients receive comprehensive and effective care.

nutrients Substances found in food that are used by the body to promote growth, maintenance and repair.

nutrition The process by which the body ingests, absorbs, transports, uses and eliminates food.

nystagmus Rapid involuntary eye movements.

obesity An excess of body fat (adipose tissue).

obstructive shock Shock caused by an obstruction in the heart or great vessels that either impedes venous return or prevents effective cardiac pumping action.

occult bleeding Hidden bleeding.

oedema Accumulation of fluid in the body's tissues; an excess accumulation of fluid in the interstitial space.

oesophageal varices Enlarged, thin-walled veins that form in the submucosa of the oesophagus.

oesophagojejunostomy Removal of the entire stomach with anastomosis of the distal oesophagus to the jejunum.

oestrogen Hormone produced by the ovary.

oliguria Urine output of less than 400 mL in 24 hours.

oncogene Gene capable of triggering cancerous characteristics.

oncology The study of cancer.

opioid A chemical that works by binding to opioid receptors, which are found principally in the central nervous system and the gastrointestinal tract.

oral mucositis Inflammation and ulceration of the oral mucosa.

orchitis Infection or inflammation of the testicle.

orthopnoea Difficulty breathing when supine.

orthostatic hypotension A decrease in systolic blood pressure of more than 10 to 15 mmHg and a drop in diastolic blood pressure on standing

osmosis The process by which water moves across a selectively permeable membrane from an area of lower solute concentration to an area of higher solute concentration.

ossification The process of bone formation.

osteoarthritis (OA) (degenerative joint disease) The most commonly occurring of all forms of arthritis. This disease is characterised by loss of articular cartilage in articulating joints and hypertrophy of the bones at the articular margins.

osteomalacia (adult rickets) Metabolic bone disorder characterised by inadequate mineralisation of bone matrix.

osteomyelitis Infection within the bone that can lead to tissue death and necrosis.

osteoporosis Literally defined as 'porous bones', a metabolic bone disorder characterised by loss of bone mass, increased bone fragility and an increased risk of fractures.

ostomy General term for an operation in which an artificial opening is created.

otitis externa Inflammation of the ear canal, commonly known as *swimmer's ear*.

otitis media Inflammation or infection of the middle ear.

otosclerosis Abnormal bone formation in the osseous labyrinth of the temporal bone causing the footplate of the stapes to become fixed or immobile in the oval window. The result is a conductive hearing loss.

ovarian cycle The female cycle that occurs from puberty until menopause in which the production of ova occur.

oxyhaemoglobin The combined form of haemoglobin and oxygen; found in arterial blood, it carries oxygen to body tissues.

pacemaker A pulse generator used to provide an electrical stimulus to the heart when the heart fails to generate or conduct on its own a rate that maintains the cardiac output.

$PaCO_2$ Partial pressure of carbon dioxide in arterial blood.

Paget's disease A skeletal disorder that results from excessive osteoclastic activity. Paget's disease is characterised by bone deformity, especially of the long bones of the lower limbs, the pelvis, the lumbar vertebrae and the skull.

pain tolerance The amount of pain a person can endure before responding to it.

palliative care An area of care that has evolved out of the hospice experience, but exists outside of hospice programs and is not restricted to the end of life. Palliative care is focused on the relief of physical, mental and spiritual distress for individuals who have an incurable illness and is used earlier in the disease experience than hospice care. The goal of palliative care is to prevent and relieve suffering by early assessment and treatment of pain and other physical, psychosocial and spiritual needs to improve the person's quality of life.

pallor Lack of colour; paleness of skin.

pancreatitis Inflammation of the pancreas.

pandemic The worldwide spread of a disease.

PaO_2 Partial pressure of oxygen in arterial blood.

paracentesis Aspiration of fluid from the peritoneal cavity.

paralytic ileus Impaired propulsion or forward movement of bowel contents.

paraplegia Paralysis of the lower portion of the body, sometimes involving the lower trunk.

parenchyma The key elements of an organ essential to its functioning, as distinct from the capsule that encompasses it and other supporting structures.

parenteral nutrition (PN) Intravenous administration of carbohydrates (high concentrations of dextrose), protein (amino acids), electrolytes, vitamins, minerals and fat emulsions.

Parkinson's disease (PD) Progressive, degenerative neurological disease characterised by non-intention tremor, bradykinesia and muscle rigidity.

paroxysmal nocturnal dyspnoea (PND) Attacks of acute shortness of breath that occur at night, waking up the person

partial gastrectomy Removal of a portion of the stomach, usually the distal half to two-thirds

partial-thickness burn Burn that involves the entire dermis and the papillae of the dermis (superficial partial-thickness burn) or extends into the hair follicles (deep partial-thickness burn).

passive immunity Temporary protection—provided by antibodies produced by other people or animals—against disease-producing antigens. Protection is gradually lost when these acquired antibodies are used up either by natural degradation or by combining with the antigen.

pathogens Virulent organisms rarely found in the absence of disease.

pediculosis An infestation with lice, parasites that live on the blood of an animal or human host.

pelvic inflammatory disease (PID) A term used to describe infection of the pelvic organs.

penetrance The percentage or likelihood that an individual who has inherited a gene mutation will actually express the disease signs and symptoms in his or her lifetime.

penetrating trauma Occurs when a foreign object enters the body, causing damage to body structures.

peptic ulcer An ulcer that occurs in any area of the gastrointestinal tract exposed to acid-pepsin secretions, including the oesophagus, stomach or duodenum.

peptic ulcer disease (PUD) A break in the mucous lining of the gastrointestinal tract where it comes in contact with gastric juice.

perforation Penetration of ulcer through mucosal wall.

pericarditis Inflammation of the pericardium.

perioperative nursing A highly skill, specialised area of nursing practice incorporating a number of sub-specialties.

peripheral obesity Obesity characterised by a waist-to-hip ratio of less than 0.8, more commonly seen in women.

peripheral vascular disease (PVD) Impaired blood supply to peripheral tissues, particularly the lower extremities.

peristalsis Alternating waves of contraction and relaxation of involuntary muscle.

peritoneal dialysis Procedure in which electrolytes, waste products and excess water are removed from the body by diffusion using the peritoneum surrounding the abdominal cavity as the dialysing membrane.

peritonitis Inflammation of the peritoneum.

pernicious anaemia Anaemia resulting from failure to absorb dietary vitamin B_{12} due to lack of intrinsic factor.

persistent (chronic) pain Ongoing and prolonged pain, not always associated with an identifiable cause but often arising from an acute cause.

persistent vegetative state (PVS) Condition of complete unawareness of self and the environment.

personal responsibility Admitting responsibility for choices made.

person-centred care A holistic approach to the planning, delivery and evaluation of healthcare that is grounded in mutually beneficial partnerships between healthcare professionals, patients and families. Person-centred care is underpinned by the principles of trust, empathy, dignity, autonomy, respect, choice, transparency and desire to help individuals lead the life they want.

pertussis (whooping cough) A highly contagious acute upper respiratory infection cause by the bacterium *Bordetella pertussis*.

phagocytosis A process by which a foreign agent or target cell is engulfed, destroyed and digested. Neutrophils and macrophages, known as phagocytes, are the primary cells involved in phagocytosis.

phantom limb syndrome (phantom pain) A confusing pain syndrome that occurs following surgical or traumatic amputation of a limb. The person experiences pain in the missing body part even though there is complete mental awareness that the limb is gone.

pharmacogenetics The study of how genetic factors influence drug action.

pharyngitis Acute inflammation of the pharynx.

phenotype The expression of a person's entire physical, biochemical and physiological make-up, as determined by the individual's genotype and environmental factors.

pheochromocytoma Tumours of chromaffi in tissues in the adrenal medulla. These tumours, which are usually benign, produce catecholamines (adrenaline or noradrenaline, also known as epinephrine and norepinephrine) that stimulate the sympathetic nervous system.

phimosis Constriction of the foreskin so that it cannot be retracted over the glans penis.

photophobia Sensitivity to light.

plasmapheresis (plasma exchange) Removal of the plasma component from whole blood.

pleural effusion Collection of excess fluid in the pleural space.

pleuritis Inflammation of the pleura.

pneumonia Inflammation of the lung parenchyma (the respiratory bronchioles and alveoli).

pneumothorax Results when air enters the pleural space due to blunt and penetrating injuries to the chest.

polycystic kidney disease (PKD) A hereditary disease characterised by cyst formation and massive kidney enlargement.

polycythaemia (erythrocytosis) Excess red blood cells characterised by a haematocrit higher than 55%.

polydipsia Excessive thirst.

polymorphisms DNA sequences that have many forms but give the genetic 'directions' for the same thing.

polymyositis A systemic connective tissue disorder characterised by inflammation of connective tissue and muscle fibres leading to muscle weakness and atrophy.

polyphagia Excessive eating.

polyuria A condition where increased blood volume increases renal blood flow and the hyperglycaemia acts as an osmotic diuretic, thereby increasing urine output.

portal hypertension Elevated pressure in the portal venous system that causes rerouting of blood to adjoining lower pressure vessels.

portal systemic encephalopathy Impaired consciousness and mental status due to the accumulation of toxic waste products in the blood (ammonia in particular) as blood bypasses the congested liver.

positioning Exposes the operative site in conjunction with access for anaesthesia administration. Proper positioning is imperative to prevent injury to the person.

postoperative phase Period when a procedure or surgery has been completed and the person is recovering from the stress associated with the surgery.

postpoliomyelitis syndrome A complication of a previous infection by the poliomyelitis virus.

preload The amount of cardiac muscle fibre tension or stretch that exists at diastole, just before ventricular contraction.

premenstrual syndrome (PMS) Complex of symptoms characterised by irritability, depression, oedema and breast tenderness preceding the monthly menses.

preparedness Having a comprehensive disaster plan in place that coordinates efforts among many people, agencies and levels of government.

preoperative phase Time when preparation of the person for surgery is conducted and completed.

presbycusis Age-related loss of the ability to hear high-frequency sounds; may occur because of cochlear hair cell degeneration or loss of auditory neurons in the organ of Corti.

presbyopia Impaired near vision resulting from a loss of elasticity of the lens related to ageing.

prescription medication misuse Non-medical use of pharmaceuticals or use for genuine medical purposes but without a valid prescription, or when prescribed in excessive quantities or frequencies, or when an iatrogenic dependence has developed.

pressure injury Ischaemic lesion of the skin and underlying tissue caused by external pressure that impairs the flow of blood and lymph.

pretibial myxoedema Also known as thyroid dermopathy, pretibial myxoedema refers to lesions of the skin resulting from the accumulation of hyaluronic acid, as a result of thyroid disease.

priapism Sustained, painful erection that lasts at least 4 hours and is not associated with sexual arousal.

primary care A clinical perspective that provides first contact services for individuals and families.

primary healthcare (PHC) Involves communities, public policy and social and environmental determinants of health.

primary hypertension (idiopathic, essential) A persistently elevated systemic blood pressure.

primary survey An initial assessment of a person to determine if there is serious compromise to airway, breathing or circulation.

procedural pain A type of breakthrough pain that is predictable because it is associated with movement such as turning or coughing.

progesterone Hormone produced by the ovary; works with oestrogen to control the menstrual cycle.

proptosis Forward bulging of one or both eyes.

prostatitis Inflammation of the prostate gland.

protein energy malnutrition (PEM) The state of decreased body pools of protein with or without fat depletion or a state of diminished functional capacity, caused at least partly by inadequate nutrient intake relative to nutrient demand, and/or which is improved by nutritional repletion.

proteinuria Abnormal proteins in the urine.

proximal determinants Determinants that have a more direct impact on health, and include lifestyle and behavioural factors as well as underlying health conditions.

pruritus Subjective itching sensation producing an urge to scratch.

psoriasis Chronic, non-infectious skin disorder that is characterised by raised, reddened, round circumscribed plaques covered by silvery white scales.

psychosis A mental health condition in which there is a loss of contact with reality.

psychostimulants A diverse group of natural and synthetic drugs with a wide range of psychological and physical effects, including euphoria, increased energy and irregular heartbeat.

ptosis Drooping of the eyelid.

pulmonary embolism Sudden occlusion of a pulmonary artery resulting in disruption of blood supply to the lung parenchyma.

pulmonary hypertension Condition in which the pulmonary arterial pressure is elevated to an abnormal level.

pulmonary oedema An abnormal accumulation of fluid in the interstitial tissue and alveoli of the lung.

pulmonic valve One of the semilunar valves, separating the ventricles from the great vessels.

pulse Rhythmic pressure waveform that can be felt over an artery.

pulse pressure The difference between the systolic and diastolic blood pressure.

puncture wound Wound that occurs when a sharp or blunt object penetrates the integument.

pupillary light reflex Reflex in which the pupil contracts in response to a bright light.

pyelonephritis Upper urinary tract inflammation affecting the kidney and renal pelvis.

pyuria (bacteriuria) Pus in the urine.

quadriplegia Injury to cervical segments of the cord thus impairing function of the arms, trunk, legs and pelvic organs.

rabies Viral (rhabdovirus) infection of the central nervous system transmitted by infected saliva that enters the human body through a bite or an open wound.

radiation therapy Therapy that uses radiation to kill a tumour, to reduce its size, to decrease pain or to relieve obstruction.

rapid cycling Having four or more mood episodes within a 12-month period.

Raynaud's disease Disorder characterised by episodes of intense vasospasm in the small arteries and arterioles of the fingers and possibly the toes; has no identifiable cause.

Raynaud's phenomenon Disorder characterised by episodes of intense vasospasm in the small arteries and arterioles of the fingers and possibly the toes; occurs secondarily to another disease.

reactive arthritis (Reiter's syndrome) An acute, non-purulent inflammatory arthritis that complicates a bacterial infection of the genitourinary or gastrointestinal tracts.

recovery The final phase of an emergency; the period when the emergency is under control and the community starts to rebuild.

Recovery A recognised and accepted paradigm, related to a personal journey, that has significant implications for people who have mental health problems, their carers, mental health professionals and mental health services.

referral Timely consultation and handing over of clinical care of people to the appropriate personnel and facility for ongoing management.

reflux, urinary Backflow of urine towards the kidneys.

refraction The bending of light rays as they pass from one medium to another medium of different optical density.

regional anaesthesia Anaesthesia that desensitises a particular area but does not involve the full central nervous system or cause sedation.

regional and remote health workforce A statistical representation of nurses working in identified regional and remote areas which includes the number of currently employed nurses, acknowledging their age, experience and qualifications.

regurgitation (valvular) Backflow of blood through an incompletely closed valve into the area it just left.

renal artery stenosis Narrowing of the renal artery.

renal colic Acute, severe, intermittent pain in the flank and upper outer abdominal quadrant generally associated with acute obstruction of a ureter and resulting ureteral spasm.

renal insufficiency Any condition in which the kidneys are unable to remove accumulated metabolites from the blood, leading to altered fluid, electrolyte and acid–base balance.

respiratory failure Inability of lungs to oxygenate the blood and remove carbon dioxide adequately to meet the body's needs, even at rest.

response Occurs in the emergency stage and after a disaster event has occurred.

retinal detachment Separation of the retina or sensory portion of the eye from the choroid.

retrieval Specialised transfer of people with needs exceeding the capacity of their current location to a clinical facility providing a higher level of specialised healthcare.

retrograde ejaculation Seminal fluid discharged into the bladder.

rheumatic disorders Refers to diseases of the muscles and bones as well as the joints.

rheumatic fever A systemic inflammatory disease caused by an abnormal immune response to pharyngeal infection by group A beta-haemolytic streptococci. The condition is characterised by acute inflammation, joint pain, fever and cardiac valve scarring.

rheumatic heart disease (RHD) Slowly progressive valvular deformity following acute or repeated attacks of rheumatic fever; characterised by rigid and deformed valve leaflets; fused valve commissures and fibrosis of chordae tendineae.

rheumatoid arthritis A chronic systemic autoimmune disease that causes inflammation of connective tissue, primarily in the joints.

rhinitis Inflammation of the nasal cavities.

rhinoplasty Surgical reconstruction of the nose.

risk factors Defined as individual or environmental variables that are related to the increased likelihood that a negative outcome will occur.

sarcoidosis Systemic disease characterised by granulomas in the lungs, lymph nodes, liver, eyes, skin and other organs.

scabies Parasitic infestation caused by the mite *Sarcoptes scabiei*.

schizophrenia A mental disorder characterised by abnormalities in the perception or expression of reality.

sciatica Pain over the sciatic nerve.

scleroderma Hardening of the skin; a chronic condition characterised by the formation of excess fibrous connective tissue and diffuse fibrosis of the skin and internal organs.

scoliosis A lateral curvature of the spine.

scope of practice The roles, functions, responsibilities, activities and decision-making capacity that nurses are educated, competent and authorised to perform.

sebum An oily substance secreted from sebaceous glands; softens and lubricates the skin and hair, and decreases water loss from the skin in low humidity. Sebum also protects the body from infection by killing bacteria.

secondary hypertension Elevated blood pressure resulting from an identifiable underlying process.

secondary survey A head-to-toe assessment of a person that includes all body systems.

seizure An episode of excessive and abnormal discharge of electrical activity within the central nervous system.

semen Contains sperm and fluids secreted by the male reproductive system glands.

septic arthritis Develops when a joint space is invaded by a pathogen.

septic shock One part of a progressive syndrome called systemic inflammatory response syndrome. Beginning with an infection, septic shock progresses to bacteraemia, then sepsis, then septic shock and finally multiple organ failure syndrome.

septicaemia Systemic disease associated with the presence of bacteria or their toxins in the blood.

seroconversion Antibody response to a disease or vaccine.

serum bicarbonate (HCO_3^-) Reflects the renal regulation of acid–base balance. It is often called the metabolic component of arterial blood gases.

severe acute respiratory syndrome (SARS) Lower respiratory illness of unknown aetiology; spread by close person-to-person contact.

sex chromosome A chromosome responsible for determining the sex of an individual.

sexually transmitted infection (STI, sexually transmitted disease, venereal disease) Any infection transmitted by sexual contact, including vaginal, oral and anal intercourse.

shingles See *herpes zoster*.

shock A clinical syndrome characterised by a systemic imbalance between oxygen supply and demand. This imbalance results in a state of inadequate blood flow to the peripheral tissues, causing life-threatening cellular dysfunction, hypotension and oliguria.

sickle cell anaemia A hereditary, chronic haemolytic anaemia characterised by episodes of sickling, during which red blood cells become abnormally crescent shaped.

sinusitis Inflammation of the mucous membranes of one or more of the sinuses.

Sjögren's syndrome An autoimmune disorder that causes inflammation and dysfunction of exocrine glands throughout the body.

skin tear A traumatic wound occurring principally on the extremities of older adults, as a result of friction alone or shearing and friction forces that separate the epidermis from the dermis (partial-thickness wound), or which separate both the epidermis and the dermis from underlying structures (full-thickness wound).

sleep apnoea Absence of airflow through the upper airways for 10 or more seconds.

social determinants of health The social factors that influence the health status and health outcomes of individuals and communities.

social model of health A model of health which views health as multifaceted, focusing on social rather than biological determinants of health. This model emphasises health equity and prevention of illness or injury, as well as collaboration and empowerment. The social model of health is also referred to as new public health or the social ecological model.

solvents Produce a depressant effect on the central nervous system and comprise a range of products producing vapours which, when inhaled through the nose or mouth, may cause an intoxicated feeling and lead to an altered state of consciousness.

somatic cell Any cell in the body that is not a sex cell (ova and sperm).

Somogyi phenomenon A morning rise in blood glucose to hyperglycaemic levels following an episode of nocturnal hypoglycaemia and a counter-regulatory hormone response.

spasticity Increased muscle tone in disease of the corticospinal motor tract.

spermatocoele A mobile, usually painless mass containing dead spermatozoa that forms in the epididymis.

spinal cord injury (SCI) Injury to spinal cord, usually due to trauma and classified according to systems.

spinal shock Temporary loss of reflex function below the level of injury.

sprain Tearing or stretching of a ligament that results from a twisting motion.

sprue A chronic primary disorder of the small intestine in which the absorption of nutrients, particularly fats, is impaired.

squamous cell carcinoma Malignant tumour of the squamous epithelium of the skin or mucous membranes.

starvation Inadequate dietary intake; the condition of being without food for long periods of time.

status asthmaticus Severe, prolonged asthma that does not respond to routine treatment. Without aggressive therapy, status asthmaticus can lead to respiratory failure with hypoxaemia, hypercapnia and acidosis.

steatorrhoea Greasy, frothy, yellow stools resulting from excess fat in the faeces.

stem cells (haemocytoblasts) Bone marrow precursor cells for all blood cells.

stem cell transplant (SCT) Infusion of donor stem cells to replace the recipient's blood cell lines (white blood cells, red blood cells and platelets).

stenosis Condition where valve leaflets fuse together and are unable to open or close fully.

steroids Often used illegally to build muscles and enhance exercise performance; also known as performance- and image-enhancing drugs (PIEDs).

stigma Severe social disapproval.

stoma Surface opening.

Strain Stretching injury to a muscle or a muscle–tendon unit caused by mechanical overloading.

stress-induced (erosive) gastritis See *erosive gastritis*.

striae A line above or below tissue that differs in colour and texture from surrounding tissue.

stridor High-pitched, harsh inspiratory sound indicative of upper airway obstruction.

stroke (brain attack, cerebrovascular accident, CVA) A condition in which neurological deficits occur as a result of decreased blood flow to a focal (localised) area of brain tissue.

stroke volume (SV) The amount of blood pumped into the aorta with each contraction of the left ventricle.

subacute thyroiditis Inflammation of the thyroid gland.

subdural haematoma A localised mass of blood that collects between the dura mater and the arachnoid mater.

subluxation Partial separation (or dislocation) of the bones of a joint.

substance dependence A severe condition occurring when the use of a chemical substance is no longer under an individual's control for at least 3 months. Continued use of the substance usually persists despite adverse effects on the person's physical condition, psychological health and interpersonal relationships (used interchangeably with 'addiction').

substance-induced disorder A reversible substance-specific syndrome related to the type of drug used.

substance-related disorder Maladaptive patterns of substance use leading to clinically significant impairment or distress.

substance use The use of any chemical in a fashion inconsistent with medical or culturally defined social norms despite physical, psychological or socially adverse effects.

substance use disorder A medical condition in which the use of one or more substances leads to a clinically significant impairment characterised by a range of mental, physical and behavioural symptoms that often cause problems related to one's personal life, relationships and work, as well as increasingly hazardous use, tolerance and withdrawal.

sudden cardiac death (SCD) Unexpected death occurring within 1 hour of the onset of cardiovascular symptoms.

sundowning A behavioural change in Alzheimer's disease characterised by increased agitation, time disorientation and wandering during afternoon and evening hours.

superficial burn Burn involving only the epidermal layer of the skin; most often results from damage from sunburn, ultraviolet light, minor flash injury (from a sudden ignition or explosion) or mild radiation burn associated with cancer treatment.

surfactant A lipoprotein produced by the alveolar cells; interferes with adhesion of water molecules, reducing surface tension and helping to expand lungs.

surgery An invasive medical procedure performed to diagnose or treat illness, injury or deformity. Although surgery is a medical treatment, the nurse assumes an active role in caring for the person before, during and after surgery.

surgical debridement The process of excising a wound to the level of fascia (fascial excision) or sequentially removing thin slices of a burn wound to the level of viable tissue (sequential excision).

syndrome of inappropriate ADH secretion (SIADH) Characterised by high levels of antidiuretic hormone (ADH) in the absence of serum hypo-osmolality, and most often caused by the ectopic production of ADH by malignant tumours.

synovitis Inflammation of the synovial membrane lining the articular capsule of a joint.

syphilis A sexually transmitted infection caused by a spirochaete that may invade almost any body tissue or organ. It enters the body through a break in the skin or mucous membranes and can be transferred to the fetus through the placental circulation.

systemic lupus erythematosus (SLE) A chronic inflammatory immune complex connective tissue disease.

systolic blood pressure This arterial pressure wave produced by ventricular contraction (systole) averages 120 mmHg in healthy adults.

T lymphocytes (T cells) Type of lymphocyte that matures in the thymus gland.

tachypnoea Abnormally rapid respiratory rate.

telehealth A broad term that refers to the use of technology to contribute to the provision of healthcare, usually at a distance.

tendonitis Inflammation of a tendon

tension pneumothorax A condition in which an injury to the chest allows air to enter but not escape the pleural cavity.

terrorism An action, or threat of action, that causes harm or interference, and is made with the intention of advancing a political, religious or ideological cause.

test sensitivity How specifically a test identifies (positive test result) individuals who are affected and/or who have a disease phenotype.

test specificity How specifically a test does not identify (negative test result) individuals who are unaffected or do not have a disease phenotype.

testicular torsion Twisting of the testes and spermatic cord.

testosterone Male hormone produced in the testes.

tetanus Disorder of the nervous system caused by a neurotoxin elaborated by *Clostridium tetani.*

tetany Tonic muscular spasms.

thalassaemia An inherited disorder of haemoglobin synthesis in which either the alpha or beta chains of the haemoglobin molecule are missing or defective.

therapeutic relationship A relationship that aims to empower the person with the knowledge and ability to recover from their illness.

third spacing The accumulation and sequestration of trapped extracellular fluid in an actual or potential body space as a result of disease or injury.

thoracentesis Invasive procedure in which fluid (or occasionally air) is removed from the pleural space with a needle.

thought content The actual content of what a person is thinking.

thrill Palpable vibration over the precordium or an artery.

thromboangiitis obliterans (Buerger's disease) An occlusive vascular disease involving inflammation, spasm and clot formation in small and medium-sized peripheral arteries.

thrombocytopenia A platelet count of less than 100,000 per millilitre of blood.

thromboembolus A thrombus that breaks loose from the arterial wall.

thrombus A blood clot that adheres to a vessel wall.

thyroid crisis An extreme state of hyperthyroidism that is rare today because of improved diagnosis and treatment methods. Also called thyroid storm.

thyroid gland A gland situated at the front of the throat which secretes thyroid hormones (thyroxine (T_4) and triiodothyronine (T_3)) to regulate the body's metabolic process.

thyroid storm *See thyroid crisis.*

thyroidectomy A procedure performed to treat cancer of the thyroid.

thyrotoxicosis See *hyperthyroidism.*

tidal volume (TV) The amount of air (approximately 500 mL) moved in and out of the lungs with each normal, quiet breath.

tinnitus Perception of sound such as ringing, buzzing or roaring in the ears.

titrate To determine the concentration of (a solution) by titration or perform the operation of titration.

tolerance A cumulative state in which a particular dose of a chemical elicits a smaller response than before. With increased tolerance, the individual needs higher and higher doses to obtain the desired effect.

tonsillitis Acute inflammation of the palatine tonsils.

tophi Small white nodules in subcutaneous tissue composed of urate deposits resulting from gout.

total gastrectomy Removal of the entire stomach.

total peripheral vascular resistance (TPVR) The opposing forces or impedance to blood flow as the arterial channels become more and more distant from the heart.

toxic multinodular goitre A tumour characterised by small, discrete, independently functioning nodules in the thyroid gland tissue that secrete excessive amounts of thyroid hormone.

trachoma A chronic conjunctivitis caused by *Chlamydia trachomatis*, and a significant preventable cause of blindness worldwide.

transdermal Medication absorbed through the skin without injection.

transdisciplinary Transdisciplinary approaches in health involve partnerships and strategies that cross many health and other professional discipline boundaries to create a holistic approach, addressing multiple influences.

transfusion An infusion of blood or blood components.

transient ischaemic attack (TIA) Brief period of localised cerebral ischaemia that causes neurological deficits lasting for less than 24 hours.

transjugular intrahepatic portosystemic shunt (TIPS) Used to relieve portal hypertension and its complications of oesophageal varices and ascites.

translocation The joining of a part of or a whole chromosome to another separate chromosome.

trauma An injury to human tissues and organs resulting from the transfer of energy from the environment

traumatic brain injury (TBI) A traumatic insult to the brain capable of causing physical, intellectual, emotional, social and vocational changes.

tremor Rhythmic movement.

triage Means 'sorting'. Triage is the process by which all people presenting to an ED for care are assessed and their care prioritised according to actual or potential severity of illness or injury.

triage in regional and remote areas Clinical determination of the acuity of the presenting health problems for people seeking healthcare in regional and remote areas.

trichomoniasis A sexually transmitted infection caused by a parasite passed from person to person.

tricuspid valve A valve between the right atrium and ventricle of the heart; prevents blood from flowing backwards into the atrium.

trigeminal neuralgia (tic douloureux) A chronic disease of the trigeminal cranial nerve (cranial nerve V) that causes severe facial pain.

triglycerides Molecules of glycerol with fatty acids used to transport and store fats in body tissues.

trisomy Possessing three chromosomes instead of the usual two, as in trisomy 21 or Down syndrome.

Trousseau's sign Contraction of the hand and fingers in response to occlusion of the blood supply by a blood pressure cuff; caused by decreased blood calcium levels.

tuberculosis (TB) Chronic, recurrent infectious disease caused by *Mycobacterium tuberculosis*; usually affects the lungs, although any organ can be affected.

tumour marker A protein molecule detectable in serum or other body fluids. This marker is used as a biochemical indicator of the presence of a malignancy.

Turner's syndrome A chromosomal abnormality in which all or part of one of the sex chromosomes is absent.

twilight sedation Anaesthesia that provides analgesia and amnesia, but in which the person remains conscious. People are able to breathe independently and are cardiovascularly stable.

tympanoplasty Surgical reconstruction of the middle ear.

type 1 diabetes mellitus The result of pancreatic islet cell destruction and a total deficit of circulating insulin.

type 2 diabetes mellitus Results from insulin resistance with a defect in compensatory insulin secretion.

ulcer A lesion of the skin or mucous membranes.

ulcerative colitis Chronic inflammatory bowel disorder of the mucosa and submucosa of the colon and rectum.

ultrafiltration Removal of excess body water using a hydrostatic pressure gradient.

uraemia Literally, 'urine in the blood'; the syndrome or group of symptoms associated with end-stage kidney disease.

urea An end product of protein metabolism and, along with water, the main constituent of urine.

ureteral (or ureteric) stent Thin catheter inserted into the ureter to provide for urine flow and ureteral support.

ureteroplasty Surgical repair of a ureter.

urgency A sudden, compelling need to urinate.

urinary calculi Calculi or 'stones' in the urinary tract.

urinary diversion Procedure to provide for urine collection and drainage following cystectomy. The most common urinary diversion is the ileal conduit.

urinary drainage system The ureters, urinary bladder and urethra.

urinary incontinence Involuntary urination.

urinary retention Incomplete emptying of the bladder.

urticaria Hives.

vaccine Suspensions of whole or fractionated bacteria or viruses that have been treated to make them non-pathogenic.

Valsalva manoeuvre Closing the glottis and contracting the diaphragm and abdominal muscles to increase intra-abdominal pressure to facilitate expulsion of faeces.

valvular heart disease Interference of blood flow to, within and from the heart.

varicocoele Dilation of the pampiniform venous complex of the spermatic cord.

varicose veins Irregular, tortuous veins with incompetent valves.

vasoconstriction Smooth muscle contraction that narrows the vessel lumen.

vasodilation Smooth muscle relaxation that expands the vessel lumen.

vasogenic shock See *distributive shock*.

venous stasis Occurs when venous blood collects and stagnates in the lower leg.

venous thrombosis (thrombophlebitis) Blood clot (thrombus) formation on the wall of a vein, accompanied by inflammation of the vein wall and obstructed venous blood flow.

vertigo Sensation of whirling or rotation.

very-low-kilojoule diet (VLKD) A protein-sparing modified fast (1,700 to 3,500 kilojoules/day or less) under close medical supervision that may be used to treat significant obesity.

vital capacity The sum of TV (tidal volume) 1 IRV (inspiratory reserve volume) 1 ERV (expiratory reserve volume); approximately 4,500 mL in healthy people.

vitiligo Abnormal loss of melanin in patches.

volatile acids Acids eliminated from the body as a gas.

Volkmann's contracture A common complication of elbow fractures; can result from unresolved compartment syndrome. Arterial blood flow decreases, leading to ischaemia, degeneration and contracture of the muscle.

voluntary assisted dying (VAD) The assistance provided to a person by a health practitioner to end their life.

vomiting The forceful expulsion of the contents of the upper gastrointestinal tract resulting from contraction of muscles in the gut and abdominal wall.

warts (verrucae) Lesions of the skin caused by the human papillomavirus.

weaning Process of removing the person from ventilator support and re-establishing spontaneous, independent respirations.

wheeze Continuous, musical sound caused by narrowing of the lumen in a respiratory passage.

wild-type gene The most common type of gene; designated as normal.

withdrawal Cessation of use of a substance to which an individual has become addicted.

xenograft A transplant from an animal species to a human.

xerosis Dry skin.

xerostomia Excessive dryness of the mucous membranes (due to chemotherapy or radiation).

X-linked dominant Any gene found on the X chromosome or traits determined by such genes; also refers to the specific mode of inheritance of such genes. One altered gene on an X chromosome in a male can produce disease, such as haemophilia.

X-linked recessive The result of an altered gene on the X chromosome.

Zollinger–Ellison syndrome Peptic ulcer disease caused by a gastrinoma, or gastrin-secreting tumour of the pancreas, stomach or intestines.

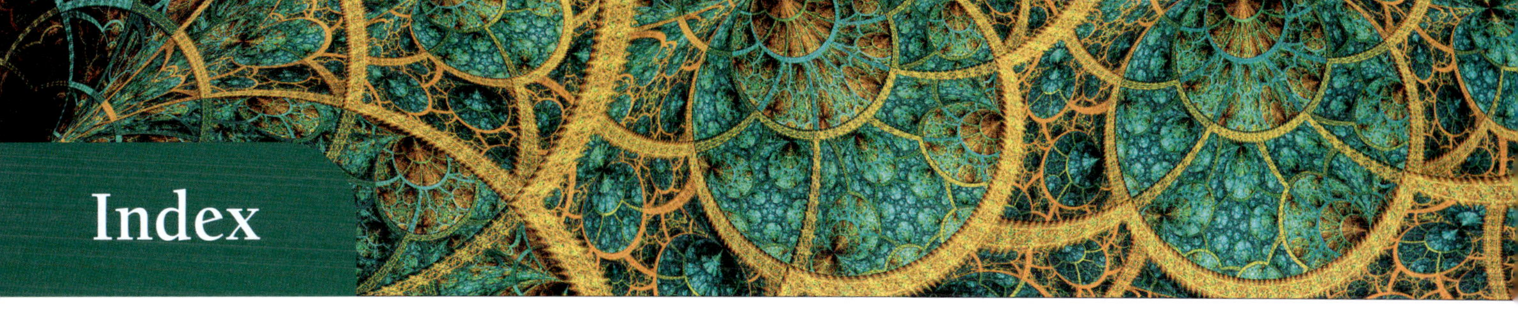

Index

Page numbers in **bold** indicate definitions of key terms.

F

S